The
American Psychiatric Press
Synopsis of Psychiatry

Editorial Board

The
American Psychiatric Press
Synopsis of Psychiatry

Edited by

ROBERT E. HALES, M.D., M.B.A.
Professor and Vice Chair,
Department of Psychiatry,
University of California, Davis,
School of Medicine and Medical Center;
Medical Director, Sacramento County Mental Health Division
and Treatment Center,
Sacramento, California

STUART C. YUDOFSKY, M.D.
D. C. and Irene Ellwood Professor and Chairman,
Department of Psychiatry and Behavioral Sciences,
Baylor College of Medicine;
Chief, Psychiatry Service,
The Methodist Hospital,
Houston, Texas

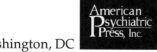

Washington, DC   London, England

Note: The authors have worked to ensure that all information in this book concerning drug dosages, schedules, and routes of administration is accurate as of the time of publication and consistent with standards set by the U.S. Food and Drug Administration and the general medical community. As medical research and practice advance, however, therapeutic standards may change. For this reason and because human and mechanical errors sometimes occur, we recommend that readers follow the advice of a physician who is directly involved in their care or in the care of a member of their family.

Books published by the American Psychiatric Press, Inc., represent the views and opinions of the individual authors and do not necessarily represent the policies and opinions of the Press or the American Psychiatric Association.

Diagnostic criteria included in this textbook are reprinted, with permission, from the *Diagnostic and Statistical Manual of Mental Disorders*, 4th Edition. Copyright 1994, American Psychiatric Association.

Copyright © 1996 American Psychiatric Press, Inc.
ALL RIGHTS RESERVED
Manufactured in the United States of America on acid-free paper
99 98 97 96   4 3 2 1
First Edition

American Psychiatric Press, Inc.
1400 K Street, N.W., Washington, DC   20005

Library of Congress Cataloging-in-Publication Data

American Psychiatric Press synopsis of psychiatry / edited by Robert E. Hales and Stuart C. Yudofsky.
        p.   cm.
    Condensed information from: American Psychiatric Press textbook of psychiatry. 2nd ed. 1994.
    Includes bibliographical references and index.
    ISBN 0-88048-889-1
    1. Psychiatry.   I. Hales, Robert E.   II. Yudofsky, Stuart C.
III. American Psychiatric Press textbook of psychiatry.
    [DNLM: 1. Mental Disorders.   2. Psychiatry.   WM 100 S9935 1996]
    RC454.S95   1996
    616.89—dc20
    DNLM/DLC
for Library of Congress   93-48305
                                                                     CIP

British Library Cataloguing in Publication Data

A CIP record is available from the British Library.

To the women in our lives
Dianne and Julia Hales
Beth, Elissa, Lynn, and Emily Yudofsky

Contents

Section I: Theoretical Foundations

Section II: Assessment

Section III: Psychiatric Disorders

Section IV: Psychiatric Treatments

Section V: Special Topics

Contributors

W. Stewart Agras, M.D.
Professor of Psychiatry, Director of Outpatient Psychiatry Services, Behavioral Medicine Program, Stanford University School of Medicine, Stanford, California

Nancy C. Andreasen, M.D., Ph.D.
Andrew H. Woods Professor of Psychiatry, Department of Psychiatry, University of Iowa College of Medicine; Mental Health Clinical Research Center, University of Iowa Hospitals and Clinics, Iowa City, Iowa

Aaron T. Beck, M.D.
University Professor of Psychiatry, Department of Psychiatry, University of Pennsylvania; Director, Center for Cognitive Therapy, Philadelphia, Pennsylvania

Judith V. Becker, Ph.D.
Professor of Psychiatry and Psychology, University of Arizona Health Sciences Center, Tucson, Arizona

Robert I. Berkowitz, M.D.
Philadelphia Child Guidance Center, Philadelphia, Pennsylvania

Donald W. Black, M.D.
Associate Professor of Psychiatry, Department of Psychiatry, University of Iowa College of Medicine, Iowa City, Iowa

Dan Blazer, M.D., Ph.D.
J. P. Gibbons Professor of Psychiatry, Dean of Medical Education, Duke University Medical Center, Durham, North Carolina

Jonathan F. Borus, M.D.
Psychiatrist-in-Chief, Brigham and Women's Hospital, Boston, Massachusetts; Associate Professor of Psychiatry, Harvard Medical School, Boston, Massachusetts; Editor, *Academic Psychiatry*

Jack D. Burke, Jr., M.D., M.P.H.
Professor and Head of the Department of Psychiatry and Behavioral Science, Texas A&M University Health Science Center; Chairman of the Department of Psychiatry at Scott and White Clinic and Hospital, Temple, Texas

Stephen F. Butler, Ph.D.
Director, Department of Psychology, Northeast Psychiatric Associates/Brookside Hospital, Nashua, New Hampshire

John F. Clarkin, Ph.D.
Professor of Clinical Psychology in Psychiatry, Cornell University Medical College; Director of Psychology, New York Hospital—Westchester Division, White Plains, New York, and Payne Whitney Clinic, New York, New York

Joseph T. Coyle, M.D.
Eben S. Draper Professor of Psychiatry and Neuroscience, Chair of the Consolidated Department of Psychiatry, Harvard Medical School, Boston, Massachusetts

C. Deborah Cross, M.D.
Assistant Professor of Psychiatry, Albany Medical College; Assistant Psychiatrist, Albany Medical Center Hospital, Albany, New York

Mina K. Dulcan, M.D.
Head, Department of Child Psychiatry, Osterman Professor of Child Psychiatry, Children's Memorial Hospital, Chicago, Illinois; Chief of Child and Adolescent Psychiatry, Northwestern University School of Medicine, Evanston, Illinois

Joe G. Fagan, M.D.
Department of Psychiatry, Walter Reed Army Medical Center, Washington, D.C.

Richard J. Frances, M.D.
Director, Department of Psychiatry, Institute for Psychotherapy and Counseling of Hackensack Medical Center, Hackensack, New Jersey; Professor of Clinical Psychiatry, University of Medicine and Dentistry of New Jersey, New Jersey Medical School, Newark, New Jersey

John E. Franklin, Jr., M.D.
Department of Psychiatry and Behavioral Science, Northwestern Memorial Hospital, Chicago, Illinois

George Fulop, M.D.
Assistant Professor, Division of Behavioral Medicine and Consultation Psychiatry, Department of Psychiatry, Mount Sinai School of Medicine, New York, New York

T. B. Ghosh, M.D.
Medical Director, Anxiety and Mood Disorders Clinic, California Pacific Medical Center, San Francisco, California

Carlos A. González, M.D.
Assistant Professor of Psychiatry, Department of Psychiatry, Yale University School of Medicine, New Haven, Connecticut

Jack M. Gorman, M.D.
Professor of Clinical Psychiatry; Director, Department of Clinical Psychobiology, Columbia University College of Physicians and Surgeons and New York State Psychiatric Institute, New York, New York

Kevin F. Gray, M.D.
Assistant Professor of Psychiatry, University of Texas Southwestern Medical Center, Dallas, Texas

John H. Greist, M.D.
Distinguished Senior Scientist, Dean Foundation of Health, Research and Education; Clinical Professor of Psychiatry, University of Wisconsin Medical School, Madison, Wisconsin

Ezra E. H. Griffith, M.D.
Professor of Psychiatry and of African and Afro-American Studies, Department of Psychiatry, Yale University School of Medicine; Director, Connecticut Mental Health Center, New Haven, Connecticut

John G. Gunderson, M.D.
Associate Professor of Psychiatry, Harvard Medical School, Boston, Massachusetts; Director, Personality and Psychosocial Research Program, McLean Hospital, Belmont, Massachusetts

Katherine A. Halmi, M.D.
Professor of Psychiatry, Cornell University Medical College; Director, Eating Disorders Program, Cornell Medical Center—Westchester, White Plains, New York

Margaret E. Hertzig, M.D.
Associate Professor of Psychiatry, Cornell University Medical College; Director, Child and Adolescent Outpatient Department, Payne Whitney Clinic, New York, New York

Eric Hollander, M.D.
Vice-Chairman, Psychiatry, Mount Sinai School of Medicine, Queens Hospital Center, Jamaica, New York

Gerald I. Hurowitz, M.D.
Assistant Clinical Professor of Psychiatry, Columbia University College of Physicians and Surgeons; Director of Psychopharmacology, McKeen Behavioral Service, Columbia-Presbyterian Medical Center, New York, New York

Stephen W. Hurt, Ph.D.
Associate Professor of Clinical Psychology in Psychiatry, Cornell University Medical College; Associate Attending Psychologist, New York Hospital—Westchester Division, White Plains, New York

Steven E. Hyman, M.D.
Associate Professor of Psychiatry and Neuroscience; Director, Division on Addictions, Harvard Medical School; Director of Research, Department of Psychiatry, Massachusetts General Hospital, Boston, Massachusetts

James W. Jefferson, M.D.
Distinguished Senior Scientist, Dean Foundation for Health, Research and Education; Clinical Professor of Psychiatry, University of Wisconsin Medical School, Madison, Wisconsin

Charles A. Kaufmann, M.D.
Associate Professor of Clinical Psychiatry, Department of Psychiatry, Columbia University College of Physicians and Surgeons, New York, New York

Richard J. Kavoussi, M.D.
Assistant Professor of Psychiatry, Medical College of Pennsylvania, Philadelphia, Pennsylvania

Stuart L. Keill, M.D.
Professor and Vice Chairman for Clinical Affairs, Department of Psychiatry, School of Medicine, University of Maryland, Baltimore, Maryland

Steven A. King, M.D.
Associate Director, Pain Clinic; Associate Professor, Department of Psychiatry and Human Behavior, Jefferson Medical College, Philadelphia, Pennsylvania

James A. Knowles, M.D., Ph.D.
Assistant Professor of Clinical Psychiatry, Department of Psychiatry, Columbia University College of Physicians and Surgeons, New York, New York

David J. Kupfer, M.D.
Professor and Chairman, Department of Psychiatry, University of Pittsburgh School of Medicine, Pittsburgh, Pennsylvania

H. Richard Lamb, M.D.
Professor of Psychiatry, Department of Psychiatry and the Behavioral Sciences, University of Southern California School of Medicine, Los Angeles, California

Hanna Levenson, Ph.D.
Director, Brief Psychotherapy Program, California Pacific Medical Center, San Francisco, California

James L. Levenson, M.D.
Professor of Psychiatry, Medicine and Surgery, Medical College of Virginia, Richmond, Virginia

Stephen S. Marmer, M.D., Ph.D.
Assistant Clinical Professor, UCLA Neuropsychiatric Institute, Department of Psychiatry and Biobehavioral Medicine, University of California at Los Angeles; Faculty, Southern California Psychoanalytic Institute, Los Angeles, California

Ronald L. Martin, M.D.
Chairman, Department of Psychiatry, University of Kansas School of Medicine, Wichita, Kansas

Steven Mattis, Ph.D.
Associate Professor of Clinical Psychology in Psychiatry, Cornell University Medical College; Associate Attending Psychologist, New York Hospital—Westchester Division, White Plains, New York

J. Stephen McDaniel, M.D.
Assistant Professor of Psychiatry, Emory University School of Medicine, Atlanta, Georgia

Lee Monroe, M.S.
Communications Director at The Institute of Living; Vice President of the Board of Directors, Connecticut Halfway Houses, Inc., Hartford, Connecticut

Michael G. Moran, M.D.
Associate Professor of Psychiatry, University of Colorado School of Medicine, Denver, Colorado

John M. Morihisa, M.D.
Professor and Chairman, Department of Psychiatry, Albany Medical College, Albany, New York

Jeffrey Newcorn, M.D.
Division of Child and Adolescent Psychiatry, Department of Psychiatry, Mount Sinai School of Medicine, New York, New York

Thomas C. Neylan, M.D.
Medical Director, Inpatient Psychiatry, California Pacific Medical Center, San Francisco, California

Katharine A. Phillips, M.D.
Instructor in Psychiatry, Harvard Medical School, Boston, Massachusetts; Assistant Psychiatrist and Director, Body Dysmorphic Disorder Clinic, McLean Hospital, Belmont, Massachusetts

John M. Plewes, M.D.
Chief of Psychiatry and Neurology, USA Medical Center, Ft. Bragg, North Carolina

Charles W. Popper, M.D.
Clinical Instructor in Psychiatry, Harvard Medical School, Boston, Massachusetts; Editor, *Journal of Child and Adolescent Psychopharmacology*

Stephen Rachlin, M.D.
Chairman, Department of Psychiatry and Psychology, Nassau County Medical Center, East Meadow, New York; Professor of Clinical Psychiatry, School of Medicine, State University of New York at Stony Brook

Darrel A. Regier, M.D., M.P.H.
Director of the Division of Epidemiology and Services Research, National Institute of Mental Health, Rockville, Maryland

Charles F. Reynolds III, M.D.
Professor of Psychiatry and Neurology, Department of Psychiatry, University of Pittsburgh School of Medicine, Pittsburgh, Pennsylvania

Ronald O. Rieder, M.D.
Associate Director of Education, Department of Psychiatry, Columbia University College of Physicians and Surgeons, New York, New York

John S. Rolland, M.D.
Clinical Associate Professor of Psychiatry; Co-Director, Center for Family Health, Pritzker School of Medicine, University of Chicago, Chicago, Illinois

Richard B. Rosse, M.D.
Associate Professor of Psychiatry, Georgetown University School of
Medicine; Chief, Georgetown Teaching Service, Washington Veterans
Administration Medical Center, Washington, D.C.

Bruce S. Rothschild, M.D.
Director, Consultation/Liaison Services, St. Francis Hospital and Medi-
cal Center, Hartford, Connecticut; Assistant Professor of Psychiatry,
University of Connecticut School of Medicine, Farmington, Connecticut

Stephen C. Scheiber, M.D.
Executive Vice President, American Board of Psychiatry and Neurology, Inc., Deerfield, Illinois; Adjunct Professor, Department of Psychiatry, Northwestern University School of Medicine, Evanston, Illinois;
Adjunct Professor, Department of Psychiatry, Medical College of Wisconsin, Milwaukee, Wisconsin

Theodore Shapiro, M.D.
Professor of Psychiatry and Professor of Psychiatry in Pediatrics, Cornell University Medical College; Director, Child and Adolescent Psychiatry, Payne Whitney Clinic, New York, New York

Edward K. Silberman, M.D.
Clinical Professor of Psychiatry and Human Behavior; Director of Residency Education, Jefferson Medical College of Thomas Jefferson University, Philadelphia, Pennsylvania

Jonathan M. Silver, M.D.
Associate Professor of Clinical Psychiatry, Columbia University College
of Physicians and Surgeons; Director of Neuropsychiatry, Columbia-
Presbyterian Medical Center, New York, New York

Daphne Simeon, M.D.
Assistant Professor of Psychiatry, Mount Sinai School of Medicine,
Queens Hospital Center, Jamaica, New York

Robert I. Simon, M.D.
Clinical Professor of Psychiatry; Director, Program in Psychiatry and
Law, Georgetown University School of Medicine, Washington, D.C.

William H. Sledge, M.D.
Professor and Associate Chairman for Education, Department of Psychiatry, Yale University School of Medicine, New Haven, Connecticut

David Spiegel, M.D.
Professor of Psychiatry and Behavioral Sciences, Stanford University School of Medicine, Stanford, California

Ronald J. Steingard, M.D.
Assistant Professor of Psychiatry, Harvard Medical School; Director of Psychopharmacology, Children's Hospital, Boston, Massachusetts

Nada L. Stotland, M.D.
Associate Professor, Departments of Psychiatry and Obstetrics and Gynecology, University of Chicago, Chicago, Illinois

Alan Stoudemire, M.D.
Professor of Psychiatry, Emory University School of Medicine, Atlanta, Georgia

James J. Strain, M.D.
Director, Division of Behavioral Medicine and Consultation Psychiatry, Department of Psychiatry, Mount Sinai School of Medicine, New York, New York

Kenneth Tardiff, M.D., M.P.H.
Professor of Psychiatry; Medical Director, Payne Whitney Clinic, New York Hospital—Cornell Medical Center, New York, New York

John G. Tierney, M.D.
Assistant Professor of Psychiatry, Emory University School of Medicine; Chief of Consultation Liaison Services, Emory Clinic, Atlanta, Georgia

Robert J. Ursano, M.D.
Professor of Psychiatry and Neuroscience; Chairman, Department of Psychiatry, Uniformed Services University of the Health Sciences, Bethesda, Maryland

Bruce S. Victor, M.D.
Director, Psychopharmacology Department, California Pacific Medical Center, San Francisco, California

Sophia Vinogradov, M.D.
San Francisco VA Medical Center, San Francisco, California

Froma Walsh, Ph.D.
Professor, SSA and Department of Psychiatry; Co-Director, Center for Family Health, Pritzker School of Medicine, University of Chicago, Chicago, Illinois

William L. Webb, Jr., M.D.
Psychiatrist-in-Chief Emeritus of The Institute of Living, Hartford, Connecticut; Professor of Psychiatry, University of Connecticut School of Medicine, Farmington, Connecticut

Janet B. W. Williams, D.S.W.
Professor of Clinical Psychiatric Social Work (in Psychiatry and Neurology), Biometrics Research, Department of Psychiatry, Columbia University College of Physicians and Surgeons, New York, New York

Michael G. Wise, M.D.
Clinical Professor of Psychiatry, Louisiana State University and Tulane School of Medicine, Metairie, Louisiana

Dennis Wolf, M.D.
Division of Behavioral Medicine and Consultation Psychiatry, Department of Psychiatry, Mount Sinai School of Medicine, New York, New York

Jesse H. Wright, M.D., Ph.D.
Professor, Department of Psychiatry and Behavioral Sciences, University of Louisville School of Medicine; Medical Director, Norton Psychiatric Clinic, Louisville, Kentucky

Irvin D. Yalom, M.D.
Professor of Psychiatry; Psychotherapy, Group Therapy, and Existential Therapy Program, Stanford University School of Medicine, Stanford, California

Stuart C. Yudofsky, M.D.
D. C. and Irene Ellwood Professor and Chairman, Department of Psychiatry and Behavioral Sciences, Baylor College of Medicine; Chief, Psychiatry Service, The Methodist Hospital, Houston, Texas

Sean H. Yutzy, M.D.
Assistant Professor of Psychiatry, Department of Psychiatry, Washington University School of Medicine, Washington University, St. Louis, Missouri

Preface

The first edition of *The American Psychiatric Press Textbook of Psychiatry,* published in 1988, was widely used by psychiatry residents and practicing clinicians, and received enthusiastic reviews in JAMA, the *New England Journal of Medicine,* and the *American Journal of Psychiatry.* Because of the rapid growth of the knowledge base of our field, 18 new contributors and eight new members of the editorial board were added for the second edition. As a result, the second edition was approximately 20% larger than the first edition, with a total of 1,694 pages.

Directors of medical student education communicated to us that the second edition contained more information than was required at the medical student level and that the cost of the textbook was prohibitive for many students. In addition, residency training directors in several other medical disciplines suggested that a condensed version of the second edition would be valuable for beginning residents in psychiatry and for those in primary care specialties and neurology. For all these reasons, we have prepared for publication the *Synopsis of Psychiatry.*

The goal of the *Synopsis of Psychiatry* is to condense and distill the most relevant information from every chapter of the second edition of the *Textbook of Psychiatry* and to present the information in a cohesive, interesting, and clinically applicable format. Each of the authors of the original chapters contained in the *Textbook of Psychiatry* recommended what material they believed could be deleted without damaging the overall purpose and educational content of the chapters. Working together with the authors, our text editor, Jude Berman, Ed.D., did a marvelous job integrating the sections within each chapter. As a professional educator, Dr. Berman provided invaluable assistance in helping the chapter authors and us reduce by 50% the size of the *Textbook of Psychia-*

try. Every effort was made to retain as many tables and figures in the synopsis as possible, since residents and educators have indicated that these formats have been particularly useful for coursework and review.

Carol Nadelson, M.D., Ron McMillen, and the excellent staff at the American Psychiatric Press were extremely helpful and responsive to us. We thank, in particular, Claire Reinburg, the Editorial Director, for facilitating this project. We also express gratitude to the many psychiatrists, other mental health professionals, and students at all levels who made suggestions and have encouraged us to publish the *Synopsis of Psychiatry*. We hope that the synopsis will serve as a useful resource to clinicians in assessing and treating patients who suffer from mental disorders and to residents and students at all levels in their learning about psychiatry and the people whom we serve.

Robert E. Hales, M.D., M.B.A.
Sacramento, California

Stuart C. Yudofsky, M.D.
Houston, Texas

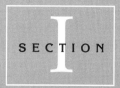

SECTION

I

Theoretical Foundations

CHAPTER 1

The Neuroscientific Foundation of Psychiatry

Steven E. Hyman, M.D.
Joseph T. Coyle, M.D.

Advances in research on the brain have occurred with a rapidly increasing pace over the last 20 years, reaching the point that neuroscience can justifiably be considered the biomedical foundation of psychiatry. Neuroscience research offers important opportunities to psychiatry in the interest of the care of patients and, in the long term, for the better understanding of human experience and behavior. Thus, it is essential for psychiatry to harness this rapidly evolving area of knowledge.

■ FUNCTIONAL ANATOMY OF THE NEURON

The *neuron* is a cell type that is highly specialized, both anatomically and biochemically, to carry out the functions of information processing and signaling. Within the nervous system, hundreds of types of neurons serve specialized functions. In contrast with many other cell types that are capable of cell division throughout the life of the individual, neurons do not divide once they are fully mature. This inability of most mature neurons to undergo mitosis has obvious implications for the irreversible effects of damage to the nervous system.

The neuron can be divided into four distinct components, the *cell body* (or *perikaryon*), the *dendrites*, the *axon*, and the *presynaptic terminal* (Figure 1–1). The synthesis of proteins and other structural components

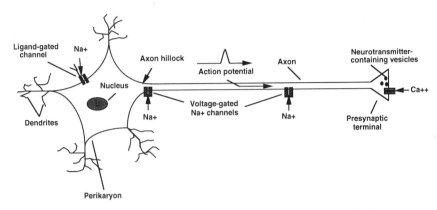

Figure 1–1.   Schematic representation of a neuron. A ligand-gated channel, possibly a glutamate receptor, is shown permitting Na^+ entry into the cell body of a neuron. If the balance of positive to negative charges is adequate to depolarize the neuron to threshold in the region of the proximal axon or axon hillock, voltage-gated Na^+ channels will open, generating an action potential. The action potential propagates down the axon because of the sequential opening of Na^+ channels. When the action potential invades the presynaptic terminal, voltage-gated Ca^{++} channels open, and the entry of Ca^{++} causes neurotransmitter release (see discussion in text). Repolarization of the neuron results from the opening of voltage-gated K^+ channels in rapid succession after Na^+ entry.

of neurons generally occurs in the perikaryon. Situated within the perikaryon of the neuron is the nucleus, which contains the genetic material in the form of deoxyribonucleic acid (DNA). The information for protein synthesis is encoded by genes contained within the DNA; this genetic information is read out by a process called *transcription*, in which DNA serves as a template for the synthesis of ribonucleic acid (RNA). The resulting primary RNA transcripts are then processed to yield mature messenger RNA (mRNA) that is exported out of the nucleus into the cytoplasm of the perikaryon. There the mRNA is translated into proteins on organelles called *ribosomes*. The rich concentration of RNA-protein synthetic machinery surrounding the nucleus in the perikaryon accounts for the "Nissl substance" observed with certain classical stains of neurons in brain tissue. Protein translation occurs largely within the perikaryon, but active ribosomes have recently been detected in dendrites, raising the possibility that local control of protein translation by neural signaling processes may occur.

The *axon* is a fine tubular extension from the neuronal cell body down which electrical impulses are conducted to the nerve terminals. Neurons generally send out only a single axon, the length of which varies from less than a millimeter for interneurons to over a meter for motor neurons innervating the extremities. As it approaches its terminal field of innervation, the axon may branch to varying degrees, depending on the number of neurons with which it makes synaptic contact.

Dendrites are multiple fine tubular extensions of the neuronal cell body that serve as the primary structure for the reception of synaptic contacts from other neurons. Neurons are generally involved in the integration of multiple synaptic inputs. Neurons such as the Purkinje cells in the cerebellum and components of the reticular core of the brain stem, which have marked integrative functions, possess very extensive dendritic "trees" that receive synaptic input from thousands of neurons.

The *synapse* is a specialized structure involved in the transmission of information from one neuron to another; transmission is generally accomplished by chemical messengers called *neurotransmitters,* but in some cases it may be electrical. Structurally, the synapse consists of an outpouching of the terminal portion of the axon of the *presynaptic neuron,* known as a "bouton," which is firmly attached to the dendritic membrane of the adjacent *postsynaptic neuron* by specialized contacts. The dendritic membrane at the synapse is markedly enriched with receptors that respond to the neurotransmitter released by the terminal bouton of the presynaptic neuron. The presynaptic terminal contains a number of cellular structures that allow it to remain metabolically and functionally somewhat independent of the neuronal cell body. The terminal contains mitochondria—the power packs of the cell that generate adenosine triphosphate (ATP) from the aerobic metabolism of glucose—enzymes involved in the synthesis and degradation of neurotransmitters, and the storage vesicles that maintain substantial concentrations of the neurotransmitter in a protected state, awaiting release.

The fundamental property that permits neurons to function in information processing and signaling is the excitable nature of their membrane. This property derives from the membrane's specialized nature: it maintains a voltage gradient between the interior of the neuron and the extracellular fluid, and selectively gates the transmembranal flow of ions. Two types of proteins are primarily responsible for the regulation of ion distribution and hence voltage across the neuronal membrane: the transmembrane *ion pumps* and the *voltage-gated ion channels.*

Pumps critical in establishing the physiological gradient of ions found across the neuronal membrane are an energy (ATP)-dependent pump, the sodium-potassium ATPase, which moves two Na^+ ions out of the cell for every K^+ ion it allows in; and pumps that remove Ca^{++} from the cell. At rest, there are high relative concentrations of Na^+ and Cl^- outside the neuron and a high relative concentration of K^+ inside the cell. The major source of negative charge inside the cell is derived from negatively charged amino acids. Overall, the membrane is polarized, with a voltage difference across the membrane of about −70 mV with respect to the outside. This is called the *resting membrane potential.*

When the neuronal membrane is depolarized to about −35 mV, an *action potential* occurs, which represents cell "firing" and is the fundamental mechanism of neuronal signaling. Specifically, as the interior of the cell becomes more positive, specialized voltage-gated Na^+ channels open, permitting more positive ions to flow into the cell (Figure 1–1). The action potential represents the spread of depolarization by the vectorial opening of adjacent voltage-gated Na^+ channels. Because each Na^+ channel that opens in succession provides the positive charge to bring the next segment of the axon up to threshold for opening of its Na^+ channels, the action potential is self-regenerating; once begun, it propagates down the axon without fail. When the action potential arrives in the presynaptic terminal, it causes opening of the unique voltage-gated Ca^{++} channels found there. Ca^{++} entry initiates a series of complex biochemical processes that cause the neurotransmitter-containing vesicles to fuse with the presynaptic membrane and release their contents into the synapse, thus permitting synaptic transmission. Because the entry of positive charge depolarizes the membrane, bringing the neuron closer to threshold for firing an action potential, neurotransmitter receptors that permit entry of cations such as Na^+ or Ca^{++} are excitatory, and those that cause entry of anions such as Cl^- or the exit of cations such as K^+ are inhibitory.

Neuronal dendrites and cell bodies are continuously summating excitatory and inhibitory inputs to determine whether a neuron will generate an action potential. The innervation of the neuron is not random but highly organized. Excitatory inputs are generally concentrated at the distal end of dendrites, whereas inhibitory inputs are located primarily at the proximal end of dendrites and around the perikaryon. This spatial distribution means that inhibitory inputs play a predominant role in determining whether a neuron will generate an action potential. Because the action potential is self-regenerating, the decision to fire an action potential is an all-or-none process. Once the balance is struck toward adequate depolarization in the region of the proximal axon (i.e., axon hillock), where the density of voltage-gated Na^+ channels is high, an action potential is generated (Figure 1–1).

■ NEUROTRANSMITTERS

Neurotransmitters in the brain can be divided conceptually into two classes: the classical small molecule neurotransmitters, such as norepinephrine, are locally synthesized in nerve terminals, and the neuropeptide neurotransmitters, such as the endorphins, are synthesized in the perikaryon (Table 1–1 and Table 1–2).

Table 1–1. "Classical" neurotransmitters

Acetylcholine	Aspartic acid
Histamine	Gamma-aminobutyric acid
Serotonin	Glutamic acid
Dopamine	Glycine
Norepinephrine	Homocysteine
Epinephrine	Taurine

Table 1–2. Selected neuropeptide neurotransmitter candidates

Adrenocorticotropic hormone (ACTH)	Gastrin
Angiotensin II	Glucagon
Atriopeptin	Insulin
Beta-endorphin[a]	Leu-enkephalin[a]
Bombesin	Luteinizing hormone–releasing factor
Bradykinin	Met-enkephalin[a]
Calcitonin gene–related peptide (CGRP)	Neurotensin
	Neuropeptide Y
Carnosine	Somatostatin
Cholecystokinin	Substance P
Corticotropin-releasing factor	Thyrotropin-releasing hormone (TRH)
Dynorphin[a]	Vasoactive intestinal peptide (VIP)
Galanin	Vasopressin

[a]Members of the endorphin family.

☐ Classical Neurotransmitters

Among the small molecule neurotransmitters, the catecholamines, which include dopamine, norepinephrine, and epinephrine, have served as important models of synthesis, release, and metabolism. While each acts as a neurotransmitter in its own right, the catecholamines are products of sequential steps in a single biosynthetic pathway (Figure 1–2). The enzymes responsible for catecholamine synthesis are synthesized in the cell perikaryon and are transported down axons to presynaptic terminals. Neurons that utilize dopamine as their neurotransmitter possess the only the first two enzymes in this pathway, tyrosine hydroxylase and dopa decarboxylase. Neurons that release norepinephrine express a third enzyme, dopamine beta-hydroxylase, and neurons that produce epinephrine express a fourth enzyme, phenylethanolamine-N-methyl-transferase (PNMT). Because tyrosine hydroxylase is a tightly controlled

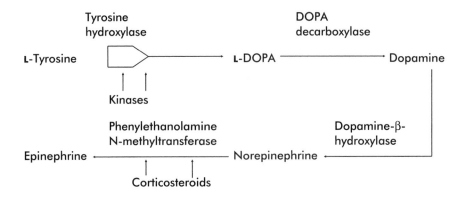

Figure 1–2. The biosynthetic pathway for catecholamines. Note that tyrosine hydroxylase is activated by phosphorylation by protein kinases, and the synthesis of phenylethanolamine-N-methyltransferase is regulated by corticosteroids.

rate-limiting enzyme, important regulatory mechanisms that determine neurotransmitter availability are common to this entire group of neurotransmitters.

The synthetic pathways for classical neurotransmitters generally, although not invariably, involve the conversion of an informationally inert precursor to an informationally "charged" neurotransmitter. In the case of the catecholamines, the amino acid L-tyrosine serves as the precursor. Tyrosine hydroxylase, the rate-limiting enzyme in the synthesis pathway, is virtually saturated by the ambient levels of tyrosine in the brain. Therefore, increasing levels of this amino acid in the brain would not significantly affect catecholamine biosynthesis. In order to prevent a vicious cycle of catecholamine synthesis and degradation, tyrosine hydroxylase is subject to end-product inhibition. Accordingly, when the concentration of catecholamines in the nerve terminal exceeds their storage capacity, the excess catecholamines inhibit the activity of tyrosine hydroxylase, thereby preventing further synthesis of catecholamines. Thus, when the catecholaminergic neurons are silent, further synthesis of catecholamines is arrested. On the other hand, when catecholamines are released and the stores are depleted, this inhibitory feedback is removed and the rate of synthesis increases.

With neural activity, however, other mechanisms come into play that are biologically even more significant. Repeated firing of the catecholamine neuron causes activation of second messenger systems and therefore of protein kinases (see below). Phosphorylation of tyrosine hydroxylase, by protein kinases, reduces its sensitivity to feedback inhibition and, in addition, increases its affinity for a critical co-factor, pterin

(Nose et al. 1985). Periods of prolonged, increased catecholaminergic neuronal activity brings into play a second mechanism, the synthesis of additional enzyme molecules in the biosynthetic pathway for catechol-amines. This second process is regulated at the level of the catechola-minergic cell body where additional mRNA encoding for tyrosine hydroxylase is transcribed from the nuclear DNA. Thus, the synthesis of catecholamines is under dynamic regulation that is tightly coordinated by the activity of the catecholaminergic neuron.

After the enzymatic synthesis of catecholamines occurs within the cytosol of the nerve terminal, the catecholamines are concentrated in vesicles, small membranous sacs within the nerve terminal. Vesicular storage of catecholamines is an active process that is inhibited by the antihypertensive drug reserpine. The storage vesicles serve two pur-poses. First, they protect the catecholamines from enzymatic degrada-tion by the enzyme monoamine oxidase (MAO). This catabolic enzyme is localized on the outer membrane of the mitochondria. Interference with vesicular storage by treatment with reserpine releases catecholamines within the nerve terminal so that they are rapidly degraded by MAO. Second, the vesicles mediate the quantal release of catecholamines by exocytose when an action potential reaches the nerve terminal.

In addition to the intracellular enzyme MAO, a second enzyme that inactivates catecholamines is located on the outer surface of the neuronal membrane as well as on the outer surface of many other cell types. This enzyme, catechol-O-methyltransferase (COMT), catalyzes the inactiva-tion of catecholamines by methylating one of the ring hydroxyl groups. However, these enzymatic mechanisms are not the most significant mechanism by which the action of catecholamines in the synapse is ter-minated. The most critical mechanisms include diffusion out of the syn-apse and active reuptake of the catecholamines into the nerve terminal that released them via a specific transporter protein driven by the gradi-ent of sodium across the neuronal membrane (Pacholczyk et al. 1991). The dopamine and norepinephrine transporters are members of a large gene family of proteins that also includes the serotonin and GABA trans-porters (Giros and Caron 1993).

Figure 1–3 summarizes processes involved in the synthesis, storage, release, and inactivation of classical neurotransmitters. These interre-lated processes ensure a steady availability of the neurotransmitter in the nerve terminals that can be regulated by neural activity, and the inac-tivation of the released neurotransmitter so that it does not produce un-desired effects on neighboring neurons. Similar mechanisms act, to a variable degree, for the other classical neurotransmitters, including sero-tonin, acetylcholine, and histamine. The amino acid neurotransmitters, however, represent an important exception from the principle that neurotransmitters are synthesized from neurophysiologically inactive

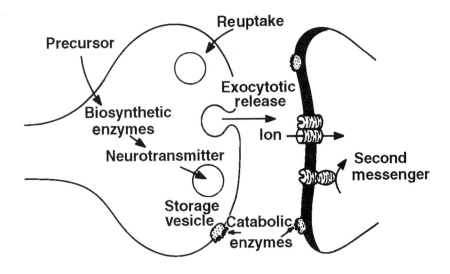

Figure 1–3.   Schematic representation of the processes involved in the synthesis, synaptic action, and inactivation of classical neurotransmitters.

precursors. The amino acids glutamate and aspartate appear to be the predominant excitatory neurotransmitters in the brain; the amino acids GABA and glycine appear to be major inhibitory neurotransmitters. These molecules are present in plasma and are important precursors for protein synthesis, characteristics that would seem to be incompatible with the role of a neurotransmitter, which must have highly restricted spatial and temporal actions. However, the brain expends considerable energy on selective transport processes and catabolic enzymes to maintain extremely low concentrations of these amino acid neurotransmitters in the extracellular space of the brain.

☐ Neuropeptides

The fact that small proteins (peptides) are used in the body as signals has long been known based on their role as hormones in the pituitary and other endocrine organs. The potential role of peptides as neurotransmitters derived from the discovery that the releasing factors controlling the secretion of several pituitary hormones were, in fact, peptides synthesized by neurons in the arcuate nucleus of the hypothalamus. Although it was originally believed that a neuron uses only one neurotransmitter, it has recently become apparent that neurons usually release more than one neurotransmitter. Most investigations have demonstrated co-localization of a classical neurotransmitter and one or more neuropeptides, although two classical neurotransmitters (e.g., serotonin and GABA) may co-exist in the same neuron.

Unlike the small molecule neurotransmitters synthesized by enzymatic processes located within the nerve terminal, the neuropeptides are synthesized within the neuronal cell body. This reflects the fact that synthesis of neuropeptides, being small proteins, is directed by mRNA, which has been transcribed from DNA within the nucleus. It is now known that single genes often give rise to multiple active peptides, and further, that the array of peptides produced from a single gene may vary in cell type. The generation of such diversity begins following transcription of the gene that encodes the peptide precursor. In eukaryotic cells most genes have their protein coding sequences (called *exons*) interrupted by noncoding sequences (called *introns*). When a gene is transcribed, the primary transcript is co-linear with the DNA and therefore contains both exons and introns. Before the RNA leaves the nucleus to be translated, the introns are removed and the exons are "spliced" to form a mature mRNA. The primary transcript of certain neuropeptide genes is spliced in alternate ways in different cell types. By including or excluding particular exons in the mature cytoplasmic mRNA, mRNAs encoding distinctly different peptides can be produced. For example, calcitonin and calcitonin gene-related peptide (CGRP) are the products of the same gene derived by such alternate splicing.

The mature mRNAs encoding neuropeptides are translated on the rough endoplasmic reticulum (ER) to give rise to large precursors called *polyproteins*. These precursors (e.g., pre-proopiomelanocortin or pre-proenkephalin) contain a sequence, almost always at the amino terminus of the protein, that targets the protein to the neuron's secretory pathway. This *leader sequence,* or "pre" sequence, is rapidly cleaved by an endopeptidase, leaving the remainder of the precursor (e.g., proopiomelanocortin or proenkephalin). This precursor then undergoes further proteolytic cleavage and subsequent chemical modification (e.g., glycosylation, amidation, acetylation, or phosphorylation) within the ER and Golgi to yield numerous biologically active peptides for release. Just as alternate splicing of mRNAs permits the generation of multiple signaling molecules for a single gene, differential processing of peptide precursors permits the generation of multiple signaling molecules from a single peptide precursor. Within peptide precursors pairs of basic amino acid residues (lysine or arginine) are recognized by processing enzymes as sites for cleavage.

Among the peptide neurotransmitters, the endogenous opioid peptides are the best studied and have clear relevance to psychiatry because of their role in the stress response, motivated behavior, and analgesia. Approximately 20 active opioid peptides have been isolated and characterized from mammalian brain, pituitary, and adrenal glands. All of these endogenous opioids contain the same four amino acids at their amino terminus, Tyr-Gly-Gly-Phe, followed by either Met or Leu (Met-enkephalin, Leu-enkephalin). All of the opioid peptides derive from one of three large polyprotein precursors, each encoded by a separate gene. The precursors are proenkephalin (which encodes six copies of the Met-enkephalin sequence and one of the Leu-enkephalin sequence), pro-dynorphin (precursor of the endogenous opioid dynorphin and related peptides), and proopiomelanocortin (POMC). POMC is particularly interesting because it contains the sequences of active peptides with apparently different biological function, the opioid peptide, beta-endorphin, and adrenocorticotropic hormone (ACTH), and because it is processed to yield different active peptides in different tissues.

■ RECEPTORS

The identification, characterization, and, more recently, molecular cloning of neurotransmitter receptors has been a major advance in neuroscience that has had considerable impact on the understanding of information processing in the brain and the sites of action of neuroactive substances, including psychotropic drugs. Although neurotransmitters are commonly described as excitatory or inhibitory, as if this action were inherent to their molecular structure, the nature of neuronal responses to a neurotransmitter ultimately depends upon the presence of a receptor linked to a transducer. For this reason, depending upon the receptors and transducers located on a given neuron, a neurotransmitter might exert inhibitory, excitatory, or more complicated "modulatory" effects.

Neurotransmitter receptors are proteins that span the neuronal membrane. These proteins have ligand binding regions that are accessible to extracellular messengers and other regions involved in transducing the binding interaction into an intercellular effect. The reversible binding of the neurotransmitter to the receptor causes a conformational change that triggers the transmembrane signaling event. The known neurotransmitter receptors can activate two different general classes of effects: they can directly control or gate the opening of an ion channel that is an intrinsic part of the receptor molecule itself, or they can act by regulating the function of a signal transducing *G-protein* (see below) that is associated with the inner surface of the membrane. Receptors that gate an intrinsic ion channel are called *ligand-gated channels;* receptors that act via G-proteins are called *G-protein–linked receptors.* As is the case for other important classes of molecules discussed above, such as the voltage sensitive ion channels and the neurotransmitter transporters, the ligand-gated channels, the G-protein–linked receptors, and the G-proteins themselves each form independent large families of molecules with homologous structures. Each of these large *gene families* is thought to have begun with a single primitive ancestor (e.g., an ancestral ligand-gated channel) that, through gene duplication and mutation, gave rise to a large number of genes and hence proteins with specific but related functions, permitting increasing complexity of neural signaling during evolution.

Receptors bind their specific ligand in an avid, specific, reversible, and saturable (i.e., the number of receptor sites are limited) fashion; neuroscientists have taken advantage of these characteristics to label receptors with radioactive ligands. If the avidity of a specific interaction between the radioligand and receptor is sufficiently high, the radioligand can be caught in the act of binding to the receptor long enough so that the radioactive complex can be isolated. This strategy has greatly facilitated studies to determine the characteristics of these neurotransmitter-receptor interactions and their localization within the nervous system. For example, the relative affinity of drugs or neurotransmitter analogs for a receptor can be determined by their potency at preventing the binding of the radioactive ligand to its receptor.

☐ Ligand-Gated Channels

The ligand-gated channels are proteins that contain a neurotransmitter binding site and a channel pore. To form the pore, the protein traverses the membrane four times. Activation of this class of receptors, which contain rapidly responsive intrinsic ion channels, is responsible for fast "point-to-point" information transfer in the brain. The major excitatory neurotransmitter in the brain appears to be glutamate. A subset of its receptors directly gate Na^+ channels so that when glutamate binds to the receptor, transmembrane channel within the receptor molecule opens to permit the influx of sodium, hence depolarizing the neuron. Other important excitatory ligand-gated channels in the nervous system include the nicotinic acetylcholine receptors. The major inhibitory neurotransmitter in the brain is GABA, and in the spinal cord the closely related amino acid glycine. When GABA or glycine stimulate their receptors, intrinsic channels admit Cl^-, resulting in hyperpolarization of the neuronal membrane.

☐ G-Protein–Linked Receptors

Fast excitatory neurotransmission in the brain appears to be subserved by a small number of neurotransmitters, especially glutamate. In contrast, with only one known exception (the 5-HT$_3$ receptor), the receptors for all the monoamines and neuropeptides do not directly gate ion channels, but act via membrane-associated signal-transducing proteins called

G-proteins. G-protein–linked receptors are involved in a constant process of modulation of the responsiveness of neural circuits, adding further complexity to the rapid transmission of excitatory and inhibitory impulses by glutamate, GABA, and related neurotransmitters throughout the neural network.

The G-protein–linked receptors that have been structurally analyzed to date by molecular cloning studies have a common overall structure, crossing the neuronal membrane seven times. The ligand binding domain appears to be in a pocket produced by these transmembrane domains within the plane of the membrane. Coupling to intracellular signaling mechanisms occurs on the cytoplasmic side of the neuronal membrane. G-proteins, so named because they bind guanine nucleotides, are associated with the inside of the neuronal membrane. Binding of ligand to the receptor causes a change in its conformation that produces activation of the G-proteins. The G-proteins, in turn, transduce the receptor-mediated signal into intracellular effects.

G-proteins are heterotrimers (i.e., proteins made up of three different subunits denoted α, β, and γ). With few exceptions the α subunits, which are very diverse, are the specific effectors of G-protein activation (Figure 1–4). In the inactive state the α, β, and γ subunits are bound together and a molecule of guanosine diphosphate (GDP) is bound to the α subunit. When activated by a receptor, the GDP is replaced by a guanosine triphosphate (GTP) on the α subunit and the α subunit dissociates from its complex with β and γ. This active α subunit remains associated with the membrane where it can cause the opening or closing of specific voltage-gated ion channels or the activation or inhibition of enzymes that produce intracellular second messengers. The particular action depends on which α type of subunit is activated by a given receptor. The effects of G-proteins on ion channels alter the responses of neurons to subsequent stimulation by excitatory or inhibitory neurotransmitters, such as glutamate and GABA. In addition, G-proteins regulate enzymes that produce second messengers. For example, G_s-linked receptors activate adenylate cyclase to increase cyclic AMP production; G_i-linked receptors inhibit adenylate cyclase.

Although the number of second messengers found within cells is large, their mechanism of action can be generalized. With few exceptions (e.g., cyclic AMP can independently gate certain ion channels within the olfactory system), second messengers exert their major biological effects via specific protein kinases. Protein kinases are enzymes that transfer phosphate groups from adenosine triphosphate (ATP) to specific protein substrates. Based on their charge and size, phosphate groups alter the conformation of proteins and hence their function. Because phosphorylation is a covalent modification, it can act over a very long time scale. Substrates for second messenger-activated phosphorylation include ion

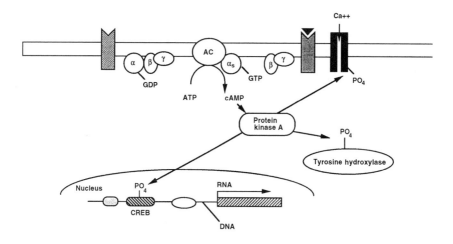

Figure 1–4.   The adenylate cyclase second messenger system. Shown at top is a schematic of a neuronal membrane. Neurotransmitter receptors (stippled), voltage-gated channels (a Ca^{++} channel is shown in black), and adenylate cyclase (AC) are integral membrane proteins. The subunits of heterotrimeric G-proteins (see text)—α, β, and γ—are associated with the inner surface of the membrane. An unoccupied receptor is shown at left; in this circumstance, the α subunit is bound to GDP and the G-protein subunits are fully associated. With binding of neuro-transmitter (black triangle) shown at right, the receptor can activate the G-protein. GDP is exchanged for GTP, and the α subunit dissociates from β and γ. Here α_s is shown at center activating adenylate cyclase that catalyzes the synthesis of the intracellular second messenger cyclic AMP (cAMP) from adenosine triphosphate (ATP). Cyclic AMP activates protein kinase A (which is shown phosphorylating the calcium channel), the neurotransmitter-synthesizing enzyme tyrosine hy-droxylase, and the transcription factor CREB within the nucleus of the cell.

channels, receptors, neurotransmitter synthesizing enzymes, cytoskele-tal proteins, and proteins that control gene transcription. By activating protein phosphorylation, G-protein–linked receptors regulate diverse functions within the cell, and by regulating gene expression they even regulate the cell's protein constituents. Phosphorylation, which may, for example, inactivate receptors or increase or decrease the likelihood of voltage gated ion channel opening, will alter the way that neurons pro-cess information, thus altering the behavior of brain circuits in significant ways. Clearly, then, the brain is not simply a hard-wired network relay-ing information via excitatory and inhibitory potentials. The brain is con-stantly modifying how the neurons within it process information. Such plasticity of neural functioning is required for processes such as learning and memory, and is also likely involved in the onset of psychopathology (e.g., the state changes that occur with onset of depression) and the mechanism of action of many psychotropic drugs.

■ SYSTEMS NEUROBIOLOGY

□ Ascending Monoamine Systems and Acetylcholine

Among the neuronal systems directly relevant to psychiatric disorders and psychotropic drugs are chemically coded neurotransmitter systems with their cell bodies found within the reticular core of the brain stem and its rostral extension in the basal forebrain (Coyle 1986). These include neurons utilizing the neurotransmitters norepinephrine, dopamine, serotonin, histamine, and acetylcholine. The reticular core neurons are not involved in conveying specific information but rather modulate more global neuronal function via G-protein–linked receptors. Instead, they are thought to be involved in the control of arousal, attention, vigilance, and mood.

Noradrenergic Neurons

Norepinephrine is the principal neurotransmitter of an important class of neurons within the reticular core of the brain stem. The synthetic pathway for norepinephrine is shown in Figure 1–2. The principle noradrenergic nucleus is the *locus coeruleus,* so named because of its bluish color in fresh brain sections. The locus coeruleus is located bilaterally on the floor of the fourth ventricle (Figure 1–5). Additional noradrenergic (norepinephrine-releasing neurons) nuclei are scattered in the medulla and pons and primarily innervate the brain stem. The estimated 40,000 neurons in the human locus coeruleus are the primary source of noradrenergic innervation for most of the CNS, including the forebrain, cerebellum, and spinal cord. Like the other ascending monoamine neurons, the noradrenergic axons are fine, unmyelinated processes that contain neurotransmitter throughout their extent. Beaded varicosities along the axons are sites of specialized synaptic contacts known as *synapsis en passage.* As best exemplified in the cerebral cortex, individual noradrenergic axons make synaptic contacts with thousands of neurons, and the axonal arbor appears as a dense meshwork ramifying throughout all cortical layers (Figure 1–5). Furthermore, individual noradrenergic neurons send axons that innervate functionally diverse regions of the brain (e.g., cerebral cortex and cerebellum).

   The effects of norepinephrine are mediated in the brain by two classes of receptors: α- and β-adrenergic receptors. These classes are further subdivided, based upon pharmacological characteristics and physi-

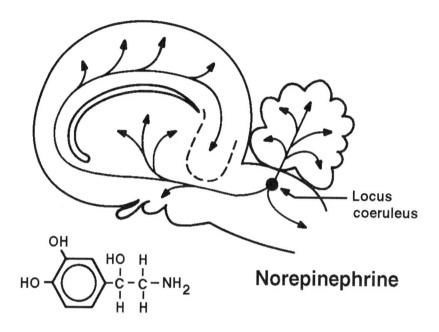

Figure 1–5. The primary projections of the noradrenergic locus coeruleus.

ologic effects, into α_1 and α_2, and β_1 and β_2 receptors. Stimulation of α_1 receptors results in activation of phosphoinositide turnover. α_2 receptors are linked via G_i / G_o to inhibition of adenylate cyclase and opening of a K^+ channel. These actions tend to decrease neuronal firing. The α_2 receptors on the noradrenergic cell body, which can be stimulated via recurrent noradrenergic collaterals, slow the firing rate of noradrenergic neurons. In addition, when activated, α_2 receptors on noradrenergic terminals decrease the amount of norepinephrine released, presumably by reducing the influx of calcium during the depolarization of the nerve terminal. Clonidine is an agonist at α_2 receptors; thus clonidine inhibits locus coeruleus firing. This accounts for its efficacy in attenuating physical symptoms of acute withdrawal from opiates.

β_1 and β_2 receptors are distinguished principally by the lower intrinsic activity of norepinephrine at the latter receptor and the differential sensitivity to certain antagonists. In brain, the β_1 receptors appear to have a high degree of localization on neurons whereas the β_2 receptors are predominantly, although not exclusively, associated with non-neuronal elements such as the glial cells. Activation of β receptors results in stimulation of adenylate cyclase via G_s and the elevation of the intracellular levels of cyclic AMP. Thus, the cellular responses to beta agonists reflect the activation of cyclic AMP–dependent protein kinases. Desensitization of cortical beta-adrenergic receptors is a general effect of antidepressants.

Serotonergic Neurons

The cell bodies of serotonin-releasing neurons are located in the raphe nuclei found near the midline of the brain stem (Figure 1–6). Like the locus coeruleus noradrenergic neurons, the serotonergic neurons provide a highly collateralized innervation to virtually all areas of the CNS. Nevertheless, components of the raphe nuclei provide more regionally discrete patterns of innervation. Serotonergic neurons display a distinctive slow (1 to 5 spikes per second) and highly regular rate of spontaneous activity that varies with behavioral state. Endogenous "pacemaker" ion channels in serotonergic neurons are responsible for this regular rate of firing, which occurs in the absence of excitatory input. This tonic activity means that serotonin is nearly always found in the synaptic cleft, although the amount of serotonin depends on such factors as the phase of the sleep-wake cycle, level of arousal, and timing of the circadian cycle. Serotonin receptors with a high affinity for serotonin are tonically acti-

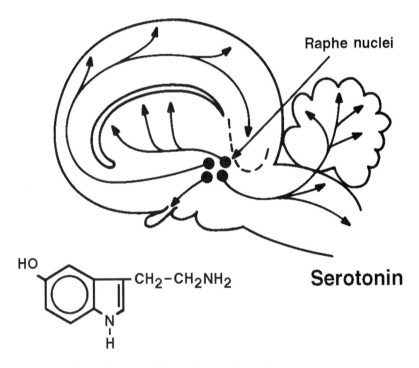

Figure 1–6. The pathways of the raphe serotonergic neurons.

vated while those with a lower affinity are only phasically activated during times of increased firing.

The synaptic effects of serotonin are mediated by a large number of pre- and postsynaptic receptors. Current pharmacologic and cloning studies suggest seven types of 5-HT receptors with multiple subtypes, numbering 14 in all. Those directly relevant to psychopharmacology include the 5-HT$_{1A}$ receptor, which is largely presynaptic and the apparent site of action of the anxiolytic drug buspirone and the 5-HT$_{1D}$ receptor, which is found on vascular endothelium and is the site at which the new antimigraine drug sumatriptan is an agonist. The 5-HT$_2$ receptor is postsynaptic and appears to be the key site of action for LSD, mescaline, and related hallucinogens. In the striatum, the 5-HT$_{2C}$ receptor may be important in the extrapyramidal control of movement. The atypical antipsychotic drug clozapine is a 5-HT$_{2C}$ receptor antagonist (along with antagonist properties at many other receptors), and risperidone is a mixed D$_2$ and 5-HT$_{2C}$ receptor antagonist.

5-HT$_{1A}$ and 5-HT$_{1D}$ receptors inhibit adenylate cyclase and activate a voltage sensitive K$^+$ channel via G$_i$. 5-HT$_{1C}$ and 5-HT$_2$ receptors activate the inositol triphosphate/diacyglycerol second messenger pathways. The 5-HT$_3$ receptor is the only known monoamine receptor that is a ligand-gated channel. The novel antiemetic drug odansetron antagonizes the excitatory effects of serotonin at its 5-HT$_3$ reception in the chemotrigger zone of the medulla. (The other significant receptor type on these neurons are dopamine D$_2$ receptors; thus older antiemetics are all dopamine receptor antagonists.) Serotonergic neurons, through their innervation of the thalmus and cerebral cortex, have been associated with regulation of alertness. Serotonin effects in the limbic system may have a role in control of mood, anxiety, and aggression, and in the spinal cord with modulation of pain.

Dopaminergic Neurons

Three major dopaminergic systems have been of particular interest for psychiatric research (Figure 1–7). Large pigmented dopaminergic neurons located in the substantia nigra within the midbrain provide a remarkably dense innervation of the caudate and putamen that account for approximately 15% of the synapses in these structures. This highly collateralized pathway of unmyelinated axons arborizes into a fine filigree of varicosity-laden axons, providing thousands of *synapses en passage*. The nigrostriatal dopaminergic projection is intimately involved in the initiation and smooth execution of the motor activities and may play a comparable role in cognitive function, reflecting the major projection from the frontal cortex to the caudate. Degeneration of the nigrostriatal dopamine projections causes the symptoms of Parkinson's disease; and,

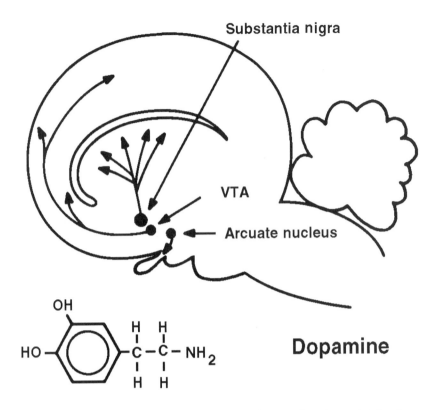

Figure 1–7. The three major dopaminergic pathways: the nigrostriatal pathway, the mesocorticolimbic pathway (originating in the ventral tegmental area [VTA]), and the arcuate nucleus pathway to the infundibulum.

the blockade of dopamine receptors by neuroleptic drugs causes clinically similar extrapyramidal side effects, reflecting impaired striatal dopaminergic neurotransmission.

The more medially localized dopaminergic neuronal cell bodies in the ventral tegmental area (VTA) provide innervation to the nucleus accumbens, a pivotal arena of limbic circuitry, as well as to the neocortex, cingulate cortex, amygdala, and hippocampus. Whereas in the rat, dopamine innervation of the cortex is sparse and limited to prefrontal regions, in primates there appears to be significant innervation of the entire cerebral cortex by VTA dopamine neurons. The dopamine projection of the VTA to the nucleus accumbens has been implicated as a "brain reward" circuit, mediating the positively reinforcing effects of drugs of abuse, including cocaine, amphetamine, and probably opiates The cortical dopaminergic projections may be implicated in attention, "working memory," and, by inference, cognitive integration. Based on the dopamine antagonist properties of antipsychotic drugs (see below), dysfunction of meso-corticolimbic dopamine circuits has been hypothesized to occur in schizophrenia and other psychotic disorders. Finally, a group of dopaminergic neurons located in the arcuate nucleus of the hypothalamus send axons that terminate in the venous sinuses of the pituitary. This tubero-infundibular dopamine projection inhibits the release of the pituitary hormone prolactin.

The synaptic effects of dopamine appear to be mediated by several pharmacologically and physiologically distinct receptors. It is likely that not all dopamine receptor types have been discovered, and at present the nomenclature is unsettled. Based on their structure (deduced from molecular cloning) and their pharmacologic properties, there appear to be two families of dopamine receptors called D_1-like (the D_1 and D_5 receptors, also called D_{1A} and D_{1B}) and D_2-like (the D_2, D_3, and D_4 receptors, also called D_{2A}, D_{2B}, and D_{2C}). In addition, a long and a short form of the D_2 receptor have been found based on alternative splicing of the D_2 receptor mRNA, but no obvious functional differences between the forms have been found. The different receptor types have overlapping but nonidentical distributions in brain regions innervated by dopamine fibers. The D_1 and D_5 receptors activate adenylate cyclase via G_s. The D_2 receptor inhibits adenylate cyclase and activates a voltage sensitive K^+ channel via G_i. The precise second messenger effects of D_3 and D_4 receptors are not yet clear. The antipsychotic drugs are antagonists of D_2, D_3, and D_4 receptors.

Cholinergic Neurons

The major source of cholinergic innervation to the cerebral cortex, hippocampus, and limbic structures is a complex of large neurons located in the basal forebrain (Figure 1–8). The nucleus basalis of Meynert, a somewhat dispersed group of cholinergic cell bodies located in the ventral and medial aspects of the globus pallidus, sends axons that innervate the cerebral cortex. The more anteriorly located diagonal band of Broca and medial septal nucleus innervate the hippocampal formation and cingulate cortex. The terminal arbor of the cholinergic afferents provides a meshwork of randomly oriented fibers distributed to all layers of the cerebral cortex, whereas in the hippocampal formation a much more laminar-specific distribution is apparent, especially in the dentate gyrus. The dense cholinergic innervation of the caudate and putamen is not provided by these ascending projections but by local circuit neurons whose axonal arbors are restricted to the basal ganglia.

The postsynaptic effects of acetylcholine in the forebrain appear to be mediated by both muscarinic and nicotinic receptors. The nicotinic receptors in the brain are ligand-gated channels, somewhat different from

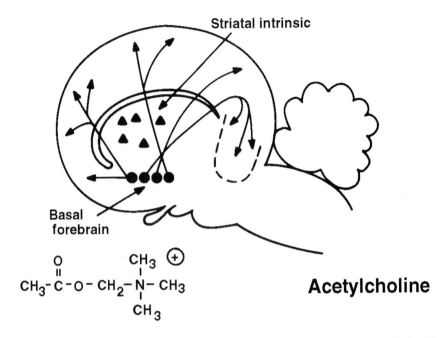

Figure 1–8. The forebrain cholinergic neurons. Cholinergic neurons in the basal forebrain, including the nucleus basalis of Meynert, the diagonal band of Broca, and the medial septal nucleus, innervate the cerebral cortex, hippocampus, and limbic structures. The striatum contains local circuit cholinergic interneurons.

those mediating the effects of acetylcholine at the neuromuscular junction in that several brain-specific receptor subunits have been found. Aside from the central psychotropic effects of nicotine itself, the role of nicotinic receptors in the brain remain relatively poorly understood.

At least four types of muscarinic cholinergic receptors have been identified by pharmacological and cloning studies (M_1–M_4). A fifth muscarinic receptor identified by cloning has not yet been established as functional. The muscarinic receptors mediating the effects of acetylcholine for the cortical and hippocampal cholinergic projections play an integral role in higher cognitive functions, especially learning and memory. Drugs that block these receptors, such as scopolamine or atropine, and processes that destroy the basal forebrain cholinergic projections in experimental animals produce selective deficits in memory functions. Notably, striking losses of cortical and hippocampal cholinergic axons seem to be a consistent defect in Alzheimer's disease and may contribute to the cognitive impairments in this disorder (Coyle et al. 1983). The cholinergic system has also been implicated in control of mood states because muscarinic receptor antagonists have mood enhancing effects in humans, whereas the centrally active acetylcholinesterase inhibitor physostigmine has been reported to provoke depressed mood. Finally, cholinergic projections have a role in sleep, especially REM sleep when locus coeruleus noradrenergic neurons are tonically inhibited while cholinergic neurons are active. Cholinergic drugs promote REM, and anticholinergic drugs antagonize it. The observation that REM latency is decreased in major depression (consistent with hyperactivity of cholinergic neurons) is further evidence that cholinergic systems may play a role in regulation of mood and mood disorders.

☐ Amino Acids

The primary excitatory and inhibitory neurotransmitters in the brain are the amino acids L-glutamate and GABA. This broad role in information processing indicates that they are localized to a large number of different neuronal systems throughout the brain, unlike the reticular core neurons whose cell bodies are restricted primarily to discrete nuclei within the brain stem.

GABA

GABAergic neurons are particularly relevant to psychiatry because the benzodiazepines, the barbiturates, many anticonvulsants, and possibly ethyl alcohol exert their primary effects through activation of the GABA receptors (see below). Within the cerebral cortex, hippocampus, and limbic structures, GABAergic neurons are predominantly local circuit neurons that have their cell bodies and axonal terminal arbors entirely contained within the structures (Figure 1–9). In fact, GABAergic inhibitory neurotransmission dominates in these structures since pharmacologic blockade of GABA receptors with bicuculline causes diffuse disinhibition and seizures. GABAergic neurons are also found as long projection neurons in other areas of the brain. For example, the main output of the caudate-putamen projecting to the globus pallidus and the substantia nigra are GABAergic neurons. The vulnerability of subsets of these striatal GABAergic neurons in Huntington's disease contributes to the abnormal movements that characterize that disorder. The cerebellar efferent neurons, the Purkinje cells, are also long GABAergic projection neurons. The cerebellar signs such as ataxia that result from excessive doses of barbiturates or ethanol likely reflect potentiation of GABAergic neurotransmission via these cerebellar efferents.

Glutamate

Glutamate is the most important excitatory neurotransmitter in the brain; well-studied examples of neurons that use glutamate include the

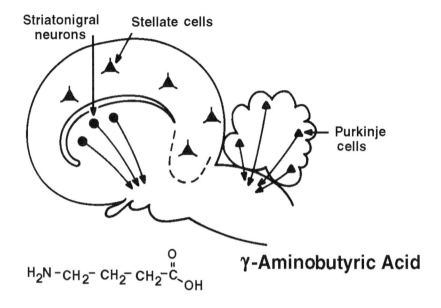

Figure 1–9.   Major GABAergic pathways. The inhibitory neurotransmitter GABA is synthesized by local circuit stellate cells within the cerebral cortex, by the cerebellar Pirkinje cells, and by striatonigral neurons.

pyramidal cells in the cerebral cortex and in the hippocampal formation (Figure 1–10), and primary sensory afferents. Most fast excitatory neurotransmission in the brain is subserved by glutamate receptors that are ligand-gated channels. These receptors have been named for their pharmacologic agonists, kainate, AMPA, and N-methyl-D-aspartate (NMDA). Subtypes of these receptors are currently a matter of intense research based on the molecular cloning of novel receptor subunits (Nakanishi et al. 1990). There are also glutamate receptors that activate G-proteins, currently referred to as "metabotropic" glutamate receptors. Cloning studies have identified multiple diverse subtypes of these receptors as well.

Binding of glutamate causes kainate and AMPA receptors to open an intrinsic Na^+ channel; in addition certain subtypes may also admit Ca^{++}. NMDA receptors are unique in that their channel, which can permit both Na^+ and Ca^{++} entry, is blocked by Mg^{++} under resting conditions. Activation of NMDA receptors can only occur when two events occur simultaneously: glutamate must bind to the receptor and the membrane must be depolarized (e.g., by activation of surrounding non-NMDA glutamate receptors) which permits Mg^{++} to exit the channel. Because two simultaneous events are required for NMDA receptor activation (i.e., the recep-

Pyramidal cells

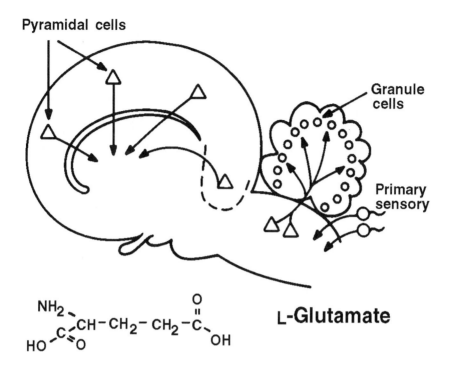

Granule cells

Primary sensory

L-Glutamate

Figure 1–10.   Major glutamatergic pathway. The excitatory neurotransmitter L-glutamic acid is released by a number of neurons including cortical and hippocampal pyramidal cells, cerebellar granule cells, cerebellar climbing fibers, and primary sensory afferents.

tor is a coincidence detector), NMDA receptors have been considered a possible substrate for associative learning.

Glutamate has been implicated in an increasing number of neurologic and psychiatric disorders. A striking finding relevant to psychiatry is that the psychotomimetic effects of phencylidine (PCP) and related compounds are due to their abilities to block the NMDA receptor channel (Martin and Lodge 1985). Since glutamate is the neurotransmitter of cortical and hippocampal pyramidal neurons, it has been hypothesized that the dissociative and psychotomimetic effects of PCP may reflect interference with glutamatergic neurotransmission in these brain regions.

Olney (1969) first demonstrated that peripheral injection of glutamate into neonatal animals produced a selective pattern of neuronal degeneration that affected neurons in the arcuate nucleus of the hypothalamus, the circumventricular organs of the brain, and the inner layers of the retina. He proposed that neurotoxicity of glutamate resulted from an overwhelming depolerization of the neurons mediated by excitatory glutamate receptors. Subsequent studies revealed that intracerebral injection of agonists at three major types of glutamate receptors (i.e., the kainate, AMPA, and NMDA receptors) killed neurons in proximity to the injection site but spared axons from distant neurons and nonneuronal elements such as glia. Depending upon the site of brain injection, these "excitotoxins" can produce models of several neurodegenerative disorders including Huntington's disease, temporal lobe epilepsy, and spinocerebellar degeneration (Schwarz and Meldrum 1985).

These observations raised the question of whether glutamate and related endogenous excitatory neurotransmitters might cause neuronal degeneration in the brain under certain circumstances, as a result of excessive release or insufficient inactivation. With the development of potent and specific antagonists for NMDA receptors, recent findings have validated this hypothesis (Choi and Rothman 1990). Accordingly, treatment with NMDA antagonists prevents degeneration of neurons in the limbic system as a consequence of persistent seizures, degeneration of neurons in the striatum as a consequence of profound hypoglycemia, and prevention of degenerations of neurons in the hippocampus as a result of ischemia. These results hold the promise for the development of new classes of "neuroprotective" medications that may prevent or markedly decrease brain damage consequent to hypoxemia and ischemia, the most frequent causes of morbidity and death following stroke and myocardial infarction (Robinson and Coyle 1988).

☐ Purines

Just as certain amino acid building blocks of proteins (e.g., glutamate, glycine) can act as signaling molecules in the nervous system, it has been found that certain purine building blocks of nucleic acids can also act as neurotransmitters. The purine *adenosine* acts via two types of G-protein–linked receptors. It has been established that the behavioral stimulant effects of caffeine result from its action as a competitive antagonist of adenosine receptors. In addition, it appears that adenosine triphosphate (ATP), the main source of energy for cells, may also act as a neurotransmitter. One type of ATP receptor has been shown to be a ligand-gated channel.

☐ Endorphins

This family of neuropeptides was originally discovered in studies to determine whether there were endogenous substances in the brain that served as agonists at opiate receptors. The pentapeptides Met-

and Leu-enkephalin were the first endogenous opioid peptides discovered, although subsequent studies have revealed a whole family of these peptides with differential effects at subclasses of opioid receptors (Table 1–2).

The enkephalins are found primarily in local circuit neurons in several regions of the central nervous system, but are also found in projection neurons. Enkephalin-containing interneurons within the periaqueductal gray matter, the raphe nuclei, and the dorsal horn of the spinal cord are critical components of endogenous analgesic systems. Enkephalin-containing interneurons that release VTA dopaminergic neurons from tonic inhibition by GABAergic neurons may present part of the substrate of opiate-induced brain reward and therefore of opiate abuse and addiction. Enkephalin neurons are also found in high concentrations in the caudate, putamen, and globus pallidus, where they appear to be involved in motor function.

The larger endogenous opioid peptide, beta-endorphin, has a dual localization. Beta-endorphin is contained within a group of neurons within the hypothalamus that send axons that project to limbic areas. In addition, beta-endorphin is secreted by the corticotrophs in the anterior pituitary. The co-localization of ACTH and beta-endorphin reflects the common source of these two peptides from the precursor, POMC (see above). During periods of stress, the release of both ACTH and beta-endorphin may contribute to stress-related analgesia.

■ MOLECULAR NEUROBIOLOGY

Perhaps the most exciting development in neuroscience research has been the increasing exploitation of molecular biological techniques (Hyman and Nestler 1993). These strategies offer considerable hope for bridging the gap between clinical genetics in psychiatry and the molecular processes that regulate brain structure and function.

☐ Regulation of Protein Phosphorylation and Neural Gene Expression by Neurotransmitters and Drugs

One of the most important properties of the nervous system is its plasticity: it can adapt to changes in the environment and it can learn. A good example of adaptation was described above in the discussion of tyrosine hydroxylase, the rate-limiting enzyme in catecholamine biosynthesis. Under circumstances in which norepinephrine- or dopamine-expressing neurons must fire at high rates, they adapt by increasing the activity of tyrosine hydroxylase and, in addition, they produce more molecules of tyrosine hydroxylase. The former adaptation is due to protein phosphorylation and the latter to regulation of gene expression. Together, these are the most significant mechanisms regulating long-term adaptation, and, in all likelihood, all forms of memory, in the nervous system. Regulation of neural gene expression by neurotransmitters, hormones, and drugs can potentially produce long-lasting alterations in virtually all aspects of a neuron's functioning by altering levels of neurotransmitter-synthesizing enzymes, peptide neurotransmitters, receptors, ion channels, signal transduction proteins, cytoskeletal components within the cells, and other critical neural proteins.

Protein phosphorylation and regulation of gene expression are often related: in most cases, protein kinase-dependent phosphorylation couples environmental stimuli to changes in neural gene expression. (The other important mechanism regulating neural gene expression is via steroid hormones, described below.) While gene expression is regulated at many levels, control of the initiation of transcription appears to be the major mechanism gating the flow of information from the genome into the production of cellular proteins. The regulation of transcription initiation involves two critical processes, positioning of *RNA polymerase,* the enzyme that transcribes DNA into RNA, at the correct start site of genes, and controlling the efficiency of initiations to produce the appropriate transcriptional rate. These control functions are subserved by short stretches of DNA (*cis-regulatory elements*) within genes that act as specific binding sites for proteins that regulate transcription, generally called *transcription factors.* Mutational analyses have shown that each gene has a particular combination of cis-regulatory elements. The cis-regulatory elements are mediated via the transcription factors that bind to them, and the nature, number, and spatial arrangement of these elements determine a gene's unique pattern of expression, including the cell types in which it is expressed, the times during development at which it is expressed, the basal levels at which it is expressed, and its responsiveness to environmental stimuli.

As described above, stimulation of G-protein–linked receptors activates or inhibits second messenger systems and, in turn, protein kinases. When activated, certain protein kinases not only act in the cell cytoplasm, but translocate into the nucleus of the cell where they can phosphorylate transcription factors. Those transcription factors that are activated (or inactivated) by phosphorylation can couple stimulation of neurotransmitter receptors with changes in gene expression.

Those cis-regulatory elements that bind transcription factors that are physiologically regulated (e.g., by phosphorylation) and therefore confer neurotransmitter, hormone, or second messenger responsiveness on genes are often called "response elements." Perhaps the best characterized example of a second messenger response element is one that confers activation by cyclic AMP (and therefore cyclic AMP-dependent protein kinase) on those genes in which it is found. The discovery and analysis of *cyclic AMP response elements* (CREs) within many genes depended on the ability to mutate DNA sequences "in vitro" and then to reintroduce them into cells in culture (a process called "transfection"). The effects of the mutations in the DNA sequences on the ability of cyclic AMP to activate the gene could then be observed. Using such approaches, it was discovered that CREs contain the DNA sequence CGTCA or closely related sequences, and that this sequence of nucleotides could bind a protein called CREB (CRE binding protein). When bound to a CRE, CREB activates transcription when it is phosphorylated by cyclic AMP-dependent protein kinase. Many additional response elements and transcription factors have been characterized.

☐ Steroid Hormone Receptors

An important family of DNA response elements that do not involve phosphorylation are the glucocorticoid response elements (GREs) and other steroid hormone response elements. Unlike neurotransmitters or peptide hormones, which bind to cell surface receptors, glucocorticoids and other steroid hormones are fat soluble and directly enter cells. They act by binding to specific receptors within the cell cytoplasm. Cytoplasmic steroid receptors include glucocorticoid receptors, estrogen receptors, mineralocorticoid receptors, and the like. Since steroid hormones diffuse widely, the specificity of response depends upon the presence or absence of specific receptors within particular cells. When activated by hormone binding, steroid receptors translocate into the nucleus where they bind to GREs (or other steroid hormone response elements) contained within particular genes. The binding of the receptor to the DNA then increases or decreases the rate at which these target genes are transcribed. Thus steroid hormone receptors act as hormone-sensitive transcription factors. Most of the known effects of glucocorticoids, gonadal steroids, thyroid hormone, and vitamin D on cellular function are mediated via their actions on gene expression.

■ MOLECULAR PSYCHOPHARMACOLOGY

The discovery of drugs that selectively reduce the symptoms of psychiatric disorders has yielded a productive set of pharmacological probes to study the potential roles of specific neural systems in the pathophysiology of psychiatric disorders. Of course, it cannot be assumed that the molecular or cellular site of action of a psychotropic medication localizes the pathophysiologic defect responsible for the disorder. It is entirely possible that the neuronal system affected by the drug is only secondarily involved, and that the pharmacologically induced alteration in its function compensates for a primary defect elsewhere in the nervous system. Nevertheless, our ability to identify the molecular targets and neural systems on which psychotropic drugs act has given rise to important pathophysiological theories and has provided the impetus for important discoveries in basic neuroscience.

☐ Antipsychotic Drugs

The discovery that both reserpine and the phenothiazine chlorpromazine reduced the agitation, hallucinations, and delusions of psychotic patients ushered in the modern era of psychopharmacology 35 years ago. Several disparate observations implicated forebrain dopamine neurons in the mechanism of action of neuroleptics in the early 1960s. Hornykiewicz (1966) had just demonstrated that Parkinson's disease was associated with a profound loss of dopamine in the substantia nigra and in the caudate-putamen. Reserpine, an antipsychotic structurally unrelated to the phenothiazines, was found to cause a marked depletion of biogenic amines, including dopamine, in the brains of experimental animals. The most common neurological side effects observed with all the effective antipsychotic medications were parkinsonian symptoms.

In studies with chlorpromazine and haloperidol, Carlsson noted that while these antipsychotics did not deplete dopamine from the brain, like reserpine, they did produce a marked increase in the turnover of dopamine. Carlsson proposed that antipsychotic medications may exert their therapeutic effects by blocking the brain receptors for dopamine (Carlsson and Lindqvist 1963). When the full range of clinically effective neuroleptics were examined, a remarkably high correlation was observed between their clinical potency as antipsychotics and their affinity for the D_2 dopamine receptor binding site, but not other neurotransmitter receptors (Creese et al. 1976). Recent molecular cloning studies have identified at least three additional dopamine receptors and raised doubts about whether D_2 antagonism is necessary or even sufficient for antipsychotic drug action. The atypical antipsychotic drug clozapine, which may have unique efficacy in schizophrenia but is relatively free of extrapyramidal effects, binds with low affinity to D_2 receptors, but with high affinity to the newly discovered D_4 receptor (Van Tol et al. 1991). Almost all drugs that interact with D_2 receptors also interact with D_3 and D_4 receptors. Clozapine's uniquely low affinity for the D_2 receptor explains its lack of extrapyramidal side effects, and perhaps its unique efficacy in treating "negative" symptoms of schizophrenia (e.g., withdrawal) that may actually be caused by D_2 receptor antagonism.

All antipsychotic drugs require weeks of administration before achieving their maximum therapeutic effect. Patients on clozapine may continue to improve for months, suggesting that blockade of dopamine receptors (of whatever type eventually turns out to be most important) represents the initial interaction of antipsychotic drugs with the nervous system. However, some as yet unknown, slow-onset adaptive response of the nervous system to dopamine receptor blockade represents the actual mechanism by which antipsychotic symptoms are relieved. Mechanisms thought most likely focus on the possibility that dopamine receptor blockade leads to significant changes in proteins (e.g., ion channels, receptors, enzymes) contained by target neurons (which may be the dopaminoceptive neuron itself or other neurons one or more synapses removed). Such delayed onset, long-lasting changes in neural functioning are likely to involve second messenger-mediated changes in gene expression.

□ Antidepressants

The first clues to the mechanism of action of the antidepressant drugs resulted from an experiment to monitor the catabolism of radioactive norepinephrine in vivo, in which a small portion of the systematically administered norepinephrine was retained unmetabolized in peripheral tissues (Axelrod et al. 1959). The amount of radioactive norepinephrine sequestered in these tissues was proportionate to the degree of sympathetic innervation. In subsequent studies, Axelrod demonstrated that noradrenergic neurons possessed a high affinity transport process to take up norepinephrine and that tricyclic antidepressant drugs were potent inhibitors of this transport process. Central noradrenergic, dopaminergic, and serotonergic neurons were subsequently found to possess specific transporter proteins for their neurotransmitters. These transporters, which have now been cloned, are the primary mechanism for the termination of action of these neurotransmitters after release into the synaptic cleft.

Detailed studies over the years have revealed that the cyclic antidepressants are potent blockers of the norepinephrine and/or serotonin transporters and thereby potentiate the action of these two neurotransmitters in the synaptic cleft. More recently, selective serotonin uptake inhibitors such as fluoxetine and sertraline have been introduced. Studies of the tricyclic antidepressants and newer serotonin-selective reuptake inhibitors have verified the important distinction between identifying the initial site of action of a drug and understanding its mechanism of therapeutic action. Whereas the inhibition of reuptake and therefore potentiation of noradrenergic and serotonergic neurotransmission is a fairly immediate consequence of administration of antidepressants, there is substantial delay in the onset of symptomatic improvement in major depressive disorder. This delay is reminiscent of the action of antipsychotic drugs mentioned above.

The delay in onset of clinical effects prompted investigators to search for effects of antidepressants that only appeared with chronic drug administration. The first such delayed-onset effect to be observed was desensitization of beta-adrenergic receptors in rat cortex. This desensitization occurs in response to virtually all effective antidepressant treatments, even antidepressants highly specific for the serotonin transporter and repeated electroconvulsive seizures. It was subsequently demonstrated that selective destruction of brain serotonergic neurons prevents antidepressant-induced beta-receptor desensitization, demonstrating a functional linkage between serotonergic and noradrenergic systems (Janowsky et al. 1982). Subsequently it has been shown that some, but not all, antidepressant treatments desensitize α_2-adrenergic receptors and serotonin 5-HT$_2$ receptors.

As evidence has accumulated, it appears likely that these alterations in receptor sensitivity are markers of chronic antidepressant effect, but probably do not represent the mechanism of therapeutic action. The receptor findings, however, suggest feasible research strategies. For example, it is now known that beta-adrenergic receptor desensitization is due to increases in activity of cyclic AMP–dependent protein kinases, including a kinase with high specificity for the beta receptor itself. Activation of these kinases probably results from increased noradrenergic stimulation of the beta receptors themselves resulting from the initial actions of antidepressants (e.g., blockade of reuptake or inhibition of monoamine oxidase). Thus, beta-receptor desensitization is a cellular marker showing that chronic antidepressant administration leads to increased activation of cyclic AMP dependent protein kinases within noradrenergically innervated neurons.

☐ Lithium

The precise mechanism of action of lithium in treating manic-depressive illness is unknown, but it appears that uniquely among psychiatric drugs, lithium acts directly on G-proteins and second messenger systems. Many neurotransmitter receptors, including adrenergic and 5-HT$_2$ serotonergic receptors, are linked via G-proteins (most likely G$_q$) to activation of phospholipase C, an enzyme that hydrolyzes a membrane phospholipid, phosphatidylinositol bisphosphate (PIP$_2$), to yield two second messengers, diacylglycerol and inositol triphosphate (IP$_3$). Lithium inhibits certain steps in the phosphatidylinositol cycle; it has been hypothesized that these actions are responsible for lithium's antimanic and antidepressant effects.

Lithium alters the coupling of a number of neurotransmitter receptors to G-proteins, which alters the function of multiple neurotransmitter-signal transduction pathways in the brain. However, this is not believed to cause specific effects on manic and depressed states.

☐ Anxiolytics

Although the prototypical benzodiazepine chlordiazepoxide was discovered serendipitously, the remarkable properties of this and subsequently synthesized benzodiazepines, and their superiority over barbiturates as sedatives and anxiolytics, soon became apparent. The benzodiazepines have a far more favorable ratio between anxiolytic action and sedative effects than the barbiturates, a greater therapeutic index, and less risk for dependence and serious withdrawal symptoms.

Understanding the molecular sites of action of benzodiazepines as well as barbiturates depended upon the elucidation of the physiologic and receptor mechanisms mediating the effects of GABA, the major inhibitory neurotransmitter in the brain. Local application of GABA to individual neurons results in inhibition of their firing, caused by opening of chloride channels in the neuronal membrane, thus hyperpolarizing the neuron. Using ligand binding techniques with radioactive GABA, a GABA receptor was detected within brain membranes. Moreover, using radioactive diazepam, it was possible to directly label the recognition sites for benzodiazepine. With additional investigation it was established that the benzodiazepine receptor represented a binding site on the $GABA_A$ receptor, a large multisubunit protein that serves as the main type of receptor for GABA in the central nervous system.

The $GABA_A$ receptor contains at least three major binding sites relevant to psychopharmacology. The binding site for GABA resides on the β subunit of the receptor; benzodiazepines bind to the α subunit. However, the α subunit is unable to bind benzodiazepines unless a γ subunit is present in the complex. Benzodiazepines do not directly open the receptor chloride channel. Rather, they act by increasing the affinity of the GABA binding site on the β subunit for GABA and thereby enhance the synaptic actions of GABA. Barbiturates also bind to the $GABA_A$ receptor, but at a site physically distinct from benzodiazepines; thus, both drugs can be bound to the receptor at once. Barbiturates exert a similar influence on receptor function to benzodiazepines, increasing the affinity of the receptor for GABA and thereby increasing the ability of GABA to activate the receptor Cl^- channel. Unlike the benzodiazepines, however, higher doses of barbiturates can directly cause opening of the Cl^- channel in the absence of GABA. This may explain why barbiturates cause more serious CNS depression (with greater likelihood of lethality) than benzodiazepines when taken in overdose. In addition to increasing the affinity of the $GABA_A$ receptor for GABA, benzodiazepines and barbiturates increase the affinity of the receptor for each other.

■ REFERENCES

Axelrod J, Weil-Malherbe H, Tomchick R: The physiological disposition of ^{3}H-epi-nephrine and its metabolite, metanephrine. J Pharmacol Exp Ther 127:251–256, 1959

Carlsson A, Lindqvist M: Effect of chlorpromazine and haloperidol on formation of 3-methoxytyramine and normetanephrine in mouse brain. Acta Pharmacol Toxicol 20:140–144, 1963

Choi DW, Rothman SM: The role of glutamate neurotoxicity in hypoxic-ischemic neuronal death. Annu Rev Neurosci 13:171–182, 1990

Coyle JT: Aminergic projections from the reticular core, in Diseases of the Nervous System. Edited by Asbury A, McKhann G, McDonald W. Philadelphia, PA, WB Saunders, 1986, pp 880–889

Coyle JT, Price DL, DeLong MR: Alzheimer's disease: a disorder of cholinergic innervation of cortex. Science 219:1184–1190, 1983

Creese I, Burt DR, Snyder SH: Dopamine receptor binding predicts clinical and pharmacological potencies of antischizophrenic drugs. Science 192:481–483, 1976

Giros B, Caron MG: Molecular characterization of the dopamine transporter. Trends Pharmacol Sci 14:43–49, 1993

Hornykiewicz O: Dopamine and brain function. Pharmacol Rev 18:925–964, 1966

Hyman SE, Nestler EJ: The Molecular Foundations of Psychiatry. Washington, DC, American Psychiatric Press, 1993

Janowsky AJ, Okada F, Applegate C, et al: Role of serotonergic input in the regulation of the beta-adrenoreceptor coupled adenylate cyclase system in brain. Science 218:900–901, 1982

Martin D, Lodge D: Ketamine acts as a non-competitive N-methyl-D-aspartate antagonist on frog spinal cord in vitro. Neuropharmacology 24:999–1006, 1985

Nakanishi N, Shneider NA, Axel R: A family of glutamate receptor genes: evidence for the formation of heteromultimeric receptors with distinct channel properties. Neuron 5:569–581, 1990

Nose PS, Griffith LC, Schulman H: Ca^{2+}-dependent phosphorylation of tyrosine hydroxylase in PC 12 cells. J Cell Biol 101:1182–1190, 1985

Olney JW: Brain lesions, obesity and other disturbances in mice treated with monosodium glutamate. Science 164:719–721, 1969

Pacholczyk T, Blakely RD, Amara SG: Expression cloning of a cocaine- and antidepressant-sensitive human noradrenaline transporter. Nature 350:350–354, 1991

Robinson, Coyle JT: Glutamate and related acidic neurotransmitters: from basic science to clinical practice. FASEB J 1:446–455, 1988

Schwarz R, Meldrum B: Excitatory amino acid antagonists provide a therapeutic approach to neurologic disorders. Lancet 2:140–143, 1985

Van Tol HMV, Bunzow JR, Guan HC, et al: Cloning of the gene for a human dopamine D_4 receptor with high affinity for the antipsychotic clozapine. Nature 350:610–614, 1991

Genetics

Ronald O. Rieder, M.D.
Charles A. Kaufmann, M.D.
James A. Knowles, M.D., Ph.D.

At the core of psychiatric genetics has been the investigation of the genetic contribution to psychiatric disorders. These core studies, however, have led researchers into many related areas, such as the search for environmental etiological factors, the refinement of psychiatric nosology, the investigation of normal and abnormal psychological/behavioral traits, and the development of effective methods for the prevention and treatment of psychiatric disorders.

The goals of genetic investigation in psychiatry are as follows:

1. To establish and specify the genetic component of the etiology of psychiatric syndromes, and thus determine a) to what extent a psychiatric disorder is genetically caused; b) the DNA rearrangement of the genetic contribution; c) the biopsychosocial abnormalities associated with the gene or genes involved; and d) the processes by which genetic abnormalities lead to symptoms.
2. To establish and specify the nongenetic component of the etiology of psychiatric syndromes, and thus identify environmental factors that, acting independently of or interacting with vulnerable genotypes, produce or increase the likelihood of a disorder.

This work was supported in part by National Institute of Mental Health (NIMH) Research Scientist Development Award K02 MH 00682 (CAK) and NIMH Schizophrenia Research Training Grant MH 18870 (ROR, JAK).

3. To validate the boundaries of diagnostic entities and subtypes within entities by determining a) the genetic associations between disorders, or between subtypes of a disorder, to establish groupings of genetically related disorders (e.g., a schizophrenia spectrum), or to split disorders established on clinical phenomenology (e.g., different subtypes of schizoaffective disorder); and b) the characteristics (e.g., severity, subject's age at onset) of a disorder that increase its heritability, thereby helping to identify diagnostic boundaries that more closely correspond to biological boundaries.
4. To specify the genetic contribution to traits and psychological symptoms, independent of their role as components of defined psychiatric syndromes.
5. To develop methods of preventing or treating psychiatric disorders based on knowledge of genetic and environmental factors in their etiology. These methods include genetic counseling, alteration of the necessary/permissive environment for persons at risk, and gene therapy.

■ METHODS

Research methods have evolved for each of the aims of genetic investigation. The methodologies have over the past two decades been especially productive in determining to what extent a psychiatric disorder is genetically caused (Table 2–1). New techniques hold the promise of determining the location, nature, and product of the genetic contribution to many disorders. Genetic investigation of a psychiatric disorder attempts to answer a sequence of questions:

- Is the illness familial?
- Is this familiality caused by genetic factors?
- What are the various clinical expressions of the abnormal gene(s)?
- What are the earliest manifestations of this predisposition to illness?
- What environmental variables increase or decrease the chances of predisposed individuals developing the disorder?
- What is the mode of transmission?
- Where is (are) the abnormal gene(s)?
- What is the biological, physiological, and psychological outcome of the genetic abnormality?

Different techniques, each with its own advantages and disadvantages, as described below, are used to attempt to answer these questions.

☐ Is the Illness Familial?—Family Risk Studies and Epidemiological Studies

Family risk studies are designed to determine to what extent an illness runs in families, because all genetic illnesses have increased rates of illness among relatives (though not all familial traits are genetic [e.g., language]). Research by the pioneers of psychiatric genetics in the early part of the 20th century demonstrated that there were higher rates of schizophrenia and manic-depressive illness among family members of affected individuals than in the general population. As diagnostic criteria have been developed and validated, such studies have continued, both for the psychoses and for other diagnostic entities (schizophrenia [Kendler et al. 1985], affective disorders [Andreasen et al. 1987], panic disorder [Noyes et al. 1986], simple phobias [Fyer et al. 1990], anorexia nervosa [Gershon et al. 1984]).

Calculation of the extent of psychiatric disorders among the relatives of probands begins with the rates as determined through the process of family interviews. Because some family members will not have passed through the age of risk for the disorder, it would be an underestimate of the eventual rate of psychopathology among relatives to assume that these individuals will remain well. Therefore, the data are usually reported in terms of *lifetime morbid risk*, which is an estimate of the eventual rate of illness among relatives, were they to be followed through the age of risk.

When the lifetime morbid risks for first-degree relatives of ill and control probands are determined, a *relative risk* for first-degree relatives of ill probands can be calculated. As seen in Table 2–2, this relative risk varies from approximately 3 to 25 for the psychiatric disorders studied, indicating significant familial aggregation for all of them. From these data it appears that bipolar disorder, schizophrenia, bulimia nervosa, panic disorder, and alcoholism are the most familial.

However, such rates of illness may be influenced by environmental conditions shared by family members. Thus, the extent to which a disorder is familial cannot be immediately taken as an indication of the extent to which it is genetically determined. There also may be *assortative mating*, which is the tendency for those with a psychiatric disorder to mate preferentially, usually with those who have similar psychopathology, or in other nonrandom ways, thus increasing the likelihood of the children inheriting a genetic predisposition to the disorder beyond what would be the case were only one parent affected. Unless recognized, this could lead to a familial pattern that overestimates the genetic effect.

Large-scale epidemiological studies, such as the National Institute of Mental Health (NIMH) Epidemiologic Catchment Area (ECA) study (Robins et al. 1984), can contribute to the value and interpretation of the

Table 2–1. Evidence in support of genetic transmission of various psychiatric disorders

Illness	Genetic transmission supported by				Comments
	Family risk studies	Twin studies	Adoption studies	Linkage studies	
Schizophrenia	+	+	+	+	
Bipolar disorder	+	+	+		
Major depression	+	+	(+)		
Panic disorder and agoraphobia	+	+			Increased panic disorder among relatives of agoraphobic patients but not vice versa.
Generalized anxiety disorder	+	+			
Simple phobia	+	+			
Social phobia	+	+			
Obsessive-compulsive disorder	(+)				Familial increase of other disorders—anxiety and depressive disorders—and obsessive symptoms.
Posttraumatic stress disorder		+			
Anorexia nervosa	+	+			More relatives have affective disorders than eating disorders.
Briquet's syndrome/somatization disorder and sociopathy	+	(+)	+		Male family members tend to have sociopathy; female members, somatization disorder.
Alcoholism	+	(+)	+		Familial transmission more evident among males than females.

	1	2	3	4	Comments
Personality disorders					
Antisocial	+	+			
Schizotypal	+	+			Schizotypal personality disorder is increased in relatives of schizophrenic probands, and perhaps in relatives of affective disorder probands as well.
Borderline		+			
Avoidant	+	+			
Dependent	+	+			
Huntington's disease	+		(+)	+	
Alzheimer's disease	+		(+)	+	Linkage studies show heterogeneity.

Note. Evidence discussed, with references, in text. + indicates most or all findings support genetic transmission; (+) indicates some findings support genetic transmission, but others do not.

Table 2–2.   Relative risk for psychiatric disorders

Disorder	Relative risk	Reference
Bipolar disorder	24.5	Weissman et al. 1984a
Schizophrenia	18.5	Kendler et al. 1985
Bulimia nervosa	9.6	Kassett et al. 1989
Panic disorder	9.6	Crowe et al. 1983
Alcoholism	7.4	Merikangas 1989
Generalized anxiety disorder	5.6	Noyes et al. 1987
Anorexia nervosa	4.6	Strober et al. 1985
Simple phobia	3.3	Fyer et al. 1990
Social phobia	3.2	Fyer et al. 1993
Somatization disorder	3.1	Cloninger et al. 1986
Major depression	3.0	Weissman et al. 1984
Agoraphobia	2.8	Crowe et al. 1983

Note. Other studies may have relative risk ratios that differ considerably from those in these studies, especially if different diagnostic criteria were used. However, the methodological soundness of studies referenced here prompted our selection of them for discussion in the text and in this comparison.

familial data. With the use of structured interview schedules and standardized diagnostic criteria, estimates of the population prevalence of disorders can be determined and compared with the data obtained from the family studies. Some studies blend the techniques of epidemiology and family risk, studying geographic, ethnic, or cultural isolates (Egeland et al. 1987).

In isolated populations we expect greater genetic homogeneity for the psychiatric disorder present, because all or most cases of the disorder may stem from a common progenitor who is the single source of the pathogenic gene(s). There may also be a higher prevalence of certain disorders in such populations. These elevated rates may be caused by an increased frequency of the abnormal genotype or a higher rate of expression of the gene (i.e., increased penetrance). Isolated kindreds showing a high incidence of the disorder provide the best samples for the segregation and linkage analytic techniques, described below, which can demonstrate and localize a potent genetic contributory factor.

☐ Do Genetic Factors Contribute to the Illness?— Twin and Adoption Studies

After a psychiatric disorder has been found to be familial, twin and adoption studies are used to dissect the relative contributions of genetics and environment to the etiology of the disorder.

Twin Studies

Twin studies examine the concordance, or the co-incidence, of a disorder in monozygotic, genetically identical (MZ) and in dizygotic, fraternal (DZ) twins, the latter sharing, on average, one-half their genes, as do siblings. One strategy involves comparing concordance in MZ pairs and same-sex DZ pairs. If only the rearing environment has predisposed an index case to illness, then the co-twin, whether MZ or DZ, should also be at risk, and the rates for both MZ and DZ twins should be elevated (compared with the population rate) and equal. If, on the other hand, pathogenic genes have predisposed the index twin to illness, then a MZ co-twin would be at a higher risk than would a DZ co-twin. The concordance rate for MZ twins would be higher than that for DZ twins, and the latter should be similar to the concordance rate for siblings.

One assumption of this strategy is that the MZ and DZ twins have the same degree of similarity of the familial environment—in other words, that MZ twins do not share more environmental similarity than do DZ twins in ways that would increase the MZ concordance for psychiatric disorders. It is obvious that in some ways MZ twins are treated more similarly (e.g., being dressed alike). It is also clear that in many families MZ twins receive very similar emotional and attitudinal input from their parents. However, to indicate the complexity of this issue, there is evidence that the temperamental characteristics of the MZ twins (which may be genetic in origin) generate this similarity in rearing.

Because it is difficult to determine the degree to which shared environment could account for the increased MZ concordance rates of twins raised in the same home, studies of twins raised apart in uncorrelated (i.e., randomly assigned) environments would be useful. Ideally, the concordance rates of MZ and DZ pairs raised apart could be compared, but even having only such a sample of MZ twins would allow for comparison of their concordance rates to those of MZ twins raised in the same home. Systematic samples of such twins are hard to obtain, however, and case reports of concordance are more likely to be noted and published than are those of discordant pairs.

A third way to use the concordance rates for twins to address the question of genetic versus environmental factors is to examine the extent to which MZ twins are discordant for a disorder. Given that MZ twins are genetically identical, any degree of discordance implies that there are nongenetic etiological factors that can either produce or unmask the disorder. For example, these findings could result from "phenocopies," cases that appear to have the disorder in question but have an environmentally determined, pathogenically distinct illness that mimics the genetically determined disease. Another possibility is that environmental conditions might be necessary to add to or to interact with genetic factors to produce the illness, leading to MZ twins being both predisposed genetically for the disorder but discordant on the basis of having experienced different environments. Huntington's disease has a nearly 100% MZ concordance rate, whereas common psychiatric disorders such as schizophrenia and bipolar disorder have rates that approximate 50% and 65%, respectively.

The twin strategies described above produce quantitative data that are tempting to translate into estimates of the extent to which a disorder is genetically or nongenetically caused. The *heritability* of a psychiatric disorder is defined as the portion of a trait's variation in the population that is accounted for by genetic factors.

Calculations of heritability use such data as the concordance rates of twins or morbid risk among other relatives, but these calculations are dependent on a presumed mode of inheritance as well as other assumptions. For almost all psychiatric disorders, the mode of inheritance is unknown, and the heritability values calculated with different mode of transmission assumptions, even using the same rates of MZ-DZ concordance, can differ widely. However, the data can be safely interpreted in a qualitative way by seeing if the simplest-case hypotheses can be rejected. The simplest-case situations are when causation is either purely genetic or purely through shared environment. In other words, if the 95% confidence limits of the MZ-DZ concordances do not extend to their being equal, then the data are consistent with the disorder having a significant genetic causation (without proving such). Similarly, if the 95% confidence limits for the MZ concordance rate do not extend to 100%, then it can be assumed that environmental factors are likely in some way to be etiological contributors, although it may be that this occurs only through the production of phenocopies.

Questions regarding the interpretation of MZ twin concordance rates may be resolved by another twin strategy, the study of the offspring of discordant MZ twins. If the ill twin has a purely environmentally caused disorder, then the offspring of the well co-twin should not be at elevated risk (unless they are exposed to the pathogenic environmental insults that their aunt/uncle, but not their parent, experienced). On the other hand, if the ill and well twins share a genetic predisposition to the illness, but one had not experienced certain precipitating or contributing environmental insults, then the well co-twin will be a carrier of liability for the illness and his or her offspring will be at elevated risk. This strategy was pioneered by Fischer (1971), and extended by Gottesman and Bertelsen (1989), who found that the offspring of nonschizophrenic MZ co-twins and the offspring of their ill co-twins had an equal morbid risk for the illness, suggesting that much of the discordance between the twins could be attributed to differential exposure to environmental factors.

Adoption Studies

Adoption studies are based on the fact that adoption separates the two major influences parents have on their children, namely, genes and rearing. It offers researchers a naturalistic "experiment" that has the potential to answer the questions of whether a disorder is familial because of genetic transmission or the shared environment. Four types of adoption studies have been employed:

1. *Adoptee study method:* the study of adopted-away children of a parent with a disorder.
2. *Cross-fostering strategy:* the study of children born of nondisordered parents adopted into a family with a disordered parent.
3. *Adoptee's family method:* the study of the adoptive and the biological relatives of disordered adoptees.
4. *MZ twins reared apart:* the study of MZ twins reared apart, as discussed above.

Such research is much easier to conceptualize than to execute. State-of-the-art investigations using these strategies must employ systematic sampling, adoptee control subjects, careful attention to make diagnoses blind to the diagnosis of the index case, and the use of operationalized diagnostic criteria. Adoption studies have been done for affective disorders, alcoholism, sociopathy, obesity, and other psychiatric conditions, as well as for IQ and personality variables. Although adoption offers an ideal separation of genetic from environmental influences, this research has methodological pitfalls. Because few children are adopted away immediately after birth, there are usually some familial environmental influences of undetermined significance that are difficult to measure. Also, "environment" does not begin at birth; the uterine environment of an affected mother may be significant in the transmission of the illness, which may be examined by comparing the risk to the children of affected mothers versus affected fathers, or, in the adoptee's family method, the risk to paternal half-siblings versus maternal half-siblings.

☐ What Are the Various Clinical Expressions of the Abnormal Gene(s)?—Spectrum Studies

In most of the family studies done on the major psychiatric disorders, investigators have found an increase not only in the disorder in question but also in other types of psychopathology. At times, this increase has been in milder or related syndromes of the major disorder, such as dysthymia in the relatives of patients with major depression, or unipolar depression in the relatives of patients with bipolar disorder. In other illnesses, more distant syndromes have appeared—an increase of affective disorders in the relatives of eating disorder patients, and of sociopathy in the relatives of patients with somatization disorder.

As evidence has accumulated suggesting that genetic factors account for the increased familial incidence of the major psychiatric disorders, the hypothesis has been put forth that the other syndromes found to be increased among relatives are also the result of this same genetic predisposition. This concept has been expressed as the "spectrum" of disorders related to, for example, schizophrenia or bipolar disorder. As discussed below, the former is said to include schizotypal personality, paranoid personality, schizoaffective disorder (as in DSM III-R [American Psychiatric Association 1987]) and atypical psychosis; the latter, bipolar-II disorder, recurrent major depressive disorder, cyclothymia, dysthymia, schizoaffective disorder (Research Diagnostic Criteria [RDC; Spitzer et al. 1978] bipolar type), and possibly others.

The diagnostic trend in American psychiatry, prominently represented in DSM-III (American Psychiatric Association 1987) and subsequent manuals, has been to narrow the boundaries of Axis I disorders and to develop alternative categories (e.g., atypical psychosis, psychosis not otherwise specified [NOS]), for less severe or mixed-symptom cases. It was hoped that these restrictions would produce more symptomatically and etiologically homogeneous categories, an especially appropriate development for the study of treatment effects and biological markers, for which a sample of "pure" cases could thus be recruited.

For many types of genetic studies, however, determining who in the family is ill and who is well, for all family members, is often of the utmost importance. Studies attempting to determine the mode of transmission (i.e., segregation analysis) and linkage studies are most obviously affected by misclassification. Because there are problems posed by both overinclusion and overexclusion, the issue of which phenotypic syndromes are manifestations of the genotype is essential. In practice, the spectrum of disorders found in the current or prior studies to be increased in the family members of index cases, as compared with similarly diagnosed control families, are often entered into one or more data analyses as alternative manifestations of the genotype. In genetic research studies, then, the spectrum concept is not only developed but also employed.

The problems of employing spectrum diagnoses become even greater when this genetic causation is assumed to apply in a clinical situation. For heterogeneous illnesses the etiological factors most often at work in index families may not be those represented in the population at large. Thus, whereas a schizophrenic patient's first-degree relative with a schizotypal personality disorder may very likely share the genetic predisposition to schizophrenia, the schizotypal individual without such a family history may be much less likely to have this same genetic makeup. The determination of the extent to which a spectrum illness is associated with the "index" disorder must include identification of that spectrum illness in family studies of other index disorders, and in family studies that take the spectrum diagnosis as the index disorder. An example of this process has occurred with schizotypal personality disorder, first described as occurring in the families of schizophrenic patients, and thus classified as part of the schizophrenic spectrum. More recently an equal increase of schizotypal personality disorder in the families of affective disorder patients has been shown (Squires-Wheeler et al. 1989). Family studies now being done of schizotypal disorder itself (Siever et al. 1990) may help in determining the extent of schizotypal personality disorder's associations with both disorders, or its independent transmission.

☐ What Are the Early Manifestations of and Environmental Risk Factors for the Illness?—High-Risk Studies

High-risk research, or the study of children at risk, is a strategy that begins with a factor of known or putative importance for the development of psychopathology and examines, through controlled studies, the influence of that factor on exposed infants or children. Such a design has been used to delineate the effects of maternal alcohol consumption during pregnancy and low birth weight. It has also been used to identify the early development of psychopathology among the offspring of parents with psychiatric disorders. This strategy entails selection of parent probands with an accurately diagnosed disorder, evaluation of psychopathology in the co-parents, and usually a longitudinal evaluation of the children, using a battery of psychological and biological measures, as well as a record of environmental conditions during development. These studies can investigate 1) presymptomatic differences between the high-risk group and the control group, and whether such abnormalities predict later psychopathology; 2) early manifestations of psychopathology in subjects who later develop the same disorder that their parents experienced; 3) the childhood psychopathological syndromes that may be genetically related to the adult psychiatric disorders of either or both parents; and 4) environmental variables that are associated with the development of illness in the genetically predisposed group.

Investigating presumably predisposed individuals in the well state for hidden psychological or physiological differences that could play a role in their development of the illness (e.g., psychological or physiological differences in the response of sons of alcoholic parents to alcohol) avoids one of the major pitfalls of studies of already-ill individuals—namely, that abnormalities found in ill subjects may be sequelae of the illness or of its treatment rather than aspects of an intrinsic vulnerability. Investigations of the first manifestations of an illness (such as attentional deficits in the children of schizophrenic parents) may be helpful in establishing the nature of a genetically determined "core deficit" in evolving illnesses such as schizophrenia. Examining the rates of specific childhood disorders in the at-risk group (e.g., the rates of separation anxiety in the children of parents with panic disorder) can establish links between childhood and adult syndromes in the same way that family and adoption studies can identify a spectrum of adult disorders with a possibly shared genetic causation.

With the advent of methods, such as linkage analysis, for establishing the location of the genes or genes involved in psychiatric disorders and the presence or absence of the abnormal genotype among offspring, there will be a new generation of high-risk studies that can be used to better explore the early manifestations of the genotype and the influence of environmental factors.

☐ What Is the Mode of Transmission?— Segregation Analysis

When family, twin, and adoption studies show that genetic factors play a role in the pathogenesis of a disorder, then *segregation analysis* is used to attempt to determine the mode of transmission of these genetic factors. This is done by studying the pattern of inheritance of the disorder in a collection of families. Mutations at any single gene are inherited in a dominant or recessive manner and may be autosomal or sex-linked. If the disorder is transmitted in families in one of these patterns, it is likely due to a single gene.

For example, approximately 50% of the offspring of parents affected with one of the dominant monogenic disorders (Huntington's disease or acute intermittent porphyria) are themselves affected. Affected offspring always have an affected parent (unless the offspring's condition represents a new mutation, which is rare). If a group of families with a particular disorder all display this pattern of transmission, then it is concluded that the disorder is caused by a single dominant gene. For the recessive disorders (e.g., phenylketonuria), each affected individual will have unaffected parents who must nonetheless be carriers, and approximately 25% of the offspring of two carrier parents will be affected. There is often an increased incidence of consanguineous marriages (inbreeding) in these families. In the sex-linked recessive disorders (e.g., DMD), all of the daughters of an affected father are unaffected carriers, and 50% of their sons in turn will be affected. Furthermore, no father-to-son transmission occurs.

Segregation analysis was originally developed as a test for recessive inheritance: segregation ratios in sibships were observed and compared with the 25% affected–to–75% unaffected ratio predicted by Mendel's first law. Subsequently, this modest approach has been expanded into a sophisticated mathematical analysis. Qualitative notions such as dominant and recessive inheritance have given way to quantitative estimates of gene frequency, gene transmission probability, and genotype penetrance. Moreover, the laws of Mendelian inheritance have been replaced by models for single-gene transmission that incorporate intermediate types of gene effect. When these estimates and models are varied, they predict different phenotypic resemblances between different classes of relatives (MZ twins, DZ twins, full sibs, half sibs, and parents and offspring). These predictions are then statistically compared with the observed concordance between relatives, allowing the investigator to determine "best fit" models. If there is an extremely close fit between the predictions and the observations, then the model's mode of inheritance and quantitative estimates are supported. If, on the other hand, even the best-fit model for a certain mode of transmission shows little resemblance to the observed concordances, then it can be ruled out as a possible mode of transmission. However, it is important to note that segregation analysis relies on pooled data from many nuclear families and assumes genetic homogeneity across these families. This assumption is not always warranted (disorders may be phenotypically identical but etiologically distinct) and may lead to spurious results, such as the false rejection of monogenic transmission.

At present, more than 3,000 monogenic disorders are recognized; not infrequently they affect mental functioning (McKusick 1992). Approximately 25% of recessive and sex-linked disorders, such as phenylketonuria and Lesch-Nyhan syndrome, respectively, are associated with mental retardation. Unfortunately, segregation analyses of common psychiatric disorders do not confirm one of the simple Mendelian or sex-linked patterns described above (Matthysse and Kidd 1976). For this reason the psychiatric disorders belong to the group of "complex" (i.e., non-Mendelian) genetic disorders.

Complex patterns can arise from multiple genetic phenomena. The first of these is *genetic heterogeneity*. If a disorder can be caused by an abnormal gene at two (or more) genetic loci, and one of these causes the disorder in a recessive pattern and the other in a dominant pattern, then a segregation analysis of all those with the disorder will support neither model. Genetic heterogeneity is suspected because it has been shown in so many other medical disorders for which the genetics have been determined. Complex patterns may also occur because of environmental influences. There may be individuals who have the disorder but do not have any genetic predisposition. These individuals are said to have a phenocopy of the genetic form of the disorder. The psychiatric disorders are thought to exhibit many of the above phenomena, complicating segregation analysis. All of the major psychiatric disorders can be mimicked by medical illnesses, and thus other phenocopies, indistinguishable clinically, are suspected.

Another cause of complex inheritance patterns is termed *polygenic* or *multifactorial inheritance.* Such findings occur if multiple genes, none of which is of much significance by itself, interact with one another to cause the disorder (polygenic inheritance), or if multiple genes (some of which might have a major effect) and various environmental factors all contribute (multifactorial inheritance [Kidd 1981]). Because polygenic and multifactorial models have many variables, they produce a wide variety of possible values for familial concordances and thus can often fit quite closely with the observed data. In other words, monogenic disorders can be characterized by specific segregation ratios (i.e., rates of disorder in relatives), whereas polygenic disorders cannot.

There are a few predictions stemming from polygenic models that differ from those of monogenic models. In polygenic disorders (e.g., cleft lip/palate), relatives of affected probands are at greater risk of being affected, with increasing severity of illness in the proband and with greater numbers of other affected relatives. In addition, risk of illness drops off precipitously as one moves from MZ twins to first- and second-degree relatives (Risch 1990), and there are often affected relatives on both maternal and paternal sides (Gottesman and Shields 1982). Also, known monogenic disorders have low population prevalences. This suggests that common diseases (i.e., those occurring in more than 1% of the population) are likely to be polygenic, as are many traits that have been genetically studied (e.g., intelligence, height, skin color).

☐ Where Is the Abnormal Gene?—Genetic Linkage Analysis and Association Studies

Two general approaches to discovering genetic factors responsible for the pathogenesis of disease have been employed. In the first approach, *functional (gene) cloning,* an abnormal gene product (e.g., a defective enzyme) is identified and the abnormal gene coding for that product is delineated. To illustrate this approach, consider the Lesch-Nyhan syndrome. Excessive urinary excretion of uric acid in patients with the disorder led to the identification of a specific deficiency in a critical enzyme, hypoxanthine phosphoribosyltransferase (HPRT). Subsequently, DNA sequences complementary to HPRT mRNA were cloned and then used to localize and analyze the abnormalities in the structural gene for the deficient enzyme. A variety of molecular defects were identified in different patients, including single-base mutations, gene deletions, and gene rearrangements. Depending on the specific type of molecular defect, the patient's clinical phenotype may vary from simple gout to full-blown Lesch-Nyhan syndrome.

This approach has achieved considerable success in the study of recessive and X-linked disorders that are associated with an abnormal accumulation of metabolites in well-established biochemical pathways. For the major neuropsychiatric disorders, unfortunately, there are currently no proven metabolic abnormalities. For this reason a second approach, called *positional cloning*, has been applied to cloning the disease genes. In this alternative strategy the broad location of an abnormal gene is identified, without reference to the abnormal protein for which it codes, by the use of genetic linkage and association studies. More refined molecular analysis then allows for the identification of first the specific gene and then the gene product that underlie the disease. Researchers using the positional cloning approach have elucidated the pathogenesis of cystic fibrosis, NF1, DMD, and some forms of familial Alzheimer's disease. The gene for Huntington's disease has been localized to chromosome 4 but has not yet been cloned.

Genetic linkage analysis is a technique based on exceptions to Mendel's second law (Cox and Suarez 1985). This empirical observation, also known as the *law of independent assortment*, states that alleles (specific gene configurations) at different genetic loci are inherited independently of one another. This clearly applies to loci lying on different chromosomes. This law also often applies to loci lying on the same chromosome because of the exchange of genetic material between homologous chromosomes that occurs during the meiotic phase of gametogenesis in a process known as *crossing over*. This phenomenon is illustrated in Figure 2–1.

Genetic association studies look for correlations between certain alleles at a locus and the population of individuals with a disease. Although certain allele pairings of linked loci are likely to be disproportionately represented within any given kindred, as recombination occurs, this eventually will result in an even distribution of disease-marker allele combinations within the population at large. When the disease gene and marker loci are relatively far apart, such distribution will occur over the course of a few generations. On the other hand, if marker loci are close to a mutation that has spread through the population, this equilibrium may not have occurred. Thus an association between a disease and a particular allele within the population (linkage disequilibrium) suggests that the location of the disease gene and the marker locus are within a small genetic region. The advantage of this method over linkage analysis is that it

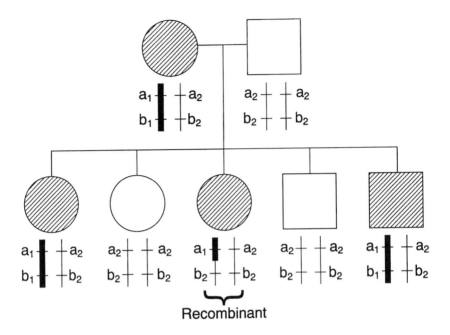

Figure 2–1. Genetic linkage and recombination. Depicted is a hypothetical family (circles: females; squares: males) transmitting an autosomal dominant disease. The disease locus A (containing either the defective allele a_1, or its normal counterpart a_2) lies close to a marker locus B (containing marker alleles b_1 and b_2). The mother is affected with the disease (solid symbol) and is heterozygous at both the disease and marker loci. The father is unaffected (open symbol) and is homozygous at both loci. Because the disease and marker loci are genetically linked (i.e., they lie near each other), crossing over rarely occurs between them. Most children who inherit the disease allelle a_1 also receive the b_1 marker allele from their mother. Occasionally, a recombination event (i.e., "crossing over") occurs in the mother, and she transfers a chromosome bearing the b_2 marker allele along with the disease allele (as occurred in the daughter labeled "recombinant"). The frequency of such recombinants increases as the distance between the disease and marker locus increases.

may be sensitive to genes with small phenotypic effects. The drawback of this method is that the ability to detect a genetic association falls off rapidly as genetic distance increases. The choice of the genetic control group is also critical. If those with the illness are from different genetic backgrounds than the control subjects with whom they are compared, the observed differences in allele frequencies may be due to racial differences rather than to differences in disease status (population stratification). Newer statistical approaches have been developed to address this potential artifact.

Historically, a variety of marker loci have been used for genetic linkage mapping. The first markers were blood antigens from both erythrocytes (ABO, Rh, MNS) and leukocytes (HLA) that could be measured serologically; serum proteins and isoenzymes that could be measured electrophoretically; and common anomalies such as color blindness. The major shortcomings of these marker loci were their paucity (about 30 known) and their irregular distribution throughout the genome. In the early 1980s the first markers using DNA polymorphisms, the restriction fragment length polymorphisms (RFLPs), came into use. The RFLP markers detect variations in DNA sequence that cause the presence or absence of sites for enzymes that cut specific sequences of DNA (i.e., restriction endonucleases). Because a restriction endonuclease site is either present or absent in a given chromosome (i.e., there are only two possible alleles), the RFLP markers limit the frequency of heterozygotes to 50%. This limitation, and the cumbersome technique required to generate the RFLP data (i.e., Southern blots), have been the stimulus to develop the microsatellite markers. These markers utilize the naturally occurring variations in the length of dinucleotide (also tri-, tetra-, pentanucleotide) DNA repeat sequences.

☐ Problems of Diagnosis and Classification in Genetic Investigations

Most genetic studies are greatly impeded by any ambiguity in knowing who has and who does not have the illness being studied. For example, accurate diagnosis of all family members is essential for all forms of segregation analysis and for almost all studies of linkage. (Changes in the diagnoses of pedigree members can have profound effects on the evidence for linkage, as described below for studies of bipolar disorder.)

The various versions of research diagnostic criteria recently developed for psychiatric disorders have not solved the diagnostic problems that exist for genetic investigation. These criteria often exclude ambiguous cases, rather than clarify their status. Also, although reliable criteria have been constructed for many psychiatric disorders, validation of the diagnostic categories as specific entities has not been established.

The high prevalence rates of psychiatric disorders and the existence of many known medical disorders that can produce the major psychiatric syndromes are reasons to believe that most psychiatric diagnostic categories are clinical syndromes, identifying patients with a variety of etiological abnormalities. A diagnosis of Huntington's disease or DMD is known to specify a group with a specific etiology and pathogenesis, whereas a diagnosis of schizophrenia or major depressive disorder is not. If the diagnostic entities psychiatry has established are not etiologically homogeneous, then searching for the modes of transmission or genetic linkages of these disorders may be likened to the genetic study of pneumonia, renal failure, or dropsy. Thus, even the most reliable criteria available for psychiatric disorders, validated to the best of our current ability, may fail to identify certain individuals having the disease (especially those with milder or deviant forms) and may also fail by identifying as affected some individuals with a "similar disease" (if there are multiple diseases that lead to a common clinical picture).

Most psychiatric disorders are probably complex in origin, with multiple interacting genetic and environmental contributors (i.e., polygenetic or multifactorial inheritance). In these cases, for linkage studies to succeed, the diagnostic schema must identify a group in which most patients share some specific abnormal genetic component, and this may not be the case with the current nomenclature. Psychiatric nosology has of course aimed at identifying illnesses with the specificity needed by genetic analysis, and it has explored the validity of various diagnostic systems, using broad versus narrow definitions, exclusion criteria, definitions of "functional impairment" and "secondary cases," and correction factors for diagnostic instability. The relative failure of this attempt may be inevitable for a nosology based on clinical phenomenology, and greater knowledge of the biological pathogenesis of psychiatric disorders may be necessary. To make use of the new advances in genetic methodology, it may be necessary for psychiatry to discover subtypes of current diagnostic categories that have one or more specific measurable biochemical or physiological traits (e.g., precipitation of panic attacks with lactate infusion, association of schizophrenia with deviant eye tracking) in addition to the symptoms of the illness. This development may be fostered by the emerging advances in neuroradiography, neurophysiology, neurochemistry, and the specification of cognitive deficits.

However, certain aspects of psychiatric disorders will continue to make accurate diagnosis problematic, such as late age at onset, intermittent expression of symptoms, variation in symptomatology over time (e.g., major depressive disorder becoming bipolar disorder), and the influence of environmental factors on the emergence (i.e., penetrance) of these disorders or in producing phenocopies. Also, there are mild or intermediate forms for all the major conditions, and such cases may at times represent formes frustes that are genetically associated with the major disorder. There are benefits to counting these cases as affected in genetic studies, but there is likely to be even more etiological heterogeneity in these milder/intermediate syndromes than in the major ones, and considering such cases as affected can result in misleading results regarding specific genetic determinations.

■ GENETICS OF PSYCHIATRIC DISORDERS

☐ Schizophrenia

Older studies consistently demonstrated elevated morbid risks for schizophrenia in the first-degree relatives of schizophrenic probands (parents, mean = 5.6%; sibs, 10.1%; children, 12.8%) compared with those in the general population (0.9%), which suggests that schizophrenia is familial (Gottesman and Shields 1982). More recent studies that have satisfied modern criteria for the collection of family data have corroborated these earlier findings (Kendler 1986). The relatively lower risk to parents is at odds with Mendelian inheritance—all first-degree relatives, sharing 50% of their genes, should show equal risk—but may reflect the reproductive fitness effects. It would appear that schizophrenia, both broadly and narrowly defined, is familial. Furthermore, schizoaffective disorder (as in DSM-III-R), paranoid disorder, atypical psychosis, and schizotypal personality disorder also aggregate in the relatives of schizophrenic probands, indicating the possible boundaries of the phenotypic spectrum (Kendler et al. 1985).

In all, 817 MZ twin pairs and 1,016 same-sex DZ twin pairs have been studied, with weighted mean probandwise concordances of 59.2% and 15.2%, respectively, being reported (Kendler 1986). Nonetheless, estimates of probandwise concordance have varied, possibly reflecting differences in diagnostic criteria, case sampling, and zygosity assessment across studies (Walker et al. 1991). The risk of schizophrenia in MZ co-twins of affected probands is at least three times that in DZ co-twins and some 40 to 60 times the risk in the general population. Approximately half of MZ twin pairs are discordant for schizophrenia despite genetic identity. Although many nonschizophrenic MZ co-twins of affected probands show a variety of psychiatric disorders, including "neurotic" and character disorders and "schizoid" conditions, many appear normal. The offspring of nonschizophrenic MZ co-twins may be at as high a risk for schizophrenia as are the offspring of their affected sibs (Fischer 1971; Gottesman and Bertelsen 1989; Kringlen and Cramer 1989), implying that these co-twins carry the schizophrenic genotype despite their "normal" appearance. These findings suggest a range of phenotypes compatible with the schizophrenic genotype, and highlight the importance of epigenetic (environmental) factors in the pathogenesis of the disorder.

The affected members of discordant MZ twin pairs show left hemisphere hypodensity on computed tomography (CT) scan (Reveley et al. 1987), smaller anterior pes hippocampi on magnetic resonance imaging (MRI) (Suddath et al. 1990), and diminished activation of the dorsolateral prefrontal cortex while performing the WCS, as measured by regional cerebral flood flow (Weinberger et al. 1992).

All four varieties of adoption study have been applied to schizophrenia: adoptee study method, cross-fostering, adoptee's family method, and the study of MZ twins reared apart. Heston (1966) found a significantly greater risk for schizophrenia among the offspring of schizophrenic mothers separated at birth than among the adopted-away offspring of control mothers. This finding was replicated in a Danish sample by Rosenthal et al. (1968), in a study that has withstood blind reanalysis using DSM-III criteria; and in a Finnish sample by Tienari et al. (1987), in a study that has incorporated such modern techniques as direct, blind interview of adoptees and detailed examination of adoptive families, the latter permitting an analysis of genotype-environmental interactions (Tienari 1991).

The sole cross-fostering study to date found equivalent rates of severe psychiatric illness among adoptees from biological parents without psychiatric illness, regardless of whether the adoptees were reared by adoptive parents with schizophrenia or without the illness: both adoptee groups had rates of illness significantly lower than those in a group of adoptees from biological parents with schizophrenia and related disorders (Wender et al. 1974). In addition to providing evidence for the etiological importance of genetic factors in schizophrenia, this study argues against a causative role for rearing factors associated with parent psychosis, except, perhaps, in the presence of a susceptible genotype.

In studies employing the adoptee's family method schizophrenia and related disorders were found to be more common in the biological relatives of 34 schizophrenic adoptees, while the rates for these disorders did not differentiate the adoptive relatives of either adoptee group, being low in both. The Danish adoption study has withstood reanalysis using DSM-III criteria (Kendler and Gruenberg 1984) and has been replicated with a second cohort of 41 index and control adoptees (Kety 1988). The biological relatives of schizophrenic adoptees have shown higher rates not only of schizophrenia but also of DSM-III diagnosed schizotypal and paranoid personality disorders, again expanding the boundaries of the schizophrenic syndrome (Kendler and Gruenberg 1984). Finally, two studies of monozygotic twins reared apart have shown high pairwise concordance for schizophrenia, providing further evidence for a genetic component in the etiology of this disorder (Gottesman and Shields 1982).

High-risk studies have examined both early characteristics that distinguish the offspring of schizophrenic parents from control subjects and premorbid features that predict which of those offspring will go on to develop schizophrenia. By 1 year of age, high-risk infants were more likely than control infants to show "anxious" attachment behavior and sensorimotor deficits. By 2 years of age, they were seen to be more passive and less attentive in play. Later, they had less social competence.

These findings have been taken as evidence of an inherited neurointegrative defect in schizophrenia (Fish et al. 1992).

Older high-risk children have demonstrated defective emotional rapport and disturbed cognition in unblinded clinical interviews (Parnas et al. 1982), diminished attention on measures such as the Continuous Performance Test (Watt et al. 1984), and greater impairment on the aforementioned psychometric index derived from the MMPI (Moldin et al. 1990a). These abnormalities support the Bleulerian notion of a primary affective, associational, and attentional disturbance in schizophrenia. Moreover, because these abnormalities characterize high-risk individuals who go on to develop either schizophrenia or schizotypal personality disorder, they support the genetic relatedness of these disorders. Because the abnormalities described herein affect only about 10% to 25% of high-risk offspring (Watt et al. 1984), they appear to be somewhat removed from a core monogenic defect (if present) in schizophrenia. On the other hand, smooth pursuit eye movement dysfunction has been reported to characterize approximately 50% of the teenage children of schizophrenic parents and thus may more closely reflect the schizophrenic diathesis (Mather 1985).

Premorbid predictors of schizophrenia (versus schizotypal personality disorder) among high-risk children have included obstetrical complications; soft neurological signs such as impaired balance, left-right confusion, and motor overflow in childhood; and autonomic hypoarousal in adolescence (Cannon et al. 1990). Moreover, adult correlates of schizophrenia (versus schizotypal personality disorder) among high-risk offspring have included ventricular enlargement (especially of the third ventricle) on CT scan (Dykes et al. 1992). It is tempting to speculate that these clinical and radiological findings reflect a common perinatal neurological insult that contributes to disease expression. This speculation is also supported by retrospective studies of schizophrenic patients and by studies of discordant MZ twins. In these studies, poorer outcome has been associated with the triad of obstetrical complications, neurological dysfunction, and ventricular enlargement.

Several models for the genetic transmission of schizophrenia have been proposed, including monogenic/single major locus, oligogenic, and polygenic/multifactorial models. Monogenic models have difficulty accounting for the sharp drop in risk for schizophrenia as one moves from MZ twins to first- and second-degree relatives. Oligogenic models involving the epistatic interaction of two or three gene loci may better account for these data (Risch 1990). Likewise, monogenic models are hard pressed to account for the observed increased risk of schizophrenia in relatives, given either increased severity in the proband or a greater number of other affected relatives (Gottesman and Shields 1982). These observations, on the other hand, are compatible with a polygenic/multifactorial model. Furthermore, O'Rourke et al. (1982) have argued against a single-locus, two-allele model by citing its inability to account for the observed distribution in the rates of schizophrenia among four classes of relatives of schizophrenia probands (parents, siblings, MZ, and DZ co-twins) in 21 studies meeting criteria of adequacy. Finally, several segregation analyses have similarly rejected monogenic models or, at least, have been unable to reject polygenic models (Risch and Baron 1984; Vogler et al. 1990).

These results are not incompatible, however, with a so-called mixed model involving a major locus in the setting of a multifactorial background (Tsuang et al. 1991). Moreover, they do not preclude the possibility that major loci underlie certain aspects of the schizophrenia phenotype. Thus, admixture analysis, a strategy complementary to segregation analysis that examines the population distribution of a quantitative phenotype for multimodality (each mode presumably reflecting the mean phenotypic consequence of a particular genotype), has provided preliminary evidence for a major gene underlying the aforementioned psychometric index derived from the MMPI (Moldin et al. 1990b) and smooth pursuit eye movement dysfunction (Clementz et al. 1992).

Chromosome 5 (5q11.2-13.3) has been widely investigated as the location of a potential major susceptibility locus for schizophrenia following a report of an uncle/nephew pair with neuroleptic-responsive DSM-III-R schizophrenia (Bassett et al. 1988) and a partial trisomy of the long arm of chromosome 5. A third family member with a balanced translocation involving the trisomic region was phenotypically normal. Sherrington et al. (1988) examined five Icelandic and two English pedigrees and found linkage between 5q and schizophrenia, schizophrenia "spectrum" disorders, and a variety of other psychiatric disorders. Numerous subsequent studies, however, have failed to replicate this initial linkage finding (Crowe et al. 1991; Hallmayer et al. 1992; Macciardi et al. 1992; McGuffin et al. 1991).

Candidate genes have also been examined for linkage to schizophrenia. The regulatory gene homeobox 2 (chromosome 17p) appears not to be linked to the schizophrenia locus in the aforementioned northern Swedish isolate. Similarly, the neurochemical gene proopiomelanocortin (2p) appears not to be linked in families segregating schizophrenia (Feder et al. 1985). Other neurochemical genes, such as those for tyrosine hydroxylase (11p; Kennedy et al. 1988), the dopamine D_2 receptor (11q; Moises et al. 1991), and the serotonin 5-HT_2 receptor (13q; Hallmayer et al. 1992), were excluded in the Swedish pedigree. Recently, linkage has been excluded between all five dopamine receptors (D_{1-5}) and schizophrenia (as well as the P50 quantitative definition of the schizophrenia phenotype) in nine multigenerational pedigrees (Coon et al. 1993). There is preliminary evidence from two independent samples, however, that homozygosity at the dopamine D_3 receptor gene (3q) is associated with schizophrenia. It is conceivable that this represents an example of heterozygote advantage (Crocq et al. 1992).

Molecular studies of schizophrenia have included quantitation of known mRNAs for specific candidate proteins, screening of unknown mRNAs through in vitro translation and two-dimensional gel electrophoresis, and direct sequencing of genomic DNA. In an example of the first approach, Harrison et al. (1991) found decreased non-NMDA glutamate receptor mRNA in the hippocampus of patients with schizophrenia, suggesting a role for aberrant glutaminergic function in the disorder. In an example of the second approach, Perrett et al. (1992) identified over 200 products coding for mRNA from postmortem tissue. One novel 26-kilodalton protein was specifically decreased in schizophrenia brain (18% of control level). In an example of the third approach, Sarkar et al. (1991) directly sequenced the dopamine D_2 receptor gene from 14 patients with schizophrenia and found no significant sequence differences in seven functionally significant regions.

☐ Mood (Affective) Disorders

The major mood disorders, bipolar disorder and major depression, have been found to be highly familial in a number of European and American studies. First-degree relatives of bipolar probands have an elevated morbid risk for both bipolar and major depressive illness, whereas relatives of major depression probands have an elevated risk for major depression but not bipolar disorder (Weissman et al. 1984). Schizoaffective disorder, especially schizoaffective disorder with manic symptoms, also has frequently been found to be associated with a high rate of bipolar disorder among relatives.

In addition to finding these high familial rates of affective disorder, a number of studies have found that the risk for family members and the morbid risk in the population have increased for those born in later versus earlier decades of the 20th century (Gershon et al. 1987; Klerman et al. 1985). This has been termed an "age-period-cohort effect," and it has been found to be present in many countries (Weissman et al. 1992).

The results of a large NIMH collaborative study reported by Andreasen et al. (1987) for interviewed relatives found that schizoaffective probands with depressive features had a somewhat elevated rate (2.5%) of schizophrenia in first-degree relatives, and a zero prevalence of bipolar-I disorder. These findings were quite different from those of schizoaffective disorder, bipolar type, providing evidence that certain types of schizoaffective disorder may not be related to bipolar disorder. In this study, the authors decided to report rates of illness rather than morbid risk figures.

Early age at onset (under age 20) has been shown, in more than six studies with depressed and/or bipolar probands, to be associated with an increased rate of illness among adult relatives 2- to 3-fold (versus relatives of other depressed probands). The increase is even greater for early-onset cases among relatives (Kupfer et al. 1989). The corresponding increase in a study of prepubertal depression was 14-fold (Weissman et al. 1988). In two studies, reduced REM latency was also associated with higher familial rates (Giles et al. 1988; Mendlewicz et al. 1989).

Twin studies have supported the importance of genetic factors in the transmission of the major affective disorders. Summed data from older twin studies give a 65% pairwise concordance rate for MZ twin pairs and a 14% rate for DZ pairs (Nurnberger and Gershon 1982). The MZ rate for bipolar disorder is higher than that for major depression. Older studies had an average MZ concordance of 72% for bipolar probands, with a Danish study, using strict criteria, finding an MZ rate of 79% versus 19% for DZ pairs (Bertelsen et al. 1977). This study found MZ and DZ rates of 54% and 24%, respectively, for major depression probands. Two recent twin studies of major depression by Kendler et al. (1992d) and McGuffin et al. (1991) both found substantial evidence for genetic factors, but differed on whether the environmental contribution to the disorder was from shared environmental (e.g., familial) factors or from experiences not shared by the twins.

The few adoption studies of major affective disorders have produced somewhat conflicting data that are confounded by differences in sampling. The one study of adopted-away offspring found that the children of mothers with bipolar disorder or major depression had a higher rate of major affective disorder than did the adopted-away children of mothers with other psychiatric conditions (Cadoret 1978). Mendlewicz and Rainer (1977) found a significantly increased risk for affective illness in the biological parents of bipolar adoptee probands, compared with their adoptive parents or with the biological parents of control subjects. Wender et al. (1986) studied a group of adoptees with mixed affective disorder diagnoses and found an increase in suicide and some affective disorders among their biological, but not their adoptive, relatives when each was compared to his or her corresponding control subject. Conversely, von Knorring et al. (1983) found no differences between the biological parent groups, and noted an excess of psychiatric illness in the adoptive parents of the index cases, who were primarily adoptees with nonbipolar depression.

Many psychiatric disorders have been associated with bipolar disorder and/or major depression in family studies, including dysthymia, cyclothymia, schizoaffective disorder (RDC criteria), alcoholism, eating disorders, attention-deficit disorder, and migraine. In addition, certain personality traits, such as rigidity, appear to be increased among relatives (Maier et al. 1992). However, preferential mating between those persons with affective disorders, plus the frequency of secondary depressions complicating almost all severe illnesses, makes it difficult to determine whether these associations actually reflect joint etiological determinants.

High-risk studies of children of parents with major affective disorders have quite consistently found high rates of social and psychiatric impairment. Controlled studies of specific diagnoses have noted an increased prevalence of major depression, conduct disorder, attention-deficit disorder, anxiety disorder, and substance abuse, as well as poorer social functioning and more school problems, among these children. The age at onset of depression in these high-risk offspring was earlier (mean ages 12 to 13) than among depressed control subjects whose parents were not depressed (mean age at onset of 16 to 17).

The promise of DNA polymorphisms and linkage analysis initially inspired hopes of rapidly solving the questions of the chromosomal location of any major genetic contribution to bipolar disorder and other mood disorders, as well as the mode of inheritance and the extent of heterogeneity.

☐ Anxiety Disorders

The recent prospective NIMH epidemiological study of 1-year prevalence rates found anxiety disorders, at 12.6%, to be the most common category of illness (Regier et al. 1993). Diagnostic terms and concepts in the area of anxiety disorders have changed considerably over the past decade, diminishing the relevance of older studies in this area. However, whenever studied, "anxiety neurosis" was found to be highly familial, with up to two-thirds of families showing cases in first-degree relatives. Studies using DSM-III-R diagnostic categories have reported increased familial rates for panic disorder and agoraphobia, generalized anxiety disorder, and simple and social phobias, but not for other anxiety disorders.

A family study of panic disorder by Crowe et al. (1983) found a 17.3% risk for panic disorder in first-degree relatives and an additional risk of 7.4% for "probable panic disorder." Control rates were 1.8% and 0.4%, respectively. Noyes et al. (1986) found high risk for panic disorder (definite plus probable) both in the relatives of panic disorder probands (17.3%) and in the relatives of agoraphobic probands (8.3%), compared with 4.2% in the relatives of control subjects. They also found that the risk for agoraphobia was increased among the relatives of agoraphobic probands (11.6%), but not the relatives of panic disorder probands (1.9%), when compared with control subjects (4.2%). All agoraphobic probands and relatives had panic attacks as well. Both studies showed no increase of generalized anxiety disorder in the relatives of the index cases. Noyes et al. concluded that their findings are consistent with agoraphobia being a more severe variant of panic disorder, and that these two disorders are unrelated to generalized anxiety disorder. These findings have been supported by studies that have concluded that the risk for panic disorder among first-degree relatives is increased fivefold (Hopper et al. 1987), and that agoraphobia is increased in the families of agoraphobic patients, but not in those of patients having only panic disorder (Gruppo Italiano Disturbi d'Ansia 1989).

Determining the relationship of panic disorder to both alcoholism and depression is more complicated. The Crowe-Noyes studies mentioned above reported increased alcoholism among the probands' relatives. However, alcoholism may occur secondarily, from self-medicating efforts to alleviate the panic attacks and/or agoraphobia. With regard to depression, both of these studies failed to show an increase of major depression among relatives of panic disorder cases, which would argue for panic disorder and agoraphobia being etiologically separate from the mood disorders. Other studies have indicated that there may be a common predisposition to depression and anxiety disorders (Leckman et al. 1983). Thus, the issue of the familial/genetic relationship between panic disorder and major depression has not been resolved.

The possibility of a genetic relationship between adult and childhood anxiety disorders has been prompted by the high rates of separation anxiety and school phobia reported by adults with panic disorder. Some family studies have shown elevated rates of separation anxiety in the children of parents with panic disorder/agoraphobia, but others have concluded that childhood school phobias are related to adult neurotic illness in general rather than specifically to adult agoraphobia. Family studies of generalized anxiety disorder, simple phobias, and social phobia have found familial aggregation. Noyes et al. (1987) noted that the increased rates of generalized anxiety disorder were specific and that they were not found among the relatives of panic disorder patients. Fyer et al. (1990) reported a rate of 31% for simple phobia in first-degree relatives, compared with 11% in controls. For social phobia, two studies (Fyer et al. 1993; Reich et al. 1988) found a threefold increase in this disorder in the relatives of probands, the latter reporting rates of 16% vs. 5% in the control group.

The findings with obsessive-compulsive disorder (OCD) are inconsistent with regard to familiality (Black et al. 1992). Some studies have linked OCD with Gilles de la Tourette syndrome (Leckman and Chittenden 1990). No increase of posttraumatic stress disorder (PTSD) was found in the families of PTSD probands studied (using family history methodology) by Davidson et al. (1989).

Twin studies have now been done on each of the major anxiety disorders. Torgersen (1983) found that 4 of 13 MZ co-twins (31%) were concordant for panic disorder and/or agoraphobia, compared with 0 of 16 DZ co-twins. Kendler et al. (1992c) found evidence for a significant genetic contribution to agoraphobia, social phobia, and animal phobia in a study of female twins. These authors also found evidence for the importance of environmental factors: some factors predisposed to all phobias, but other environmental experiences had a more specific effect, especially for simple phobias. Kendler et al. (1992b) also conducted a twin study of generalized anxiety disorder, finding MZ-DZ concordances of 28% and 17%, concluding that this disorder, too, was moderately familial and heritable. These authors estimated that the important environmental factors were not those shared by twins.

Other twin studies of anxiety disorders (i.e., PTSD and OCD) do not show familial aggregation. True et al. (1993) reported that genetic factors provided a substantial contribution to all the symptoms of PTSD (but did not report MZ-DZ concordance rates). Goldberg et al. (1990), who studied monozygotic males only and thus were unable to estimate the genetic influence, discovered that those twins with military service in Southeast Asia, especially those twins with high levels of combat experience there, had a much greater incidence of the disorder than did their co-twins (17.6% to 4.8%). For OCD, Carey and Gottesman (1981) found significant MZ-DZ differences (87% vs. 47%, respectively), which is similar to results found earlier in a Japanese investigation. These twin studies of OCD indicate that genetic factors may be involved, although familial aggregation has not been shown.

Of the anxiety disorders, only panic disorder has had findings from linkage studies reported in the literature. Crowe et al. (1990) examined multiple candidate genes (i.e., tyrosine hydroxylase, adrenergic receptors, proopiomelanocortin) and did not find any evidence of genetic linkage.

☐ Eating Disorders

Anorexia nervosa and bulimia nervosa have been studied with the techniques of psychiatric genetics, although not as extensively as have other major disorders. Family studies of anorexia nervosa have shown an increased rate of anorexia itself as well as bulimia and subclinical anorexia nervosa. In one study, first-degree female relatives had lifetime risks for these disorders of 2.3%, 2.3%, and 5.4%, respectively, compared with control risks of 0.5%, 1.0%, and 0% (Strober et al. 1985). Most notably, however, many studies have found an increased risk for affective disorders among the first-degree relatives of anorexic patients, a risk exceeding that for eating disorders and equaling the risk among the relatives of patients with major depression (Winokur et al. 1980). Another study found a morbid risk of approximately 13% for major depression, plus a risk of approximately 8% for bipolar or schizoaffective disorder, in first-degree relatives of probands with anorexia nervosa, with control rates of 5.8% and 0.9%, respectively (Gershon et al. 1984). Family studies of bulimia have also found high rates of mood disorders and eating disorders (Kassett et al. 1989). The high rates of mood disorders in this study were found among the relatives of bulimic patients regardless of whether the relatives had mood disorders themselves.

Twin studies have been reported for anorexia and bulimia. Holland et al. (1988) found 56% of 25 MZ anorexic twin pairs and 5% of 20 DZ pairs to be concordant for the disorder. For bulimia, Kendler et al. (1991) found concordances of 23.9% for MZ and 8.7% for DZ twin pairs, as well as an increased risk for bulimia-like syndromes that appeared to be milder versions of the same illness caused by the same factors. Both research groups interpreted their data to show large genetic effects. Various studies have also reported increasing rates of both eating disorders, in the population and among family members, for those born later versus earlier in this century.

Because anorexia nervosa and bulimia nervosa have such high rates of familial affective disorder, determining the nature of the relationship between all of these entities is an area of current investigation and theorizing. One important issue that awaits determination is whether or not only those anorexic and bulimic patients with depression have high rates of depression among relatives. If even those patients without depression show high rates of depression among relatives, there may be major genetic factors shared between the eating disorders and mood disorders, with the phenotypic variations based only on modifying genes and environment.

☐ Somatoform Disorders and Sociopathy

The DSM-IV (American Psychiatric Association 1994) criteria for somatization disorder are a shortened and simplified version of the criteria for Briquet's syndrome (Guze 1970). Most of the studies reviewed here are of Briquet's syndrome rather than of somatization disorder, as this latter concept is relatively new. Studies have shown strong overlap of the two concepts, but also the possibility of greater severity and/or greater homogeneity for patients meeting the full Briquet's criteria, as indicated by higher rates of familial aggregation. The prevalence of Briquet's syndrome in first-degree female relatives has been found to be 7.7%, compared with 2.5% in control subjects (Cloninger et al. 1986).

The connection between Briquet's syndrome and antisocial personality disorder was first recognized by finding the coincidence of these two disorders in many samples, especially among women. (Histrionic personality disorder has been associated with these two disorders as well.) Family studies have repeatedly shown a link, most consistently by finding Briquet's syndrome among female relatives of probands (male or female) who are sociopaths or criminals, but also by finding elevated rates of sociopathy in the first-degree relatives of Briquet's or somatization subjects (Lilienfeld et al. 1986).

Adoption studies have given support more to genetic than to environmental determinants of the associations between these disorders. Some studies, using the adoptee study method, have shown an increase of somatic symptoms without medical explanation, as well as antisocial symptoms, among female adoptees of biological parents having antisocial personality. The largest study, using the adoptee's family method, comprising 144 female adoptee "somatizers" (identified by having two or more sick leaves per year), identified two types of the disorder, each having a link to a form of criminality among the subjects' fathers. One type, termed "diversiform somatization," was linked to a syndrome of alcoholism plus criminal behavior in biological fathers, with the finding of increased alcohol abuse among adoptive fathers as well. The other type, "high-frequency somatizers," had biological fathers with a recurrent history of arrest for violent crimes but no history of alcoholism, and no increase of psychopathology among adoptive fathers (Cloninger et al. 1984).

Older twin studies of hysteria found higher MZ than DZ rates of concordance, but the pairwise MZ rates were low enough (averaging 21%) to question the importance of genetic factors. A more recent twin study examined a mixed group of somatoform disorders and found an MZ concordance of 29% and a DZ concordance of 10% for the group of disorders as a whole (Torgersen 1986).

Multifactorial models of transmission allow for the possibility of linking clinically discrete illnesses on a continuum of shared liability. Such a model was proposed by Cloninger et al. (1975), in which Briquet's syndrome in women, sociopathy in men, and sociopathy in women were considered to be increasingly severe expressions of the same multifactorial determinants. This model adequately fits the available data on the risks to first-degree relatives of probands having the various disorders.

Most twin and adoption studies of criminality and antisocial personality have focused on the transmission of these conditions per se and their relationship with alcohol abuse, rather than on their relationship with somatization disorder. A genetic component has consistently been supported (Cloninger and Gottesman 1987), as well as environmental factors. The largest of these studies (Bohman et al. 1982) delineated two types of criminality, each showing genetic predisposition without significant overlap. One was associated with alcoholism and more violent, repeated offenses. The other, associated with petty crimes, appeared to be caused by a genetic predisposition independent of alcoholism as well as by environmental factors that differed for the two sexes. The specific nature of gene-environment interaction is now being investigated, revealing the importance of exposure to alcoholism, antisocial behavior, and other factors associated with low socioeconomic status for those who are genetically predisposed (Cadoret et al. 1990).

☐ Alcoholism

The rates of alcoholism in the population vary greatly by definition and by sex. The 6-month prevalence rates found in the ECA study, in which broad criteria were used, were 8.2% to 10.4% for males and 1.0% to 1.9% for females (Robins et al. 1984). Alcoholism has also been shown to be highly familial in many studies, which show the risk to first-degree relatives to be increased approximately sevenfold. Pitts and Winokur (1966), using modern family study methods and strict diagnostic criteria for severe alcoholism, found a risk of 16% in the fathers and 7% in the sibs of alcoholic subjects, versus risks of 1.6% and 0.5% for the relatives of matched control subjects. As with mood disorders and eating disorders, the risk among family members, and in the general population, appears to be rising (Reich et al. 1988).

Adoption studies that have provided evidence that genetic factors, as well as environmental ones, are involved in the etiology of alcoholism. Goodwin (1979) showed that alcoholism in the biological parents predicted alcoholism in their male offspring, even when the latter were raised by unrelated adoptive parents. Cadoret et al. (1980) reported similar results. The results for female offspring were less clear. Goodwin (1979) found elevated rates of alcoholism among both the adopted-away daughters of alcoholic persons and the control adoptees, while Cadoret et al. (1985) found higher rates in the daughters of the index cases compared with control subjects. Data from a large Swedish sample also support a genetic predisposition to alcoholism in both women and men (Cloninger et al. 1981), as well as the possible importance of certain environmental factors (such as lower occupational status of the adoptive father). In all of these studies, alcoholism in the adoptive environment was not shown to increase the risk for alcoholism among the adoptees. However, Cadoret et al. (1985) found that alcoholism in the adoptive family more broadly defined (to include all adoptive first- and second-degree relatives) increased the rates of alcohol abuse among adoptees. Because alcohol abuse frequently coexists with antisocial personality and depression, these studies examined the question of the specificity of inheritance. They suggest that one subtype of alcoholism may relate to criminality and antisocial personality, but that depression is not genetically related.

The twin studies of alcoholism have led to inconsistent findings. This inconsistency is probably the result of the MZ-DZ concordance ratio being relatively low (1.0–2.0), and of variations in the severity of illness of probands in the various studies. Though some studies have found no differences in the concordance rate (e.g., 29% for MZs, 33% for DZs [Gurling et al. 1984]), the two most recent studies have each found MZ rates greater than DZ rates for both male and female twins, if the diagnosis was restricted to more severe cases. Pickens et al. (1991) found that for alcohol dependence these rates were 59% versus 36% for males and 25% versus 5% for females; Kendler et al. (1992a) reported 26% versus 12% for female twins with similar diagnostic criteria. Another finding, that of Kaprio et al. (1984), highly implicates genetic factors: MZ concordances were found to be greater than DZ concordances for heavy alcohol use whether or not the twins were raised together.

If alcoholism were heterogenous, with a significant percentage of cases having a major genetic causative influence, then alcoholism in persons having alcoholic parents or other first-degree relatives may differ from that in nonfamilial cases. Also, the offspring (sons) of alcoholic persons may differ from the offspring of nonalcoholic control subjects. Such studies have in fact shown that familial alcoholic persons have earlier and more severe alcoholic-related problems, early development of physical dependence, and poorer treatment outcome (Goodwin 1984). High-risk studies of sons of alcoholic persons, compared with control subjects, have shown a decreased intensity of subjective feelings of intoxication, reduced objective signs of intoxication, and differences in plasma cortisol and prolactin following ethanol challenge (Schuckit and Gold 1988).

☐ Personality Traits and Disorders

Because personality can be described by so many attributes, researchers have worked to condense these into a few "dimensions," usually by factor analytic techniques. Those that have emerged as most replicable and most used in genetic studies are extraversion and neuroticism, originally derived by Eysenck (1981). The dimensions of harm avoidance, reward dependence, and novelty seeking, as defined by Cloninger (1986, 1987), plus the additional dimensions of persistence, self-directedness, cooperativeness, and self-transcendence, are now also widely used for personality research.

The extensive family, twin, and adoption studies of extraversion and neuroticism give strong evidence for a genetic effect, but the extent of the genetic contribution, measured as heritability estimates, is greater in twin studies than in family studies, in which values of approximately one-half those in twin studies have been reported. A possible interpretation, as discussed by Plomin et al. (1990), is nonadditive genetic variance, an allelic interaction that makes identical twins quite alike but does not "breed true" for first-degree relatives, because only one of the alleles can be passed on from a parent.

Reich (1989) found avoidant and dependent personality disorders to be significantly familial, and this held true for the disorders when grouped as Cluster C ("anxious cluster") as well. In a later report, Reich (1991) found that the increase in anxious cluster personality diagnoses among relatives was also found for probands with mixed anxiety and depression who did not have personality disorders. Relatives of Cluster B ("flamboyant cluster") personality disorders showed a high level of personality disorder psychopathology, but of a diverse nature. Borderline personality disorder has also been found to be modestly familial. We have already discussed the familiality of Cluster A personality disorders in the section above on schizophrenia.

☐ Alzheimer's Disease

Epidemiological studies reveal an increased prevalence of dementia in the family members of Alzheimer's patients. Family studies are hindered by the late age at onset, because individuals can die from other conditions or develop a dementia from a different etiology. St. George-Hyslop et al. (1989) reported that estimates of the increase in Alzheimer's disease risk to family members vary widely and may be small (10%–14.4% for parents; 3.8%–13.9% for siblings). Life table studies that adjust for deaths not due to Alzheimer's disease find that the risk of Alzheimer's disease may be as high as 50% in family members by age 90 and only 10% in control subjects (Breitner et al. 1986; Mohs et al. 1987). The increased family prevalence of Alzheimer's disease may occur predominantly in an early-onset group (Li et al. 1995), although it may be that such cases are just more easily ascertained.

Only a small number of twin studies have been published (Cook et al. 1981; Embry and Bruyland 1985; Nee et al. 1987). The concordance rates, thus far, are similar in MZ and DZ pairs (about 40%), with some pairs having quite disparate ages at onset. These twin studies support a large environmental influence on the etiology of Alzheimer's disease.

The occurrence of neuropathological changes indicative of Alzheimer's disease in individuals with Down's syndrome initially directed a search for an Alzheimer's disease locus on chromosome 21. This chromosome also contains the locus for the amyloid precursor protein (APP), the precursor of amyloid, itself a major constituent of the senile plaques of Alzheimer's disease. However, linkage was not found in pedigrees evaluated by others. A mutation in the APP gene has been identified that co-segregated with Alzheimer's disease in two unrelated chromosome 21–linked early-onset families (Goate et al. 1991). This finding supports, but does not prove, a role for this abnormality and amyloid deposition in at least some families with Alzheimer's disease.

Schellenberg et al. (1992) described linkage to chromosome 14q in nine early-onset pedigrees. This region of chromosome 14 contains several candidate genes (e.g., proteases, protease inhibitors, transcriptional regulators) that may be involved in APP processing. A genetic contribution to the more frequent late onset type of this illness was reported by Corder et al. (1993). There is an association of the illness, and the early onset of the illness, with the presence of the type 4 allele of the apolipoprotein E gene located on chromosome 19. Apolipoprotein E transports amyloid, and thus also might be involved in its deposition. This finding could allow individuals to determine whether they were at increased risk for developing Alzheimer's disease at a certain age.

☐ Gilles de la Tourette Syndrome

The familial nature of Tourette syndrome was described by Gilles de la Tourette himself in 1885 when he observed that mild cases of the disorder occurred in the same families as more classic cases (Baraitser 1990). The risk of Tourette syndrome in the first- and second-degree relatives of patients with Tourette syndrome is 3.6% (Zausmer and Dewey 1987). (Compare this risk with the population prevalence of 0.029%.) The Tourette syndrome spectrum may include chronic motor tics and, in at least some pedigrees, transient tic disorder (Kurlan et al. 1988). Other studies have suggested that patients not infrequently have relatives with marked obsessive-compulsive behavior. Conversely, there is a significantly increased rate of tics in patients with OCD and their relatives (Pitman et al. 1987).

In a systematically conducted twin study utilizing strict diagnostic criteria, the monozygotic concordance for Tourette syndrome was 53% and the dizygotic concordance 8%, suggesting a role for genetic factors in the disorder (Price et al. 1985). A large Mennonite kindred has been described in which 54 of 159 members had Tourette syndrome or chronic motor tics, and in which these phenotypes demonstrated an autosomal dominant mode of transmission. Pauls et al. (1990) have conducted a formal segregation analysis of Tourette syndrome in a large multigenerational kindred. The analysis was consistent with an autosomal dominant mode of inheritance with nearly complete penetrance under three definitions of illness (Tourette syndrome alone, Tourette syndrome or chronic tics, and Tourette syndrome or chronic tics or OCD).

■ PSYCHOPHARMACOGENETICS

Psychopharmacogenetics refers to the study of genetic differences in the behavioral response to pharmacological agents. Behavioral differences may result from both pharmacokinetic variability (i.e., genetic differences in the absorption and degradation of drugs) and pharmacodynamic variability (i.e., genetic differences in tissue sensitivity to drugs).

Pharmacokinetic studies have focused on antidepressants (both tricyclics and monoamine oxidase inhibitors [MAOIs]), neuroleptics, ethanol, and amphetamine. Plasma levels of one of the tricyclics, nortriptyline, appear to be under genetic control: MZ twins exhibit more comparable concentrations than DZ twins following identical oral doses (Alexanderson et al. 1969). The responsible genetic factor appears to be under polygenic control. Plasma levels of the MAOI phenelzine are also under genetic control: a polymorphism in the hepatic enzyme N-acetyltransferase that is responsible for degradation of the drug has been identified and appears to be inherited in a Mendelian fashion. Individuals with the less active isoenzyme ("slow acetylators") appear to be more prone to side effects from phenelzine (Price-Evans et al. 1965) and, in at least one study, have shown greater therapeutic response to moderate doses of the drug. There is also evidence to suggest that the tendency to respond to a specific class of antidepressants (tricyclic vs. MAOI) is familial (Pare et al. 1962). While this might reflect the aforementioned pharmacokinetic differences in the rates of metabolism of these drugs, it is equally plausible that there are genetically distinct biological types of depression associated with different drug responses.

Genetic factors also appear to be important in the likelihood of developing an agranulocytotic reaction to the atypical neuroleptic clozapine. Lieberman et al. (1990) found increased frequencies of the HLA antigens B38, DR4, and DQw3 in Ashkenazi Jews who developed agranulocytosis.

Ethanol detoxification occurs via the oxidative enzyme alcohol dehydrogenase (ADH). This process may be under genetic control. Following a test dose of ethanol, relatives of alcoholic subjects show higher levels of the metabolic product of ADH, acetaldehyde, than do relatives of nonalcoholic subjects matched for drinking history (Schuckit and Rayses 1979). Moreover, there are significant ethnic differences in ADH activity between individuals of European or Asian ancestry, which may contribute to observed differences in their tolerance to ethanol. It has been reported that electroencephalographic changes following oral administration of ethanol are more similar in MZ than in DZ twins; blood ethanol levels, on the other hand, are not more similar in MZ than in DZ twins (Propping 1977).

Finally, Nurnberger et al. (1981) have indicated that psychiatrically normal MZ twin pairs show heritable differences in central nervous system noradrenergic function, as evidenced by differences in excitation, early morning motor activity, attention, and growth hormone and prolactin release following intravenous administration of amphetamine. These differences were not correlated with plasma amphetamine levels.

Their study suggests that pharmacological probes, such as amphetamine, might be used to investigate genetically caused differences in neurophysiology that may be related to psychopathology.

■ GENETIC COUNSELING

With the increasing awareness among patients, families, psychiatrists, and the general public of the genetic aspects of psychiatric illness, interest in genetic counseling has developed. However, the aims of those seeking genetic counseling for psychiatric disorder are manifold, and these, as well as the data and techniques involved, must be understood by physicians before attempting such an endeavor or referring patients for it.

It is often not the patient who seeks genetic counseling; or, if such is the case, it may be at the insistence of others. Family members and prospective spouses frequently ask for genetic information 1) to learn about the risk for themselves or their offspring, 2) to obtain advice on decisions of marriage or pregnancy, 3) to gain an understanding of a devastating illness in a family member, or 4) to reduce their sense of guilt or to ascribe guilt to others. Patients themselves, when they do seek this type of help, usually do so in the context of an ongoing therapeutic relationship. They may be seeking to understand the cause of their illness, to discover the implications it has for their descendants (present and future), or to determine whether it is curable. The components, or stages, of counseling, as described by Tsuang (1978), are as follows:

- Diagnosis
- Family history
- Estimation of the risk of recurrence
- Evaluation of the aims, intelligence, and emotions of the counselee
- Helping the counselee understand the risk of recurrence in the context of the burden of the disorder
- Formation of a plan of action
- Follow-up

Accurate diagnosis is essential, and careful review of the patient's history as well as diagnostic interviews with relatives may reveal diagnostic issues that have genetic implications. With the diagnosis established, there are various methods of estimating the risk of recurrence. Risk rates for siblings, offspring, and other classes of relatives are available. These, however, are averages that are known not to apply under certain circumstances. For example, the risk for schizophrenia is increased in families by severity of the proband's illness, the presence of schizophrenic relatives besides the proband, and psychiatric illness in the proband's mate (Gottesman and Shields 1982). More sophisticated analyses can take into account information such as the number of ill relatives, subclinical or "spectrum" illnesses, and the age of risk for onset of illness, but such computerized programs need to assume an underlying mode of transmission. The mode of transmission is not known for most psychiatric disorders, and such assumptions can affect risk estimates greatly (up to 10-fold). Thus, establishing accurate risk estimates in family members for most psychiatric disorders is not currently possible, and counseling must proceed in the face of considerable uncertainty.

The genetic counselor, especially one who is psychiatrically trained, has an opportunity to provide much important aid beyond estimating the risks of recurrence. This includes evaluating and helping the counselee, especially by reducing the amount of misinformation, confusion, guilt, and fear regarding the illness. The counselor may also be able to offer a plan with the potential for reducing or preventing the transmission of the illness, but should recognize that counseling, though often successful in its educational goals, is unlikely to affect reproductive decisions (Kessler 1989). In doing this work, the counselor must combine the skills of geneticist, internist, psychiatrist, psychotherapist, marital counselor, and family therapist. Within psychiatry and in other fields, especially pediatrics, expertise and training programs have developed in this area, and such specialized training is a prerequisite for success in this task.

■ REFERENCES

Alexanderson B, Price-Evans DA, Sjoqvist F: Steady-state plasma levels of nortriptyline in twins: influence of genetic factors and drug therapy. BMJ 4:764, 1969

American Psychiatric Association: Diagnostic and Statistical Manual of Mental Disorders, 3rd Edition, Revised. Washington, DC, American Psychiatric Association, 1987

American Psychiatric Association: Diagnostic and Statistical Manual of Mental Disorders, 4th Edition. Washington, DC, American Psychiatric Association, 1994

Andreasen NC, Rice J, Endicott J, et al: Familial rates of affective disorder: a report from the National Institute of Mental Health Collaborative Study. Arch Gen Psychiatry 44:461–469, 1987

Baraitser M: The Genetics of Neurological Disorders, 2nd Edition. New York, Oxford Medical, 1990

Bassett AS, Jones B, McGillivray BC, et al: Partial trisomy chromosome 5 cosegregating with schizophrenia. Lancet 1:799–801, 1988

Bertelsen A, Harvald B, Hauge M: A Danish twin study of manic-depressive disorders. Br J Psychiatry 130:330–351, 1977

Black DW, Noyes R Jr, Goldstein RB, et al: A family study of obsessive-compulsive disorder. Arch Gen Psychiatry 49:362–368, 1992

Bohman M, Cloninger CR, Sigvardsson S, et al: Predisposition to petty criminality in Swedish adoptees, I: genetic and environmental heterogeneity. Arch Gen Psychiatry 39:1233–1241, 1982

Breitner JCS, Murphey EA, Folstein MF: Familial aggregation of Alzheimer dementia, II: clinical genetic implications of age dependent onset. J Psychiatr Res 20:45–55, 1986

Cadoret RJ: Evidence for genetic inheritance of primary affective disorder in adoptees. Am J Psychiatry 135:463–466, 1978

Cadoret RJ, Cain CA, Grove WM: Development of alcoholism in adoptees raised apart from alcoholic biologic relatives. Arch Gen Psychiatry 37:561–563, 1980

Cadoret RJ, O'Gorman TW, Troughton E, et al: Alcoholism and antisocial personality: interrelationships, genetic and environmental factors. Arch Gen Psychiatry 42:161–167, 1985

Cadoret RJ, Throughton E, Bagford J, et al: Genetic and environmental factors in adoptee antisocial personality. Eur Arch Psychiatry Clin Neurosci 239:231–240, 1990

Cannon TD, Mednick SA, Parnas J: Antecedents of predominantly negative- and predominantly positive-symptom schizophrenia in a high-risk population. Arch Gen Psychiatry 47:622–632, 1990

Carey G, Gottesman II: Twin and family studies of anxiety, phobic, and obsessive disorders, in Anxiety: New Research and Changing Concepts. Edited by Klein DF, Rabkin J. New York, Raven, 1981, pp 117–136

Clementz BA, Grove WM, Iacono WG, et al: Smooth-pursuit eye movement dysfunction and liability for schizophrenia: implications for genetic modeling. J Abnorm Psychol 101:117–129, 1992

Cloninger CR: A unified biosocial theory of personality and its role in the development of anxiety states. Psychiatric Developments 4:167–226, 1986

Cloninger CR: A systematic method for clinical description and classification of personality variants: a proposal. Arch Gen Psychiatry 44:573–588, 1987

Cloninger CR, Gottesman II: Genetic and environmental factors in antisocial behavior disorders, in The Causes of Crime: New Biological Approaches. Edited by Mednick SA, Moffitt TE, Stack SA. New York, Cambridge University Press, 1987, pp 92–109

Cloninger CR, Reich T, Guze SB: The multifactorial model of disease transmission, III: familial relationship between sociopathy and hysteria (Briquet's syndrome). Br J Psychiatry 127:23–32, 1975

Cloninger CR, Bohman M. Sigvardsson S: Inheritance of alcohol abuse: cross-fostering analysis of adopted men. Arch Gen Psychiatry 38:861–868, 1981

Cloninger CR, Sigvardsson S, von Knorring A-L, et al: An adoption study of somatoform disorders, II: identification of two discrete somatoform disorders. Arch Gen Psychiatry 41:863–871, 1984

Cloninger CR, Martin RL, Guze SB, et al: A prospective follow-up and family study of somatization in men and women. Am J Psychiatry 143:873–878, 1986

Cook RH, Schneck SA, Clark DB: Twins with Alzheimer's disease. Arch Neurol 38:300–301, 1981

Coon H, Byerley W, Holik J, et al: Linkage analysis of schizophrenia with five dopamine receptor genes in nine pedigrees. Am J Hum Genet 52:327–334, 1993

Corder EH, Saunders AM, Strittmatter WJ, et al: Gene dose of apolipoprotein E type 4 allele and the risk of Alzheimer's disease in late onset families. Science 261:921–923, 1993

Cox NJ, Suarez BK: Linkage analysis for psychiatric disorders, II: methodological considerations. Psychiatric Developments 3:369–382, 1985

Crocq M-A, Mant R, Asherson P, et al: Association between schizophrenia and homozygosity at the dopamine D3 receptor gene. J Med Genet 29:858–860, 1992

Crowe RR, Noyes R [Jr], Pauls DL, et al: A family study of panic disorder. Arch Gen Psychiatry 40:1065–1069, 1983

Crowe RR, Noyes R Jr, Samuelson S, et al: Close linkage between panic disorder and α-haptoglobin excluded in 10 families. Arch Gen Psychiatry 47:377–380, 1990

Crowe RR, Black DW, Wesner R, et al: Lack of linkage to chromosome 5q11-q13 markers in six schizophrenia pedigrees. Arch Gen Psychiatry 48:357–361, 1991

Davidson J, Smith R, Kudler H: Familial psychiatric illness in chronic posttraumatic stress disorder. Compr Psychiatry 30:339–345, 1989

Dykes KL, Mednick SA, Machon RA, et al: Adult third ventricle width and infant behavioral arousal in groups at high and low risk for schizophrenia. Schizophr Res 7:13–18, 1992

Egeland JA, Gerhard DS, Pauls DL, et al: Bipolar affective disorders linked to DNA markers on chromosome 11. Nature 325:783–787, 1987

Embry C, Bruyland S: Presumed Alzheimer's disease beginning at different ages in two twins. J Am Geriatr Soc 33:61–62, 1985

Eysenck HJ: A Model for Personality. New York, Springer, 1981

Feder J, Gurling HMD, Darby J, et al: DNA restriction fragment analysis of the proopiomelanocortin gene in schizophrenia. Am J Hum Genet 37:286–294, 1985

Fischer M: Psychoses in the offspring of schizophrenic monozygotic twins and their normal co-twins. Br J Psychiatry 118:43–52, 1971

Fish B, Marcus J, Hans SL, et al: Infants at risk for schizophrenia: sequelae of a genetic neurointegrative defect. A review and replication analysis of pandysmaturation in the Jerusalem Infant Development Study. Arch Gen Psychiatry 49:221–235, 1992

Fyer AJ, Mannuzza S, Gallops MS, et al: Familial transmission of simple phobias and fears: a prelimary report. Arch Gen Psychiatry 47:252–256, 1990

Fyer AJ, Mannuzza S, Chapman TF, et al: A direct interview family study of social phobia. Arch Gen Psychiatry 50:286–293, 1993

Gershon ES, Schreiber JL, Hamovit JR, et al: Clinical findings in patients with anorexia nervosa and affective illness in their relatives. Am J Psychiatry 141:1419–1422, 1984

Gershon ES, Hamovit JH, Guroff JJ, et al: Birth-cohort changes in manic and depressive disorders in relatives of bipolar and schizoaffective patients. Arch Gen Psychiatry 44:314–319, 1987

Giles DE, Biggs MM, Rush AJ, et al: Risk factors in families of unipolar depression, I: psychiatric illness and reduced REM latency. J Affect Disord 14:51–59, 1988

Goate AM, Chartier-Harlin MC, Mullan M, et al: Segregation of a missense mutation in the amyloid precursor protein gene with familial Alzheimer's disease. Nature 349:704–706, 1991

Goldberg J, True WR, Eisen SA, et al: A twin study of the effects of the Vietnam War on posttraumatic stress disorder. JAMA 263:1227–1232, 1990

Goodwin DW: Alcoholism and heredity: a review and hypothesis. Arch Gen Psychiatry 36:57–61, 1979

Goodwin DW: Studies of familial alcoholism: a review. J Clin Psychiatry 45:14–17, 1984

Gottesman II, Bertelsen A: Confirming unexpressed genotypes for schizophrenia: risks in the offspring of Fischer's Danish identical and fraternal discordant twins. Arch Gen Psychiatry 46:867–872, 1989

Gottesman II, Shields J, Schizophrenia: The Epigenetic Puzzle. Cambridge, UK, Cambridge University Press, 1982

Gruppo Italiano Disturbi d'Ansia: Familial analysis of panic disorder and agoraphobia. J Affect Disord 17:1–8, 1989

Gurling HM, Oppenheim BE, Murray RM: Depression, criminality and psychopathology associated with alcoholism: evidence from a twin study. Acta Genet Med Gemellol (Roma) 33:333–339, 1984

Guze SB: The role of follow-up studies: their contribution to diagnostic classification as applied to hysteria. Seminars in Psychiatry 2:392–402, 1970

Hallmayer J, Kennedy JL, Wetterberg L, et al: Exclusion of linkage between the serotonin$_2$ receptor and schizophrenia in a large Swedish kindred. Arch Gen Psychiatry 49:216–219, 1992

Harrison PJ, McLaughlin D, Kerwin RW: Decreased hippocampal expression of a glutamate receptor gene in schizophrenia. Lancet 337:450–452, 1991

Heston LL: Psychiatric disorders in foster home reared children of schizophrenic mothers. Br J Psychiatry 112:819–825, 1966

Holland AJ, Sicott N, Treasure J: Anorexia nervosa: evidence for a genetic basis. J Psychosom Res 32:561–571, 1988

Hopper JL, Judd FK, Derrick PL, et al: A family study of panic disorder. Genet Epidemiol 4:33–41, 1987

Kaprio J, Koskenvuo M, Langinvainio H: Finnish twins reared apart, IV: smoking and drinking habits. A preliminary analysis of the effect of heredity and environment. Acta Genet Med Gemellol 33:425–433, 1984

Kassett JA, Gershon ES, Maxwell ME, et al: Psychiatric disorders in the first-degree relatives of probands with bulimia nervosa. Am J Psychiatry 146:1468–1471, 1989

Kendler KS: Genetics of schizophrenia, in American Psychiatric Association Annual Review, Vol 5. Edited by Frances AJ, Hales RE. Washington, DC, American Psychiatric Press, 1986, pp 25–41

Kendler KS, Gruenberg AM: An independent analysis of the Danish adoption study of schizophrenia, VI: the relationship between psychiatric disorders as defined by DSM-III in the relatives and adoptees. Arch Gen Psychiatry 41:555–564, 1984

Kendler KS, Gruenberg AM, Tsuang MT: Psychiatric illness in first-degree relatives of schizophrenic and surgical control patients: a family study using DSM-III criteria. Arch Gen Psychiatry 42:770–779, 1985

Kendler KS, MacLean C, Neale M, et al: The genetic epidemiology of bulimia nervosa. Am J Psychiatry 148:1627–1637, 1991

Kendler KS, Heath AC, Neale MC, et al: A population-based twin study of alcoholism in women. JAMA 268:1877–1882, 1992a

Kendler KS, Neale MC, Kessler RC, et al: Generalized anxiety disorder in women: a population-based twin study. Arch Gen Psychiatry 49:267–272, 1992b

Kendler KS, Neale MC, Kessler RC, et al: The genetic epidemiology of phobias in women: the interrelationship of agoraphobia, social phobia, situational phobia, and simple phobia. Arch Gen Psychiatry 49:273–281, 1992c

Kendler KS, Neale MC, Kessler RC, et al: A population-based twin study of major depression in women: the impact of varying definitions of illness. Arch Gen Psychiatry 49:257–266, 1992d

Kennedy JL, Giuffra LA, Moises HW, et al: Evidence against linkage of schizophrenia to markers on chromosome 5 in a Northern Swedish pedigree. Nature 336:167–170, 1988

Kessler S: Psychological aspects of genetic counseling, VI: a critical review of the literature dealing with education and reproduction. Am J Med Genet 34:340–353, 1989

Kety SS: Schizophrenic illness in the families of schizophrenic adoptees: findings from the Danish national sample. Schizophr Bull 14:217–222, 1988

Kidd KK: Genetic models for psychiatric disorders, in Genetic Research Strategies for Psychobiology and Psychiatry. Edited by Gershon ES, Matthysse S, Breakefield XO, et al. Pacific Grove, CA, Boxwood Press, 1981, pp 369–382

Klerman GL, Lavori PW, Rice J, et al: Birth cohort trends in rates of major depressive disorder among relatives of patients with affective disorder. Arch Gen Psychiatry 42:689–693, 1985

Kringlen E, Cramer G: Offspring of monozygotic twins discordant for schizophrenia. Arch Gen Psychiatry 46:873–877, 1989

Kupfer DJ, Frank E, Carpenter LL, et al: Family history in recurrent depression. J Affect Disord 17:113–119, 1989

Kurlan R, Behr J, Medved L, et al: Transient tic disorder and the spectrum of Tourette's syndrome. Arch Neurol 45:1200–1201, 1988

Leckman JF, Chittenden EH: Gilles de La Tourette's syndrome and some forms of obsessive-compulsive disorder may share a common genetic diathesis. Encephale 16:321–323, 1990

Leckman JF, Weissman MM, Merikangas KR, et al: Panic disorder and major depression: increased risk of depression, alcoholism, panic, and phobic disorders in families of depressed probands with panic disorder. Arch Gen Psychiatry 40:1055–1060, 1983

Li G, Silverman JM, Smith CJ et al: Age at onset and familial risk in Alzheimer's disease. Am J Psychiatry 152:424–430, 1995

Lieberman JA, Yunis J, Egea E, et al: HLA-B38, DR4, DQw3 and clozapine-induced agranulocytosis in Jewish patients with schizophrenia. Arch Gen Psychiatry 47:945–948, 1990

Lilienfeld SO, VanValkenburg C, Larntz K, et al: The relationship of histrionic personality disorder to antisocial personality and somatization disorders. Am J Psychiatry 143:718–722, 1986

Macciardi F, Kennedy JL, Ruocco L, et al: A genetic linkage study of schizophrenia t chromosome 5 markers in a northern Italian population. Biol Psychiatry 31:720–728, 1992

Maier W, Lichtermann D, Minges J, et al: Personality traits in subjects at risk for unipolar major depression: a family study perspective. J Affect Disord 24:153–163, 1992

Mather JA: Eye movements of teenage children of schizophrenics: a possible inherited marker of susceptibility to the disease. J Psychiatr Res 19:523–532, 1985

Matthysse SW, Kidd KK: Estimating the genetic contribution to schizophrenia. Am J Psychiatry 133:185–191, 1976

McGuffin P, Katz R, Rutherford J: Nature, nurture and depression: a twin study. Psychol Med 21:329–335, 1991

McKusick V: Mendelian Inheritance in Man, 10th Edition. Baltimore, MD, Johns Hopkins University Press, 1992

Mendlewicz J, Rainer JD: Adoption study supporting genetic transmission in manic depressive illness. Nature 268:327–329, 1977

Mendlewicz J, Sevy S, deMaertelaer V: REM sleep latency and morbidity risk of affective disorders in depressive illness. Neuropsychobiology 22:14–17, 1989

Merikangas KR: Genetics of alcoholism: a review of human studies, in Genetics of Neuropsychiatric Diseases. Edited by Wetterberg I. London, Macmillan, 1989, pp 269–280

Mohs RC, Breitner JCS, Silverman JM, et al: Alzheimer's disease: morbid risk among first-degree relatives approximates 50% by 90 years of age. Arch Gen Psychiatry 44:405–408, 1987

Moises HW, Gelernter J, Giuffra LA, et al: No linkage between D_2 dopamine receptor gene region and schizophrenia. Arch Gen Psychiatry 48:643–647, 1991

Moldin SO, Rice JP, Gottesman II, et al: Psychometric deviance in offspring at risk for schizophrenia, II: resolving heterogeneity through admixture analysis. Psychiatry Res 32:311–322, 1990a

Moldin SO, Rice JP, Gottesman II, et al: Transmission of a psychometric indicator for liability to schizophrenia in normal families. Genet Epidemiol 7:163–176, 1990b

Nee LE, Eldridge R, Sunderland T, et al: Dementia of the Alzheimer type: clinical and family study of 22 twin pairs. Neurology 37:359–363, 1987

Noyes R Jr, Crowe RR, Harris EL, et al: Relationship between panic disorder and agoraphobia: a family study. Arch Gen Psychiatry 43:227–232, 1986

Noyes R Jr, Clarkson C, Crowe RR, et al: A family study of generalized anxiety disorder. Am J Psychiatry 144:1019–1024, 1987

Nurnberger JI Jr, Gershon ES: Genetics, in Handbook of Affective Disorders. Edited by Paykel ES. New York, Guilford, 1982, pp 126–145

Nurnberger JI Jr, Gershon ES, Jimerson DC, et al: Pharmacogenetics of D-amphetamine response in man, in Research Strategies for Psychobiology and Psychiatry. Edited by Gershon ES, Matthysse S, Breakefield XO, et al. Pacific Grove, CA, Boxwood Press, 1981, pp 257–268

O'Rourke DH, Gottesman II, Suarez BK, et al: Refutation of the general single locus model for the etiology of schizophrenia. Am J Hum Genet 34:630–649, 1982

Pare CMB, Ress L, Sainsbury MJ: Differentiation of two genetically specific types of depression by the response to antidepressants. Lancet 2:1240–1343, 1962

Parnas J, Schulsinger F, Schulsinger H, et al: Behavioral precursors of schizophrenia spectrum: a prospective study. Arch Gen Psychiatry 39:658–664, 1982

Pauls DL, Pakstis AJ, Kurlan R, et al: Segregation and linkage analyses of Tourette's syndrome and related disorders. J Am Acad Child Adolesc Psychiatry 29:195–203, 1990

Perrett CW, Whatley SA, Ferrier I, et al: Changes in brain gene expression in schizophrenic and depressed patients. Schizophr Res 6:193–200, 1992

Pickens RW, Svikis DS, McGue M, et al: Heterogeneity in the inheritance of alcoholism: a study of male and female twins. Arch Gen Psychiatry 48:19–28, 1991

Pitman RK, Green RC, Jenike MA, et al: Clinical comparison of Tourette's disorder and obsessive-compulsive disorder. Am J Psychiatry 144:1166–1171, 1987

Pitts FN, Winokur G: Affective disorder, VII: alcoholism and affective disorder. J Psychiatr Res 4:37–50, 1966

Plomin R, DeFries JC, McClearn GE: Behavioral Genetics: A Primer, 2nd Edition. San Francisco, CA, WH Freeman, 1990

Price RA, Kidd KK, Cohen DJ, et al: A twin study of Tourette syndrome. Arch Gen Psychiatry 42:815–820, 1985

Price-Evans DA, Davison K, Pratt RTC: The influences of acetylator phenotype on the effects of treating depression with phenelzine. Clin Pharmacol Ther 6:430–433, 1965

Propping P: Genetic control of ethanol action on the central nervous system: an EEG study of twins. Hum Genet 35:309–334, 1977

Regier DA, Narrow WE, Rae DS, et al: The de facto US mental and addictive disorders service system: Epidememiologic Catchment Area prospective 1-year prevalence rates of disorders and services. Arch Gen Psychiatry 50:85–94, 1993

Reich JH: Familiality of DSM-III dramatic and anxious personality clusters. J Nerv Ment Dis 177:96–100, 1989

Reich J[H]: Using the family history method to distinguish relatives of patients with dependent personality disorder from relatives of controls. Psychiatry Res 39:227–237, 1991

Reich T, Cloninger CR, Van Eerdewegh P, et al: Secular trends in the familial transmission of alcoholism. Alcoholism 12:458–464, 1988

Reveley MA, Reveley AM, Baldy R: Left cerebral hemisphere hypodensity in discordant schizophrenic twins: a controlled study. Arch Gen Psychiatry 44: 625–632, 1987

Risch N: Linkage strategies for genetically complex traits, I: multilocus models. Am J Hum Genet 46:222–228, 1990

Risch N, Baron M: Segregation analysis of schizophrenia and related disorders. Am J Hum Genet 36:1039–1059, 1984

Robins LN, Helzer JE, Weissman MM, et al: Lifetime prevalence of specific psychiatric disorders in three sites. Arch Gen Psychiatry 41:949–958, 1984

Rosenthal D, Wender PH, Kety SS, et al: Schizophrenics' offspring reared in adoptive homes. J Psychiatr Res 6:377–391, 1968

Sarkar G, Kapelner S, Grandy DK, et al: Direct sequencing of the dopamine D_2 receptor (DRD2) in schizophrenia reveals three polymorphisms but no structural change in the receptor. Genomics 11:8–14, 1991

Schellenberg GD, Bird TD, Wijsman EM, et al: Genetic linkage evidence for a familial Alzheimer's disease locus on chromosome 14. Science 258:668–671, 1992

Schuckit MA, Gold EO: A simultaneous evaluation of multiple markers of ethanol/placebo challenges in sons of alcoholics and controls. Arch Gen Psychiatry 45:211–216, 1988

Schuckit MA, Rayses V: Ethanol ingestion differences in blood acetaldehyde concentrations in relatives of alcoholics and controls. Science 203:54–55, 1979

Sherrington R, Brynjolfsson J, Petursson H, et al: Localization of a susceptibility locus for schizophrenia on chromosome 5. Nature 336:164–167, 1988

Siever LJ, Silverman JM, Horvath TB, et al: Increased morbid risk for schizophrenia-related disorders in relatives of schizotypal personality disordered patients. Arch Gen Psychiatry 47:634–640, 1990

Spitzer RL, Endicott J, Robins E: Research Diagnostic Criteria: rationale and reliability. Arch Gen Psychiatry 35:773–782, 1978

Squires-Wheeler E, Skodol AE, Bassett A, et al: DSM-III-R schizotypal personality traits in offspring of schizophrenic disorder, affective disorder, and normal control parents. J Psychiatr Res 23:229–239, 1989

St George-Hyslop PH, Myers R, Haines JL, et al: Familial Alzheimer's disease: progress and problems. Neurobiology of Aging 10:417–425, 1989

Strober M, Morell W, Burroughs J, et al: A controlled family study of anorexia nervosa. J Psychiatr Res 19:239–246, 1985

Suddath RL, Christison GW, Torrey EF, et al: Anatomical abnormalities in the brains of monozygotic twins discordant for schizophrenia. N Engl J Med 322:789–794, 1990

Tienari P: Interaction between genetic vulnerability and family environment: the Finnish adoptive family study of schizophrenia. Acta Psychiatr Scand 84:460–465, 1991

Tienari P, Lahti I, Sorri A, et al: The Finnish adoptive family study of schizophrenia. J Psychiatr Res 21:437–445, 1987

Torgersen S: Genetic factors in anxiety disorders. Arch Gen Psychiatry 40:1085–1089, 1983

Torgersen S: Genetics of somatoform disorders. Arch Gen Psychiatry 43:502–505, 1986

True WR, Rice J, Eisen SA, et al: A twin study of genetic and environmental contributions to liability for posttraumatic stress symptoms. Arch Gen Psychiatry 50:257–264, 1993

Tsuang MT: Genetic counseling for psychiatric patients and their families. Am J Psychiatry 135:1465–1475, 1978

Tsuang MT, Gilbertson MW, Faraone SV: Genetic transmission of negative and positive symptoms in the biological relatives of schizophrenics, in Positive vs. Negative Schizophrenia. Edited by Marneros A, Tsuang MT, Andreasen N. New York, Springer-Verlag, 1991, pp 265–291

Vogler GP, Gottesman II, McGue MK, et al: Mixed-model segregation analysis of schizophrenia in the Lindelius Swedish pedigrees. Behav Genet 20:461–472, 1990

von Knorring A-L, Cloninger CR, Bohman M, et al: An adoption study of depressive disorders and substance abuse. Arch Gen Psychiatry 40:943–950, 1983

Walker E, Downey G, Caspi A: Twin studies of psychopathology: why do the concordance rates vary? Schizophr Res 5:211–221, 1991

Watt NF, Anthony EJ, Wynne LC, et al (eds): Children at Risk for Schizophrenia: A Longitudinal Perspective. Cambridge, UK, Cambridge University Press, 1984

Weinberger DR, Berman KF, Suddath R, et al: Evidence of dysfunction of a prefrontal-limbic network in schizophrenia: a magnetic resonance imaging and regional cerebral blood flow study of discordant monozygotic twins. Am J Psychiatry 149:890–897, 1992

Weissman MM, Gershon ES, Kidd KK, et al: Psychiatric disorders in the relatives of probands with affective disorders: the Yale University–National Institute of Mental Health Collaborative Study. Arch Gen Psychiatry 41:13–21, 1984

Weissman MM, Warner V, Wickramaratne P, et al: Early-onset major depression in parents and their children. J Affect Disord 15:269–277, 1988

Weissman MM, Members of the Cross-National Collaborative Group: The changing rate of major depression: cross-national comparisons. JAMA 268:3098–3105, 1992

Wender PH, Rosenthal D, Kety SS, et al: Crossfostering: a research strategy for clarifying the role of genetic and experiential factors in the etiology of schizophrenia. Arch Gen Psychiatry 30:121–128, 1974

Wender PH, Kety SS, Rosenthal D, et al: Psychiatric disorders in the biological and adoptive families of adopted individuals with affective disorders. Arch Gen Psychiatry 43:923–929, 1986

Winokur A, March V, Mendels J: Primary affective disorder in relatives of patients with anorexia nervosa. Am J Psychiatry 137:695–698, 1980

Zausmer DM, Dewey ME: Tics and heredity: a study of the relatives of child tiqueurs. Br J Psychiatry 150:628–634, 1987

CHAPTER 3

Epidemiology of Mental Disorders

Jack D. Burke, Jr., M.D., M.P.H.
Darrel A. Regier, M.D., M.P.H.

Psychiatric epidemiology is the quantitative study of the distribution of mental disorders in human populations. *Clinical epidemiology* is unusual among clinical disciplines in focusing on populations rather than on individuals, a characteristic that has led it to be called the basic science of *public health.* By using the concept of a population as a starting point for investigations, clinical researchers can reduce, or at least identify, sources of selection bias. By providing *quantitative* methods to study populations, epidemiology fosters precision in estimating the importance of risk factors, the performance of diagnostic tests, and the effectiveness of new treatments. These applications of epidemiological methods extend far beyond the traditional concern about the importance of measuring community rates of illness and assessing the extent of unmet need in the population.

Once the *distribution* of mental disorders in the population has been determined quantitatively, epidemiologists can identify high-risk groups in whom the study of risk factors may lead to important clues about the etiology of a disorder. Epidemiological techniques are powerful in dealing with multifactorial risks for clinical disorders; a new field of *genetic epidemiology* has grown in the past decade to combine molecular genetics and epidemiological studies of human populations. By taking *specific mental disorders* as the focus of study, psychiatric epidemiology deals with clinical entities that have immediate relevance to clinical research and practice whether the population is in the community or in clinical settings. Epidemiological studies are helpful in a clinical discipline that is concerned with improving its nosology, because it is a natural aim of epidemiological methods to examine the full spectrum of clinical illness, including subclinical variants, and to consider such problems as the threshold of severity to set for a disorder (i.e., number of symptoms for a diagnosis). Longitudinal epidemiological studies are useful in examining the course of illness, and epidemiology has developed experimental methods to test the effect of clinical or preventive interventions on the outcome of illness.

■ USES OF PSYCHIATRIC EPIDEMIOLOGY

Seven uses of epidemiology have been described by Morris (1964) (Table 3–1). These types of studies can be broadly grouped according to the level of investigation of particular study designs. *Descriptive* studies provide estimates of the rate of disorder in a population; *analytic* studies explore variations in rates among different groups to identify risk factors; and *experimental* studies assess the effect of preventive or therapeutic interventions designed to alter the development or outcome of illnesses.

At the broad descriptive level, epidemiological data on the rates of illness in a community can be combined with information about use of health services to determine the extent of untreated illness in the community population, to identify possible barriers to obtaining proper care, and to help in planning the most efficient allocation of public and private resources. At the analytic level, epidemiological methods have been used both to assess the performance of diagnostic tests and to identify patients who are at greatest risk of side effects (e.g., development of tardive dyskinesia after neuroleptic medication). At the experimental level, controlled trials of therapeutic agents, including both medication and psy-

---

Table 3–1.   Uses of epidemiology

Descriptive studies
  Community diagnosis
  Completion of the clinical picture
  Identification of syndromes
Analytic studies
  Assessment of individual risks
  Historical study
Experimental studies
  Identification of causes
  Assessment of the working of health services

---

chotherapy, are used to determine whether a particular treatment regimen has any significant beneficial effects.

☐ Descriptive Level

For a broad range of purposes, from major policy decisions on providing community-based services for mentally ill individuals to more personal decisions such as locating a new private practice or hospital, some of the most important questions about the nature of illness in the community population can be difficult to answer. For example, how many people in the community have a clinically significant mental disorder? Which disorders are most common? To what extent are the treatment needs of these individuals being met?

Some aspects of mental disorders are difficult to study if the subjects can only be drawn from treatment settings. For example, careful study of the early development of mental disorders can usually best be accomplished before the individual has sought clinical care. For some disorders such as agoraphobia, which might reduce the likelihood that a person will be seen in treatment, epidemiological studies of the community appear to be especially important. Other questions of increasing importance, such as the co-occurrence of multiple disorders and the ascertainment of familial risks, can best be accomplished through an epidemiological framework. Ideally, epidemiological studies that use clinically based procedures for assessing potential cases can also contribute to clinical knowledge through identification of new, previously unrecognized conditions of clinical interest.

☐ Analytic Level

Knowing the rates of illness for the population at large provides the epidemiologist with a powerful springboard to identification of groups in that population who have especially high risks of developing the illness. Once these high-risk groups have been determined, it is possible to design more highly targeted studies to characterize the particular characteristics that place members of the group at higher risk. For this purpose, it is possible to investigate biological, genetic, environmental, infectious, or other factors that help explain the increased rate of illness in the more highly affected groups. Statistical techniques developed by epidemiologists provide estimates of the magnitude of elevated risk, and help establish the relative importance of individual risk factors when more than one factor has been identified.

In searching for possible risk factors and trying to establish their relative importance, investigators in psychiatric epidemiology have been especially interested in historical trends. For example, there has been some suggestive evidence that depressive illness may be occurring more commonly in younger generations, or perhaps having an onset at an earlier age, through the second half of this century (Klerman and Weissman 1989). Similarly, efforts to understand the apparent increase in adolescent drug abuse and adolescent suicide have used historical trends to try to elucidate specific risk factors.

☐ Experimental Level

Once possible risk factors have been identified and a likely causal chain has been proposed, it is possible to design interventions and test how effective they are in reducing the clinical problem of interest. For example, community-based interventions to reduce cigarette smoking may lead to a reduction in subsequent development of lung cancer. In psychiatry, two disorders that have been identified as particularly suitable for possible preventive interventions are depression and drug abuse.

■ EPIDEMIOLOGICAL METHODS

This overview of statistical and analytic methods parallels the discussion of the three broad categories of epidemiological studies.

☐ Descriptive Methods

Population Sampling

One distinguishing feature of epidemiological studies is the explicit use of a "population" from which the study subjects are drawn. Although the popular notion that epidemiologists deal with community populations is often correct, the epidemiological approach of using an explicit population can be demonstrated as easily in a clinical setting as in a community setting. For example, clinical research on schizophrenia may be conducted on patients who are most convenient for the research team to enroll in the study. Often these subjects may be those who are closest at hand, for example, long-term residents of a chronic state hospital. Or they may be those with particular relatives or other involved people who encourage the subject to participate in the study, or even those who feel most involved with the research or clinical team, for example, in gratitude for effective treatment. It is quite possible for such a study sample to be useful and to produce valid results. However, in such a sample of convenience there is always a danger of "selection bias," which arises when some particular characteristic associated with the variables of interest has led to higher or lower participation in the study.

Technical aspects of drawing the sample are relatively easy to describe. The simplest case is the *simple random sample,* which consists of using random numbers to draw subjects from a list of the entire study population, for example, to select cases for a study from a series of consecutive admissions to a hospital. A more complicated design includes drawing samples randomly from within different subgroups of the study population. For example, if men are much less commonly admitted to a particular hospital than women, it may be desirable to draw cases separately from male and female admissions. This technique, known as *stratified random sampling,* entails the use of an adjustment factor to correct for the fact that men and women will be sampled at different proportions. For example, 10% of female admissions but 50% of male admissions may be recruited into the study. The resulting sample needs to be adjusted by these different sampling fractions whenever the results are referred back to the study population of consecutive admissions to the hospital. A third type of sampling design, called *cluster sampling,* is more convenient whenever individual cases cannot be easily rostered, for example, when patients are drawn from different clinics within a large medical center. Although this sampling technique is usually more economical, it provides for less precise estimates.

Whatever technique is used to draw the sample from the study population, the very fact of drawing a sample means that the study results are only estimates for the data that would have been obtained if the entire study population had been examined. For that reason, it is common to report whether results are statistically significant, or only represent sampling variation. This report can be provided in terms of an interval showing how imprecise the sample estimate is, or whether any differences observed are within the range expected for that study design. Well-known methods based on the standard error of a particular estimated value, such as a mean or a proportion, are used to derive either *confidence intervals* or *tests of statistical significance.*

Diagnostic Assessment

At the heart of any epidemiological study, whether within a community or a clinical population, is a determination of the disease status of the subjects in the study. Four characteristics of diagnostic instruments are especially important.

1. The *safety* of any diagnostic procedure in human populations must be established, whether for psychiatric interviews or for more invasive procedures.
2. The *feasibility* of a diagnostic procedure is especially important for investigators in terms of the proposed sample size and difficulty in gaining access to subjects.

3. Demonstrating *reliability,* or consistency, in diagnostic assessment between examiners or between examinations has become a standard requirement that research assessments have been expected to meet.
4. Ideally, the diagnoses produced in any clinical or research setting would be accurate, that is, would demonstrate *validity.* However, the fact that there is no absolute standard for establishing a definitive diagnosis, and the fact that even skilled clinicians have low reliability for their routine diagnoses, make it difficult to assess validity. New assessment procedures are often tested by comparison to existing well-known procedures or to diagnostic judgments of "senior clinicians," although, it is generally recognized that neither of these comparisons provides an authoritative basis for assessing validity.

Measuring Reliability

Any diagnostic procedure should be able to produce consistent results when used to assess the same phenomena, either by different examiners or on different occasions. These measures of consistency, called *inter-rater reliability* and *test-retest reliability,* are essential characteristics of any diagnostic test (Figure 3–1).

The simplest measure of agreement is simply the percentage of times both tests agree that the subject is positive or that the subject is negative. This figure, known as *percentage agreement,* is commonly used but is no longer recommended. Because some agreements will occur by chance, the percentage agreement figure tends to overstate the reliability of a diagnostic procedure. The most widely used measure of agreement for reliability studies is *kappa,* a measure that corrects for the proportion of chance agreements to give an indication of agreement achieved beyond what would have occurred by chance alone. Guidelines for interpreting kappa suggest that values above 0.75 are excellent, values between 0.40 and 0.75 (inclusive) are good, and values below 0.40 are poor. One difficulty arises when the condition being assessed is rare; if this occurs, the kappa value is attenuated (Fleiss 1981).

Validity

Several types of validity have been described. *Face validity,* which refers to a judgment by "experts" that the items or procedure of a test "make sense," may be helpful in persuading clinicians to employ the test, but it may have no relationship to the accuracy of the test results. *Content validity* refers to a judgment by experts that the items of the test cover the appropriate domains of knowledge relevant for the test's purposes. While it is important to know if content validity does not exist, simply providing adequate coverage of relevant items does not guarantee that the test results will be accurate.

	Examiner A		
	Positive	Negative	
Examiner B			
Positive	a = 14	b = 16	$B_1 = 30$
Negative	c = 22	d = 148	$B_2 = 170$
	$A_1 = 36$	$A_2 = 164$	n = 200

P_o = proportion of agreement observed

$$= \frac{a + d}{n} = 0.81$$

P_c = proportion of agreement by chance

$$= \left[\left(\frac{A_1}{n} \right) \times \left(\frac{B_1}{n} \right) \right] + \left[\left(\frac{A_2}{n} \right) \times \left(\frac{B_2}{n} \right) \right]$$

$$= 0.724$$

$$\text{Kappa} = \frac{(P_o - P_c)}{(1 - P_c)}$$

$$= (0.81 - 0.724)/(1 - 0.724) = 0.31$$

Figure 3–1. Calculation of kappa.

In the absence of a definitive standard for establishing accuracy in an authoritative way, current practice in psychiatry is to use another, usually well-known, test with a similar purpose as a comparison instrument, for *criterion validity*. In assessing diagnostic interviews, for example, a comparison could be another psychiatric interview that has already been shown to have adequate reliability, or a panel of "expert clinicians" whose consensus judgment is considered the best composite picture of clinical knowledge for a given subject.

In studies of criterion validity, several measures of interest have been developed. *Sensitivity* is a measure of the number of true cases who are detected by the instrument being evaluated; the false negative rate is generally considered the number of true cases who are missed by the instrument. *Specificity* is the number of true noncases who are accurately assessed by the new instrument; the false positive rate commonly is considered the number of true noncases who are mistakenly called cases by the diagnostic instrument (Figure 3–2). Another measure, *positive predictive value,* is especially useful to clinicians who are assessing the potential value of a new test. This measure estimates the number of positive subjects on the new test who truly represent cases of the disorder.

	"Truth"		
	Disorder present	Disorder absent	
New instrument			
Positive	a = 70	b = 16	a + b = 86
Negative	c = 10	d = 104	c + d = 114
	a + c = 80	b + d = 120	n = 200

Sensitivity = a/(a + c) = (70/80) = 0.875

Specificity = d/(b + d) = (104/120) = 0.867

Figure 3–2. Calculation of sensitivity and specificity.

Prevalence Rates

The *prevalence rate* is the proportion of a population who have the disorder at a given time. If the population sampling has been performed adequately, the sampling design allows estimation of the denominator for this proportion, and the case assessment procedure allows estimation of the numerator, or number of cases. Most commonly, prevalence rates are reported as of a given point, such as a day on the calendar or the day of interview in a study. In this case, the measure is known as the *point prevalence rate*. Another measure, *lifetime prevalence rate*, is the proportion of a population who have ever had the illness at any point in their lives. As with any proportion from an adequate sampling design, it is possible to calculate the standard error, so prevalence rates should be accompanied by information about the confidence interval or the standard error to allow tests of significance for differences between prevalence rates.

☐ Analytic Methods

To identify risk factors, a first step is to examine subgroups in the population to determine where the rates of illness are higher than usual. Although it would be relatively easy to use point prevalence rates for this purpose, the conclusions based from that kind of analysis would likely be flawed because these rates represent all subjects who are ill at a given time, regardless of how long they have had the disorder. As a result, chronic cases tend to be overrepresented in such a cross-sectional study, and some groups may have higher rates of illness because the disorder has been present for a longer time. To overcome the uncertainty introduced by chronic cases, risk factors for developing an illness are best examined by comparing rates of new cases, *incidence rates*, in the population. Study designs involving incidence rates need to be more complex than for prevalence surveys because the development of new cases usually requires passage of time.

Prospective Longitudinal Studies

An excellent way to assess incidence rates in a population would be to form a sample of persons from the population who are younger than the typical age at onset of the disorder of interest, and to assess them for a variety of characteristics that are potential risk factors to be considered in the study. Diagnostic assessments, to exclude anyone from the sample who has already developed the illness, are undertaken also at the outset of the study. After a reasonable amount of time has passed, typically 1 year, subjects are reexamined to determine who has developed the illness. The incidence rate is calculated with the number of new cases in the numerator and the total number of persons at risk at the beginning of the time period in the denominator. For a 1-year period, this estimate would be the annual incidence rate. To assess elevated risks, the incidence rates in different groups could be compared. In this kind of study, if persons below the poverty line have twice the incidence rate of those above the poverty line, the ratio of incidence rates would be 2.0, and this ratio is taken as a measure of the *relative risk.* This figure indicates that those in the poverty group would have twice the rate of developing illness as those above the poverty line. Note that prevalence rates cannot be used to estimate relative risk for developing an illness, because prevalence includes both onset and duration; a chronic illness will have a higher prevalence than a short-lived one even if both have the same incidence rate.

Case Control Studies

Because prospective longitudinal studies are difficult and often expensive to conduct, and because they are even more difficult in the case of rare disorders, in which the incidence rate is low, an alternative study design is often used. This design is especially useful in the exploratory stage before putative risk factors have been identified well enough to justify undertaking a prospective longitudinal study. In this design, known cases are identified, for example, from hospital or medical records, and individuals who are similar in age, sex, socioeconomic status, or other relevant characteristics and are known not to have the illness are matched to these cases as a comparison group. Some assessment is then made of personal characteristics that existed before the time the cases would have developed the illness. However, if the populations from whom the cases or the subjects in the comparison group have been drawn are not specified, an alternative measure to incidence rate ratios, called the *odds ratio,* can provide a reasonable estimate of relative risk.

Bias

Besides selection bias, these cross-sectional studies are subject to additional types of bias. First, the examiner who attempts to establish the risk factor status by inquiring about the subject's past history may have clues, perhaps even from the subject's clinical condition at the time, that the subject is in the case or comparison group; as a result, the examiner may probe more or less deeply to establish the presence of a particular risk factor and thus may inadvertently help to confirm the study's hypothesis. Such a possibility is called *observer bias* and is especially problematic for studies in which retrospective assessments are needed. Another potential problem is *confounding bias,* which occurs when an unexamined characteristic is associated both with the suspected risk factor and with the disorder and is the true underlying cause of the disorder.

☐ Experimental Methods

The experimental method developed in the natural sciences has also been applied to study the onset and course of illness. The central feature of the experimental method is *random assignment* of subjects to either the experimental intervention group or the control group without the intervention. This process of assigning subjects at random is expected to prevent selection bias and also to reduce possible confounding bias, because any unknown underlying causes would be equally distributed between the control and experimental groups, at least when large enough numbers are considered. The practice of having examiners and subjects "blind" to their assignment in experimental or control groups is expected to minimize observer bias. This experimental methodology has been used in clinical trials of treatments, both pharmacological and psychotherapeutic, to determine their effectiveness for psychiatric patients. Similar methodology has also been developed for preventive interventions, to test the effectiveness of preventive programs in preventing the onset of illness in high-risk groups. One problem in designing these intervention trials is to determine how many subjects are needed to show that any differences in the two groups' outcomes are *true* differences, that is, statistically significant above the level expected from sampling variation. Because larger numbers of subjects provide more precise estimates from sampling, a key issue for clinical and epidemiological intervention trials is to estimate how many subjects are needed to be able to detect a true difference as large as the one expected by the investigator.

■ ADVANCES IN PSYCHIATRIC EPIDEMIOLOGY: DIAGNOSTIC ASSESSMENTS

Three major sources of potential error can make it difficult to achieve reliability in diagnostic assessments, both in clinical studies and in epidemiology. *Information variance* refers to the fact that different examiners, or even the same examiner on different occasions, may solicit different information from the subject and therefore use a different data base for assessing potential disorders and classifying them. *Observer variance* suggests that different examiners may interpret the same data differently, either reported symptoms such as depressed mood or clinical signs such as blunted affect. *Criterion variance* refers to the problem that different examiners, even when using the same data base, may have different criteria for assigning a subject to a particular diagnostic category.

One of the largest and best-known studies of variability of psychiatric diagnosis, conducted in the late 1960s in London and New York, was the U.S.-U.K. Diagnostic Project (Cooper et al. 1972). Its principal aim was to examine whether the apparently higher rates of schizophrenia in the United States represented a true difference from those in Europe, or whether the apparent difference resulted only from variability in diagnostic practices. A major advance of that study was the application of standardized protocols guiding the psychiatric interview of subjects, such as the Present State Examination (PSE; Wing et al. 1974). These interview protocols specified exactly the information to be obtained by the examiner, and a glossary and full course of training were provided to ensure that examiners would be consistent in the way they interpreted the information from the psychiatric interview. In the diagnostic project, criterion variance was minimized by having panels of judges review all of the information available on cases to make consensus ratings of diagnosis.

In 1972, researchers from Washington University in St. Louis proposed a new way of controlling criterion variance in research by publishing a set of specified criteria to be used in assigning diagnoses to research subjects (Feighner et al. 1972). These two approaches—an interview protocol and a set of explicit criteria—were linked in the mid-1970s by the development of a new set of criteria, the Research Diagnostic Criteria (RDC), and the simultaneous development of a standardized interview based on these criteria, the Schedule for Affective Disorders and Schizophrenia (SADS; Endicott and Spitzer 1978). This combined approach of using a standardized interview schedule with fully specified criteria guiding assignment to a particular diagnostic category made it possible for researchers to achieve a new standard of reliability in diagnostic assessments. This feature made its use widespread, a fact that also yielded the advantage of providing comparability in research studies across different centers and over time.

When the DSM-III criteria were published in 1980 (American Psychiatric Assocation 1980), they represented an extension and elaboration of the approach of specifying criteria to be met for each psychiatric disorder. From the extensive experience with previous interview schedules, confidence developed that a fully specified set of questions for an interview schedule could be written so that even nonclinicians could administer them. With support from senior officials of the National Institute of Mental Health (NIMH), an interview schedule was commissioned that would be suitable for large-scale epidemiological studies in community populations. The resulting instrument, the NIMH Diagnostic Interview Schedule (DIS; Robins et al. 1981), contains the exact wording of questions intended to meet the DSM-III criteria of the most important disorders thought to exist in community populations. A careful probe system was also developed for use with positive responses to be sure that the phenomenon being assessed was not attributable to drugs or alcohol or to medical illness or injury, and was significant enough that it could contribute toward accumulating evidence for a psychiatric disorder. Computer scoring programs were developed to handle the large amount of data that would be gathered on each subject in the large-scale survey, and the resulting system was used as the basis for a new multisite epidemiological study called the NIMH Epidemiologic Catchment Area Program (ECA; Regier et al. 1984).

■ SURVEYS OF CLINICAL AND COMMUNITY POPULATIONS

Epidemiological surveys of patients seen in treatment settings as well as of the broader population of community residents have been conducted over the past four decades in the United States and abroad.

☐ Clinical Populations

National Reporting Program

The National Reporting Program is a series of periodic surveys of patients and facilities in the mental health delivery system. These surveys include an annual census of state and county mental hospitals, an inventory of specialty mental health facilities, and a sample survey of patients drawn from the universe of mental health facilities. One use of such data on treatment services is to examine the extent of service provided in different locations.

Social Class and Mental Illness

A classic study based on detailed information from mental health treatment settings in New Haven, Connecticut, was conducted by Hollingshead and Redlich (1958) in the 1950s. Within the New Haven area, every mental health facility and private office practice psychiatrist was surveyed to determine the number of patients seen in these different settings. The investigators estimated that patients in treatment within a 6-month period for any mental disorder represented 8 per 1,000 residents in the community. They demonstrated that the rate in the highest social classes ranged from 5 to 7 per 1,000, compared to 17 per 1,000 in the lowest social class, V.

Primary Care Settings

Studies conducted in the United Kingdom in the mid-1960s demonstrated that patients seen in general practice settings had rates of diagnosable mental disorders as high as 15%. Studies conducted in the United States subsequently demonstrated that the rate of disorder among those visiting a general physician over a 3- to 6-month period of time were even higher (i.e., up to 28%) when standardized psychiatric interviews such as the lifetime version of the SADS (SADS-L) or DIS were used instead of relying on the chart diagnosis. The most common disorders in these primary care patients have been depressive illnesses, anxiety illnesses, and mixed conditions including substance abuse (Kamerow et al. 1986; Katon and Schulberg 1992). At the same time, more recent studies have demonstrated that the general physician commonly does not record a diagnosis of a mental disorder in the patient's chart, does not report it on special inquiries conducted during the research, and does not provide treatment or referral to a specialty mental health clinician.

☐ Community Populations

Stirling County Study

Leighton et al. (1963) surveyed 1,010 adult residents in a rural Canadian county of 20,000 people. They estimated that 20% of the adult population were in need of psychiatric attention for a diagnosable mental disorder, although 57% had evidence of symptom patterns corresponding to the major categories of illness in DSM-I. One of the intriguing findings of that study was that high rates of illness were found in areas of social and economic deterioration, although the variables leading to this higher association were not identifiable.

Midtown Manhattan Study

In an area of midtown Manhattan with 110,000 adults, Srole et al. (1962) sampled 1,660 persons. Psychologists and social workers interviewed respondents according to a structured schedule, and the information was subsequently interpreted by two psychiatrists. There have been continuing controversies about the way this diagnostic information was presented, particularly because some observers have been concerned that it implied the existence of a single spectrum of illness, without allowance for specific psychiatric disorders. This impression was reinforced by the most widely publicized version of the findings, which noted that 81.5% of the population were shown to have at least mild impairment from psychological symptoms, although only 23.4% had significant impairment. There was widespread skepticism in both the scientific community and the public about a field that claimed that fewer than 20% of the population were "mentally healthy."

☐ NIMH Epidemiologic Catchment Area Program

The ECA was conducted at sites in five areas: New Haven, Connecticut; Baltimore, Maryland; St. Louis, Missouri; Durham, North Carolina; and Los Angeles, California. At each site, clearly specified geographic areas based on the catchment areas that had been developed through the Community Mental Health Act of 1963 were sampled so that a minimum of 3,000 adults aged 18 and older from each area would be interviewed at the initial examination. In addition, residents of institutions such as prisons, nursing homes, and chronic care hospitals were also sampled, and 500 respondents from these institutional settings were interviewed.

Besides the DIS, which was used to generate psychiatric diagnoses, extensive questions were asked about use of health and mental health services in the 6 to 12 months preceding the interview. Another interview 6 months after the initial examination, conducted by telephone in four of the five sites, inquired about subsequent use of health and mental health services after that first interview. A follow-up personal interview was conducted about 12 months after the initial visit, and the DIS and the Health Service questions were repeated at that time (Robins and Regier 1991).

The onset, recency, and clustering of symptoms were determined using the DIS, which made it possible to produce prevalence rates of disorders occurring in the past 1 month, 6 months, 1 year, and over the lifetime of all individuals in the sample. Because retrospective data on outpatient service use were obtained for the previous 6 months, 6-month period prevalence rate data have conventionally been presented when an analytic objective has been to compare prevalence and service use data. To generate estimates of mental illness in the community, data from the 18,572 subjects in the community samples at the five sites were pooled and standardized by age, sex, and race/ethnicity to the 1980 U.S. Census of the noninstitutionalized population (Regier et al. 1988; Robins and Regier 1991). For the major DSM-III disorders covered by the DIS, estimates for the 6-month prevalence rates from the pooled data, standardized to the U.S. population, are presented in Table 3–2.

Use of health and mental health services for those persons with specific disorders and with any DIS disorder is represented in Table 3–3. For individuals with any DIS/DSM disorder in the past 6 months, 17.6% sought some type of mental health treatment from either a medical physician or a mental health specialist during the prior 6 months. There is marked variation in level of service use by type of mental disorder diagnosis. More recent estimates of the annual prevalence of mental disor-

Table 3–2. Estimate of 6-month prevalence of DIS/DSM-III disorders in the United States

Disorder	Rate per 100 population	
Any DIS disorder covered	19.1%	(0.4)
Any DIS disorder except cognitive impairment and substance abuse	13.7	(0.4)
Substance use disorders	6.0	(0.3)
Alcohol abuse/dependence	4.7	(0.2)
Drug abuse/dependence	2.0	(0.1)
Schizophrenic/schizophreniform disorders	0.9	(0.1)
Schizophrenia	0.8	(0.1)
Schizophreniform disorder	0.1	(0.0)
Affective disorders	5.8	(0.3)
Manic episode	0.5	(0.1)
Major depressive episode	3.0	(0.2)
Dysthymia[a]	3.3	(0.2)
Anxiety disorders	8.9	(0.3)
Phobia	7.7	(0.3)
Panic disorder	0.8	(0.1)
Obsessive-compulsive disorder	1.5	(0.1)
Somatization disorder	0.1	(0.0)
Personality disorder (antisocial personality disorder)	0.8	(0.1)
Cognitive impairment[a] (severe)	1.3	(0.1)

Note. Data based on five Epidemiologic Catchment Area sites, standardized to 1980 U.S. census. DIS = Diagnostic Interview Schedule (Robins et al. 1981); DSM-III = *Diagnostic and Statistical Manual of Mental Disorders,* 3rd Edition (American Psychiatric Association 1980). Numbers in parentheses are standard errors.
[a]Because no recent information exists, the rates are the same for all prevalence time periods.

Table 3–3.   Estimate of any visit for mental health reasons to mental health specialist or medical physician over a 6-month period for persons with 6-month diagnosis of mental disorders

Diagnosis	Any mental health visit	
No mental disorder	4.5%	(0.2)
Any DIS/DSM-III disorder	17.6	(0.9)
Any DIS/DSM-III disorder except cognitive impairment or substance abuse	22.0	(1.2)
Substance use disorder	12.4	(1.3)
Alcohol abuse/dependence	12.7	(1.5)
Drug abuse/dependence	11.0	(2.0)
Schizophrenia/schizophreniform disorders	48.1	(5.5)
Schizophrenia	48.6	(5.9)
Schizophreniform	43.8	(15.3)
Affective disorders	30.5	(2.1)
Manic episode	32.8	(6.9)
Major depressive episode	38.2	(2.8)
Dysthymia	24.2	(2.5)
Anxiety disorders	20.1	(1.3)
Phobia	18.6	(1.4)
Panic disorder	50.4	(5.4)
Obsessive-compulsive disorder	26.5	(4.2)
Somatization disorder	60.9	(9.0)
Personality disorder (antisocial personality disorder)	17.3	(4.0)
Severe cognitive impairment	6.6	(1.5)

Note.   DIS = Diagnostic Interview Schedule (Robins et al. 1981); DSM-III = *Diagnostic and Statistical Manual of Mental Disorders,* 3rd Edition (American Psychiatric Association 1980). Numbers in parentheses are standard errors.

ders have been calculated based on the ECA data. Regier et al. (1993) estimate that 28.1% of the adult population have a mental disorder during any 1 year, compared with the earlier estimate of 15% of the population. Of this group with a 1-year disorder, only about one in four (28.5% of those with a 1-year DIS disorder) sought mental health or chemical dependency services. When the entire adult population is considered, 14.9% sought mental health or chemical dependency services.

Analysis of reported onset of the major disorders covered by the DIS indicated that younger generations are experiencing earlier onset and higher rates of both major depression and drug abuse and dependence. This evidence is especially important in suggesting a possible causal link between adolescent depression and subsequent drug abuse. In fact, analysis of this link for young adults in the ECA suggested that early depression or anxiety doubled the subsequent risk of drug abuse/dependence (Christie et al. 1988).

Another striking finding has been the demonstration that for several disorders, peak onset occurs at earlier ages than had been thought. While there are limitations to using retrospective recall of onset in a cross-sectional study, systematic examination of reported onset among ECA respondents with a history of a disorder suggests that adolescence and early adulthood are important time periods for development of many major mental disorders (Burke et al. 1990; Table 3–4).

Findings of an increased co-occurrence of DSM-III disorders (Boyd et al. 1984) were amplified in an examination of the co-occurrence of mental disorders with alcohol and other drug use disorders. Among respondents with an alcohol disorder, 37% had a comorbid mental disorder; among those respondents with abuse or dependence of another drug besides alcohol, more than 50% had a comorbid mental disorder. In particular, respondents with schizophrenia, bipolar disorder, or antisocial personality disorder had elevated rates of both alcohol and drug use disorders. About 20% of individuals with a mental disorder who were seen in a specialty mental health clinic setting had a current diagnosis of substance abuse or dependence (Regier et al. 1990).

■ RISK FACTORS FOR SPECIFIC DISORDERS

For several major groups of disorders, critical comparisons of epidemiological research in the past decade have helped identify high-risk groups, and sometimes the magnitude of associated risk factors has been quantified as well.

□ Schizophrenia

In reviewing epidemiological studies of schizophrenia conducted in Europe, Jablensky (1986) concluded that point prevalence rates can be estimated to vary from 2.5 to 5.3 per 1,000, and annual incidence rates from 0.2 to 0.6 per 1,000. These figures represent a definitive summary of

Table 3–4.   Median age at onset of selected mental disorders

Disorder	Age (years)
Major depression (unipolar)	25
Bipolar illness	19
Panic disorder	24
Obsessive-compulsive disorder	23
Phobias	13
Drug abuse/dependence	18
Alcohol abuse/dependence	21

literature published in a variety of languages. Several studies outside Europe are consistent with these findings. An independent clinical examination of DSM-III schizophrenia in a sample derived from the NIMH ECA in Baltimore found a point prevalence of 6.4 per 1,000 adults, including both active and remitted cases at time of interview (von Korff et al. 1985). In a multinational study conducted in 10 countries, Sartorius et al. (1986) found an annual rate of first service contact for a "broad" definition of schizophrenia ranging from 0.15 to 0.42 per 1,000 population at risk, which is consistent with earlier estimates of annual disease incidence.

Torrey (1980) has suggested that the disorder may be related to some aspect of modern industrialized life (e.g., easier transmission of viruses). The evidence has been inconsistent, but an intriguing finding from some studies has been the suggestion that development of schizophrenia is related to maternal exposure to influenza in the second trimester (O'Callaghan et al 1991b; Sham et al. 1992). Some studies have indicated that individuals with schizophrenia have a predominance of winter births (O'Callaghan et al. 1991a). Others have suggested that the apparent increase in recognition of the disorder over the past two centuries could be explained more easily as a result of the change in disease concepts, in both psychiatry and society (Jablensky 1986). In social terms, Cooper and Sartorius (1977) hypothesized that industrialization removes the relatively benign influence of preindustrialized life on the family and social structures that could support the individual with this disorder, so the disease becomes more apparent in industrialized societies.

In general, prevalence rates have been roughly equal for males and females, although there is evidence that males have an earlier age at onset (Flor-Henry 1985). Possibly the best-known risk factor is genetic, as first-degree relatives have been shown to have a higher risk of developing schizophrenia themselves. The genetic contribution was first distinguished from possible environmental influences by Kety et al. (1968), who used a case control design to study offspring of schizophrenic parents who had been adopted early and raised away from their biological parents. Even these genetic studies do not, however, provide an exhaustive explanation. Monozygotic twins share the illness in only about 40% to 50% of cases, according to one of the most rigorous studies of this topic (Gottesman and Shields 1972).

☐ Depressive Illness

Examining the literature on prevalence of affective disorders just before the ECA began, Boyd and Weissman (1981) found generally consistent prevalence rates in studies within industrialized nations. They reported the point prevalence of unipolar depression as about 3 per 100 adult males and about 4 to 9 per 100 adult females.

While considerable research on risk factors and genetic transmission has been conducted in clinical populations for both unipolar depression and bipolar illness, epidemiological studies of community populations have suggested two intriguing leads for more research. In a variety of studies, prevalence rates of unipolar depression for females have been approximately twice as high as those for men. Because this female predominance is shown in community as well as in clinical settings, it cannot be attributed to a greater tendency for females to visit clinical facilities. At present, the range of possible explanations for this female predominance extends from hypotheses about the socioeconomic status of women in industrialized societies to hormonal, genetic, and other biological factors. Specific work by Brown and Harris (1978) has implicated the occurrence of adverse life events as a contributing factor to depression, and ECA data suggest an interaction between adverse events and early childhood experiences such as parental separation/divorce (Landerman et al. 1991). One analysis of ECA data has suggested that poor outcome in women, especially older women, may also contribute to the higher prevalence rates in women (Sargeant et al. 1990). In further analysis of the New Haven data, Weissman (1985) found the highest rates of depressive illness among unhappily married men and women, and Bruce et al. (1990) found higher rates of depressive episodes and dysphoria following conjugal bereavement.

A second hypothesis from epidemiological data is that depression may be increasing among younger generations. Skeptics have suggested that it is not illness that is increasing in the young, but pessimism in their elders. However, analysis of several data sets has suggested that depressive illness has occurred more frequently, or has had onset at an earlier age, in generations born since World War II (Burke et al. 1991; Klerman and Weissman 1989).

☐ Anxiety Disorders

Recent epidemiological studies of anxiety disorders have provided evidence of the high frequency of these disorders in the general population. In a comprehensive review of major community surveys, Marks (1986) found that point prevalence rates for all anxiety disorders ranged from 2.9 to 8.4 per 100. In terms of specific disorders, the rates ranged from 1.2 to 3.8 per 100 for agoraphobia; 4.1 to 7.0 per 100 for simple phobia; 1.8 to 2.5 per 100 for obsessive-compulsive disorder; and 0.4 to 3.1 per 100 for panic disorder.

One striking point about these figures is that anxiety disorders appear to be more common in community populations than in clinical settings. This finding reflects evidence like that from the ECA indicating that only 15% to 23% of those with an anxiety disorder in the prior 6 months received any clinical care for their condition. In the case of obsessive-compulsive disorder, for example, Karno et al. (1988) have noted that the epidemiological data suggest that this disorder is 25 to 60 times more common than had been thought on the basis of studies in clinical populations. In addition, the low rate of treatment changes the impression of the relative importance of particular anxiety disorders. For example, Marks notes that in one study agoraphobia accounted for 50% of cases of anxiety seen in treatment settings, but only 8% of cases in the general population of that area. The existence of large groups of individuals with diagnosable anxiety disorders makes it difficult to generalize results from studies using only patient populations.

☐ Substance Abuse

Several studies have attempted to identify risk factors for drug use and abuse. Adolescents with a cluster of interpersonal difficulties, such as social isolation, have been reported by Newcomb et al. (1986) to have higher rates of drug use than do their peers. Using data from the ECA, Christie et al. (1988) have shown that young adults with a history of major depression or anxiety disorders have about twice the risk of subsequent DSM-III drug abuse and dependence as do those without these prior disorders. By studying adoptees, Cadoret et al. (1986) provided evidence that adults with drug abuse were more likely to have had biological parents with alcohol problems or antisocial personality, or adoptive parents who divorced or had psychiatric problems. For alcohol abuse and dependence, Helzer et al. (1990) found wide variation among different cultures in the standardized lifetime prevalence of alcohol dependence (from 1.5% in Taiwanese metropolitan areas to 11.3% in Edmonton, Alberta, Canada). But they found similarity in age at onset, symptoms, and risk factors such as male gender, antisocial personality, and major depression.

☐ Personality Disorders

Epidemiological study of personality disorders has been hampered by the difficulty in assessing these conditions, especially when using standardized instruments in nonclinical populations (Burke and Burke 1992). The only personality disorder studied in the ECA was antisocial personality, as the original DSM-III criteria permitted assessment by a structured interview like the DIS. The 6-month prevalence rate was 0.8%, with predominance in males under age 45.

Risk factors for antisocial personality have been examined in a variety of longitudinal studies, especially in view of the probable but not inevitable continuity between childhood conduct disorder and adult antisocial personality (American Psychiatric Association 1980; Robins and Price 1991). Using data from the ECA, Robins and Price have suggested that a reported history of childhood conduct problems leads to higher rates of many psychiatric disorders in both men and women. Because the ECA also suggested that conduct problems in childhood have been more common in younger cohorts, these authors raised the possibility that increased rates of major depression may be related to the apparent rise in childhood conduct problems (Robins and Price 1991). Analysis of a Danish cohort of 18- to 21-year-old males born in the period from 1959 to 1961 suggested that having an alcoholic father did not raise the risk of adult antisocial personality, but that having been physically abused as a child was a risk factor for aggressive and antisocial behaviors (Pollock et al. 1990). Findings from these two studies suggest that interventions in childhood to reduce physical abuse and conduct problems may be helpful in reducing the development of antisocial personality disorder in adulthood.

One Axis II disorder that may be specified well enough for epidemiological study is histrionic personality disorder. Psychiatrists from the Baltimore ECA team conducted a separate interview with respondents chosen from the ECA sample, and reported a current prevalence of 2.1% for this disorder. They did not find any difference in rates between males and females. Women in this sample given diagnoses of histrionic personality disorder also had an elevated rate of major depression and of unexplained medical symptoms; men had elevated rates of substance use disorders (Nestadt et al. 1990). In the same study, obsessive-compulsive personality disorder was ascertained, and an overall rate of 1.7% was found (Nestadt et al. 1991).

■ REFERENCES

American Psychiatric Association: Diagnostic and Statistical Manual of Mental Disorders, 3rd Edition. Washington, DC, American Psychiatric Association, 1980

Boyd JH, Weissman MM: Epidemiology of affective disorders: a reexamination and future directions. Arch Gen Psychiatry 38:1039–1046, 1981

Boyd JH, Burke JD Jr, Gruenberg E, et al: Exclusion criteria of DSM-III: a study of co-occurrence of hierarchy-free syndromes. Arch Gen Psychiatry 41:983–989, 1984

Brown GW, Harris T: Social Origins of Depression: A Study of Psychiatric Disorder in Women. Tavistock, London, 1978

Bruce ML, Kim K, Leaf PJ, et al: Depressive episodes and dysphoria resulting from conjugal bereavement in a prospective community sample. Am J Psychiatry 147:608–611, 1990

Burke JD Jr, Burke KC: Diagnostic interviews in psychiatric epidemiology (Chapter 23), in Psychiatry. Edited by Michels R. Philadelphia, PA, JB Lippincott, 1992

Burke KC, Burke JD Jr, Regier DA, et al: Age at onset of selected mental disorders in five community populations. Arch Gen Psychiatry 47:511–518, 1990

Burke KC, Burke JD Jr, Rae DS, et al: Comparing age at onset of major depression and other psychiatric disorders by birth cohorts in five US community populations. Arch Gen Psychiatry 48:789–795, 1991

Cadoret RJ, Troughton E, O'Gorman TW, et al: An adoption study of genetic and environmental factors in drug abuse. Arch Gen Psychiatry 43:1131–1136, 1986

Christie KA, Burke JD, Regier DA, et al: Epidemiologic evidence for early onset of mental disorders and higher risk of drug abuse in young adults. Am J Psychiatry 145:971–975, 1988

Cooper J[E], Sartorius N: Cultural and temporal variations in schizophrenia: a speculation on the importance of industrialization. Br J Psychiatry 130:50–55, 1977

Cooper JE, Kendell RE, Gurland BJ, et al: Psychiatric Diagnosis in New York and London: A Comparative Study of Mental Hospital Admissions. London, Oxford University Press, 1972

Endicott J, Spitzer RL: A diagnostic interview: the Schedule for Affective Disorders and Schizophrenia. Arch Gen Psychiatry 35:837–844, 1978

Feighner JP, Robins E, Guze SB, et al: Diagnostic criteria for use in psychiatric research. Arch Gen Psychiatry 26:57–63, 1972

Fleiss JL: Statistical Methods for Rates and Proportions, 2nd Edition. New York, Wiley, 1981

Flor-Henry P: Schizophrenia: sex differences. Can J Psychiatry 30:319–322, 1985

Gottesman II, Shields J: Schizophrenia and Genetics: A Twin-Study Vantage Point. New York, Academic, 1972

Helzer JE, Canino GJ, Yeh E-K, et al: Alcoholism—North America and Asia: a comparison of population surveys with the Diagnostic Interview Schedule. Arch Gen Psychiatry 47:313–319, 1990

Hollingshead AB, Redlich FC: Social Class and Mental Illness: A Community Study. New York, Wiley, 1958

Jablensky A: Epidemiology of schizophrenia: a European perspective. Schizophr Bull 12:52–73, 1986

Kamerow DB, Pincus HA, Macdonald DI: Alcohol abuse, other drug abuse, and mental disorders in medical practice: prevalence, costs, recognition, and treatment. JAMA 255:2054–2057, 1986

Karno M, Golding JM, Sorenson SB, et al: The epidemiology of obsessive-compulsive disorder in five US communities. Arch Gen Psychiatry 45:1094–1099, 1988

Katon W, Schulberg HC: Epidemiology of depression in primary care. Gen Hosp Psychiatry 14:237–247, 1992

Kety SS, Rosenthal D, Wender PH, et al: The types and prevalence of mental illness in the biological and adoptive families of adopted schizophrenics, in The Transmission of Schizophrenia. Edited by Rosenthal D, Kety SS. Oxford, UK, Pergamon, 1968, pp 345–362

Klerman GL, Weissman MM: Increasing rates of depression. JAMA 261:2229–2235, 1989

Landerman R, George LK, Blazer DG: Adult vulnerability for psychiatric disorders: interactive effects of negative childhood experiences and recent stress. J Nerv Ment Dis 179:656–663, 1991

Leighton DC, Harding JS, Macklin DB, et al: The Character of Danger: Psychiatric Symptoms in Selected Communities. New York, Basic Books, 1963

Marks IM: Epidemiology of anxiety. Social Psychiatry 21:167–171, 1986

Morris JN: Uses of Epidemiology, 2nd Edition. Baltimore, MD, Williams & Wilkins, 1964

Nestadt G, Romanoski AJ, Chahal R, et al: An epidemiological study of histrionic personality disorder. Psychol Med 20:413–422, 1990

Nestadt G, Romanoski AJ, Brown CH, et al: DSM-III compulsive personality disorder: an epidemiological survey. Psychol Med 21:461–471, 1991

Newcomb MD, Maddahian E, Bentler PM: Risk factors for drug use among adolescents: concurrent and longitudinal analyses. Am J Public Health 76:525–531, 1986

O'Callaghan E, Gibson T, Colohan HA, et al: Season of birth in schizophrenia: evidence for confinement of an excess of winter births to patients without a family history of mental disorder. Br J Psychiatry 158:764–769, 1991a

O'Callaghan E, Sham P, Takei N, et al: Schizophrenia after prenatal exposure to 1957 A2 influenza epidemic. Lancet 337:1248–1250, 1991b

Pollock VE, Briere J, Schneider L, et al: Childhood antecedents of antisocial behavior: parental alcoholism and physical abusiveness. Am J Psychiatry 147:1290–1293, 1990

Regier DA, Myers JK, Kramer M, et al: The NIMH Epidemiologic Catchment Area Program: historical context, major objectives, and study population characteristics. Arch Gen Psychiatry 41:934–941, 1984

Regier DA, Boyd JH, Burke JD Jr, et al: One-month prevalence of mental disorders in the United States—based on five Epidemiologic Catchment Area sites. Arch Gen Psychiatry 45:977–986, 1988

Regier DA, Farmer ME, Rae DS, et al: Comorbidity of mental disorders with alcohol and other drug abuse: results from the Epidemiologic Catchment Area (ECA) Study. JAMA 264:2511–2518, 1990

Regier DA, Narrow WE, Rae DS, et al: The de facto US Mental and Addictive Disorders Service System: Epidemiologic Catchment Area prospective 1-year prevalence rates of disorders and services. Arch Gen Psychiatry 50:85–94, 1993

Robins LN, Price RK: Adult disorders predicted by childhood conduct problems: results from the NIMH Epidemiologic Catchment Area Project. Psychiatry 54:116–132, 1991

Robins LN, Regier DA (eds): Psychiatric Disorders in America: The Epidemiologic Catchment Area Study. New York, Free Press, 1991

Robins LN, Helzer JE, Croughan J, et al: National Institute of Mental Health Diagnostic Interview Schedule: its history, characteristics, and validity. Arch Gen Psychiatry 38:381–389, 1981

Sargeant JK, Bruce ML, Florio LP, et al: Factors associated with 1-year outcome of major depression in the community. Arch Gen Psychiatry 47:519–526, 1990

Sartorius N, Jablensky A, Korten A, et al: Early manifestations and first-contact incidence of schizophrenia in different cultures. Psychol Med 16:909–928, 1986

Sham PC, O'Callaghan E, Takei N, et al: Schizophrenia following pre-natal exposure to influenza epidemics between 1939 and 1960. Br J Psychiatry 160:461–466, 1992

Srole L, Langner TS, Michael ST, et al: Mental Health in the Metropolis: The Midtown Manhattan Study. New York, McGraw-Hill, 1962

Torrey EF: Schizophrenia and Civilization. New York, Jason Aronson, 1980

von Korff M, Nestadt G, Romanoski A, et al: Prevalence of treated and untreated DSM-III schizophrenia: results of a two-stage community survey. J Nerv Ment Dis 173:577–581, 1985

Weissman MM: Presentation of the 1985 Rema Lapouse Mental Health Epidemiology Award at the special award session of the American Public Health Association Annual Meeting, Washington, DC, November 1985

Wing JK, Cooper JE, Sartorius N: Measurement and Classification of Psychiatric Symptoms. New York, Cambridge University Press, 1974

CHAPTER 4

Normal Child and Adolescent Development

Theodore Shapiro, M.D.
Margaret E. Hertzig, M.D.

The current focus in modern psychiatry on descriptive nomenclatures, diagnosis, and treatment does not necessarily include a developmental point of view. On the other hand, there are strong historical and clinical reasons why any student of personality and pathology within a medical framework should be interested in what is known about the normal developmental process.

■ HISTORICAL BACKGROUND

The understanding of psychiatrists such as Pinel—who recorded longitudinal histories of French asylum patients—that psychopathology in adulthood might have something to do with life history is deeply ingrained in the notion of "humane treatment." In the United States, Adolf Meyer, founder of the concept of psychobiology, emphasized the life event chart as a mainstay of clinical knowledge. While these trends in general psychiatry held sway, Freud (1905/1953) elaborated the idea that the first five years of life had a determining effect on later psychopathology.

From a more general medical vantage point, pediatrics was split off from general medicine. Most pediatricians consider themselves practitioners of developmental medicine. Outside of medicine, the language of developmental psychology derives from Darwin's linking of variation in forms of life to their survival value in evolution. Darwin's formulations then led to Ernst Haeckel's biogenetic law that "ontogeny recapitulates phylogeny." Concepts such as maturation, development, differentiation, pleiomorphism, and organizers all have been borrowed from embryology and have enriched our understanding of how children start to be, beginning with gametization, embryogenesis, and then birth, and progressing to later developmental stages that can be observed and staged.

■ DEVELOPMENTAL PRINCIPLES

The terms *growth, maturation,* and *development,* although used imprecisely in common parlance, connote a direction from more global reactiveness to more specified reactiveness and from a less complex organization to a more complex state of organization. *Growth* usually refers to the simple accretion of tissue (i.e., an increase in size or in the number of cells). Changes in height and weight are examples of growth. *Maturation* is a convenient fiction that has a somewhat teleological implication of a direction toward which the individual is headed in accord with his or her functions, abilities, structures, and competencies. In its most narrow meaning, the term suggests that there is a natural unfolding of genetic potential toward an end that is known as "maturity." The concept does not invoke the variation that may occur in certain special ecologies. *Development,* on the other hand, includes whatever the maturational potential provides plus the variations in social and environmental influence. This concept refers to the changing structure of behavior and thought over time.

Normative studies suggest a cephalocaudal developmental sequence, with the head end of the organism at the beginning of life being a more highly differentiated functional entity than the tail end. Biological forces such as myelinization of the central long tracts progressing from head to toe help us to understand that regardless of the cultural variation in the early months, most human children begin to walk between the ages of 10 and 18 months (Gesell and Amatruda 1947). Similarly, the landmarks of language development occur in a lockstep sequence. Moreover, no matter what language is spoken by the parent, by the time the child is 2 years old, he or she usually can string together two- and sometimes three-word utterances with some understanding of grammatical format. Any errors that are made derive from overgeneralization of grammatical rules and are not random. However, to add complexity, each line of development may mature independently, such as in a limited cerebral palsy affecting only the small section of the cortex that controls limb motor pathways.

From the developmental vantage, these maturational regularities are acted upon by social nurturing influences; the achievements are not entirely innate. For example, if a child is tied down or forced to remain recumbent, the maturational event of walking surely will be delayed because of muscular disuse. Similarly, although the capacity for language and grammar may be built-in, children will not achieve speech and language in the usual manner if they are deaf or if they are not spoken to.

☐ Differentiation and Integration

Maturation within individual systems also requires that we consider another central theme in development, *differentiation.* Just as the blastosphere differentiates into endoderm, ectoderm, and mesoderm, and these further mature into more highly differentiated tissues, so, analogously, do psychological and social systems differentiate. In a psychological sense, the general arousal of infants differentiates selectively into responses signifying that the child distinguishes between human and nonhuman, mother and nonmother, friend and foe.

Integration also emerges between and among the varying senses. In the beginning the eye sees what impinges on it; the hand grasps that which is put into it. At 3 or 4 months, if the child sees the hand and the thing to be grasped in the same visual field, he or she will grasp. It is not until some time later that the child reaches for that which he or she sees even if the hand is not in the visual field. At a psychological level, the capacity to put together good and bad experiences with a person and also to change set in relation to varying exposures requires integration. As the infant, showing more differentiated and integrated functioning, moves from the more global apprehension of the world, he or she may also lose some functions that were natively available.

☐ Hierarchic Reorganization and Critical Periods

As each stage unfolds, the question arises as to whether it could unfold without the child having had to pass through the prior stage. *Epigenesis* is the concept of sequential steps influencing subsequent steps. Each stage in that model is highly dependent on resolution of the experiences of the prior stage. The epigenetic vantage point permits, but does not necessarily include, another model known as *hierarchic reorganization* (Werner 1957). According to this concept, each new integration of biological and neuronal function meshes with psychocognitive capacities that are more than the sum of their parts. Each stage is truly a new structure permitting functions and adaptations that are not easily predicted from their precursors. These reorganizations permit the next level of behavior and competence as the child pulls himself or herself along the chronological ladder.

Invoking a hierarchically reorganized sequence permits consideration of *critical periods,* which require that an environmental releaser stimulate the emergence of a developmental capacity that is inborn and ready for use only within a limited time period. If no release occurs, the function is said to *involute.* However, such releasers may not adequately describe the way in which human biological development takes place since the time lines are not as critically limited as in other mammals.

■ DEVELOPMENTAL PSYCHOLOGIES

Most psychiatrists are well versed in the retrospective reconstructive attitude of the Freudian developmental system. The *genetic point of view* was Freud's attempt to retrospectively divine the infantile roots of adult behavior and pathology. His assumptions of polymorphously perverse infantile sexuality and the maturational sequences described in libido theory were based on retrospective reconstructions of how men and women seem to organize their fantasy lives. Later psychoanalytic thinkers (e.g., Mahler et al. 1975; Spitz 1965) created their own developmental systems that elaborated Freud's system.

The behavioral vantage point, which was well outlined in the initial work of Watson (1919) and then B. F. Skinner (1953), is based on learning theory and takes a Lockean philosophical position in which experience is said to be inscribed on a blank slate of mind, thereby transforming it. No competence becomes possible that is not learned. Furthermore, nothing can be learned that is not within the capacity of the species, which in turn determines the limits of responsiveness. The virtue of a learning model for development is that such a model can be empirically apprehended and there is little inferred substructure and very few intervening variables.

Jean Piaget (Piaget and Inhelder 1969) set out to determine how intelligent behavior evolves. Calling himself a "genetic epistomologist" concerned only with non-affect-laden behavior, he addressed the issue of how children strategically arrive at right or wrong answers utilizing their native capacities and regularized sequence of stages. The normative developmental theory of Arnold Gesell (Gesell and Amatruda 1947) is more closely related to the learning theorists, but within the medical framework. Gesell attempted to unify the biological and neurodevelopmental principles that were available at that time from embryogenesis and the normative sequences of observed behaviors. Gesell's studies inspired others to examine large numbers of children "cross-sectionally" in order to find out what they do at each chronological age. Normative, cross-sectional studies, however, do not tell how one progresses (i.e., the process) throughout the longitudinal cycle from one stage to another. *Longitudinal* studies more easily address such issues. Although longitudinal studies are not generally reported in terms of how child A responds at point X and then at point Y, investigators in such studies do have the potential to do just that: to track developmental facts in individual subjects at varying stages, looking for outcomes from past behaviors and checking on retrospective suggestions.

☐ Psychoanalytic Developmental Viewpoint

The psychoanalytic view of childhood (Table 4–1) derives from two sources. The first source (i.e., *genetic*) uses retrospective and reconstructive inferences about the patient's past to construct a coherent and plausible sequenced history. The other source (i.e., *developmental*), based on the prospective studies by psychoanalytically oriented observers, attempts to observationally flesh out the models of development derived from the genetic point of view.

The Freudian Perspective

Freud's initial view of childhood as a period of polymorphously perverse infantile sexuality grew out of his observation that adult disorder reveals certain constant, compelling features. Adult sexuality consists not only of coitus and gametization, but of erotic arousal that depends on stimulation of a variety of bodily zones. Perverse activity and normal foreplay both led to arousal and orgasmic behavior. Moreover, neurotic individuals did not dare think about the things that perverse individuals perpetrated. On these grounds, Freud suggested that repression was the prime mechanism that both hid and modified early sexual thoughts from the conscious minds of neurotic individuals. Libido theory was introduced to describe the maturational sequence that children were expected to traverse en route to adulthood. The theory included the active and passive aims of children seen retrospectively in relation to their primary objects, mother and father. These aims became what Erikson (1963) called the enactments and fantasies of the tragedies and comedies that occur around the orifices of the body.

Psychopathology was viewed by Freud as the result of either a fixation at (i.e., an arrest in the progress of psychosexual maturation) or a regression to (i.e., a symbolic or functional return to earlier ways of acting or thinking) one or another of these stages. As Erikson (1963) noted, the body zones and modes of function are analogous to other behaviors in life. For example, ingesting and spitting out as bodily acts were

Table 4–1. Psychoanalytic theories of development

Period	Freud	Erikson	Spitz	Mahler	Stern
Infancy (approximately 0–12 months)	Oral	Trust vs. mistrust	Smiling response (1st organizer, 6 weeks); stranger anxiety (2nd organizer, 7 months)	Normal autism (0–2 months); normal symbiosis (2–6 months); separation-individuation: subphase 1, differentiation (6–10 months)	Sense of an emergent self (throughout life span); sense of a core self (2 months throughout life span); sense of a subjective self (7 months throughout life span)
Toddler (approximately 12–36 months)	Anal	Autonomy vs. shame and doubt	"No" (3rd organizer, 15 months)	Subphase 2, practicing period (10–15 months); subphase 3, rapprochement (16–24 months); subphase 4, consolidation and resolution (24–36 months)	Sense of a verbal self (15 months throughout life span)
Preschool (approximately 3–5 years)	Phallic Oedipal	Initiative vs. guilt Initiative vs. guilt			
School-age (approximately 5–12 years)	Latency	Industry vs. inferiority			
Adolescence (approximately 12 years and up)		Identity vs. role confusion			

thought to become introjection and projection as mental defenses, and so forth.

Freud took a strongly developmental position in response to the challenge of Otto Rank, who wrote that birth anxiety was at the center of symptom formation. Freud suggested that anxiety functions as a signal that a dangerous situation is at hand in response to the emergence of specific thoughts as they threaten to break into consciousness. According to Freud's hierarchy of threats, helplessness is the first signal of danger. Separation occurring somewhere between 7 and 24 months follows, and then castration anxiety (or body integrity anxiety) takes over from the third to the sixth years. Finally danger of punishment by guilt ensues from an internalized value system embodied in the superego, which is an agency of the tripartite mind of the new structural model.

The Perspective of Ego Psychology

Freud's work was followed by empirical observations by others who moved away from depth psychology toward what was called *ego psychology.*

Spitz's genetic field theory.   René Spitz's (1965) genetic field theory was derived from direct observation of infants. He invoked the concept of the "organizer" in the development of human behavior, of which three have significance for the differentiation process. The concept of an organizer was derived from the embryological model that prescribes a formative fixing element in maturation that interferes with the pluripotentiality of protoplasm.

Spitz's first organizer, the *smiling response,* includes a consistent and repeatable social smile in response to a full face or a moving oval with darkened areas representing eyes. The format of the human face entailed here suggests that this is the first "not-me" object to be appreciated by an infant. This generalized other is smiled at sometime around 6 weeks. This maturational landmark links outside experience and autonomous function, supporting the notion of a regularly responsive internalization en route to what psychoanalysts call *object constancy.*

The next organizer, the *stranger response,* occurs at about 7 months. The child now turns away from the stranger with apprehension, terminating what Anna Freud (1965) has called the period of "need satisfying object." This second organizer marks the attachment to a specific other. The third organizer, the *development of the signal for no,* then signifies a fully internalized and individuated human toddler who now can undo with a verbal signal.

Mahler's separation-individuation theory.   Mahler's separation-individuation theory continues the process of development into the postuterine period, involving the "hatching" of human consciousness, with the toddler as a separate, discrete autonomous agency. In Mahlerian terms the child moves from an autistic to a symbiotic stage in which he or she is initially enmeshed psychologically with the mother as though he or she were not separate from the mother (Mahler et al 1975).

During the *differentiation* subphase, psychological birth occurs under the rubric of hatching, which is characterized by a permanently alert sensorium in which visual and manual examination of the external world become central. Next emerges the *practicing* subphase, characterized by increased curiosity. The child now appears as if he or she were omnipotent and as if an internal agency were not dissociated from an external agency. Only with the understanding that the mother is separate, during the next subphase, does the child arrive at what is called "object constancy," which ensues at about 25 months to 3 years. Relative independent action can take place after the child is able to keep a stable mental image of the important caregiver.

Anna Freud's multilinear theory.   Anna Freud (1974) described a series of developmental lines according to which the child moves 1) from being nursed to rational eating, 2) from wetting and soiling to bowel and bladder control, 3) from egocentricity toward companionship with peers, 4) from play to the capacity to work, 5) from physical to mental pathways of discharge of drives, 6) from animate to inanimate objects, and 7) from irresponsibility to guilt. One can infer from these observations and their variations that a central theme evolves concerning how the child organizes behavior in an affective climate and in relation to others. This has become the observational groundwork of what now is called *object-relations theory* in psychoanalysis, in which the object referred to is the child's mental representation of significant adults such as parents.

☐ Normative Cross-Sectional Development

Cross-sectional developmental observers determine what children can do at varying ages and seek to construct sequential maps consisting of stages. Gesell divides behavior into four sectors: adaptive, language, and personal-social (Gesell and Amatruda 1947). He tracked these behavioral observations over the long period of infancy and described a normative timetable. The essential question asked is does the child at age X achieve behavior in accord with what most children at age X can do? Gesell's organizing principle was neurodevelopmental integrity. He watched the child in the supine and prone positions give way to the sitting position and then to the standing and walking position. Nonetheless, Gesell matches Freud when he states that the developmental span that lies between birth and 5 years is formative and of major significance for the entire life of the human organism. The developmental quotient (i.e., maturational age divided by chronological age and then multiplied by 100 [(MA/CA) x 100]) gives a rough index of what the child tested can do at each stage.

Other cross-sectional schemes of childhood pertain largely to the development of intelligence. Binet invented the IQ (intelligence quotient) measure for that purpose. His test was revised in the United States as the Stanford-Binet Intelligence Test, which has been in continuous use as the IQ standard ever since. It has become, with revisions, a normative outline of what children are, on the average, capable of at each age. The most recent studies of cross-sectional behavior have tried to include a large sector of behaviors other than verbal behavior. Thus, the Wechsler Intelligence Scale for Children (WISC) was designed to include both verbal and performance scales.

☐ Piagetian Cognitive Development

Piaget took a unique stance when he noted that getting the right answer is only one aspect of intelligence. He wished instead to understand how it is that children come to know what they seem to know. Piaget found the regularities in sequence that permit abstract intelligent behavior.

Piaget proposes that the infant is born with two kinds of reflexes: those that remain fixed through life and those that are plastic in response to experience. The experiential world impinges on the child reflexively, and gradually a mental organization, called a *schema*, develops around repeated interactions. The *process* of development remains the same throughout life, but the *structures* change. The repeated process involves a reexperiencing in *assimilation*, but the assimilative schemas can change as they *accommodate*, leading to *adaptation*. For Piaget, assimilation is the incorporation of a structure of action that the subject judges to be equivalent into existing schemas. Accommodation, in turn, occurs when the schema must change to appreciate new objects and differentiate them from old assimilatory forms. Around this universal complementary functional format, the child then passes through four stages: sensory-motor, preoperational, concrete operational, and formal operational.

During the *sensory-motor stage*, no behavior and its schema is separated into sensory and motor components. A thing to be acted upon is appreciated as the thing acted upon. It does not exist as a sensorily discrete entity without action. It is as if the infant were constantly embedded in a trial-and-error world.

As the infant strips away the motor component, he or she can, between the ages of 18 months and 2 years, maintain a stable mental representation and create a representational world. This inaugurates the *preoperational* period, during which things are worked upon in accord with how effective the child is.

The *concrete operational stage*, from 7 to 14 years, introduces a series of functional components suggesting that behavior becomes more rule-governed and that the rules permit decentering. When the child decenters he loses his literal egocentricity—that is, he can generalize. However, he cannot yet generalize from data. Conservation becomes possible, and change in surface appearance does not necessarily signify basic change as in the concepts of volume or weight. Reversal operations may become possible, and trial and error are superseded by mental work employed to solve problems in one's mind, as in equation reversibility.

The stage of *formal operations* involves reasoning from empirical observations that then can be abstracted as general rules that can be used to dictate future actions. The child is now sufficiently decentered to take on another's vantage point, and reversibility is well established. The rules of logic of language are established. Piaget wrote also about imagination, dreams, and language as functions with logical structures.

☐ Ethological Development

Bowlby (1969) recognized the nature of human ties as an organizing precursor to later mature development. Reviewing the nature of the maternal tie, he established what he called a component instinctual response system that bore some similarity to Freud's 1905 theory. The infant is described as having five components that make up attachment behavior. Experiences are integrated to create a unified mental representation. The activated reflexes of *sucking, clinging,* and *following* have representation in other species, but are also present in the human. *Crying* and *smiling* achieve their ends by reciprocal maternal behavior: they bring the mother to the child. Each of these component instincts is considered to be an inborn response that is activated by an external caregiver (e.g., the mother). The evolutionary basis for this attachment is accounted for in the survival value and the natural selection for these responses.

Protest, despair, and *grief* were repeatedly observed upon separation, and then, if these responses were carried on too long, *denial* of need ensued. These behaviors serve as negative indicators that the normal process of the attached state has been interrupted. The research of Bowlby and others indicates that children who have been poorly attached later develop untoward consequences. Recent studies (e.g., Fonagy et al. 1991) have demonstrated that the mother's attachment profile extracted from a carefully structured interview (Main et al. 1985) is highly correlated with security of attachment of the child. This finding places great weight on the interactive nature of early behavior.

■ NORMAL GROWTH AND DEVELOPMENT: BIRTH TO PREPUBERTY

We now will traverse the developmental span from birth to preadolescence, and then consider adolescence separately, in order to provide an overview of physical, neurological, sensory-motor, and cognitive development. Following this, we will then discuss the development of emotion in an interpersonal context. Finally, we will look at adolescence as a way station to youth and middle age that offers the integrations necessary for later life. Although we stress the early years, a truly developmental perspective includes the entire life span.

☐ Neurodevelopmental and Cognitive Organization

Biodevelopmental Reorganizations in the First Two Years of Life

The human infant is born with a largely prewired nervous system, and many capacities designed for survival are already built into the organism (Stern 1985). The variations in the environment seem to influence the central nervous system (CNS) and neuronal networks largely through increases and decreases in the proliferation of synaptic connections and dendritic growth. There is a general proliferation of neural connections through the sixth and seventh year of life, followed by a decline, so that at puberty the network appears less dense (however, not as sparse as that found in the human brain at birth) (Huttenlocher 1979).

Changes on the electroencephalogram (EEG), clinical neurological status, and cognitive levels also can be cited to document periods of radical change. These latter observations have led to formulations on the psychobehavioral level known as *discontinuities in development,* or as *biodevelopmental shifts* by other developmentalists intent on bringing the behavioral level into relation with the substrate (Emde et al. 1976; Shapiro and Perry 1976).

Neurological organization.   The first suggestion of a biodevelopmental shift occurs at the time of the first social organizer, the social smile, signaling the recognition of an external stimulus of the human face as a releaser. The EEG becomes reorganized at a physiological level. Moreover, the rapid heartbeat of early infancy during disposition of attention gives way to slowing of the heartbeat with attentive staring after 2 months.

The six or seven regularly recurring REM periods during adult sleep only gradually emerge, evolving from early infancy (less than 3 months), when light sleep (Stages 1 and 2) dominates the EEG (Roffwarg et al. 1966). Moreover, sleep EEGs of premature infants show that up to 70% of sleep time is spent in a Stage-1 REM pattern. Sleep spindles appear only at 3 to 4 months, and by 3 months the infantile form of going to sleep that is characterized by rapid shifts from Stage 1 to Stage 4 recedes. These changes parallel the behavioral characteristics known as *settling*, when 70% of babies become night sleepers, rescinding their former pattern of waking at 3- to 4-hour intervals. By the end of the first year of life, the adult pattern of sleep is established.

Motoric behavior.   Gesell emphasizes the capacity to turn over, sit upright, and, finally, use bipedal locomotion as developmental markers of maturation. These achievements are signs of the integration of CNS structures. Not only do they subsume the progression from cephalic dominance to the importance of manual dexterity and locomotion in human children. They also mark the growing capacity of the child to become separate from the caretaking parent on the grounds of motor competence.

Behaviorally the infant at birth lies in a "fencer" position (tonic neck reflex) and during alert wakeful times can be stimulated to focus, grasp, and respond reflexively to rooting and sucking, all of which are adaptive for survival. These behaviors later give way to lying in a supine position and beginning to use both hands for grasping and mouthing objects as hand-mouth integrations become possible. Only by 10 months does the infant grasp objects in both hands and bring them to the midline. Symmetrical use of limbs and axial support become essential to the child's being able to turn over at 4 months and, ultimately, to achievement of the sitting position at 6 months. As these neuromuscular achievements take hold, other developing systems are also evident.

Linguistic behavior.   The vocal apparatus is used to produce protolinguistic expressions attracting the environment to the child. Even at this stage, infants seem to be prepared to selectively attend to congruent visual and acoustic signals. Infants' babbling begins to take on meaning and significance as it differentiates into the speech of their mothers. Sapir (1921) suggests that in the beginning the child is overheard. Buhler (1934) suggests that the infant moves from expression to appeal to propositionalizing. However, we now understand that the child can distinguish phonetic contrasts in a highly refined manner (Eimas et al. 1971). This refinement may undergo both specialization and involution as development proceeds so that appreciated distinctions that are important in one language involute if the infant hears another language (Kuhl 1992).

Cognitive behavior.   The cognitive substructures that subsume representational reality and thus constancy are dependent upon the achievement of the passage through the Piagetian sensory-motor period to the preoperational and early concrete operational stages. During the first year of development, the child is undergoing major cognitive shifts in his of her capacity to apprehend the external environment in a manner consonant with commonsense cultural reality. The period from birth to 18 months, from the standpoint of the development of intelligent action, concerns the development of a representational reality that spans the six stages of sensory-motor intelligence, as described by Piaget.

The first and second stages refer to *heterologous and practical groups* in which no behavior pattern relative to vanished objects is observed and each event in time and space does not seem to be connected to its contiguous event. The infant may focus on the red ball held in the air in a reflexive manner, but when the ball is dropped, he or she will focus at the first position rather than following the ball's trajectory. It is as if the experience is fragmented, or cut into frames. As noted, sensory impressions are intimately entwined with motor activity, hence the term sensory-motor intelligence. In fact, paradoxically, our adult concept of a distinctive perceptual sensory experience apart from motor activity should be viewed as an achievement of development. Recent work indicates that earliest memories are stored as procedural sequences, only later to be translated into nominal and verbal propositions. The latter changes are related to hippocampal development (Cohen et al. 1985).

The third stage of cognitive development is presumed when the child *extends movements already started,* which indicates that there is some sense of "thing permanence" so that, for example, the child follows the trajectory of the dropped ball to a vanishing point. The fourth stage is characterized by *reversible operations* of seeking and finding with an active search for the vanished object. However, the child is not yet able to take into account the *sequential displacements* that go on out of sight.

By the fifth stage, *objective groups* are established and there is some sense of the permanence of the object that is extended into the sixth and final stage, that of *representative groups.* Only then can the child imagine invisible displacements. The "thing" finally exists as a mental property, naively but practically assumed to be in the world. From age 16 to 18 months, "things" are freed of their motor components. The child can begin to mentally retrace movements. The possibility of a mental world has become established on purely cognitive grounds.

The establishment of a representational world has some bearing on other matters of representations that touch emotions. For example, how does the child represent the mother? How does the child keep an image alive as a mental property even in the absence of a stimulus? What are the precursors to fantasying, imagining, and, finally, projecting the future? These features are abstracted in Piaget's model into the minimum set of achievements that are required in the mental schemata that lead to the accession of well-established representations of the external world.

Toddler and Preschool Years: Language and Cognition

From 3 years of age on, the toddler can begin to copy geometric forms, name them, and progressively begin to represent the human figure. The 3-year-old, full of exuberance, is also a language user. He or she can participate at table and can behave in limited social situations. Attendance at nursery school, with its routinized group demands of sharing and taking turns, becomes possible. Fantasy pretend play emerges in the early socialization process as well. During the preoperational period, the child is still not able to decenter or imagine the vantage point from different positions in a room. There is no conservation of weight or volume and no cardinality of number or reversibility.

Qualitative differences between developmental stages may not be as clear-cut as formerly thought. An uncanny experiment suggests that some abilities are present early but must reemerge later during the age period of 2 to 6 years with new cognitive underpinnings. If one puts a cube in an infant's mouth and then presents different shaped objects visually, the child focuses on the cube. Other synesthesias have been described as well. For example, certain vowel sounds are regularly associated with certain colors (e.g., \a\ with red). The fact that these synesthesias do not last throughout the life cycle indicates some involution of inbuilt propensities. Certain children at 3 or 4 years of age can solve some conservation problems, but these problems must be presented in relatively simple terms. This indicates that perhaps some of the failures and difficulties of younger children are due to the kind of language that was used in the initial experiments.

Social referencing (Klinnert et al. 1986) is one area in which an early relationship influences cognitive performance. A young child who is capable of crawling (i.e., age 8 months and older) can recognize a "visual cliff" (i.e., an illusion that there is a drop-off, although a transparent plexiglass plate covers the drop). The child stops crawling at the cliff margin. However, if the mother is at the other end encouraging him or her, the child will proceed in accord with the afforded confidence.

As the child moves into the toddler years, much of what takes place in the cognitive sphere well into the beginnings of school rests upon the acquisition of language and communicative ability. The emotional and social climate of learning also becomes very important, and we tend to take the neurodevelopmental aspects and cognitive aspects more for granted until the changes that occur at ages 6 and 7 years. Language competence and performance develop at a rapid pace. The 2-year-old rapidly achieves telegraphic speech of two words, then adds grammatical morphemes (i.e., small endings on words that signify tense, person, etc.). These rapid shifts occur sequentially, in an orderly manner, in accord with the language that is spoken. By 3 years of age the child is a fairly competent speaker, with a three- to six-word mean length of utterance (MLU).

Although it was formerly thought that the first 50-word corpus consisted of only nouns, some children have a higher concentration of prepositions and verbs that refer to rather complicated concepts (Nelson 1981). Moreover, what we thought of as concreteness during the 1- to 3-word stage may represent a more canny understanding of the world than our prior understanding would admit. There is general agreement that the child may imitate before he or she comprehends, and that production follows; thus, there is a greater constraint developmentally on expression-production than on understanding. A most remarkable finding that undoes some of the mechanical presuppositions about language development concerns the early detection of narrative lines in children's learning, even with children at ages 2 or 3 years (Bretherton 1989; Nelson 1986).

The remarkable achievement of deixis suggests a very early capacity to distinguish a "this" from a "that," or "I" from "you," from "me." These distinctions are regularly achieved by 2 years. Similarly, concreteness begs for explanation. The child of limited vocabulary who designates his or her dog "Rex" may then see a horse or a sheep and call either "Rex." The child may exhibit concreteness in other ways because of a limited understanding of the nuances of language. This is most apparent in the adult concept of the *joke*. Jokes told by 5- to 10-year-olds tend to be puns or restatements of naughty words and are not very funny to adults. The child practices with the laughter that goes with the presumed joke. He or she also seems to thrive on repetition.

Although the cognitive and neurodevelopmental capacities necessary for independence may be present before 7 years of age, the maturity of the mental apparatus and judgments about the world are not sufficient for the child to take his or her place in the larger social world. We have instituted nursery schools for day care and kindergartens since the late 19th century, but these are generally places where socialization occurs and manipulative skills are stressed. Although variation is apparent early in life and may persist, most cultures have decided that formal schooling should take place somewhere between 6 and 7 years.

The Second Biodevelopmental Shift

Every level of study, from the neurodevelopmental to the cognitive and social, suggests a discontinuity at age 7 years that would correspond to a second biodevelopmental shift. The brain attains its adult format and reaches the asymptote of its maximum weight at 7 years. Neuronal dendrites are most dense at this age. Moreover, it is after age 7 that children begin to understand that their feelings, intuitions, and thoughts may be of interest to others and, more important, may be thought about by others. Children of age 7 have had the experience of viewing the actions of others in terms of separate motivation, and they can infer feelings. They also seem to begin to understand cause-and-effect relationships. They can grasp the concept of conservation of weight (despite how much a piece of clay is distorted in shape), of volume (despite container shape), or of number (despite, for example, the length of a line of coins).

Children aged 7 years and older may also develop rigidities. They become rule bound and even moralistic about rules, outreasoning their parents in accord with the rules they have been taught. They chastise parents for smoking or for minor infractions of the law. Although they expect devotion and rigor from their parents, children this age sometimes break rules too. Children at this age are exceedingly fickle in friendships, but at the same time demand absolute allegiance. "Best friends" may turn out to be different individuals each day. Children during this period tend to set up clubs with complicated rule structures. Rituals are also rampant.

The period that Freud called *latency*, and is now more neutrally named *middle childhood*, becomes a time of mastering a great number of facts and skills. The period through fourth grade is considered a time of skill development. Self-righteousness and preoccupation with being admired and cared for, and acceptance of the ministrations of parents, are the hallmark of this stage. This also is a period when games are paramount and when persistence at games and collecting are central concerns.

☐ Affective-Interactive Organization

The Newborn Infant

From the first moments of life the infant's physical characteristics and behavioral patterns attract the caring attention of the people in its environment. Bowlby (1969) proposed that attachment originates in inherited species-characteristic behavior called "inborn response systems." By clinging, sucking, vocalizing, crying, smiling, and following, the infant brings or keeps the caregiver close. Human babies initially follow with their eyes and cling as part of a grasp reflex, and suck to obtain nutrition needed for survival. The behavioral patterns of the newborn ensure the proximity of the caretaker that is necessary for sheer physical survival.

Among these inborn response systems, *affectivity* is essential. For the first 2 months of life, the care of the infant is primarily concerned with the regulation and stabilization of sleep-wake and hunger-satiation cycles. The parents of newborns are focused on the tasks of responding to signals of distress: of feeding, changing, and getting the infant to sleep.

The newborn infant seeks sensory stimulation in periods of quiet alertness. The world of the newborn is not the blooming, buzzing confusion postulated by William James. Between birth and 2 months of age infants select out the movement and size attributes of visual stimuli. As noted earlier, these very young infants are capable of recognizing similarities and differences not only within sense systems but across sensory modalities as well. By 6 weeks of age babies tend to look more closely at faces that speak, and in experimental situations they focus longer on faces that move in ways consistent with, rather than discrepant from, a simultaneously presented auditory stimulus.

Infants can perceive persons as unique forms from the very beginning. Newborns act differently when scanning live faces than when scanning inanimate patterns; they vocalize more and their movement patterns are smoother and more coordinated (Brazelton et al. 1974). Neonates have consistently been shown to be able to discriminate the mother's voice from that of another woman reading the same material (DeCasper and Fifer 1980), and infants as young as 2 days have been found to be able to reliably imitate an adult model who either smiled, frowned, or showed a surprise face (Field et al. 1982). Babies are particularly receptive to the ways in which people interact with them. Mothers have little difficulty in deciding whether their babies are content or distressed, and only somewhat more difficulty in attaching specific affective labels to facial expressions.

Emergence of Emotional Experience

Emotional experiences require a sense of self—an "I" to evaluate changes in "me"—as well as the cognitive capacity to perceive, discriminate, recall, associate, and compare. From this perspective, the very young baby's emotional expressions tell us little of his or her emotional experience. In Stern's (1985) view, an emergent sense of self—in relation to others—is present from birth. The affects, perceptions, sensorimotor events, memories, and other cognitions that accompany social interactions become increasingly integrated over time, providing a framework for the further elaboration of both a sense of self and an awareness of and attachment to others.

During the first 2 months of life, the baby is in a state of quiet alertness for only very short periods of time. Gesell and Amatruda (1947) noted that the 4-week-old child sleeps for as many as 20 hours each day. Often it is only in the late afternoon (typically between four and six o'clock) that there is a more sustained opportunity for social interaction. By 2 months of age, biobehavioral transformations affecting the nature and quality of social interactions are well underway (Emde et al. 1976). Sleep and activity cycles have stabilized, motor patterns are more mature, and altered visual scanning patterns permit new strategies for attachment to the world. Symmetry, complexity, and novelty are becoming salient attributes of visual stimuli. Learning occurs more rapidly and more inclusively. The perceptual preferences for the human face and voice, present at birth, are fully operative. The social smile is well established, vocalizations directed at persons entering the infant's range of vision have begun, and mutual gaze is actively sought.

The period between 2 and 7 months is perhaps the most exclusively social period of life. Typically, caregivers repeat their exaggerated facial expressions, gestures, and vocalizations with minor variations, which serve to regulate the infant's level of arousal and excitation within a tolerable range. Infants, too, are able to regulate their level of social engagement, using gaze aversion to cut out stimulation that has risen above an optimal range, and vocalizations and alterations of facial expression to invite new levels of stimulation when excitation has fallen too low. Infants draw upon these daily life experiences to consolidate a sense of a core self as a separate, cohesive, bounded physical unit. During this period, babies are increasingly able to recognize relations between actions and reactions, to engage in voluntary activities, and to anticipate the consequences of such activities.

Emergence of Seven-Month Wariness (Stranger Anxiety)

The development of a core sense of self is paralleled by an increasing ability to engage in social discriminations. Between 4 and 6 months the baby begins to respond to more than one person at a time. At about this time a wariness of strangers first becomes apparent (Schaffer and Emerson 1964). The baby appears cautious and watchful in the presence of strangers. Often wariness is combined with expressions of interest and curiosity. Although facial expressions of fear begin to be noted at 6 months of age (Cicchetti and Sroufe 1978), outright fear in the presence of a stranger is not regularly observed until somewhat later (8 to 12 months), and even then it is dependent on the situation. Fear is most likely when strangers intrude rapidly and seek to pick up the infant (Horner 1980).

Affective Attunement

Infants of 9 months appear to be capable of joint attention. Not only will they visually follow the direction of the mother's pointing finger beyond her hand to the target, but after their gaze reaches the target they will look back at the mother and appear to use the feedback from her face to confirm that they have arrived at the intended goal. Similarly, babies at this time are increasingly capable of communicating intention and of sharing affective experiences.

Stern (1985) provides rich behavioral descriptions of the process of affective sharing that characterizes attunement. *Attunement* refers to that dimension of the caregiver's behavior that matches not behavior per se, but some aspect of the behavior that appears to underscore the baby's feeling state. In attunements, the matching is largely cross-modal—that is, the modality of expression used by the mother to match the infant's behavior is different from that used by the infant. These experiences play a role in the infant coming to recognize that internal feeling states are forms of human experience that are shareable with others. The baby's behavior is also beginning to be influenced by the emotional expressions of others—a phenomenon called *social referencing*. Taken together, Stern's sense of a core self and his sense of intersubjective self correspond to what self psychologists term the "subjective" or "existential self"—the "me" (Harter 1983).

Selective Attachment

By 10 months of age most infants not only exhibit wariness of strangers but also have developed selective attachments to a small number (usually three or four) of specific persons. There is usually a marked hierarchy among these various attachments, with the mother at top. Once attachment has developed, babies actively seek proximity and contact with the mother, particularly when faced with an unfamiliar or frightening situation. When they are with their mother they tend to comfortably play and explore the environment, but when mother is out of sight, the infants will very likely follow or protest, either immediately or after a short while. The term *separation anxiety* has been used to describe the distress exhibited by the baby when mother is unavailable.

The Strange Situation

Ainsworth et al. (1978) developed a research method for assessing the quality of attachment in 12- to 18-month-old children. The *strange situation* procedure involves a set series of 3-minute separations and reunions with a caregiver and with a stranger in an unfamiliar room. Children who show mild protest following the departure, who seek the mother when she returns, and who are easily placated by her (about two-thirds of a sample of middle-class 1-year-old American children) are considered the most *securely attached*. Infants who do not protest maternal departure and who do not approach the mother when she returns (about one-quarter of the sample) are characterized as *avoidant*. Children who become markedly upset by departure and who resist the mother's efforts to comfort them when she returns (about a tenth of the sample) are described as *resistant* or *anxiously attached*. Babies designated as showing *secure* attachments tend later to exhibit greater social competence and better peer relationships (Sroufe and Fleeson 1984).

The 1-year-old child's behavior in the strange situation provides a prototype for many of the social developmental changes during the next 2 years. The child's capacity to physically explore the environment, to engage in social interactions, to comfort himself or herself, and to derive comfort from others in the absence of the mother increases dramatically.

Separation-Individuation

In the period between approximately 10 and 16 months the child devotes considerable energy to practicing locomotor skills and exploring the environment. Early in this period, the infant will search for the absent mother or repeat "Mama." Later the child shows a greater tolerance for separation and may seem unconcerned with the mother's whereabouts.

Between 16 to 24 months, ambivalence is often intense. The child seems to want to be united with but at the same time be separate from the mother. Temper tantrums, whining, sad moods, and intense separation reactions are at their peak. Mahler suggests that during this *rapprochement subphase* the mental image of mother is considered to be insufficiently strong to provide comfort in periods of upset.

Between 24 and 36 months, *negativism, willfulness,* and *contrariness* give way to a new realization of social demands. Disappointment, frustration, and absence of mother become better tolerated as the child's mental representation of the mother develops more stability. Not only is the mother clearly perceived as a separate person in the outside world, but the internal representations of her "good" and "bad" aspects are more solidly integrated. The availability of a secure and reliable internal representation of mother affords comfort when she is absent.

Between 18 months and 3 years, the development of language contributes to the further organization of the sense of self and the sense of others. Language provides the self and other with a new medium for exchange with which to create shared meanings. With the advent of what Stern (1985) refers to as the "verbal self," children begin to see themselves objectively. By 18 months of age they are able to recognize themselves in mirrors, still pictures, and videotapes. By 2 years they begin to use "I" to refer to themselves, and shortly thereafter to call other people "you." Genetic, prenatal-hormonal, pubertal-hormonal, and socialization factors all contribute to the determination of subsequent sexual status and orientation, but for most children, gender identity becomes established as well.

Emotions in Toddlers and Middle Childhood

The recognition and labeling of the basic emotions of joy, sadness, anger, and fear develop earlier than those of emotions such as contempt and shame. By 2 years of age, children can dissimulate emotions and pretend to assume emotional states. Between 2 and 4 years of age, children produce increasingly appropriate facial expressions when provided with a verbal label, while between 3 and 4 years they begin to be able to designate what emotions are appropriate to particular situations. Emotional experiences become increasingly more clearly defined through the interaction of children with their social environment.

By 3 years of age, children have developed a well-articulated sense of both the subjective self and the objective self. The advent of language facilitates the capacity for symbolic play reflective of daily life experiences, as well as the identification and sharing of affective states. Children come to know the names of their feelings and when to display what affects, and increasingly to experience empathy. Between 3 and 5 years of age, the concept of a private self that is not observable by others begins to be elaborated. Expressed emotions, which encompass a full range of affects, fluctuate easily at age 4 but have become more stable by age 5. The ability to use language to distinguish among affects expands, as does the capacity to identify situation-appropriate emotions. Relationship patterns become more complicated, and rivalries, jealousies, secrets, and envy begin to emerge. Fantasies become increasingly complex. Behavioral differentiation of the sexes is minimal when children are observed or tested individually. Sex differences emerge primarily in social situations, and their nature varies with the gender composition of dyads and groups.

The period of middle childhood is marked by changes in the ability to regulate and modulate affects. Six-year-olds can be highly emotional, and angry outbursts are frequent. By age 7, children may appear to be moody and sulky, and complain that they are unliked and that people are mean and unfair. By age 8, children are described as impatient and demanding, frequently bursting into tears or laughing uproariously. Humor begins to play a role in the modulation of affects. A sense of right and wrong emerges, and children may feel guilty and inwardly unhappy and frankly sad if they have failed to live up to a standard. First-graders have come to appreciate that they cannot change—say, become an animal or a child of the opposite sex—and that the self is continuous from past to future (Guardo and Bohan 1971).

During this period children are also interested in defining their place in the family. Children fluctuate between love for family and worries about not belonging. Fantasies of having been adopted and having rich and powerful natural parents are frequent. The relationship between siblings is distinctive in its emotional power and intimacy. Studies of siblings throughout childhood and adolescence report a marked range of individual differences between sibling pairs in measures of friendliness, conflict, rivalry, and dominance.

During middle childhood, interests in relationships with peers and teachers expand. Childhood games with rules emerge as does a capacity for intimacy with a "best friend." However, the two sexes engage in fairly different kinds of activities and games. Boys play in somewhat larger groups, on the average, and their play is rougher and more expansive. Girls tend to form close, intimate friendships with one or two other girls, and these friendships are marked by the sharing of confidences. Boys' friendships are more oriented around mutual interests in activities. The breakup of girls' friendships is usually accompanied by more intense emotional reactions than is the case for boys. Boys in groups are more likely than girls in all-girl groups to interrupt one another, refuse to comply with another child's demand, heckle a speaker, or call another child names. Girls in all-girl groups are more likely than boys to express agreement with what another speaker has just said, pause to give another girl a chance to speak, and acknowledge a point made by another speaker (Maccoby 1990).

Between 9 and 10 years of age, children still define themselves in terms of concrete objective categories such as address, physical appearance, possessions, and play activities. Self-criticism is prominent, but children are also beginning to be able to accept jokes by others about themselves. The concept of family continues to be important to most children, although they often prefer to be either on their own, with friends, or with other adults who, like the parents, may serve as role models. There are well-developed capacities for empathy, love, compassion, and sharing, as well as outbursts of person-directed anger, self-evaluative depression, and self-centered righteousness.

■ ADOLESCENCE

☐ What Is Adolescence?

Adolescence has come to represent the developmental bridge between middle childhood or latency and adulthood. It also marks a discontinuity in development based upon biological, psychological, and social factors that set this period apart from both childhood and adulthood. Modern theorists suggest that developmental processes continue throughout the life cycle and that each phase or period may be subjected to a developmental analysis. In that sense this chapter on development is incomplete. Adolescence stands out because of the disruptions in behavior, the moodiness, and the difficulties in living, as well as the conflicts and strife with families that have been considered normative.

These popular opinions are striking in view of the fact that adolescence is relatively new on the developmental scene, partly so because there remains some uncertainty as to how to define adolescence and whether adolescence existed in preindustrial society or exists in non-Western communities (Esman 1990). From a sociological vantage point, the rites of passage that mark the terminus of childhood represent entry into adulthood rather than into an intermediate phase. More recent work seeks to define adolescence as a distinct subculture with its own lore and rules.

☐ Puberty

Biologically, puberty refers to attaining the capacity to procreate as a mature member of a species. The notion of puberty as a phase in the biological life cycle is more important from a psychosocial vantage point because the external characteristics (i.e., secondary sexual characteristics) of both sexes become prominent social signs. In females puberty occurs 2 years earlier than in males, and the first signs are breast buds, followed by the growth of pubic and axillary hair and the attainment of a feminine body habitus with broadening of the hips (Tanner 1968). In the United States, girls achieve menarche at a mean age of 12.7 years (Zacharias et al. 1970), with 5% beginning at 11 to 11.5 years, 25% at 12 to 12.5, and 60% by age 13. Nine percent of normal females experience menarche up to 5 years after the beginning of breast development. A height spurt also begins to take place at age 11 that peaks at 12 and then falls off at 14 or 15. Menarche is frequently followed by irregular anovulatory periods for 12 to 18 months, at which time a more regular menstrual cycle ensues (Tanner 1968).

In boys, the height spurt begins somewhat later, at age 12, peaking at around 14 years, and begins to fall by age 16 or 17. Correspondingly, the penis and the testes are already on their way to achieving adult size and form. Pubic and axillary hair likewise begin to be prominent, as does the masculine habitus, and there is deepening of the voice.

In both sexes these primary and secondary sexual changes correspond to activation of hypothalamic functions that in turn stimulate the gonadotropic hormones of the pituitary. These hormones stimulate both estrogen and luteinizing hormone at the periphery as well as testosterone, especially in boys. These changes are thought to be coordinated with maturation of the hypothalamic cells. They become less sensitive to the feedback dampening effect of circulating sex hormones. In males nocturnal emissions are observed to occur about a year after the secondary sexual characteristics develop, and mark the beginning of the capacity to procreate.

The regular trend toward earlier puberty, especially in girls, in European and American populations has been attributed to better diet. There is also some suggestion that menarche and physical maturity may have long historical cycles so that the early onset of puberty in our time may be a temporary event.

☐ Cognitive Organization in Adolescence

Piaget (1952) suggests that operational intelligence gained at age 7 is advanced *abstract* intelligence in adolescence. Achievement of the landmark of abstract intelligence, however, does not occur as uniformly at the age of 14 as previously thought. There are data to suggest that only 10% of 14-year-olds, and 35% of 16- to 17-year-olds, achieve formal operations. Sixty percent of those classified as gifted adolescents attain formal operations.

☐ Social Determinants of Adolescence

The social significance of adolescence did not take hold until economic gain became attached to long periods of education and continuation of economic dependency. One of the by-products of adolescence is the conflict experienced by biologically mature organisms who are still dependent on family support both socially and psychologically. At the same time, changing social patterns may affect youngsters from ages 12 to 18. For example, there are more than eight million one-parent families in the United States. In addition, divorce rates peak early in the first 2 years of marriage but then again just when families are rearing young teenagers. Other social forces involving the women's movement have changed family patterns, with both parents going out to work and women beginning or finishing their education just as their children can begin to be physically, but not psychologically, able to care for themselves. Poverty continues to have a major effect as well. Sociopathy, drug use, and legal entanglements associated with psychiatric disorder have much higher representation in the lower-socioeconomic-status classes.

☐ Psychology of Adolescence: Normative Studies

Adolescence was largely ignored by analysts until Anna Freud described a rapid oscillation between excess and asceticism during adolescence. She viewed the rapid swings of behavior and mood as secondary to the surgent effect on behavior of the drives stimulated by sexual maturity and the hormones of puberty. The instability of the newly stressed defenses against impulse was seen as the ego's contribution to the erratic behaviors being manifested.

Erikson's (1959) concept of "adolescent turmoil" and his concomitant notion of "identity diffusion" became the hallmarks of our view of normal adolescence. Although Erikson cautioned that diffusion was a maladaptive, temporary state, he implied that we all traverse the stage more or less. Only now do we generally accept the formulations of Offer and Offer (1975), who showed that, by and large, adolescence is more quiescent than was formerly thought. Offer and Offer studied two Midwestern middle- and upper-middle-class community high schools. Their findings, although based on only adolescent males, were later extended and verified by others (see Emde 1985; Hauser et al. 1991). The young men in Offer and Offer's sample were 14 years old and entering high school in 1962. Those individuals who were within at least one standard deviation from the mean in 9 of 10 scales of personal and social adjustment were the subjects of the study. Sixty-one adolescents were then studied more intensively by a questionnaire technique and were followed well into later life to determine outcome. To convey the advantaged status of the sample, it is worth noting that 74% went to college during the first year after high school graduation. They came largely from intact families, and through the 8 years of study, from 1962 to 1970, there were no serious drug problems or any major delinquent activity, and no one was arrested for political sit-ins. The group showed no visible generational gap or difference in basic values from their parents.

☐ Varieties of Adolescent Psychological Development

The Offers found three developmental routes, which they designated as *continuous growth* (23% of the sample), *surgent growth* (35%), and *tumultuous growth* (21%). The remaining 21% were not easily classified but were closer to the first two categories than the third. In the continuous growth group, major separation, death, and severe illness were less frequent. Parents were described as encouraging independence, and the adolescents showed a capacity for what was described as good human relationships. They were able to achieve Eriksonian intimacy and to display shame and guilt, and had few problems of major intrapsychic complexity as far as the methods of investigation could provide. The surgent group were "late-bloomers," as the term implies. They were not as action-oriented as the first group and were given to more frequent depressive and anxious moments. They were often successful but tended to be less introspective and reported more areas of disagreement between parents about child raising. Finally, the tumultuous group reported recurrent self-doubt and conflict with their families and came from less stable backgrounds. Academically this group preferred the arts, humanities, and social sciences to professional and business careers.

The results of studies such as the Offers' (Offer and Offer 1975) and those of Block and Haan (1971) and Vaillant (1977) tend to negate the notion that turmoil is necessary for adolescent development. Block and Haan (1971) showed a persistence of character style as individuals develop. The 84 males and 86 females in the study were divided into five and six types, respectively. Among the males the following groups were isolated:

1. *Ego-resilient adolescents*
2. *Belated adjustors* (similar to Offer's surgent group)
3. *Vulnerable over-controllers*
4. *Anomic extroverts* (with less inner life and relatively uncertain values)
5. *Unsettled undercontrollers* (given to impulsivity)

The categories represented by these individuals are not meant to refer to pathological entities but rather to styles of adaptation. Block divided the cohort of females into six categories. As students of development, we can recognize the culture-bound stereotypes used:

1. *Female prototype* (obeying stereotyped descriptions of what the authors thought of as feminine in the 1980s)
2. *Cognitive type* (intellectualized in the way in which they negotiate problems)
3. *Hyperfeminine repressors* (close in description to persons with hysterical personality disorders)
4. *Dominating narcissists*
5. *Vulnerable undercontrollers*
6. *Lonely independents*

Hauser et al. (1991) studied a sample of 133 14-year-olds longitudinally. Almost half the sample had been inpatients in a psychiatric hospital. However, these authors' mode of study did not show crucial differences in the outcome of this largely middle-class group through their teen years. An ego scale was used that describes stages in maturation with designations such as preconformist, conformist, and postconformist. The authors found three paths of progression from the steady conformist group: early, advanced, and dramatic. This central group of progressive development represents the "team players" of adolescence and constitutes one-third of the group. Only 6 teenagers attained the level designated as a stage of integrity and conscience, the highest level on the scale. Their parental environment was of a model sort, but as a group they did not differ significantly from the steady conformists in the measures taken.

☐ Developmental Themes of Adolescence

Dependence Versus Independence

The *dependence/independence* interaction refers to the intrapsychic struggle for a sense of emancipation from the nuclear family that permits goals to be formed as a personal claim. Adolescents feel that they must extricate themselves from the caretaking hold of parents. They see their elders as either exacting gratitude or inducing guilt and shame as internal controls over individual action. On the other hand, these actions may strike families as egocentric and selfish.

In contrast to nuclear families, children growing up in collectivist societies, where the group rather than the parents is the controlling social force, find it very difficult to move into the larger society where independent individualized action seems to be required (Ainsworth 1962). The notion of an individual achiever and self-starter seems to be related to social values, and these values then become the prominent dynamism in regard to what Blos (1985) called a second separation-individuation phase. This is achieved only with ambivalence and conflict in many families.

License Versus Intellectualized Control

The conflict between *license* and *intellectualized control* is probably best exemplified by Anna Freud's descriptions. Adolescence may be a period of experimentation regarding sexuality, drug use, general disobedience, and other opportunities seen as temptations. Newly formed cognitive skills also permit intellectuality to be used as a controlling mechanism both on a defensive basis and as an interpersonal tool to resist indulgence of wishes and to help define one's goals during adolescence.

Family Versus Peer Group

The third theme, *group formation* in adolescence, is intimately related to the first two themes. Large or small peer group formation brings the adolescent's attempt at removal from family life into sharp focus. Whether this removal is used as a substitution for or regression from family life depends on how the group is used. During the juvenile period just prior to adolescence, or in early adolescence, Sullivan (1953) described the "chumship" as a time of same-sex social companionship and interest in which sharing and comparing of personal secrets take place. During this initial small group formation the adolescent is gradually made aware that companionship, companionableness, and the inner life can some-how now be translated into intimate relations with same-age, same-sex peers for developmental advantage. These small groups of two then gradually develop into larger groups.

Phenomenologically, young women begin to wear the same clothes and share the same style, and young men belong to a team and exhibit the common expressions of individuality in pairs, bringing to light a kind of twinning effect that then proceeds into larger group formation. The larger groups may be clubs, teams, or social groups. If these new social groups take on an antifamily stance or become indifferent to the values of the community, they may become degenerated groups or gangs. However, each adolescent in the group may then bolster his or her indi-vidual pride in the new group identity. New peer leadership is estab-lished as well that seems to the adolescent to be more caring and more responsive to his or her needs than parents have been in the past.

Among girls the adolescent breakaway from the family may center on romantic fantasies that another peer's parent(s) is more ideal than one's own parent(s). This "family romance" fantasy, which seems to be universal among both sexes at ages 6 and 7, is revived in adolescence. Together the young women plan together, discuss crushes, and plot strategies about romantic concerns. The sense of community that is gen-erated sometimes expands into threesomes, foursomes, and small group formation, or is manifested in better-organized group activities such as dancing, gymnastics, or intellectual clubs.

Normalization Versus Privacy

The *normalizing function of adolescent community* must be contrasted with the need for privacy. These two issues are sometimes, but not always, in opposition to each other. The normalizing function addresses issues of what the adolescent can tell a peer, what is private, and what the adoles-cent must feel is either sacred to the family or sacred to himself or herself. The tempting possibility of sharing a special fantasy with somebody in-volves risk taking for the adolescent and is an essential part of learning where he or she fits into the expanding world. Even as the adolescent clings to groups, he or she also craves privacy. The closed door, secret telephone conversations, diaries, and music blasting through earphones are but a few examples of the need to counteract the adolescent's urge to tell with his or her need to hide.

Idealization Versus Devaluation

While attempting to normalize his or her experience, the adolescent often spends a great deal of time in *idealizing and devaluing adults or peers.*

Crushes, pinups, and hero worship are the hallmark of the adolescent. Indeed, sometimes one's parent or parents may be temporarily idealized. The usual, expected adolescent sequence involves devaluing one's parents while at the same time idealizing a public figure or special teacher. Such idealization and devaluation, however, are fragile and frequently lose their power as rapidly as they are constructed. The slightest hurt or presumed injury is significant. A crush on a teacher or the longing wish to be a superstar quarterback or a prima ballerina may help the young adolescent to take the appropriate steps in the fulfillment of building ego ideals against which his or her own developmental progress may be measured.

Identity, Role, and Character

Identity, role, and *character* have been associated in the developmental literature with the name of Erik Erikson (1963), who contended that the sense of ego identity is "the accrued confidence that the inner sameness and continuity prepared in the past are matched by the sameness and continuity of one's meaning for others, as evidenced in the tangible promise of a 'career'" (pp. 261–262). The adolescent seeks to establish continuity with the past and to mentally work over the various and sometimes fragmentary idealizations and identifications to ultimately form a coherent unity in character. Thus, identity not only extends backward, but is projected forward in the form of establishment of goals, aims, and anticipated career and life-style. Identity contains many of the elements that might be addressed under concepts such as character and personality. It is important to note that adolescence is a period involving the rapid establishment of these presumed structures. If a failure occurs, there may be a functional breakdown akin to what Erikson called "identity diffusion," a condition that is marked by doubt, confusion, insecurity, and aimlessness.

Sexuality: Identity, Role, and Partner

Sexuality may be seen as a substructure of identity, but it is important during the adolescent period not only in terms of role establishment but in terms of matching one's core sexual identity with sexual role and sexual object choice. The early phases of sexual functioning are characterized by a recrudescence of masturbation, especially in males. It is only as the teenager moves into the second part of adolescence (ages 15 to 20) that the overuse of masturbation as a discharge channel gives way to more differentiated sexual activity that is guided by fantasies about others with a clearer determination of mental parties in pleasure. Whether this object is heterosexual or homosexual, the maturational thrust is in the direction of permitting one's sexuality to be expressed as a bid for an affiliation that ultimately will bind affection and bodily pleasure. One of the important aspects of masturbatory activity in adolescence concerns the idiosyncratic establishment of the masturbation fantasy created to satisfy many features of past problems and current understanding. In short, the adolescent can in fantasy be active and passive, sadistic and compliant, tender and vigorous, male and female. In fact, he or she can be an observer or exhibitor as well.

As adolescents move into the world and attempt to express their sexuality, they seek a person who more or less matches their mental object. Adolescents then attempt to work out the varying aspects of what is arousing and what creates a human interaction and brings the elements of satisfaction and security together. Sexual experimentation may take place. Adolescence is a time of dating, going together, and experimentation with others. Even if sexual intercourse or its arousing foreplay is not accomplished, it is on the mind of the adolescent. If the sexuality is enacted during adolescent turmoil and rebellion, developmental conflicts that correspond to issues concerning dependence and independence, license and intellectualization, and removal from family groups with sexual alliance are the themes of the enactment. Choosing someone who is the opposite of one's mother or father in appearance or removed from one's ethnic group may be an example of reaction formation in the face of threatened oedipal impulses. Nonetheless, choices too close to home may have the same meaning of oedipal patterning and dependency.

Young men, accustomed to counterdominance and competitive reactions to their own power assertions, may find themselves relating to women who agree with them and otherwise offer enabling responses. Young women, in interactions with men, are less likely to receive the reciprocal agreement and opportunities to talk that they have learned to expect from other women. Whereas the behavior of men in mixed-sex and same-sex groups tends to be similar, women's behavior in mixed groups is more complex. Some women become more like men—raising their voices, interrupting, and otherwise becoming more assertive than they would be when interacting with women only. Others appear to act as they do in same-sex groups, sometimes in exaggerated form, and may end up speaking less and smiling more than they would in a women's group.

Although patterns of mutual influence can become more symmetrical in intimate male-female dyads, the distinctive styles of the two sexes still persist (Maccoby 1990). On balance, the interactive styles of girls and women appear to put them at a disadvantage in cross-sex encounters, a factor of increasing importance as more and more women enter the workplace in traditionally male occupations. Moreover, the centrality of interdependence and caring relationships in the lives of girls and women tends to be viewed pejoratively by those persons, including many wo-men themselves, who stress the importance of self-actualization through competitive success (Gilligan 1982).

Reshuffling of Defenses (Style)

In the beginning of adolescence there is a tendency to project outward and to make adaptations that are alloplastic (i.e., externalized). The world, not the adolescent's inner wishes or aims, becomes the reason why the adolescent acts the way he or she does. Blame is placed outside of the individual; responsibility for actions are seen as exterior to the self. This tendency toward denial and projection has led some investigators to suggest that the adolescent acts in a way that may be dystonic to con-sensual reality. In other adolescents identifications take hold early in a firmer way, and reaction formations and repression begin to help the individual to cut loose from earlier oedipal ties. We begin to see in ado-lescents a clear establishment of defensive operations in line with pro-ductive work and adaptation using their idealized images as guides to planning future aims.

■ REFERENCES

Ainsworth MDS: The effects of maternal deprivation: a review of findings and controversy in the context of research strategy, in Deprivation of Maternal Care: A Reassessment of Its Effects. Public Health Papers No 14. Geneva, World Health Organization, 1962

Ainsworth MDS, Blehar MD, Waters E, et al: Patterns of Attachment: A Psycho-logical Study of the Strange Situation. Hillsdale, NJ, Erlbaum, 1978

Block J, Haan N: Lives Through Time. Berkeley, CA, Bancroft Books, 1971

Blos P: Son and Father: Before and Beyond the Oedipus Complex. New York, Free Press, 1985

Bowlby J: Attachment and Loss, Vol 1: Attachment. New York, Basic Books, 1969

Brazelton TB, Koslowski B, Main N: The origins of reciprocity: the early mother-infant interaction, in The Effect of the Infant on Its Caregiver. Edited by Lewis M, Rosenblum L. New York, John Wiley, 1974, pp 49–76

Bretherton I: Pretense: the form and function of make-believe play. Developmen-tal Review 9:383–401, 1989

Buhler K: Sprachtheorie. Jena, Fischer Verlag, 1934

Cicchetti D, Sroufe LA: An organizational view of affect: illustration from the study of Down's syndrome infants, in The Development of Affect. Edited by Lewis M, Rosenblum LA. New York, Plenum, 1978, pp 309–335

Cohen NJ, Eichenbaum H, Deacedo BS, et al: Different memory systems underly-ing acquisition of procedural and declarative knowledge. Ann N Y Acad Sci 444:54–71, 1985

DeCasper A, Fifer W: Of human bonding: newborns prefer their mothers' voices. Science 208:1174–1176, 1980

Eimas PD, Squeland ER, Josczyk P, et al: Speech perception in infants. Science 171:303–306, 1971

Emde RN: From adolescence to midlife: remodeling the structure of adult development. J Am Psychoanal Assoc 33(suppl):59–112, 1985

Emde RN, Gaensbauer T, Harmon R: Emotional Expression in Infancy: A Bio-Behavioral Study. New York, International Universities Press, 1976

Erikson E: Growth and Crises of the Healthy Personality. New York, International Universities Press, 1959

Erikson E: Childhood and Society, 2nd Edition, Revised and Expanded. New York, WW Norton, 1963

Esman A: Adolescence and Culture. New York, Columbia University Press, 1990

Field M, Woodson R, Greenberg R, et al: Discrimination and imitation of facial expressions by neonates. Science 218:179–181, 1982

Fonagy P, Steele H, Steele M: Maternal representations of attachment during pregnancy predict the organization of infant-mother attachment at one year of age. Child Dev 62:891–905, 1991

Freud A: The Assessment of Normality in Childhood. New York, International Universities Press, 1965

Freud A: A psychoanalytic view of developmental psychopathology. Journal of the Philadelphia Association for Psychoanalysis 1:7–17, 1974

Freud S: Three essays on the theory of sexuality (1905), in The Standard Edition of the Complete Psychological Works of Sigmund Freud, Vol 7. Translated and edited by Strachey J. London, Hogarth Press, 1953, pp 123–245

Gesell AL, Amatruda CS: Developmental diagnosis, in Normal and Abnormal Child Development: Clinical Methods and Psychiatric Applications, 2nd Edition. New York, Hoeber, 1947, pp 3–14

Gilligan C: In a Different Voice: Psychological Theory and Women's Development. Cambridge, MA, Harvard University Press, 1982

Guardo CJ, Bohan JB: Development of a sense of self-identity in children. Child Dev 42:1909–1921, 1971

Harter S: Developmental perspectives on the self-system, in Handbook of Child Psychology, Vol 4: Socialization, Personality, and Social Development. Edited by Hetherington EM. New York, Wiley, 1983, pp 275–385

Hauser ST, Powers S, Noam GG: Adolescents and Their Families. New York, Free Press, 1991

Horner TM: Two methods of studying stranger reactivity in infancy: a review. J Child Psychol Psychiatry 21:203–219, 1980

Huttenlocher PR: Synaptic density in human frontal cortex: developmental changes and effects of aging. Brain Res 163:195–205, 1979

Klinnert MD, Emde RN, Butterfield P, et al: Social referencing: the infant's use of emotional signals from a friendly adult with mother present. Developmental Psychology 22:427–432, 1986

Kuhl P: Linguistic experience alters phonetic perception in infants by six months. Science 255:606–608, 1992

Maccoby EE: Gender and relationships: a developmental account. Am Psychol 45:513–520, 1990

Mahler MS, Pine F, Bergman A: The Psychological Birth of the Human Infant: Symbiosis and Individuation. New York, Basic Books, 1975

Main M, Kaplan N, Cassidy J: Security in infancy, childhood and adulthood: a move to the level of representation, in Growing Points of Attachment Theory and Research (Monogr Soc Res Child Dev 50 [1–2, Ser No 209]). Edited by Bretherton I, Waters E. 1985, pp 66–106

Nelson K: Individual differences in language development. Developmental Psychology 17:170–187, 1981

Nelson K: Event Knowledge: Structure and Function in Development. Hillsdale, NJ, Erlbaum, 1986

Offer B, Offer JB: From Teenage to Young Manhood: A Psychological Study. New York, Basic Books, 1975

Piaget J: The Origins of Intelligence in Children. Translated by Cook M. New York, International Universities Press, 1952

Piaget J, Inhelder B: The Psychology of the Child. New York, Basic Books, 1969

Roffwarg H, Muzio J, Dement W: Ontogenetic development of the human sleep-dream cycle. Science 152:604–619, 1966

Sapir E: Language: An Introduction to the Study of Speech. New York, Harcourt, Brace, and World, 1921

Schaffer HR, Emerson PE: The development of social attachments in infancy. Monogr Soc Res Child Dev 29 (3, Ser No 94), 1964

Shapiro T, Perry R: Latency revisited: the age 7 plus or minus 1. Psychoanal Study Child 31:79–105, 1976

Skinner BF: Science and Human Behavior. New York, Macmillan, 1953

Spitz RA: The First Year of Life: A Psychoanalytic Study of Normal and Deviant Development of Object Relations. New York, International Universities Press, 1965

Sroufe LA, Fleeson J: Attachment and the construction of relationships, in Relationships and Development. Edited by Hartup W, Rubin Z. New York, Cambridge University Press, 1984, pp 51–71

Stern DN: The Interpersonal World of the Infant: A View From Psychoanalysis and Development Psychology. New York, Basic Books, 1985

Sullivan HS: Interpersonal Theory of Psychiatry. Edited by Perry HS, Gawel ML. New York, WW Norton, 1953

Tanner JM: Growth of bone, muscle and fat during childhood and adolescence, in Growth and Development of Mammals. Edited by Lodge ME. London, Butterworths, 1968

Vaillant GE: Adaptation to Life. Boston, Little, Brown, 1977

Watson J: Psychology From the Standpoint of a Behaviorist. Philadelphia, PA, JB Lippincott, 1919

Werner H: Comparative Psychology of Mental Development. New York, International Universities Press, 1957

Zacharias L, Wurtman RJ, Shatzoff M: Sexual maturation in contemporary American girls. Am J Obstet Gynecol 108:833–846, 1970

CHAPTER 5

Theories of the Mind and Psychopathology

Stephen S. Marmer, M.D., Ph.D.

■ THE PSYCHOANALYTIC TRADITION

☐ Freud's Theories

So powerful is the influence of the theories of Sigmund Freud that it is nearly impossible to think about personality or about psychotherapy absent of Freudian considerations. Even the proponents of most alternative theories accept parts of the Freudian legacy that were hotly contested a century ago.

Pre-Psychoanalytic Theories

Charcot's work in hysteria opened for Freud the path that eventually led to psychoanalysis. Rejecting that patients suffering from hysteria were either malingering or had a "wandering uterus," Charcot emphasized the link between their symptoms and traumatic events. That hysterical symptoms followed popular rather than anatomically correct malfunction of sensation or movement meant that symbolic factors were importantly involved. Further, Charcot demonstrated the role that hypnosis played in the treatment of hysteria. For him, hysteria was caused by trauma in susceptible individuals, yet the condition was also receptive to influence by treatment in the realm of ideas. Words, concepts, and symbols could be curative.

Freud's theory of hysteria implied a theory of the mind. At first, Freud thought that hysteria was caused by actual events, generally traumatic, the memories of which do not fade away in the usual fashion. After a traumatic event, painful memory is repressed. However, because of a memory's powerful emotional charge, hysterical phenomena are the direct result of reproductions or enactments of the traumatic event. Hypnosis was employed to get rid of the pathological memory.

Here several problems arose that forced expansion of the theory. First, it was nearly always the case that the removal by *abreaction,* or emotional release through discharge of painful affect, of a single memory rarely brought about cure. Every symptom had a multiplicity of "overdetermined" causes. Second, Freud was an indifferent hypnotist, and some patients found that talking freely was more effective. Some patients developed powerful emotional attachments to their doctors, which would eventually lead Freud to elaborate his theory of *transference.* Finally, Freud developed the theory that actual traumatic events, generally seductions, were not at the root of hysteria, although he never totally abandoned this view as a possibility in selected cases. This turned Freud from an exploration of actual traumatic experience toward an exploration of the world of inner fantasy. These latter two revisions, transference and fantasy, heralded central aspects of what was to become *psychoanalysis.*

Besides shifting from a direct trauma theory to one emphasizing fantasy, Freud also revised his thinking on the manner in which traumatic events influence the neurotic symptomatic response. Charcot had emphasized that trauma itself caused hysteria in susceptible individuals. In "The Neuro-psychoses of Defence" (1894/1962), Freud stated that it was not the trauma itself, but rather the defense against the recollection of the memory of the trauma and its affects that caused neurosis. Predisposition or susceptibility was deemphasized. What was defended against was the linkage of the memory and the affect. In hysteria, the affect could undergo "conversion" to a motor or sensory symptom that, although determined symbolically by the memory's ideational content, allowed for the removal of the idea itself from consciousness. "Obsessional neurotics" could not "convert" in this manner, and in these individuals both the affect and the memory data remained in consciousness but separated from each other. The significance here lies in the recognition of *defense* and in the acknowledgment that neurotic processes are at work in a variety of symptomatic situations. Moving from a directly causal trauma theory to one that employed the concept of defense enriched Freud's notion of mental life.

Topographical Model

Freud recognized that the bulk of psychic life lies outside of consciousness. It was his major contribution to psychiatric thinking to elaborate and illuminate unconscious mental life. Freud regarded this contribution as one of the two hypotheses fundamental to his psychoanalytic theory. The second, related hypothesis was that of "psychic determinism," which held that all mental events were causally linked to others in an associative network. These hypotheses were in turn bolstered and modified by Freud's discoveries about dreams (1900/1953).

The *topographical model* introduces the three "areas" of the mind: conscious, preconscious, and unconscious (Table 5–1). The conscious mind was already conceptualized within existing psychiatric and neurological theories. The enduring significance of the topographical model was to define unconscious mental processes as the field of psychoanalytic investigation and treatment. Freud's first concept of unconscious processes has been called the *descriptive unconscious.* By this, Freud was referring to the fact that mental life could not be limited to conscious or cognitive processes alone. The fact that comatose patients could report registering events that took place while they had been unconscious was enough to suggest that mental life continued even during periods when consciousness was interrupted. Similar proofs included the phenomena of posthypnotic suggestion, the very act of dreaming, and patients with dual or multiple personality. The concept of the "descriptive unconscious," which filled in the gaps in mental life and accounted for well-observed phenomena such as sleep or coma, predates Freud and aroused relatively little controversy.

Freud asserted that there are forces at work that keep mental processes and mental content unconscious, or that work to push the content of the unconscious into consciousness (Freud 1915a/1957, 1915b/1957). These forces constitute the *dynamic unconscious.* It is not merely that there is a neutral continuity of mental life at all times. Rather, the placement of mental content in consciousness or in the unconscious is a matter of the relative strength of powerful forces. Evidence of the power of these forces could be taken from examples of what Freud called the "psychopathology of everyday life" in his work of the same name (Freud 1901/1960). Examples would be a slip of the tongue that betrays one's true feelings in a setting where polite dissembling would be in order, or a behavior that reveals deeper disavowed feelings, such as a bridegroom stopping at a green light on the way to his wedding. In the clinical setting resistance to remembering is evidence that forces are at work to keep mental content out of the patient's awareness. Yet the memories, ideas, and affects that are repressed exert their effect through symptoms that symbolically express what was to remain unconscious.

Perhaps even more important than the dynamic unconscious is the theory of the "system unconscious." The system unconscious, which Freud abbreviated as the system *UCs,* works by a different internal logic than does the conscious mind. In this theory, consciousness, or more properly the system conscious (system *Cs*), is linked to sensation and

Table 5–1. The topographical model

	Operating system	Motivation principle	Descriptive position	Dynamic position	"System" position
Conscious	Secondary process	Reality principle	Within awareness	Not repressed; easily accessible	Word oriented; denotative; linear; time bound; declarative
Preconscious	Secondary process	Reality principle	Outside of awareness	Not repressed; can have relatively easy access when attention is focused	Word oriented; denotative; linear; time bound; can be poetic
Unconscious	Primary process	Pleasure principle	Outside of awareness	Repressed; difficult access; available in dreams and symptoms	Image oriented; connotative; nonlinear; not time bound; symbolic

perception, as well as to speech and the association with words. The apparatus of perception records events, which are then stored as representations, or mnemic images. The storage system arranges these images in a chronological sequence, and also into an associative system that connects related subjects. This unconscious storage system records "thing-presentations" that are related to memory traces, which may be linked to other "thing-presentations" according to the various affects and attributes that the "thing-presentation" possesses. Associative links are made by means of a logic system specific to the system UCs, called "primary process."

Primary process.   *Primary process* is the set of rules that govern the workings of the system UCs. Primary process is motivated by what Freud first called the "unpleasure principle," and later renamed the "pleasure principle" (Freud 1915b/1957). In the pleasure principle, unpleasure is avoided at all times, and drives seek discharge. Thus, under the pleasure principle, the motivation of the system UCs is to fulfill wishes and to discharge instinctual drives. Attachment to a particular mental content moves freely from one association to another, in what is called a "mobile cathexis," a terribly awkward neologism describing the concept of investment or binding of psychic energy. In primary process, time flows equally in both directions, permitting the blending of past, present, and future; an idea and its opposite may coexist, and mental contents are condensed and displaced freely.

Condensation is the representation of multiple ideas, memories, and affects in a single symbol. *Displacement* is the operation of taking attributes, affects, or aspects of one thing and attaching them to another. *Symbolization* is often listed as a third attribute of primary process. Since the system UCs operates on the basis of "thing-presentations," symbols rather than words constitute its language.

Secondary process.   The so-called system preconscious (or system PCs) and the system Cs work by the rules of *secondary process*. The basic motivating force in secondary process is the "reality principle," according to which gratification is delayed for other purposes. This delay of gratification required by the reality principle is made possible by, and in turn makes possible, delays in discharge of drives. Thus, attention moves more slowly from one thing to another in the associative path of secondary process. What has come to be known as "Aristotelian logic" is followed: time moves in forward linear direction, contradictions may not exist simultaneously, and thinking is more concerned with the content and logic of ideas than with their emotional intensity. The vocabulary of the system PCs and the system Cs consists of both "thing-presentations" and "word-presentations." Freud felt that an indispensable ingredient of consciousness was this linkage between the imagistic, visual thinking of thing-presentations and the linguistic, auditory thinking of word-presentations. This notion underlies the emphasis on psychoanalysis as a "talking cure," and on the power of verbal associations and verbal interpretations. It is precisely because thing-presentations, governed by the primary process in the system *UCs*, can be translated into verbal word-presentations, governed by secondary process in the system *Cs*, that conscious influences can gradually assert transforming control over the unconscious part of mental life.

Dreams and dreaming.   Dreams have always had a special place in the development of psychoanalytic theory, and Freud said that whenever he began to doubt the direction of his work, he would return to the bedrock of dream theory for renewed certainty. He called dreams "the Royal Road to the Unconscious." Through the analysis and self-analysis of dreams, Freud discovered the main points of his theory.

Dreams, according to Freud (1900/1953, 1917[1915]/1957), were the outstanding example of unconscious mental activity. Dreamers reported what Freud called the "manifest dream": the conscious rendition of what the dreamer had experienced during the act of dreaming. But even manifest dreams revealed imagistic content, with improbable actions, and frequent blending of past and present. Freud theorized that every dream contains several elements: *day residue,* which consists of the memories of events of the preceding day that retain unconscious emotional charge; and *nocturnal stimuli,* which may be noises within the area where the dreamer is sleeping, or may be enteroceptive awareness of bodily states (e.g., a full bladder). These relatively conscious elements are blended with *unconscious wishes* and the childhood memories associated with such wishes. Together, these constitute the *latent dream.*

In the process of sorting through the day residue and the nocturnal stimuli, the associative files to repressed unconscious childhood (or "infantile") wishes are stimulated. With the ability of the system *UCs* to make rapid associative links via the mobile cathexis of primary process, elements from different periods can easily be mixed. Because the dreamer is asleep, motoric discharge for these infantile drives and wishes is blocked, producing a dream experienced as a visual hallucination. The mere fact of exposure to these otherwise repressed wishes ordinarily would create anxiety, and in so doing might awaken the dreamer. Therefore, through the capacity of the system *UCs* to use the primary process operations of condensation and displacement, together with the innate symbolizing inherent in thing-presentations, the dream is disguised. The disguised dream affords the dreamer maximum expression of forbidden infantile wishes with minimum discovery. In this respect, dreams work the same way as Freud understood neurotic symptoms to work. They are both *compromise formations,* which simultaneously express and disguise, reveal and conceal, the underlying unconscious mental content, with its memories, associations, and drives.

The process of turning the latent dream into the manifest dream is called *dream work.* To the initial actions of condensation, displacement, and symbol formation is added the transformation of the dream after the dreamer awakens. This smoothing out of the logical contradictions in the dream to make it conform more to the rules of secondary process and conscious narration is called *secondary elaboration* or *secondary revision.*

The psychoanalytic approach to understanding a dream involves reversing the disguises of this dream work. Under the assumption of psychic determinism, every part of the dream comes into being for a reason related to the latent content of the dream and the dream censorship. Through the process of free association, the dreamer inexorably will be led back across the associative network to the original repressed memories and drives that stimulated the dream in the first place. The reliance on free association to understand dreams places emphasis on the individual's personal use of symbols. Although dreamers from a common culture or era have similarities that would lead them to use common symbols, Freud emphasized that it was the individual's own personal free associations, not a standardized "dream dictionary," that would lead to the latent dream meaning.

Instinctual Drives

Earlier in his work, Freud explained the cause of psychopathology in terms of his theory of trauma, particularly sexual trauma. When that theory was no longer tenable, Freud continued to preserve the central role of sexuality in the genesis of neurosis. He was able to reason that his patients had not universally been traumatized, but rather that they universally had sexual fantasies. This conclusion Freud deduced from his patients' dreams and associations, and most importantly from the transference.

Transference, which will be described more fully later on in this chapter, is the phenomenon whereby feelings and relationships from the past bend our perceptions and reactions in the present. For Freud, it was the capacity of individuals under the influence of transference to recreate their fantasies within the treatment situation that made him downplay actual trauma and emphasize fantasy in his theory of neurosis.

Instinctual drives are the form that physiological forces take in mental life. When the organism is stimulated, instinctual drives must be satisfied or relieved according to the basic principle of constancy. Thus, instinctual drives of all types become mentally significant as psychic energy. This energy has an innate tendency toward discharge, but may become attached ("cathected") to various mental representations on its way to achieving ultimate discharge, or may become bound or redirected.

Every instinctual drive has a pressure (or quantitative strength), a source, an object, and an aim. Because it was the maldischarge of sexual instinct that presented itself clinically in his earliest patients, Freud turned his attention to those instinctual drives first. Noting the frequency of childhood sexual fantasies, Freud postulated that sexuality begins not at puberty, as the then-prevailing view had it, but in childhood. For the adult, the source of sexual energy was excitation of the genital area, the aim was genital orgasm, and the object was a person who possessed the complementary genitals of the opposite sex. Matters were not so simple with childhood sexuality.

Sexuality can be broken down into component instincts (Freud 1905/1953). The first would be sucking. The pleasure that the infant gets from sucking is considered by Freud to be sexual in nature, and is termed "autoerotic." Soon the infant distinguishes the differences between sucking at the breast and autoerotic sucking. This is the phase of *orality*. In this phase the erotogenic zone is the mouth, and the aim is not only to nurse at the breast but to do all the things that a mouth is capable of doing, such as taking in, savoring, swallowing, digesting, and (later) biting, spitting, and remaining closed. As the child matures, the principal erotogenic zone moves to *anal* and *urethral* areas. Once again, what starts as direct pleasure in the sensation of urination and defecation generalizes to pleasure in what those zones can do, including such things as retaining, controlling, making orderly, expelling, and withholding. Sexuality next organizes in the *phallic stage*. Finally, childhood sexuality is bound during *latency*, when its energy is stripped for the next half-dozen years of its intense pleasurable affect and displaced onto other activities. It is this displacement that makes it possible for the child during latency to become absorbed with the cognitive tasks of school. Sexuality again reappears in its direct form in the true *genital phase*, which begins with puberty and goes on to adulthood.

Freud justified expanding his notion of sexuality beyond that of adult heterosexual intercourse for several reasons. There was the evidence of his early patients and their fantasies of childhood sexual experiences and yearnings. The transference, in which things that were not explicitly sexual in themselves took on intense sexual charge, also provided further evidence. Still further justification for Freud's expanded notion of sexuality could be found in the perversions. Finally, Freud noted the component instincts in normal foreplay: "oral" sexuality, such as visual stimulation and kissing; "anal" sexuality, such as mastery, control, and domination, and the switching back and forth between activity and passivity; and "phallic" sexuality, with its focus on the penis itself, concomitant with exhibitionistic activity and an emphasis on exaggerated masculine and feminine roles. These component instincts seen in foreplay lead to and heighten genital sexuality if the participants are normally sexually healthy.

In expanding the concept of sexuality, Freud was very explicit about the fact that his was not a theory of pansexuality. There was always an alternate category of instincts. In the earlier stages of Freud's work, the opposing categories of instincts were sexuality, also called "libido," and life-preservation, also called "ego instincts." At birth these two are joined in the "anaclitic" relationship between infant and mother. That is, the sexual pleasure in sucking is joined with the survival instinct in suckling. Freud hypothesized that, at first, the infant cannot distinguish between autoerotic sucking, the hallucination of the breast, and the real experience of sucking at the breast. As the infant makes this distinction, the survival ego-instinct and the pleasurable libidinal activity of the sexual instinct undergo a dysjunction, which, in turn, makes possible the beginnings of object relations.

Death instinct. The subject of the death instinct has been difficult and controversial for the psychoanalytic tradition. Freud acknowledges the hypothetical nature of his theory of instinctual drives; but the view that instinctual life consisted of libido in opposition to ego-instincts did not adequately explain such phenomena as sadism, masochism (Freud 1924/1961), or negative therapeutic reaction (i.e., when the patient gets worse the closer the treatment gets to the heart of the patient's issues). Nor could such a view explain the extremes of melancholia, excessively aggressive behavior in patients, or the symptoms of traumatic neurosis.

To further understand the dilemma Freud faced, we should review his reliance on the pleasure principle as demonstrated in his theory of dreams. Recall that dreams were regarded by Freud as the disguised fulfillment of an infantile wish. According to the pleasure principle, unacceptable anxiety-producing wishes emerge from the unconscious during sleep and are transformed by the mechanism of dream work into a manifest dream that allows the dreamer to continue to sleep by taking anxiety below the threshold of awakening. The purpose of the dream is to bring pleasure through maximum tolerable expression of a wish. If dreams were under the influence of the pleasure principle alone, how then could we explain the persistent existence of painful traumatic dreams repeated over and over again? We cannot unless we go "beyond the pleasure principle" (1920/1955) to another principle. In this second principle, the "nirvana principle," drive discharge is sought for the purpose of reestablishing quiescence and using stimulus barriers to restore the organism to an undisturbed state. The pleasure principle explains the rules governing the operation of libido, and the nirvana principle explains and underlies the operation of the death instinct.

The new instinctual drive, termed the "death instinct," consisted of three elements: 1) aggression and the tendency to create destruction and disorder; 2) the compulsion to repeat patterns and memories, even without constructive purpose; and 3) the establishment of stimulus barriers to achieve a state of quiescence. All three elements were seen to arise independent of the pleasure principle, but, "luckily," as Freud (1933[1932]/ 1964) noted, "the aggressive instincts are never alone but always alloyed with the erotic ones" (p. 111). The death instinct was a broad concept that Freud used to explain the phenomena of ambivalence, aggression, sadism, masochism, and severe melancholia, and the general operation of instinctual drives by the nirvana principle to establish stimulus barriers and to create a state of quiescence.

Narcissism and Object Relations

The topics of narcissism and object relations emerged naturally from Freud's instinct theory. Freud had indicated that every instinctual drive has a source, an aim, and an object. The object of an instinct is that through which the instinct is able to achieve its aim. It seems that Freud is implying that objects serve the purpose of providing satisfactory ways of achieving satisfaction for instinctual drives. Clearly the pleasure-seeking aspects predominate. However, as soon as we look carefully at what is involved in satisfaction of instincts, the situation becomes more complicated, because our way of relating to objects, though initially instinctually driven, soon becomes separated from the initial instinctual need.

Instincts start out in their component forms. Sexuality, for example, is expressed orally, tactilely, and visually, and is only later consolidated into a multifaceted whole. By the same token, the objects of these component instincts also start out as *part objects.* Mother's breast is the part object of the oral component of sexuality; her face is the part object of the visual component. The drives become progressively more consolidated, and the objects become progressively more whole, as development progresses. The biologically driven instinctual needs merge under the phase of so-called genital organization, and the child's ability to make out of his or her experiences with part objects a relationship with a complex, whole object is one of the main tasks of maturity in childhood.

The notion of object relations tends to emphasize the interplay or interrelationship between the subject and the object. On the one hand, objects are entirely fungible. One is as good as another as long as it can fulfill an instinctual aim. Presumably for a newborn, any nipple would be equally as good, and any bottle, any formula equally as good. On the other hand, during the course of development, the modes of relating to objects and our specific history with them leave a trail in our identity that is not at all fungible but highly particular. Freud, on the one hand, thought that objects were the easiest part of a drive complex to vary, and yet, on the other hand, he indicated that we never actually find objects, but that we indeed only re-find them. The psychoanalytic tradition demands that object relationships be thought of in terms of internal fantasy life as well as the real relationship.

In object relations the infant starts in a state of autoerotism, attached to the self and oblivious of external objects. As the ego develops, there is a stage of primary narcissism in which the individual is concerned with and in love with himself or herself. From this stage the child moves to a state of object relatedness that starts out as need related but in the course of frustration of these needs returns for defensive purposes to a focus on the self, called secondary narcissism. In secondary narcissism, the individual makes object choices of persons like himself or herself. These later object choices are narcissistic object choices in that we are drawn to people who are like the way we would want to be, or who in some respect help define who we are. We are then ever after influenced by our lost narcissistically held object.

Primary narcissism (Freud 1914a/1957) is a state in which the infant takes itself and its perceptions as a love object. This stage precedes the full acknowledgment of the external world as having a reality of its own beyond the infant. If development proceeds optimally, the child will become less self-absorbed and less omnipotent and will develop the capacity to love others for themselves. The child will also retain some reserve of primary narcissism to fuel self-confidence and self-esteem. In unfavorable development, which can come from neglect, conflict, or trauma, the child will develop narcissistic ties to others based on their ability to do things for the child or to maintain his or her self-esteem. In the resonating valence of secondary narcissism the child, in lieu of legitimate self-esteem, relies on others to define his or her very being and existence.

Anxiety

As Freud originally conceived it, anxiety resulted from an accumulation of sexual tension or dammed-up libido. Freud then believed that neurosis originated in the holding back from libido. Later in his thinking, Freud began to consider some of the differences between realistic anxiety and neurotic anxiety, anxiety as an affect, anxiety as a physiological reaction, and anxiety as connected with fear and fright. Anxiety can be bodily movements, an awareness of unpleasure, and an autonomic reaction.

Freud (1926/1959) concluded that psychological anxiety was in fact a signal phenomenon, and that neurotic anxiety starts as the remembrance of realistic anxiety. A real danger is one that threatens a person with an external reality. A neurotic danger is one that threatens him or her from a fantasy or from an instinctual internal demand. If an individual feels overwhelmed, he or she is placed in a traumatic situation. Also, if the person feels overwhelmed by an object on whom he or she depends for instinctual satisfaction or for survival, he or she is in a traumatic situation. Each stage of life has age-appropriate determinants of anxiety, beginning with the fear of birth, and moving through the fear of separation from the mother and the fear of castration. The fear of the superego is experienced initially as fear of its anger or punishment, and then as fear of its loss of love, and ultimately as fear of death. Generally speaking, when faced with a realistic anxiety, we fight or we flee. Faced with an internal neurotic anxiety, we generally act against the internal source; thus, we displace the anxiety by doing something with the drive to make it no longer dangerous to us.

Various forms of neurotic anxiety express themselves as phase-appropriate or age-appropriate prototypes, but earlier ones continue to underlie later ones, and later fears can revive earlier ones. This accounts for great complexity in our neurotic lives and is in turn accounted for by the fact that time flows in both directions in primary process. Indeed, anxiety produces repression and other defenses, rather than repression producing anxiety. The various transference neuroses can be understood in terms of the type of neurotic anxiety from which they emerged.

The Structural Model

In the structural model Freud proposed the division of the mind into id, ego, and superego. It should be emphasized that the structural and topographical points of view are neither incompatible nor exactly complementary; they are two different approaches to understanding the mechanisms of mental functioning.

According to the structural theory, the organism starts out as a poorly organized collection of drives. These drives are initially intensely physiologically driven. During this phase, the need to survive and the path to pleasure lean on each other. According to the original version of the structural theory, the ego does not exist at this phase, but the potential for the ego to exist begins immediately with perception. In fact, the ego owes its origin to and starts out from its activity of perception. In the course of perceiving, the ego discerns differences between internal and external; differences between pleasurable and unpleasurable; and differences between those perceptions that can be changed by body movement, those that can be made to disappear solely through mental acts, and those that the organism cannot influence. Thus the ego starts out as a function of the body that defines the mental image of the body; first and foremost the ego is a bodily ego.

One way the ego learns the difference between internal and external is through the sense of touch. This unique sensory modality is the earliest one in which the ego is simultaneously the organ that does the touching and the organ that is aware that it is being touched. Touching one's own skin thus becomes the beginning of learning who one is and what one's boundaries are. The distinction between the hallucinated dream or wish for the breast and the actual breast constitutes another way of distinguishing between internal and external, between real and hallucinated. The feeling of satiation that comes from the hallucinated breast does not last, in contrast to the feeling of satiation that comes from the real breast. Dreamed or wished mental content comes and goes for internal reasons. The mother and other objects in the world come and go of their own external volition. Thus the ego, in the course of its formation, begins to establish the *reality principle.* Rooted in perception, the ego is also anchored in reality, while the id, rooted in drives, is anchored in the pleasure principle.

The goal and mission of the id is to provide maximum pleasure through maximum fulfillment of the instinctual drives. The goal of the ego is to attain clarity of perception, accuracy of interpretation of the perceptions, and the greatest possible consonance with reality. Early on, the id learns, so to speak, that the hallucinations, dreams, and wishes of the pleasure principle are not ultimately as satisfying as the accuracy of the perceptions of the reality principle. The id forms an alliance with the ego, subordinating itself and its energy to the ego in return for the ego's help in focusing the organism's behaviors around the reality principle for maximum satisfaction of instinctual drives. Thus, during this period of cooperation, the ego gains enormous strength from the id.

The reality principle requires that drive discharge must be postponed, deferred, or redirected in order to meet the constraints of reality. The pleasure principle works on the basis of primary process, with mobile cathexis and rapid movement from one strategy to another so as to get immediate gratification. Thus, although the ego and the id start out as allies, they frequently find themselves working at cross-purposes, with the impatient id wanting immediate results, and the cautionary ego insisting upon delay. The ego's "weapon" against the id could be the refusal to cooperate for the purpose of achieving the id's goals; doing so, however, would defeat the ego's goals as well, for the reality principle is also a more sophisticated and comprehensive version of the pleasure principle in that it too wishes gratification. Through its capacity to understand time and to delay discharge, the ego understands that the shortest path is not always the most efficient one. The ego then inflicts anxiety upon the id, creating unpleasure for the id. The avoidance of such unpleasure is a paramount consideration for the id. One can say, in somewhat anthropomorphic terms, that the id starts out wanting fulfillment; finds an ally in the ego, which has access to valuable perceptions;

and engages in cooperation with the perceptual ego in order to accomplish its ends. However, the id, having soon enough given more power to the ego than it originally anticipated, now finds itself the recipient of unpleasure from its ally.

In the course of its evolution, the ego deals with an environment that more than any other single thing consists of the actions of the parents. The ego needs the parents and their cooperation and alliance every bit as much as the id needed the ego's perceptual cooperation. Thus, the successful pursuit of its mission to maximize pleasure according to the constraints of the reality principle requires that the ego understand and ultimately mold itself to the actions of the parents. In doing so, the ego becomes like the parents through identification. It needs the parents, but the parents, being separate individuals, are not always available. The ego takes the parents in and then has permanent mental representations of these important figures upon which it can rely in their absence. The expectations of the parents and the ego's knowledge of what it needs to do to get maximum cooperation from the parents form the basis of the *ego ideal*. The realistic awareness of those things that bring the ego unpleasure and diminish the cooperation between the ego and the parents becomes the basis of the *superego*.

The superego is initially auditory, coming from the perception of the word "no." The ego finds itself in relation to the ego ideal and superego in very much the position that the id found itself in relation to the ego earlier. The superego and ego ideal enforce a reality principle of an advanced form, a kind of moral reality principle rather than a purely perceptual reality principle, upon the ego. In similar fashion the ego offers some of its energy to the superego for maximum clarity of moral reality. The superego in turn uses its capacity to inflict anxiety to keep the ego in line. Thus, we have a finely tuned network in which the ego stands in relation to an id driven by the pleasure principle, reality understood by the reality principle, and the identification with important figures in the environment as a superego.

The superego starts out as harsh because the cognitive ability of the young child to understand the subtleties of the reason for prohibitions is absent. For example, the early, or "archaic," superego is extremely harsh because the small infant about to stick his finger into an electrical outlet is greeted with a loud "No!" from the parent, who might in addition slap the child's hand. The superego then is blunt, direct, harsh, and unequivocal. The archaic superego is incapable of a calm lecture on the dangers of electricity, but over the course of time a more mature superego might indeed function like that. In the resolution of the oedipal phase, the ego ideal and the harsh archaic superego blend to form a more mature superego, containing both punitive and loving elements, guiding the individual both for what not to do in order to avoid unpleasure and for what to do in order to gain maximum pleasure and self-regard.

The strength and harshness of the superego do not rest upon the actual harshness or gentleness of the parents during the oedipal period. Rather, the superego is an amalgam of real parental prohibitions, real parental approval, the ability of the child to overcome splitting defenses, the nature and power of the child's drives and fantasies, and the style with which the child metabolizes those fantasies.

Freud maintained that although there were in some respects no differences between ego and id, and that indeed they were parts of each other, a key difference had to do with the ways in which they were organized. The ego is the organized aspect of the id. The superego is a further organized aspect of the ego and thus the id too. At times it appears as though the ego is stronger than the id, in that it can cause repression and can inflict anxiety. Yet the ego is also powerless over the id. They react against one another and yet they are the same as each other, one being organized more along the lines of secondary process and the reality principle, the other being organized more along the lines of primary process and the pleasure principle. It is also important to remember that from the point of view of the descriptive unconscious, most of the functions of ego, superego, and id are unconscious. Occasionally, bits of the id emerge in consciousness and a bit more of the ego and the superego is also accessible to consciousness. Their forces interact with one another out of ordinary awareness.

Mechanisms of Defense

In order to function smoothly, the ego has to have a set of automatic operations with which to deal with the competing memories, perceptions, external realistic needs, drives, and anxieties that it faces. These automatic operations by which the ego balances its competing interests are known as *defense mechanisms*. Each defense mechanism employs capacities of the mind to alter mental content.

Freud listed nine defense mechanisms, and Anna Freud (1936/1946) slightly modified the list, adding a tenth. Valenstein (Bibring et al. 1961) generated a "glossary of defenses" that contained 24 basic mechanisms and 15 more complex ones. Vaillant (1977) discussed pathological defense mechanisms and adaptive coping mechanisms, expanding the list manyfold.

However we organize the list, it is important to remember that defenses not only ward off unacceptable mental content but are themselves mental content with accompanying fantasies (Wallerstein 1983). Defenses also yield pleasure by allowing a degree of discharge while simultaneously warding off the drive through negation or fantasy. We must analyze in detail the fantasy contained within any particular defense, remembering as well that there can be defenses not only against unwelcome mental contents but against other defenses (Wälder 1936). Thus defenses exist in hierarchical layers.

Each kind of psychopathology demonstrates its characteristic specific clusters of defenses. For example, in hysteria, repression and conversion are prominent defenses. In obsessive-compulsive disorder, isolation, reaction formation, regression, and undoing are the primary mechanisms. In paranoia and psychosis, introjection and projection are the primary mechanisms of defense. If one can know the diagnosis, one can infer the defense mechanisms most likely to be encountered in the treatment. Conversely, if one observes certain defensive operations in action, one can infer the diagnosis. One can also predict the form in which the transference will unfold by knowing the principal defense mechanisms utilized by a particular patient. The classical defense mechanisms as enumerated by Freud are briefly discussed in the following subsections.

Repression.   Repression is the defense that keeps from consciousness unwanted affects, memories, or drives on an unconscious basis. When something is successfully repressed, it is barred from access to consciousness, but it is also no longer amenable to further modification by the ego and can take on a life of its own in the form of a symptom complex or a portion of character structure.

Regression.   When the defense of regression is employed, we return to an earlier level of maturational functioning. We see mild regression in medically ill patients, and in college students when they return home on vacations.

Isolation.   Isolation separates affect from memory. It is a defense mechanism that is frequently employed by obsessional persons and, in its more common form, consists of both ideational content and affect having access to consciousness, but not at the same time. What is blocked is the link between ideational content and affect. In its extreme forms, patients who utilize isolation may be unable to feel too much emotion of any kind. Thoughts or affects are treated as though they were untouchable and therefore require distance.

Reaction formation.   In reaction formation, another defense mechanism frequently found in obsessional persons, affects are transformed into their opposites and ambivalence is resolved in the opposite manner from which it arises.

Undoing.   In undoing, a behavior is engaged in or a series of fantasies are indulged in that atone for a forbidden fantasy, affect, or memory.

Projection.   Projection is a complex defense mechanism that can operate at a more primitive or a more advanced level. Projection involves the fantasy of spitting, throwing, or in some other way hurling from ourselves some unacceptable mental content. This defense mechanism is prevalent in paranoia. The advantage for the person who is using projection is that he or she rids himself or herself of unwelcome thoughts and affects; the disadvantage, however, is that the projecting person then lives in a world of others who harbor toward him or her the unacceptable affects and fantasies that he or she wishes to disown. Once the affect is projected, one's ability to modify the content of the projection is severely diminished.

A more primitive form of projection is *projective identification,* in which not just unacceptable affect or pieces of mental content but rather identity itself is projected. Thus there is confusion between the identity of the person engaged in the projective identification and the person who is the recipient. An additional attribute of projective identification is that the recipient of this process, rendered especially open by virtue of empathy or intimacy, experiences the projective identification as a confusing identity-disturbing introjection of his or her own (Segal 1973).

Introjection and identification.   Identification is both a defense and a normal mechanism of growth. Important objects are taken in to avoid the pain of losing or being separated from them. When the identification is primitive, it is called *introjection,* more closely resembling unconscious imitation. When a child develops a low frustration tolerance and becomes irritable as a result of an angry parent's interactions, the child is "swallowing whole" this image of the angry parent and growing into it himself or herself. When the characteristics of a parent become the child's own in a way that allows the child to modify them as he or she matures, this is *identification.* Incorporation entails partial blending of the external object and the self. Identification implies that the traits of the individual no longer remain bound to specific memories but are acquired as one's own.

Turning against the self.   Any drive can be directed toward its object or turned back against the self or both at once. This is the basis of secondary narcissism and explains how sadism and masochism can be two sides of the same coin.

Reversal.   The defense of reversal is the process by which the aim of an instinct is transformed into its opposite, as in activity changing to passivity or passivity changing into activity. It is part of the elaboration of how sadism and masochism can alternate with each other. It is a defense very closely related to turning against the self.

Denial. Denial is the invalidation of an unpleasant or unwanted piece of information, and involves living one's life as though it did not exist. It is a more severe form of defense related to repression. It denies access to consciousness, but is more thoroughgoing and costly in that a piece of reality has to be not only ignored as in repression but actually invalidated. Thus, reality testing is diminished. Milder forms of denial may exist in transient ways.

Splitting. In splitting, aspects of mental content are kept separate. Initially this consists of keeping pleasurable affects and memories, and the "good objects" with which they are associated separate from unpleasurable affects and memories, and the "bad objects" to which they are linked. At a phase when the infant would be overwhelmed by unpleasure, splitting helps the child form good objects and an idea of a good self. In adulthood, splitting severely interferes with all important ego functions. Splitting creates "alternating univalences" rather than integrated ambivalence or a state of wholeness in which self and other can be seen as possessing good and bad aspects simultaneously. This defense is often seen in patients with borderline personality disorder as they alternate between overidealizing those who meet their needs and devaluing those who frustrate them.

Sublimation. Sublimation occurs when the ego functions to achieve maximum satisfaction of drives with minimum anxiety and minimum disruption of the environment.

Technique

If the cause of any psychopathology is the existence of unconscious forces at work, and if the mind works primarily in unconscious ways through unconscious defense mechanisms, then, in order to make proper diagnosis and treatment, one must look for ways in which unconscious forces reveal themselves to observation. It is in the transference that unconscious processes are revealed as indirect light reveals dust in a room or as a cloud chamber permits us to infer the existence of subatomic particles by the trail they leave behind (Freud 1912/1958, 1913/1958, 1914b/1958; Gill 1979).

The therapeutic alliance. A precondition for treatment is the establishment of a *working alliance* or *therapeutic alliance* (Greenson 1967). The patient is encouraged to associate freely, and the analyst is encouraged to have free-floating attention but to reserve interventions to one kind only: interpretations. The function of the analyst is to listen, accept, and interpret. Analysis is the interpretation of transference and resistance in the context of a therapeutic alliance.

Transference.   Transference is the relationship arising in the analytic setting to fill the gaps of the mild sensory deprivation that occurs in the analyst's office. We know that in full-scale sensory deprivation people will hallucinate to fill the void. In the very mild, carefully titrated, unilateral communicative freedom that exists in the psychoanalytic situation, the patient supplies through fantasy the missing or withheld judgments of the analyst. By not discussing reality, personal opinions, private reflections, or details of personal biography, the analyst leaves the field open for the patient to supply the missing details, and the transference emerges like a projective test. The style with which the patient reports material to the analyst, therefore, becomes a clue about how the unconscious processes of that patient work.

Transference is the set of feelings, beliefs, convictions, fantasies, and reactions that the patient brings into the analysis. We can infer that the patient brings those reactions to many important relationships and situations. Because of the analytic situation, the transference is allowed to flourish, is not diluted or diffused by ordinary conversation, and ultimately becomes the central focus of both the patient and the analyst in the form of the transference neurosis. This becomes the one event to which patient and analyst are witness in real time, giving it a status greater than either contemporaneous events of external life or the historical past. When present experiences and historical events of the patient's past are replicated in the analysis through the transference, one can have maximum confidence that one is dealing with the central and relevant features of that patient's mental structure.

Resistance.   Resistance is the phenomenon by which the patient does not participate in the analysis. Originally this meant resistance to free association, when the patient would not disclose what he or she was thinking. Now resistance means that the patient is in the act of resisting the ongoing nature of the analytic process of unfolding of the transference, free communication of mental content, and free flow of affect. Or he or she is trying to transform the relationship into something other than analysis by turning it into a friendship, into advice giving, or into problem solving (Schafer 1973).

Interpretation.   Interpretation is the articulation on the part of the analyst, and eventually on the part of the patient, of the connections and meaning of what is going on during the process of analysis. Interpretations are strongest and most comprehensive when, as in the example given earlier, they link the historical past to the current life situation and to phenomena within the analysis such as the transference.

To the extent that a treatment relies on the interpretation of transference and resistance, it comes closer to psychoanalysis. To the extent that it relies more on explanation, on theory, on construction of the historical past in lieu of the unfolding of the transference, on formulae for decoding rather than living through defense mechanisms, it moves into the realm of psychoanalytic psychotherapy or psychodynamic psychotherapy. To the extent that it focuses more on confrontation, on specific problem solving, or on teaching of techniques, it becomes more cognitive or behavior therapy. To the extent that the patient comes to treatment for direct solutions to problems, it most closely resembles counseling.

☐ Followers of Freud

Object Relations and the Self

Freud had included a theory of object relations in his classical theory. Instincts had a source, an aim, and an object. The oedipal period depended on the actual relationship with the parents, and Freud (1917 [1915]/1957), attempting to distinguish between the depression of normal mourning and the pathological depression of melancholia, talked about the influence of object relations. The word "object" of course is in contrast to the word "subject." Critics of psychoanalysis who point to use of the term "object relations" and contend that therefore psychoanalysis is not concerned with human beings simply misunderstand the usage of this term.

Freud (1917[1915]/1957) said that ordinarily when a significant object is lost to us, we enter a period of mourning, but that if the object relation was more of a narcissistic object choice than a true object relation, and if it was filled with intense ambivalence, then "the shadow of the object falls upon the ego." In other words, through identification we take in qualities of the object that then influence our ego state. Thus, a narcissistic object choice develops, in which others are not viewed in their own right but rather in terms of the extent to which they fulfill our needs. Thus, when they are lost, we have to incorporate them into ourselves in order not to feel that we are lost. Then the negative half of the ambivalence that we felt toward the object we now direct toward the self, hence melancholia. Freud never completed the elaboration of his object-relational theory—a task that was left to his successors (Greenberg and Mitchell 1983; Sutherland 1980).

Melanie Klein.   Melanie Klein (Klein et al. 1973) paid substantial attention to the process of pathological identification and to the fate of the incorporated object. She placed her emphasis on the discharge of the aggressive drives, and was less concerned with the source and the aim and more concerned with the object of the drives. Noting the child's tendency to split experience into good and bad, Klein postulated that the child first has relations with part objects and that only later in development does the child have relations with whole objects. Her theory said that this tendency to engage in projective identification, to get rid of our unwelcome impulses and our unwelcome incorporation of part objects, causes our internal mental life to be populated by chimeras and distorted and incomplete versions of objects; the more pathological splitting there was, the more split we would be in our internal mental life and the more vulnerable to ongoing distortion.

Fairbairn. W. R. D. Fairbairn was the first true object-relations theorist (Fairbairn 1972). Whereas Freud felt that the drive was primary and the objects were interchangeable, Fairbairn felt that the objects were primary and the drives were interchangeable. If for Freud anyone could satisfy the baby's hunger, for Fairbairn we were given hunger so that we could have a reason to make a human bond. For Fairbairn the ego is present at birth. Because it is immature and it cannot tolerate the intensity of stimuli, this pristine ego is then rendered asunder, splitting into a libidinal ego (which has an association with the exciting object) and an antilibidinal ego (which has an association with a rejecting object). The course of maturity, then, is to undo the split and reintegrate into a more robust central ego.

Winnicott. D. W. Winnicott pointed out that it is neither conceptually nor clinically proper to conceive of a baby without the mother as well. This viewpoint restores an interpersonal balance to psychoanalysis. A "good-enough" mother (Winnicott 1965) will respond to the baby's communications, meeting its needs within an optimal zone of frustration and gratification. Imposing her own needs, a pathological mother will force the baby to create a "false self" to protect its "true self." On the other hand, a mother who accepts increasing autonomy in gradual stages permits the child to have its own agenda while still remaining dependent on her. Under such circumstances the child can be himself in the presence of a mother who can be herself while they are still together. Winnicott called this "the capacity to be alone" in the presence of someone else. Winnicott also postulated an intermediate stage of separation-individuation during which the infant relates to "transitional objects" (Winnicott 1953) that are neither self nor other but form an intermediate zone.

Kohut. Heinz Kohut also placed emphasis on the relationship between self and object. Kohut (1971) postulated two lines of development, one involving the libido and conflict, and the other involving the development of the self. The development of a cohesive self requires optimal empathy that consists of mirroring and idealization. Mirroring is the experience wherein children define themselves by observing themselves in the gleam in their mother's eye. Kohut felt that the development of a cohesive self is more important than instincts.

Kohut's sensitivity to absences of phase-appropriate mirroring and idealization led him to emphasize deficiencies of emotional nutrients over conflicts as a cause of pathology. The narcissistic dilemma comes from object relations that were arrested in a phase during which others are seen in terms of how they help to define us. Kohut (1977) characterized this phase with the term "selfobjects."

With the introduction of "selfobjects," a new school within psychoanalysis began. The theory of self psychology emphasized the absence of crucial "emotional vitamins" as the main pathogenic feature of childhood. On the assumption that "a well-regulated self can manage its drives," repair of an incoherent self was seen as the task of psychotherapy. Interpretation of childhood manifestations in adult action came to be seen as less important than empathic understanding of the transference-expressed needs of the patient at that moment. Affective attunement between patient and therapist superseded genetic interpretations, and deficiency superseded conflict.

As self psychology has matured, new emphasis has been focused on the intersubjective nature of psychotherapy (Stolorow and Brandschaft 1987; Stolorow and Lachmann 1980). This new focus can be seen in technique, in which therapists influenced by self psychology are more likely to take personal responsibility for negative affects in the transference and are more likely to address the patient's experience of hurt than the patient's active role in his or her life frustrations (Fine and Fine 1990).

Kernberg.   Otto Kernberg's (1976) contribution to object-relations theory was to emphasize that affect, self representation, and an object representation always appear together. The infant is born unable to distinguish between internal and external and is only able to distinguish between pleasurable and unpleasurable experience. At first the child has difficulty distinguishing between realistic experiences and dreamed or hallucinated experiences. However, the infant can distinguish between experiences that feel good and experiences that feel bad—termed "passive splitting," so called because it occurs as a result of the maturational phase of the infant rather than an affirmative mental effort. Eventually, as the infant begins to distinguish between inner and outer, he or she develops active splitting, based on the fear that if the good and the bad were to get too close together the bad would destroy the good. Finally, the infant, growing into a child, begins to be aware of whole objects, to distinguish between internal and external, and to fuse good and bad. This fusion into a whole self and a whole object coincides with the maturation of the superego and the fusion between the old, archaic superego and the ego ideal. Tremendous energy is liberated as a result of this fusion because the energy necessary to keep splits apart can now be employed for other purposes.

Theories of Development

It is known that physically and cognitively the child grows in phases after birth until it reaches adulthood. Developmental theories assume that psychological growth also proceeds in phases, and the emotional capability of the child and his or her capacity for dealing with mental content, even the definition of what constitutes mental content, change according to the maturational stage. Developmental arrests, fixation points, and points of regression have an impact on the development of the particular psychological system at greatest risk at any given age. The correlation of psychopathology in adults with the developmental stage of presumed trauma during childhood was an important extension of the concept that childhood events influence adult states.

The classical theory of Freud and Abraham. The classical theory of Freud (1905/1953, 1925/1961) and Abraham (1968) holds that, at birth, the infant is in a state of autoerotism, in which the infant is attached only to itself, for a psychological sense of self per se does not yet exist. Gradually, through the experience of frustration as well as the emergence of the ego and the beginnings of the reality principle associated with the maturation of perception, the child begins to recognize that there is a distinction between internal and external, and a rudimentary form of object relations emerges.

The child's first main modality for relating is oral, meaning literally the mouth, lips, and tongue importantly involved in nursing. But orality also includes taking in of perceptions and "swallowing" the world of sensory perceptions. If there is excessive frustration, the child will retreat from early object-relatedness and establish a state of secondary narcissism. If frustration is moderate and optimal, the child will begin to recognize bit by bit that the objects of the world are not under his or her full control, nor is he or she under their full control. As the child matures, libidinal interest leaves the initial oral phase and enters an aggressive oral phase in which swallowing and taking in are replaced by biting and spitting. The child learns to say no, and this signals a crucial step in the differentiation of the child from others and the growing establishment of a sense of self (see Spitz 1965).

Next comes the anal phase in which questions of control over bodily contents and the nature of bodily contents are paramount. These issues are both literal in terms of weaning and toilet training, and metaphorical in terms of the functions that an anus is supposed to fulfill, namely control of time, delay of discharge, containment, making sure that everything is in its proper place, yielding to authority, and making judgments about whether one's internal contents are good or bad. Difficulties in this area will result in fixation at the anal phase and yield an anal character type, with overemphasis on parsimony, orderliness, and obstinacy. Disorders characterized by obsessive-compulsive behaviors are thought to result from fixations at the anal phase.

The third phase of development is the phallic phase, expressed by means of interest in the penis itself, which, according to the classical theory, for boys results in exhibitionism, and for girls a feeling of envy and inferiority. Modern theorists have importantly modified this aspect of classical theory.

Exhibitionism and its grandiosity lead to a heightened rivalry with the same-sex parent and usher in the oedipal phase. This oedipal period shows its earliest beginnings in 3- to 4-year-olds and culminates in 5- to 6-year-olds. The oedipal phase was seen as preeminent in neurosis because it was 1) the culmination of childhood libidinal development, 2) a multiperson interaction on which future social relatedness would be based, and 3) the hypothesized period of solidification for the superego—the time when gender identity was fixed and sexual object choice was decided. Moving from a two-person to a three-person world was momentous because it prepared the child to relinquish the fantasy of centrality in the universe. Conventions of society, values of culture, the ability to share, the roots of sublimation—all converge at this time. Oedipal issues were felt to be universal and would eventually emerge in every psychoanalysis. Neurosis was believed to be crystallized at this time. A latency period follows, interrupted by puberty and followed by adolescence.

Klein and Fairbairn.   Melanie Klein felt that the critical issue at birth was that the infant relies on introjection, projective identification, and splitting, and sees the world in terms of what she called "part objects." Aggression is preeminent and uncontrollable and cannot be neutralized. If successful, the child then moves to the depressive position by age 6 months when the realization occurs that objects are not entirely split but that they are indeed whole, and when the realization of the imperfection of the world and of the power of aggression takes hold.

Fairbairn (1972) felt that the ego is present from birth and that the child is object seeking, not pleasure seeking. According to Fairbairn a child is born with a pristine ego, but owing to conflict the child is forced to split off the unacceptable object relations and ego states. Thus, an "id" is created as a result of splitting the pristine ego and repressing the libidinal ego and its associated exciting objects. A "superego" is created by splitting off the antilibidinal ego and its associated rejecting objects. To the extent that these splits are deep and profound, the remaining central ego is impoverished and depleted with little in the way of mature object relations. The task of treatment and of maturity becomes restoring as much as possible to the central ego and reducing the libidinal ego and its exciting objects and the antilibidinal ego and its rejecting objects.

Bowlby.   John Bowlby, agreeing with Fairbairn that the child at birth was object seeking, asserted that there was a primary independent bonding drive that was not anaclitic, leaning on physiological survival, but autonomous and independent and had phases of its own. Bowlby (1958) offered five responses that make up attachment behavior: sucking, clinging, following, crying, and smiling, which are behavior patterns specific to man. Working quasi-independently but synergistically, each one has a specific trajectory and reaches its height during different months of the first 3 years of life. The components of attachment behavior influence the development of the cognitive sphere as well as the formation of character structure. In Bowlby's theory parent-child relationships are central and object relations are placed parallel rather than subservient to the necessity for instinctual drive discharge.

Balint.   Michael Balint described a stage of development in his more severely disturbed patients in which they developed a "basic fault" (Balint 1968). Balint adopted this term to indicate that some form of integration was missing in much the way an earthquake faultline would reveal the lack of integration of tectonic plates. The problem was one of integration, of something missing, rather than drives that were frustrated in their inability to find expression. Balint felt that this basic fault was caused by a failure of fit between the response of the mother and the needs of the child. Those persons who suffer from this basic fault will slip into one of two types of object relations: "ocnophilia," in which the relations with others are filled with great intensity and deep dependence, or "philobatism," in which objects are avoided and the inner world is intensely clung to. These two developmental alternatives then characterize the organizing principles for the reaction to the inadequate mother-child relationship.

Erikson.   Erik Erikson (1963) postulated eight phases of development, spanning the entire life and serving as nodal points for adaptation to the age-appropriate requirements of any phase of development, adding the concept of zones and modes. The zone of development is the organ system or cluster of physical and conceptual skills that the organism has at its disposal to deal primarily with that particular phase of development and its requirements. The mode has to do with the manner in which the developmental task is undertaken. For example, one might say that the zone of the oral phase is the mouth. The mode is that of taking in, of swallowing, and of digesting, spitting, or vomiting. When the oral mode is emphasized, we have issues of dependency and of neediness, hunger, and starvation that might operate quite independent of the oral zone.

Instead of using bodily zones to serve as signposts for his theory, Erikson chose the developmental task that exists at any particular age. *Basic trust versus mistrust* is the stage of acquisition of sense that the universe is reliable and that our most important object relations are consistent and available. *Autonomy versus shame and doubt* addresses the question of how much control of our body and our thinking can we attain, and how much will we be a disappointment to those around us and to ourselves. The phase of *initiative versus guilt* coincides with the issues of the oedipal phase for Freud and Abraham. During the stage of *industry versus inferiority* the child deals with latency and school. During puberty and adolescence is the phase of *identity versus role confusion*, our opportunity to clarify issues of personal identity and the depersonification of internal representations. Psychopathology around areas of identity confusion appears at this time. The young adulthood phase of *intimacy versus isolation* opens the task of rediscovering attachment and mature bonding. In midadulthood, the issue is *generativity versus stagnation*, and in maturity the questions concern *ego integrity versus despair*.

Margaret Mahler.   For Mahler (Mahler et al. 1975), the issue was not the progress of libidinal development but rather phases of separation and individuation. The key question of development was, To what extent does the infant, who is originally born without identity, acquire a sense of separate identity?

During the period from birth to 2 months, sleep-like states of the newborn and very young infant far outweigh states of arousal and are reminiscent of the primal states that prevailed during intrauterine life. The enhanced awakening and the increased perceptual experience of the infant permit a gradual distinction between what is inside and what is outside, and what is pleasurable and what is unpleasurable. Mahler feels that the mechanism of splitting arises in its first form during the *symbiotic phase*. The essential feature of this phase is an omnipotent fusion with the representation of the mother and a delusion of a common boundary between two physically separate individuals. The symbiotic phase reaches its peak at about 4 to 5 months of age, when it starts to decline as the beginnings of differentiation emerge.

Differentiation starts as a "hatching process" that coincides with a more permanently alert sensorium. The infant's attention during the first few months had been primarily inward; now it becomes more outward. It is at this phase that transitional objects become important. At about 7 to 8 months, the baby is beginning to move away from the mother, but can do so only for brief periods of time and then has to check back with the mother visually or tactilely. The stranger reaction and stranger anxiety of 7 to 8 months indicate the progress of the differentiation phase.

Practicing occurs from about 10 months to 16–18 months. The enormous expansion of the child's ability to be autonomous during this phase creates a state of imperviousness to disappointment that makes the child appear to be in love with the world. The child's ability to walk and to move away from the mother, together with the beginning of representational cognition (the precursor of speech), makes the child a more separate and autonomous person. By 18 months, the infant has matured sufficiently to recognize in a new way his or her dependency. During the practicing phase, the child had been preoccupied with all of the new skills he or she was acquiring that permitted greater separation. Now there is greater susceptibility to frustration, greater fears of object loss, and more awareness of separation and consequently greater anxiety. Mahler believes that the child alternates between periods of great need for closeness and periods of need for distance. During this subphase of *rapprochment,* the child needs to be refueled by intimate bodily contact and other kinds of communication. He or she will shadow the mother and will dart away and then come back and dart away again. Disturbances in this phase leave the child confused about autonomy; lacking a solid, cohesive self; and preoccupied with the dangers of separation—all of which might result in a clinging, dependent pattern or in a pattern of defiant, defensive disengagement.

The next subphase Mahler called the *consolidation of individuality* and the beginnings of emotional *object constancy.* This stage begins at 24 to 30 months and lasts in a major way for 2 to 3 more years and in a subtler way for the rest of one's life. In this subphase the child takes the progressive steps toward object integration, affective stability, and a synthesis between the previously separated good and bad experiences.

Psychopathology and Character States

The weakest part of psychoanalytic theory is that of psychopathology. Psychoanalysts have generally striven to understand the entire workings of the mind. Symptoms are regarded as signs of malfunction of internal mental processes rather than as diagnostic entities themselves. Hence, a phenomenological approach has never played the important role for psychoanalysis that it has for psychiatry in general.

When Freud began treating patients, most of whom presented with hysteria, he found that the repression of unacceptable mental content was the central feature causing the symptoms. He postulated that the symptom was like a dream in that it was a compromise formation that allowed partial expression of a repressed idea or affect. The obvious therapeutic course, therefore, was to make the unconscious conscious. This Freud could do relatively quickly, and in the early days of psychoanalysis treatment was very brief, perhaps sometimes only a few weeks in length. Over time it became increasingly clear that symptoms could not be separated from character structure. The shift from analyzing id content to analyzing ego mechanisms solidified this change of emphasis from symptom neurosis to character.

Abraham (1968) attempted to organize character according to the presumed stage of development that was malformed. Wilhelm Reich (1972) tended to classify character according to the predominant form that the neurosis took. Thus, for Reich there were phallic characters, passive characters, dependent characters, obsessional characters, hysterical characters, etc. The goal, according to Reich, was to strive for a genital character. Reich's extremely important contribution to psychoanalysis was to emphasize the way in which character structure reveals itself directly and indirectly in the transference, which helped to shift psychoanalytic technique away from interpreting mental *content* in favor of interpreting mental *process.*

Classification of character states.   To understand an individual patient, one has to conduct a careful review of systems based on the patient's functional capacities and style of mental action. Within each of these categories one can make judgments about diagnosis and presumed underlying dynamics. There are six main areas that one must understand so as to classify properly a patient's character pathology (Table 5–2, derived from Kernberg's [1976] work).

Diagnoses.   Having done a review of systems, to evaluate a patient's character structure and psychopathology, one will reduce the likelihood of mistakenly being drawn astray by overreliance on the presenting symptoms. There is a spectrum of character pathology, from the individual who is primarily psychotic through persons with low, medium, and high levels of character structure, up through persons in the normal range. Those persons with borderline and narcissistic disorders, those who have an infantile personality, those with multiple sexual perversions without stable object relations or ongoing partners, hypomanic persons, schizoid persons, those persons with a paranoid personality, some persons who abuse substances, and those persons who are antisocial, chaotic, and impulse-ridden—all fall into the category of low character function and severe character pathology. Passive-aggressive persons, sadomasochistic persons, some of the better-functioning infantile and

Table 5–2. A classification of character states

Category	Psychotic organization	Low level of organization	Medium level of organization	Higher level of organization	Healthy organization
Instinctual development		Preponderance of pathological condensation of genital and pregenital strivings, with excess primitive aggression.	Pregenital, especially oral; regression and fixation points predominate.	Genital primacy attained.	
Ego and its defenses	Lack of good, consistent reality testing.	Splitting and related defenses (e.g., primitive dissociation, denial, idealization, devaluation, omnipotence, projective identification).	Uses repression-type defenses, but reverts to splitting-type defenses under stress.	Repression and related defenses (e.g., intellectualization, rationalization, undoing, projection).	Considerable conflict-free energy. Sublimation.
		Excessive splitting impairs ego's synthetic function.	Reaction formations coexist with partial expression of rejected impulses.	Inhibitions and reactive traits predominate. Constricted ego.	
		Direct expression of instincts is linked with defenses.	Inconsistent self.		
		Self not cohesive or integrated; mix of grandiose, and contemptible and shameful.			

(continued)

Table 5–2. A classification of character states *(continued)*

Category	Psychotic organization	Low level of organization	Medium level of organization	Higher level of organization	Healthy organization
Superego		Archaic unintegrated superego precursors.	Lack of integration; sadistic, with overidealization in ego ideal.	Integrated, though severe, harsh, and perfectionistic.	Less severe superego, more realistic ego ideal, integration between them.
Internalized object relations	Difficulty distinguishing between self and object. Fusion, symbiosis, or autistic thinking.	Part objects predominate; object constancy not fully established. Inability to love an object who frustrates. Self not stable. Good and bad self images not integrated. Identity diffusion. Inner world inhabited by caricatures of good and bad aspects of important objects.	Stable self and object world, but with severe conflictual relationships. May fragment under severe stress.	Stable self, stable representational world. Whole objects predominate.	Mostly whole objects, and a consistent, cohesive self.
Affect		Impaired capacity for guilt or mourning. Basis for self-evaluation constantly fluctuating between harsh criticism	Severe mood swings (according to relationship with superego and ego ideal).	Can experience guilt and mourning. Wider range of affects.	Wide range of possible affects.

	...and overidealized aspirations of grandiose notions.			
	Sexual and aggressive drives partially inhibited.	"Structured impulsivity."	Impulsive. Contradictory repetitive behaviors seen.	Sadistic, polymorphously perverse infantile drives.
	Good empathic powers. Able to love and to mourn. Excellent anxiety tolerance and frustration threshold.	Can have fairly deep and stable object relations, with genuine concern. Considerable empathy. Better anxiety tolerance.	Modest empathy. Slight anxiety tolerance.	Little empathy. Little conflict-free energy. Very poor tolerance of affects, especially anxiety.
Interpersonal	Moderate impairment of social adaptation. Problems may appear only in closest relationship (e.g., spouse, children).		Lasting, though turbulent relationships, sometimes promising intimacy that cannot be sustained.	Relationships tend to be need-gratifying or threatening. Chronic work failure and creative failure. Not nurturing to others when under stress.

(continued)

Table 5–2. A classification of character states *(continued)*

Category	Psychotic organization	Low level of organization	Medium level of organization	Higher level of organization	Healthy organization
Diagnostic groups		Infantile personality. Many of the narcissistic disorders. Most borderline patients. Antisocial, as-if, chaotic impulse-ridden, inadequate, and self-mutilating.	Passive-aggressive, sadomasochistic. Better-functioning infantile and hysteroid types. Many narcissistic, some borderline persons. Persons with stable sexual deviations with relatively stable object relations.	Hysterical characters, obsessive-compulsive, depressive-masochistic persons.	
		Persons with multiple sexual perversions, especially those without stable object relations or ongoing partners.	Cyclothymic persons.		
		Paranoid personalities, hypomanic, schizoid.	Some persons who abuse substances (especially food and alcohol).		
		Some persons who abuse substances (including gambling, eating, alcohol and drugs).			

hysteroid–type persons, many persons with narcissistic personalities, some persons with borderline disorders, some persons with some of the more stable sexual deviations with relatively stable object relations, some cyclothymic persons, and some persons who abuse substances, particularly those who abuse substances that are not illegal such as food and alcohol—all fall into the category of medium character function. The higher level of character function includes the persons with hysterical characters, obsessive-compulsive persons, depressive-masochistic persons, and the assortment of neurotic persons whose complaints are lack of sufficient creativity, difficulties in achieving intimacy, and inability to sustain creativity.

Borderline and narcissistic states.   Although there is general agreement that the borderline and narcissistic states are related to each other, investigators in the field nevertheless have considerable differences of opinion with regard to the details of these two states. Kohut wrote almost as if to imply that in his conceptualization nearly all of these patients have narcissistic disorders, and the tiny few who are so badly damaged that they cannot be treated with psychoanalysis are consigned to the borderline category. Kernberg seemed to conceptualize these persons primarily as suffering from the mechanisms of borderline personality organization and suggests that perhaps some of the most well-functioning group who have the lowest levels of aggression resemble those patients whom Kohut referred to as narcissistic. Masterson (1981) and Rinsley (1980) felt that there are many more borderline patients than there are narcissistic ones. Rinsley believes that the fixation point for narcissism is late in the rapprochement phase, because these are patients who generally have a higher level of function and more signs of maturity. Masterson felt that the predominance of grandiosity in these patients indicates that they are fixated in the practicing phase, as though stuck in the grandiose time warp characteristic of that phase.

The significance of one's point of view is that it will influence the sequence in which interpretations are given. For instance, Masterson advocated confrontation for borderline patients and interpretation for narcissistic patients, because the borderline patients lack a sense of identity and therefore will coalesce around the clarifying aspect of a confrontation, whereas the narcissistic patients will disintegrate if their fragile hold on well-being is punctured.

The Rediscovery of Trauma

The most exciting development for theory of the mind and psychopathology in the 1980s and 1990s has been the rediscovery of the role trauma plays in shaping personality and creating symptoms. Many authors (Davis 1990; Edelson 1990; Erdleyi 1990) have commented on the central role of trauma in the theories of the 19th century. Trauma was the linchpin for Charcot's theory of hysteria and Janet's notion of the role of dissociation in his theory of the mind.

It is not entirely clear what characteristics of the 1980s were responsible for this rediscovery. The posttraumatic stress disorders of the veterans of the war in Vietnam made a dramatic impact on American psychiatrists. The capacity of real trauma to have prolonged influence on symptoms and a debilitating effect on personality and adaptation forced us to rethink our assumptions about the relationship between trauma and the ability to function. Long-lasting dissociation and physiological instability in these patients could not be ascribed simply to preexisting conditions or to fantasy.

From the perspective of physical findings, pediatrics had become aware in the 1970s of the "battered child." In the 1980s, the awareness of the psychiatric findings exploded into public consciousness. Incest was found to be much more frequent than had been believed, and the results of childhood sexual and physical abuse were found to be longer lasting and more profound than previously thought. Whether the survivors of hijacking, hostage taking, kidnapping, or escape from religious or political cults, patients emerging from traumatic scenarios represented certain characteristic findings that challenged the field of psychiatry.

Both acute trauma (Herman 1992) and chronic trauma (Herman 1992; Horowitz 1991; Kluft 1985; Putnam 1985; Spiegel 1990) can cause psychopathology, and both can warp the formation of personality. Acute trauma is more likely to be limited to the traditional symptoms of posttraumatic stress disorder: flashbacks, numbing, and hypervigilance. Chronic trauma leads to an increase in dissociative defenses that place the memory of the full impact of the trauma at a distance. Somatization may be one result, with physical symptoms expressing the psychic pain of the trauma, as in the phenomenon known as alexithymia. The alexithymic person is unable to feel affect as emotions and instead feels it in the form of body sensations. Memory problems ranging from reduced concentration to amnesia can be another response.

Perhaps the most important finding in the rediscovery of trauma was the awareness of the profound impact and widespread nature of the defense of dissociation. Dissociative responses can range from feelings of partial unreality in the form of depersonalization and derealization, all the way to such profound identity disturbances as multiple personality disorder (Kihlstrom and Hoyt 1990; Marmer 1991). Although it appears that Freud (1920/1955) thought of dissociation as a basic defense unto itself, we now usually think of dissociation as a defense mechanism combining denial, repression, and isolation to detach the person from unbearable awareness—both ideational and emotional—of trauma and of the person's reaction to it. The effects of growing up in a dissociated state are severe and profound and can interfere with all aspects of cognitive and psychological development. Any part of the experience may be dissociated, or dissociation itself can become an organizing principle. In the latter case, thoughts, affects, body feelings, perceptions, memory, or concentration can be disconnected, singly or in combination. How the individual develops will depend on which combinations of the dissociative process predominate.

The thread that all these responses have in common is the organization of the mind that keeps the traumatic memory and its emotion out of awareness. All people develop the structure of their mind under the influence of nature, nurture, and fate (Winnicott 1988). Likewise, all people develop their personalities and their psychopathology in response to conflict, deficiency, and trauma. Traditional psychoanalytic theory emphasizes the concept of conflict, with different mental forces battling against each other, and fantasy struggling with reality. Self-psychology emphasizes deficiency, noting the effects on the formation of a coherent self when an insufficient supply of empathy is available during childhood. To these viewpoints is now being added an awareness of real trauma and the mind's reaction to it to form symptoms of somatization, alexithymia, flashbacks, numbing, hypervigilance, depersonalization, amnesia, dissociation, and repetition of trauma.

The pendulum of theory has a way of swinging too far in one direction, then too far in the other. Charcot and Janet focused on the innate vulnerability of some persons to real trauma. Freud called our attention to the complex way our fantasies can alter our perceptions and shape our personalities. Kohut and his followers make the question of lack of empathy their theory's fulcrum. Now a new wave of theorists in the tradition of Janet are again reminding us of the pivotal role of trauma. The student of psychiatric theory must remember that conflict and fantasy, deficiency and empathy, and trauma and dissociation are all present in everyone. The art is to see the correct proportion in each person.

■ DYNAMIC PSYCHIATRY

□ Jung

Carl Jung is one of the most voluminous writers in dynamic psychiatry, and the primary rival of Freud. Jungians have had only an indirect influence on general psychiatry and psychology, but have had a large influence in academic settings where psychoanalysis and depth psychology are taken seriously, as well as a substantial influence on psychotherapy in general and their own movement in particular.

Jung originally was a member of Freud's circle. However, several years after their collaboration began the two drifted apart permanently and irrevocably. Jung had had a wide background in philosophy, religion, and anthropology, as well as considerable psychiatric experience working with psychotic patients prior to and following his contact with Freud. The first significant difference between Freud (1925[1924]/1959) and Jung (1961) came on the question of libido and psychic energy. Freud had contended that libido was sexual, whereas Jung considered the libido to be the unitary force of psychic energy, not explicitly sexual, nor even limited to being sensual, but something closer to the *élan vital* of Henri Bergson.

Freud and Jung also disagreed about the nature of the unconscious. For Freud, the content of the unconscious was the product of the individual's personal history. Although the unconscious contained innate drives, its specific content consisted of the introjects, identifications, fantasies, memories, affects, and associations accumulated over a life span. For Jung (1966), the unconscious mind consisted of a collective unconscious, which was the storehouse of latent memories of our cultural past, our racial memory, the entire history of *homo sapiens,* and even prehuman memory, shared by all human beings as the psychic residue of evolution. Jung conceptualized the personal unconscious as constituting only a small portion of the total unconscious. In Jung's view, the ego was similar to the conscious mind.

The structure of the unconscious consisted of component archetypes. Jung (1964) conceptualized them as innate ideas (or preformatting) that ready us for real experiences. For instance, there is an innate idea of the mother that readies us for our real life experience with our mother. There are innate ideas of father, of hero, of leader, and so forth. These archetypes originate in the mind as a permanent deposit accreted over the generations as the categories into which human symbolic thought is preordained to be experienced. Archetypes are also dynamic systems that can act with partial independence.

Five archetypes define personality organization. The *persona* is the outward mask which balances the demands of society with internal needs. An individual may have both a public and a private persona. *Anima* and *animus* are the feminine and masculine prototypes within each of us. The *shadow* is the representation of animal instincts that human beings have as their legacy of evolution from lower animals. The shadow concept gives us passion, vitality, and zest as well as our concept of evil, devil, or enemy. The *self* holds everything together and attempts to produce unity, equilibrium, and stability by balancing various archetypes and complexes.

The mind has four functions or operations: thinking, feeling, sensing, and intuiting, which may be directed primarily to the inner world of subjective reality (i.e., introversion), or to the external world of objective reality (i.e., extroversion). *Thinking* is verbal and ideational, and consists of logic and reasoning. *Feeling* permits pleasure and pain, anger and joy, love and loss. It is also the faculty with which we make judgments about good and bad. Through *sensation* we acquire facts. *Intuition* is perception by means of unconscious processes, involving the essence of reality that lies beyond thoughts, perceptions, and feelings. Each faculty within the individual is either in unity or in opposition, or acts in compensation for weaknesses in another realm. Thus, the purpose of treatment is to restore balance and promote unity by means of understanding the component parts.

In keeping with the ontogenetic point of view emphasizing personal history, Freud held that the dream is the unique idiosyncratic product of the dreamer and reflects an amalgam of current life situations, recent events, and infantile wishes from important periods of childhood. From the phylogenetic perspective, Jung contended that the dream reveals imbalances in the unity of the self and is understood by identifying the archetypal meaning of the symbols in question.

■ REFERENCES

Abraham K: Selected Papers on Psychoanalysis. Translated by Bryan D, Strachey A. New York, Basic Books, 1968

Balint M: The Basic Fault. London, Tavistock, 1968

Bibring GL, Dwyer TF, Huntington DS, et al: A study of the psychological processes in pregnancy and of the earliest mother-child relationship. Psychoanal Study Child 16:9–72, 1961

Bowlby J: The nature of the child's tie to his mother. Int J Psychoanal 39:350–373, 1958

Davis PJ: Repression and the inaccessibility of emotional memories, in Repression and Dissociation: Implications for Personality Theory, Psychopathology, and Health. Edited by Singer JL. Chicago, IL, University of Chicago Press, 1990, pp 387–403

Edelson M: Defense in psychoanalytic theory: computation or fantasy? in Repression and Dissociation: Implications for Personality Theory, Psychopathology, and Health. Edited by Singer JL. Chicago, IL, University of Chicago Press, 1990, pp 33–60

Erdleyi MH: Repression, reconstruction, and defense: history and integration of the psychoanalytic and experimental frameworks, in Repression and Dissociation: Implications for Personality Theory, Psychopathology, and Health. Edited by Singer JL. Chicago, IL, University of Chicago Press, 1990, pp 1–31

Erikson E: Childhood and Society, 2nd Edition, Revised and Enlarged. New York, WW Norton, 1963

Fairbairn WRD: Psychoanalytic Studies of the Personality. London, Routledge & Kegan Paul, 1972

Fine S, Fine E: Four psychoanalytic perspectives: a study of differences in interpretive interventions. J Am Psychoanal Assoc 38:1017–1048, 1990

Freud A: The Ego and the Mechanisms of Defence (1936). Translated by Baines C. New York, International Universities Press, 1946

Freud S: The neuro-psychoses of defence (1894), in Standard Edition of the Complete Psychological Works of Sigmund Freud, Vol 3. Translated and edited by Strachey J. London, Hogarth, 1962, pp 41–68

Freud S: The interpretation of dreams (1900), in Standard Edition of the Complete Psychological Works of Sigmund Freud, Vol 4. Translated and edited by Strachey J. London, Hogarth, 1953

Freud S: The psychopathology of everyday life (1901), in Standard Edition of the Complete Psychological Works of Sigmund Freud, Vol 6. Translated and edited by Strachey J. London, Hogarth, 1960

Freud S: Three essays on the theory of sexuality, I: the sexual aberrations (1905), in Standard Edition of the Complete Psychological Works of Sigmund Freud, Vol 7. Translated and edited by Strachey J. London, Hogarth, 1953, pp 135–172

Freud S: Recommendations to physicians practising psycho-analysis (1912), in Standard Edition of the Complete Psychological Works of Sigmund Freud, Vol 12. Translated and edited by Strachey J. London, Hogarth, 1958, pp 109–120

Freud S: On beginning the treatment (further recommendations on the technique of psycho-analysis I) (1913), in Standard Edition of the Complete Psychological Works of Sigmund Freud, Vol 12. Translated and edited by Strachey J. London, Hogarth, 1958, pp 121–144

Freud S: On narcissism: an introduction (1914a), in Standard Edition of the Complete Psychological Works of Sigmund Freud, Vol 14. Translated and edited by Strachey J. London, Hogarth, 1957, pp 67–102

Freud S: Remembering, repeating and working-through (further recommendations on the technique of psycho-analysis II) (1914b), in Standard Edition of the Complete Psychological Works of Sigmund Freud, Vol 12. Translated and edited by Strachey J. London, Hogarth, 1958, pp 145–156

Freud S: Repression (1915a), in Standard Edition of the Complete Psychological Works of Sigmund Freud, Vol 14. Translated and edited by Strachey J. London, Hogarth, 1957, pp 141–158

Freud S: The unconscious (1915b), in Standard Edition of the Complete Psychological Works of Sigmund Freud, Vol 14. Translated and edited by Strachey J. London, Hogarth, 1957, pp 159–215

Freud S: Mourning and melancholia (1917[1915]), in Standard Edition of the Complete Psychological Works of Sigmund Freud, Vol 14. Translated and edited by Strachey J. London, Hogarth, 1957, pp 237–260

Freud S: Beyond the pleasure principle (1920), in Standard Edition of the Complete Psychological Works of Sigmund Freud, Vol 18. Translated and edited by Strachey J. London, Hogarth, 1955, pp 1–64

Freud S: The economic problem of masochism (1924), in Standard Edition of the Complete Psychological Works of Sigmund Freud, Vol 19. Translated and edited by Strachey J. London, Hogarth, 1961, pp 155–170

Freud S: Some psychical consequences of the anatomical distinction between the sexes (1925), in Standard Edition of the Complete Psychological Works of Sigmund Freud, Vol 19. Translated and edited by Strachey J. London, Hogarth, 1961, pp 241–258

Freud S: An autobiographical study (1925[1924]), in Standard Edition of the Complete Psychological Works of Sigmund Freud, Vol 20. Translated and edited by Strachey J. London, Hogarth, 1959, pp 1–74

Freud S: Inhibitions, symptoms and anxiety (1926), in Standard Edition of the Complete Psychological Works of Sigmund Freud, Vol 20. Translated and edited by Strachey J. London, Hogarth, 1959, pp 75–175

Freud S: New introductory lectures on psycho-analysis (1933[1932]) (Lectures XXIX–XXXV), in Standard Edition of the Complete Psychological Works of Sigmund Freud, Vol 22. Translated and edited by Strachey J. London, Hogarth, 1964, pp 1–182

Gill MM: The analysis of the transference. J Am Psychoanal Assoc 27(suppl):263–288, 1979

Greenberg JR, Mitchell SA: Object Relations in Psychoanalytic Theory. Cambridge, MA, Harvard University Press, 1983

Greenson RR: The Technique and Practice of Psychoanalysis, Vol 1. New York, International Universities Press, 1967

Herman JL: Trauma and Recovery. New York, Basic Books, 1992

Horowitz MJ (ed): Person Schemas and Maladaptive Interpersonal Patterns. Chicago, IL, University of Chicago Press, 1991

Jung CG: Memories, Dreams, Reflections. New York, Vintage, 1961

Jung CG: Man and His Symbols. New York, Dell, 1964

Jung CG: Two Essays on Analytical Psychology. Princeton, NJ, Princeton University Press, 1966

Kernberg O: Object-Relations Theory and Clinical Psychoanalysis. New York, Jason Aronson, 1976

Kihlstrom JF, Hoyt IP: Repression, dissociation and hypnosis, in Repression and Dissociation: Implications for Personality Theory, Psychopathology, and Health. Edited by Singer JL. Chicago, IL, University of Chicago Press, 1990, pp 181–208

Klein M, Heimann P, Isaacs S, et al: Developments in Psycho-Analysis. London, Hogarth/Institute of Psycho-Analysis, 1973

Kluft RP (ed): Childhood Antecedents of Multiple Personality. Washington, DC, American Psychiatric Press, 1985

Kohut H: The Analysis of the Self: A Systematic Approach to the Psychoanalytic Treatment of Narcissistic Personality Disorders. New York, International Universities Press, 1971

Kohut H: The Restoration of the Self. New York, International Universities Press, 1977

Mahler MS, Pine F, Bergman A: The Psychological Birth of the Human Infant: Symbiosis and Individuation. New York, Basic Books, 1975

Marmer SS: Multiple personality disorder: a psychoanalytic perspective. Psychiatr Clin North Am 14:677–693, 1991

Masterson JF: The Narcissistic and Borderline Disorders: An Integrated and Developmental Approach. New York, Brunner/Mazel, 1981

Putnam FW Jr: Dissociation as a response to extreme trauma, in Childhood Antecedents of Multiple Personality. Edited by Kluft RP. Washington, DC, American Psychiatric Press, 1985, pp 65–97

Reich W: Character Analysis, 3rd Edition. New York, Farrar, Straus & Giroux, 1972

Rinsley DB: Treatment of the Severely Disturbed Adolescent. New York, Jason Aronson, 1980

Schafer R: The idea of resistance. Int J Psychoanal 54:259–285, 1973

Segal H: Introduction to the Work of Melanie Klein. London, Hogarth/Institute of Psycho-Analysis, 1973

Spiegel D: Hypnosis, dissociation, and trauma: hidden and overt observers, in Repression and Dissociation: Implications for Personality Theory, Psychopathology, and Health. Edited by Singer JL. Chicago, IL, University of Chicago Press, 1990, pp 121–142

Spitz RA: The First Year of Life: A Psychoanalytic Study of Normal and Deviant Development of Object Relations. New York, International Universities Press, 1965

Stolorow R, Brandschaft B: Developmental failure and psychic conflict. Psychoanalytic Psychology 4:241–253, 1987

Stolorow R, Lachmann R: The Psychoanalysis of Developmental Arrests. New York, International Universities Press, 1980

Sutherland JD: The British object relations theorists: Balint, Winnicott, Fairbairn, Guntrip. J Am Psychoanal Assoc 28:829–860, 1980

Vaillant GE: Adaptation to Life. Boston, MA, Little, Brown, 1977

Wälder R: The principle of multiple function: observations on over-determination. Psychoanal Q 5:45–62, 1936

Wallerstein R: Defense, defense mechanisms, and the structure of the mind. J Am Psychoanal Assoc 31 (suppl):201–225, 1983

Winnicott DW: Transitional objects and transitional phenomena. Int J Psychoanal 34:89–97, 1953

Winnicott DW: The Maturational Processes and the Facilitating Environment. London, Hogarth/Institute of Psycho-Analysis, 1965

Winnicott DW: Human Nature. New York, Schocken Books, 1988

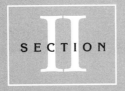

SECTION

II

Assessment

CHAPTER 6

The Psychiatric Interview, Psychiatric History, and Mental Status Examination

Stephen C. Scheiber, M.D.

The *psychiatric interview* is the essential vehicle for assessment of the psychiatric patient. The patient reveals what is troubling him or her in the context of a confidential patient-doctor relationship. The psychiatrist listens and then responds so as to obtain as clear an understanding of the patient's problems in the context of the patient's culture and environment as possible. The more accurate the diagnostic assessment, the more appropriate is the treatment planning (Halleck 1991).

The *psychiatric history* includes information about the patient as a person, the chief complaint, the present illness, the premorbid adjustment, the past history, the history of medical illnesses, a family history of psychiatric and medical disorders, and a developmental history of the patient. The psychiatrist obtains as much history as needed to arrive at a differential diagnosis. With subsequent interviews, the psychiatrist refines his or her working diagnosis and examines the influences of biological, psychological, cultural, familial, and social factors on the patient's life. During the course of taking a psychiatric history, the patient's perceptions of himself or herself and his or her experiences are evaluated, as well as the patient's perspectives on his or her problems, the goals of treatment, and the desired treatment relationship.

The *mental status examination* is a cross-sectional summary of the patient's behavior, sensorium, and cognitive functioning. Information pertaining to the mental status of the patient is obtained informally during a psychiatric interview as well as through formal testing. Informal information is based on the psychiatrist's observations of the patient and his or her listening to what the patient says. Categories of such information include appearance and behavior, eye contact, mode of relating, mood, affect, quality and quantity of speech, thought content, thought processes, and use of vocabulary.

Formal testing considers orientation, attention and concentration, recent and remote memory, fund of information, vocabulary, abilities to abstract, judgment and insight, and perception and coordination. The need for and specificity of formal testing are based on information and clues derived from the psychiatric interview (Othmer and Othmer 1989).

■ THE PSYCHIATRIC INTERVIEW

The single most important method of arriving at an understanding of the patient who exhibits the signs and symptoms of a psychiatric disorder is by the psychiatric interview. Common features of both the psychiatric interview and the medical interview include identifying data regarding the patient, the chief complaint, the history of the present illness, the significant past history, and the social history and family history. Distinctive features of the psychiatric interview include examining feelings about significant events in the individual's life, identifying significant persons and their relationship to the patient in the course of his or her life, and identifying and tracing the major influences on the biological, social, and psychological development of the individual. The interviewer gathers cross-sectional data related to the signs and symptoms of primary psychiatric disorders, such as anxiety disorders, mood disorders, schizophrenic disorders, and organic brain disorders—that is, those categorized under Axis I of the five axes of DSM-IV (American Psychiatric Association 1994). The interviewer simultaneously is examining for lifetime patterns of the individual's adaptation and relation to the environment in the form of character traits and, at times, character disorders that are described formally under Axis II of DSM-IV.

In the course of a thorough medical/psychiatric examination, the clinician elicits historical information, including genetic and family predispositions that may influence the type of problems that the patient presents, and completes a physical examination with appropriate laboratory and roentgenographic examinations to ascertain the patient's medical problems. Such problems are listed under Axis III of the DSM-IV. Axes IV and V are used to supplement the psychiatric diagnoses and estimate, respectively, the severity of psychosocial stressors and the highest level of adaptive functions currently and in the past year. As such, these axes have potential value in planning treatment and assessing the prognosis of the patient's condition.

The psychiatrist in the course of the interview assesses whether the patient exhibits psychotic thinking and/or behavior and whether the patient is harboring suicidal or homicidal thoughts or plans. The patient's capacity to control impulses is also assessed. If in the course of an interview it is determined by the psychiatrist that a patient may be a danger to himself or herself or to others by virtue of a major mental disorder, then the psychiatrist is obligated to consider psychiatric hospitalization to protect the patient and/or society.

In addition to being a process of eliciting information for the analysis of cross-sectional data to arrive at a formal diagnosis and to obtain information regarding the growth and development of the individual, the psychiatric interview is also a potentially healing event in which a patient, a suffering individual with psychiatric signs and symptoms, gains relief from his or her symptoms by revealing himself or herself in the context of a trusting, nonjudgmental relationship with his or her psychiatrist. During the course of a diagnostic interview the psychiatrist assesses which of several modalities of therapy could benefit the patient.

☐ General Considerations

Initiation

The initial contact for setting up a psychiatric interview is usually by telephone. The psychiatrist elicits enough information to determine whether the patient is in need of an immediate assessment and examination for a psychiatric hospitalization. If the psychiatrist judges that the patient may need hospitalization, the psychiatrist tells the patient to go to the emergency room, and then the psychiatrist either goes to the emergency room himself or herself or arranges for someone to evaluate (not admit) the caller.

Coordinating care with a referring physician is important, particularly when there are overlapping medical/psychiatric problems and when medications are prescribed. Many medications will alter the mental status of the patient (e.g., antianxiety agents, antihypertensive agents, anticholinergic drugs). Psychotropic medications can influence medical conditions (e.g., lithium and renal disease). The patient's physician is also an excellent resource from whom the psychiatrist may obtain objective information. If the patient agrees to psychiatric treatment, the primary physician is informed of this. The psychiatrist sends the referring physician a summary of his or her clinical findings, conclusions, and recommendations upon conclusion of the evaluation.

In initial contacts with a patient, the psychiatrist should ascertain whether the patient's presenting problems are appropriate for the psychiatrist's field of expertise. If the patient requests a particular treatment and the psychiatrist does not have experience with or believe in the efficacy of that treatment, he or she offers to refer the patient to a colleague with specific expertise. In addition to listening to the patient's problems, the psychiatrist advises the patient about what to expect when coming for an interview. The psychiatrist inquires about when the patient would be available to come for an evaluation and sets up a time that is mutually agreeable (Table 6–1).

Requests for appointments with a psychiatrist are also initiated by third parties. These can include relatives, treating physicians, judges, lawyers, employee health services, student health services, and others. In every instance, it is essential for the psychiatrist to learn what the patient has been told about requests for a psychiatric consultation or evaluation and to find out what the patient expects from seeing a psychiatrist. The purpose of the examination should be explicit. If a relative is calling it is important not only to ascertain what the patient knows of the call but to find out the reasons why the patient is not calling directly. The psychiatrist does everything possible to dissuade a family member from using deception in getting the patient to agree to an appointment. Third-party callers should also be advised of what information they can expect following a psychiatric examination. In most instances, without the patient's consent, no information will be shared. In the case of a minor, the information may be shared with the parent. If the purpose of an examination is to collect information as an expert witness in a court of law, then the patient is advised at the onset of the interview that everything he or she says may be used as part of the psychiatrist's expert testimony.

Table 6–1. Initial steps of the psychiatric interview

Background information	Determination of urgency
Reason for call	Primary physician's name and
Location of patient	phone number
How caller can be reached	
Presenting complaints	**Expectations**
Referral source's name and	Time for assessment
telephone number	Cost of evaluation
Treatment history	Purpose of assessment
Concurrent medical conditions	Psychiatrist's availability for
What patient hopes to gain	treatment

Time

The amount of time set aside for an initial psychiatric outpatient evaluation varies, ranging from 45 minutes for some evaluations to 90 minutes for others. If the evaluation is conducted at the bedside on a medical service, the length of the interview is often shorter, because of the patient's medical condition, and more frequent, brief visits may be necessary. In emergency room settings, the evaluation may be prolonged, particularly if hospitalization is in question and supporting data are needed from resources not immediately available, such as from relatives and treating physicians who have to be reached by telephone. If a patient is exhibiting psychotic behaviors during an outpatient appointment, the interview may be abbreviated if, in the judgment of the psychiatrist, prolonging the interview will aggravate the patient's condition.

Among the psychiatrist's first observations of the patient will be the patient's handling of time. A patient who arrives an hour early for an appointment usually is very anxious. Those arriving very late are very often conflicted about coming. Psychiatrists can learn much about patients' handling of time by exploring with patients the reasons for their tardiness. Psychiatrists need to be aware and conscious of their own handling of time as well.

Setting

The most important space consideration for a psychiatric interview is establishing privacy so that the interview proceeds in a setting where confidentiality can be assured. In academic settings, where audiovisual equipment and one-way viewing mirrors are used for teaching purposes, the patient is owed an explanation by the resident about the purposes for which recording devices are being used. The patient has the right of refusal regarding the use of such devices. Most patients attending a clinic in a teaching institution expect that part of going to such an institution for help will involve using teaching aids for residents.

The setting should promote comfort for both patient and psychiatrist. The height of chairs should be approximately equal in size so that neither party is looking down on the other. There should be no barriers between the patient and doctor such as a desk, and there should be sufficient lighting. Background sounds should be minimized. Hospital bedside consultations are difficult to conduct while assuring privacy; the psychiatrist should check with the nursing staff to see whether the patient's condition will permit his or her being moved to a quiet room. In hospital emergency room settings, a "quiet" room should be available with a mattress and no removable (potentially dangerous) objects. For a potentially agitated paranoid patient, unimpeded access to an exit door is important. For young children, a playroom setup with toys for the children to express themselves is preferable for diagnostic interviewing. Much formal training, skill, and experience are needed to appropriately evaluate a child in a playroom setting (Kestenbaum 1991).

Note Taking

The purpose of taking written notes during a psychiatric interview is for the psychiatrist to have accurate information to prepare his or her report of the interview. Neophyte interviewers tend to take extensive notes, because they are lacking in knowledge and experience regarding what is pertinent and relevant and what is not. If preoccupied with taking notes, the psychiatrist will often miss the patient's important nonverbal messages and will not pursue important leads in the interview. Another problem with extensive note taking is the failure to notice important aspects of the mental status examination, such as appearance and behavior. If the patient's resentment about note taking interferes with the interview, the psychiatrist refrains from doing so.

The psychiatrist should summarize his or her notes, observations, and conclusions as soon after the interview as possible. Prompt recording of data and information while still fresh in the psychiatrist's mind maximizes the accuracy of the information and minimizes distortions and gaps in the data base that will result when the psychiatrist delays his or her recording. The notes that are incorporated in the patient's record are necessarily more comprehensive following initial interviews than subsequent ones, because all of the data constitute new information. With subsequent interviews, only new, pertinent information needs to be recorded.

Interruptions

The time set aside and agreed upon for a patient interview is viewed as sacred and protected time for the patient. Calculated measures are taken to discourage interruptions, such as a sign hung on the door. Incoming telephone calls are screened by a secretary and the callers informed that the psychiatrist is with a patient. Sessions are interrupted only for emergencies.

Relatives or Friends Accompanying the Patient

When relatives arrive with the patient, the psychiatrist always interviews the patient first and indicates to relatives that he or she may wish to talk with them later. In the course of the patient's interviews, the psychiatrist can indicate his or her desire to speak with the relatives and explore the patient's feelings about the psychiatrist's doing so. The patient must grant permission before relatives are interviewed. If the patient refuses, the psychiatrist must respect the patient's wishes. Patients must also grant permission before the psychiatrist discusses their case with any other party.

An exception to this rule occurs when the psychiatrist judges the patient to be in imminent danger of hurting self or others and when the patient refuses voluntary hospitalization. In such an instance, the patient must be told why the psychiatrist is obliged to talk to a third party without the patient's permission. If the psychiatrist wants to meet with the patient's relatives, he or she must advise the patient whether this will be done with the patient present or alone. If in doubt, the psychiatrist opts to have the patient present. If the psychiatrist chooses to see relatives without the patient present, the ground rules need to be established with relatives that the psychiatrist is not at liberty to share any information obtained from the patient in confidence without the patient's permission but is at liberty to share with the patient information that relatives reveal.

Sequence

The formal assessment of the patient begins with the psychiatrist's initial observations of the patient. The psychiatrist observes the patient's appearance and behavior in the waiting area. At the beginning of the interview, the psychiatrist encourages the patient to speak as spontaneously and openly as possible about the reasons for his or her coming at this time. The psychiatrist establishes a primary posture of listening, allowing the patient to tell his or her story with minimal interruptions or direction. In the early part of the interview, if the patient stops talking, the psychiatrist encourages him or her to continue with comments such as "Tell me more about [a particular incident]." If the patient describes a significant event in his or her life and expresses no emotion, the psychiatrist inquires, "How do you feel about this?" The psychiatrist establishes that he or she is interested in not only the chronology of events that led to the the patient's coming but also the feelings that accompany such events, and encourages the patient's expression of these feelings. At times, when the expression of feelings is too overwhelming for the patient, the psychiatrist must not push the patient beyond his or her tolerance to express them. Once the psychiatrist has a grasp of the essentials of the present illness and accompanying feelings, he or she then shifts the focus to other subjects.

In the middle portion of the interview, the psychiatrist tries to learn about the patient as a person. There are numerous areas of the patient's life to explore: significant relationships, multigenerational family history, current living situation, occupation, avocations, education, value systems, religious and cultural background, military history, social history, medical history, developmental history, sexual history, and legal history, to name a few. The breadth of material requires several interview sessions for the psychiatrist to gather the pertinent data. As a rule, the psychiatrist moves from areas assumed to be of positive value to those of neutral interest and, finally, to those that the psychiatrist anticipates will be more emotionally charged for the patient. Throughout these initial inquiries, the psychiatrist is ascertaining the patient's strengths and weaknesses and is monitoring the responses to ascertain potential areas of conflict for the patient. The psychiatrist's follow-up inquiries will be guided by the responses to the initial questions.

In the concluding portion of the interview, the psychiatrist indicates to the patient the remaining time left. The patient is asked whether there are any important areas that the patient has not talked about. The psychiatrist asks whether the patient has any questions. The psychiatrist then answers each of the patient's questions. If the psychiatrist has insufficient information to answer a question, he or she tells the patient just that. At this time the psychiatrist shares with the patient his or her clinical impressions in words that the patient understands. The psychiatrist then presents a treatment plan to the patient. Psychiatrists have the ethical responsibility to try and assist patients to receive optimal care. On the other hand, patients must decide within the limitations of their physical abilities what is feasible for themselves and their families.

If records and information are available from other sources, the psychiatrist requests written permission to obtain medical records from hospitals or other physicians. If the psychiatrist wishes to contact others by telephone, he or she obtains permission from the patient before doing so. If the patient is receiving medical care from other physicians, the psychiatrist obtains consent to contact them. If the patient is reluctant to grant permission, the psychiatrist explains his or her reasons for wanting to initiate these contacts.

It is important to solicit patients' reactions to as well as agreement with a given treatment plan. Patients are entitled to know the various treatments that are available for their disorder. The psychiatrist shares with the patient his or her specific recommendations for treatment and responds to the patient's questions as to why the psychiatrist believes these suggestions are best for the patient. If the patient wishes an alternative plan, it would be best for the psychiatrist to postpone implementation of specific treatment until there is mutual agreement. There is a better likelihood for patient compliance when the patient understands a treatment plan and agrees to it (Nurcombe and Fitzhenry-Coor 1982).

☐ The Physician-Patient Relationship

Transference

Transference is a process whereby the patient unconsciously projects his or her emotions, thoughts, and wishes related to significant persons in his or her past life onto people in his or her current life and, in the context of the psychiatrist-patient relationship, onto the psychiatrist. It is as if the patient is reacting to the psychiatrist as if the psychiatrist were part of the patient's past. Whereas the reaction patterns may have been appropriate in an earlier life situation, they are inappropriate when applied to figures in the present, including the psychiatrist. This theoretical construct is borrowed from the psychoanalytic literature.

It is important for the psychiatrist to recognize these patterns and to treat them as distortions and not to respond in kind. An ultimate understanding of such unconscious behaviors is one of the goals of insight-oriented psychotherapy. In the early training of a psychiatrist, the psychiatric supervisor devotes considerable time to the resident's understanding of the process of transference so that the resident will not treat these reaction patterns as personal assaults.

Countertransference

Countertransference is a process whereby the psychiatrist unconsciously projects his or her emotions, thoughts, and wishes from his or her past onto the patient's personality or onto the material that the patient is presenting, thus expressing unresolved conflicts and/or gratifying the psychiatrist's own personal needs. These reactions are inappropriate in the patient-doctor relationship. In this instance, the patient assumes the role of an important person from the psychiatrist's earlier life.

One of the values of personal psychoanalysis for psychiatrists is to enhance their awareness of their unconsciously motivated behaviors so that they can better use their countertransference reactions to understand their patients. In their training, residents will be helped by a supervisor to examine their countertransference reactions so that these reactions will not interfere with patients' treatment but will aid the residents in understanding their patients.

Therapeutic Alliance

The therapeutic alliance is a process whereby the patient's mature, rational observing ego is used in combination with the psychiatrist's analytic abilities to advance his or her understanding of the patient. The basis for such an alliance is the trusting relationship established in early

life between the child and the mother, as well as other significant trusting relationships from the patient's past. The psychiatrist encourages the
development of this alliance, and both persons must invest in cultivating
the alliance so that the patient can benefit. The psychiatrist enhances this
alliance by his or her professional conduct and attitudes of caring, concern, and respect.

Psychiatrists accept and respect patients' value systems and their integrity as persons. Without a therapeutic alliance, patients cannot reveal
their innermost thoughts and feelings. Psychiatrists must never exploit
patients sexually nor gain financial advantages as the result of the doctor-patient relationship. They must never victimize patients by exploiting their role as physician healers.

Resistance

Resistance is a theoretical construct that reflects any attitude or behaviors
that run counter to the therapeutic objectives of the treatment. Freud described several types of resistance, including conscious resistance, ego resistance, id resistance, and superego resistance. Conscious resistance by
patients occurs for a variety of reasons, such as lack of trust of psychiatrists, shame on the part of patients in revealing certain events and aspects of themselves or feelings that they are experiencing, or fear of
displeasing or risking rejection by psychiatrists. One form of resistance
by patients is silence. The psychiatrist must acknowledge the difficulties
the patient is experiencing and encourage the patient to verbalize material that is difficult to express.

One form of ego resistance is *repression resistance,* whereby, for
mostly unconscious reasons, the same forces that led to the patient's
symptoms keep him or her from developing an awareness of the
underlying conflicts. A second type of ego resistance, *transference resistance,* can take many forms. Such resistance may occur when the patient
projects undesirable feelings onto the psychiatrist and ascribes these
feelings to the psychiatrist. This, in turn, can lead to the patient's attacking the psychiatrist, and a negative transference can result. A third type
of ego resistance is *secondary-gain resistance.* A patient's symptoms will
elicit nurturing responses from significant figures and will gratify his or
her dependency needs. Patients unconsciously resist giving up their
symptoms.

Resistance takes many forms. These include patients' censoring of
what they are thinking, intellectualization, generalization, preoccupation with one phase of life, concentration on trivial details while avoiding important topics, affective displays, frequent requests to change
appointment times, using minor physical symptoms as an excuse to
avoid sessions, arriving late or forgetting appointments, forgetting to

pay bills, competitive behaviors with the psychiatrist, seductive behaviors, asking for favors, and "acting out" (MacKinnon and Michels 1971).

Confidentiality

Psychiatrists are bound by medical ethical principles to not divulge any information that is revealed to them without patients' consent. They must protect patients and assume responsibility for seeing that no harm will come to patients by virtue of the patients' revealing information about themselves. If patients refuse to give permission to psychiatrists to reveal information, whether it be to a referring physician or in filling out an insurance form, psychiatrists must respect the patients' wishes.

In hospital or clinic settings, the patient is told about the types of information that will be recorded and who may have access to the information. When psychiatrists record information in the general hospital record, they record only those data that are pertinent to the overall care of the patient. In general hospital settings, it is preferable to have separate psychiatric records that can be housed and locked in an area separate from the general hospital records and to which only trained psychiatric personnel will have access. Only when patients are in danger of hurting themselves or others by virtue of their mental illness is the psychiatrist obliged to reveal such information in order to institute involuntary hospitalization. When third-party carriers are seeking psychiatric information, psychiatrists review with patients the information that has been prepared for the carrier and obtain patients' permission to submit reports.

☐ Interview Technique

Facilitative Messages

The most important component in the psychiatrist-patient relationship is the interest psychiatrists convey in their patients. The most important element in the psychiatric interview of patients is for psychiatrists to allow patients to tell their stories in an uninterrupted fashion. Psychiatrists assume an attentive listening posture; they do not ask excessive questions that would interrupt the flow of the interview. Some techniques to facilitate communication are described below (Table 6–2).

Open-ended questions.   An open-ended question reflects a topic that the psychiatrist is interested in exploring but leaves it to the patient to choose the areas he or she believes are relevant and important to share. The psychiatrist attempts to get the patient to relate in his or her own words, as much as possible, the most significant aspects of his or her

Table 6–2. Facilitative messages

Type	Example
Open-ended questions	"Tell me about . . ."
Reflections	"You're anxious about succeeding."
Facilitation	"Uh huh."
Positive reinforcement	"Good. That helps me understand you."
Silence	Long pause allowing patient to take distance from verbal material.
Interpretation	"When you can't perform the way you think you should, you try to do something to please."
Checklist questions	"When you feel 'nervous,' do you develop sweaty palms? heart palpitations? rapid breathing? butterflies in your stomach?"
"I want" messages	"We should explore other topics besides your depression. Tell me about your family."
Transitions	"Now that you've told me about your job, tell me what a typical day is like."
Self-disclosure	"When I've been in similar situations, I feel terrified."

problem. The psychiatrist may return later in the interview to fill in specific details if the patient fails to do so spontaneously.

Reflections.   The psychiatrist often wants to draw patients' attention to the affective concomitants of their verbal productions. One way of doing this is by rephrasing what the patient has stated and stressing the feelings that accompany a reported event. By restating the patient's verbalizations, the psychiatrist provides the patient with an opportunity to correct any misconceptions that the psychiatrist may have about the patient's condition.

Facilitation.   The psychiatrist uses body language and minimal verbal cues to encourage and reinforce the patient's continuing along a particular line of thought with minimal interruptions in the patient's flow of verbalizations. Examples of these cues include nodding of the head, or comments such as "Uh huh," raising of eyebrows, and leaning toward the patient. Facilitations indicate to the patient that the psychiatrist is interested in the particular train of thought and that he or she is attentive to what the patient is saying.

Positive reinforcement.   The subjects that the psychiatrist explores with the patient are frequently ones that the patient is unaccustomed to talking about and finds difficult to explain. When the patient has struggled with a particular topic and is then able to communicate clearly, the psychiatrist signals his or her approval by using positive reinforcement. Explicit statements of approval encourage the patient to verbalize more as he or she explores other areas of his or her life.

Silence.   The judicious use of silence when interviewing a patient is an important component of the psychiatrist's repertoire of interviewing techniques. Silences allow patients to take some distance from what they have been saying and can help patients place some order or enable them to better understand the psychological meaning and context of what has transpired in the interview. Patients often try to please the psychiatrist by continuously verbalizing in the belief that the psychiatrist wishes to have them speak continuously. It is often necessary for the psychiatrist to educate patients that silences are desirable.

Interpretation.   The psychiatrist works with patients to try and help them understand their motivations and the meanings of their thoughts, feelings, and actions. The psychiatrist examines repeated patterns of behaviors and draws inferences regarding these patterns. The psychiatrist may lead the patient in the direction of self-interpretation by taking certain pieces of data that the patient assumes are unrelated and helping him or her identify certain patterns. The patient can then piece together these seemingly unrelated events and feelings and draw inferences for himself or herself. Another way of interpreting is when the psychiatrist both presents the patterns of behavior and draws the inferences for the patient as a tentative hypothesis that the patient can then either accept or reject.

Checklist questions.   The psychiatrist spells out a list of potential responses for a patient when the patient is unable to describe or quantify to the degree of specificity that the psychiatrist believes is important to know in particular situations. A checklist of questions can be useful when open-ended questions do not yield the necessary information.

"I want" messages.   When the psychiatrist senses that an interview has failed to progress because of the patient's need to focus on a single theme, the psychiatrist asserts that they need to move on to other areas of inquiry. The psychiatrist is firm with the patient that sufficient information has been obtained about the single theme and that he or she understands the patient's concerns and feelings about that particular topic.

Transitions.   Once sufficient information regarding a particular part of a patient's history is obtained, the psychiatrist then signals to the patient his or her satisfaction with the understanding of that portion of the interview and invites the patient to move on to another area. These transitions allow the psychiatrist to guide the patient from one significant topic to another while signaling to the patient the areas that are important for the psychiatrist to learn about.

Self-disclosure.   The psychiatrist, at times, will judge that it is in the patient's best interest for the psychiatrist to disclose certain thoughts, feelings, or actions about himself or herself. This self-disclosure may be in response to the patient's questions, or it may occur when the psychiatrist believes that sharing his or her own experiences will benefit the patient.

Obstructive Messages

Obstructive messages tend to interfere with the uninterrupted flow of the patient's verbalizations and stand in the way of the establishment of a trusting relationship between psychiatrist and patient (Table 6–3). These communications are interview techniques that should be avoided. Some were learned in medical school, and psychiatric residents need to be coached in how to avoid using them.

Excessively direct questions.   Excessive direct questions represent the antithesis of open-ended questions. They occur when the psychiatrist directs the patient to a single response. This technique lends itself to the patient's answering only what is on the psychiatrist's list of questions. It presupposes that the psychiatrist alone knows the issues, priorities, and relevant information. The patient thus becomes a passive recipient of the psychiatrist's inquiries and fails to become an equal partner with the psychiatrist.

Preemptive topic shifts.   Rather than responding to the patient's cues about meaningful events, the psychiatrist moves from one topic to another, seemingly insensitive to what is important to the patient. Rather than focusing on the patient's shaky feelings and exploring this area in depth, the psychiatrist shifts to other areas that he or she wants to cover and fails to investigate issues that are of immediate concern to the patient. The patient is left feeling that the psychiatrist is unconcerned about the patient's troubles.

Premature advice.   The psychiatrist may assert his or her authority by telling the patient what to do without sufficient information and without engaging the patient in seeking solutions to his or her own problems. Rather than pursuing what may be the etiology of the patient's complaint and getting details of what may be going on in the patient's life,

Table 6–3. Obstructive messages

Type	Example
Excessively direct questions	**Psychiatrist:** What's making you sad? **Patient:** I've lost a girlfriend. **Psychiatrist:** Do you cry a lot? **Patient:** Probably not. **Psychiatrist:** Did you grieve inadequately? **Patient:** I'm not sure.
Preemptive topic shifts	**Patient:** I feel suicidal. **Psychiatrist:** Are you feeling despondent? **Patient:** I'm terribly depressed. **Psychiatrist:** Are you having trouble with your marriage? **Patient:** I can't say.
Premature advice	**Patient:** I have an upset stomach. **Psychiatrist:** You may want to try antacids and warm milk at bedtime and six meals a day.
False reassurance	**Psychiatrist:** You need not worry about your phantom pain—lots of persons with amputations experience the same problem.
Doing without explanation	**Psychiatrist:** I know what your problem is. You're suffering anxiety from too much stress. Cut back your hours of study. Take these pills three times a day. Start eating three meals a day.
Put-down questions	**Psychiatrist:** How can you continue to complain about your academic inadequacies when you have all A's and just made Phi Beta Kappa?
"You are bad" statements	**Psychiatrist:** You keep crying when you mention your mother—hysterics are known to do that.
Trapping patients with their own words	**Psychiatrist:** You just said you were pleased with your progress; now you are complaining that you're still depressed.
Nonverbal messages of resentment	Psychiatrist turns away from patient, shuffles papers on desk, and closes eyes when patient repeats same verbalization.

the psychiatrist advances a series of solutions that may be totally inappropriate for the patient. Such premature advice leads the patient to react with resentment and hinders his or her relationship with the psychiatrist.

False reassurance.   When the psychiatrist tells the patient that something will or will not occur and either has insufficient information to draw that conclusion or the clinical situation suggests that just the opposite may happen, then the psychiatrist is giving the patient false reassurance. Such responses serve to undermine the patient's trust in the psychiatrist.

Doing without explaining.   When psychiatrists do something to or for patients without reviewing their rationale and without getting the patients' consent, they falsely assume that patients accept their authority without question and are passive recipients of their ministrations. Other than in life-threatening emergency situations, psychiatrists as physicians are obligated to describe what they plan to do for or to patients and not only obtain consent in advance but elicit patients' cooperation as well.

Put-down questions.   Although the psychiatrist may pose a question, the underlying message is one of criticism, derision, or annoyance with the patient. Although there is no justification for ever attacking a person's appearance, couching disapproval in the form of a question is an indirect way for the psychiatrist to express his own feelings.

"You are bad" statements.   Another form of derision of a patient is when the psychiatrist, falsely believing that he or she is making an interpretation, makes a statement critical of the patient. The psychiatrist then places the patient in a defensive posture, while falsely believing he or she is interpreting the patient's behavior.

Trapping patients with their own words.   The psychiatrist may focus on contradictions in the patient's verbalizations to the point of trapping the patient. Confronting the patient with a contradiction in his verbalizations is counterproductive.

Nonverbal messages of resentment.   A psychiatrist may be annoyed or disapprove of a patient's behaviors. Rather than dealing directly with the patient, he or she uses body language to signal disapproval. Because of the psychiatrist's behavior, the patient experiences diminished self-esteem and feels demeaned.

☐ Specific Interviewing Situations

Interviewing the Delusional Patient

The psychiatrist's examination of the patient's delusional beliefs yields significant information regarding the patient's underlying psychodynamic conflicts. The psychiatrist can also observe how the patient defends against painful realities in his or her life and uses his or her delusional system as a form of protection. The psychiatrist looks for the precipitating stresses in the patient's life that led to the formation of these delusions.

The delusional patient is most often brought to treatment by third parties against his or her will. It is important for the psychiatrist to empathically acknowledge the patient's wishes not to be a patient, but also to point out how the psychiatrist may be helpful to the patient and to encourage the patient to communicate with him or her. Very often, as the patient's overall clinical condition improves, he or she stops talking about his or her delusional beliefs. It is not necessary for the psychiatrist to raise questions about the delusions, even though he or she may be curious about how steadfast the patient is in retaining the delusions.

Interviewing the Depressed and Potentially Suicidal Patient

The assessment of depression begins with the patient's appearance and behavior. The psychiatrist observes the patient's general demeanor and posture to be slowed. The patient walks slowly, holding his or her head down, and lacks in spontaneity. Some patients present with an anxious or an agitated depression, with the wringing of hands and pacing. Others exhibit a retarded depression, with a paucity of spontaneous movements. The pace of the interview itself is usually slow, with the patient responding to questions with long pauses and short answers. Very often there is a blunted range of facial expressions, and, at other times, the patient may cry or fight back tears. Not all patients will verbalize feeling depressed. They will often give clues through their verbalizations that indicate a sense of giving up and of not wanting to go on. A depressed patient's thinking and verbalizations are also slowed. Voice intonation patterns are often monotonal. Thinking often reveals excessive guilt, feelings of loss of self-esteem and self-confidence, and a general lack of interest in activities that the patient had previously participated in. These patients exhibit low energy, and their social contacts are diminished as well.

Because the patient often has a number of physical manifestations that are part of the depression, the psychiatrist explores problems with sleep, appetite, bowel habits, sexual functioning, and pain syndromes, among others. The psychiatrist explores the nature of these disturbances and how they have interfered with the patient's functioning. In exploring the origins of a depression, the psychiatrist looks for significant losses and separations in the patient's life. The psychiatrist should also explore anniversary phenomena, namely, depression that occurs on the anniversary of a significant loss.

The psychiatrist takes an active role when interviewing the depressed patient. The patient is encouraged to verbalize what he or she is experiencing. The psychiatrist empathizes with the patient's pain and mental anguish. Prolonged silences on the part of the psychiatrist are rarely helpful with these patients and should be discouraged. It is essential that the psychiatrist find out what kinds of thoughts the patient has had regarding suicide and whether the patient has ever acted on these thoughts, what plans he or she currently has, and what has kept him or her from acting on these plans. By pursuing the topic of suicide the psychiatrist arrives at a clinical judgment about the imminent danger of suicide in the patient's life. He or she also learns about what suicide means to an individual patient.

Interviewing the Psychosomatic Patient

Psychosomatic patients may interpret psychiatric consultation as a signal that their primary physician has given up on them. It is important for the psychiatrist to discuss with the referring physician what the patient has been told about the consultation and to ascertain what clinical questions the referring physician wants the psychiatrist to address in the consultation. Before seeing the patient, the psychiatrist reviews the patient's medical history, including medications and medical procedures, and the results of any tests.

After introducing and identifying himself or herself as a psychiatrist, the consultant psychiatrist reviews with the patient the complaints that led to the patient's seeking care. The psychiatrist then explores with the patient his or her understanding of the reasons for the primary physician's wanting a psychiatric consultation. The psychiatrist establishes his or her interest in the patient's physical complaints as well as any emotional concomitants, and also follows up with the patient in clarifying any misunderstandings about the psychiatrist's role as a consultant.

While reviewing the patient's medical history with the patient, the psychiatrist looks for clues of any psychological stresses that may be accompanying the patient's physical symptoms. The psychiatrist checks for autonomic signs of distress during the interview and inquires about the patient's feelings at these points. As the interview progresses, the psychiatrist reviews the specific circumstances that were occurring in the patient's life when he or she first became symptomatic, any significant antecedent events, and the range of feelings that the patient experienced with the onset of the illness.

The psychiatrist inquires as to how the patient's symptoms may be interfering with the patient's level of functioning, and looks for both the primary and the secondary gains of the symptoms. The psychiatrist explores what the patient feels is wrong with himself or herself, what he or she fears will happen as a result of the illness, and in what ways the symptoms will interfere with the patient's future life. Because the patient's presenting complaints are physical, the psychiatrist establishes that he or she is interested in these complaints and that in no way is his or her intention to minimize the significance of the complaints. The psychiatrist acknowledges that subjective complaints are real and that his or her inquiries about emotional concomitants are necessary to gain a better understanding of the patient.

Interviewing the Elderly Patient

Elderly patients often need special attention during a psychiatric interview. Psychiatrists usually need to slow the pace of the interview and may need several short interviews instead of one prolonged interview. They need to pay special attention to any physical limitations, whether they be sensory, motor, coordination, extrapyramidal, or other. The physical status of elderly patients needs special attention so that those with cardiac or respiratory limitations are not overly stressed in an individual interview session. The psychiatrist needs to review medications prescribed and those taken over the counter so that he or she is especially attuned to any drug interactions and aware of the influences of these medications on the elderly patient's mental status and behavior.

Interviewing the Violent Patient

Patients exhibiting violent behavior are most frequently seen in a hospital emergency room setting. One of the first judgments that psychiatrists must make is the safety of removing physical restraints from patients. If the patients are judged to be unable to communicate verbally or out of touch with reality, then the psychiatrists, before proceeding with their interview, request that the patients be placed in a quiet room where they may be restrained. If patients exhibit any hostile or belligerent behavior when the restraints are being removed, psychiatrists then request that the restraints remain in place until patients are calmer. The interview is often conducted with a security officer present, as the officer's uniform is often a deterrent for patients acting out their impulses. Psychiatrists emphasize to patients that the restraints are needed for both the patients' safety and for the safety of those persons in the immediate area.

Psychiatrists never confront or challenge violent patients. They let patients know when they are frightened by the patients' behavior, and seek assistance in placing potentially violent patients in a safe setting. On inpatient units, a seclusion room is used as a temporary placement for violent patients until their behavior is judged not to be dangerous to themselves or others. Psychiatrists work with available staff to maintain the safety of the patient, the staff, and other patients.

Interviewing Relatives

The psychiatrist can share any material with the patient that a relative presents. It is of vital importance to consider involving family members and other significant persons in the treatment of most (but not all) patients. Relatives' observations of the patient's presenting problems, their impressions of his or her current living situation, their understanding of the family, their knowledge of the patient's past history, and their recital of developmental milestones can aid in the diagnosis and add to the psychiatrist's understanding of the patient. Relatives can also participate in treatment and aid with compliance, such as with medications, and they can work with the patient and psychiatrist in noting significant changes in the patient's condition. The more serious the psychiatric condition, the more likely the patient will benefit from a relative's participation in assessment and/or treatment. The relative's participation is contingent upon the knowledge and agreement that the psychiatrist cannot without obtaining consent divulge to a relative material that the patient presented in confidence to the psychiatrist.

■ PSYCHIATRIC HISTORY

When recording the patient's history, a specific format is used, including patient identification, circumstances of referral, chief complaint, history of present and past illness, and history involving family, alcohol and drug use, sexuality, and medical background (Table 6–4).

☐ Identification of the Patient

The psychiatrist begins with a brief report of who the patient is, including the following:

- Full name
- Age
- Race
- National/ethnic origin
- Religious affiliation
- Marital status and number of children
- Current employment (past employment if the patient is unemployed)
- Living situation
- Total number of hospitalizations (and in each case the name of the hospital), including nonpsychiatric hospitalizations
- Total number of hospitalizations *for the presenting problem* (if the patient had been hospitalized)
- Name and phone number of the patient's primary physicians
- Name and number of the nearest living relative

Table 6–4.   Order of recording psychiatric history

1. Patient identification
2. Circumstances of referral
3. Chief complaint
4. History of present illness
5. Past psychiatric history
6. Alcohol and drug history
7. Family history
8. Past personal history
   a. Prenatal history
   b. Infancy and early childhood development
   c. Middle childhood
   d. Late childhood and adolescence
   e. Adult history
9. Sexual history
10. Medical history

☐ Circumstances of Referral

The psychiatrist describes how the patient came to see him or her, who referred the patient, and how the patient was transported. If a patient is referred by a professional, the name and phone number of the referring agent are recorded. If a third party brought the patient, the psychiatrist notes who this is and what the third party's relationship is to the patient. The psychiatrist records his or her judgment of the reliability of the third-party informant.

☐ Chief Complaint

The psychiatrist records verbatim the patient's reasons for seeking help at the time of the initial interview. If the patient is too disturbed to verbalize his or her reasons for being seen, a statement from a third party is recorded and the informant is identified. The chief complaint is not always evident in the first interview, particularly in patients with long, complex histories.

☐ History of Present Illness

The psychiatrist records the chronology of events that occurred from the onset of symptoms up to the present. With patients who can give a coherent account of their problems, the psychiatrist inquires when the symptoms began. The patient's highest level of functioning is established and a description is made of how the patient's problems are interfering with his or her optimal functioning. The psychiatrist examines the patient's functioning in the biological, psychological, and social spheres. The psychiatrist documents all the relevant symptoms and notes the precipitating stressors at the time the patient became symptomatic.

☐ Past Psychiatric History

The psychiatrist inquires about the first time the patient was aware of any psychiatric problems. The psychiatrist asks whether any help was sought at that time and, if so, inquires about the nature of the treatment, any medications, and the reason for discontinuing treatment. Significant events such as hospitalizations, as well as information on where they took place, which treatment modalities were used in these settings, and the length of stay, should also be noted.

☐ Alcohol and Drug History

The psychiatrist obtains history from the patient on the consumption of alcohol and drugs. Inquiries are made about the precise amounts that are consumed, frequency of use, and the method of administration. The psychiatrist learns about the patient's reasons for using drugs. Tolerance for drugs such as sedatives or narcotics is ascertained. The psychiatrist asks whether the patient has ever considered drug taking or alcohol consumption a problem and, if so, whether the patient has 1) overdosed on drugs, 2) lost consciousness in the past, and 3) ever suffered from withdrawal effects from drugs. Any previous efforts of withdrawal from addicting substances are noted including any problems such as delirium tremens with alcohol withdrawal. The psychiatrist also notes whether the patient has been in psychiatric treatment or has been treated in separate chemical dependency programs including self-help groups. The effects of alcohol consumption and drug taking on the patient's life are also evaluated. These effects include the patient's ability to maintain employment, his or her ability to maintain social relationships, and whether the patient has had any trouble with the law such as charges of driving while intoxicated.

☐ Family History

The psychiatrist reviews and records a family tree and lists names and ages of living relatives and names, ages, and time of death of deceased relatives. Any emotional problems as well as organic diseases in family members are indicated. Family histories are particularly useful in families who seem to have a genetic vulnerability for psychiatric or organic diseases, including schizophrenia, major affective disorders, Huntington's chorea, and epilepsy. The family history also describes who the significant relatives have been in the patient's life, what they were like as persons, how the patient related to them, and what roles they played in the patient's upbringing, as well as a description of current significant relationships.

☐ Past Personal History

The psychiatrist obtains information on the patient's past personal history in order to help determine a psychodynamic formulation of the patient's problems. The psychiatrist seeks to understand the critical past events that have led the patient to be the way he or she is today as a person. The clues regarding relevant areas to explore are gleaned from the patient's presentations of the present illness.

Prenatal History

The psychiatrist records information on the patient from conception to birth. The principal family members are described, and the environment and the household before the patient was born are noted. Data about any problems with the delivery, such as a caesarean section and the reasons for it, and any defects at birth are also important to record. Drugs taken by the mother, whether prescribed, over the counter, or illicit, are important to know.

Infancy and Early Childhood Development

The psychiatrist describes the early infant-mother relationship, noting any problems in feeding and sleep patterns, as well as developmental milestones and illnesses. Symptoms of unusual rocking behaviors, head banging, screaming, thumb sucking, temper tantrums, bed wetting, and nail biting are explored and recorded. Delays of motor activities, speech development, and socialization are noted. The psychiatrist examines the child's play activities. Independent behaviors and the capacity to concentrate and to look for social interactions are assessed. The psychiatrist also ascertains who the significant people were in the caregiving of the baby and what particular influences each had on the child's development. A description is given of each sibling and of how early sibling relationships developed.

Middle Childhood (Ages 3 to 11)

The psychiatrist inquires about nursery school experiences and how the child adapted to social situations. The child's reactions to first going off to school and leaving home are noted. The psychiatrist inquires about important figures in the patient's life, as well as about recreational, athletic, and cultural activities. The psychiatrist also records any prolonged illnesses, surgeries, and accidents with injuries and the influence of these medical/surgical events on the patient's life. The psychiatrist learns who meted out punishment and assesses the effects that these behaviors had on the child's development. The psychiatrist also explores any significant personal losses or separations during this period. Symptoms reflecting emotional distress are noted, such as enuresis, nail biting, night terrors, and excessive masturbation.

Late Childhood and Adolescence

The psychiatrist traces the biological development in terms of major body changes and their influence on the individual, and inquires about the child's interests and activities, participation in organized sports, hobbies, church activities, introduction to civic responsibilities, work history, social network, and the influence of religious instruction and the commonalities and differences of the child's belief systems with those of his or her family. In addition to academic achievements, the psychiatrist studies the child's areas of special interest, and his or her peer group relationships. The psychiatrist examines areas that have led to psychological stress, such as problems in relationships with authority figures, with peers, and with siblings. The psychiatrist also inquires about eating disorders, sleep disturbances, periods of depression, suicidal ideation, alcohol and drug intake, and problems that relate to the personal identity of the teenager.

Adult History

The psychiatrist explores the patient's capacities for intimacy, development of friendships, social networks, adult educational history, employment record, intellectual pursuits, recreational activities, and avocational interests. The patient's military history, civic responsibilities, religious affiliations, value systems, political involvements, fiscal security, vacation habits, and relationship with his or her family are also reviewed. The psychiatrist documents what the patient's plans are for the future, whether such plans are achievable, and how the patient intends to implement them.

☐ Sexual History

The psychiatrist inquires about the patient's early life experiences related to sexual development. The psychiatrist inquires about what and how the patient learned about sexual activities, conception, and pregnancy, and who was responsible for the learning. The psychiatrist also inquires about a history of sexual abuse. The psychiatrist asks both male and female patients about their experiences in puberty. With female patients, the inquiries begin with menarche. The female patient is asked about who prepared her for menses, what she was told about what to expect, what the meaning of menses was to the patient, and what the parents' reactions to the menarche were. For both male and female patients, a masturbatory history is obtained with explorations about fantasies that accompanied masturbation. Descriptions of sexual experiences, both heterosexual and homosexual, are elicited. Attitudes of the patient toward heterosexual and homosexual fantasies and experiences are noted.

The psychiatrist then explores adulthood attitudes and behaviors. Also recorded are expectations regarding children, as well as the different stages of development of existing children. Marital crises and threats, or actual separations and/or divorces, are also subjects of inquiry. Areas of sexual conflict or sexual dysfunctions are examined. Patients are reluctant to discuss some, if not all, of these topics regarding sexuality because of accompanying shame, embarrassment, or discomfort.

☐ Medical History

The psychiatrist reviews the patient's medical history, including common as well as chronic childhood illnesses, conditions leading to frequent medical consultation and treatment, and those requiring emergency room visits as well as those leading to hospitalizations. The psychiatrist also reviews the patient's surgical experiences and those requiring the administration of anesthesia. The history of accidents and orthopedic interventions is recorded. The psychological meaning of illnesses and interventions is explored in terms of the patient's feelings about injury to body parts, effects on body image, and fears and concerns about invalidism and death. The psychiatrist reviews adult-onset illnesses, medical interventions, and surgical and obstetrical events. The effects of these on the patient's functioning at work and at play, on the families, and on interpersonal relationships are noted. The psychiatrist also assesses the patient's motivations for and capacities to assist in recovery, his or her levels of denial of the impact of serious illnesses on functioning and longevity, and the coping mechanisms that the patient employs. Inquiries are made about support systems that the patient has used to aid in the recovery from past illnesses, including the availability of these systems and the willingness of the patient to use them to help with the current situation.

■ MENTAL STATUS EXAMINATION

The mental status examination is a description of all the areas of mental functioning of the patient. It serves the same function for psychiatrists as the physical examination does for the primary care physician. Psychiatrists follow a structured format in recording their findings. These descriptive data are then used to support the psychiatrists' diagnostic conclusions. An outline of the component parts of the mental status examination follows (Engel 1979; Keller and Manschreck 1981; Reiser and Schroder 1980; Small 1981; Tilley and Hoffman 1981).

☐ General Description

Appearance

The psychiatrist records in detail the prominent physical features of the individual, including facial features, height, weight, cleanliness, posture, clothing, level of eye contact, and an estimate of how old the patient looks compared with chronological age.

Motor Behavior

The psychiatrist describes the patient's gait and freedom of movement, noting the firmness and strength of handshake. The psychiatrist observes any involuntary or abnormal movements, such as tremors, tics, mannerisms, lip smacking, akathisias, or repeated stereotyped movements.

Speech

The psychiatrist listens for the patient's rate of speech, the spontaneity of verbalizations, the range of voice intonation patterns, the volume in terms of loudness, defects with verbalizations such as stammering or stuttering, and any aphasias.

Attitudes

The psychiatrist summarizes how the patient related to him or her in the course of the interview, focusing on any shifts in attitude. It is also helpful for the psychiatrist to keep track of his or her own attitudes toward the patient.

☐ Emotions

Mood

When describing a mood, the psychiatrist records how deeply it is felt, the length of time that it prevails, and how much it fluctuates. Anxious, panicky, terrified, sad, depressed, angry, enraged, euphoric, and guilty are moods frequently described.

Affective Expression

The psychiatrist observes and records the patient's nonverbal behaviors such as facial mobility, voice intonation patterns, and body movements to assess affective expression. Range of expression and feeling tones are described, and any incongruities are noted.

Appropriateness

The psychiatrist judges whether the affective tone and expression are appropriate to the subject matter being discussed in the context of the patient's thinking. Disharmonies between affective expression and thought content are worthy of exploration with the patient.

☐ Perceptual Disturbances

Hallucinations and Illusions

A *hallucination* is a perceptual distortion that a patient experiences for which there is no external stimulus. An *illusion* is a false impression that results from a real stimulus.

Depersonalization and Derealization

Depersonalization describes patients' feelings that they are not themselves, that they are strange, or that there is something different about themselves for which they cannot account. *Derealization* expresses patients' feeling that the environment is somehow different or strange but they cannot account for these changes.

☐ Thought Process

Stream of Thought

The psychiatrist records the quantity and rate of the patient's thoughts. The psychiatrist notes whether there is a retardation or an acceleration.

The psychiatrist also examines the patient for the goal directedness and continuity of thoughts. *Circumstantiality* is a disorder of associations in which the patient exhibits lack of goal directedness, incorporates tedious and unnecessary details, and has difficulty in arriving at an end point. *Tangentiality* describes a thought process whereby the patient digresses from the subject under discussion and introduces thoughts that seem unrelated, oblique, and irrelevant. A sudden cessation in the middle of a sentence at which point a patient cannot recover what he or she has said or complete his or her thoughts is an example of *blocking*. *Loose associations* describe a jumping from one topic to another with no apparent connection between the topics. *Perseveration* refers to the patient's repeating the same response to a variety of questions and topics, with an inability to change his or her responses or to change the topic.

Marked abnormalities of thought processes include neologisms, word salad, clang associations, and echolalia. *Neologisms* are words that patients make up and are often a condensation of several words that are unintelligible to another person. *Word salad* is an incomprehensible mixing of meaningless words and phrases. In *clang associations* the connections between thoughts may be tenuous, and the patient uses rhyming and punning. *Echolalia* describes a patient's irreverent parroting of what another person has said.

Thought Content (Delusions, Obsessions, Compulsions, Preoccupations, Phobias)

One important area the psychiatrist inquires about is whether the patient has suicidal thoughts. This is particularly true in patients who signal feelings of helplessness, hopelessness, worthlessness, or giving up. In addition to the description of delusions, the psychiatrist assesses the degrees of organization of the delusion. Ideas of reference and influence are also described in detail. The psychiatrist notes any obsessions the patient may have. Phobias are often not spontaneously conveyed in the interview, and the psychiatrist should make specific inquiries about their presence (Campbell 1981; Thompson 1979).

Abstract Thinking

Several methods are used to test abstract, or categorical, thinking. These include testing similarities, differences, and the meaning of proverbs. Concreteness of responses on formal testing reflects intellectual impoverishment, cultural deprivation, and organic brain disease. Bizarre and inappropriate responses to proverbs reflect schizophrenic thinking.

Education and Intelligence

Intelligence is best measured in the clinical interview by the patient's use of vocabulary. The expectations of levels of intelligence are influenced by the level of education of the patient. Specific testing for intelligence is only used when deficits are anticipated based on the interview.

Concentration

In the interview, troubles with concentration are reflected in the patient's inability to pay attention to the questions that he or she is being asked. He or she may be distracted by external or internal stimuli. When the patient's concentration is impaired, the psychiatrist often has to repeat his or her questions. Formal testing for concentration includes serial 7s, where the patient is asked to subtract 7 from 100 and keep subtracting 7 from each answer. Serial 3s or counting backward from 20 can be substituted if the patient has cognitive difficulties performing serial 7s. If the patient has been asked to do serial 7s repeatedly, he or she should start subtracting from 101 rather than 100 to avoid giving learned responses.

Immediate recall and concentration abilities often overlap. One way to test for immediate recall is to ask the patient to repeat digits forward and backward. The patient is instructed that the psychiatrist is going to recite numbers and then ask the patient to repeat them.

☐ Orientation (Time, Place, Person, Situation)

Testing for time includes asking the patient the month, the day of the month, the year, the day of the week, and the time of day and the season of the year. Orientation to place includes the patient's knowing the name of the place where he or she is currently located and the name of the city and state. Orientation to person includes the patient's knowing his or her own name and the names and roles of persons in his or her immediate surrounding. Orientation to situation indicates the patient's present circumstances and why he or she finds himself or herself in such circumstances. This is often an important clue toward the competency of individuals to give informed consent. Patients who have deficits in all three orientation spheres are commonly suffering from an organic brain disease.

☐ Memory

Remote Memory

The psychiatrist tests for remote memory by asking where the patient grew up, where he or she went to school, and what his or her first job was, and inquires about significant people from the past (e.g., naming of presidents) and also significant events (e.g., the Vietnam War).

Recent Past Memory

To test for recent past memory, the psychiatrist inquires about what the patient ate for breakfast or what he or she read in the newspaper, or asks for details about what the patient watched on television the night before.

Recent Memory

The psychiatrist tests recent or short-term memory by asking the patient to repeat the names of three unrelated objects and then informing him or her that they will go on to discuss other subjects and that in 5 minutes the patient will be asked to name the three objects.

☐ Impulse Control, Judgment, Insight, and Reliability

Impulse control is the ability to control the expression of aggressive, hostile, fearful, guilty, affectionate, or sexual impulses in situations where their expression should be maladaptive. A loss of control can reflect a low frustration tolerance (Yudofsky et al. 1986).

Judgment refers to the patient's capacity to make appropriate decisions and appropriately act on them in social situations. An assessment of this function is best made in the course of obtaining the patient's history. There is no necessary correlation between intelligence and judgment. Formal testing is rarely helpful.

The capacity of the patient to be aware and to understand that he or she has a problem or illness and to be able to review its probable causes and arrive at tenable solutions is referred to as *insight*. Emotional insight refers to the patient's awareness of his or her motivations, and, in turn, his or her feelings, so that the patient can change long-standing, ingrained patterns of behavior. Self-observation alone is insufficient for insight. Emotional insight must be applied for change to occur (Ross and Leichner 1984).

Upon completion of an interview, the psychiatrist assesses the *reliability* of the information that has been obtained. Factors affecting reliability include the patient's intellectual endowment, his or her honesty and motivations, the presence of psychosis or organic defects, and the patient's tendency to magnify or understate his or her problems.

◼ PSYCHODYNAMIC FORMULATION

At the conclusion of the interview, history taking, and mental status examination, the psychiatrist documents a psychodynamic formulation of the patient. The psychiatrist describes the key elements of the patient's personality structures, principal psychological conflicts, and healthier, adaptive abilities. The psychiatrist assesses the ego functions of the patient, including defense mechanisms used, regulation and control of drives, relationships to others, self-representation, stimulus regulation, adaptive relaxation, reality testing, and synthetic integration. By reviewing the patient's developmental history, the psychiatrist assesses the patient's typical drives, impulses, wishes, and anxieties at each stage of development. The psychiatrist can then establish the origins of each of the patient's conflicts and how they carry over to successive periods of development. The psychiatrist focuses on the major adaptive problems of the patient and on how earlier developmental deficits help explain the patient's current difficulties (Pruyser 1979; Wallerstein 1983; Yudofsky et al. 1986).

Psychiatrists thus trace from early development to the present patients' major conflicts, evolving symptoms, character traits, and defenses. They then organize these data in a psychodynamic formulation (MacKinnon and Yudofsky 1986).

■ REFERENCES

American Psychiatric Association: Diagnostic and Statistical Manual of Mental Disorders, 4th Edition. Washington, DC, American Psychiatric Association, 1994

Campbell RJ: Psychiatric Dictionary, 5th Edition. New York, Oxford University Press, 1981

Engel IM: The mental status examination in psychiatry: origin, use and content. Journal of Psychiatric Education 3:99–108, 1979

Halleck SL: Evaluation of the Psychiatric Patient: A Primer. New York, Plenum, 1991

Keller MB, Manschreck TC: The bedside mental status examination—reliability and validity. Compr Psychiatry 22:500–511, 1981

Kestenbaum CJ: The clinical interview of the child, in Textbook of Child and Adolescent Psychiatry. Edited by Wiener JM. Washington, DC, American Psychiatric Press, 1991, pp 65–73

MacKinnon RA, Michels R: The Psychiatric Interview in Clinical Practice. Philadelphia, PA, WB Saunders, 1971

MacKinnon RA, Yudofsky SC: The Psychiatric Evaluation in Clinical Practice. Philadelphia, PA, JB Lippincott, 1986

Nurcombe B, Fitzhenry-Coor I: How do psychiatrists think? Clinical reasoning in the psychiatric interview: a research and education project. Aust N Z J Psychiatry 16(1):13–24, 1982

Othmer E, Othmer SC: The Clinical Interview Using DSM-III-R. Washington, DC, American Psychiatric Press, 1989

Pruyser PW: The Psychological Examination: A Guide for Clinicians. New York, International Universities Press, 1979

Reiser DE, Schroder AK: Patient Interviewing: The Human Dimension. Baltimore, MD, Williams & Wilkins, 1980

Ross CA, Leichner P: Residents training in the mental status examination. Can J Psychiatry 29:315–318, 1984

Small SM: Outline for Psychiatric Examination. East Hanover, NJ, Sandoz Pharmaceuticals, 1981

Thompson MGG (ed): A Resident's Guide to Psychiatric Education. New York, Plenum, 1979

Tilley DH, Hoffman JA: Mental status examination: myth or method? Compr Psychiatry 22:562–564, 1981

Wallerstein RS: Defenses, defense mechanisms, and the structure of the mind. J Am Psychoanal Assoc 31(suppl):207–225, 1983

Yudofsky, SC, Silver JM, Jackson W, et al: The Overt Aggression Scale for the objective rating of verbal and physical aggression. Am J Psychiatry 143:35–39, 1986

CHAPTER 7

Psychiatric Classification

Janet B. W. Williams, D.S.W.

■ GENERAL PURPOSES OF CLASSIFICATION SYSTEMS

There are three general purposes to having a diagnostic classification system, as well as many specific clinical, administrative, legal, and research functions. First, such a system provides a language with which all mental health professionals can communicate. Generally agreed-upon names for the various mental syndromes serve as a shorthand way of describing the entities that mental health professionals deal with, enabling efficient communication. Second, in order to study the natural history of a particular disorder and develop an effective treatment, it is necessary to define the characteristics of that disorder and have an understanding of how it differs from other, similar disorders. To the extent that a relationship between diagnosis and treatment has been established for a particular category, the proper diagnosis of a person's condition can indicate the most effective treatment.

Finally, the ultimate purpose of classification is to develop an understanding of the causes of the various mental disorders. Knowing the cause of a disorder usually leads to the development of an effective treatment. The etiology or pathophysiological process for most of the mental disorders in DSM-IV is unknown, except for those disorders that are due to a general medical condition and those few disorders (e.g., posttraumatic stress disorder, adjustment disorder) for which the etiology is included in the definition. For most of the DSM-IV disorders, however, etiological theories abound, formulated by clinicians and researchers of differing theoretical orientations. However, despite differing etiological

211

theories about how these disorders come about, it has become clear that clinicians and researchers can agree on what the disorders look like. Therefore, in DSM-III, DSM-III-R, and DSM-IV, a descriptive approach to classification has been taken that includes definitions of the various disorders without reference to their etiology, except for those disorders for which the etiology or pathophysiological process is known.

■ MENTAL DISORDER: DEFINITION

In order to develop and refine a diagnostic classification system of mental disorders, it is necessary to have some definition of the concept "mental disorder." For many years, sociologists, psychologists, philosophers of science, and members of the legal profession have struggled with defining the concept (Spitzer and Williams 1982). It was not until the early 1970s, when the issue of whether or not to classify homosexuality as a mental disorder was confronted, that psychiatry began to struggle with the issue. This effort eventually resulted in a definition of mental disorder in DSM-III that has been retained, in refined form, in DSM-III-R and DSM-IV:

> In DSM-IV, each of the mental disorders is conceptualized as a clinically significant behavioral or psychological syndrome or pattern that occurs in an individual and that is associated with present distress (a painful symptom) or disability (impairment in one or more important areas of functioning) or with a significantly increased risk of suffering death, pain, disability, or an important loss of freedom. In addition, this syndrome or pattern must not be merely an expectable and culturally sanctioned response to a particular event, e.g., the death of a loved one. Whatever its original cause, it must currently be considered a manifestation of a behavioral, psychological, or biological dysfunction in the individual. Neither deviant behavior, e.g., political, religious, or sexual, nor conflicts that are primarily between the individual and society are mental disorders unless the deviance or conflict is a symptom of a dysfunction in the individual, as described above. (American Psychiatric Association 1994)

It is recognized that more precise boundaries for the concept "mental disorder" cannot be specified, just as they cannot for "physical disorder." A common misunderstanding about the disorders in DSM-IV is that each category represents a discrete entity with distinct boundaries between it and other mental disorders, and between it and normality. Also, it must be made clear that the objects of the classification are conditions that persons have, rather than the persons themselves (Spitzer and Williams 1979). Thus, for example, there should be no reference to "a schizophrenic" or "a depressive," but rather to "a person with schizophrenia," or someone "who has depression."

■ DEVELOPMENT OF THE *DIAGNOSTIC AND STATISTICAL MANUAL* SYSTEM: PROCESS AND CONTROVERSIES

☐ DSM-I

The first version of the diagnostic manual was published by the American Psychiatric Association (APA) in 1952 and was called at that time *Diagnostic and Statistical Manual, Mental Disorders.* The major significance of this book was that, for the first time, it provided descriptions for the mental disorder categories it listed.

☐ DSM-II

In 1965 the APA decided that a new edition of the DSM should be published to coincide with the eighth revision of the World Health Organization (WHO) international system, International Classification of Diseases (ICD). Although it did not differ substantially from the first DSM, DSM-II was published in 1968.

☐ DSM-III

In the years since DSM-II was published, a major revolution took place in psychiatry with the development of diagnostic criteria. Beginning in 1972 with the publication of the Feighner criteria (Feighner et al. 1972), research was greatly enhanced by the availability of specific definitions of diagnostic categories. Further, it was demonstrated that such criteria increased the reliability with which these diagnoses could be made (Spitzer et al. 1978a). The Feighner criteria were revised and expanded in 1978 into the Research Diagnostic Criteria (RDC; Spitzer et al. 1978b), covering 21 categories. The greatest challenge to the developers of DSM-III was the creation of specified criteria for over 150 diagnostic categories.

For the first time in the development of a standard diagnostic manual, an extensive field trial was conducted with the proposed DSM-III prior to its adoption (Spitzer et al. 1979). In the course of this project, 670 adults and 126 children were evaluated in a test of the reliability of the drafted diagnostic criteria. Although the method of this reliability study was less than ideal because of uncontrollable field conditions, the study did demonstrate that improvements had been made in our ability to reliably diagnose most of the major mental disorders.

The impact of DSM-III was remarkable. Soon after its publication, it became widely accepted in the United States as the common language of mental health clinicians and researchers for communicating about the disorders for which they have professional responsibility. All major textbooks of psychiatry and other textbooks that discuss psychopathology either made extensive reference to DSM-III or largely adopted its terminology and concepts, and it was used as a major teaching tool in medical student education and residency training programs (Williams et al. 1985).

☐ DSM-III-R

Work on DSM-III-R was begun in 1983, just three years after the publication of DSM-III. New data had accumulated that indicated the need for changes in some of the DSM-III definitions, and experience with the criteria had revealed many instances in which they were not entirely clear, were inconsistent across diagnostic categories, or were even contradictory.

☐ DSM-IV

Work on DSM-IV proceeded in three major phases. First, each work group developed extensive literature reviews bearing on controversial issues in its field, and considered recent scientific findings that might suggest changes in the classification, text, or criteria for DSM-IV (Widiger et al. 1990). Second, a series of analyses of data from studies that had already been completed or were in progress was funded by the John D. and Catherine T. MacArthur Foundation to answer specific nosological questions. Finally, 12 field trials were funded by the National Institute of Mental Health (NIMH), the National Institute on Drug Abuse (NIDA), and the National Institute on Alcohol Abuse and Alcoholism (NIAAA), to study the impact of changes that were being considered for inclusion in DSM-IV (Frances et al. 1991).

■ DIAGNOSTIC RELIABILITY

The reliability of a diagnostic category puts an upper limit on its usefulness (i.e., validity). The extent to which a diagnostic category is reliable is the extent to which clinicians can agree with each other on the identification of the disorder; this includes agreement on when the disorder is or is not present. A series of cases with different diagnoses is necessary in order to assess reliability, and the degree to which clinicians can correctly discriminate the diagnostic differences is measured.

☐ Assessment Methods and Sources of Unreliability

There are several methods for testing reliability, each having its own advantages and disadvantages. The easiest but least powerful way is to ask two clinicians to diagnose independently a series of cases based on written case records, or on audio- or videotapes of diagnostic interviews with the subjects.

There are two methods of assessing "live" reliability. The first is the *joint method,* so named because it involves two or more clinicians jointly observing the same interview. One of the clinicians conducts the interview, and often the other may ask additional questions. In the *test-retest method,* each clinician independently conducts his or her own interview, one after the other. An advantage of this procedure is that it more closely approximates the model of interchangeable interviewers, because a reliable diagnosis is one that can be made in the same patients by different people. As expected, reliability assessed by this method is generally lower than that obtained by joint assessments because of the increase in information variance (Spitzer and Williams 1985). Despite the fact that the test-retest method requires subjects to undergo more interviews and may be more difficult to coordinate logistically, this expense is usually worth the increase in generalizability of the results.

Even when both clinicians observe the same patient interview, they may pay attention to different things, resulting in *observation variance.* For example, one clinician may notice that the subject has psychomotor agitation, whereas the other clinician may not. *Interpretation variance* is when clinicians differ in the way they interpret the signs and symptoms exhibited by the patient. An example of this would be differing interpretations of the content of a patient's delusions, such that one clinician decides the delusions are bizarre, and the other does not. Observation variance can be minimized with training; interpretation variance is minimized when both clinicians use the same definitions of psychopathological symptoms.

A final source of variance that affects diagnostic reliability is *criterion variance,* resulting when clinicians use differing rules for summarizing their observations into diagnoses. As discussed above, standard sets of specified diagnostic criteria have been available since the early 1970s. Criterion variance is minimized when clinicians use the same diagnostic criteria.

☐ Statistical Indices of Reliability

Generally, one is interested in knowing the reliability of a single diagnostic category (e.g., How good is agreement on the diagnosis of schizophrenia?), a diagnostic class (e.g., How good is the agreement on a diagnosis of any mood disorder?), or an entire classification of disorders (e.g., What is the average reliability of all DSM-IV Axis I disorders?). One way of calculating agreement is simply to calculate the percentage of cases in the sample on which there is agreement.

In 1960, Cohen proposed the use of the *kappa statistic* for indexing agreement among clinicians, correcting for chance agreement. The values of kappa vary from −1.0 (total disagreement) to +1.0 (perfect agreement), with a kappa of 0 indicating no more than chance agreement. It is generally agreed that a kappa value of 0.70 and above is quite good, between 0.50 and 0.70 is fair, and below 0.50 is poor (Perry 1992; Spitzer and Fleiss 1974). Kappa is calculated as follows:

$$\text{kappa} = \frac{P_{\text{observed}} - P_{\text{chance}}}{1 - P_{\text{chance}}}$$

■ TYPES OF VALIDITY

☐ Diagnostic Validity

The *validity* of a diagnosis is the extent to which it serves the multiple purposes for which it is intended. There are four major types of validity that are applied to psychiatric diagnoses: face, descriptive, predictive, and construct.

Face validity is the extent to which, on the face of it, the definition of a disorder seems reasonable as a description of a particular clinical entity and allows professionals to communicate about the disorder. *Descriptive validity* is the extent to which the defining features of a diagnostic category are unique to that category. If a diagnosis has high *predictive validity*, it is useful for predicting the natural history and treatment response of a person with the disorder. Finally, *construct validity* is the highest form of validity and the form for which most of the mental disorders have the least evidence. Construct validity is the extent to which we understand the etiology or pathophysiological process of a disorder. Evidence for the construct validity of a disorder includes evidence of a genetic factor, a biological mechanism, and social and environmental factors that cause the disorder.

☐ Procedural Validity

When evaluating the usefulness or accuracy (i.e., validity) of a particular diagnostic test or procedure, it is necessary to evaluate it against some standard procedure that is assumed to be valid. This is referred to as *procedural validity* and should not be confused with diagnostic validity (discussed previously) (Spitzer and Williams 1985).

There are basically three important indices with which a new test or procedure can be evaluated, using some standard test or procedure as the criterion: sensitivity, specificity, and predictive power. The *sensitivity* of a diagnostic procedure is calculated as the percentage of "true" cases it correctly identifies as having the diagnosis (i.e., its *true-positive* rate). The *specificity* is the percentage of noncases that it correctly identifies as *not* having the diagnosis (i.e., its *true-negative* rate). Finally, the *predictive power* of a test is the percentage of total cases in which the test agrees with the standard—that is, the total number of cases that both tests agree have the diagnosis plus the total number of cases that both tests agree do not have the diagnosis, all divided by the total number of cases. The predictive power of a test can be broken down into positive predictive power and negative predictive power. A test's total predictive power is a summation of these two statistics.

■ STRUCTURED INTERVIEWS

In recent years, psychiatric research has been greatly facilitated by the evolution of specified diagnostic criteria and by structured diagnostic interviews keyed to these criteria (Spitzer et al. 1992b; Stangl et al. 1985). Such interviews have many advantages: 1) they enhance the reliability with which diagnoses are made, 2) they facilitate the recording of which specific symptoms are present and which are absent, and 3) they enable even relatively junior clinicians to make reliable psychiatric diagnoses.

Standardized interview schedules that are specifically designed to yield a range of the major psychiatric diagnoses represent a more recent advance. Those in most widespread use are described below; undoubtedly, all will be adapted to accommodate DSM-IV criteria. A growing number focus on one or more personality disorders (Stangl et al. 1985; Zanarini et al. 1987). It should also be noted that similar interview guides have now been developed to cover diagnoses often made in children and adolescents (Gutterman et al. 1987; Hodges 1993).

☐ Present State Examination (PSE)

The PSE, the "grandparent" of structured diagnostic interviews, was developed 20 years ago in England (Wing et al. 1967). It consists of a structured interview schedule that generally focuses on symptoms that have occurred during the past month. Diagnoses are made by a computer program called CATEGO. The latest version of this interview schedule, PSE-10, has been incorporated into a new system known as SCAN (Schedules for Clinical Assessment in Neuropsychiatry; Wing et al. 1990). SCAN is a comprehensive procedure that enables a clinician to assess many of the DSM-III-R categories, with optional sections for further characterizing certain aspects of psychopathology and other clinical variables. Its development was sponsored by the WHO, and it was specifically designed for worldwide use.

☐ Schedule for Affective Disorders and Schizophrenia (SADS)

The Schedule for Affective Disorders and Schizophrenia (SADS; Endicott and Spitzer 1978) has been widely used in this country and abroad for making diagnoses according to the RDC described in an earlier section of this chapter. Diagnoses are made by the clinician following the interview, in consultation with the RDC criteria. Mini six-point rating scales are provided for most of the symptoms, which generate extensive descriptive information and a mechanism for charting change over time, but make the administration of the instrument lengthy. Several versions of the SADS have been developed, including the SADS-L (lifetime version), which is used for community subjects and patients' relatives (Endicott and Spitzer 1978), and the SADS-LA[R] (revised lifetime version for anxiety disorders specifically), which focuses on a detailed history of anxiety symptoms (Schleyer et al. 1990).

☐ NIMH Diagnostic Interview Schedule (DIS) and WHO-ADAMHA Composite International Diagnostic Interview (CIDI)

The Diagnostic Interview Schedule (DIS; Robins et al. 1981) was explicitly developed for use by nonclinicians to facilitate the screening of a large number of community subjects in the Epidemiologic Catchment Area survey (Regier et al. 1984). The Composite International Diagnostic Interview (CIDI; Robins et al. 1988), a revision and expansion of the DIS, was developed for international cross-cultural epidemiological studies and comparative studies of psychopathology. Although these instruments have been used in some studies by clinical interviewers, they are fully structured to minimize the amount of judgment required to administer them; thus they do not make use of the skills of an experienced clinical interviewer, which many believe is essential to ensure the validity of the diagnostic assessments (Spitzer 1983).

☐ Structured Clinical Interview for DSM-IV (SCID)

The Structured Clinical Interview for DSM-IV (SCID) is designed to enable clinicians to gather the appropriate information to make Axis I and II diagnoses according to DSM-IV (Spitzer et al. 1992b; Williams et al.

1992). Modeled on a clinical diagnostic interview, the SCID begins with an overview of the present illness and past episodes of psychopathology. It then proceeds to inquire systematically about specific symptoms, beginning with screening questions to rule in or rule out specific disorders. The SCID is designed for use in a modular fashion so that an investigator can select for a particular study only those diagnostic modules that are relevant for the sample of subjects in that study. Several versions of the SCID for Axis I disorders have been developed: the SCID-P for use with psychiatric patients, the SCID-OP for psychiatric outpatients only, and the SCID-NP for community subjects, patients' relatives, primary care patients, and other persons not identified as psychiatric patients. The SCID-II, for making personality disorder diagnoses, is designed to be used with a self-report questionnaire that the subject completes just before the interview. The clinician then focuses on the positive responses to the questionnaire in reviewing the personality disorder symptoms.

■ DSM-IV: GENERAL FEATURES

☐ Diagnostic Criteria

Specified diagnostic criteria are included in DSM-IV for every specific category. These criteria have been revised from those in DSM-III-R, based on continued clinical experience and new empirical findings.

☐ Descriptive Approach

One of the most important and successful features of DSM-III was its generally atheoretical, or descriptive, approach to defining the mental disorders. For a few of the DSM-III mental disorders, notably the organic mental disorders, the etiology or pathophysiological process is known or presumed, or included in the definition (as in adjustment disorder). For most of them, however, the etiology is unknown, although there may be many theories about the causes of the various disorders. The developers of DSM-III recognized that, by and large, clinicians could agree on the defining features of most of the mental disorders despite their disagreement about their causes. For this reason, except for those disorders for which the etiology is known, the mental disorders in DSM-III, DSM-III-R, and DSM-IV are defined without reference to etiological theories. This approach does not inhibit the belief in specific etiological theories or the creation and study of new ones, and it does at least encourage the study of homogeneous groups of patients in the pursuit of data supporting such theories.

☐ Diagnostic Hierarchies

In DSM-III-R most of the diagnostic hierarchies were removed; those that remain in DSM-IV largely follow two principles:

1. Disorders due to a general medical condition and substance-induced disorders preempt the diagnosis of any other disorder that could produce the same symptoms, if an etiological general medical condition or substance can be identified. For example, a patient with a major depressive syndrome could be diagnosed as having either major depressive disorder, mood disorder due to hypothyroidism, or hallucinogen mood disorder. If the history or laboratory tests reveal that the depression began during the course of hypothyroidism, or during hallucinogen intoxication, the clinician should consider one of the two latter diagnoses rather than major depressive disorder. However, if no etiological general medical condition or specific substance intoxication or withdrawal is identified, and the criteria for a major depressive disorder are met, it is the mood disorder that should be diagnosed.

2. When a more pervasive disorder commonly has essential or associated symptoms that are the defining symptoms of a less pervasive disorder, only the more pervasive disorder is diagnosed if its diagnostic criteria are met. For example, when chronic mild depression is present only when the essential features of schizophrenia are also present, only schizophrenia is diagnosed rather than schizophrenia and dysthymic disorder (to account for the chronic mild depression), because depressive symptoms are commonly associated with schizophrenia.

☐ Multiaxial System for Evaluation

The DSM-III took a major step forward by incorporating, for the first time in an official diagnostic system in this country, a multiaxial system for evaluation. The basic concept of such a system is that several different domains of information that are assumed to be of high clinical value are evaluated for each person. Use of a multiaxial system ensures that attention is given to certain types of disorders, aspects of the environment, and areas of functioning that might be overlooked if the focus were on assessing a single presenting problem. Although not empirically demonstrated, it is assumed that a multiaxial evaluation is more useful for treatment planning and evaluating prognosis, because it better reflects the interrelated complexities of the various biological, psychological, and social aspects of a person's condition (Williams 1985a, 1985b).

The DSM-IV multiaxial system consists of five axes. All of the mental disorders are included in the first two axes: Axis I is for "Clinical Disorders and Other Conditions That May Be a Focus of Clinical Attention," and Axis II is for "Personality Disorders" and "Mental Retardation." The provision of a separate axis for personality disorders and mental retardation ensures that consideration is given to the possible presence of such disorders that might otherwise be overlooked when attention is directed to the usually-more-florid Axis I disorders.

Axis III is for listing current general medical conditions that the clinician believes are potentially relevant to the understanding or management of the case. General medical conditions can be related to mental disorders in a variety of ways. In some cases it is clear that the general medical condition is directly etiological to the development or worsening of a mental disorder (e.g., anxiety disorder due to hyperthyroidism), and that the mechanism for this effect is physiological. In other instances the general medical disorder may not seem to be etiological but is important in the overall management of the case (e.g., a person with diabetes mellitus admitted to the hospital for an exacerbation of schizophrenia for whom insulin management must be monitored). Sometimes a general medical disorder has important prognostic or treatment implications for the mental disorder, as, for example, a case involving both major depressive disorder and arrhythmia, in which the choice of pharmacotherapy is influenced by the general medical condition.

The fourth axis provides a checklist for recording psychosocial and environmental problems that may affect the diagnosis, treatment planning, and prognosis of the individual's mental disorders (on Axes I and II). A psychosocial or environmental problem may be a negative life event, an environmental difficulty, an interpersonal stress, an inadequacy of social supports or personal resources, or another problem that describes the context in which a person's difficulties have developed. In general, only those problems that have been present during the year prior to the evaluation should be noted; in many cases it is appropriate to record more than one problem. When a psychosocial or environmental problem is the primary focus of clinical attention, it is also recorded on Axis I with its corresponding code from the section listing "Other Conditions That May Be a Focus of Clinical Attention."

The Global Assessment of Functioning (GAF) Scale on Axis V summarizes psychological, social, and occupational functioning on a continuum of mental health-illness. The GAF ratings are made for current functioning and generally reflect the present need for treatment or care. Ratings may be made for other time periods (e.g., past year) for special purposes.

☐ Systematic Descriptions

The DSM-IV includes standard categories of information in order to offer a complete description of the features of the various disorders. The description of each category begins with its *diagnostic features,* the clinical signs and symptoms that are required in order to make the diagnosis. This is followed by a discussion of the disorder's *associated features and disorders,* which can include 1) descriptive features and mental disorders that are often associated with the disorder but are not essential for making the diagnosis; 2) associated laboratory findings that may be diagnostic, confirmatory of the construct of the disorder, or merely associated with the complications of the disorder; and 3) associated symptoms, physical examination signs, and general medical conditions that may be of diagnostic significance but are not essential to the diagnosis, or that are merely associated conditions.

A section addressing *specific age, cultural, or gender features* provides guidance for the clinician concerning variations in the presentation of the disorder that may be attributable to the individual's developmental stage, cultural setting, or gender. This section also includes information on differential prevalence rates. Under *prevalence and incidence* data are provided on point and lifetime prevalence and incidence of the disorder. These data are provided for different clinical settings when known.

The section on *predisposing factors* describes the characteristics of a person that can be identified before the development of the disorder and that increase the risk of that person developing the disorder. The section on *course* describes the typical lifetime patterns of presentation and evolution of the disorder. This may include information on the usual age at onset, mode of onset, chronicity, typical duration of episodes, and progression over time. Under *complications* is a description of the types of serious morbidity that may occur as a result of having the disorder. The *familial pattern* section provides data on the frequency of the disorder among first-degree biological relatives of those persons with the disorder as compared with the general population. Finally, each category also includes a discussion of *differential diagnosis,* describing how to distinguish the disorder in question from other disorders that have some similar presenting characteristics.

☐ Cross-Cultural Considerations

The DSM-III has been translated into many languages and has been widely used in other parts of the world. Somewhat surprisingly, its use in cultures vastly different from those of most of the people who were mainly responsible for developing it was generally successful (Spitzer et al. 1983). In DSM-IV this issue received even more attention. Three additional innovative features were added to DSM-IV. First, because of evidence suggesting that the symptoms and course of a number of DSM-IV disorders are influenced by local cultural factors, a new section that describes specific cultural features was added to the text for many disorders. Second, descriptions of some "culture-bound syndromes" were added as examples to "not otherwise specified" categories (e.g., possession trance added as an example to dissociative disorder not otherwise specified). Finally, an appendix to DSM-IV provides a guideline for cultural formulation and a glossary of culture-bound syndromes.

☐ Relational Disturbances

An often-made criticism of DSM-III focused on the fact that it includes only those mental disorders that are conceptualized as occurring in the individual, restricting usefulness in the diagnosis and treatment of problems that occur in the family and other relational units (Wynne 1987). Early in the development of DSM-IV, the Coalition on Family Diagnoses was formed to consider possible changes that might be made in DSM-IV. This collaboration resulted in several new features, including the addition of a group of "relational problems" to the section entitled "Other Conditions That May Be a Focus of Clinical Attention." This new grouping includes relational problems related to a mental disorder or general medical condition, parent-child relational problems, partner relational problems, sibling relational problems, and relational problems not otherwise specified. In addition, an optional axis, called the Global Assessment of Relational Functioning (GARF) Scale, appears in an appendix to DSM-IV.

☐ Appendixes

The DSM-IV contains a number of appendixes, many of which are designed to make the manual more user-friendly. As in DSM-III and DSM-III-R, a small forest of "decision trees" are provided to make the differential diagnostic process easier. Using one of these trees, a clinician can follow a series of questions to rule in or out various disorders. A glossary of technical terms that are included in the criteria of DSM-IV has been retained as an appendix. In order to highlight the changes made in DSM-III-R, an annotated listing of changes made for DSM-IV specifies the corresponding categories in each manual, with a brief discussion of the reasons for major changes. A numerical listing of the codes and an alphabetical listing of the diagnostic categories are included as separate appendixes, as are listings of selected ICD-9 codes for general medical conditions, and corresponding ICD-10 codes for DSM-IV disorders.

■ DSM-IV: OVERVIEW OF THE MAJOR CLASSES

In the following subsections, the major classes of DSM-IV are described, without detailed discussion of the way they differ from those in DSM-III-R.

Categories that were added to DSM-IV and those that were deleted since DSM-III-R are listed in Table 7–1 and discussed in more detail in an appendix to DSM-IV entitled "Annotated Listing of Changes in DSM-IV."

☐ Disorders Usually First Diagnosed in Infancy, Childhood, or Adolescence

Those disorders usually first diagnosed in infancy, childhood, or adolescence are divided into a number of minor classes: mental retardation, learning disorders, motor skills disorder, pervasive developmental disorders, attention-deficit and disruptive behavior disorders, feeding and eating disorders of infancy or early childhood, tic disorders, communication disorders, elimination disorders, and other disorders of infancy, childhood, or adolescence. All of the childhood disorders are recorded on Axis I, except mental retardation, which is recorded on Axis II.

Table 7–1.   Summary of major changes from DSM-III-R to DSM-IV

Categories added
  Rett's disorder
  Childhood disintegrative disorder
  Asperger's disorder
  Bipolar II disorder
  Substance persisting disorder
  Substance-induced sexual dysfunction disorder
  Sexual dysfunction due to general medical condition
  Acute stress disorder
  Narcolepsy
  Breathing-related sleep disorder

Categories deleted
  Cluttering
  Identity disorder
  Transsexualism
  Gender identity disorder of adolescence or adulthood, nontranssexual type
  Avoidant disorder of childhood or adolescence
  Overanxious disorder
  Alcohol (and other drug categories) idiosyncratic intoxication
  Adjustment disorder subtypes of: physical complaints, withdrawal, and
    work (or academic) inhibition
  Passive aggressive personality disorder (moved to Appendix B)

☐ Delirium, Dementia, Amnestic, and Other Cognitive Disorders

The next three sections in DSM-III-R were grouped together as "organic mental disorders." However, because this term implies that the "nonorganic" mental disorders in DSM do not also have a biological basis, it has not been used in DSM-IV. Instead, the so-called cognitive disorders are grouped together. The mental disorders due to general medical conditions and the substance-related disorders are referenced and described within the diagnostic classes with which they share phenomenology. This makes the classification more user-friendly because it references in one place all of the disorders that a clinician must consider when making a differential diagnosis, for instance, of anxiety symptoms (Spitzer et al. 1989, 1992a).

The cognitive disorders include deliria, dementias, and amnestic disorders due to general medical conditions and substances. A category of cognitive disorder not otherwise specified (NOS) has been added for disorders characterized by cognitive dysfunction presumed to be due to either substance use or a general medical condition, but that do not meet criteria for any of the specific delirium, dementia, or amnestic disorder categories.

☐ Mental Disorders Due to a General Medical Condition Not Elsewhere Classified

This section of DSM-IV includes categories for catatonic disorder, personality change, and mental disorder NOS, all of which are due to a general medical condition.

☐ Substance Related Disorders

This major class of disorders includes categories for dependence, abuse, intoxication, and withdrawal for the specific substance groups, as well as the criteria for hallucinogen persisting perception disorder. The text descriptions and criteria for substance-induced delirium and dementia, and those for amnestic, psychotic, mood, anxiety, sexual dysfunction, and sleep disorders, appear in the sections for those disorders with which they share phenomenology.

Single sets of criteria for dependence and abuse apply across all of the substance groups. *Substance dependence* is defined by a maladaptive pattern of substance use leading to clinically significant impairment or distress. This maladaptive use may include tolerance or withdrawal, and other symptoms that indicate loss of control of substance use and continued use of the substance despite adverse consequences. *Substance abuse,* which describes the consequences of maladaptive substance use, is defined with a lower threshold than substance dependence and is only appropriate when the criteria for substance dependence have never been met. The substances themselves are divided into 11 specific groups: alcohol, amphetamine, caffeine, cannabis, cocaine, hallucinogen, inhalant, nicotine, opioid, phencyclidine, and sedative, hypnotic, or anxiolytic. A category for polysubstance dependence is also included.

☐ Schizophrenia and Other Psychotic Disorders

This major class includes schizophrenia and its subtypes, schizophreniform disorder, schizoaffective disorder, delusional disorder, brief psychotic disorder, shared psychotic disorder, psychotic disorder due to a general medical condition, substance-induced psychotic disorder, and psychotic disorder not otherwise specified.

The diagnosis of *schizophrenia* requires both a period of active symptoms (delusions, hallucinations, disorganized speech, grossly disorganized or catatonic behavior, and negative symptoms), and a total duration of the disturbance of at least 6 months. This duration usually includes a period of prodromal symptoms in which there is deterioration in functioning, an active phase of psychotic symptoms, and a residual phase during which there is impairment in functioning but not the florid psychotic symptoms characteristic of the active phase. The symptoms of the active phase must be present for a signficant portion of time during a 1-month period, unless they are successfully treated.

Schizophreniform disorder is phenomenologically the same as schizophrenia, except that the disturbance has had a duration of less than 6 months (but of at least 1 month). There is a provision for clinicians to indicate whether or not the condition is associated with good prognostic features (e.g., good premorbid functioning, acute onset). Such cases are particularly unlikely to go on to meet the criteria for schizophrenia.

In *schizoaffective disorder* there is an uninterrupted period of illness during which, at some time, there is a major depressive or manic episode concurrent with psychotic symptoms characteristic of schizophrenia, and during the same period of illness there have been delusions or hallucinations for at least 2 weeks in the absence of prominent mood symptoms. Further, symptoms meeting criteria for a mood episode are present for a substantial portion of the total duration of the active and residual periods of the illness. Schizoaffective disorder must be distinguished from schizophrenia on the one hand, and psychotic mood disorders on the other.

The essential feature of *delusional disorder* is the presence of nonbizarre delusions of at least 1 month's duration, that are not due to any other mental disorder such as schizophrenia or a mood disorder, or to a general medical condition or use of a substance. The following delusional types are recognized: erotomanic, grandiose, jealous, persecutory, somatic, mixed, and unspecified.

Brief psychotic disorder may occur following a marked stressor (in which case it is equivalent to the DSM-III-R category of brief reactive psychosis), or without a marked stressor. This disorder is characterized by psychotic symptoms lasting from 1 day to 1 month, with the person's eventual full return to his or her premorbid level of functioning.

In *shared psychotic disorder* there is a delusion that develops in one person in the context of a close relationship with another person who has an already-established delusion. The same delusion is at least partly shared by both persons.

Psychotic disorder due to a general medical condition has been added to this group of disorders. Although the general medical condition is listed on both Axis I and Axis III, it should be coded only on Axis III. *Substance-induced psychotic disorder* has also been added to this part of the classification.

Finally, the category of *psychotic disorder NOS* is used when there are psychotic symptoms present but there is inadequate information to make a more specific diagnosis, when there is contradictory information, or when none of the full criteria for any of the specific psychotic disorders above are met.

☐ Mood Disorders

The mood disorders are divided into depressive disorders (i.e., major depressive and dysthymic disorders), and bipolar disorders (i.e., bipolar I, bipolar II, and cyclothymic disorders). The depressive disorders are characterized by one or more periods of depression, and the absence of a history of manic or hypomanic episodes. *Dysthymic disorder* is a form of chronic depression of at least 2 years' duration that is distinguished from a chronic major depressive disorder by its lesser severity.

In *bipolar I disorder* there is one or more manic episodes, and although the diagnosis does not require a history of a major depressive episode, in virtually all cases such an episode eventually develops (Nurnberger et al. 1979). *Bipolar II disorder*, newly added to the classification, does require one or more major depressive episodes, at least one hypomanic episode, and the absence of a history of manic or mixed episodes (Endicott et al. 1985). Manic episodes are distinguished from hypomanic episodes by their duration and marked impairment in social or occupational functioning or the need for hospitalization. *Cyclothymic disorder* is a chronic mood disturbance of at least 2 years' duration that involves numerous periods with hypomanic symptoms and numerous periods with depressed mood or loss of interest or pleasure.

A "seasonal pattern" can be indicated for major depressive episodes when there is a regular temporal relationship between the onset of the mood episodes and a particular time of the year; full remissions also must occur at a characteristic time of the year. This specification makes use of the accumulated evidence regarding the validity of a seasonal sub-type of mood disorder (Rosenthal et al. 1984; Terman et al. 1989). Clinicians can also indicate if a major depressive or manic episode developed within 4 weeks after giving birth ("with postpartum onset").

☐ Anxiety Disorders

In DSM-IV the disorders in which anxiety is experienced directly, or in which there is avoidance behavior due to anxiety, are grouped together in the class of anxiety disorders. In *panic disorder* there are recurrent un-expected panic attacks, with at least one of the attacks being followed by a month or more of persistent concern about having additional attacks, or worry about the implications of the attack or its consequences, or a significant change in behavior related to the attacks. Many cases of panic disorder are complicated by the presence of agoraphobia, which is anxi-ety about being in places or situations from which escape might be diffi-cult or in which help might not be available if one has another panic attack; in such cases the diagnosis of *panic disorder with agoraphobia* is made.

Agoraphobia without history of panic disorder is exceedingly rare in clini-cal settings, because agoraphobia typically develops out of fear of hav-ing another panic attack and the resulting avoidance behavior. *Specific and social phobias* both involve marked and persistent fear of a situation or stimulus with consequent avoidance behavior (or intense anxiety or distress when enduring the situation or stimulus). In *obsessive-compulsive disorder* there are either true obsessions or compulsions that cause marked distress, are time-consuming, or significantly interfere with daily functioning.

Posttraumatic stress disorder follows a traumatic event in which the person has experienced an event that involved actual or threatened death or serious injury or a threat to the physical integrity of himself or herself or others. This event is reexperienced by the person, along with other characteristic symptoms, for more than a month. Examples of symptoms specific to children are included. *Acute stress disorder* is a new category added to DSM-IV for a posttraumatic syndrome that lasts for at least 2 days but no longer than 4 weeks.

Finally, *generalized anxiety disorder* involves excessive anxiety and worry, lasting at least 6 months, about a number of events or activities. The person finds it difficult to control the worry, and it is associated with physical symptoms of anxiety, such as restlessness, difficulty concentrating, and sleep disturbance. The prevalence and validity of this diagnosis are unclear (Brown et al. 1994).

Categories for *anxiety disorder due to general medical condition, substance-induced anxiety disorder,* and *anxiety disorder NOS* also appear in this section.

☐ Somatoform Disorders

Somatoform disorders all involve physical symptoms that, while suggesting a general medical disorder, cannot be accounted for by any known general medical condition. Thus, this diagnostic class includes *somatization disorder,* a chronic illness with recurrent and multiple physical complaints; *conversion disorder,* in which there is one or more symptoms or deficits affecting voluntary motor or sensory function; *hypochondriasis,* a preoccupation with fears of having, or the idea that one has, a serious disease based on the person's misinterpretation of bodily symptoms; *body dysmorphic disorder,* in which there is preoccupation with an imagined defect in appearance; *pain disorder,* in which pain is the predominant focus of the clinical presentation and psychological factors are judged to have an important role in the onset, severity, exacerbation, or maintenance of the pain; and *undifferentiated somatoform disorder,* which is characterized by one or more chronic physical complaints that cause clinically significant distress or impairment in social, occupational, or other important areas of functioning.

☐ Factitious Disorders

Individuals who simulate physical or psychological symptoms in such a way that their simulation is not discovered, and who therefore appear to voluntarily produce illness, have disorders that are classified as *factitious disorders.* These individuals' actions are compulsive and voluntary in the sense that they are intentionally produced or feigned, but not in the sense that they can be controlled. The prototypical *factitious disorder with predominantly physical signs and symptoms* is also referred to in the literature as Munchausen syndrome.

☐ Dissociative Disorders

Dissociative disorders all involve a disturbance or alteration in the normally integrative functions of identity, memory, or consciousness. The disturbance or alteration may be sudden or gradual, and transient or chronic. If it occurs primarily in identity, the person's customary identity is temporarily forgotten and a new identity is assumed or imposed (as in *dissociative identity disorder,* formerly called "multiple personality disorder"), or the customary feeling of one's own reality is lost and is replaced by a feeling of unreality (as in *depersonalization disorder*). If the disturbance occurs primarily in memory, important personal events cannot be recalled (as in *dissociative amnesia* and *dissociative fugue*).

☐ Sexual and Gender Identity Disorders

Sexual dysfunctions, paraphilias, and gender identity disorders are included in this diagnostic class. In the *sexual dysfunctions* there is inhibition in sexual desire or in the psychophysiological changes of the sexual response cycle. *Paraphilias* all involve sexual arousal in response to objects or situations that are not part of normative arousal-activity patterns. Further, the behavior, sexual urges, or fantasies cause clinically significant distress or impairment in social, occupational, or other important areas of functioning. Finally, in *gender identity disorder* there is a strong and persistent cross-gender identification, with persistent discomfort with one's sex or a sense of inappropriateness in that gender role.

☐ Eating Disorders

Anorexia nervosa and bulimia nervosa are the two specific categories in this class of disorders. In *anorexia nervosa* there is a refusal to maintain one's body weight at or above a minimally normal weight for age and height, with an intense fear of gaining weight or becoming fat. This fear is accompanied by a disturbance in the way in which the individual experiences his or her body weight or shape. *Bulimia nervosa* is characterized by recurrent episodes of binge eating accompanied by recurrent inappropriate compensatory behaviors in order to prevent weight gain, such as self-induced vomiting, fasting, or excessive exercise.

☐ Sleep Disorders

This diagnostic class includes disorders of sleep that are chronic, rather than the transient disturbances of sleep that are commonly experienced. Sleep disorders are divided into the *dyssomnias,* in which there is a disturbance in the amount, quality, or timing of sleep; the *parasomnias,* in which the hallmark is an abnormal event that occurs either during sleep or at the threshold between wakefulness and sleep; *sleep disorders related to another mental disorder,* in which insomnia or hypersomnia is judged to be related to another Axis I or II disorder, but is sufficiently severe to warrant independent clinical attention; and *other sleep disorders,* which include sleep disorder due to a general medical condition and substance-induced sleep disorder.

The dyssomnias include *primary insomnia,* in which there is difficulty initiating or maintaining sleep, or nonrestorative sleep, for at least 1 month, with consequent clinically significant distress or impairment in functioning; *primary hypersomnia,* characterized by complaint of excessive sleepiness for at least 1 month, also resulting in clinically significant distress or impairment in functioning; *narcolepsy* (added in DSM-IV), with irresistible attacks of refreshing sleep occurring daily over at least 3 months, cataplexy, and intrusions of REM sleep into the transition between sleep and wakefulness (e.g., sleep paralysis); *breathing-related sleep disorder,* in which there is sleep disruption leading to excessive sleepiness or insomnia that is due to a sleep-related breathing disorder such as sleep apnea; and *circadian rhythm sleep disorder,* a persistent or recurrent pattern of sleep disruption leading to excessive sleepiness or insomnia that is due to a mismatch between the sleep-wake schedule required by a person's environment and his or her circadian sleep-wake pattern.

The parasomnias include *nightmare disorder,* characterized by repeated awakenings from sleep with detailed recall of extended and extremely frightening dreams; *sleep terror disorder,* in which there are also recurrent awakenings from sleep, but these are accompanied by intense anxiety and signs of autonomic arousal such as tachycardia and sweating, and yet no detailed dream is recalled; and *sleepwalking disorder,* in which the individual repeatedly walks about during sleep and is relatively unresponsive during the episodes. In both sleep terror and sleepwalking disorders, there is later amnesia for the episode. Finally, *insomnia or hypersomnia related to [Axis I or Axis II disorder]* may be diagnosed when the sleep disturbance is sufficiently severe to cause clinically significant distress or impairment in social, occupational, or other important areas of functioning.

☐ Impulse Control Disorders Not Elsewhere Classified

The impulse control disorders not elsewhere classified involve disturbances in impulse control that do not satisfy the criteria for other diagnostic categories (e.g., substance-related disorders or paraphilias). These disorders are characterized by 1) recurrent failure to resist an impulse, drive, or temptation to perform some act that is harmful to oneself or others; 2) an increasing sense of tension before committing the act; and 3) a sense of either pleasure, gratification, or relief at the time of committing the act. Included in this class of disorders are *intermittent explosive disorder, kleptomania, pyromania, pathological gambling,* and *trichotillomania* (a disorder characterized by impulsive pulling out of one's own hair).

☐ Adjustment Disorder

Adjustment disorder is a clinically significant reaction to an identifiable stressor that occurs within 3 months of the onset of the stressor and persists for no longer than 6 months after the termination of the stressor or its consequences. This category is not diagnosed if the disturbance meets the criteria for another specific Axis I disorder, or is merely an exacerbation of a preexisting Axis I or Axis II disorder.

☐ Personality Disorders

The diagnostic criteria for each of the 10 specific personality disorders are in the form of a brief summary description of the disorder followed by an index of specific behaviors, no single one of which is required to make the diagnosis. A residual category, personality disorder NOS, is provided for 1) disorders of personality functioning that do not meet the criteria for any specific personality disorder, and 2) other specific personality disorders not included in this classification.

In differentiating a personality disorder from an Axis I disorder, the clinician must consider several factors. First, a personality disorder is characteristic of the person's current and long-term functioning and is not limited to episodes of illness; that is, it represents a pervasive pattern of disturbance that is present in a variety of contexts in the person's life. Second, in distinguishing a personality disorder from a personality trait, the clinician must determine that the behaviors are above a certain threshold in terms of causing either subjective distress or significant impairment in social or occupational functioning, and of having enough criteria met. Finally, the disturbance must begin by early adulthood, and usually is apparent by adolescence.

☐ Other Conditions That May Be
a Focus of Clinical Attention

Other conditions may be a focus of clinical attention but are not considered mental disorder diagnoses. A list of such conditions (e.g., medication-induced movement disorders, relational problems, problems related to abuse or neglect, bereavement, occupational problems, malingering, and phase-of-life problem) is included for use when no mental disorder diagnosis is appropriate but help is needed, or when there is a mental disorder related to one of these conditions but the condition is sufficiently severe to warrant independent clinical attention. In addition, there are codes for indicating that the diagnosis is deferred on Axis I or Axis II, or that there is no diagnosis or condition on these axes.

■ REFERENCES

American Psychiatric Association: Diagnostic and Statistical Manual: Mental Disorders. Washington, DC, American Psychiatric Association, 1952

American Psychiatric Association: Diagnostic and Statistical Manual of Mental Disorders, 2nd Edition. Washington, DC, American Psychiatric Association, 1968

American Psychiatric Association: Diagnostic and Statistical Manual of Mental Disorders, 3rd Edition, Revised. Washington, DC, American Psychiatric Association, 1987

American Psychiatric Association: Diagnostic and Statistical Manual of Mental Disorders, 4th Edition. Washington, DC, American Psychiatric Association, 1994

Brown TA, Barlow DH, Liebowitz MR: The empirical basis of generalized anxiety disorder. Am J Psychiatry 151:1271–1280, 1994

Cohen J: A coefficient of agreement for nominal scales. Educational and Psychological Measurement 20:37–46, 1960

Endicott J, Spitzer RL: A diagnostic interview: the Schedule for Affective Disorders and Schizophrenia. Arch Gen Psychiatry 35:837–844, 1978

Endicott J, Nee J, Andreasen N, et al: Bipolar II: combine or keep separate? J Affect Disord 8:17–28, 1985

Feighner JP, Robins E, Guze SB, et al: Diagnostic criteria for use in psychiatric research. Arch Gen Psychiatry 26:57–63, 1972

Frances A, Davis WW, Kline M, et al: The DSM-IV field trials: moving toward an empirically derived classification. European Psychiatry 6:307–314, 1991

Gutterman EM, O'Brien JD, Young JG: Structured diagnostic interviews for children and adolescents: current status and future directions. J Am Acad Child Adolesc Psychiatry 26:621–630, 1987

Hodges K: Structured interviews for assessing children. J Child Psychol Psychiatry 34:49–68, 1993

Nurnberger J Jr, Roose SP, Dunner DL, et al: Unipolar mania: a distinct clinical entity? Am J Psychiatry 136:1420–1423, 1979

Perry JC: Problems and considerations in the valid assessment of personality disorders. Am J Psychiatry 149:1645–1653, 1992

Regier DA, Myers JK, Kramer M, et al: The NIMH Epidemiologic Catchment Area program: historical context, major objectives, and study population characteristics. Arch Gen Psychiatry 41:934–941, 1984

Robins LN, Helzer JE, Croughan J, et al: National Institute of Mental Health Diagnostic Interview Schedule: its history, characteristics, and validity. Arch Gen Psychiatry 38:381–389, 1981

Robins LN, Wing J, Wittchen HU, et al: The Composite International Diagnostic Interview: an epidemiologic instrument suitable for use in conjunction with different diagnostic systems and in different cultures. Arch Gen Psychiatry 45:1069–1077, 1988

Rosenthal NE, Sack DA, Gillin JC, et al: Seasonal affective disorder: description of syndrome and preliminary findings with light therapy. Arch Gen Psychiatry 41:72–80, 1984

Schleyer B, Aaronson C, Mannuzza S, et al: SADS-LA[R]. New York, Anxiety Disorders Clinic, New York State Psychiatric Institute, 1990

Spitzer RL: Psychiatric diagnosis: are clinicians still necessary? Compr Psychiatry 24:399–411, 1983

Spitzer RL, Fleiss JL: A re-analysis of the reliability of psychiatric diagnosis. Br J Psychiatry 125:341–347, 1974

Spitzer RL, Williams JBW: Dehumanizing descriptors (letter)? Am J Psychiatry 136:1481, 1979

Spitzer RL, Williams JBW: The definition and diagnosis of mental disorder, in Deviance and Mental Illness (Sage Annual Reviews of Studies in Deviance, Vol 6). Edited by Gove WR. Beverly Hills, CA, Sage, 1982, pp 15–31

Spitzer RL, Williams JBW: Classification of mental disorders, in Comprehensive Textbook of Psychiatry/IV, 4th Edition, Vol 1. Edited by Kaplan HI, Sadock BJ. Baltimore, MD, Williams & Wilkins, 1985, pp 591–613

Spitzer RL, Endicott J, Robins E: Reliability of clinical criteria for psychiatric diagnosis, in Psychiatric Diagnosis: Exploration of Biological Predictors. Edited by Akiskal H, Webb W. New York, Spectrum, 1978a, pp 61–73

Spitzer RL, Endicott J, Robins E: Research Diagnostic Criteria: rationale and reliability. Arch Gen Psychiatry 35:773–782, 1978b

Spitzer RL, Forman JBW, Nee J: DSM-III field trials, I: initial interrater diagnostic reliability. Am J Psychiatry 136:815–817, 1979

Spitzer RL, Williams JBW, Skodol AE (eds): International Perspectives on DSM-III. Washington, DC, American Psychiatric Press, 1983

Spitzer RL, Williams JBW, First MB, et al: A proposal for DSM-IV: solving the "organic/nonorganic" problem (editorial). J Neuropsychiatry Clin Neurosci 1:126–127, 1989

Spitzer RL, First M[B], Williams JBW, et al: Now is the time to retire the term "organic mental disorders." Am J Psychiatry 149:240–244, 1992a

Spitzer RL, Williams JBW, Gibbon M, et al: The Structured Clinical Interview for DSM-III-R (SCID), I: history, rationale, and description. Arch Gen Psychiatry 49:624–629, 1992b

Stangl D, Pfohl B, Zimmerman M, et al: A structured interview for the DSM-III personality disorders: a preliminary report. Arch Gen Psychiatry 42:591–596, 1985

Terman M, Terman JS, Quitkin FM, et al: Light therapy for seasonal affective disorder: a review of efficacy. Neuropsychopharmacology 2:1–22, 1989

Widiger TA, Frances AJ, Pincus HA, et al: DSM-IV literature reviews: rationale, process, and limitations. J Psychopathology and Behavioral Assessment 12:189–202, 1990

Williams JBW: The multiaxial system of DSM-III: where did it come from and where should it go? I: its origins and critiques. Arch Gen Psychiatry 42:175–180, 1985a

Williams JBW: The multiaxial system of DSM-III: where did it come from and where should it go? II: empirical studies, innovations, and recommendations. Arch Gen Psychiatry 42:181–186, 1985b

Williams JBW, Spitzer RL, Skodol AE: DSM-III in residency training: results of a national survey. Am J Psychiatry 142:755–758, 1985

Williams JBW, Gibbon M, First MB, et al: The Structured Clinical Interview for DSM-III-R (SCID), II: multisite test-retest reliability. Arch Gen Psychiatry 49:630–636, 1992

Wing JK, Birley JLT, Cooper JE, et al: Reliability of a procedure for measuring and classifying "present psychiatric state." Br J Psychiatry 113:499–515, 1967

Wing JK, Babor T, Brugha T, et al: SCAN: Schedules for Clinical Assessment in Neuropsychiatry. Arch Gen Psychiatry 47:589–593, 1990

World Health Organization: International Classification of Diseases, 10th Revision. Geneva, World Health Organization, 1992

Wynne LC: A preliminary proposal for strengthening the multiaxial approach of DSM-III: possible family-oriented revisions, in Diagnosis and Classification in Psychiatry: A Critical Appraisal of DSM-III. Edited by Tischler GL. Cambridge, UK, Cambridge University Press, 1987, pp 477–488

Zanarini MC, Frankenburg FR, Chauncey DL, et al: The Diagnostic Interview for Personality Disorders: interrater and test-retest reliability. Compr Psychiatry 28:467–480, 1987

CHAPTER 8

Psychological and Neuropsychological Assessment

John F. Clarkin, Ph.D.
Stephen W. Hurt, Ph.D.
Steven Mattis, Ph.D.

The proliferation of both assessment devices and treatment options in recent years has given rise to the need for a structure to define criteria for referral for testing, selection of tests, and utilization of the resulting information. In this chapter, after reviewing the general issues related to the definition and development of psychological tests, we discuss the goals of psychological assessment and provide a heuristic structure for considering the main areas of such an assessment. We review the best existing tests within this structure and provide a clinical decision tree that relates both to the referral of patients for testing and the selection of appropriate tests.

■ DEFINITION AND DEVELOPMENT OF PSYCHOLOGICAL ASSESSMENT INSTRUMENTS

Three types of instruments are currently utilized in the assessment of patient functioning: psychological tests, rating scales, and semistructured interviews.

Psychological tests are standardized methods of sampling behaviors in a reliable and valid way. The test stimuli, the method of presenting these stimuli, and the method of scoring the responses are carefully standardized to ensure reliability. The actual test stimuli can be constructed in numerous ways. For example, test items on the Wechsler Adult Intelligence Scale—Revised (WAIS-R; Wechsler 1981), a widely used intelligence test, include factual questions (e.g., What does ponder mean?), and each answer is scored 2 (i.e., to contemplate), 1 (i.e., to wonder), or 0 (i.e., to fret). The restandardized Minnesota Multiphasic Personality Inventory–2 (MMPI-2; Butcher et al. 1989), a highly developed and widely used symptom and personality test, consists of questions about presence or absence of feelings, thoughts, and experiences (e.g., "I usually feel that life is worthwhile," an item on Scale 2) in a true/false format. Test stimuli on the Rorschach (Rorschach 1949), a widely used projective test of personality styles and characteristics, are amorphous inkblots. The patient is asked to tell the examiner what it looks like or what it reminds the patient of. The response is recorded verbatim and scored with a standardized system.

Behavior rating scales are standardized devices that allow various informants or observers (e.g., therapist, nurse on a clinical inpatient unit, relatives, trained observers) to rate the behavior of the patient in specified areas. To aid the observer in a reliable rating of the behavior, anchor points are provided in one of several ways. For example, on the Brief Psychiatric Rating Scale (BPRS; Overall and Gorham 1962), somatic concern, defined as the "degree of concern over present bodily health," is rated by the interviewer on a 7-point scale from *not present* to *extremely severe.*

Semistructured interviews are standardized by controlling the questions, including specifying what kind of probes can be used, and standardizing the scoring of the patient's response, often by using rating scales as described above. Although developed for research, these interviews have clinical usefulness in the reliable assessment of diagnostic criteria. As an example of a semistructured interview item, the following is a question from the Schedule for Affective Disorders and Schizophrenia (SADS; Endicott and Spitzer 1978): "Have you felt depressed (sad, blue, moody, down, empty, as if you didn't care)?" The patient's answer is scored on a rating scale provided in the instrument from 1 (not at all) to 5 (severe [e.g., most of the time feels "wretched"]) to 7 (very extreme [e.g., constant, unrelieved, extremely painful feeling of depression]).

The science of assessment depends upon the development of instruments that meet certain standards. Chief among these standards are those for reliability and various types of validity.

Standardization of administration and scoring to minimize the influence of factors unrelated to the area of assessment is essential for establishing *reliability.* The degree to which a test meets acceptable standards for reliability is evaluated by readministering the test at later times to determine if individual scores remain stable; developing alternative forms of the test that, when compared, provide roughly equivalent scores for an individual; and demonstrating that any subgroup of items from the test yields a score comparable to an equivalent number of items in any other subgroup of items. These procedures for establishing reliability are generally referred to as *test-retest reliability, alternate form reliability*, and *split-half reliability*, respectively.

Establishing a test's *validity* requires a demonstration that a test measures what it is intended to measure. Three major types of validity can be assessed: 1) content validity, 2) criterion-related validity, and 3) construct validity. *Content validity* can be achieved only if the content of the test can be said to adequately sample the area of interest. For example, an intelligence test must contain items that tap several areas of intellectual functioning, such as knowledge of words, arithmetic ability, abstracting ability, knowledge of social conventions, and so forth, in order to meet acceptable standards for content validity. *Criterion-related validity* refers to the test's relationship to independent criteria of an individual's ability in a particular area (i.e., concurrent validity) or to the ability of the test to make predictions about future behavior (i.e., predictive validity). For example, a test of the severity of depressive symptoms would achieve concurrent validity if scores on the test were closely related to a trained observer's rating of the severity of the depression, and would achieve predictive validity if scores on the test were found to be related to the likelihood that a given individual would respond to a specific treatment for reducing depressive symptoms. *Construct validity* can be achieved only by demonstrating that the test specifically measures a theoretical construct of interest and that scores on the test are unrelated to similar areas.

■ GOALS OF ASSESSMENT

The role of assessment has always been closely linked to the need to plan and implement successful intervention strategies for the remediation of psychological disorders. As a consequence, the goals of assessment should constantly be revised as new treatment aims and methods are developed. Common assessment goals are listed in Table 8–1.

Diagnostic assessment remains the primary reason for clinical psychiatric referral. DSM-IV (American Psychiatric Association 1994), the revision of the diagnostic nomenclature of the American Psychiatric Association's DSM-III-R (American Psychiatric Association 1987), continues to provide a focus for diagnostic issues and both capitalizes on and fuels a growing interest in the issues of accurate diagnosis. Much of the

Table 8–1.   Specific objectives of assessment

1. To clarify diagnostic uncertainty following clinical interview.
2. To specify the severity of symptoms and other difficulties.
3. To assess patient strengths (e.g., intelligence, personality traits).
4. To inform differential treatment assignment.
5. To develop a role consistent with a therapeutic alliance.
6. To monitor the impact of treatment.

research stimulated by the development and implementation of DSM-III and DSM-III-R focused on the sensitivity and specificity of the diagnostic criteria in light of the need to identify homogeneous groups of symptoms that are optimally responsive to a growing armamentarium of psychiatric and psychological interventions.

■ MAJOR AREAS OF ASSESSMENT

To further the overall goal of clinical assessment (i.e., differential treatment planning), one must consider the most important content areas of assessment. The assessment procedures chosen should depend upon the nature of the patient's difficulties revealed or suspected during routine psychiatric examination. They should be carried out in the context of the major dimensions of human functioning relevant to diagnosis and treatment planning. The areas or dimensions of human functioning that seem most central for diagnosis and treatment planning include 1) symptoms and related Axis I disorders, 2) cognitive functioning, 3) personality traits and disorders, 4) psychodynamics, and 5) environmental demands and social adjustment. In the subsections that follow we review the best available instruments in each of these five areas.

☐ Assessment of Axis I Constellations and Related Symptoms

As psychiatric nomenclature has undergone revision, assessment tools have been developed that rely on interviews and self-reports (Table 8–2), providing data that are immediately relevant to diagnosis.

The SADS represents this tradition. Developed in the 1970s at the New York State Psychiatric Institute, the SADS was designed as a semistructured interview instrument to gather information pertinent to the classification of psychiatric disorders. Its primary purpose was to provide information that was sufficient to classify patients into relatively homogeneous subgroups for the purposes of research (Endicott and Spitzer 1979). These classifications were explicated using the Research Diagnostic Criteria (RDC; Feighner et al. 1972), which specified explicit symptomatic criteria for 23 psychiatric disorders. These criteria served as the forerunner to DSM-III and have, in the main, been incorporated into that version of psychiatric nomenclature.

The SADS takes approximately 2 hours to complete, and some training in the formal assessment of psychopathology is required. Considered in relation to the DSM-III, the SADS provides extensive (major depressive disorder, dysthymic disorder, schizophrenia, anxiety disorders) but incomplete coverage of the Axis I disorders, pays little attention to Axes II and IV, and utilizes a separate scale, the Global Assessment Scale (GAS; Endicott et al. 1976) to provide information relevant to Axis V. These difficulties in establishing a uniform relationship between the SADS and DSM-III have led Spitzer and his associates to revise the SADS.

Omnibus Measures of Symptoms

There are a number of instruments that have been developed for the assessment of a wide variety of symptoms (Table 8–3). These measures depend on either self-report or interview methods for gathering data.

Minnesota Multiphasic Personality Inventory. The Minnesota Multiphasic Personality Inventory (MMPI; Hathaway and McKinley 1967), along with its recent successor, the MMPI-2, is probably the most widely used assessment instrument in existence. There are a number of reasons for its extensive use, including its efficiency (the patient spends 1 to 2 hours taking the test, which can then be computer scored), the extensive data accumulated with the test, its normative base, and the use of validity scales that indicate the patient's test-taking attitude. Although labeled as a "personality test," the MMPI was constructed to assess what are now categorized as DSM-III Axis I conditions and, to a lesser extent, a few dimensions of personality that are not represented on DSM-III Axis II.

Using this method of criterion-keyed scoring, McKinley and Hathaway constructed nine clinical scales: hypochondriasis (Hs, or Scale 1), depression (D, or Scale 2), hysteria (Hy, or Scale 3), psychopathic deviance (Pd, or Scale 4), masculinity-femininity (Mf, or Scale 5), paranoia (Pa, or Scale 6), psychasthenia (Pt, or Scale 7), schizophrenia (Sc, or Scale 8), and mania (Ma, or Scale 9). Items were worded so that persons with an elementary school education could take the test, and norms were established for determining the degree of disturbance typical of psychopathological groups. For example, an item on Scale 2 (i.e., depression) reads as follows: "I find it hard to keep my mind on a task or job (True)."

In addition to the clinical scales, validity scales were developed to

Table 8–2.   Assessment of DSM-III-R Axis I disorders

Instrument	General classification	Description	Scoring features
Schedule for Affective Disorders and Schizophrenia (SADS)	Semistructured interview	7-point rating scales of symptoms	Oriented to diagnosis using RDC
Structured Clinical Interview for DSM-III-R (SCID)	Semistructured interview	3-point rating scales of symptoms	Oriented to diagnosis using DSM-III-R

Note.   RDC = Research Diagnostic Criteria.

Table 8–3.   Instruments for the assessment of symptom patterns

Instrument	General classification	Description	Scoring features
Minnesota Multiphasic Personality Inventory–2 (MMPI-2)	Self-report	566-item checklist, true/false format	T scores for 13 criterion scales
Personality Assessment Inventory (PAI)	Self-report	344 items, true/false format	4 validity scales, 10 clinical scales covering symptoms and severe personality disorders
Hopkins Symptoms Checklist–90 (SCL-90)	Self-report	90-item checklist, 5-point intensity scales	T scores for 9 symptom clusters
Brief Psychiatric Rating Scale (BPRS)	Clinical interview	16 items, 7-point severity scales	5 factor scores and total scores
Millon Clinical Multiaxial Inventory–II (MCMI-II)	Self-report	175 items, true/false format	3 validity scales, 22 clinical scales covering Axis I and Axis II areas

assess the test-taking attitudes of the patient. McKinley, Hathaway, and Meehl (1948) focused on the assessment of defensiveness or of minimizing symptoms and problems ("faking good") and maximizing or exaggerating problems ("faking bad"). Validity scales were constructed to evaluate these dimensions, which are helpful in interpreting the severity of symptomatic complaints on the clinical scales.

The MMPI has been revised and restandardized as the MMPI-2 (Butcher et al. 1989). Revisions include the deletion of objectionable items and the rewording of other items to reflect more modern language usage, as well as the addition of several new items focusing on suicide, drug and alcohol abuse, Type A behavior, interpersonal relations, and treatment compliance. Restandardization of the norms was based on a randomly solicited national sample of 1,138 males and 1,462 females.

The MMPI and MMPI-2 are good examples of psychological tests, because both were developed with careful attention to issues of reliability and validity. Both the severity and the pattern of symptomatic disturbance are considered, and a large body of literature relevant to these tests' predictive validity has developed. Moreover, the MMPI and MMPI-2 provide information on the response style of the individual taking the test, a personality attribute that is essential in interpreting the clinical scales.

Personality Assessment Inventory.   The Personality Assessment Inventory (PAI; Morey 1991), focuses on clinical syndromes that have been staples of psychopathological nosology and have retained their importance in contemporary diagnostic practice. Items were written with careful attention to their content validity, which was designed to reflect the phenomenology of the clinical construct across a broad range of severity. An initial pool of 2,200 items was generated from the research literature, classic texts, the DSM, and other diagnostic manuals and from the clinical experience of practitioners who participated in the project. This pool of items was finally reduced to 344 items covering 4 validity scales, 11 clinical syndromes, 5 treatment planning areas, and the two major dimensions of the interpersonal complex. All items are rated based on a 4-point Likert-type response format. For example, on the borderline scale is the following item: "I'm too impulsive for my own good." Final clinical validation was carried out on the data from 235 subjects from 10 clinical sites and 2 community and 2 college student samples.

Hopkins Symptom Checklist–90.   The Hopkins Symptom Checklist–90 (SCL-90; Derogatis 1977) is another example of a self-report instrument designed to provide information about a broad range of complaints typical of individuals with psychological symptomatic distress. Briefer than the MMPI-2 and the PAI, the SCL-90 contains only 90 items and can be administered in 30 minutes and scored by computer. These items are combined into nine symptom scales: 1) somatization, 2) obsessive-compulsive behavior, 3) interpersonal sensitivity, 4) depression, 5) anxiety, 6) hostility, 7) phobic anxiety, 8) paranoid ideation, and 9) psychoticism. In addition, three global indices are compiled: 1) general severity, 2) positive symptom distress index, and 3) total positive symptoms.

A companion instrument, the Hopkins Psychiatric Rating Scale (HPRS; Derogatis et al. 1974), can be used to rate material obtained through direct interview of the patient on each of the nine symptom dimensions of the SCL-90. No structured interview procedure is associated with the HPRS, so formal training in the interview assessment of psychopathology is essential to the accuracy of the assessment. Eight additional dimensions are covered in the interview.

Brief Psychiatric Rating Scale.   Another widely used rating scale for a range of psychiatric symptoms is the Brief Psychiatric Rating Scale (BPRS; Overall and Gorham 1962), which was developed mainly for the assessment of symptoms with an inpatient population. Areas rated include somatic concern, anxiety, emotional withdrawal, conceptional disorganization, guilt, tension, mannerisms and posturing, grandiosity, depressive mood, hostility, suspiciousness, hallucinatory behavior, motor retardation, uncooperativeness, unusual thought content, blunted affect, excitement, and disorientation.

Other rating scales for inpatient settings.   There are a number of rating scales for the assessment of general areas of psychopathology that can be used most efficiently in inpatient settings by personnel who make routine observations of patient behavior (Raskin 1982). The best-known scales of this type are the Inpatient Behavioral Rating Scale (IBRS; Green et al. 1977), patterned after the BPRS, and the Nurses' Observation Scale for Inpatient Evaluation–30 (NOSIE-30; Honigfeld and Klett 1965).

Specific Areas of Symptomatology

In addition to the omnibus measures of symptomatology, there are a number of instruments that assess one area of symptomatology in depth (Table 8–4).

Substance abuse.   The need for the assessment of substance abuse potential is reflected in omnibus symptom rating scales such as the MMPI-2, which contains an item key, the MacAndrew Alcoholism Scale (MacAndrew 1965), for identifying patients who have histories of alcohol abuse or who have the potential to develop problems with alcohol (Hoffmann et al. 1974). A more thorough instrument, the Alcohol Use

Table 8–4. Selected instruments for the assessment of specific symptom areas

Instrument	General classification	Description	Scoring features
Substance abuse			
Alcohol Use Inventory (AUI)	Self-report	228 items rated on 2- to 6-point scales	17 primary scales in four areas and 7 second-order factor scales
Eating Disorders Inventory–2 (EDI-2)	Self-report	91 forced-choice items rated on a 6-point frequency scale	8 subscales and 3 provisional scales for issues and features pertinent to eating disorders
Affects			
State-Trait Anxiety Inventory (STAI)	Self-report	Two 20-item scales, 4-point frequency ratings	Total scores for state and trait anxiety
S-R Inventory of Anxiousness	Self-report	14-item responses on 5-point severity scales to 11 situations	Focus on intensity and quality of situations arousing anxiety
Anxiety Disorders Interview Schedule	Semistructured	Items pertinent to DSM-III-R anxiety and depressive disorders	Clinical judgment and application of DSM-III-R decision rules
Fear Questionnaire	Self-report	17 items reflecting specific phobias rated on 9-point avoidance scales	Total scores for agoraphobia, social phobia, and blood and injury phobias
Beck Depression Inventory (BDI)	Self-report	20 items, 4-point intensity scales	Total score
Hamilton Rating Scale for Depression (Ham-D)	Clinical interview	17 to 24 items, 3- to 5-point severity scales	Total score

(continued)

Table 8–4. Selected instruments for the assessment of specific symptom areas (*continued*)

Instrument	General classification	Description	Scoring features
Affects (*continued*)			
Dyadic Adjustment Scale (DAS)	Self-report	40 items, 7-point scales	Total score
Manic-State Rating Scale (MSRS)	Observer rating	26 items, each scored for frequency and intensity	Total score
Suicidal behavior			
Suicide Intent Scale (SIS)	Self-report	15 items, 3-point categorical scales	Total score
Index of Potential Suicide	Self-report or semistructured interview	50 items, 5-point severity scales	Total score and 6 subscores
Reasons for Living Inventory (RFL)	Self-report	6 factors	Total score
Thought disorder			
Schedule for Affective Disorders and Schizophrenia (SADS)	Semistructured	Severity ratings of hallucinations and delusions	Oriented to diagnosis using RDC
Thought Disorder Index	Content rating	22 categories at 4 levels of severity	Total score

Note. RDC = Research Diagnostic Criteria.

Inventory (AUI; Horn et al. 1986), is a self-administered test standardized on over 1,200 admissions to an alcoholism treatment program. It contains 24 scales that measure alcohol-related problems, and considers the subjects' responses in four separate domains: benefits from drinking, style of drinking, consequences of drinking, and concerns associated with drinking.

Garner developed an inventory to assess attitudes and behaviors associated with anorexia nervosa. This inventory, the Eating Disorders Inventory–2 (EDI-2) (Garner 1992), consists of 91 items rated on 6-point frequency scales. The items were chosen to reflect important clinical aspects of anorexia and were retained if they successfully discriminated between anorexic, normal-weight, and obese males and females. Internal reliability, construct validity, and treatment response data have been reported, and the EDI-2 can be a useful screening instrument for identifying inpatients with potentially serious eating disorders.

Affects.   The content, range, and management of emotional expression constitute a symptomatic area of focus for the evaluation of psychopathology and are important in the differential diagnosis of a wide variety of psychiatric disorders. The main affects of interest are anxiety, depression, and elation.

As one factor in the larger context of the total personality, anxiety can be assessed with the 16–Personality Factor Inventory (16-PF; Cattell et al. 1970), the Eysenck Personality Inventory (EPI; Eysenck and Eysenck 1969), and the Taylor Manifest Anxiety Scale (TMAS; Taylor-Spence and Spence 1966), a scale derived from the MMPI. The Anxiety Status Inventory (ASI) is a rating scale for anxiety developed for clinical use following an interview guide, and the Self-Rating Anxiety Scale (SRAS) is a companion self-report instrument, both developed by Zung (1971). Both scales assess a wide range of anxiety-related behaviors: fear, panic, physical symptoms of fear, nightmares, and cognitive effects. These scales are recommended for the serial measurement of the effects of therapy on anxiety states. Hamilton (1959) devised an anxiety rating scale parallel to the Ham-D but less frequently utilized. The Endler S-R Inventory of Anxiousness (Endler et al. 1962) is a self-report measure of the interaction between the patient's anxiety and environmental situations such as interpersonal, physically dangerous, and ambiguous situations. This instrument has been widely used as a therapy outcome measure and is recommended as an instrument that may be helpful in tailoring treatment to the specific circumstances of the patient's anxiety.

A semistructured interview, the Anxiety Disorders Interview Schedule (ADIS; Di Nardo et al. 1983), is used to differentiate subcategories of anxiety disorders as well as to rule out affective disorders and other major problems. From a differential treatment point of view, it is important to distinguish between agoraphobia with panic, generalized anxiety disorder, and panic disorder, because they are optimally treated with different therapeutic approaches.

The Fear Questionnaire (Marks and Mathews 1979) is a brief paper-and-pencil instrument that yields scores on scales of agoraphobia, social phobia, and blood and injury phobia. The Beck Depression Inventory (BDI; Beck et al. 1961) is administered concurrently, because many patients with agoraphobia are also depressed. Finally, the Dyadic Adjustment Scale (DAS; Spanier 1976) is administered to assess the marital context of the agoraphobia, an important clinical factor. In addition, the patient is asked to keep a weekly record for the purpose of self-monitoring the type and amount of outside activity on a daily basis.

Another prototype of an assessment program linked to a specific patient population defined by a symptom complex is that described by Aaron Beck for the outpatient treatment of depressive disorders. Initial screening is focused on the presence, type, and severity of any depressive disorders (DSM-III Axis I) and personality disorders (DSM-III Axis II). In addition, the patient is given the BDI so that the severity of the depression may be assessed and the specific depressive symptoms highlighted. The Young Loneliness Inventory (Young 1982) is used to assess the possible absence of friendships and intimate ties, a factor closely linked to depression. The Dysfunctional Attitude Scale (Weissman and Beck 1978) is given to the patient to assess maladaptive underlying assumptions or attitudes that are directly related to the mediating goals of Beck's cognitive treatment for depression.

The Manic-State Rating Scale (MSRS; Beigel et al. 1971) is a 26-item observer-rated scale that is useful with patients with bipolar depression. Eleven items reflecting elation-grandiosity and paranoid-destructive features of manic patients have produced the most consistent results and have been applied successfully in the prediction of inpatient length of stay (Young et al. 1978). The scale demonstrated adequate reliability and concurrent validity, and reflects clinical change (Janowsky et al. 1978). Secunda et al. (1985) used similar item content from several instruments employed in the National Institute of Mental Health Clinical Research Branch Collaborative Program on the psychobiology of depression to develop indices for responsiveness to lithium treatment in manic patients. A newer rating scale, the Internal State Scale (ISS; Bauer et al. 1991), is a self-report instrument that allows individuals to rate the present state of 17 items reflecting bipolar symptomatology on a 100-millimeter line.

The Buss-Durkee Hostility Inventory (Buss and Durkee 1957) is a 75-item self-report questionnaire that measures different aspects of hostility and aggression. Megargee et al. (1967) developed an overcontrolled hostility scale using MMPI items. A review of the number of studies involving this scale (Greene 1991) suggests that it can be used to screen for patients who display excessive control of their hostile impulses and are socially alienated. Spielberger developed a State-Trait Anger Expression Inventory (STAEI; Spielberger et al. 1976), a self-report instrument that takes about 15 minutes to complete. This 44-item scale divides behavior into state anger (i.e., current feelings) and trait anger (i.e., disposition toward angry reactions), and the latter area has subscales for angry temperament and angry reaction.

Suicidal behavior.   Self-report instruments that focus specific and detailed attention on known predictors of suicidal behavior are sometimes clinically useful. The Suicide Intent Scale (SIS; Beck et al. 1974), the Index of Potential Suicide (Zung 1974), and the Suicide Probability Scale (SPS; Cull and Gill 1986) are three widely used instruments. A complementary approach has been taken, culminating in the development of the Reasons for Living Inventory (RFL; Linehan et al. 1983).

Thought disorder.   The test most widely used in examinations for thought disorders has been the Rorschach Inkblot Test, which was developed by the Swiss psychiatrist Hermann Rorschach. In this test, a relatively ambiguous stimulus (a colored or achromatic "inkblot") is used, and, without additional instruction, individuals are asked to state what the blot looks like to them. Responses are scored for location (i.e., the area of the card that elicits a response), determinants (i.e., form, movement, color, and shading), form quality (i.e., the degree to which percepts are congruent with the area chosen), and content (e.g., human, animal, object). Exner (1978) developed a scoring system that attempts to integrate the best aspects of prior systems. The relationship of various forms of thought disorder and its severity to psychiatric diagnosis and treatment has been examined extensively (Solovay et al. 1986). Although the scoring scheme can be applied to any record of verbal production, its most frequent application has been in the context of verbal records from the administration of such tests as the WAIS and the Rorschach.

☐ Assessment of Cognitive Functioning

One assesses specific cognitive abilities in psychiatric patients for several reasons: 1) to document disorders in cognitive skills referable to primary or concomitant neurogenic disorder (e.g., discriminating between a thought disorder and a language disorder or the mnemonic deficits of a depression versus a dementia), or 2) to document a specific disorder in cognition referable to a specific class of psychiatric disorders (e.g., intrusion into thought of task-irrelevant items in patients complaining of delusional or obsessive ideation, or disturbances in recall in patients with major affective disorders).

Common clinical questions in a psychiatric setting with a neuropsychological focus include 1) dementia in the elderly, 2) toxicity in substance-abusing individuals, and 3) specific learning disabilities in children and adolescents. In clinical psychiatric populations, the possibly confounding influences of behavioral impairment because of the nature and severity of the emotional disturbance and the impact of concurrent pharmacological treatments must be carefully assessed in order to reduce the rate of false-positive diagnoses of organic mental disorder. In one form or another, most neuropsychological assessments of cognitive processes evaluate the presence of disorders in the following abilities:

- General intelligence
- Attention and concentration
- Memory and learning
- Perception
- Language
- Conceptualization
- Constructional skills
- Executive motor processes
- Affect

In many clinical settings, the areas of higher cortical functions of interest are assessed by a formal battery of tests. Two such standardized batteries are the Halstead-Reitan (Boll 1981) and the Luria-Nebraska (Golden et al. 1978) neuropsychological batteries (Table 8–5). The Halstead-Reitan is a composite battery of tests originally developed by Ward Halstead and his former student, Ralph Reitan. In its present form, the Halstead Neuropsychological Test Battery consists of five tests that yield seven summary scores and a total impairment index. The five tests are a category test, a tactile perception test, a speech sounds perception test, the Seashore rhythm test, and a finger oscillation test. A group of tests referred to as the allied procedures are frequently included as a part of the total examination. The entire examination typically takes from 4 to 6 hours depending on the number of ancillary procedures (i.e., intelligence and academic performance) included. The reliability and validity of the tests are well established, and normative data for most comparisons of interest in clinical psychiatric populations are available.

A second widely used battery of procedures has been developed from the work of Luria (1973). Christensen (1975) was instrumental in bringing Luria's stimuli and procedures to the attention of neuropsychologists outside the former Soviet Union. Golden et al. (1978) have been the primary proponents and developers of a standardized neuropsychological instrument using Christensen's published material. In its present form, the Luria-Nebraska covers the areas of motor function,

Table 8–5. Instruments for the assessment of cognitive functioning

Instrument	Focus of assessment	Description	Scoring features
Halstead-Reitan	Neuropsychological battery	Items sampling intellectual, tactual, auditory, and kinesthetic functions	7 summary sources for clinical interpretation
Luria-Nebraska	Neuropsychological battery	269 items sampling intellectual, motor, sensory, and expressive skills	14 T scores for clinical interpretation
Wechsler Adult Intelligence Scale–Revised	General intellectual abilities	166 items sampling intellectual skills	Full scale, verbal and performance IQs
Wechsler Intelligence Scale for Children–III	General intellectual abilities	187 items sampling intellectual skills	Full scale, verbal and performance IQs
Wechsler Preschool and Primary Scale of Intelligence	General intellectual abilities	Taps 6 verbal areas and 5 performance	Full scale, verbal and performance IQs
Wide Range Achievement Test	Academic achievement	Reading, spelling, arithmetic achievement	Standard score
Mini Mental State Exam	Brief assessment of general cognitive impairment	30 items sampling orientation, memory, and drawing skills	Total number correct
Dementia Rating Scale	Brief assessment of general cognitive impairment	144 items sampling attention, memory, abstraction, drawing, executive motor skills	5 subscale scores, total scores, percentile score relative to dementia patients
Continuous Performance Test	Attention	Test of vigilance	Hits, false alarms, reaction time

(continued)

Table 8–5.   Instruments for the assessment of cognitive functioning (*continued*)

Instrument	Focus of assessment	Description	Scoring features
Wechsler Memory Scale—Revised	Memory	Attention, verbal and nonverbal memory	Subscale scores on attention, verbal and nonverbal memory
Benton Test of Visual Retention	Memory	Reproduction of geometric figures	Total number correct, total number of errors
Benton Line Orientation Test	Perception	Target lines at given orientations detected from among a radial display of lines	Total number correct
Benton Face Recognition Test	Perception	Target face detected from among similar faces	Total number of correct detections
Goldman-Fristoe-Woodcock Auditory Battery	Perception	Auditory perception measured under 3 different conditions of ambient noise	Total number correct
Multilingual Aphasia Battery	Language	8 subtests	Percentiles obtained for each subtest
Neurosensory Center Comprehensive Examination for Aphasia	Language	24 subtests (20 language, 4 control)	Percentiles obtained for each subtest
Conceptual Level Analogies Test	Conceptualization	Verbal analogies	Number correct
Raven Progressive Matrices Test	Conceptualization	Spatial analogies test using patterned visual stimuli	Number correct
Category Test (booklet)	Conceptualization	Concept formation task	Total number of errors
Wisconsin Card Sorting Test	Conceptualization	Concept formation task	Total number of categories obtained, total number of perseverative errors
Trail Making Test	Set sequencing	Connect dots in ascending numeric order, then in alternating alpha-numeric order	Time to completion
Purdue Pegboard	Fine motor	Fine motor task	Number of pegs placed in 30 seconds

rhythm (and pitch) skills, tactile and visual functions, receptive and expressive speech, writing, reading and arithmetic skills, memory, and intelligence. The complete examination consists of 269 items that yield raw scores in each area. Three additional scores for right- and left-hemisphere impairment and a pathognomonic score are also computed. These 14 raw scores are plotted as T scores for the purposes of interscale and interindividual comparison. The present literature on the Luria-Nebraska includes studies of brain-damaged, medical control, and chronically schizophrenic groups. The results of these studies established the preliminary validity of the battery; no reliability data have been published.

Premorbid Intelligence

Premorbid intelligence may be estimated by assessing those cognitive abilities that do not rapidly deteriorate with dementing processes. These include the general fund of information and vocabulary as measured by the respective subtests of the WAIS, or reading recognition as measured by the Wide Range Achievement Test reading subtest (Jastak and Wilkinson 1981) or the Nelson Adult Reading Test (Nelson 1982), which has new North American norms and with which reasonable validity has been demonstrated. It is also common to estimate premorbid intelligence on the basis of educational and vocational background.

General Intellectual Abilities

The most frequently used instrument, the WAIS-R, has been described in an earlier section. Because of the length of administration, abbreviated versions of this measure are often employed either by using only some of the subtests or by using fewer of the specific items and weighting each response. Alternatively, different, briefer measures may be employed—for example, the Ammons Quick Test (Ammons and Ammons 1962) or the Shipley-Hartford Test (Shipley 1946).

Most tests of general intellectual abilities obtain normative data from an unimpaired population and therefore are sensitive instruments in detecting individuals whose performance lies at the extremes of the normal range. Such instruments lose sensitivity to discriminate among patient populations whose performance falls outside this range. There are a number of instruments in broad use for the assessment of general cognitive abilities in patient populations. All such instruments have skewed distributions in normal populations (i.e., a decided floor effect) but distribute well in the atypical population. Perhaps the most commonly used instrument in a psychiatric setting is the Mini-Mental State Exam (MMSE) (Folstein et al. 1975), a 10-minute test generating 30 points, in which a score below 24 is considered to be good evidence of clinically significant cognitive impairment. A commonly used instrument is the Dementia Rating Scale (Mattis 1988), a 20- to 30-minute instrument generating 144 points with greater sensitivity at the upper levels that better enables detection of progressive changes of dementia over several years (Haxby et al. 1992).

Attentional Disorders

Attentional processes are most commonly measured by the WAIS-R subtests constituting the "distractibility" triad (i.e., digit span, mental arithmetic, and digit symbol). In digit span the patient is asked to repeat a string of digits of increasing length and then, in a separate administration, repeat a string of digits in reverse of the order in which they were presented. The digit string cannot be repeated by the examiner, so lapses in attention by the patient result in repetition of only the shorter strings. In the mental arithmetic subtest, the patient is asked to solve arithmetic problems of increasing difficulty without the aid of pencil and paper. Selection and monitoring of the appropriate arithmetic operation while storing partial solutions are easily disrupted by alterations in arousal and attention. The digit symbol subtest presents the patient with the digits 1 through 9 and gives each digit a separate, very simple geometric design. The digits are then randomly sequenced in rows across the page, and the patient must draw the appropriate design beneath each digit. The number of designs correctly drawn in 90 seconds is noted. This task not only is affected by impairment of the attentional system but is very sensitive to fine motor tremor and extrapyramidal impairment secondary to neurotoxins.

With increasing use of computer-assisted examinations, a popular continuous performance test developed by Rosvold can be employed (Mirsky and Kornetsky 1964; Rosvold et al. 1956). In this task, the patient is presented with a randomly selected letter in midscreen at fixed intervals and directed to push a button (or press the space bar) when a given letter is presented. The number of correct responses (i.e., hits), misses, false alarms (i.e., the number of times the bar is pressed in response to a nontarget item), and correct rejections is then noted. The advantage to this computer-assisted approach to the measure of attention lies in its flexibility and the accuracy with which responses can be recorded and stimuli presented. The reaction time of each response can be measured and fluctuations in reaction time noted over the duration of the task. Stimulus characteristics such as stimulus duration, speed of presentation, or even size of target and duration of task can be systematically altered.

Research in attentional processes has demonstrated the efficacy of a procedure called *dichotic stimulation* (Kimura 1967), which presents dissimilar auditory stimuli simultaneously to each ear and requires the patient to report both stimuli. Thus the patient might simultaneously hear the number "1" in the right ear and "4" in the left ear. Strings of three such pairs might be presented to the adult patient and he or she asked to report all six digits. The competing stimuli can be matched for such stimulus characteristics as time of onset, offset, peak amplitude, and so forth, making it a very difficult speech sound discrimination task as well as an attentional measure.

Memory Disorders

The memory disorder of particular interest to the clinician is the one that affects "recent" memory and that is generally referrable to impairment of limbic system functioning. Operationally, one seeks to present the patient with a specific set of information or events and then divert attention so that it cannot be rehearsed, and then require the patient to demonstrate that the target information has been encoded and stored by either reproducing the material or recognizing it among distractor items. Thus recall of brief paragraphs or reproduction of geometric designs from memory is often used to assess mnemonic processes. Among the most commonly used standard tests of memory are the Wechsler Memory Scale—Revised (Wechsler 1987), which presents both verbal and nonverbal material as the items to be remembered, and the Benton Test of Visual Retention (Benton 1955), which presents only geometric designs. Free recall of recent events has been found to be among the most sensitive functions of the memory process. Unfortunately, in many instances free recall has been found to be quite fragile and vulnerable to disruption because of affective arousal, depression, and motivational factors, and therefore may present many "false positives" when being used to discriminate between neurogenic and psychogenic diagnostic considerations. It has been suggested that mechanisms other than free recall might be employed to assses the integrity of encoding and storage processes. Recognition memory techniques, in which the patient is asked to detect a recently presented word or design from among distractor items, have been successfully used to discriminate patients with major affective disorders from those with organic amnesias such as progressive dementia.

The well-designed instruments assessing both recall and recognition memory generally present the patient with a list-learning task requiring free recall and, subsequent to that, a recognition memory probe in which the patient must detect the target from distractor items. Most of the instruments introduce either an interpolated list or a significant time delay before presentation of the final recall and recognition trials. Among the most widely used instruments are the Rey Auditory Verbal Learning Test (Geffen et al. 1990) and the California Verbal Learning Test (Delis et al. 1987). Several instruments have multiple forms that are useful in the serial examination of patients—for example, the Hopkins Verbal Learning Test (Brandt 1991) and the Mattis-Kovner Verbal Learning Test (Mattis et al. 1978).

Perceptual Disorders

Very little evidence exists for a significant prevalence of perceptual deficits in a psychiatric population when care is taken to exclude significant problem-solving components from the task and the presence of concurrent toxic metabolic disorders in the patients. Nonetheless, it is probably a good idea to rule out the presence of perceptual deficits. Visual perceptual processes can be assessed with tasks such as the Benton Line Orientation Test (Benton et al. 1975), which requires the patient to match a target line at a given orientation to true vertical with alternative lines presented at various orientations. Another such test is the Benton Face Recognition Test (Benton and Van Allen 1968), in which a photograph of a face is presented as the target and the patient is requested to detect this face from alternatives.

Auditory perception tends to be difficult to assess without hardware. However, at present the fidelity available in small portable "walkman"-type tape recorders with earphones affords the clinician a wide range of excellent auditory stimuli. Tests such as the Goldman-Fristoe Test of Speech Sound Discrimination (Goldman et al. 1976) allow for the assessment of the efficiency of speech sound detection with and without background noise.

Language Disorders

Perhaps the most specific index of neurogenic impairment is the presence of a language disorder. For almost all right-handed individuals and half of left-handed individuals, focal or diffuse impairment of the left hemisphere is likely to result in an aphasia (i.e., a disorder of language comprehension and/or usage). In general, the aphasia examination will consist of specific measures of disorders of linguistic processes well correlated with focal brain lesion. Most such batteries will contain measures of verbal labeling or word-finding skills, language comprehension, imitative speech, and motor-expressive speech. Many such tests also include specific measures of reading and writing. Among the most commonly used multifactorial instruments are the Multilingual Aphasia Examination (Benton and Hamsher 1976), the Neurosensory Center Comprehensive Examination for Aphasia (Spreen and Benton 1977), and the Boston Diagnostic Aphasia Examination (Goodglass and Kaplan 1972). Among the most widely used screening instruments for the assessment of aphasia is the Halstead-Wepman Aphasia Screening Test (Halstead and Wepman 1959).

Conceptualization Disorders

Perhaps the most direct measure of the concept of abstract or categorical thinking is the similarities subtest of the WAIS-R, which presents the patient with perceptually dissimilar items and asks him or her to determine the category to which they both belong (e.g., "How are North and West alike?"). Proverb explanation has a long history in the psychiatric mental status examination as a task designed to measure abstract reasoning and is included among the items of the comprehension subtest of the WAIS-R (e.g., "Shallow brooks are noisy"). However, some consider explanation of proverbs too dependent on general intellectual abilities and socio-cultural factors to be a specific measure of concretization of thought. Analogistic reasoning can also be gauged using such tasks as the Conceptual Level Analogies Test (Willner 1971) for verbal reasoning and the Raven Progressive Matrices Test (Raven 1960) for nonverbal or spatial analogistic reasoning.

Two measures of concept formation arising from the neuropsychological literature have been applied to psychiatric patients. The data thus far indicate that schizophrenic patients, like patients with frontal lobe lesions, have particular difficulty with the booklet form of the Category Test (DeFillipis et al. 1979) and the Wisconsin Card Sorting Test (Heaton 1981). Both tests require the patient to induce a concept or rule of organization from patterned visual stimuli.

Constructional Disorders

Perhaps the quickest estimate of the integrity of the CNS can be obtained by asking the patient to draw a complex figure. Posterior sensory, central spatial, and anterior planning, monitoring, and simple motor skills must all be intact, integrated, and appropriately sequenced for this task to be successfully completed. One can alter the degree to which psychological and dynamic factors, and initiative or executive planning, play a role by modulating both task structure and design complexity. For example, asking the patient to draw a person in his or her family requires a maximum level of planning, initiative, and decision making; does not put any limit on the degree of complexity of the figures; and involves a subject matter fraught with complex feelings and attitudes. Patients without structural impairment but with conflictual feelings about family or disordered thinking that affects planning and execution will have difficulty on such tasks. However, asking a patient to draw a clock, setting the hands to a specific time (e.g., 10 to 11), also requires complex planning and initiative but without the conflictual overlay. Contrasting the patient's figure drawing to his or her clock and copy of geometric figures often allows valid inferences as to presence and locus of CNS impairment and the degree to which affective and psychiatric factors impair otherwise intact cognitive skills. Quite often, construction tasks other than drawing, such as the block design and object assembly subtests of the WAIS-R, are used for the same assessment goals.

Disorders in Executive Motor Skills

In general, in assessing disorders in executive skills, one is alert to the presence of perseveration in motor activity, thought, and affect. Perseveration of motor activity is often elicited by starting the patient on a simple repeated task and then altering one of the motor components. Thus, having the patient perform a simple diadochokinetic task such as alternating palm up–palm down and then presenting as the next task palm up–palm down–fist, may result in repeated performance of only two components of the task. Similarly, asking the patient to write, in script, alternating "m"'s and "n"'s will also elicit simple motor perseveration. Perseveration of thought or set is often quickly elicited by shifting task instruction.

Disorders in evolving or shifting more complex ideas can also be measured quite accurately. Concept formation tasks such as the booklet form of the Category Test and the Wisconsin Card Sorting Test differ in specific directions and stimuli but present a series of specific examples of a class of events and require the patient to induce the concept or rule of which they are an exemplar. The rule changes over time. Thus, one might observe the failure of the patient to induce the first concept or perseverate the same rule well past its utility. The number of perseveration errors is among the scores obtained on both tests.

Disorders in Motor Skills

Examination of simple motor skill disorders is usually exceptionally brief and the results quite reproducible and valid. One can measure line quality parameters of copied geometric drawings (Mattis et al. 1975). One can, in addition, present simple fine-motor coordination tasks such as the Purdue Pegboard (Costa et al. 1963) or the Grooved Pegboard. The Purdue Pegboard measures the number of slim cylinders (i.e., pegs) one can insert in a row of holes in 30 seconds. One notes the number of 1) pegs placed with the right hand alone, 2) pegs placed with left hand alone, and 3) pairs of pegs placed using both hands simultaneously. The number of pegs placed simultaneously has proven to be a sensitive measure of frontal dysfunction. The Grooved Pegboard has pegs that contain a flange on one side so that the pegs fit into a keyhole-shaped opening. The keyholes are placed in differing orientations on the board. One notes the total time to place all the pegs with each hand alone. Given the greater fine-motor component to the grooved pegs, the Grooved Pegboard tends to be a more sensitive measure of tremor than is the Purdue.

☐ Assessment of Personality Traits and Disorders

In developing a treatment plan for a specific patient, the psychiatrist must assess personality traits for various reasons: personality traits or disorders may 1) be the focus of intervention, 2) exacerbate or be related to the incidence of certain symptoms (e.g., depression), or 3) either help or hinder the development of a therapeutic relationship with the patient.

Dimensional Assessment of Personality

Several widely used and psychometrically sound instruments are available for the assessment of personality (Table 8–6). Such tests include the 16-PF, the EPI, the California Psychological Inventory (CPI; Gough 1956), and the Personality Research Form (PRF; Jackson 1974). These instruments were designed for the validation of personality constructs rather than for the assessment of psychopathology, although they have been employed in clinical settings with limited success. These instruments and their designers, however, have not been oriented toward psychopathology, and there is no explicit theory of personality disorder that underlies the interpretation of results from these tests.

The NEO–Personality Inventory (NEO-PI), a carefully constructed instrument measuring five central facets of personality, has gained in recognition (Wiggins and Pincus 1992). The revised version, the NEO-PI-R (Costa and McCrae 1992), provides a measure of five facets of personality: neuroticism, extraversion, openness, agreeableness, and conscientiousness. Each of the facets also includes six subscales. For example, the six facets of neuroticism include anxiety, anger/hostility, depression, self-consciousness, impulsiveness, and vulnerability.

Benjamin (1974) developed an instrument for the assessment of interpersonal behavior, the Structural Analysis of Social Behavior (SASB), and a computer-based scoring system marketed under the trade name INTREX, which is self-administered. The SASB can also be used by clinicians to record their impressions about the patient. A related coding scheme has been developed for use by trained observers to record the patient's actual interactions with others, such as family members, during the course of treatment.

Assessment of Personality Disorders

A relatively new approach to the assessment of personality disorders is to construct instruments, either self-report or semistructured interviews, that evaluate the presence or absence of specific personality traits described in Axis II of DSM-III-R. DSM-III-R neither defines nor develops from any particular theory of personality. Instead, it identifies clusters (in most cases those with little empirical validation) of personality traits

Table 8–6. Instruments for the assessment of personality traits and disorders

Instrument	General classification	Description	Scoring features
16-Personality Factor Inventory (16-PF)	Self-report	3 equivalent forms of 106–187 items each	Scaled scores for 16 personality traits
Eysenck Personality Inventory (EPI)	Self-report	57 yes/no items, parallel forms	Scores on extraversion and neuroticism
California Personality Inventory (CPI)	Self-report	468 items	Scores on 18 scales and 4 special scales
Personality Research Form (PRF)	Self-report	352 items	Scores on 22 personality traits
NEO–Personality Inventory—Revised (NEO-PI-R)	Self-report	240 items, 5-point scale	Five domain scales and 30 facet scales
Structural Analysis of Social Behavior (SASB)	Self-report	36–72 statements of interpersonal behavior, true/false format	Internalized attitudes regarding self and significant others
Structured Clinical Interview for DSM-III-R (SCID)	Semistructured interview	3-point rating scales of personality traits	Yields Axis II diagnoses
Personality Disorders Examination	Semistructured interview	Semistructured interview for patient and self-report by family member on the patient	Dimensional and categorical scales on DSM-III-R Axis II personality disorders
Millon Clinical Multiaxial Inventory–II (MCMI-II)	Self-report	175 items, true/false format	Base rate scores on 22 clinical scales
Structural Interview for the DSM-III-R Personality Disorders (SIDP)	Semistructured interview	3-point rating scales	Yields DSM-III-R Axis II diagnoses

that are considered sufficiently maladaptive to warrant the designation "personality disorder." Personality traits that are inflexible and maladaptive and cause either significant impairment in social or occupational functioning or subjective distress are defined as a personality disorder in DSM-III-R. The most promising instruments of this type include the Personality Diagnostic Questionnaire (PDQ; Hurt et al. 1984), the Millon Clinical Multiaxial Inventory (MCMI; Millon 1983), the SCID, the Personality Disorders Examination, and the Structural Interview for the DSM-III Personality Disorders (SIDP; Stangl et al. 1985).

The PDQ is a self-report inventory of Axis II traits, and the test yields scores on each of the 13 personality disorder categories of DSM-III. Preliminary investigation of the instrument suggests that patients typically report a number of traits and will often meet criteria for several diagnostic categories; the PDQ may, however, be useful for screening (Hurt et al. 1984).

The MCMI is a 175-item true-false self-report instrument that yields scores on 11 personality disorder dimensions closely related to the personality disorder diagnoses of DSM-III Axis II, and 9 clinical syndromes. Probably the major difficulty with this instrument is psychometric in nature, as there is much item overlap in the scales. In the MCMI-II (Millon 1987), a revision of the original scale, two new personality disorder scales were introduced and two prior personality scales were modified. An item-weighting system has been introduced into the MCMI-II to reflect item differences related to the strength of each item's supporting validation data.

There are three semistructured interviews that have been designed to assess, via the patient's report and the clinical judgment of the interviewer, the presence of Axis II disorders: the Personality Disorders Examination (PDE), the Structural Interview for the DSM-III Personality Disorders, and the Structured Clinical Interview for DSM-III-R. The PDE (Loranger 1988) is a semistructured interview that yields both dimensional and categorical scores for DSM-III Axis II criteria. An important feature of this semistructured interview, which takes approximately 1 to 2 hours to administer, is that the criteria are assessed in related clusters such as self-concept, affect expression, reality testing, impulse control, interpersonal relations, and work. The instrument is likely to be widely used. In fact, it has been translated into several languages and was used in an international study approved by the World Health Organization and the then Alcohol, Drug Abuse, and Mental Health Administration (Loranger et al. 1991).

The SIDP consists of a semistructured interview form that provides 160 questions pertinent to the diagnostic criteria of Axis II of DSM-III. The questions are organized into 16 assessment areas, such as low self-esteem/dependency, egocentricity, ideas of reference and magical thinking, and hostility/anger. The questions are keyed to the DSM-III criteria for Axis II disorders. A rating form provides a 3-point rating scale for each criterion. Ratings are based on the clinical assessment of the interview data. SCID-II is concerned with the assessment of Axis II personality disorders. The interview format is determined by the DSM-III-R disorders and provides no guide for elaborating the assessment of the criteria.

☐ Assessment of Psychodynamics

The assessment of factors relevant to psychodynamic and psychoanalytic theory and treatment approaches has a long history in the clinical psychological literature. The development of the "standard battery," including the WAIS, Rorschach, and Thematic Apperception Test (Table 8–7), has its origins in the efforts of clinical psychologists to provide an assessment of such psychodynamic factors as drives, unconscious wishes, conflicts, and defenses. For those clinicians committed to the psychodynamic model, assessments that focus exclusively on overt behaviors will be less than totally satisfactory.

The most widely used assessment procedure for the examination of patients over a range of ego functions and dynamic factors is the Rorschach Inkblot Test described earlier. Scoring systems have been developed by many authors, and, more recently, Exner developed a scoring system that attempts to integrate the best aspects of the prior systems. From these scores, inferences are drawn concerning the patient's self-image, identity, defensive structure, reality testing, affective control, amount and degree of fantasy life, degree of thought organization, and potential for impulsive acting out.

The Thematic Apperception Test (TAT) is another widely used projective process for assessing the patient's self-concept in relation to others. Originally developed by Murray (1943), the test consists of a set of 30 pictures depicting one or more individuals. The patient is asked to make up a story based on each picture. The stories generated are then scored for the individual's needs as reflected in the feelings and impulses attributed to the major character in each story and the interactions with the environment leading to a resolution.

☐ Assessment of Environmental Demands and Social Adjustment

The interaction between the patient and the pressures of the environment is now acknowledged in the standard diagnostic system (DSM-IV) by a rating on Axis IV. Probably the most substantiated area with empirical data indicating the impact of the patient-environment interaction is the investigation of expressed emotion (EE) and its influence on the course of schizophrenia. This work suggests that certain elements in the home environment of a schizophrenic patient can adversely affect the course of the illness. EE can be assessed by the Camberwell Family Interview (Brown and Rutter 1966), a 1-hour semistructured interview of a relative of the patient. The scoring scheme for this instrument is not readily accessible and is therefore not usable in standard clinical situations.

In measuring both stress and the patient's ability to cope with stress, one can assess the stimuli, the individual's response to the stimuli, or the interaction of the person with stressful stimuli (see Table 8–8). The Jenkins Activity Survey (JAS; Jenkins et al. 1967) is the prototype of an interaction-based measure of stress, focusing on the cognitive and perceptual characteristics of the individual that mediate responses to stress. This instrument has been shown to have predictive validity in studies of reaction to coronary heart disease. The Derogatis Stress Profile (DSP; Derogatis 1982) is useful in evaluating stimuli from work and home, and can be used to assess health, as well as characteristic attitudes and coping mechanisms.

The term *social adjustment* refers to the skill of an individual in handling interpersonal situations, whether at home, in school, or in the work setting. Notable assessment instruments for use with psychiatric patients include the Katz Adjustment Scale—Relative's Form, the Social Adjustment Scale—Self-Report, and the Dyadic Adjustment Scale (DAS; Spanier 1976). The Katz Adjustment Scale—Relative's Form (KAS-R) (Katz and Lyerly 1963) is a relative's self-report inventory of the patient's symptomatic behavior and social adjustment in the community. The scale has sections on symptoms and social behavior, performance of socially expected tasks, relative's expectation for the performance of these tasks, the patient's free-time activities, and the relative's satisfaction with the performance of these free-time activities. The Social Adjustment Scale—Self-Report (SAS-SR) (Weissman and Bothwell 1976) contains 42 questions covering instrumental and affective qualities in role performance, social and leisure activities, relationships with extended family, marital role, parental role, family unit, and economic independence.

■ CLINICAL DECISION TREE

In clinical psychiatric settings, assessment is most often requested to aid in reducing uncertainty regarding diagnosis and in evaluating the severity of specific symptoms or symptom complexes (e.g., depression, suicide intent, or thought disorder). Such an assessment plays an important role in providing information on patients that can be usefully generalized by facilitating comparisons between patients or by tracking the severity of

Table 8–7. Instruments for the assessment of psychodynamics

Instrument	General classification	Description	Scoring features
Rorschach Inkblot Test	Unstructured or projective test	10 ambiguous inkblots, responses scored on multiple criteria	Accuracy of form, location, use of color, shading, etc., provide summary scores
Thematic Apperception Test (TAT)	Unstructured or projective test	30 ambiguous scenes	Affects, outcomes, and other qualities

Table 8–8. Instruments for the assessment of environmental stressors

Instrument	General classification	Description	Scoring features
Jenkins Activity Survey (JAS)	Self-report	52 items, multiple choice	Scores on 4 scales: Type A behaviors, speed and impatience, job involvement, and hard drive and competitiveness
Derogatis Stress Profile (DSP)	Self-report	77 items	T scores for 11 dimensions
Katz Adjustment Scale	Observer rating	127 items, 4-point frequency scale	12 clusters of behaviors
Social Adjustment Scale—Self-Report (SAS-SR)	Self-report	42 questions, rated on 5-point scale of severity	Mean score for 7 areas and an overall score
Dyadic Adjustment Scale (DAS)	Self-report	31 items, 4 dimensions	Total score
Marital Satisfaction Inventory	Self-report	280 items	T scores on 11 scales

symptoms under the impact of treatment. This assessment may form the basis for recommended treatments, help in establishing goals for the general treatment plan, or help in determining treatment progress and the need for further intervention.

With medical care costs soaring due in part to an indiscriminate use of laboratory tests, psychiatrists should be clear about the precise areas for assessment before referring a patient for testing. Likewise, the clinical psychologist should pursue the testing with efficiency and utilize instruments that will answer the referral questions with precision, reliability, and validity. Both psychiatrist and psychologist should utilize a clinical decision tree that informs their differential therapeutic procedures.

■ REFERENCES

American Psychiatric Association: Diagnostic and Statistical Manual of Mental Disorders, 3rd Edition, Revised. Washington, DC, American Psychiatric Association, 1987

American Psychiatric Association: Diagnostic and Statistical Manual of Mental Disorders, 4th Edition. Washington, DC, American Psychiatric Association, 1994

Ammons RB, Ammons CH: The Quick Test (QT): provisional manual. Psychol Rep 11:111–161, 1962

Bauer MS, Crits-Christoph P, Ball WA, et al: Independent assessment of manic and depressive symptoms by self-rating: scale characteristics and implications for the study of mania. Arch Gen Psychiatry 48:807–812, 1991

Beck AT, Ward CH, Mendelson M, et al: An inventory for measuring depression. Arch Gen Psychiatry 4:561–571, 1961

Beck AT, Schuyler D, Herman I: Development of suicidal intent scales, in The Prediction of Suicide. Edited by Beck AT, Resnick HLP, Lettieri DJ. Bowie, MD, Charles Press, 1974, pp 45–56

Beigel A, Murphy DL, Bunney WE Jr: The Manic-State Rating Scale: scale construction, reliability, and validity. Arch Gen Psychiatry 25:256–262, 1971

Benjamin LS: Structural analysis of social behavior. Psychol Rev 81:392–425, 1974

Benton AL: Visual Retention Test. New York, Psychological Corporation, 1955

Benton AL, Hamsher K: Multilingual Aphasia Examination. Iowa City, IA, University of Iowa, 1976

Benton AL, Van Allen MW: Impairment in facial recognition in patients with cerebral disease. Cortex 4:344–358, 1968

Benton AL, Hannay HJ, Varney NR: Visual perception of line direction in patients with unilateral brain disease. Neurology 25:907–910, 1975

Boll TJ: The Halstead-Reitan Neuropsychology Battery, in Handbook of Clinical Neuropsychology. Edited by Filskov SB, Boll TJ. New York, Wiley, 1981, pp 577–607

Brandt J: The Hopkins Verbal Learning Test: development of a new memory test with six equivalent forms. The Clinical Neuropsychologist 5:125–142, 1991

Brown GW, Rutter M: The measurement of family activities and relationships: a methodological study. Human Relations 19:241–263, 1966

Buss AH, Durkee A: An inventory for assessing different kinds of hostility. Journal of Consulting Psychology 21:343–349, 1957

Butcher JN, Dahlstrom WG, Graham JR, et al: Manual for the Restandardized Minnesota Multiphasic Personality Inventory (MMPI-2): An Administrative and Interpretive Guide. Minneapolis, MN, University of Minnesota Press, 1989

Cattell RB, Eber HW, Tatsuoka MM: Handbook for the Sixteen Personality Factor Inventory. Champaign, IL, Institute for Personality and Ability Testing, 1970

Christensen AL: Luria's Neuropsychological Investigation: Manual. New York, Spectrum, 1975

Costa LD, McCrae RR: NEO PI-R: Professional Manual. Odessa, FL, Psychological Assessment Resources, 1992

Costa LD, Vaughan HG, Levita E, et al: Perdue Pegboard as a predictor of the presence and laterality of cerebral lesions. Journal of Consulting Psychology 27:133–137, 1963

Cull JG, Gill WS: Suicide Probability Scale (SPS) Manual. Los Angeles, CA, Western Psychological Services, 1986

DeFillipis NA, McCambell E, Rogers P: Development of a booklet form of the Category Test: normative and validity data. Journal of Clinical Neuropsychology 1:339–342, 1979

Delis DC, Kramer J, Kaplan E, et al: California Verbal Learning Test (CVLT), Research Edition Manual. New York, Psychological Corporation, 1987

Derogatis LR: The SCL-90R. Baltimore, MD, Clinical Psychometric Research, 1977

Derogatis LR: Self-report measures of stress, in Handbook of Stress. Edited by Goldberger L, Breznitz S. New York, Free Press, 1982, pp 270–294

Derogatis LR, Lipman RS, Rickels K, et al: The Hopkins Symptom Checklist (HSCL): a measure of primary symptom dimensions, in Psychological Measurements in Psychopharmacology, Vol 7: Modern Problems of Pharmacopsychiatry. Edited by Pichot P. Basel, S Karger, 1974, pp 79–110

Di Nardo PA, O'Brien GT, Barlow DH, et al: Reliability of DSM-III anxiety disorder categories using a new structured interview. Arch Gen Psychiatry 40:1070–1074, 1983

Endicott J, Spitzer RL: A diagnostic interview: the Schedule for Affective Disorders and Schizophrenia. Arch Gen Psychiatry 35:837–844, 1978

Endicott J, Spitzer RL: Use of the Research Diagnostic Criteria and the Schedule for Affective Disorders and Schizophrenia to study affective disorders. Am J Psychiatry 136:52–56, 1979

Endicott J, Spitzer RL, Fleiss J, et al: The Global Assessment Scale: a procedure for measuring overall severity of psychiatric disturbance. Arch Gen Psychiatry 33:766–771, 1976

Endler NS, Hunt J McV, Rosenstein AJ: An S-R inventory of anxiousness. Psychol Mono: Gen Applied 76(monogr no 536, issue no 17):1–31, 1962

Eysenck HJ, Eysenck SB: The Structure and Measurement of Personality. San Diego, CA, RR Knapp, 1969

Exner JE Jr: The Rorschach: A Comprehensive System, Vol 2. New York, Wiley, 1978

Feighner JP, Robins E, Guze SB, et al: Diagnostic criteria for use in psychiatric research. Arch Gen Psychiatry 26:57–63, 1972

Folstein MF, Folstein SE, McHugh PR: Mini-mental state: a practical method for grading the cognitive state of patients for the clinician. J Psychiatr Res 11:189–198, 1975

Garner DM: Eating Disorder Inventory 2: Professional Manual. Odessa, FL, Psychological Assessment Resources, 1992

Geffen G, Moar KJ, O'Hanlon AP, et al: Performance measures of 16- to 86-year-old males and females on the Auditory Verbal Learning Test. The Clinical Neuropsychologist 4:45–63, 1990

Golden CJ, Hammeke TA, Purisch AD: Diagnostic validity of a standardized neuropsychological battery derived from Luria's neuropsychological tests. J Consult Clin Psychol 46:1258–1265, 1978

Goldman R, Fristoe M, Woodcock RW: Auditory Skills Test Battery. Circle Pines, MN, American Guidance Service, 1976

Goodglass H, Kaplan E: Assessment of Aphasia and Related Disorders. Philadelphia, PA, Lea & Febiger, 1972

Gough HG: California Psychological Inventory. Palo Alto, CA, Consulting Psychologists Press, 1956

Green RA, Bigelow L, O'Brien P, et al: The Inpatient Behavior Rating Scale: a 26-item scale for recording nursing observations of patients' mood and behavior. Psychol Rep 40:543–549, 1977

Greene RL: The MMPI-2/MMPI: An Interpretive Manual. Needham Heights, MA, Allyn and Bacon, 1991

Halstead WC, Wepman JM: The Halstead-Wepman Aphasia Screening Test. Journal of Speech and Hearing Disorders 14:9–15, 1959

Hamilton M: The assessment of anxiety states by rating. Br J Med Psychol 32:50–55, 1959

Hathaway SR, McKinley JC: Minnesota Multiphasic Personality Inventory Manual, Revised Edition. New York, Psychological Corporation, 1967

Haxby JV, Raffaele K, Gillete J, et al: Individual trajectories of cognitive decline in patients with dementia of the Alzheimer type. J Clin Exp Neuropsychol 14:575–592, 1992

Heaton RK: Wisconsin Card Sorting Test Manual. Odessa, FL, Psychological Assessment Resources, 1981

Hoffmann H, Loper RG, Kammeier ML: Identifying future alcoholics with MMPI alcoholism scales. Quarterly Journal of Studies on Alcohol 35:490–498, 1974

Honigfeld G, Klett CJ: The Nurses' Observation Scale for Inpatient Evaluation: a new scale for measuring improvement in chronic schizophrenia. J Clin Psychol 21:65–71, 1965

Horn JL, Wanberg KW, Foster FM: Alcohol Use Inventory. Minneapolis, MN, National Computer Systems, 1986

Hurt SW, Hyler SE, Frances A, et al: Assessing borderline personality disorder with self-report, clinical interview, or semistructured interview. Am J Psychiatry 141:1228–1231, 1984

Jackson DN: Personality Research Form Manual. Goshen, NY, Research Psychologists Press, 1974

Janowsky D, Judd L, Huey L, et al: Naloxone effects on manic symptoms and growth hormone levels. Lancet 2:320, 1978

Jastak S, Wilkinson GS: The Wide Range Achievement Test—Revised. Wilmington, DE, Jastak Associates, 1981

Jenkins CD, Rosenman RH, Friedman J: Development of an objective psychological test for the determination of the coronary-prone behavior pattern in employed men. Journal of Chronic Diseases 20:371–379, 1967

Katz MM, Lyerly SB: Methods for measuring adjustment and social behavior in the community, I: rationale, description, discriminative validity and scale development. Psychological Reports Monograph 13:503–535, 1963

Kimura D: Functional asymmetry of the brain in dichotic listening. Cortex 3:163–178, 1967

Linehan MM, Goodstein JL, Nielson SL, et al: Reasons for staying alive when you are thinking of killing yourself: the Reasons for Living Inventory. J Consult Clin Psychol 51:276–286, 1983

Loranger AW: Personality Disorder Examination (PDE) Manual. Yonkers, NY, DV Communications, 1988

Loranger AW, Hirschfeld RMA, Sartorius N, et al: The WHO/ADAMHA international pilot study of personality disorders: background and purpose. Journal of Personality Disorders 5:296–306, 1991

Luria AR: The Working Brain: An Introduction to Neuropsychology. Translated by Haigh B. New York, Basic Books, 1973

MacAndrew C: The differentiation of male alcohol outpatients from nonalcoholic psychiatric patients by means of the MMPI. Quarterly Journal of Studies on Alcohol 26:238–246, 1965

Marks IM, Mathews AM: Brief standard self-rating for phobic patients. Behav Res Ther 17:263–267, 1979

Mattis S: Dementia Rating Scale: Professional Manual. Odessa, FL, Psychological Assessment Resources, 1988

Mattis S, French JH, Rapin I: Dyslexia in children and young adults: three independent neuropsychological syndromes. Dev Med Child Neurol 17:150–163, 1975

Mattis S, Kovner R, Goldmeier E: Different patterns of mnemonic deficits in two organic amnestic syndromes. Brain Lang 6:179–191, 1978

McKinley JC, Hathaway SR, Meehl PE: The MMPI, VI: K scale. Journal of Consulting Psychology 12:20–31, 1948

Megargee EI, Cook PE, Mendelsohn GA: Development and validation of an MMPI scale of assaultiveness in overcontrolled individuals. J Abnorm Psychol 72:519–528, 1967

Millon T: Millon Clinical Multiaxial Inventory, 3rd Edition. Minneapolis, MN, Interpretive Scoring Systems, 1983

Millon T: Millon Clinical Multiaxial Inventory–II: Manual for the MCMI-II. Minneapolis, National Computer Systems, 1987

Mirsky AF, Kornetsky C: On the dissimilar effects of drugs on the Digit Symbol Substitution and Continuous Performance Tests: a review and preliminary integration of behavioral and physiological evidence. Psychopharmacologia 5:161–177, 1964

Morey LC: Personality Assessment Inventory. Odessa, FL, Psychological Assessment Resources, 1991

Murray HA: Thematic Apperception Test Manual. Cambridge, MA, Harvard University Press, 1943

Nelson HE: National Adult Reading Test (NART) Test Manual. Berkshire, MA, NFER-Nelson, 1982

Overall JE, Gorham DR: The Brief Psychiatric Rating Scale. Psychol Rep 10:799–812, 1962

Raskin A: Assessment of psychopathology by the nurse or psychiatric aide, in The Behavioral Assessment of Psychiatric Patients: Quantitative Techniques for Evaluation. Edited by Burdock EI, Sudilovsky A, Gershon S. New York, Marcel Dekker, 1982, pp 143–175

Raven JC: Guide to the Standard Progressive Matrices. London, HK Lewis, 1960

Rorschach H: Psychodiagnostics. New York, Grune & Stratton, 1949

Rosvold HE, Mirsky AF, Sarason I, et al: A continuous performance test of brain damage. J Consult Clin Psychol 20:343–350, 1956

Secunda SK, Katz MM, Swann A, et al: Mania: diagnosis, state measurement and prediction of treatment response. J Affect Disord 8:113–121, 1985

Shipley WC: The Institute of Living Scale. Los Angeles, Western Psychological Services, 1946

Solovay MR, Shenton ME, Gasperetti C, et al.: Scoring manual for the Thought Disorder Index. Schizophr Bull 12:483–496, 1986

Spanier GB: Measuring dyadic adjustment: new scales for assessing the quality of marriage and similar dyads. Journal of Marriage and the Family 38:15–28, 1976

Spielberger CD, Gorsuch RL, Luchene RE: Manual for the State-Trait Anxiety Inventory. Palo Alto, CA, Consulting Psychologists Press, 1976

Spreen O, Benton AL: Neurosensory Center Comprehensive Examination for Aphasia. Victoria, BC, University of Victoria, 1977

Stangl D, Pfohl B, Zimmerman M, et al: A structured interview for the DSM-III personality disorders: a preliminary report. Arch Gen Psychiatry 42:591–596, 1985

Taylor-Spence JA, Spence KW: The motivational components of manifest anxiety: drive and drive stimuli, in Anxiety and Behavior. Edited by Spielberger CD. New York, Academic, 1966, pp 291–326

Wechsler D: Wechsler Adult Intelligence Scale—Revised. New York, Psychological Corporation, 1981

Wechsler D: The Wechsler Memory Scale—Revised. New York, Psychological Corporation, 1987

Weissman A, Beck AT: Development and validation of the Dysfunctional Attitude Scale. Paper presented at the annual meeting of the American Association of Behavior Therapists, Chicago, 1978 [Address requests to Center for Cognitive Therapy, Room 602, 133 South 36th St., Philadelphia, PA 19104.]

Weissman MM, Bothwell S: Assessment of social adjustment by patient self-report. Arch Gen Psychiatry 33:1111–1115, 1976

Wiggins JS, Pincus AL: Personality: structure and assessment. Annu Rev Psychol 43:473–504, 1992

Willner AE: Towards development of more sensitive clinical tests of abstraction: the analogy test. Proceedings of the 78th Annual Convention of the American Psychological Association 5:553–554, 1971

Young JE: Loneliness, depression, and cognitive therapy, in Loneliness: A Sourcebook of Current Theory, Research, and Therapy. Edited by Peplau LA, Perlman DA. New York, Wiley, 1982, pp 379–405

Young RC, Biggs JT, Ziegler VE, et al: A rating scale for mania: reliability, validity and sensitivity. Br J Psychiatry 133:429–435, 1978

Zung WWK: A rating instrument for anxiety disorders. Psychosomatics 12:371–379, 1971

Zung WWK: Index of Potential Suicide (IPS): a rating scale for suicide prevention, in The Prediction of Suicide. Edited by Beck AT, Resnick HLP, Lettieri DJ. Bowie, MD, Charles Press, 1974, pp 221–249

CHAPTER 9

Laboratory and Other Diagnostic Tests in Psychiatry

John M. Morihisa, M.D.
Richard B. Rosse, M.D.
C. Deborah Cross, M.D.

With the increased use of biological therapies in psychiatry, there has been a parallel increased interest in the potential application of laboratory and diagnostic test evaluations for psychiatric patients. In addition, clinical neuroscientists have been accumulating evidence for subtle neurophysiological dysfunction in many psychiatric disorders, and an effort is being made to try to characterize and elaborate some of these abnormalities. Such research findings have significantly expanded the scope of thinking concerning many disease processes and have raised the hope that if these pathophysiological abnormalities can be clearly elucidated, new and more effective treatments might be developed.

■ USE OF DIAGNOSTIC TESTS IN DETECTING PHYSICAL ILLNESS IN PSYCHIATRIC PATIENTS

DSM-IV (American Psychiatric Association 1994) has for many psychiatric diagnoses a common criterion: the necessary exclusion of any underlying physical condition that might account for the patient's symptomatology. Indeed, several studies have found that physical illnesses are quite common among psychiatric patients. In addition, many of these

271

physical disorders have been thought to be causative or exacerbating factors in the patients' psychiatric symptomatology (Hoffman and Koran 1984).

Initial suspicion of a possible organic component to a patient's psychiatric presentation can come from clues provided by a careful history and physical examination. Although there is no complete consensus as to which signs and symptoms are most "suggestive" of organic conditions, a number of investigators have proposed criteria that they feel might implicate an organic mental disorder. For example, Hoffman and Koran (1984) outlined a table of clues "suggestive" of organic mental disorders (Table 9–1). In addition, Hall et al. (1978) reported that when a review-of-symptoms checklist was used in psychiatric outpatients, those patients

---

Table 9–1. Some clues suggestive of organic mental disorders

1. Psychiatric symptoms after age 40
2. Psychiatric symptoms
   a. During a major medical illness
   b. While taking drugs that can cause mental symptoms
3. History of
   a. Alcohol or drug abuse
   b. Physical illness impairing organ function (neurological, endocrine, renal, hepatic, cardiac, pulmonary)
   c. Taking multiple prescribed or over-the-counter drugs
4. Family history of
   a. Degenerative or inheritable brain disease
   b. Inherited metabolic disease (e.g., diabetes, pernicious anemia, porphyria)
5. Mental signs including
   a. Altered level of consciousness
   b. Fluctuating mental status
   c. Cognitive impairment
   d. Episodic, recurrent, or cyclic course
   e. Visual, tactile, or olfactory hallucinations
6. Physical signs including
   a. Signs of organ malfunction that can affect the brain
   b. Focal neurological deficits
   c. Diffuse subcortical dysfunction, such as slowed speech/mentation/movement, ataxia, incoordination, tremor, chorea, asterixis, dysarthria
   d. Cortical dysfunction (e.g., dysphasia, apraxias, agnosias, visuospatial deficits, or defective cortical sensation)

Source. Reprinted from Hoffman RS, Koran RM: "Detecting Physical Illness in Patients With Mental Disorders." *Psychosomatics* 25:654–660, 1984. Copyright 1984. Used with permission.

with four or more positive responses on the checklist had a much higher incidence of abnormal laboratory results than did those who were symptom-negative. Many of these abnormal laboratory results were felt to reflect physical conditions that influenced the patients' psychiatric presentation.

For patients known to have or strongly suspected of having a medical illness, one orders the laboratory tests necessary to work up or follow up the physical condition (Hales 1986). Those physical conditions not thought to be contributing to the psychiatric presentation also need to be appropriately evaluated, because psychiatric patients with concomitant medical problems have been reported to demonstrate increased mortality secondary to their medical conditions (Karasu et al. 1980; Koranyi 1979). In addition, there is the possibility that some of the physical conditions that initially were considered to be only coincidental to the psychiatric illness might later prove to be etiological or to exacerbate the psychiatric condition. Consultation from other medical specialists might be necessary, but the consultants' impressions and recommendations all require careful scrutiny by the attending psychiatrist, who holds the ultimate responsibility for fitting together the pattern of specialized opinions. Decisions to continue or extend laboratory evaluation are often complex and generally include some type of risk-benefit analysis, as well as consideration of prevailing economic and liability issues. Good clinical judgment needs to be the final arbiter for all clinical decisions regarding choice of laboratory and diagnostic testing. Test risks that should be considered include possible physical complications, pain, or discomfort.

Most clinicians must limit studies according to some assessment of their likely utility in each individual case. Some studies of extensive laboratory testing strategies in psychiatric patients have reported that such approaches yield a relatively small amount of useful, new information (Dolan and Mushlin 1985). However, it can be argued that subclinical physical disorders can cause or possibly exacerbate psychiatric symptoms. Cognitive or behavioral symptoms usually do not signal a specific type of underlying organic problem, but rather suggest an often extensive differential diagnosis. A wide range of different psychiatric symptoms or syndromes caused by different neuromedical conditions have been described (Giannini et al. 1978). Additionally, psychiatric symptoms alone are usually inadequate for differentiating the type of underlying medical problem present. Furthermore, many specific organic factors can cause a myriad of different psychiatric symptom pictures in different patients.

Estroff and Gold (1984) suggested that psychiatrists set up specific laboratory protocols for various common psychiatric complaints, such as depression, psychosis, and anxiety. The protocols would provide the psychiatric clinician with a thorough laboratory and diagnostic test evaluation that would be based on the possible differential diagnosis for the patient's psychiatric complaints. Many of the diagnostic tests ordered would be part of a search for different areas of possible organic dysfunction.

☐ Screening Tests in Psychiatry

There is incomplete agreement as to what should constitute a "routine" screening laboratory and diagnostic test battery (see Tables 9–2 and 9–3). Some investigators recommend a very brief and selective laboratory and diagnostic test evaluation in patients with no obvious signs or symptoms of physical disease, with the choice of tests in this situation generally based on the principle of clinical relevance to the patient's particular condition. Hoffman and Koran (1984) proposed a somewhat more extensive screening battery based on a selection of the available studies of physical disorders in psychiatric patients. Investigators who argue for less exten-

---

Table 9–2.   Some potential components of a screening battery for detecting physical disease in psychiatric patients

---

Complete blood count (CBC)[a]

Chemistry panel (including serum electrolytes,[a] glucose,[a] albumin, total protein, blood urea nitrogen,[a] creatinine,[a] calcium, phosphate, aspartate aminotransferase [SGOT],[a] alanine aminotransferase [SGPT],[a] alkaline phosphatase,[a] gamma-glutamyltransferase,[a] bilirubin,[a] iron, magnesium, serum cholesterol, and triglycerides)

Thyroid function tests[a]

Screening test for syphilis (VDRL or RPR)[a]

Human immunodeficiency virus (HIV) serology in potentially high-risk patients

Serum vitamin B_{12} and folate levels[a]

Urinalysis (with dipstick for protein and glucose)[a]

Urine toxicology (e.g., for abuse substances, heavy metals, anabolic steroids)

Urine for uroporphyrins and porphobilinogen

Erythrocyte uroporphyrinogen-1-synthetase

Serum ceruloplasmin

Chest X ray

Electrocardiogram

Electroencephalogram[a]

Computed tomography or magnetic resonance imaging[a]

Note.   The important principles of informed consent should always be applied. Tables 9–2 and 9–3 are not meant to be mutually exclusive.
[a]These tests are included in the recommended screening battery for patients with new onset of dementia. Tests considered "supplemental" to the core battery are computed tomography, magnetic resonance imaging, electroencephalogram, and lumbar puncture studies.

Table 9–3. Potential supplementary laboratory and diagnostic tests to evaluate physical conditions in psychiatric patients

---

Computed tomographic scan

Magnetic resonance imaging scan

Skull films

Electroencephalogram

Blood or breath alcohol level

Drug screen (e.g., thin layer chromatography) and possible confirmatory test(s) for positive results (e.g., gas chromatography–mass spectroscopy)

Heavy-metal screen

Blood levels of medications

Sedimentation rate

Antinuclear antibodies

Lumbar puncture with cerebrospinal fluid studies

Serum and urine copper levels

Serum ceruloplasmin

Human immunodeficiency virus testing

Monospot test

Blood cultures

Skin test for tuberculosis or brucellosis

Pregnancy tests

Urine for uroporphyrins

Urine and serum osmolality

Polysomnography

Nocturnal penile tumescence

Evoked potentials

Stool tests for occult blood

Arterial blood gases

Note. The important principles of informed consent should always be applied. Tables 9–2 and 9–3 are not meant to be mutually exclusive.

---

sive, more selective routine screening batteries would probably recommend that many of these previously described laboratory and diagnostic tests be ordered only if indicated by the history, clinical, or initial laboratory evaluation. Dolan and Mushlin (1985) studied 250 psychiatric inpatients who had a mean number of routine admission laboratory tests of close to 30 and found that the mean percentage of true positive results from all the laboratory tests performed was only 1.8%, and that only 11 patients (4%) had important medical problems discovered through the routine laboratory testing described by the investigators. These authors reported that a routine battery consisting of only a CBC (hemoglobin, hematocrit, white blood cell [WBC] count, and mean cell volume); serum levels of thyroxine, calcium, aspartate aminotransferase (AST), alkaline phosphatase, and syphilis serology; and a urinalysis would have identified as requiring further evaluation all 11 psychiatric patients who had diagnoses made on the basis of the screening laboratory examination.

Economic factors and cost-benefit analyses for populations of patients are often taken into consideration in this debate (especially with the increasing emphasis on cost containment in health care). Until some consensus is reached, the psychiatrist must use his or her judgment in selecting screening protocols for patients who present without symptoms that mandate a specific laboratory strategy.

☐ Diagnostic Screening Batteries for Geriatric Psychiatric Patients

Regarding the most useful diagnostic test screening battery for geriatric patients, no complete consensus exists. For a geriatric population, Kolman (1985) suggested the use of a fairly extensive routine admission screening protocol: serum hemoglobin; a WBC count; sedimentation rate; serum B_{12} and folate levels; a biochemical profile, including serum sodium, potassium, bicarbonate, blood urea nitrogen (BUN), calcium, phosphate, alkaline phosphatase, bilirubin, thyroxine, and glucose; a urinalysis (with bacteriological culture, if appropriate); a chest X ray; a skull X ray; and an ECG.

A National Institute on Aging task force (1980) recommended a similar test battery for the evaluation of dementia; on the other hand, Larson et al. (1986) suggested that a fairly selective test-ordering strategy in the evaluation of dementia in elderly patients might not significantly compromise care and would be more cost effective. These authors' strategy utilizes a careful history and physical examination, with blood tests that initially include only a CBC, a blood chemistry battery, and TSH level.

☐ Supplementary Tests to Evaluate Physical Conditions in Psychiatric Patients

Some commonly considered supplementary laboratory and other diagnostic tests that can at times be useful to screen and evaluate physical conditions in psychiatric patients are outlined in Table 9–3. Supplementation of the routine screening battery is indicated when there are specific clues in the patient's history, physical, or laboratory examination of an underlying physical condition. For instance, in a young psychotic patient with a movement disorder, a serum and urine copper and serum ceruloplasmin might be ordered to help rule out Wilson's disease. In the case of a patient taking prescribed or over-the-counter medications, the physician might order a blood level for those medications that have meaningful therapeutic or toxic ranges. Attempts at providing recommendations for thorough laboratory test evaluations for many possible physical problems that can potentially masquerade as psychiatric illness have been outlined (Giannini et al. 1978).

Any laboratory abnormality noted on a routine or supplemental laboratory screen needs to be thoughtfully evaluated and the need for possible follow-up carefully considered. Consultation with other specialists might at times be required. Some additional tests commonly employed in the workup of some potentially significant physical conditions include lumbar puncture, urine or blood toxicology determinations, CT and magnetic resonance imaging (MRI), and EEG.

Examination of the Cerebrospinal Fluid

Any physician attempting to perform a lumbar puncture needs to a) be aware of the possible complications of the procedure and b) possess the requisite technical competence. The lumbar puncture, with subsequent examination of the obtained cerebrospinal fluid (CSF), can aid in the diagnosis of a number of important neurological diseases that can have psychiatric symptoms, including CNS syphilis, meningitis, encephalitis, and subarachnoid hemorrhage. Feinsilver (1984) discussed possible indications for a lumbar puncture, including sudden changes in mental status associated with fever or signs of meningeal irritation (e.g., Kernig sign or Brudzinski sign). Jenike (1985) outlined similar indications for the role of the lumbar puncture in the workup for dementia.

Physicians should carefully consider the indications for performing a lumbar puncture in a particular patient, because the procedure is associated with potential risks and discomfort. Some possible contraindications to a lumbar puncture include situations involving raised intracranial pressure, the presence of an intracranial mass lesion, skin infection around the lumbar puncture site, and patients' use of anticoagulants (Pryse-Phillips and Murray 1986). Common examinations of the CSF include a WBC count; sugar, protein, and chloride determinations; serology; and bacteriological studies.

Laboratory Evaluation of Suspected Drug Abuse

In certain patient populations (e.g., adolescents), illicit drug use is reportedly quite high, and it is probably best for the clinician to have a relatively low threshold for ordering a drug screen in such high-risk patients with unexplained behavioral symptoms (Gold and Dackis 1986). Some clinicians might argue that an illicit drug screen should almost always be a part of the routine screening battery for psychiatric patients, because substance-induced psychiatric disorders can frequently mimic or exacerbate idiopathic psychiatric illness. Patients with a history of illicit drug abuse or dependence probably need some type of laboratory evaluation for drug use (e.g., blood alcohol levels, urine drug screens). Historical information obtained from patients regarding recent drug use is often unreliable. In addition, routine follow-up monitoring for illicit drug use is often a necessary part of the treatment of the drug-abusing patient.

The clinician should be aware that different laboratory test methodologies exist for the detection of illicit drugs and that the various methodologies might have differing sensitivities and capacities for drug detection. Gas chromatography–mass spectroscopy (GC-MS) is perhaps the most sensitive and reliable test, but usually is also the most expensive. Detection tests for illicit drugs are either available in the form of broad drug screens, which evaluate for the presence of any number of multiple drugs, or in the form of individual tests for specific drugs, which might be designed to detect lower levels of substance use than do the tests employed in the broad drug screen (Gold and Dackis 1986). The number of *types* of drugs included in a broad screening test varies from laboratory to laboratory, and the specimens best utilized by any particular test can also be different. The number of positives detected in routine drug screens can often be increased using more specific and sensitive measurement techniques such as gas chromatography (GC), high-performance liquid chromatography (HPLC), or GC-MS. A preliminary drug screen might utilize a less expensive lab test, such as an immunoassay method, and the test results can be confirmed by a different and more sensitive test, such as GC-MS.

In some studies, drug screening tests have been reported as having significant numbers of false positive results (Panner and Christakis 1986). Factors leading to false positive results included some medically prescribed drugs that test positive for illicit drugs in certain drug tests, as well as test operator errors, equipment contamination, and sample mislabeling. In an effort to confirm positive drug screening tests, second-level confirmatory tests such as GC-MS can be utilized. Doing so can reportedly lower false positive results to as low as 1% (Panner and Christakis 1986). Conversely, true positive results may be seen for prolonged periods of time; for example, urine samples from chronic marijuana users can test positive for THC for up to 4 weeks after use of the drug (Moyer et al. 1987).

Laboratory Evaluation for Environmental Toxins

Exposure to a number of different environmental toxins has been associated with various behavioral abnormalities. Possible environmental toxins with behavioral consequences include the heavy metals, such as manganese, lead, thallium, arsenic, and mercury. In the case of suspected heavy-metal exposure, a determination of blood or urinary concentrations of these metals might be helpful (DeLisi 1984). The clinician should remain alert to the possibility of poisoning by these metals as well as other environmental toxins associated with behavioral aberrations. The appropriate laboratory tests should be ordered when the possibility of such environmental toxin exposure is high.

Computed Tomography and Magnetic Resonance Imaging in Clinical Psychiatry

Computed tomographic scanning of the head offers the clinician cross-sectional X-ray images of the brain from multiple brain levels (both cortical and subcortical). The procedure is most often employed in the evaluation of patients with suspected structural brain abnormalities (e.g., tumor, subdural hematoma, stroke, abscess). An example of a single cross-sectional CT scan image is presented in Figure 9–1. Larson et al. (1986) recommended ordering a CT scan in psychiatric patients with focal neurological findings, while others have felt that the presence of an abnormal EEG would also be a good indication for ordering a CT scan in psychiatric patients. Weinberger (1984) recommended obtaining a CT scan in those psychiatric patients whose clinical presentation includes any of the following: confusion, dementia of unknown cause, a first episode of a psychosis of unknown etiology, a movement disorder of unknown etiology, a diagnosis of anorexia nervosa, prolonged catatonia, or a first episode of major affective disorder or personality change after age 50. Emsley et al. (1986) extended these recommendations to include ordering CT scans for any patient with a history of alcohol abuse, craniocerebral trauma, or seizures.

Magnetic resonance imaging (Figure 9–2) of the brain can usefully supplement and/or replace CT in certain clinical situations, because some lesions are better appreciated on MRI than on CT scan. The MRI is usually superior to CT scan when there is suspicion of lesions in the posterior fossa, brain stem, or temporal and apical areas of the brain, because the surrounding bone can distort the CT image (Jaskiw et al. 1987) or obstruct visualization. Indeed, the CT scan, with its excellent visualization of bone and calcifications, has an important utility in the evaluation of trauma and pathological processes involving calcification. The ability to differentiate between gray and white matter, as well as CSF, gives MRI a distinct advantage over CT. MRI provides superior delineation of the pathology of and changes associated with demyelinating disease and is, as well, of special value in the investigation of pathology in the cervical spinal cord and the cervicomedullary junction (Jacobson 1988). MRI has an advantage for patients who require multiple scans over time, because there is no ionizing radiation and there are no known adverse effects of MRI studies at present. However, MRI is contraindicated in patients with ferromagnetic structures or devices that may be adversely affected by powerful magnetic fields, such as aneurysm clips (Morihisa 1991). Because of the length of time needed to complete the scan and the confining nature of the machine, some patients may be psychologically or medically unable to tolerate the procedure.

Electroencephalogram

The EEG measures brain electrical activity from electrodes placed on the scalp in standardized positions. The amplitude and frequency of the electrical activity are graphically recorded on paper by ink markers for

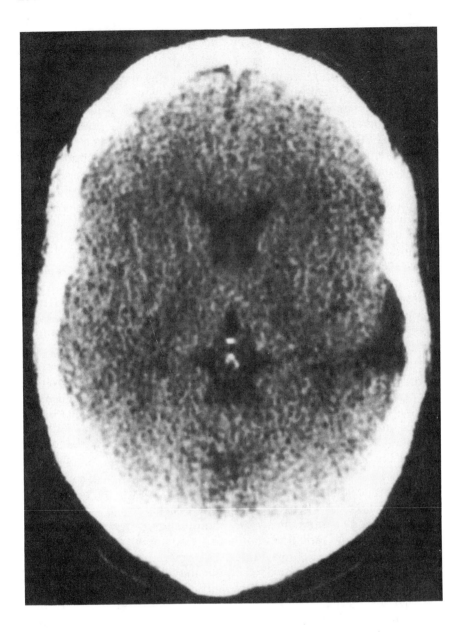

Figure 9–1. Computed tomographic scan of the head without contrast material. Image for a single brain level shown. Note hypodense area in the left temporal region adjacent to the skull. Intravenous injection of a standard roentgenographic contrast medium may be used to "enhance" a computed tomographic study for improved visualization of certain brain lesions (e.g., recent stroke, tumors, infections, abscesses).

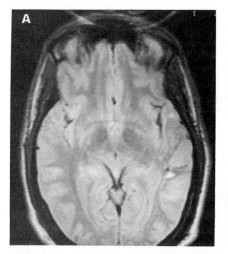

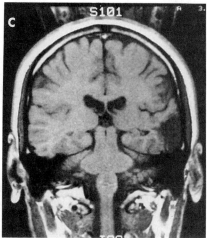

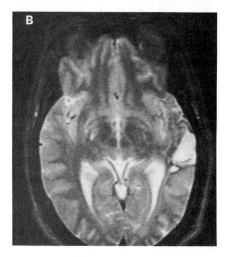

Figure 9–2. Three magnetic resonance imaging (MRI) scans from the same patient as was depicted in Figure 9–1. Each MRI here was obtained using a different scanning mode. (A) An axial "spin-echo intermediate" image. (B) A T₂-weighted image. (C) A coronal T₁-weighted image. MRI images can appear to be different depending on the scanning mode used. The signal properties of the left temporal region lesion shown in these scans suggest encephalomalacia. An MRI scan can be useful in helping to further characterize a lesion detected by computed tomography.

multiple areas of the brain surface as oscillating lines with different peaks and troughs, giving rise to the EEG tracing. The EEG frequencies have been divided into the following bands: beta activity (equal or greater than 13 Hz), alpha rhythm (between 8 and 13 Hz), theta activity (between 4 and 8 Hz), and delta activity (less than 4 Hz). The EEG is used primarily in the evaluation of epilepsy and other neurological disorders (e.g., neoplasm, trauma, stroke, metabolic or degenerative disease).

Some investigators have recommended that the EEG be a part of the routine screening battery for psychiatric patients (Hoffman and Koran 1984), especially those patients with suspected organic mental disorder. In cases where the patients have episodic behavioral disturbances that are possibly epileptic in nature, Goodin and Aminoff (1984) noted that a normal initial EEG alone cannot be used to completely exclude a diagnosis of epilepsy. Repeat EEGs or 24-hour ambulatory recordings can be obtained. Hall et al. (1980) suggested the utility of the sleep-deprived EEG, which they feel is more sensitive than a routine EEG. An increased number of various EEG abnormalities have been noted in a variety of psychiatric disorders, especially schizophrenia, although none can be considered diagnostic at this time.

Further Tests

Polysomnography.   Polysomnography involves the recording of EEG activity during sleep (or attempts at sleep) and is usually performed at night. In addition, other physiological functions that might be relevant to the evaluation of a patient's symptoms are monitored, such as electromyographic activity, electrooculographic, and electrocardiographic activity, as well as measurements of respiratory effort, airflow, and blood oxygen saturation. Polysomnography is used in the evaluation of certain sleep disorders (e.g., narcolepsy, sleep apnea, treatment-resistant insomnias). Patients being evaluated for excessive daytime sleepiness might require special daytime sleep evaluations.

Nocturnal penile tumescence studies.   Nocturnal penile tumescence (NPT) studies can be used in the evaluation of impotence. The absence of adequate erectile function during nocturnal sleep lends some diagnostic support for an organic etiology of a patient's impotence. However, abnormal NPT studies suggestive of an organic etiology have been reported in association with major depression (Thase et al. 1987).

Evoked potentials.   Evoked potential (EP) testing involves the measurement of specific brain electrical responses to discrete sensory stimuli. The evoking stimulus can be visual (as in visual EP, or VEP), auditory (AEP), or somatosensory (SSEP). In the process of EP testing, the subject is repeatedly exposed to certain stimuli (e.g., flashing lights), and the evoked brain electrical responses are added together and averaged by a computer to remove background, non–stimulus-related activity. The result is a characteristic waveform (the EP), which generally consists of negative and positive peaks spread along a time axis. EP testing can theoretically help the psychiatrist in the differentiation between some organic and functional complaints (e.g., in the evaluation of hysterical blindness using VEP). A brain-stem auditory evoked potential (BSAEP) might be ordered in cases of suspected psychogenic deafness or utilized in the evaluation of an unresponsive, mute, catatonic patient. Such a study would assess the integrity of the brain-stem structures involved in the processing of auditory stimuli. Demyelinating conditions such as multiple sclerosis can also be usefully evaluated using certain EP testing procedures. Various abnormalities of different EPs in certain psychiatric disorders have been described; however, none of these findings have been clearly demonstrated to be characteristic of any specific disorders, and their diagnostic potential is the subject of active investigation.

■ LABORATORY EVALUATION FOR SOME PSYCHIATRIC ORGANIC THERAPIES

One of the goals of the initial laboratory workup is to help provide useful baseline information for the patient who is likely to receive psychotropic medications. Many of the organic treatments are associated with adverse reactions that might be detected by changes in certain laboratory or other diagnostic test values (e.g., increasing liver function test values suggesting hepatotoxicity from a medication, or electrocardiographic changes reflecting potential cardiac toxicity from a psychotropic agent). It is therefore important to have baseline test values on a patient who is about to be exposed to an organic therapy so that future changes from these baseline values, possibly reflecting drug toxicity, can be properly assessed. When using a specific psychotropic agent, more information regarding potentially useful laboratory tests, drug-drug interactions, and possible side effects and contraindications should be reviewed in other more comprehensive publications such as the *Physicians' Desk Reference* and textbooks of psychopharmacology (e.g., Gelenberg et al. 1991; Schatzberg and Cole 1991).

☐ Tricyclic Antidepressants, Antipsychotics, and Benzodiazepines

There is no absolute consensus concerning standardized protocols for the pretreatment evaluation of most biological treatments in psychiatry. Because of the risk of agranulocytosis with clozapine, patients on this medication should have baseline and weekly WBC counts. For patients about to be started on tricyclic antidepressants (TCAs), antipsychotics, or benzodiazepine medications, Gelenberg (1983) recommended laboratory tests only as clinically indicated, based on consideration of each patient's past medical history, physical examination, previous history of adverse drug reactions, and knowledge of the potential adverse effects from the biological therapy to be utilized. For example, an ECG should be ordered in a patient with a significant history of cardiac pathology who is about to be started on an antidepressant or some of the antipsychotics, because some of these medications have been associated with potentially significant ECG abnormalities (especially the TCAs and the antipsychotic thioridazine). In the absence of a history of cardiac pathology, one might consider obtaining an ECG in a man over 30 or a woman over 40 who has not had one in the past year and is about to be started on a psychotropic medication that has been associated with potential cardiotoxicity (Gelenberg 1983).

In addition, it seems advisable to order liver function tests in patients with a history of liver disease who are about to be started on certain psychotropics that are metabolized by the liver. The clinician might need to have a lower threshold for ordering diagnostic tests in patients belonging to populations at greater risk for adverse reactions from some of the organic therapies (e.g., pediatric, geriatric, or chronically ill patients). Likewise, the follow-up laboratory evaluation for some of these organic therapies might also need to be more extensive in such vulnerable patient populations. Again, the clinician needs to be aware of the major potential adverse reactions of the organic therapies he or she employs and should use this knowledge to help guide the pretreatment and follow-up laboratory test evaluations.

☐ Pretreatment Lithium Evaluation

Lithium can have several potentially significant adverse affects, including those on the thyroid gland, kidney, heart, and developing fetus, as well as a usually benign elevation of the WBC count. Recommended pretreatment diagnostic evaluations often include a CBC, serum electrolytes, BUN, serum creatinine, thyroid function tests, urinalysis, an ECG, and, sometimes, a 24-hour urine test for creatinine clearance. For potentially pregnant patients, a pregnancy test should be ordered to clarify the patient's childbearing status.

☐ Pretreatment Anticonvulsant Evaluation

Certain anticonvulsants, such as carbamazepine, valproic acid, and clonazepam, are being increasingly employed in the treatment of patients with certain psychiatric disorders, such as in lithium-resistant or lithium-intolerant manic patients. Before the clinician utilizes any of these medications to treat a psychiatric illness, he or she should be fully aware of each of their potentially adverse effects and how they might be reflected in laboratory and other diagnostic test evaluations.

For instance, when carbamazepine is used, because of the reported risk of certain hematologic abnormalities such as aplastic anemia, leukopenia, thrombocytopenia, and anemia, it is recommended that the clinician obtain some baseline hematologic indices, which might include a

CBC and platelet count. A serum iron assay and a reticulocyte count might also be included, although clinically important hematologic toxicity with carbamazepine is felt by some to be a relatively uncommon occurrence (Hart and Easton 1982). Gelenberg (1985) recommended that a baseline laboratory screen for a patient about to start carbamazepine therapy should include a CBC, platelet count, and creatinine and liver function tests. Because carbamazepine has been reported to slow atrioventricular conduction, a pretreatment ECG might be useful in patients with a history of cardiac pathology, especially in those patients with a history of heart block.

In patients who are going to take valproic acid, baseline liver function tests are advisable because of this anticonvulsant's potential for hepatotoxicity. In patients with a clear history of liver disorder who are going to be placed on either carbamazepine or valproic acid, baseline liver function tests should be obtained. The necessary follow-up evaluation for patients on carbamazepine or valproic acid is discussed in the next section. Clonazepam has been associated with few serious side effects, and pretreatment laboratory evaluation would probably be similar to that employed for any benzodiazepine.

☐ Laboratory Evaluation Prior to Electroconvulsive Therapy

Certain laboratory and diagnostic tests are commonly completed before a patient begins ECT. The pretreatment workup often includes a CBC, blood chemistries, urinalysis, chest X ray, spinal X rays, and ECG (Sakauye 1986). In addition, a CT scan and EEG might also be ordered if indicated by medical history, physical, neurological exam, or mental status examination.

☐ Antipsychotic Blood Levels

Methodologies for the laboratory measurement of blood antipsychotic levels include gas-liquid chromatography (GLC), HPLC, GC-MS, fluorimetry, RIA, and radioreceptor assay (Creese and Synder 1977). Therapeutic levels and ranges for some of the antipsychotics have been reported (Van Putten et al. 1992), but a clear consensus concerning therapeutic levels or ranges has not yet been achieved using any measurement methodology. Interesting findings relevant to the clinical use of antipsychotic blood levels include the reports of low correlations between prescribed neuroleptic dose and subsequent serum neuroleptic levels, and reports that low neuroleptic levels for any given neuroleptic often help identify those patients who are most likely to relapse. However, patients with persistent psychotic symptoms have been reported to generally demonstrate neuroleptic levels indistinguishable from those of patients who are in remission (Brown and Laughren 1983). Specific situations in which antipsychotic blood levels might be of value include the assessment of patient compliance or the evaluation of patients taking medication but possibly achieving only low serum levels, as well as the assessment of certain drug-drug interactions.

☐ Tricyclic Antidepressant Blood Levels

There is incomplete agreement concerning the usefulness of plasma TCA levels (Kocsis et al. 1986; Simpson et al. 1983). The American Psychiatric Association (APA) Task Force on the Use of Laboratory Tests in Psychiatry (1985) concluded that plasma level measurements of imipramine, desmethylimipramine (desipramine), and nortriptyline are unequivocally useful in certain situations. Situations in which a TCA blood level might be ordered include those involving 1) patients with questionable compliance, 2) patients with a poor response to a "typical" antidepressant dose, 3) patients who experience side effects at a very low dose, 4) patients who are potentially very sensitive to side effects (e.g., medically ill or geriatric patients), and 5) patients for whom treatment is urgent and who require potentially therapeutic blood levels in as short a time possible (e.g., the severely suicidal patient).

☐ Monoamine Oxidase Inhibitors

It has been reported that therapeutic benefits from the monoamine oxidase inhibitor (MAOI) phenelzine are achieved when blood platelet monoamine oxidase (MAO) inhibition is equal to or greater than 80% (Liebowitz et al. 1984; Robinson et al. 1978). However, the techniques for measuring MAO inhibition are still evolving, and routine clinical application of this laboratory test at present is uncommon. The usefulness of this test for other MAOIs besides phenelzine is unclear.

☐ Lithium Blood Levels

Therapeutic and toxic blood levels for lithium in the treatment of bipolar affective illness have been approximated. For acute mania, Jefferson et al. (1987) reported therapeutic lithium levels from a lower range of 0.8 to 1.0 mEq/L to an upper range of 1.4 to 1.5 mEq/L. Clinicians with patients who have serum lithium levels in this upper range should be alert for possible early signs of lithium toxicity. Of course, this does not preclude the individual patients who have idiosyncratic therapeutic responses outside the generally accepted response range or patients who become toxic at relatively low serum lithium levels.

Stable, steady-state lithium levels are generally obtained about 4 to

5 days after either initiating lithium or adjusting the dose. Nevertheless, it is sometimes recommended that blood samples for lithium be drawn a couple of times a week when first initiating lithium therapy to help prevent lithium toxicity in patients requiring only small amounts of lithium to achieve therapeutic levels. Blood levels should also be drawn if the patient demonstrates any signs of possible toxicity. Blood samples for lithium determinations are generally drawn about 12 hours after the last dose of lithium.

The clinician needs to be sensitive to situations in which the serum lithium level can dramatically change—for example, in patients who are pregnant or immediately postpartum, patients who are on thiazide diuretics or are dehydrated, or patients with deteriorating renal function. If any of these or other similar situations are encountered, lithium levels might have to be drawn more frequently.

☐ Anticonvulsant Blood Levels

Therapeutic levels for anticonvulsants have been established for the use of such agents in the control of seizures. However, therapeutic blood levels for these medications in the treatment of psychiatric disorders have not been clearly developed. At this time it is unclear if the therapeutic blood serum levels described as effective in epilepsy are the same as those that are necessary for the treatment of psychiatric disorders. Emrich et al. (1984) reported that when carbamazepine or valproic acid is used in the treatment of mood disorders, the effective plasma levels are the same as those employed in the control of seizures. On the other hand, at least for carbamazepine, Post (1984) suggested that clinical monitoring of blood levels is probably only of secondary importance and seems to provide only a rough guideline of clinical efficacy. Monitoring serum carbamazepine and valproic acid levels is probably helpful in predicting possible adverse effects secondary to toxicity from the medications.

Because of the relatively rare incidence of hematologic disturbance associated with carbamazepine use, periodic follow-up of hematologic function is necessary. Hart and Easton (1982) suggested CBCs be performed biweekly for the first 2 months of carbamazepine therapy. They suggested that if no abnormalities appear during this time, counts can be obtained quarterly. Blood counts should be immediately obtained should signs or symptoms of bone marrow suppression be present.

Hyponatremia has been associated with carbamazepine therapy, so the clinician might need to order serum electrolytes if the clinical situation so warrants. Furthermore, periodic monitoring of hepatic function might be required, especially in patients with known hepatic dysfunction. Patients on valproic acid need periodic evaluation of their hepatic function (e.g., liver function tests), especially during the first 6 months of therapy (PDR 1986). Finally, carbamazepine blood levels should be carefully monitored, because this drug can increase its metabolism through induction of liver enzymes (Schatzberg and Cole 1991).

☐ Electrocardiographic Monitoring of Patients on Psychotropics

Psychotropic medications, including the TCAs, antipsychotics, and carbamazepine, have been associated with various electrocardiographic changes. The most frequently alluded-to changes are those representing a slowing of atrioventricular conduction in the heart, for example, as reflected by a widening of the QT or QRS interval on the ECG. Significantly, malignant arrhythmias have been reported in some patients taking TCAs and thioridazine. It has been suggested that a lengthening of the QT interval may prolong the period of cardiac vulnerability to potentially life-threatening arrhythmias. Patients who seem at particularly high risk of developing these potentially lethal arrhythmias are those patients with preexisting "excessively" prolonged QT intervals or those patients who develop "excessive" QT prolongation during drug treatment (Flugelman et al. 1985), as well as patients with already compromised cardiac function. Schwartz and Wolf (1978) reported that when the QT interval corrected for rate (QTc) exceeds 0.440 seconds, there is an increased risk of sudden cardiac death due to ventricular tachycardia or ventricular fibrillation.

■ BIOLOGICAL MARKER RESEARCH

Neuroscience investigators continue to search for meaningful laboratory and diagnostic tests for "functional" psychiatric disorders. These "functional," or idiopathic, disorders are those psychiatric conditions for which a clear causative or contributing neuropathophysiological lesion has yet to be identified. The proposed tests are also occasionally referred to as "biological markers," and these markers might have a number of potential future uses to psychiatrists and neuroscientists, including assistance in improving our understanding of some of the underlying neurobiology of functional disorders, in making an accurate psychiatric diagnosis, in arriving at the most appropriate treatment plan, in assessing prognosis, and in identifying those patients who are at potential risk of developing a psychiatric disorder who might benefit from preventive measures.

Some difficulties associated with the markers studied to date have been problems with sensitivity, specificity, reliability, and possible contamination from artifactual influences (e.g., concurrent illnesses, medication effects, and normal individual variation among patients). Currently, because of these and other problems, none of the markers yet seem to have the sensitivity and specificity that would make them clearly useful in routine clinical practice.

☐ Neuroendocrine Testing

Neuroendocrine testing research in psychiatry includes measurements of basal hormone levels as well as neuroendocrine challenge tests. Basal endocrine evaluation includes blood measurements of certain hormone levels (e.g., thyroid function testing or serum cortisol levels) or measurement of certain hormone metabolites in the urine. Thorough endocrine laboratory testing should be performed if the clinician suspects underlying endocrine disease. A possible example of the utility of basal hormonal measurements to the psychiatric clinician is in the case of the patient with a rapid-cycling bipolar disorder. Both clinical and subclinical hypothyroidism have been reported to be associated with a significant proportion of these patients (Cho et al. 1979; Cowdry et al. 1983). In addition, severe depression has been associated with a hypersecretion of cortisol as well as a possible loss of the normal diurnal variation of cortisol secretion (Allen et al. 1987).

Dexamethasone Suppression Test

The dexamethasone suppression test (DST) has been one of the most actively investigated of the neuroendocrine challenge tests used in psychiatric research (Allen et al. 1987; Carroll 1984). Although extensive research has been devoted to the evaluation of the clinical application of the DST, it does not appear to be appropriate for routine screening of psychiatric patients (Carroll 1986). One possible use of the DST may lie in its potential for providing biological subtypes and prognostically meaningful subgroups. For example, the DST may be useful in predicting relapse in some patients treated for depression (Nemeroff and Evans 1984).

Thyrotropin-Releasing Hormone Stimulation Test

The thyrotropin-releasing hormone stimulation test (TRHST) has been proposed as a potential biological marker of mood disorders (Loosen and Prange 1982). In major depression, a blunted TSH response to TRH has been reported to occur about 25% of the time (Loosen and Prange 1982). In another possible use of the TRHST, Targum et al. (1984) have suggested that treatment-resistant depressed patients with an "augmented"

TSH response (e.g., greater than 30 μIU/ml) might benefit from thyroid hormone medication added to their antidepressant regimen. Targum et al. (1992) also reported variability of responses to the TRH test in depressed and nondepressed elderly subjects.

Corticotropin-Releasing Hormone Stimulation Test

Another neuroendocrine challenge test perhaps related to the DST is the corticotropin-releasing hormone (CRH) stimulation test. Corticotropin-releasing hormone is normally released by the hypothalamus and acts on the pituitary to cause a release of adrenocorticotropin (ACTH). Gold et al. (1986) reported that depressed patients had basal hypercortisolism that was associated with a decreased responsiveness of ACTH to an intravenous challenge with CRH.

☐ Brain Imaging

Whereas the proposed neuroendocrine tests largely provide an indirect measure of brain activity (e.g., through central effects on endocrine function), brain imaging techniques have the potential for providing a more direct window into the functioning of the living human brain. Functional brain imaging techniques include computerized electroencephalography and evoked potential mapping, positron-emission tomography (PET), single-photon emission computed tomography (SPECT), and regional cerebral blood flow (rCBF). Magnetic resonance imaging and computed tomography are structural brain imaging techniques that can provide an anatomic view of the living human brain. Of special note, software and technical advances in MRI have allowed this technique to "evolve" into a new functional brain imaging approach, *magnetic resonance spectroscopy* (MRS). Another promising application of brain imaging technology will be the combined use of complementary brain imaging techniques (e.g., utilizing a functional brain imaging technique such as computerized EEG mapping with a structural brain imaging technique such as CT) (Morihisa and McAnulty 1985).

Positron-Emission Tomography

Whereas computerized EEG mapping provides information about brain electrical activity presumably arising from only the uppermost cortical cell layers, PET allows for the direct visualization of both cortical and subcortical (e.g., limbic system) brain functioning. Different aspects of brain functioning can be evaluated, including cerebral blood flow (CBF), brain oxygen utilization, and certain aspects of brain glucose metabolism, as well as some specific CNS neurotransmitter systems function (Figure 9–3).

Some preliminary PET findings in patients with schizophrenia and bipolar disorder have included reports of abnormalities of the anteroposterior gradient of glucose utilization (Buchsbaum 1986; Buchsbaum et al. 1984), as well as decreased absolute glucose utilization in the frontal lobes in schizophrenia (Wolkin et al. 1985). Gur et al. (1987) did not find "hypofrontality" in the schizophrenic patients studied, but reported higher subcortical/cortical glucose metabolism ratios for patients with schizophrenia as compared with normal control subjects. In another study utilizing radioisotopes capable of binding to brain dopamine D_2 receptors, D_2 receptors in the caudate nucleus were found to be higher in patients with schizophrenia than in normal control subjects (Wong et al. 1986). Tamminga et al. (1992) reported abnormalities of the limbic system, in particular the hippocampus, in schizophrenia. Attempts to correlate metabolic findings with clinical variables have thus far failed to achieve any consensus. The disparity in research design and focus has contributed to the difficulty in comparing and integrating the wide spec-

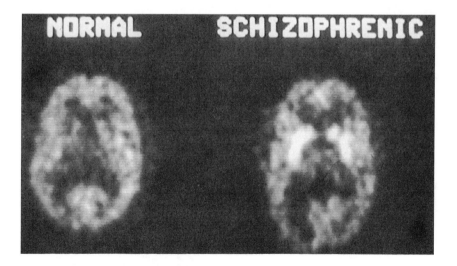

Figure 9–3. Positron-emission tomography scans utilizing radiolabeled spiperone in a normal control (*left*) and a schizophrenic patient (*right*). White areas indicate regions of maximal binding. These PET scans visualize a section of the brain that includes the basal ganglia. Note how in the schizophrenia patient the basal ganglia show a high accumulation of radiolabeled activity relative to the rest of the brain. (Courtesy of H. N. Wagner, Jr., M.D., Johns Hopkins Medical Institutions, Baltimore, Maryland.)

trum of findings. PET studies have not yet demonstrated sufficient sensitivity or specificity to elaborate a definitive role in psychiatric practice. As is the case for most brain imaging applications, PET is most accurately considered a research tool in the investigation of classical psychiatric disorders.

Single-Photon Emission Computed Tomography

Single-photon emission computed tomography can generate cross-sectional images from multiple levels of the brain and can therefore visualize the CNS in three dimensions (as can PET). SPECT utilizes radionuclides that emit gamma radiation (i.e., photons). These photons are measured by gamma detectors containing sodium iodide scintillation crystals. Information may then be calculated concerning the location in the brain and the relative amount of radionuclide at that locus. Different radiopharmaceuticals can be used to investigate different parameters of brain function.

For classical psychiatric disorders there is insufficient evidence that SPECT can yet provide the sensitivity or specificity that will be required for the development of new diagnostic or prognostic approaches (Morihisa 1991). One of the confounding variables in any attempt to consolidate SPECT findings into clinically meaningful protocols is that there is a significant discrepancy between the investigational capabilities of many SPECT systems presently in use. Nevertheless, recently developed research-grade SPECT systems feature improved resolution that can begin to rival that of PET scans, and preliminary investigations have suggested that this modality may provide complementary information in some disease entities.

Regional Cerebral Blood Flow

In rCBF, blood flow to various regions of the brain is evaluated. To accomplish this, a metabolically inert radioactive substance (usually xenon-133) is introduced into the body (usually through inhalation). The radioactive substance is carried by the blood to various parts of the brain, and radiation emanating from the brain is picked up by detectors surrounding the skull. This method of investigation of brain function depends on the close linkage between cerebral blood flow and cerebral metabolism (i.e., increased activity of a certain part of the brain is normally associated with an increase in blood flow to the area). The procedure can be performed with the subject at rest or engaging in mental activity. Unfortunately, unlike PET or SPECT, rCBF using the xenon-133 inhalation technique cannot delineate blood flow in subcortical structures.

Ingvar and Franzen (1974) reported on rCBF studies in patients with schizophrenia. They found decreased blood flow in frontal brain regions in these patients, which they did not find in their alcoholic control subjects. More recently, Weinberger et al. (1986) reported that schizophrenic subjects fail to show increased blood flow to the dorsolateral prefrontal cortex (DLPFC) during challenge by the Wisconsin Card Sorting Test, a task that is felt to require the functional integrity of the DLPFC and has been shown to be associated with increased blood flow to the DLPFC in normal subjects. This work has provided the basis for an exciting neurodevelopmental theory for the pathogenesis of schizophrenia (Weinberger 1987) and focused investigational interest on the DLPFC (Morihisa and Weinberger 1986). Furthermore, work by Weinberger et al. (1992) extended this theory to implicate dysfunction of a prefrontal-limbic neural *network* in schizophrenia.

Computed Tomography

In CT, multiple X rays are taken through the CNS that provide the basis for the elaboration of cross-sectional images of the brain. Possible indications for the use of CT in the organic workup of psychiatric patients have already been described in this chapter. Again, when CT is employed in this manner, it is generally in an effort to rule out neurological lesions, such as CNS neoplasms, that might be causing or contributing to the psychiatric symptomatology. Indeed, it would appear that it is in the evaluation of classically neurological disease processes that structural imaging techniques such as CT and MRI demonstrate their most significant utility in clinical psychiatry (Morihisa 1991).

Scientific investigators have employed CT to identify a number of subtle structural abnormalities in the CNS of patients with primary psychiatric disorders. Findings have included increased ventricular-to-brain (VBR) ratios in patients with schizophrenia (Weinberger et al. 1979) and cerebellar atrophy and third ventricle enlargement in schizophrenia (Nasrallah et al. 1985). An extensive scientific effort has been under way to attempt to correlate these structural findings with clinically relevant variables, but has thus far failed to delineate clearly any parameters that can significantly enhance our present diagnostic or treatment approach to classical psychiatric disorders. For example, it has been suggested that there may be an association between enlarged ventricles in schizophrenia and medication response, negative symptoms (Pearlson et al. 1984), and cognitive impairment (Johnston et al. 1976). The attempt to elaborate the clinical meaning of these findings is further confounded by the fact that enlarged ventricles have been reported in other psychiatric illnesses, including eating disorders, alcoholism, bipolar disorder, and dementia (Coffman 1989; Fogel and Faust 1987). It must also be emphasized that only a subpopulation of all patients with schizophrenia demonstrate significantly enlarged ventricles compared with a normal control population. Thus, it is clear that this finding is neither pathognomonic nor even characteristic of a specific psychiatric disorder (Morihisa 1991).

Magnetic Resonance Imaging

The technique of MRI provides three-dimensional visualization of the brain's structure in transverse, sagittal, and coronal planes by measuring the differential distribution of hydrogen nuclei, mainly in the water and fat of the brain. Future advances in technology will utilize MRS to image brain function, as reflected by differences in brain chemistry, for compounds that contain phosphorus-31, carbon-13, sodium-23, fluoride-19, and hydrogen, as well as the element lithium-7. In this manner, in vivo investigations of certain neurotransmitters, lipid metabolism, electrolyte balance, amino acid metabolism, high-energy phosphate metabolism, and carbohydrate metabolism may be pursued (Keshavan et al. 1991). In addition, drug studies of compounds incorporating carbon-13, lithium-7, or fluoride-19 may be possible (Guze 1991).

In the MRI technique, a magnetic field (usually 0.5 to 1.5 tesla in strength) is applied to the brain, and the spinning nuclei of hydrogen become aligned in accordance with this field. These nuclei are then exposed to brief pulses of a second field created by a radio frequency (RF) coil that causes nuclei to precess as well as spin. These pulses must "broadcast" on the characteristic resonant frequency (Larmor frequency) of hydrogen. Following the pulse, the nuclei return to their previously aligned positions and in doing so emit a characteristic electromagnetic pattern. MRI detects this characteristic signal with a radio frequency receiver. The return over time of these hydrogen nuclei to their previously aligned positions is termed *relaxation*. T_1 and T_2 (relaxation times) are measures of the rate of this return of nuclei to their original state. Adjustments in transmission parameters can emphasize (i.e., weight) certain informational characteristics in the image. For example, a T_1-weighted scan generally provides the best gray/white matter differentiation, whereas a T_2-weighted scan generally provides superior discrimination of brain tissue abnormalities (Morihisa 1991).

Some MRI studies have successfully replicated findings from previous CT research reports, and other investigators (Jernigan et al. 1991) attempted to extend the reach of structural investigations of psychiatric disorders such as schizophrenia. Most recently, MRS studies using phosphorus-31 (Pettegrew et al. 1991) have investigated CNS membrane phospholipid metabolism as well as high-energy phosphate metabolism in dorsal prefrontal cortex in schizophrenia. The authors interpreted their results as suggestive of hypoactivity in this region (supporting the Weinberger neurodevelopmental theory of schizophrenia) and also speculate that abnormalities of cell membranes may play a role in the pathogenesis of schizophrenia (Pettegrew et al. 1991).

☐ Genetic Markers

An exciting, new, and rapidly developing area is the field of genetic markers of psychiatric illness. Markers have been described for Huntington's disease (Gusella et al. 1984), and numerous reports raise the possibility of identifying clinically relevant genetic markers for psychiatric disorders. Additional strategies have included the search for genetic markers such as human leukocyte antigen (HLA) and restriction fragment-length polymorphisms (RFLPs). However, significant refinement of investigational techniques, as well as improvements in delineating the most appropriate research strategies, will be required before specific genetic markers of psychiatric disorders can be definitively demonstrated.

☐ Biochemical Markers

The laboratory has been increasingly used by physicians from all specialties to help detect, confirm, or rule out diagnoses of various physical conditions. There has also been the hope that the quantitative laboratory could similarly be used by psychiatrists and neuroscientists to help in the evaluation of patients with functional disorders. Research scientists have employed different strategies in their search for quantitative laboratory applications to psychiatry, including the examination of various potentially relevant compounds found in the blood, urine, and spinal fluid, as well as the examination of CNS enzyme and receptor systems also found in tissues outside of the brain (e.g., blood platelets, lymphocytes, skin fibroblasts). None of these strategies has yet led to any definitive biological markers for psychiatric disorders, but the tests remain important research tools and are in the process of analysis and refinement.

Body Fluid Markers

Body fluid markers include those molecular compounds found in the plasma, serum, urine, and CSF that are of particular interest to psychiatrists. Some of the biochemical markers that have been studied include neurotransmitter substances felt to be relevant to the pathogenesis of some psychiatric disorders (e.g., dopamine, serotonin, and norepinephrine), their metabolites (e.g., homovanillic acid [HVA], 5-hydroxyindoleacetic acid [5-HIAA], and 3-methoxy-4-hydroxyphenylglycol [MHPG]), various neuropeptides (e.g., endorphins, enkephalins), and biological compounds such as immunoglobulins (e.g., IgM) and plasma melatonin. Overall, most of the studies are either preliminary or have yielded mixed results.

Among some of the interesting research findings are the reported association between reduced CSF 5-HIAA and suicidal behavior (Åsberg et al. 1976) and the possibility that unipolar depressed patients may be partly differentiated from depressed bipolar patients by a lower 24-hour urinary MHPG reportedly found in some of the bipolar patients (Muscettola et al. 1984). On this latter point, however, Davis and Bresnahan (1987) did not feel that the differences were great enough to be of significant clinical utility.

Peripheral Tissue Markers

Peripheral tissue markers include those generally high-molecular-weight, complex biomolecules (e.g., neurotransmitter receptors) associated with tissues that can be obtained from outside the CNS (e.g., lymphocytes, red blood cells), as well as the in vitro study of the activity of certain peripherally obtained tissues that might serve as biological markers of psychiatric illness. From the blood, one can obtain for study several tissues rich in neurotransmitter receptors and enzymes, including platelets, lymphocytes, and red blood cells. Human platelets contain the enzyme MAO as well as $alpha_1$-adrenergic receptors, serotonin reuptake sites, ^{3}H-labeled imipramine binding sites, and dopamine receptors. Human red blood cells contain a mechanism for lithium transport and the enzyme catechol-O-methyl transferase. From the skin, one can obtain fibroblasts that contain neurotransmitter receptors and important transport systems (Stahl 1985). Abnormalities discovered in any of these peripherally derived systems might reflect defects in their counterparts found in brain. Most of the work with peripheral tissue markers is still in its infancy. Like much of the work with the biological fluid markers, peripheral tissue marker research has not produced a consistent pattern of findings.

Other potential tissue markers of interest to psychiatrists include evaluation of certain aspects of immune function, such as studies of lymphocyte responsiveness to various mitogens, measurements of natural killer cell activity, and the differences in ratios of helper lymphocytes to suppressor lymphocytes, as well as the determination of HLA in psychiatric patients. Extensive further study will be required to elucidate the clinical significance of these markers, but the role of altered immune function in psychiatric patients is an exciting arena of growing research.

☐ Provocative Tests for Panic Disorder

Intravenous lactate infusions have been reported to induce panic attacks in many patients with histories consistent with panic disorder. A commonly described procedure for this test involves the intravenous infusion of 10 ml of 0.5 M sodium lactate per kilogram of body weight over a 20-minute period (Liebowitz et al. 1985). It has been reported that approximately 70% to 90% of patients with panic disorder, compared with only 0 to 30% of control subjects, will experience a panic attack with such an infusion (Rainey and Nesse 1985). Other provocative tests of panic disorder include patient challenge with such substances as carbon dioxide, isoproterenol, beta-carboline, yohimbine, and caffeine. All of these tests remain research tools at this time.

☐ Additional Research Diagnostic Studies in Psychiatry

Polysomnography

Polysomnography, besides having demonstrated utility in the evaluation of sleep disorders (e.g., narcolepsy, sleep apneas), has also been utilized in the search for potential biological markers of psychiatric disorder. An interesting example of a research finding in this area includes the report by Kupfer et al. (1978) of an increase in the overall amount of rapid eye movement (REM) sleep and a shortened REM latency period in patients with major depression.

Neuro-ophthalmological Markers

The study of unusual eye movement patterns found more commonly among psychiatric patients compared with normal control subjects has also been an area of research for potential biological markers. One measure of an abnormal voluntary eye movement has been the evaluation of smooth pursuit eye movement (SPEM). The SPEM abnormality consists of a larger number of jerky eye movements (saccades) during the tracking of a smoothly moving object. Various eye-tracking tasks and recording techniques have been used. SPEM dysfunction has been reported in up to 85% of schizophrenic patients, 40% of bipolar patients, and about 8% of the normal population (Holzman 1985).

Computerized Electroencephalography and Evoked Potential

In computerized EEG and evoked potential mapping, computers are used to amass and process large quantities of electrophysiological data. The computers analyze the data in various ways and graphically present the data in two-dimensional, color-coded maps of brain electrical activity. Computerized EEG and EP have yet to demonstrate clear clinical utility in the diagnosis of classical psychiatric illnesses such as schizophrenia and major depression, and are most appropriately considered research tools at this time. Research investigations utilizing computerized EEG and EP approaches have added to the body of evidence suggesting brain abnormalities in schizophrenia (Morihisa 1990). Although this brain imaging technique has high chronological resolution (a window measured in milliseconds for evoked potentials), it is limited by a relatively poor spatial resolution for data collected from electrodes placed on the scalp and by vulnerability to a variety of artifacts (e.g., medication, muscle, and eye movement artifacts).

Magnetoencephalography

Magnetoencephalography (MEG) is an exciting new technique for measuring brain electrical activity (Lopes da Silva and Van Rotterdam 1982). The MEG exploits the fact that the electrical activity of the neurons of the brain generates very weak magnetic fields. By using a very sensitive instrument to measure these generated magnetic fields, the magnetic energy is converted back into an electrical signal. The detection of these very weak fields currently requires the utilization of a super quantum interference device (SQUID). The MEG can measure electrical activity in all areas of the brain (e.g., both cortical and subcortical brain tissues), in contrast to the conventional EEG and computerized EEG and EP, which are thought to reflect largely cortical surface electrical activity. The MEG is totally noninvasive, and the patient is exposed to no gamma or X irradiation.

■ REFERENCES

Allen CB, Davis BM, Davis KL: Psychoendocrinology in clinical psychiatry, in American Psychiatric Association Annual Review, Vol 6. Edited by Hales RE, Frances AJ. Washington, DC, American Psychiatric Press, 1987, pp 188–209

American Psychiatric Association: Diagnostic and Statistical Manual of Mental Disorders, 4th Edition. Washington, DC, American Psychiatric Association, 1994

American Psychiatric Association, Task Force on the Use of Laboratory Tests in Psychiatry: Tricyclic antidepressants—blood level measurements and clinical outcome: an APA Task Force report. Am J Psychiatry 142:155–162, 1985

Åsberg M, Träskman C, Thorén P: 5-HIAA in the cerebrospinal fluid: a biochemical suicide predictor? Arch Gen Psychiatry 33:1193–1197, 1976

Brown WA, Laughren TP: Serum neuroleptic levels in the maintenance treatment of schizophrenia. Psychopharmacol Bull 19:76–78, 1983

Buchsbaum MS: Brain imaging in the search for biological markers in affective disorder. J Clin Psychiatry 47 (No 10, Suppl):7–10, 1986

Buchsbaum MS, DeLisi LE, Holcomb HH, et al: Anteroposterior gradients in cerebral glucose use in schizophrenia and affective disorders. Arch Gen Psychiatry 41:1159–1166, 1984

Carroll BJ: Dexamethasone suppresion test, in Handbook of Psychiatric Diagnostic Procedures, Vol 1. Edited by Hall RCW, Beresford TP. New York, SP Medical & Scientific Books, 1984, pp 3–28

Carroll BJ: Informed use of the dexamethasone suppression test. J Clin Psychiatry 47 (No 1, Suppl):10–12, 1986

Cho JT, Bone S, Dunner DL, et al: The effect of lithium treatment on thyroid function in patients with primary affective disorder. Am J Psychiatry 136:115–116, 1979

Coffman JA: Computed tomography in psychiatry, in Brain Imaging: Applications in Psychiatry. Edited by Andreasen NC. Washington, DC, American Psychiatric Press, 1989, pp 1–65

Cowdry RW, Wehr TA, Zis AP, et al: Thyroid abnormalities associated with rapid-cycling bipolar illness. Arch Gen Psychiatry 40:414–420, 1983

Creese I, Synder SH: A simple and sensitive radioreceptor assay for antischizophrenic drugs in blood. Nature 270:180–182, 1977

Davis JM, Bresnahan DB: Psychopharmacology in clinical psychiatry, in American Psychiatric Association Annual Review, Vol 6. Edited by Hales RE, Frances AJ. Washington, DC, American Psychiatric Press, 1987, pp 159–187

DeLisi LE: Use of the clinical laboratory, in Biomedical Psychiatric Therapeutics. Edited by Sullivan JL, Sullivan PD. Boston, MA, Butterworth Publishers, 1984, pp 89–119

Dolan JG, Mushlin AI: Routine laboratory testing for medical disorders in psychiatric inpatients. Arch Intern Med 145:2085–2088, 1985

Emrich HM, Stoll KD, Muller AA: Guidelines for the use of carbamazepine and of valproate in the prophylaxis of affective disorders, in Anticonvulsants in Affective Disorders. Edited by Emrich HM, Okuma T, Muller AA. Amsterdam, Excerpta Medica, 1984, pp 211–214

Emsley RA, Gledhill RF, Bell PSH, et al: Indications for CAT scans of psychiatric patients (letter). Am J Psychiatry 143:1199, 1986

Estroff TW, Gold MS: Psychiatric misdiagnosis, in Advances in Psychopharmacology; Predicting and Improving Treatment Response. Edited by Gold MS, Lydiard RB, Carman JS. Boca Raton, FL, CRC Press, 1984

Feinsilver DL: Psychiatric diagnostic procedures in the emergency department, in Handbook of Psychiatric Diagnostic Procedures, Vol 1. Edited by Hall RCW, Beresford TP. New York, SP Medical & Scientific Books, 1984, pp 315–330

Flugelman MY, Tal A, Pollack S, et al: Psychotropic drugs and long QT syndromes: case reports. J Clin Psychiatry 46:290–291, 1985

Fogel BS, Faust D: Neurologic assessment, neurodiagnostic tests, and neuropsychiatry in medical psychiatry, in Principles of Medical Psychiatry. Edited by Stoudemire A, Fogel BS. Orlando, FL, Grune & Stratton, 1987, pp 37–77

Gelenberg AJ: Laboratory tests for patients taking psychotropic drugs. Massachusetts General Hospital Newsletter 6:5–7, 1983

Gelenberg AJ: Carbamazepine (Tegretol) for manic depressive illness: an update. Massachusetts General Hospital Newsletter 8:21–24, 1985

Gelenberg AJ, Bassuk EL, Schoonover SC: The Practitioner's Guide to Psychoactive Drugs. New York, Plenum, 1991

Giannini AJ, Black HR, Goettsche RL: Psychiatric Psychogenic and Somatopsychotic Disorders Handbook. Garden City, NY, Medical Examination Publishing, 1978

Gold MS, Dackis CA: Role of the laboratory in the evaluation of suspected drug abuse. J Clin Psychiatry 47 (No 1, Suppl):17–23, 1986

Gold PW, Loriaux DL, Roy A, et al: Response to corticotropin-releasing hormone in the hypercortisolism of depression and Cushing's disease: physiologic and diagnostic implications. N Engl J Med 314:1329–1335, 1986

Goodin DS, Aminoff MJ: Does the interictal EEG have a role in the diagnosis of epilepsy? Lancet 1:837–839, 1984

Gur RE, Resnick JM, Alavi A, et al: Regional brain function in schizophrenia, I: a positron emission tomography study. Arch Gen Psychiatry 44:119–125, 1987

Gusella JF, Tanzi RE, Anderson MA, et al: DNA markers for nervous system diseases. Science 225:1320–1326, 1984

Guze BH: Magnetic resonance spectroscopy: a technique for functional brain imaging. Arch Gen Psychiatry 48:572–574, 1991

Hales RE: The diagnosis and treatment of psychiatric disorders in medically ill patients. Milit Med 151:587–595, 1986

Hall RCW, Popkin MK, Devaul RA, et al: Physical illness presenting as psychiatric disease. Arch Gen Psychiatry 35:1315–1320, 1978

Hall RCW, Gardner ER, Stickney SK, et al: Physical illness manifesting as psychiatric disease, II: analysis of a state hospital inpatient population. Arch Gen Psychiatry 37:989–995, 1980

Hart RG, Easton JD: Carbamazepine and hematological monitoring. Ann Neurol 11:309–312, 1982

Hoffman RS, Koran LM: Detecting physical illness in patients with mental disorders. Psychosomatics 25:654–660, 1984

Holzman PS: Eye movement dysfunctions and psychosis. Int Rev Neurobiol 27:179–205, 1985

Ingvar DH, Franzen G: Abnormalities of cerebral blood flow distribution in patients with chronic schizophrenia. Acta Psychiatr Scand 50:425–462, 1974

Jacobson HG: Magnetic resonance imaging of the central nervous system: Council on Scientific Affairs Report of the Panel on Magnetic Resonance Imaging. JAMA 259:1211–1222, 1988

Jaskiw GE, Andreasen NC, Weinberger DR: X-ray computed tomography and magnetic resonance imaging in psychiatry, in American Psychiatric Association Annual Review, Vol 6. Edited by Hales RE, Frances AJ. Washington, DC, American Psychiatric Press, 1987, pp 260–299

Jefferson JW, Greist JH, Ackerman DC: Lithium Encyclopedia for Clinical Practice, 2nd Edition. Washington, DC, American Psychiatric Press, 1987

Jenike MA: Should lumbar puncture be part of the workup for dementia? Topics in Geriatrics 4:21–23, 1985

Jernigan TL, Zisook S, Heaton RK, et al: Magnetic resonance imaging abnormalities in lenticular nuclei and cerebral cortex in schizophrenia. Arch Gen Psychiatry 48:881–890, 1991

Johnston EC, Crow TJ, Frith CD, et al: Cerebral ventricular size and cognitive impairment in schizophrenia. Lancet 2:924–926, 1976

Karasu TB, Waltzman SA, Lindenmayer J-P, et al: The medical care of patients with psychiatric illness. Hosp Community Psychiatry 31:463–472, 1980

Keshavan MS, Kapur S, Pettegrew JW: Magnetic resonance spectroscopy in psychiatry: potential, pitfalls, and promise. Am J Psychiatry 148:976–985, 1991

Kocsis JH, Hanin I, Bowden C, et al: Imipramine and amitriptyline plasma concentrations and clinical response in major depression. Br J Psychiatry 148:52–57, 1986

Kolman PBR: Predicting the results of routine laboratory tests in elderly psychiatric patients admitted to hospital. J Clin Psychiatry 46:532–534, 1985

Koranyi EK: Morbidity and rate of undiagnosed physical illnesses in a psychiatric clinic population. Arch Gen Psychiatry 36:414–419, 1979

Kupfer DJ, Foster FG, Coble P, et al: The application of EEG sleep for the differential diagnosis of affective disorders. Am J Psychiatry 135:69–74, 1978

Larson EB, Reifler BV, Sumi SM, et al: Diagnostic tests in the evaluation of dementia: a prospective study of 200 elderly outpatients. Arch Intern Med 146:1917–1922, 1986

Liebowitz MR, Quitkin FM, Stewart JW, et al: Phenelzine v imipramine in atypical depression: a preliminary report. Arch Gen Psychiatry 41:669–677, 1984

Liebowitz MR, Gorman JM, Fyer AJ, et al: Lactate provocation of panic attacks, II: biochemical and physiological findings. Arch Gen Psychiatry 42:709–719, 1985

Loosen PT, Prange AJ Jr: Serum thyrotropin response to thyrotropin-releasing hormone in psychotic patients: a review. Am J Psychiatry 139:405–416, 1982

Lopes da Silva F, Van Rotterdam A: Biophysical aspects of EEG and MEG generation, in Electroencephalography: Basic Principles: Clinical Applications and Related Fields. Edited by Niedermeyer E, Lopes da Silva F. Baltimore, MD, Urban & Schwarzenberg, 1982, pp 15–26

Morihisa JM: Brain-imaging approaches in psychiatry: early developmental considerations. J Clin Psychiatry 51 (No 1, suppl):44–46, 1990

Morihisa JM: Advances in neuroimaging technologies, in Medical Psychiatric Practice. Edited by Stoudemire A, Fogel BS. Washington, DC, American Psychiatric Press, 1991, pp 3–28

Morihisa JM, McAnulty GB: Structure and function: brain electrical activity mapping and computed tomography in schizophrenia. Biol Psychiatry 20:3–19, 1985

Morihisa JM, Weinberger DR: Is schizophrenia a frontal lobe disease? An organizing theory of relevant anatomy and physiology, in Can Schizophrenia Be Localized in the Brain? Edited by Andreasen NC. Washington, DC, American Psychiatric Press, 1986, pp 17–36

Moyer TP, Palmer MA, Johnson P, et al: Marihuana testing: how good is it? Mayo Clin Proc 62:413–417, 1987

Muscettola G, Potter WZ, Pickar D, et al: Urinary 3-methoxy-4-hydroxyphenylglycol and major affective disorders: a replication and new findings. Arch Gen Psychiatry 41:337–342, 1984

Nasrallah HA, Jacoby CG, Chapman S, et al: Third ventricular enlargement on CT scans in schizophrenia: association with cerebellar atrophy. Biol Psychiatry 20:443–450, 1985

National Institute on Aging Task Force: Senility reconsidered: treatment possibilities for mental impairment in the elderly. JAMA 244:259–263, 1980

Nemeroff CB, Evans DL: Correlation between the dexamethasone suppression test in depressed patients and clinical response. Am J Psychiatry 141:247–249, 1984

Panner MJ, Christakis NA: The limits of science in on-the-job drug screening. Hastings Cent Rep 16(6):7–12, 1986

Pearlson GD, Garbacz DJ, Breakey WR, et al: Lateral ventricular enlargement associated with persistent unemployment and negative symptoms in both schizophrenia and bipolar disorder. Psychiatry Res 12:1–9, 1984

Pettegrew JW, Keshavan MS, Panchalingam K, et al: Alterations in brain high-energy phosphate and membrane phospholipid metabolism in first-episode, drug-naive schizophrenics: a pilot study of the dorsal prefrontal cortex by in vivo phosphorus 31 nuclear magnetic resonance spectroscopy. Arch Gen Psychiatry 48:563–568, 1991

Physicians' Desk Reference, 40th Edition. Oradell, NJ, Medical Economics Company, 1986

Post RM: Clinical approaches to the treatment resistant manic and depressive patient, in Psychopharmacology in Practice: Clinical and Research Update 1984. Bethesda, MD, Foundation for Advanced Education in the Sciences, 1984, pp 23–54

Pryse-Phillips W, Murray TJ: Essential Neurology, 3rd Edition. New York, Medical Examination Publishing Company, 1986

Rainey JM Jr, Nesse RM: Psychobiology of anxiety and anxiety disorders. Psychiatr Clin North Am 8:133–144, 1985

Robinson DS, Nies A, Ravaris CL, et al: Clinical pharmacology of phenelzine. Arch Gen Psychiatry 35:629–635, 1978

Sakauye KM: A model for administration of electroconvulsive therapy. Hosp Community Psychiatry 37:785–788, 1986

Schatzberg AF, Cole JO: Manual of Clinical Psychopharmacology, 2nd Edition. Washington, DC, American Psychiatric Press, Washington, DC, 1991

Schwartz P, Wolf S: QT interval prolongation as prediction of sudden death in patients with myocardial infarction. Circulation 57:1074–1077, 1978

Simpson GM, Pi EH, White K: Plasma drug levels and clinical response to antidepressants. J Clin Psychiatry 44 (No 5, Sec 2):27–34, 1983

Stahl SM: Peripheral models for the study of neurotransmitter receptors in man. Psychopharmacol Bull 21:663–671, 1985

Tamminga CA, Thaker GK, Buchanan R, et al: Limbic system abnormalities identified in schizophrenia using positron emission tomography with fluorodeoxyglucose and neocortical alterations with deficit syndrome. Arch Gen Psychiatry 49:522–530, 1992

Targum SD, Greenberg RD, Harmon RL, et al: Thyroid hormone and the TRH stimulation test in refractory depression. J Clin Psychiatry 45:345–346, 1984

Targum SD, Marshall LE, Fischman P: Variability of TRH test responses in depressed and normal elderly subjects. Biol Psychiaty 31:787–793, 1992

Thase ME, Reynolds CF, Glanz LM, et al: Nocturnal penile tumescence in depressed men. Am J Psychiatry 144:89–92, 1987

Van Putten T, Marder SR, Mintz J, et al: Haloperidol plasma levels and clinical response: a therapeutic window relationship. Am J Psychiatry 149:500–505, 1992

Weinberger DR: Brain disease and psychiatric illness: when should a psychiatrist order a CAT scan? Am J Psychiatry 141:1521–1527, 1984

Weinberger DR: Implications of normal brain development for the pathogenesis of schizophrenia. Arch Gen Psychiatry 44:660–669, 1987

Weinberger DR, Torrey EF, Neophytides AN, et al: Lateral cerebral ventricular enlargement in chronic schizophrenia. Arch Gen Psychiatry 36:735–739, 1979

Weinberger DR, Berman KF, Zec RF: Physiologic dysfunction of dorsolateral prefrontal cortex in schizophrenia, I: regional cerebral blood flow evidence. Arch Gen Psychiatry 43:114–124, 1986

Weinberger DR, Berman KF, Suddath R, et al: Evidence of dysfunction of a prefrontal-limbic network in schizophrenia: a magnetic resonance imaging and regional cerebral blood flow study of discordant monozygotic twins. Am J Psychiatry 149:890–897, 1992

Wolkin A, Jaeger J, Brodie JD, et al: Persistence of cerebral metabolic abnormalities in chronic schizophrenia as determined by positron emission tomography. Am J Psychiatry 142:564–571, 1985

Wong DF, Wagner HN, Tune, et al: Positron emission tomography reveals elevated D_2 dopamine receptors in drug-naive schizophrenics. Science 234:1558–1563, 1986

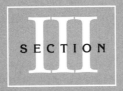

SECTION

III

Psychiatric Disorders

CHAPTER 10

Delirium, Dementia, and Amnestic Disorders

Michael G. Wise, M.D.
Kevin F. Gray, M.D.

■ DELIRIUM

Delirium was one of the first mental disorders described in medicine and is the most common psychiatric syndrome found in a general medical hospital (Lipowski 1990). It is especially common among elderly persons who are hospitalized (Francis 1992). The presence of delirium signifies impending death in 25% of identified cases (Rabins and Folstein 1982). In addition, demented or other brain-damaged patients have a lower threshold for developing a delirium and do so with greater frequency (Miller et al. 1991). Although commonly seen by physicians and associated with high mortality and morbidity, delirium remains an underresearched phenomenon. A conceptual overview of delirium is presented in Figure 10–1.

☐ Definition

More than 30 diagnostic terms have been used to describe this clinical syndrome (Francis 1992). In addition, the diagnostic criteria for delirium have changed several times since the *Diagnostic and Statistical Manual of Mental Disorders* was first published. The most recent diagnostic criteria are listed in Table 10–1 (DSM-IV, American Psychiatric Association 1994).

The DSM-IV, like its predecessors, considers different clinical presentations (i.e., hypoactive, hyperactive, and mixed states) as aspects of one entity called "delirium." This conceptualization is not accepted by

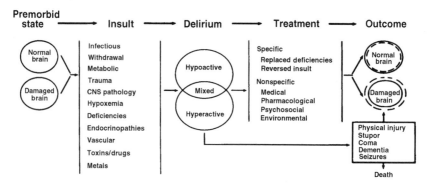

Figure 10–1.   Conceptual overview of delirium.

Table 10–1.   DSM-IV diagnostic criteria for delirium due to a general medical condition

A.   Disturbance of consciousness (i.e., reduced clarity of awareness of the environment) with reduced ability to focus, sustain, or shift attention.

B.   Change in cognition (such as memory deficit, disorientation, language disturbance, perceptual disturbance) that is not better accounted for by a preexisting, established, or evolving dementia.

C.   The disturbance develops over a short period of time (usually hours to days) and tends to fluctuate during the course of the day.

D.   There is evidence from the history, physical examination, or laboratory findings of a general medical condition judged to be etiologically related to the disturbance.

---

some medical colleagues who feel that the diagnosis of delirium should be reserved for the confused patient with agitation, autonomic instability, and hallucinations (Adams and Victor 1989). Delirium usually has a sudden onset and a brief duration, and is reversible. Therefore, delirium is herein defined as *a transient, usually reversible dysfunction in cerebral metabolism that has an acute or subacute onset and is manifest clinically by a wide array of neuropsychiatric abnormalities.*

☐ Epidemiology

Reliable research into the epidemiology of delirium is in its infancy.

Incidence and Prevalence

The frequency of delirium found within a particular population depends on the predisposition of the individuals within that population. It has been estimated that 10% to 15% of patients on acute medical and surgical wards are delirious (Engel 1967). The increasing age of the population may make this estimate low (Lipowski 1990).

Predisposing Factors

Six groups of patients are at increased risk to develop a delirium: 1) elderly patients, 2) postcardiotomy patients, 3) burn patients, 4) patients with preexisting brain damage (e.g., dementia, strokes), 5) patients with drug dependency who are experiencing withdrawal, and 6) patients with acquired immune deficiency syndrome (AIDS). Advancing age increases the risk of delirium, with an age of 60 or older usually cited as being associated with the highest risk (Francis 1992).

Dubin et al. (1979), in a thorough review of postcardiotomy delirium, reported that the frequency across studies varied from 13% to 67%. A more recent study reported a lower frequency of delirium: 8.6% of patients who received narcotic anesthesia and 5.6% who received barbiturate coma developed delirium (Nussmeier et al. 1986). Despite the generally held belief that the frequency of postcardiotomy delirium has declined with experience and improved technology, a meta-analysis of 44 studies revealed that the prevalence has remained constant at 32% (Smith and Dimsdale 1989). Smith and Dimsdale (1989) found that preoperative psychiatric intervention correlated with a decreasing occurrence of postcardiotomy delirium, which suggests that a preoperative psychiatric interview may offer some protection against delirium.

About 30% of adult burn patients have symptoms of delirium (Andreasen et al. 1972). Other studies describe an 18% incidence of delirium in burn patients (Blank and Perry 1984) and a 14% incidence of burn encephalopathy in children (Antoon et al. 1972).

The presence of preexisting brain damage, whether CNS neurological abnormalities (Folstein et al. 1991) or dementia, lowers the patient's threshold for developing a delirium (Lipowski 1990). An additional risk factor for the development of delirium is the rapid withdrawal of a drug in a patient who is physiologically dependent; this is particularly a risk in individuals who have chronically abused alcohol or benzodiazepines.

There is little evidence that psychosocial factors, sensory deprivation, or sleep deprivation alone can cause delirium (Rabins 1991). Without question, sleep-wake abnormalities are typically part of the symptomatology found in delirium. How critical sleep deprivation is to the development of the delirium remains an unanswered question. One study found that sleep disturbance developed after the score on the Mini-Mental State Exam (MMSE) decreased (i.e., after the delirium developed) but not before (Harrell and Othmer 1987). The crucial issue in sensory deprivation and sensory overload may not be the quantity of stimuli but the quality. Patients in an intensive care unit (ICU) do not lack stimulation; rather, they lack the kinds of stimuli that orient them to time and environment. Lipowski (1990) points out that "there is no evidence sensory deprivation alone can cause delirium" (p. 128).

☐ Clinical Features

Prodrome

The patient will often manifest symptoms such as restlessness, anxiety, irritability, or sleep disruption prior to the onset of a delirium. Review of the delirious patient's hospital medical chart, particularly the nursing notes, will often reveal these prodromal features.

Fluctuating Course

The clinical features of delirium are protean and, to complicate the picture further, vary rapidly over time. This variability and fluctuation in clinical findings are characteristic of delirium but can lead to diagnostic confusion among clinicians.

Attentional Deficits

It was Geschwind's belief that loss of attention was the core feature of delirium (Levkoff et al. 1991), and this concept was adopted in DSM-III-R. The delirious patient is easily distracted by incidental activities in the environment. The patient's inability to sustain attention undoubtedly plays a key role in memory and orientation difficulties.

Arousal Disturbance and Psychomotor Abnormalities

In delirium, the reticular activating system of the brain may be hypoactive, in which case patients would appear apathetic, somnolent, and quietly confused. In other patients, the brain's activating system may be hyperactive, in which case the patients are agitated and hypervigilant, and exhibit psychomotor hyperactivity. Some patients swing back and forth between hypoactive and hyperactive states (so-called mixed delirium). The patient with a hypoactive-type delirium is less apt to be diagnosed as delirious and is often labeled as depressed or uncooperative, or as having a character disorder.

The type of delirum the patient exhibits (i.e., a hyperactive or hypoactive form) may give the clinician valuable information about etiology. For example, the patient with a delirium caused by hepatic failure is virtually always hypoactive, and visual hallucinations are absent (Ross et al. 1991). In contrast, patients with delirium secondary to sedative-hypnotic withdrawal, especially alcohol withdrawal, are typically agitated, hyperactive, and hallucinating.

Sleep-Wake Disturbance

Not only is sleep-wake disturbance symptomatic of a delirium, but sleep deprivation probably exacerbates the confusion. The sleep-wake cycle of the delirious patient is often reversed. The patient may be somnolent during the day and active during the night when the nursing staff is sparse. Restoration of the normal diurnal sleep cycle is an important part of treatment.

Impaired Memory

The ability of a delirious patient to register events into memory is severely impaired. Whether because of attentional deficits, perceptual disturbances, or malfunction of the hippocampus, the patient will fail tests of immediate and recent memory. Following recovery from a delirium, some patients will be amnestic for the entire episode; others will have islands of memory for events during the episode.

Disorganized Thinking and Impaired Speech

The delirious patient's thought patterns are disorganized, and his or her reasoning is defective. The delirious patient does not understand the problem at hand and is unable to reason normally. This represents the cognitive defect that is often referred to as *clouding of consciousness.* In addition, as the severity of the delirium increases, spontaneous speech becomes incoherent and rambling (Cummings 1985).

Disorientation

The patient with a delirium, except for lucid intervals, is usually disoriented to time, often disoriented to place, but very rarely, if ever, disoriented to person. It is not unusual for a delirious patient to feel he or she is in a familiar place while also nodding agreement that he or she is being monitored in a surgical intensive care unit. The extent of the patient's disorientation will fluctuate with the severity of the delirium.

Altered Perceptions

The delirious patient will often experience misperceptions that involve illusions, delusions, and hallucinations. Virtually all patients with a delirium will have misperceptions. Patients will often weave these misperceptions into a loosely knit delusional, usually paranoid system. Visual hallucinations are common and can involve simple visual distortions or complex scenes. During a delirium, visual hallucinations occur more frequently than auditory hallucinations. Tactile hallucinations occur least frequently. In the authors' experience, most auditory and tactile phenomena that are labeled as hallucinations are, in fact, illusions.

Neurological Abnormalities

A number of neurological abnormalities are found in delirium. Testing for these signs at the bedside not only strengthens the clinician's suspicion of the diagnosis but, when added to the chart, helps other physicians recognize the presence of a confusional state. Draw a large circle on an unlined blank sheet of paper and ask the patient to draw a clock face with the hands showing 10 minutes before 11 o'clock (Figure 10–2). This, and other constructional tasks, are very sensitive indicators for the degree of confusion present. Ask the patient to name objects (testing for dysnomia) and to write a sentence (testing for dysgraphia). Dysgraphia is one of the most sensitive indicators of a delirium.

Delirious patients may not have motor system abnormalities, although many patients manifest tremor, myoclonus, asterixis, or changes in reflex and muscle tone. The tremor associated with delirium, particularly toxic-metabolic delirium, is absent at rest but apparent during movement. Myoclonus and asterixis (so-called liver flap) occur in many toxic and metabolic conditions. Symmetric reflex and muscle tone changes can also occur.

Other Features

Emotional disturbances are common in delirious patients. The intensity of the patient's emotional response to mental confusion may fluctuate relatively rapidly and may also change in character with the passage of time. The emotional responses seen in delirious patients include anxiety, panic, fear, anger, rage, sadness, apathy, and rarely—except in steroid-induced delirium—euphoria.

☐ Pathophysiology and Electroencephalographic Abnormalities

Early investigators wrote a series of classic papers that correlated the severity of delirium (i.e., cognitive dysfunction) with EEG findings (Engel et al. 1947; Romano and Engel 1944). Their clinical research established that

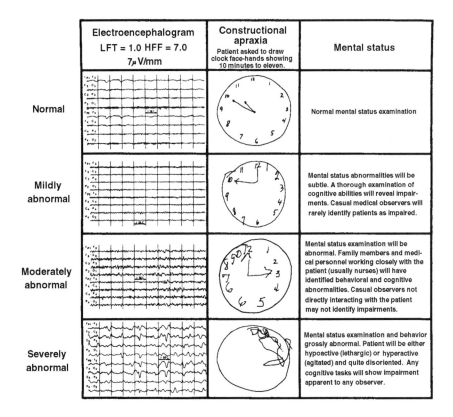

Figure 10–2. Comparison of electroencephalogram, constructional apraxia, and mental status in delirium.

1. A correlation existed between the electrical abnormality and disturbance of consciousness.
2. Changes on the EEG were reversible to the extent that the clinical delirium was reversible.
3. The character of the EEG changes appeared to be independent of the specific underlying disease process.
4. The character of the EEG changes was determined by the strength, duration, and reversibility of the noxious factors, as well as the integrity of the CNS.
5. Clinical interventions improved the EEG and also the mental status.

Spectral EEG analyses, which measure the quality of alpha, beta, theta, and delta background activity, have further supported Engel and Romano's proposed correlation between EEG slowing and cognitive deterioration. Quantitative measurement of brain electrical activity offers advantages over visual interpretation of EEG tracings. As little as 30 seconds of quantitative data can produce results representative of background frequency, compared with standard EEG techniques, which require the agitated or confused patient to lie still for 30 minutes.

Delirium is virtually always accompanied by EEG changes (Pro and Wells 1977). The EEG changes found in delirium are *not* always slowing and the pattern can be low-voltage fast activity, as in delirium tremens (Kennard et al. 1945). Low-voltage fast activity is usually found in hyperactive, agitated patients with heightened arousal (Pro and Wells 1977). EEG slowing is found in lethargic, anergic, abulic patients. The EEG slowing illustrated in Figure 10–2 is typical for delirium caused by toxic-metabolic etiologies.

Recent research has led to speculation about the role of gamma-aminobutyric acid (GABA) in delirium caused by hepatic failure, as well as delirium from other etiologies (Basile et al. 1991; Ross et al. 1991). GABAergic transmission in hepatic failure may be increased because of endogenous benzodiazepine-like compounds that cause a hypoactive delirium; on the other hand, GABAergic transmission may be decreased in sedative-hypnotic withdrawal, resulting in a hyperactive delirium. Other investigators have speculated about the importance of the cholinergic system in delirium, pointing particularly to this system's vulnerability to metabolic insults, aging, and anticholinergic drugs (Gibson et al. 1991).

☐ Differential Diagnosis

The differential diagnosis of delirium is so extensive that there may be a tendency to avoid the search for etiologies. In addition, confusional states, particularly in elderly persons, may represent the CNS's response to multiple abnormalities. Each potential contributor to the delirium needs to be pursued and addressed independently.

Nonspecific terms such as "ICU psychosis" are sometimes used as an explanation for delirium, when, in fact, these terms, with their nonspecificity, simply mask ignorance. Organic etiologies are present in a majority of delirious patients. The task for the clinician is to organize the wide array of potential causes of delirium into a usable diagnostic system.

Emergent Items

A two-tiered differential diagnostic system is very helpful when evaluating a delirious patient. The first level of this diagnostic system is represented in Table 10–2 by the mnemonic WHHHHIMP. Table 10–2 also contains many of the clinical questions that the clinician must ask to investigate the etiology.

Table 10–2.   Differential diagnosis for delirium: emergent items
(WHHHHIMP)

Diagnosis	Clinical questions
Wernicke's encephalopathy or withdrawal	Ataxia? Ophthalmoplegia? Alcohol or drug history? Increased mean corpuscular volume? Increased sympathetic activity (e.g., increased blood pressure or sweating)? Hyperreflexia?
Hypertensive encephalopathy	Increased blood pressure? Papilledema?
Hypoglycemia	History of insulin-dependent diabetes mellitus? Decreased glucose?
Hypoperfusion of central nervous system	Decreased blood pressure? Decreased cardiac output (e.g., myocardial infarct, arrhythmia, cardiac failure)? Decreased hematocrit?
Hypoxemia	Arterial blood gases (decreased Po_2)? History of pulmonary disease?
Intracranial bleeding or infection	History of unconsciousness? Focal neurological signs?
Meningitis or encephalitis	Meningeal signs? Increased white blood count? Increased temperature? Viral prodome?
Poisons or medications	Should toxic screen be ordered? Signs of toxicity (e.g., pupillary abnormality, nystagmus, or ataxia)? Is the patient on a drug that can cause delirium?

A patient with Wernicke's encephalopathy has the triad of confusion, ataxia, and ophthalmoplegia (usually lateral gaze paralysis). If Wernicke's encephalopathy is not promptly treated with parenteral thiamine, the patient will develop Korsakoff's psychosis, which is a permanent organic amnestic disorder. A check of the arterial blood gases and current and past vital signs should quickly establish whether hypoxemia or hypertensive encephalopathy is present. A number of clinical phenomena can singularly, or collectively, decrease brain perfusion. These cause "relative" hypoperfusion (relative to usual perfusion pressures), such as decreased cardiac output from a myocardial infarction, cardiac failure, arrhythmias, or anemia.

If the patient had a brief period of unconsciousness, with or without headache, and is now delirious, or if the patient had or now has focal neurological signs, suspect an intracranial bleed. Immediate neurological/neurosurgical evaluation is necessary. Especially look for urinary tract infections in a confused, elderly patient. Meningitis and encephalitis are typically acute febrile illnesses, so check vital signs for fever.

When a delirious patient is encountered in the emergency room, the clinician must consider a toxic organic reaction and order a drug screen. Pesticide or solvent poisoning is less likely, but should be considered. In hospital and emergency room patients, a very common cause of delirium is prescribed medications (Table 10–3).

Critical Items

The I WATCH DEATH mnemonic (Table 10–4) contains a comprehensive list of insults that can cause delirium. The use of the mnemonic I WATCH DEATH may sound melodramatic, but the appearance of a delirium, which is equivalent to acute brain failure, should marshal the same medical forces as failure of any other vital organ.

☐ Course Prognosis

The clinical course of a delirious patient is variable. The majority of patients who experience delirium probably have a full recovery, although the actual probability of this outcome is unknown (Lipowski 1990). Some patients will progress to stupor and/or coma and either recover (with or without chronic brain damage), become chronically vegetative, or die. Seizures can accompany delirium and are more likely to occur with drug withdrawal, particularly alcohol, and burn encephalopathy (Antoon et al. 1972). Finally, a number of patients will not completely recover; the resultant chronic brain syndrome may be global or focal (e.g., amnestic syndrome, secondary personality disorder).

Morbidity

Research indicates that hospitalization for delirium is prolonged (Francis et al. 1990). In one study, 15% of delirious postcardiotomy patients had persistent neurological signs at discharge (Tufo et al. 1970). Fernandez et al. (1989) found that only 37% of AIDS patients who became delirious had a complete recovery of cognitive function.

Delirious patients can pull out intravenous lines, nasogastric tubes, arterial lines, nasopharyngeal tubes, and intra-aortic balloon pumps. Inouye et al. (1989) reported that the risk of complications such as decubiti and aspiration pneumonia were more than six times greater in the delirious patient. Levkoff et al. (1986) projects a 1 to 2 billion dollar savings in the United States if the hospital stay of each delirious patient could be reduced by 1 day.

Table 10–3.   Drugs that can cause delirium

Antibiotic
Acyclovir (antiviral)
Amphotericin B (antifungal)
Cephalexin (Keflex)
Chloroquine (antimalarial)

Anticholinergic
Antihistamines
Chlorpheniramine (Ornade and Teldrin)
Antiparkinson drugs
   Benztropine (Cogentin)
   Biperiden (Akineton)
Antispasmodics
Atropine/homatropine
Belladonna alkaloids
Diphenhydramine (Benadryl)
Phenothiazines (especially thioridazine)
Promethazine (Phenergan)
Scopolamine
Tricyclic antidepressants (especially
   amitriptyline)
Trihexyphenidyl (Artane)

Anticonvulsant
Phenobarbital
Phenytoin (Dilantin)
Sodium valproate (Depakene)

Anti-inflammatory
Adrenocorticotropic hormone
Corticosteroids
Ibuprofen (Motrin and Advil)
Indomethacin (Indocin)
Naproxen (Naprosyn)
Phenylbutazone (Butazolidin)

Antineoplastic
5-Fluorouracil

Antiparkinson
Amantadine (Symmetrel)
Carbidopa (Sinemet)
Levodopa (Larodopa)

Antituberculous
Isoniazid
Rifampin

Analgesic
Opiates
Salicylates
Synthetic narcotics

Cardiac
Beta-blockers
Propranolol (Inderal)
Clonidine (Catapres)
Digitalis (Digoxin and Lanoxin)
Disopyramide (Norpace)
Lidocaine (Xylocaine)
Mexiletine
Methyldopa (Aldomet)
Quinidine (Quinidine, Quinaglute, and
   Duraquine)
Procainamide (Pronestyl)

Drug withdrawal
Alcohol
Barbiturates
Benzodiazepines

Sedative-hypnotic
Barbiturates (Miltown and Equanil)
Glutethimide (Doriden)
Benzodiazepines

Sympathomimetic
Amphetamines
Phenylephrine
Phenylpropanolamine

Over-the-counter
Compoz®
Excedrin P.M.®
Sleep-Eze®
Sominex®

Miscellaneous
Aminophylline
Bromides
Chlorpropamide (Diabinese)
Cimetidine (Tagamet)
Disulfiram (Antabuse)
Lithium
Metrizamide (Amipaque)
Metronidazole (Flagyl)
Podophyllin by absorption
Propylthiouracil
Quinacrine
Theophylline
Timolol ophthalmic

Table 10–4.   Differential diagnosis for delirium: critical items (I WATCH DEATH)

Infectious	Encephalitis, meningitis, and syphilis
Withdrawal	Alcohol, barbiturates, sedative-hypnotics
Acute metabolic	Acidosis, alkalosis, electrolyte disturbance, hepatic failure, and renal failure
Trauma	Heat stroke, postoperative, and severe burns
CNS pathology	Abscesses, hemorrhage, normal-pressure hydrocephalus, seizures, stroke, tumors, and vasculitis
Hypoxia	Anemia, carbon monoxide poisoning, hypotension, and pulmonary or cardiac failure
Deficiencies	Vitamin B_{12}, niacin, and thiamine and hypovitaminosis
Endocrinopathies	Hyper- or hypoadrenocortisolism and hyper- or hypoglycemia
Acute vascular	Hypertensive encephalopathy and shock
Toxins or drugs	Medications (see Table 10–3), pesticides, and solvents
Heavy metals	Lead, manganese, and mercury

Mortality

Many physicians underestimate the mortality associated with delirium. Of 77 patients who received a DSM-III diagnosis of delirium from a consultation psychiatrist, 19 (25%) died within 6 months (Trzepacz et al. 1985). Three months following diagnosis, the mortality rate for delirium is 14 times greater than the mortality rate for affective disorders (Weddington 1982).

☐ Making the Diagnosis of Delirium

Regardless of the suspected diagnosis, the evaluation of a patient follows a particular generic process. A specific diagnosis, such as delirium, follows from an appreciation of the clinical features of the syndrome and a thorough examination of the patient's mental and physical status (Table 10–5). In addition to the usual mental status examination, the examiner should, at a minimum, test for construction praxis (see Figure 10–2), writing ability, and the ability to name objects. If a delirium is present, the examiner should make every effort to identify the specific etiology (etiologies).

The gold standard for diagnosis is the clinical evaluation, and the most useful diagnostic laboratory test is the EEG. Several paper-and-pencil tests exist to aid the clinician in diagnosis. The MMSE provides a screening tool for organicity and is also used to follow the patient's clinical course serially (Folstein et al. 1975). The major problem with the

Table 10–5. Neuropsychiatric evaluation of the patient

Mental status
Interview (assessment of level of consciousness, psychomotor activity, appearance, affect, mood, intellect, and thought processes)
Performance tests (memory, concentration, reasoning, motor and constructional apraxia, dysgraphia, and dysnomia)

Physical status
Brief neurological exam (reflexes, limb strength, Babinski reflex, cranial nerves, meningeal signs, and gait)
Review of past and present vital signs (pulse, temperature, blood pressure, and respiration rate)
Review of chart (check laboratory results [e.g., VDRL and FTA-ABS]), abnormal behavior after medication started or stopped)

Laboratory examination—basic
Blood chemistries (electrolytes, glucose, calcium, albumin, blood urea nitrogen, ammonia [NH_4^+], and liver functions)
Blood count (hematocrit, white count and differential, mean corpuscular volume, sedimentation rate)
Drug levels (need toxic screen? medication blood levels?)
Arterial blood gases
Urinalysis
Electrocardiogram
Chest X ray

Laboratory—based on clinical judgment
Electroencephalogram (seizures? focal lesion? or confirm delirium)
Computed tomography (normal-pressure hydrocephalus, stroke, and space-occupying lesion)
Additional blood chemistries (heavy metals, thiamine and folate levels, thyroid battery, lupus erythematosus prep, antinuclear antibodies, and urinary porphobilinogen)
Lumbar puncture (if indication of infection or intracranial bleed)

Note. VDRL = Venereal Disease Research Laboratory; FTA-ABS = fluorescent treponemal antibody absorption.

MMSE is its lack of sensitivity (i.e., high rate of false negatives). Constructional apraxia and dysgraphia, which are usually present in a delirious patient, should be assessed (Figure 10–2).

Numerous scales are now available to help the clinician or researcher detect delirium: the Delirium Rating Scale (DRS; Trzepacz et al. 1988), Confusion Assessment Method (Inouye et al. 1990), Confusion Rating Scale (Williams et al. 1986), NEECHAM Confusion Scale (Champagne et al. 1987), Global Accessibility Scale (Anthony et al. 1982), Delirium Symptom Interview (Levkoff et al. 1991), and the High Sensitivity Cognitive Screen (Faust and Fogel 1989).

There are two levels of laboratory evaluation of a delirious patient. The basic laboratory battery (Table 10–5) is ordered for virtually every patient with a diagnosis of delirium. When information concerning the patient's history, as well as mental and physical status, is combined with the laboratory results, the specific etiology (etiologies) is often apparent. If not, the clinician should review the case and consider ordering further diagnostic studies.

☐ Treatment

After thorough evaluation of the patient, the psychiatrist is often faced with one of the following situations: 1) a specific etiology or several etiologies are identified and the patient's inappropriate behavior endangers medical care and requires immediate treatment; or 2) no specific etiology is identified and the patient's inappropriate behavior endangers medical care and requires treatment. In the former case, the clinician must systematically attempt to establish a diagnosis, because many causes of delirium have specific treatments. The goal of diagnosis is to discover reversible causes for delirium. In the event the etiology is unknown, a number of treatments are particularly applicable for the patient who is delirious. These interventions are divided into medical, pharmacological, psychosocial, and environmental categories.

Medical. In addition to ordering the laboratory tests essential to identify the cause of a delirium, one of the important roles of the psychiatrist is to raise the level of awareness of the medical and nursing staff about the morbidity and mortality associated with delirium. The patient should be placed in a room near the nursing station and vital signs closely monitored. Increased observation of the patient ensures awareness of medical deterioration and dangerous behaviors such as trying to crawl over bed rails or pulling out intravenous lines. Fluid input and output must be monitored and good oxygenation ensured. All nonessential medications should be discontinued.

Pharmacological. When a delirious patient becomes agitated, there is no consensus on the pharmacological treatment. Neuroleptic prescribing practices in delirium remain controversial; issues of rapid neuroleptization and appropriate dosage levels continue to be debated. The critical clinical issue, however, is the individual patient's situation and response to medications. Delirium is defined by its variability; thus one assessment will evoke management and medical recommendations that are time-limited in efficacy and require constant follow-up.

Review of the literature and clinical experience indicate that haloperidol is the drug of first choice when treating an agitated delirium with unknown etiology (Lipowski 1990). Haloperidol is a potent antipsychotic with virtually no anticholinergic or hypotensive properties, and it can be given parenterally. Although haloperidol is not approved by the Federal Drug Administration (FDA) for intravenous use, intravenous haloperidol has been used in very high doses in seriously ill patients without harmful side effects (Fernandez et al. 1988). Although extrapyramidal side effects are more likely with the higher-potency antipsychotic drugs, the actual occurrence rate in medically ill patients, particularly when the drug is administered intravenously, is strikingly low (Menza et al. 1987).

Other antipsychotic medications found useful in treating the positive symptom of delirium are thiothixene (Navane) and droperidol (Inapsine). Antipsychotic medications that are less potent, such as chlorpromazine and thioridazine, are not recommended because they are more likely to cause hypotension and anticholinergic side effects.

The use of benzodiazepines in delirium has its proponents. Benzodiazepines are the drugs of choice in DTs. However, the sedation that accompanies benzodiazepines may further impair the delirious patient's sensorium. In addition, some patients may be further disinhibited when given benzodiazepines. Therefore, with the exceptions of drug withdrawal states, benzodiazepines are not recommended as a sole agent in the treatment of the delirious patient. Benzodiazepines have been used with success as adjuncts to high-potency neuroleptics such as haloperidol (Adams 1984). Intravenous lorazepam in doses of 0.5 to 2.0 mg, particularly in patients who have not responded to haloperidol alone, is quite useful.

Psychosocial.   The psychological support of a patient both during and after a delirium is important. For the paranoid, agitated patient, having a calm family member remain with the patient is reassuring and can stop mishaps (e.g., pulling out arterial lines, falling out of bed). In lieu of a family member, close supervision by reassuring nursing staff is crucial. After the delirium has resolved, helping the patient understand the bizarre experience can be therapeutic (Mackenzie and Popkin 1980). An explanation to the family about delirium can reduce anxiety and calm fears.

Environmental.   Environmental interventions are sometimes helpful but should not be considered as the primary treatment. Both nurses and family members can frequently reorient the patient to date and surroundings. Placing a clock, calendar, and familiar objects in the room may be helpful. Adequate light in the room during the night will usually decrease frightening illusions. If the patient normally wears eyeglasses or a hearing aid, return of these devices to the patient may help him or her better understand the environment.

■ DEMENTIA

Dementia has emerged as a major health challenge, not only for clinicians but for society as a whole. Recent government estimates suggest that up to 4 million Americans suffer from severe dementia, and an additional 1 to 5 million individuals have mild to moderate dementia. If the elderly population grows as expected, the number of severely demented Americans is projected to increase 60% by the year 2000 and 100% by 2020 (U.S. Congress, Office of Technology Assessment 1987).

The term "dementia" is often used to describe chronic, irreversible, and progressive conditions. It must be emphasized that the diagnosis is nonspecific and should *not* automatically imply irreversibility. Indeed, reports suggest that one-third of the "demented" patients presenting for initial evaluation are found to have reversible syndromes (Rabins 1983). Therefore, dementia is defined as a syndrome of acquired, persistent intellectual impairment with compromised function in multiple spheres of mental activity, such as memory, language, visuospatial skills, emotion or personality, and cognition (Cummings et al. 1980). The principal causes of dementia are listed in Table 10–6.

A diagnostically useful way to categorize dementing disorders is into *cortical* and *subcortical* types. The clinical findings in the cortical dementias reflect dysfunction of the cerebral cortex and are characterized by amnesia, aphasia, apraxia, and agnosia. Alzheimer's disease is the classic example of a cortical dementia. Injury to subcortical structures often disrupts arousal, attention, motivation, and the rate of information processing; this manifests clinically as psychomotor retardation, defective recall, poor abstraction and strategy formation, and mood and personality alterations such as depression and apathy. Dementias due to human immunodeficiency virus (HIV) disease, Huntington's disease, and Parkinson's disease are examples of subcortical dementias (Mandell and Albert 1990).

The changes seen in patients who are demented reflect the impact of significant brain pathology, *not* normal aging. Studies by both Bamford and Crook found that memory decline in normal aging is distinct from that seen in dementia (Bamford and Caine 1988; Crook et al. 1986). Recent studies on optimally healthy elderly persons show only slowed information processing and some signs of inefficiency in finding correct problem-solving strategies (Boone et al. 1990). Naming, attention, and verbal neuropsychological tasks appear to be relatively insensitive to aging.

Table 10–6.   Etiological classification of the principal dementia syndromes

Degenerative disorders

Cortical

Alzheimer's disease
Lewy body disease
Pick's disease
Frontal lobe degeneration of
   non-Alzheimer type

Subcortical

Parkinson's disease
Huntington's disease
Progressive supranuclear palsy
Spinocerebellar degenerations
Idiopathic basal ganglia calcification
Striatonigral degeneration
Wilson's disease
Thalamic dementia

Vascular dementias

Multiple large vessel occlusions
Lacunar state (multiple subcortical
   infarctions)
Binswanger's disease (white matter
   ischemic injury)
Mixed cortical and subcortical infarctions

Myelinoclastic disorders

Demyelinating

Multiple sclerosis
Marchiafava-Bignami disease

Dysmyelinating

Metachromatic leukodystrophy
Adrenoleukodystrophy
Cerebrotendinous xanthomatosis

Traumatic conditions

Posttraumatic encephalopathy
Subdural hematoma
Dementia pugilistica

Neoplastic dementias

Meningioma (particularly subfrontal)
Glioma
Metastatic deposits
Meningeal carcinomatosis

Hydrocephalic dementias

Communicating

Normal-pressure hydrocephalus

Noncommunicating

Aqueductal stenosis
Intraventricular neoplasm
Intraventricular cyst

Basilar meningitis

Inflammatory conditions

Systemic lupus erythematosus
Antiphospholipid syndrome
Temporal arteritis
Sarcoidosis
Granulomatous arteritis

Infection-related dementias

Syphilis
Chronic meningitis
Postencephalitic dementia syndrome
Whipple's disease
Acquired immune deficiency syndrome
   (AIDS)
Jakob-Creutzfeldt disease
Subacute sclerosing panencephalitis
Progressive multifocal leukoenceph-
   alopathy

Toxic conditions

Alcohol-related syndrome
Polydrug abuse
Iatrogenic dementias
   Anticholinergic agents
   Antihypertensive agents
   Psychotropic agents
   Anticonvulsant agents
   Miscellaneous agents
Metals
Industrial solvents

Metabolic disorders

Cardiopulmonary failure
Uremia
Hepatic encephalopathy
Endocrine disorders
   Thyroid
   Adrenal
   Parathyroid
Anemia and hematological conditions
Deficiency states (vitamin B_{12}, folate)
Porphyria

Psychiatric disorders

Depression
Mania
Schizophrenia

☐ Dementia of the Alzheimer's Type

Epidemiology

Dementia of the Alzheimer's type (DAT) is the most commonly occurring dementia, accounting for approximately 50% of patients evaluated for progressive cognitive decline. Perhaps an additional 15% to 20% of patients have a combination of Alzheimer's and vascular pathology at autopsy (Cummings and Benson 1992). The risk of developing DAT increases with age. A recent community survey showed prevalence rates of 3% in individuals who were 65 to 74 years old, 19% from ages 75 to 84, and 47% over age 85 (Evans et al. 1989).

While age remains the one undisputed risk factor for DAT, several others have been proposed. For example, women are overrepresented in the DAT population. This may occur because more women live into the age of increased risk (Mendez et al. 1992). Additional proposed risk factors include a history of dementia or Down's syndrome in a first-degree relative, head injury, occupational and environmental exposures (e.g., to aluminum), electroconvulsive therapy, alcohol abuse, analgesic abuse, long-standing physical inactivity, and other medical conditions (Mendez et al. 1992). Of these, only a family history for dementia is convincingly associated with DAT; demented individuals are three to four times more likely to have an affected relative than are control subjects. Head trauma with loss of consciousness is also associated with increased risk for the development of DAT (Van Duijn et al. 1992).

Pathophysiology

On gross inspection, the brain of a patient with DAT is characterized by cortical atrophy, widened sulci, and ventricular enlargement. Microscopic examination reveals neuronal loss, neurofibrillary tangles, neuritic plaques, granulovacuolar degeneration, and amyloid angiopathy. The most severe pathological changes occur in the medial temporal lobe, including the hippocampus, amygdala, entorhinal cortex, and parahippocampal gyrus; areas of the parietotemporal and frontal lobes are involved to an intermediate degree (Pearson and Powell 1989). Tangles are located within neurons, and are composed primarily of paired helical fragments that contain abnormally phosphorylated microtubule-associated tau proteins. Plaques are located extracellularly and consist of a core of amyloid peptide and aluminosilicates, surrounded by dystrophic nerve processes, terminals, and organelles (Matsuyama and Jarvik 1989). Granulovacuolar degeneration consists of intracytoplasmic vacuoles, particularly in neurons of the hippocampus.

Amyloid angiopathy is present in nearly all cases of DAT. The amyloid found in the cerebrovasculature is identical to that in neuritic plaques; it is also present in extracerebral vessels in skin, subcutaneous tissue, and intestine (Cummings and Benson 1992). The abnormal accumulation of amyloid implies chronically enhanced production and/or decreased clearance mechanisms (Haass et al. 1992). It is important to remember that all of the neuropathological changes in DAT are found in the brains of normal, nondemented individuals; the location and number of these lesions determine the postmortem histological diagnosis (Vinters 1991).

Clinical Features

Dementia of the Alzheimer's type typically begins after age 50 and is associated with an insidious and gradually progressive decline in mental abilities. Often the patient and family members are unaware of the evolving cognitive impairment, and the onset of the illness is identified only in retrospect. Memory difficulties are manifest by the patient's forgetting tasks, repeating questions, or losing the thread of a conversation or a television program. The patient may complain about memory problems very early in the course of the disease, but insight is rapidly lost. In fact, the patient's lack of insight in the face of gross cognitive impairments is characteristic of DAT. Family members may notice that the patient is more rigid and inflexible, less adventurous, more irritable, and less spontaneous. A family vacation or trip to visit relatives often will reveal problems with orientation and memory. Intercurrent illness that requires hospitalization or anesthesia may provoke episodes of "sundowning" or delirium.

Deterioration progresses over months and years. Studies of patients with DAT consistently show a decline of 3 points per year on the MMSE. This decline in cognitive function occurs regardless of the patient's age, sex, education, or whether or not the patient resides in a nursing home (Katzman et al. 1988). Individual patients may vary in their rate of deterioration, but a dramatic decline in MMSE warrants investigation. Driving may become especially problematic, even though the patient insists he or she is competent in an automobile. Personal hygiene and grooming are neglected.

Delusional beliefs often develop (Burns et al. 1990). Patients with DAT commonly are convinced that others are trying to steal from them or harm them, that their spouse is unfaithful, that family members have been replaced by impostors (Capgras' syndrome), that their house is not really their home, or that family members are plotting to abandon them. Hallucinatory experiences may occur, with the patient hearing or talking to people who are not there. The patient may cling to family members, often not letting the caregiver out of his or her sight. The patient will pace around the house without apparent purpose, engaging in repetitive, stereotyped activities. The patient may wander from the house and get lost in familiar surroundings, or become more and more reclusive.

Well-intended attempts to assist or "force" the patient to perform tasks such as bathing or getting into a car may precipitate "catastrophic reactions." These are abrupt, possibly even violent outbursts of verbal and/or physical aggression. The overreaction in these episodes may be misinterpreted by caregivers as stubbornness, criticism, or ingratitude. Eventually, patients become unable to recognize close family members and may even misidentify their own reflection in a mirror. Late-onset seizures may appear (Romanelli et al. 1990). Primitive reflexes, such as the grasp, snout, and suck, emerge. In the final stage of the illness, the patient becomes incontinent of urine and feces, loses all intelligible vocabulary, and is unable to walk or to sit up (Reisberg 1988). Death from pneumonia or another infectious process frequently occurs during a period of total confinement in bed.

Diagnosis

The clinical diagnosis of DAT requires the gradual, progressive development of multiple cognitive deficits, including both memory impairment and cognitive disturbances (American Psychiatric Association 1994). The DSM-IV diagnostic criteria are shown in Table 10–7.

In the past, the diagnosis of DAT was one of exclusion. Fortunately, the refinement of diagnostic criteria enables clinicians to utilize specific clinical features to identify the disease. The application of modern criteria—such as the National Institute of Neurological and Communicative Disorders and Stroke-Alzheimer's Disease and Related Disorders Association (NINCDS-ARCDA) criteria—yields an accuracy rate approaching 85% compared with a postmortem diagnosis of DAT (Joachim et al. 1988).

With no laboratory test(s) yet available for DAT, diagnosis is greatly aided by the use of neuroimaging techniques. Atrophy is usually present on computed tomography (CT) and magnetic resonance imaging (MRI) in patients with DAT; however, brain atrophy of similar magnitude is sometimes found in nondemented individuals. In addition, some patients with DAT will have normal CT scans (DeCarli et al. 1990). Functional imaging using single-photon emission computed tomography (SPECT) characteristically shows bilaterally decreased cerebral blood flow in the parietal and posterior temporal lobes in patients who have DAT; frontal lobe blood flow declines in the later stages of the illness. Primary motor, sensory, visual cortices and basal ganglia maintain normal blood flow (Geaney and Abou-Saleh 1990). Positron-emission tomography (PET) also consistently shows an early and progressive hypofunction of posterior temporoparietal cortex and later involvement

---

Table 10–7.   DSM-IV diagnostic criteria for dementia of the Alzheimer's type

A. The development of multiple cognitive deficits manifested by both:
  1. Memory impairment (impaired ability to learn new information or to recall previously learned information)
  2. One (or more) of the following cognitive disturbances:
    a. Aphasia (language disturbance)
    b. Apraxia (impaired ability to carry out motor activities despite intact motor function)
    c. Agnosia (failure to recognize or identify objects despite intact sensory function)
    d. Disturbance in executive functioning (i.e., planning, organizing, sequencing, abstracting)

B. The cognitive deficits in criteria A1 and A2 each cause significant impairment in social or occupational functioning and represent a significant decline from a previous level of functioning.

C. The course is characterized by gradual onset and continuing cognitive decline.

D. The cognitive deficits in criteria A1 and A2 are not due to any of the following:
  1. Other central nervous system conditions that cause progressive deficits in memory and cognition (e.g., cerebrovascular disease, Parkinson's disease, Huntington's disease, subdural hematoma, normal-pressure hydrocephalus, brain tumor)
  2. Systemic conditions that are known to cause dementia (e.g., hypothyroidism, vitamin B_{12} or folic acid deficiency, niacin deficiency, hypercalcemia, neurosyphilis, HIV infection)
  3. Substance-induced conditions

E. The deficits do not occur exclusively during the course of a delirium.

F. The disturbance is not better accounted for by another Axis I disorder (e.g., major depressive disorder, schizophrenia).

---

of the frontal cortex; the primary motor and sensory areas appear normal (Bench et al. 1990). The stages or progression of DAT are summarized in Table 10–8.

Treatment

Therapy for DAT is divided into two main categories: 1) control of abnormal behavior associated with the illness, and 2) attempts to restore cognitive function. Behavioral disturbances such as agitation, insomnia, wandering, suspiciousness, hallucinations, and hostility often arise during the course of dementia. These are generally treated with low-dose neuroleptic medication (Schneider et al. 1990); initial treatment with low doses of a high-potency agent such as haloperidol 0.5 to 2 mg per day is

---

Table 10–8.   Principal clinical findings in each stage of dementia of the Alzheimer's type (DAT)

Stage I *(duration of disease 1 to 3 years)*
 Memory: new learning defective, remote recall mildly impaired
 Visouspatial skills: topographic disorientation, poor complex constructions
 Language: poor word list generation, anomia
 Personality: indifference, occasional irritability
 Psychiatric features: sadness or, in some cases, delusions
 Motor system: normal
 EEG: normal
 CT/MRI: normal
 PET/SPECT: bilateral posterior parietal hypometabolism/hypoperfusion

Stage II *(duration of disease 2 to 10 years)*
 Memory: recent and remote recall more severely impaired
 Visuospatial skills: poor constructions, spatial disorientation
 Language: fluent aphasia
 Calculation: acalculia
 Praxis: ideomotor apraxia
 Personality: indifference or irritability
 Psychiatric features: delusions in some cases
 Motor system: restlessness, pacing
 EEG: slowing of background rhythm
 CT/MRI: normal and ventricular dilatation and sulcal enlargement
 PET/SPECT: bilateral parietal and frontal hypometabolism/hypoperfusion

Stage III *(duration of disease 8 to 12 years)*
 Intellectual functions: severely deteriorated
 Motor: limb rigidity and flexion posture
 Sphincter control: urinary and fecal incontinence
 EEG: diffusely slow
 CT/MRI: ventricular dilatation and sulcal enlargement
 PET/SPECT: bilateral parietal and frontal hypometabolism/hypoperfusion

---

Note.   EEG = electroencephalogram; CT = computed tomography; MRI = magnetic resonance imaging; PET = positron-emission tomography; SPECT = single-photon emission computed tomography.

typically recommended. If more sedation is required, a trial with a low-potency agent such as thioridazine is recommended; in doses below 75 mg/day, this medication usually produces no detectable anticholinergic effects (Steele et al. 1986). A medication must be scheduled properly to produce the desired effects (e.g., 1 hour before bedtime to improve sleep, 1 hour prior to bathing to diminish agitation). Avoid prn ("as needed") medication, because this medicates the patient's agitation after the fact. The cautious, adjunctive use of low doses of short-acting benzodiazepines, such as lorazepam or oxazepam, may also prove beneficial. Other medications reported to help modify agitated behavior include trazodone, buspirone, and valproate. The physician must always be on the lookout for medical illnesses, such as urinary tract infections or electrolyte disturbances, that might cause sudden changes in behavior or mental status (Small 1988).

The clinician must pay close attention to the patient's environment; too much or too little stimulation may result in withdrawal or agitation. Patients with dementia do best with regular daily routines conducted in a familiar and constant environment. Clocks, calendars, nightlights, checklists, and diaries all aid in orientation and memory during the early phase of the illness. Caregivers must learn the patient's (and their own) limitations. Urge the caregivers to simplify tasks and to avoid rushing or forcing the patient to attempt things beyond his or her ability (Mace and Rabins 1991).

The discovery of profound cholinergic deficits in the brains of DAT patients led to the formulation of a "cholinergic hypothesis" analogous to the dopamine deficiency hypothesis in Parkinson's disease (Davis and Mohs 1982). As a result, various cholinomimetic strategies were tried, including the use of acetylcholine precursors, cholinergic agonists, and cholinesterase inhibitors. The therapeutic potential of these agents is limited by toxic side effects and poor penetration across the blood-brain barrier. One agent, tacrine, a centrally active, reversible cholinesterase inhibitor, has produced modest cognitive improvement in controlled trials (Davis et al. 1992). Despite the reversible hepatotoxicity seen in some patients on tacrine, this medication is now available for use in DAT. Multiple other neurotransmitter deficits are present in DAT, including norepinephrine and serotonin; thus, the utility of single neurotransmitter replacement therapy appears limited.

☐ Vascular Dementia

Vascular dementia (VaD) is the diagnostic term used when cerebral injury from vascular disease leads to multiple cognitive impairments. There is considerable heterogeneity in both the pathological and the clinical expression of VaD. Cerebral infarctions can accumulate and produce the progressive cognitive impairment called *multi-infarct dementia.* Alternatively, chronic ischemia without infarction can impair cognition or ischemic injury can coexist with other neuropathology, such as DAT (Chui et al. 1992).

Epidemiology

Vascular dementia is the second most common cause of dementia. It occurs in 17% to 29% of demented patients and is mixed with DAT in an additional 10% to 23%. The prevalence of cerebrovascular disease increases with age. VaD is most commonly encountered after age 60, and men are affected more often than women. Almost invariably, VaD is associated with stroke risk factors: hypertension, heart disease, cigarette smoking, diabetes mellitus, excessive alcohol consumption (more than three drinks per day), and hyperlipidemia.

Pathophysiology

Strokes cause dementia through several mechanisms, including the location of cerebral injury, the volume of cerebral tissue involved, the number of cerebral insults, and the co-occurrence of VaD and DAT (Tatemichi 1990). Subcortical lacunar infarctions are found in approximately 70% of patients with VaD. VaD may also result from the cumulative effects of watershed or border zone infarctions caused by critical reductions of cerebral perfusion in patients who have severe extracranial atherosclerosis; this pathology is seen in up to 40% of patients with VaD, making it the second most frequent etiology for VaD (Meyer et al. 1988). VaD may also result from the cumulative effects of multiple cerebral emboli; these embolic infarcts are found in approximately 20% of patients with VaD and represent the third most frequent cause of this dementia. Embolic infarcts are usually larger than lacunae and have bilateral hemispheric distribution. An identifiable cardiac source for the emboli is found in one-fourth of these patients.

Clinical Features

Vascular dementia is characterized by abrupt onset, stepwise progression, fluctuating course, depression, pseudobulbar palsy, a history of hypertension, a history of strokes, evidence of associated atherosclerosis, focal neurological symptoms, and focal neurological signs (Hachinski et al. 1975). These features constitute an ischemia score that helps differentiate VaD from DAT but, unfortunately, will not differentiate VaD from VaD *plus* DAT (Erkinjuntti et al. 1988).

The clinical presentation of VaD depends on the location of cerebral injury. Deep hemispheric infarction or ischemia can cause a lacunar state or Binswanger's disease and produce a subcortical dementia with pseudobulbar palsy, spasticity, and weakness. Superficial cortical infarctions can produce a cortical dementia with hemimotor and hemisensory dysfunction. Left hemisphere insults produce aphasia, acalculia, apraxia, and verbal amnesia, while right hemisphere damage causes aprosodia, disturbances in recognition of face, voice, and place, nonverbal amnesia, visuospatial deficits, and neglect of left visual field (i.e., left hemineglect). Neither the nature and prevalence of delusions nor the occurrence of hallucinations distinguishes VaD from DAT (Cummings et al. 1987). Depression is extremely common following stroke and occurs most often with left cortical and subcortical lesions. The severity of depression is positively correlated with proximity of the lesion to the left frontal pole.

Diagnosis

The DSM-IV diagnostic criteria for VaD are listed in Table 10–9. Neuroimaging plays an especially important role in diagnosis of VaD, with MRI being the most sensitive structural imaging technique (Kertesz et al. 1987). T_2-weighted MRI images are best for the detection of white matter hyperintensities that represent ischemic changes and dysmyelination (Kertesz et al. 1988). These white matter changes are not specific to VaD and may occur to some extent in DAT patients, as well as in healthy elderly control subjects. Clinical correlation is therefore essential for diagnosis (Hunt et al. 1989).

Computed tomography detects infarctions in less than half of patients with clinical evidence of VaD (Radue et al. 1978). Nonetheless, areas of decreased lucency in the white matter, called *leucoaraiosis,* are seen on CT in the majority of patients with VaD. Enlargement of the lateral and third ventricles correlates significantly with severity of cognitive impairment in VaD (Aharon-Peretz et al. 1988).

SPECT images in patients with VaD typically show a pattern of diffusely diminished cerebral blood flow with focal areas of severe hypoperfusion. This pattern could, theoretically, mimic patterns seen in other diseases; however, the presence of scattered perfusion defects (either unilateral or bilateral) located in primarily cortical areas is suggestive of VaD, especially if perfusion deficits correlate with cerebral infarcts seen on CT or MRI scans (Geaney and Abou-Saleh 1990). PET studies in patients with VaD show global reductions in cerebral metabolism, with additional focal and asymmetric areas of hypometabolism that are not limited to specific cortical or subcortical brain regions (Benson et al. 1983). This suggests that a single lesion may have extensive and distant metabolic sequelae (Metter et al. 1985). Severity of dementia correlates with the global hypometabolism and frontal cortex deficits seen on PET (Bench et al. 1990).

Treatment

The goals of treatment in VaD are to halt the progression of cognitive deterioration and to optimize remaining cognitive capacity. Therefore, therapy is focused on the management of risk factors, disease-specific interventions for medical conditions, and treatment of psychiatric illness such as depression or psychosis. Use of daily aspirin therapy (325 mg/day) to inhibit platelet aggregation is recommended (Meyer et al. 1989).

☐ Dementia Due to Pick's Disease

Pick's disease is a progressive, degenerative disorder of the frontal lobes or frontal and temporal lobes, and is perhaps the best known of a group of disorders caused by frontal lobe degeneration (FLD). FLD is more common than previously recognized, accounting for 13% to 16% of dementias in some studies. Perhaps 20% of FLD cases are diagnosed as Pick's disease; the remaining 80% are designated as FLD *of the non-Alzheimer's type*. Pick's disease is diagnosed by the presence of distinctive intraneuronal Pick bodies and ballooned Pick cells on microscopic examination; FLD of the non-Alzheimer's type lacks these distinctive histological features (Brun 1987).

Table 10–9.   DSM-IV diagnostic criteria for vascular dementia

A. The development of multiple cognitive deficits manifested by both:
    1. Memory impairment (impaired ability to learn new information or to recall previously learned information)
    2. One (or more) of the following cognitive disturbances:
        a. Aphasia (language disturbance)
        b. Apraxia (impaired ability to carry out motor activities despite intact motor function)
        c. Agnosia (failure to recognize or identify objects despite intact sensory function)
        d. Disturbance in executive functioning (i.e., planning, organizing, sequencing, abstracting)
B. The cognitive deficits in A1 and A2 each cause significant impairment in social or occupational functioning and represent a significant decline from a previous level of functioning.
C. Focal neurological signs and symptoms (e.g., exaggeration of deep tendon reflexes, extensor plantar response, pseudobulbar palsy, gait abnormalities, weakness of an extremity) or laboratory evidence indicative of cerebrovascular disease (e.g., multiple infarctions involving cortex and underlying white matter) that are judged to be etiologically related to the disturbance.
D. The deficits do not occur exclusively during the course of a delirium.

Patients with Pick's disease are clinically indistinguishable from other patients with FLD. Patients with FLD present with marked personality changes that may precede obvious cognitive decline by at least 2 years. Disinhibition and irritability are common, as are wandering, impulsivity, and poor judgment. The clinical presentation, plus the relatively late onset of memory and visuospatial disturbances in FLD, helps distinguish FLD from DAT. Frontal atrophy on CT or MRI is sometimes not apparent until late in the course of FLD, making SPECT or PET imaging useful in separating these patients from patients with DAT (Miller et al. 1991).

☐ Dementia Due to Jakob-Creutzfeldt Disease

Jakob-Creutzfeldt disease (JCD) is an uncommon neurodegenerative disease caused by a transmissible infectious agent, the "prion." Most cases arise sporadically, without any infectious source identified; familial forms, following an autosomal dominant pattern of inheritance, constitute 5% to 15% of cases. The clinical course is extremely rapid, with progressive deterioration and death within 1 year. Patients show intellectual devastation, myoclonic jerks, muscle rigidity, and ataxia. The EEG frequently shows an intermittent periodic burst pattern that is suggestive of the disease (Cummings and Benson 1992).

☐ Dementia Due to Huntington's Disease

Huntington's disease (HD) is an idiopathic neurodegenerative disorder inherited as an autosomal dominant trait with complete penetrance. Average age at onset is 40 years, with gradual progression and death about 17 years later. Pathologically, there is atrophy of the caudate nucleus and loss of the GABAergic interneurons from the striatum. The clinical triad of dementia, chorea, and a "positive" family history should suggest the diagnosis of HD. Depression is quite common in HD, and mania and schizophrenia-like persecutory delusions are also seen (McHugh and Folstein 1975). CT or MRI can demonstrate gross atrophy of the caudate nucleus in HD; functional imaging with PET shows marked caudate hypometabolism prior to any detectable loss of tissue volume (Young et al. 1986).

☐ Dementia Due to Parkinson's Disease

Parkinson's disease (PD) is characterized by progressive loss of dopaminergic neurons in the substantia nigra and other pigmented brainstem nuclei. PD is an example of a long-latency neurological disease, because the tremor, rigidity, and bradykinesia emerge when the nigrostriatal system is already 70% damaged. The pathological hallmark of

PD is the presence of Lewy bodies in the cytoplasm of the remaining nigral neurons; they likely represent an early marker for neuronal cell degeneration (Gibb 1989).

Assessment of intellectual function in patients with PD is difficult, because the clinician must consider the effects of age, depression (in perhaps half of all PD patients), and chronic disability, as well as profound motor deficits. The presentation and course of dementia in PD are variable; there appears to be an entire spectrum of Lewy body disease, ranging from cortical Lewy body dementia to Lewy bodies in the nucleus basalis associated with a cortical cholinergic deficiency and dementia. MRI studies have not demonstrated any specific pattern in demented patients with PD (Huber et al. 1989).

☐ Dementia Due to Human Immunodeficiency Virus Disease

Infection with the human immunodeficiency virus–type 1 (HIV-1) produces a dementing illness initially called the AIDS dementia complex (Navia 1990). A more recent designation is HIV-1–associated cognitive/motor complex (American Academy of Neurology AIDS Task Force 1991). HIV disease is pandemic, with an estimated 1.5 to 2 million Americans already infected. Two high-risk groups for HIV infection are bisexual/homosexual men (70% of HIV cases) and persons who abuse drugs intravenously (15%–20% of cases) (Faulstich 1987). With changes in lifestyle, teens and females are emerging as new high-risk groups.

HIV-1–associated cognitive/motor complex is separated into two disorders: a more severe form known as HIV-1–associated dementia complex, and a less severe form termed HIV-1–associated minor cognitive/motor disorder. In the latter group, only the most demanding activities of daily living reveal mild impairments in cognition, motor abilities, or behavior.

☐ Substance-Induced Dementia

The majority of patients with substance-induced dementia are alcoholic, although younger patients may become demented from chronic exposure to solvent vapors, such as spray paint that contains toluene (Filley et al. 1990). Alcoholic dementia is present in about 3% of alcoholic inpatients and is diagnosed in 7% of patients evaluated for cognitive impairment. Risk factors include female gender, age over 50, and continuous, rather than periodic, drinking (Cutting 1982). Neuropsychological deficits improve with abstinence, most dramatically in the first 10 days, with some additional limited improvement measured at 6 months (Hambidge 1990). CT imaging in abstinent chronically alcoholic persons demonstrates lateral ventricular enlargement with widening of the cortical sulci; this atrophy does not correlate with intellectual impairment and may actually improve in some patients with abstinence (Carlen et al. 1978).

☐ Dementia Syndrome of Depression

Depression is often encountered among patients evaluated for impaired cognition. Several potential relationships exist between depression and dementia: 1) depression can occur in response to the onset of cognitive impairment; 2) depression and dementia can be produced by the same underlying condition, such as stroke or Parkinson's disease; 3) symptoms of dementing illnesses may mimic those of depression and lead to the misdiagnosis of a mood disorder; and 4) depression can cause a dementia syndrome (Cummings 1989). The term "pseudodementia" is sometimes used to refer to dementia caused by depression (Caine 1981; Wells 1979). However, there is nothing "pseudo" about the cognitive impairment demonstrable in some depressed patients. In these patients, the term "dementia syndrome of depression" (DSD) is more accurate (Folstein and McHugh 1978). Currently, DSD can only be established retrospectively, as the patient recovers intellectual function following successful antidepressant therapy.

In contrast to primary dementia, the elapsed time between onset and seeking medical help is shorter in DSD and patients with DSD manifest depressed mood and delusions more than do patients with primary dementia. Sleep disturbance in DSD is more severe and involves early morning awakening. In addition, a history of previous affective disorder is reported more frequently in DSD than in primary dementia. However, behavioral deterioration in patients with primary dementia is more consistent with the severity of cognitive dysfunction than in patients with DSD (Emery and Oxman 1992).

Unlike the patient with DAT, the DSD patient retains self-awareness, has intact recognition, and has memory performance improved by prompting and organization of material. DAT patients manifest a characteristic "empty" speech, often with paraphasic errors not typically seen in DSD (Cummings 1989). Use of antidepressant or electroconvulsive therapy for DSD should be initiated on the basis of intrapsychic depressive symptoms and characteristic sleep disturbance, rather than for the mere complaint or presence of cognitive impairment (Emery and Oxman 1992).

☐ Dementia Due to Other Conditions

Serious head trauma can cause dementia and other neuropsychiatric signs or symptoms. Amnesia is the most common neurobehavioral sequela after traumatic brain injury (TBI); recovery of memory function is not always complete (Levin 1989). In addition, personality changes, attentional disturbances, and other cognitive impairments suggestive of frontal lobe damage are common (Mattson and Levin 1990). TBI also increases the risk for developing psychiatric disorders such as depression, mania, and psychosis (McAllister 1992). Even after mild head trauma, subjective symptoms such as headache, dizziness, easy fatiguability, and disordered sleep persist in some patients for several months.

A potentially reversible cause of dementia that may occur after head trauma is a *subdural hematoma*. This condition may present as a delirium or psychosis (Black 1984), and the history of head trauma may be minimal or entirely absent, especially in the elderly. Another uncommon but potentially treatable dementia associated with head trauma is *normal-pressure hydrocephalus* (NPH), which may also develop as a late complication of subarachnoid hemorrhage or intracranial infection. NPH produces a triad of clinical symptoms: 1) a *gait disturbance*, often described as "magnetic" (appears early); 2) a *subcortical dementia;* and 3) *urinary incontinence* (may appear late) (Benson 1985). Of the remaining dementia syndromes listed in Table 10–6, several are potentially reversible. These include vitamin B_{12} deficiency (O'Neill and Barber 1993), hypothyroidism (Whybrow et al. 1969), and the presence of a brain tumor (Barry and Moskowitz 1988).

■ AMNESTIC DISORDERS

Amnestic disorders are characterized by an inability to learn new information despite normal attention, an ability to recall very remote information, and no other cognitive deficits (Benson 1978). Causes of transient amnesia include epileptic convulsions, ischemic episodes, and the syndrome known as transient global amnesia (Benson and McDaniel 1991).

□ Amnestic Disorders Due to a General Medical Condition

Posttraumatic Amnesia

Head trauma is easily the most common cause of amnesia, with 400,000 to 500,000 patients hospitalized in this country each year for head injuries. Four to five times that number of head injuries occur without hospitalization (Department of Health and Human Services 1989). Posttraumatic amnesia (PTA) is the summation of several factors to include unconsciousness caused by the injury, retrograde amnesia (RGA) that ranges from a few minutes to a few years prior to the injury, and anterograde amnesia (AGA) that lingers from hours to months following recovery from unconsciousness (Levin et al. 1982). Patients with ongoing amnesia have a long period of RGA as well. As patients recover the ability to learn new information (i.e., AGA or ongoing amnesia ceases), only a short period of amnesia lasting seconds or minutes prior to the injury remains. Lishman (1968) correlated the relationship between the duration of PTA and subsequent psychiatric disability. He found that very few cases of severe psychiatric disability were seen when PTA lasted less than 1 hour, whereas PTA greater than 24 hours correlated with psychiatric disability.

Poststroke Amnesia

Amnesia can occur when a stroke damages the fornix or hippocampus. *Bilateral* posterior cerebral artery involvement with damage to the medial temporal regions commonly causes amnesia; unilateral infarction of the language-dominant hemisphere can also produce amnesia (Benson et al. 1974). There are reports of amnesia following rupture of an anterior communicating artery aneurysm (Alexander and Freedman 1984), and following bilateral medial thalamic infarction (Graff-Radford et al. 1990).

Other Causes

There are several other important clinical causes of amnesia. Both intracerebral and extracerebral *neoplasms* affecting structures critical for memory function can produce amnestic disorders. Cerebral anoxia, whether occurring as the result of an accident or an attempted suicide, or during the course of cardiopulmonary resuscitation, can produce a profound amnesia; gradual recovery is often seen over a period of months, but some residual amnesia is almost always present. *Herpes simplex encephalitis,* the most common nonepidemic encephalitis, has a unique tendency to involve the medial temporal areas of the brain. Onset is abrupt, with fever and coma evolving gradually into neurological deficits such as aphasia, hemiparesis, and a dense amnesia that persists after other deficits have cleared (Cermak and O'Connor 1983). Poorly controlled insulin-dependent diabetic individuals are at risk for amnesia because repeated or severe episodes of *hypoglycemia* can produce permanent brain injury (Sachon et al. 1992). *Surgical procedures,* including temporal lobectomy, cingulectomy, sectioning of the fornices, and injury to the mammillary bodies during removal of pituitary tumors, can result in amnestic syndromes (Cummings 1985).

Transient Amnestic Syndromes

Epileptic convulsions are a significant source of acute amnesia in clinical practice. Temporal lobe status epilepticus can produce prolonged amnestic periods, and the phenomenon known as "poriomania," an ictal or interictal state of wandering, may last for hours or even days (Mayeux et al. 1979). *Electroconvulsive therapy* (ECT) produces a period of confusion immediately following the seizure, with AGA and RGA during the course of treatment. These side effects gradually resolve over a period of weeks following cessation of treatment (Sackeim et al. 1986; Weiner et al. 1986). There may be permanent loss of specific memories for events in the months immediately preceding, during, and following a course of ECT; however, objective testing does not demonstrate that the ability to acquire new information or to remember information from the past is persistently impaired by ECT (Squire 1986). Bilateral electrode placement, excessive electrical current, closely spaced treatments, and high doses of barbiturate anesthesia may all increase the severity of cognitive side effects with ECT (American Psychiatric Association 1990b).

Transient global amnesia (TGA) is characterized by the abrupt onset of severe AGA that lasts for a period of hours. The patient returns to normal except for a dense amnestic gap during the episode (Fisher and Adams 1958). TGA occurs in middle-aged or elderly patients; focal neurological and epileptic features are absent. The etiology of TGA remains unknown.

☐ Substance-Induced Amnestic Disorder

Alcohol Persisting Amnestic Disorder

Alcohol persisting amnestic disorder, also known as Korsakoff's syndrome, is among the most common causes of amnesia and is due to thiamine deficiency associated with prolonged, heavy ingestion of alcohol (Victor et al. 1989). Korsakoff's syndrome is the chronic amnestic phase of the Wernicke-Korsakoff syndrome (WKS) and is characterized by a complete inability to learn new material and by relative sparing of remote memories. Confabulation is common in the early phases of the illness, and a variable degree of loss of insight and initiative frequently accompanies the amnesia. Other mental functions are relatively preserved. The acute phase of WKS, Wernicke's encephalopathy, is characterized by opthalmoplegia, ataxia, and confusion. The characteristic pathology of WKS involves punctate lesions of the gray nuclei in the periventricular regions surrounding the third and fourth ventricles and the Sylvian aqueduct (Victor et al. 1989). Further clinical refinement of the WKS diagnosis is needed. To date, MRI studies are unable to consistently distinguish patients with WKS from chronic alcoholic persons without cognitive impairment (Jernigan et al. 1991). Given the insidious course of WKS and the high prevalence of missed WKS diagnoses, treat *all* alcohol-dependent patients with thiamine (Blansjaar and van Dijk 1992).

☐ Benzodiazepine Persisting Amnestic Disorder

Benzodiazepines are among the most widely prescribed medications in the world. Despite valuable sedative, hypnotic, and anxiolytic properties, benzodiazepines impair memory in two distinct ways: 1) AGA following benzodiazepine administration, and 2) impairment of memory consolidation and subsequent memory retrieval (American Psychiatric Association 1990a). AGA is seen following high-dose acute intravenous benzodiazepine administration, as used in presurgical anesthesia. Amnesia is also reported following oral doses of high-potency, short-half-life benzodiazepines such as triazolam, especially when taken with alcohol (Linnoila 1990). Benzodiazepines impair memory consolidation and delay recall without affecting memory acquisition or short-term memory (Angus and Romney 1984). Benzodiazepines have no effect on the retrieval of information learned before the drug is taken (Petersen and Ghoneim 1980). High-potency, short-half-life benzodiazepines are more likely to impair memory, even after a single dose (Scharf et al. 1987). Memory impairment depends on the dose and the route of benzodiazepine administration, with higher doses and intravenous administration causing the greatest impairment. Duration of benzodiazepine treatment is also a significant factor, especially in elderly patients (American Psychiatric Association 1990a).

■ MENTAL DISORDERS DUE TO A GENERAL MEDICAL CONDITION

Unlike DSM-III-R, DSM-IV divided the "organic" diagnoses into three sections: "Delirium, Dementia, Amnestic, and Other Cognitive Disorders"; "Substance Related Disorders"; and "Mental Disorders Due to a General Medical Condition." The latter category contains diagnostic criteria for three disorders: 1) catatonic disorder due to a general medical condition, 2) mental disorder not otherwise specified due to a general medical condition, and 3) personality change due to a general medical condition. The types of personality change specified in DSM-IV include labile, disinhibited, aggressive, apathetic, paranoid, other (e.g., associated with a seizure disorder), combined (in which more than one of the preceding features predominate), and unspecified.

■ REFERENCES

Adams F: Neuropsychiatric evaluation and treatment of delirium in the critically ill cancer patient. Cancer Bulletin 36:156–160, 1984

Adams RD, Victor M: Principles of Neurology, 4th Edition. New York, McGraw-Hill, 1989

Aharon-Peretz J, Cummings JL, Hill MA: Vascular dementia and dementia of the Alzheimer type. Arch Neurol 45:719–721, 1988

Alexander MP, Freedman M: Amnesia after anterior communicating artery aneurysm rupture. Neurology 34:752–757, 1984

American Academy of Neurology AIDS Task Force: Nomenclature and research case definitions for neurologic manifestations of human immunodeficiency virus–type 1 (HIV-1) infection. Neurology 41:778–785, 1991

American Psychiatric Association: Diagnostic and Statistical Manual of Mental Disorders, 4th Edition. Washington, DC, American Psychiatric Association, 1994

American Psychiatric Association: Benzodiazepine Dependence, Toxicity, and Abuse: A Task Force Report of the American Psychiatric Association. Washington, DC, American Psychiatric Association, 1990a

American Psychiatric Association: The Practice of Electroconvulsive Therapy: Recommendations for Treatment, Training, and Privileging: A Task Force Report of the American Psychiatric Association. Washington, DC, American Psychiatric Association, 1990b

Andreasen N[J]C, Noyes R, Hartford C, et al: Management of emotional reactions in seriously burned adults. N Engl J Med 286:65–69, 1972

Angus WR, Romney DM: The effect of diazepam on patients' memory. J Clin Psychopharmacol 4:203–206, 1984

Anthony JC, LeResche L, Niaz U, et al: Limits of the 'Mini-Mental State' as a screening test for dementia and delirium among hospital patients. Psychol Med 12:397–408, 1982

Antoon AY, Volpe JJ, Crawford JD: Burn encephalopathy in children. Pediatrics 50:609–616, 1972

Bamford KA, Caine ED: Does "benign senescent forgetfulness" exist? Clin Geriatr Med 4:897–916, 1988

Barry PP, Moskowitz MA: The diagnosis of reversible dementia in the elderly: a critical review. Arch Intern Med 148:1914–1918, 1988

Basile AS, Hughes RD, Harrison PM, et al: Elevated brain concentrations of 1,4-benzodiazepines in fulminant hepatic failure. N Engl J Med 325:473–478, 1991

Bench CJ, Dolan RJ, Friston KJ, et al: Positron emission tomography in the study of brain metabolism in psychiatric and neuropsychiatric disorders. Br J Psychiatry 157 (suppl 9):82–95, 1990

Benson DF: Amnesia. South Med J 71:1221–1228, 1978

Benson DF: Hydrocephalic dementia, in Handbook of Clinical Neurology, Vol 2: Neurobehavioral Disorders. Edited by Vinken PJ, Bruyn GW, Klawans HL. New York, Elsevier, 1985, pp 323–333

Benson DF, McDaniel KD: Memory disorders, in Neurology in Clinical Practice, Vol 2. Edited by Bradley WG, Daroff RB, Fenichel GM, et al. Boston, MA, Butterworth-Heinemann, 1991, pp 1389–1406

Benson DF, Marsden CD, Meadows JC: The amnestic syndrome of posterior cerebral artery occlusion. Acta Neurol Scand 50:133–145, 1974

Benson DF, Kuhl DE, Hawkins RA, et al: The fluorodeoxyglucose ^{18}F scan in Alzheimer's disease and multi-infarct dementia. Arch Neurol 40:711–714, 1983

Black DW: Mental changes resulting from subdural hematoma. Br J Psychiatry 145:200–203, 1984

Blank K, Perry S: Relationship of psychological processes during delirium to outcome. Am J Psychiatry 141:843–847, 1984

Blansjaar BA, van Dijk JG: Korsakoff minus Wernicke syndrome. Alcohol Alcohol 27:435–437, 1992

Boone KB, Miller BL, Lesser IM, et al: Performance on frontal lobe tests in healthy, older individuals. Developmental Neuropsychology 6:215–223, 1990

Brun A: Frontal lobe degeneration of non-Alzheimer type, I: neuropathology. Archives of Gerontology and Geriatrics 6:193–208, 1987

Burns A, Jacoby R, Levy R: Psychiatric phenomena in Alzheimer's disease, I: disorders of thought content; II: disorders of perception. Br J Psychiatry 157:72–76, 1990

Caine ED: Pseudodementia: current concepts and future directions. Arch Gen Psychiatry 38:1359–1364, 1981

Carlen PL, Wortzman G, Holgate RC, et al: Reversible cerebral atrophy in recently abstinent chronic alcoholics measured by computed tomography scans. Science 200:1076–1078, 1978

Cermak LS, O'Connor M: The anterograde and retrograde retrieval ability of a patient with amnesia due to encephalitis. Neuropsychologia 21:213–234, 1983

Champagne MT, Neelon VJ, McConnell ES, et al: The NEECHAM Confusion Scale: assessing acute confusion in the hospitalized and nursing home elderly. The Gerontologist, Vol 27, No 4A, October 1987 (special issue)

Chui HC, Victoroff JI, Margolin D, et al: Criteria for the diagnosis of ischemic vascular dementia proposed by the State of California Alzheimer's Disease Diagnostic and Treatment Centers. Neurology 42:473–480, 1992

Crook T, Bartus RT, Ferris SH, et al: Age-associated memory impairment: proposed diagnostic criteria and measures of clinical change—report of a National Institute of Mental Health work group. Developmental Neuropsychology 2:261–276, 1986

Cummings JL: Amnesia, paramnesia, and confabulation, in Clinical Neuropsychiatry. Edited by Cummings JL. Orlando, FL, Grune & Stratton, 1985, pp 36–47

Cummings JL: Dementia and depression: an evolving enigma (editorial). J Neuropsychiatry Clin Neurosci 1:236–242, 1989

Cummings JL, Benson DF: Dementia: A Clinical Approach, 2nd Edition. Boston, MA, Butterworth-Heinemann, 1992

Cummings JL, Benson DF, LoVerme S Jr: Reversible dementia. JAMA 243:2434–2439, 1980

Cummings JL, Miller B, Hill MA, et al: Neuropsychiatric aspects of multi-infarct dementia and dementia of the Alzheimer's type. Arch Neurol 44:389–393, 1987

Cutting J: Alcoholic dementia, in Psychiatric Aspects of Neurologic Disease, Vol 2. Edited by Benson DF, Blumer D. New York, Grune & Stratton, 1982, pp 149–165

Davis KL, Mohs RC: Enhancement of memory processes in Alzheimer's disease with multiple-dose intravenous physostigmine. Am J Psychiatry 139:1421–1424, 1982

Davis KL, Thal LJ, Gamzu ER, et al: A double-blind, placebo-controlled multicenter study of tacrine for Alzheimer's disease. N Engl J Med 327:1253–1259, 1992

DeCarli C, Kaye JA, Horowitz B, et al: Critical analysis of the use of computer-assisted transverse axial tomography to study human brain in aging and dementia of the Alzheimer's type. Neurology 40:872–883, 1990

Department of Health and Human Services: Interagency Head Injury Task Force Report. Washington, DC, U.S. Department of Health and Human Services, February 1989

Dubin WR, Field NL, Gastfriend DR: Postcardiotomy delirium: a critical review. J Thorac Cardiovasc Surg 77:586–594, 1979

Emery VO, Oxman TE: Update on the dementia spectrum of depression. Am J Psychiatry 149:305–317, 1992

Engel GL: Delirium, in Comprehensive Textbook of Psychiatry. Edited by Freedman AM, Kaplan HI. Baltimore, MD, Williams & Wilkins, 1967, pp 711–716

Engel GL, Romano J, Ferris EB: Effect of quinacrine (atabrine) on the central nervous system: clinical and electroencephalographic studies. Archives of Neurology and Psychiatry 58:337–350, 1947

Erkinjuntti T, Haltia M, Palo J, et al: Accuracy of the clinical diagnosis of vascular dementia: a prospective clinical and post-mortem neuropathological study. J Neurol Neurosurg Psychiatry 51:1037–1044, 1988

Evans DA, Funkenstein HH, Albert MS, et al: Prevalence of Alzheimer's disease in a community population of older persons. JAMA 262:2551–2556, 1989

Faulstich ME: Psychiatric aspects of AIDS. Am J Psychiatry 144:551–556, 1987

Faust D, Fogel BS: The development and initial validation of a sensitive beside cognitive screening test. J Nerv Ment Dis 177:25–31, 1989

Fernandez F, Holmes VF, Adams F, et al: Treatment of severe, refractory agitation with a haloperidol drip. J Clin Psychiatry 49:239–241, 1988

Fernandez F, Levy JK, Mansell PWA: Management of delirium in terminally ill AIDS patients. Int J Psychiatry Med 19:165–172, 1989

Filley CM, Heaton RK, Rosenberg NL: White matter dementia in chronic toluene abuse. Neurology 40:532–534, 1990

Fisher CM, Adams RD: Transient global amnesia. Transactions of the American Neurological Association 83:143–146, 1958

Folstein MF, McHugh PR: Dementia syndrome of depression, in Alzheimer's Disease, Senile Dementia and Related Disorders. Edited by Katzman R, Terry RD, Bick KL. New York, Raven, 1978, pp 87–93

Folstein MF, Folstein SE, McHugh PR: "Mini-Mental State": a practical method for grading the cognitive state of patients for the clinician. J Psychiatr Res 12:189–198, 1975

Folstein MF, Bassett SS, Romanoski AJ, et al: The Eastern Baltimore Mental Health Survey. Int Psychogeriatr 3:169–176, 1991

Francis J: Delirium in older patients. J Am Geriatr Soc 40:829–838, 1992

Francis J, Martin D, Kapoor W: A prospective study of delirium in hospitalized elderly. JAMA 263:1097–1101, 1990

Geaney DP, Abou-Saleh MT: The use and applications of single-photon emission computerised tomography in dementia. Br J Psychiatry 157 (suppl 9):66–75, 1990

Gibb WRG: Dementia and Parkinson's disease. Br J Psychiatry 154:596–614, 1989

Gibson GE, Blass JP, Huang HM, et al: The cellular basis of delirium and its relevance to age-related disorders including Alzheimer's disease. Int Psychogeriatr 3:373–395, 1991

Graff-Radford NR, Tranel D, Van Hoesen GW, et al: Diencephalic amnesia. Brain 113:1–25, 1990

Haass CH, Schlossmacher MG, Hung AY, et al: Amyloid beta-peptide is produced by cultured cells during normal metabolism. Nature 359:322–325, 1992

Hachinski VC, Iliff LD, Zilhka E, et al: Cerebral blood flow in dementia. Arch Neurol 32:632–637, 1975

Hambidge DM: Intellectual impairment in male alcoholics. Alcohol Alcohol 25:555–559, 1990

Harrell RG, Othmer E: Postcardiotomy confusion and sleep loss. J Clin Psychiatry 48:445–446, 1987

Huber SJ, Shuttleworth EC, Christy JA, et al: Magnetic resonance imaging in dementia of Parkinson's disease. J Neurol Neurosurg Psychiatry 52:1221–1227, 1989

Hunt AL, Orrison WW, Yeo RA, et al: Clinical significance of MRI white matter lesions in the elderly. Neurology 39:1470–1474, 1989

Inouye S, Horwitz R, Tinetti M, et al: Acute confusional states in the hospitalized elderly: incidence, factors, and complications. Clin Res 37(2):524A, 1989

Inouye S, van Dyck C, Alessi C, et al: Clarifying confusion: the confusion assessment method. Ann Intern Med 113:941–948, 1990

Jernigan TL, Schafer K, Butters N, et al: Magnetic resonance imaging of Korsakoff patients. Neuropsychopharmacology 4:175–186, 1991

Joachim CL, Morris JH, Selkoe DJ: Clinically diagnosed Alzheimer's disease: autopsy results in 150 cases. Ann Neurol 24:50–56, 1988

Katzman R, Brown T, Thal LJ, et al: Comparison of rate of annual change of mental status score in four independent studies of patients with Alzheimer's disease. Ann Neurol 24:384–389, 1988

Kennard MA, Bueding E, Wortis SB: Some biochemical and electroencephalographic changes in delirium tremens. Quarterly Journal of Studies on Alcohol 6:4–14, 1945

Kertesz A, Black SE, Nicholson L, et al: The sensitivity and specificity of MRI in stroke. Neurology 37:1580–1585, 1987

Kertesz A, Black SE, Tokar G, et al: Periventricular and subcortical hyperintensities on magnetic resonance imaging. Arch Neurol 45:404–408, 1988

Levin HS: Memory deficit after closed-head injury. J Clin Exp Neuropsychol 12:129–153, 1989

Levin HS, Benton AL, Gassman RG: Neurobehavioral Consequences of Closed Head Injury. New York, Oxford University Press, 1982

Levkoff SE, Besdine RW, Wetle T: Acute confusional states (delirium) in the hospitalized elderly. Annual Review of Gerontology and Geriatrics 6:1–26, 1986

Levkoff SE, Liptzin B, Cleary P, et al: Review of research instruments and techniques used to detect delirium. Int Psychogeriatr 3:253–271, 1991

Linnoila MI: Benzodiazepines and alcohol. J Psychiatr Res 24 (suppl 2):121–127, 1990

Lipowski ZJ: Delirium: Acute Confusional States. New York, Oxford University Press, 1990

Lishman WA: Brain damage in relation to psychiatric disability after head injury. Br J Psychiatry 114:373–410, 1968

Mace NL, Rabins PV: The 36-Hour Day: A Family Guide to Caring for Persons With Alzheimer's Disease, Related Dementing Illnesses, and Memory Loss in Later Life. Baltimore, MD, Johns Hopkins University Press, 1991

Mackenzie TB, Popkin MK: Stress response syndrome occurring after delirium. Am J Psychiatry 137:1433–1435, 1980

Mandell AM, Albert ML: History of subcortical dementia, in Subcortical Dementia. Edited by Cummings JL. New York, Oxford University Press, 1990, pp 17–30

Matsuyama SS, Jarvik LJ: Hypothesis: microtubules, a key to Alzheimer disease. Proc Natl Acad Sci U S A 86:8152–8156, 1989

Mattson AJ, Levin HS: Frontal lobe dysfunction following closed head injury: a review of the literature. J Nerv Ment Dis 178:282–291, 1990

Mayeux R, Alexander MP, Benson DF, et al: Poriomania. Neurology 29:1616–1619, 1979

McAllister TW: Neuropsychiatric sequelae of head injuries. Psychiatr Clin North Am 15:395–413, 1992

McHugh PR, Folstein MF: Psychiatric syndromes of Huntington's chorea: a clinical and phenomenologic study, in Psychiatric Aspects of Neurologic Disease, Vol 1. Edited by Benson DF, Blumer D. New York, Grune & Stratton, 1975, pp 267–286

Mendez MF, Underwood KL, Zander BA, et al: Risk factors in Alzheimer's disease. Neurology 42:770–775, 1992

Menza MA, Murray GB, Holmes VF, et al: Decreased extrapyramidal symptoms with intravenous haloperidol. J Clin Psychiatry 48:278–280, 1987

Metter EJ, Mazziotta JC, Itabashi HH, et al: Comparison of glucose metabolism, x-ray CT, and postmortem data in a patient with multiple cerebral infarcts. Neurology 35:1695–1701, 1985

Meyer JS, McClintic KL, Rogers RL, et al: Aetiological considerations and risk factors for multi-infarct dementia. J Neurol Neurosurg Psychiatry 51:1489–1497, 1988

Meyer JS, Rogers RL, McClintic K, et al: Randomized clinical trial of daily aspirin therapy in multi-infarct dementia: a pilot study. J Am Geriatr Soc 37:549–555, 1989

Miller BL, Cummings JL, Villanueva-Meyer J, et al: Frontal lobe degeneration: clinical, neuropsychological, and SPECT characteristics. Neurology 41:1374–1382, 1991

Navia BA: The AIDS dementia complex, in Subcortical Dementia. Edited by Cummings JL. New York, Oxford University Press, 1990, pp 181–198

Nussmeier N, Arlund C, Slogoff S: Neuropsychiatric complications after cardiopulmonary bypass: cerebral protection by a barbiturate. Anesthesiology 64:165–170, 1986

O'Neill D, Barber RD: Reversible dementia caused by vitamin B_{12} deficiency (letter). J Am Geriatr Soc 41:192–193, 1993

Pearson RCA, Powell TPS: The neuroanatomy of Alzheimer's disease. Reviews in the Neurosciences 2:101–122, 1989

Petersen RC, Ghoneim MM: Diazepam and human memory: influence on acquisition, retrieval, and state-dependent learning. Prog Neuropsychopharmacol Biol Psychiatry 4:81–89, 1980

Pro JD, Wells CE: The use of the electroencephalogram in the diagnosis of delirium. Diseases of the Nervous System 38:804–808, 1977

Rabins PV: Reversible dementia and the misdiagnosis of dementia: a review. Hosp Community Psychiatry 34:830–835, 1983

Rabins PV: Psychosocial and management aspects of delirium. Int Psychogeriatr 3:319–324, 1991

Rabins PV, Folstein MF: Delirium and dementia: diagnostic criteria and fatality rates. Br J Psychiatry 140:149–153, 1982

Radue EW, duBoulay GH, Harrison MJG, et al: Comparison of angiographic and CT findings between patients with multi-infarct dementia and those with dementia due to primary neuronal degeneration. Neuroradiology 16:113–115, 1978

Reisberg B: Functional assessment staging (FAST). Psychopharmacol Bull 24:653–659, 1988

Romanelli MF, Morris JC, Ashkin K, et al: Advanced Alzheimer's disease is a risk factor for late-onset seizures. Arch Neurol 47:847–850, 1990

Romano J, Engel GL: Delirium, I: electroencephalographic data. Archives of Neurology and Psychiatry 51:356–377, 1944

Ross CA, Peyser CE, Shapiro I, et al: Delirium: phenomenologic and etiologic subtypes. Int Psychogeriatr 3:135–147, 1991

Sachon C, Grimaldi A, Digy JP, et al: Cognitive function, insulin-dependent diabetes and hypoglycaemia. J Intern Med 231:471–475, 1992

Sackeim HA, Portnoy S, Neeley P, et al: Cognitive consequences of low-dosage electroconvulsive therapy. Ann N Y Acad Sci 462:326–340, 1986

Scharf MB, Saskin P, Fletcher K: Benzodiazepine-induced amnesia: clinical laboratory findings. J Clin Psychiatry Monogr 5:14–17, 1987

Schneider LS, Pollock VE, Lyness SA: A metaanalysis of controlled trials of neuroleptic treatment in dementia. J Am Geriatr Soc 38:553–563, 1990

Small GW: Psychopharmacological treatment of elderly demented patients. J Clin Psychiatry 49 (No 5, Suppl):8–13, 1988

Smith LW, Dimsdale JE: Postcardiotomy delirium: conclusions after 25 years? Am J Psychiatry 146:452–458, 1989

Squire LR: Memory functions as affected by electroconvulsive therapy. Ann N Y Acad Sci 462:307–314, 1986

Steele C, Lucas MJ, Tune L: Haloperidol versus thioridazine in the treatment of behavioral symptoms in senile dementia of the Alzheimer's type: preliminary findings. J Clin Psychiatry 47:310–312, 1986

Tatemichi TK: How acute brain failure becomes chronic: a view of the mechanisms of dementia related to stroke. Neurology 40:1652–1659, 1990

Trzepacz PT, Teague GB, Lipowski ZJ: Delirium and other organic mental disorders in a general hospital. Gen Hosp Psychiatry 7:101–106, 1985

Trzepacz PT, Baker RW, Greenhouse J: A symptom rating scale for delirium. Psychiatry Res 23:89–97, 1988

Tufo HM, Ostfeld AM, Shekelle R: Central nervous system dysfunction following open-heart surgery. JAMA 212:1333–1340, 1970

U.S. Congress, Office of Technology Assessment: Losing a Million Minds: Confronting the Tragedy of Alzheimer's Disease and Other Dementias (OTA-BA-323). Washington, DC. U.S. Government Printing Office, 1987

Van Duijn CM, Tanja TA, Haaxma R, et al: Head trauma and the risk of Alzheimer's disease. Am J Epidemiol 135:775–782, 1992

Victor M, Adams RD, Collins GH: The Wernicke-Korsakoff Syndrome and Related Neurologic Disorders Due to Alcoholism and Malnutrition, 2nd Edition. Philadelphia, PA, FA Davis, 1989

Vinters HV: Pathologic issues in the diagnosis of Alzheimer disease. Bulletin of Clinical Neurosciences 56:39–47, 1991

Weddington WW Jr: The mortality of delirium: an under-appreciated problem? Psychosomatics 23:1232–1235, 1982

Weiner RD, Rogers HJ, Davidson JR, et al: Effects of electroconvulsive therapy upon brain electrical activity. Ann N Y Acad Sci 462:270–281, 1986

Wells CE: Pseudodementia. Am J Psychiatry 136:895–900, 1979

Whybrow PC, Prange AJ Jr, Treadway CR: Mental changes accompanying thyroid gland dysfunction: a reappraisal using objective psychological measurement. Arch Gen Psychiatry 20:48–63, 1969

Williams MA, Ward SE, Campbell EB: Confusion: testing versus observation. Journal of Gerontological Nursing 14:25–30, 1986

Young AB, Penney JB, Starosta-Rubinstein S, et al: PET scan investigations of Huntington's disease: cerebral metabolic correlates of neurological features and functional decline. Ann Neurol 20:296–303, 1986

CHAPTER

11

Alcohol and Other Psychoactive Substance Use Disorders

Richard J. Frances, M.D.
John E. Franklin, Jr., M.D.

In DSM-IV the term *substance-related disorders* replaces "psychoactive substance use disorders" (DSM-IV, American Psychiatric Association 1994). This change broadens the concept to include not only substances taken by individuals to alter mood or behavior but also substance-induced conditions that occur as a result of the unintentional use of a substance or as a side effect of a medication. Such cases are classified using an "Other (or Unknown) Substance Use Disorders" category. In DSM-IV the substance-related disorders place dependence, abuse, intoxication, and withdrawal syndromes in a "Substance Use Disorders" section. Disorders that were formerly in a "Psychoactive Substance-Induced Organic Mental Disorders" section, such as substance-induced delusional disorders and substance-induced mood disorders, have been moved to sections with which they phenomenologically overlap.

Specific substance-induced disorders have a three-part name (e.g., "Cocaine, Intoxication, Mood Disorder, With Manic Features") that includes the name of the substance, occurring with intoxication or withdrawal or beyond, and the phenomenological presentation, and are located both in the substance-related section and in the mood disorders section. In DSM-IV, substance dependence has not been markedly altered even though criteria related to physiological dependence have

345

been grouped differently, and there is a subtyping method of noting whether physiological dependence is part of the substance dependence (see Table 11–1).

In DSM-IV an effort is made to make a clearer distinction in the boundaries between nonpathological substance use, abuse and dependence, specific terms defining substance abuse, and the influence of cultural and situation-specific factors that impact on the definition (see Table 11–2). In DSM-IV, abuse depends on social difficulties and use in hazardous situations. In DSM-IV the diagnosis of idiosyncratic alcohol

---

Table 11–1. DSM-IV criteria for substance dependence

A maladaptive pattern of substance use, leading to clinically significant impairment or distress, as manifested by three (or more) of the following, occurring at any time in the same 12-month period:

1. Tolerance, as defined by either of the following:
    a. A need for markedly increased amounts of the substance to achieve intoxication or desired effect.
    b. Markedly diminished effect with continued use of the same amount of the substance.
2. Withdrawal, as manifested by either of the following:
    a. The characteristic withdrawal syndrome for the substance (refer to criteria A and B of the criteria sets for withdrawal from the specific substances).
    b. The same (or a closely related) substance is taken to relieve or avoid withdrawal symptoms.
3. The substance is often taken in larger amounts or over a longer period than was intended.
4. There is a persistent desire or unsuccessful efforts to cut down or control substance use.
5. A great deal of time is spent in activities necessary to obtain the substance (e.g., visiting multiple doctors or driving long distances), use the substance (e.g., chain-smoking), or recover from its effects.
6. Important social, occupational, or recreational activities are given up or reduced because of substance use.
7. The substance use is continued despite knowledge of having had a persistent or recurrent physical or psychological problem that is likely to have been caused or exacerbated by the substance (e.g., current cocaine use despite recognition of cocaine-induced depression, or continued drinking despite recognition that an ulcer was made worse by alcohol consumption).

Specify if:
With physiological dependence: evidence of tolerance or withdrawal (i.e., either item (1) or (2) is present).
Without physiological dependence: no evidence of tolerance or withdrawal (i.e., neither item (1) nor (2) is present).

Table 11–2.   DSM-IV criteria for substance abuse

A. A maladaptive pattern of substance use leading to clinically significant impairment or distress, as manifested by one (or more) of the following, occurring within a 12-month period:

1. Recurrent substance use resulting in a failure to fulfill major role obligations at work, school, or home (e.g., repeated absences or poor work performance related to substance use; substance-related absences, suspensions, or expulsions from school; neglect of children or household).

2. Recurrent substance use in situations in which it is physically hazardous (e.g., driving an automobile or operating a machine when impaired by substance use).

3. Recurrent substance-related legal problems (e.g., arrests for substance-related disorderly conduct).

4. Continued substance use despite having persistent or recurrent social or interpersonal problems caused or exacerbated by the effects of the substance (e.g., arguments with spouse about consequences of intoxication, physical fights).

B. The symptoms have never met the criteria for substance dependence for this class of substance.

---

intoxication was eliminated because it was found to be poorly researched, rare, ill defined, and overused in forensic cases.

■ ALCOHOL ABUSE AND DEPENDENCE

In DSM-IV the definitions of alcohol abuse and dependence closely follow and parallel those for other substance disorders. People vary a great deal in their tolerance to alcohol, and tolerance is difficult to measure. Withdrawal starts within several hours of stopping prolonged heavy drinking and is defined by at least *two* of the following: autonomic hyperactivity (e.g., sweating or pulse rate greater than 100); increased hand tremor; insomnia; nausea or vomiting; transient visual, tactile, or auditory hallucinations or illusions; psychomotor agitation; anxiety; or grand mal seizures.

☐ Epidemiology

Although recently there may have been a slight decline of total alcohol consumption in the United States, alcohol remains the most used and abused psychoactive chemical, with a per-person average annual consumption of 2.77 gallons of absolute alcohol by individuals age 15 and older.

In the National Institute of Mental Health Epidemiologic Catchment Area (ECA) study, which involved the use of standardized interviews in three United States cities (Robins et al. 1984), investigators found that psychoactive substance use disorders ranked first among 15 DSM-III diagnoses, with an average of 13.6% of the general population sampled having a lifetime prevalence of alcohol abuse or dependence (Myers et al. 1984). Regier et al. (1990), also using ECA data, found that in a community sample of those with an alcohol disorder and drug abuse, 53% also had a comorbid mental disorder.

Warheit and Buhl Auth (1985) found that approximately 30% of the general population are described as abstainers, 10% as heavy drinkers, and 5% to 10% as problem drinkers. In most cultures, males are represented among problem drinkers and heavy drinkers more frequently than are women, with studies showing a ratio of 4 to 1 in the United States and up to 28 to 1 in Korea (Helzer et al. 1986). Across-culture alcoholism prevalence is higher in men; women have a later onset. Alcoholic subjects have a greater than twofold comorbidity of other psychiatric disorders compared with nonalcoholic subjects. Most alcohol-related problems begin between the ages of 16 and 30, with the lowest percentage of problems in persons older than 50.

In the U.S. Department of Health and Human Services' *Fifth Special Report to the U.S. Congress on Alcohol and Health* (1984), it was estimated that 200,000 deaths per year are alcohol related. Death rates of patients with primary alcoholism have been threefold greater than those of a control group. Liver disease ranks as the fourth leading cause of death, and alcoholism presents as a major cause of liver disease. Although less than 10% of alcoholic individuals develop cirrhosis, this disease accounts for 31,500 deaths annually in the United States, with alcohol being the leading associated factor. Each year 25,000 people die and 150,000 are permanently disabled because of alcohol-related traffic accidents.

☐ Clinical Features

The early detection and treatment of alcohol abuse and dependency are complicated by denial, which tends to manifest itself in the individual, in the family, and in society as a whole. Diagnosis of alcoholism (or psychoactive substance abuse) for the patient and the physician is easier late in the course of the illness, although treatment at that point may be more complicated. Because of the widespread prevalence of alcoholism and the protean forms in which it presents, the diagnostician should always have a high index of suspicion and awareness of its signs and symptoms. The components of a basic alcohol and substance use history are listed in Table 11–3. Clinicians should be alert to the subtle signs and symptoms of early alcohol problems, including loss of communication in a marriage, frequent temper flare-ups, belligerent demands, and a loss of overall interest in the marital relationship.

The two self-administered brief screening tests most widely used for alcoholism are the Michigan Alcoholism Screening Test (MAST; Selzer 1971), a 25-question form that is 90% sensitive, and the CAGE questionnaire (Ewing 1984) (Table 11–4), a four-item test.

Personality change detected at work in the form of irritability, inability to complete projects on time, lateness, and absence may be noted. Before there are severe accidents or loss of a driver's license because of driving while intoxicated, the person may have had complaints by passengers about his or her driving. Drinking may be used to cope with depressed mood or anxiety, or as an aid to sleep. Early medical problems include morning vomiting, abdominal pain, diarrhea, gastritis, and en-

---

Table 11–3.   Components of a basic alcohol and substance use history

Chief complaint	Medical history, medications, human immunodeficiency virus (HIV) status
History of present illness	
Current medical signs and symptoms	
Substance abuse review of symptoms (ROS) for all psychoactive substances	History of past substance abuse treatment, response to treatment
	Family history, including substance abuse history
Dates of first use, regular use, heaviest use, longest period of sobriety, pattern, amount, frequency, time of last use, route of administration, circumstances of use, reactions to use	Psychiatric history
	Legal history
	Object-relations history
	Personal history

Source.   Reprinted from Frances RJ, Franklin JE: *Concise Guide to Treatment of Alcoholism and Addictions.* Washington, DC, American Psychiatric Press, 1989, p. 62. Copyright 1989, American Psychiatric Press. Used with permission.

Table 11–4.   "CAGE" screen for diagnosis of alcoholism

Have you ever:

C	thought you should CUT back on your drinking?
A	felt ANNOYED by people criticizing your drinking?
G	felt GUILTY or bad about your drinking?
E	had a morning EYE-OPENER to relieve hangover or nerves?

Note.   A score of 2 or 3 indicates a high index of suspicion of alcohol dependence, and a score of 4 is pathognomonic for dependence.
Source.   Adapted from Ewing JA: "Detecting Alcoholism: The CAGE Questionnaire." JAMA 252:1905–1907, 1984. Copyright 1984, American Medical Association. Used with permission.

larged liver. There may be an increased tendency toward accidents, bruises, blackouts, and seizures; an increase in infection; and, in those persons who smoke, the occurrence of cigarette-burned fingers. An evidence of family history should be looked for, and the possible vulnerability on a genetic basis can be explained to patients.

Adverse Physical Effects

Alcohol is primarily absorbed in the small intestine and is metabolized in the liver. Alcohol dehydrogenase (ADH), a liver enzyme, metabolizes alcohol to toxic acetaldehyde. Aldehyde dehydrogenase (AldDH) completes the transformation of acetaldehyde to acetic acid. Lactic acid, uric acid, and fat accumulation in the liver are hazardous byproducts. Alcohol dehydrogenase metabolizes 1 ounce of 86-proof spirits (or 43% alcohol) in approximately 1 hour. Alcohol is partly metabolized through the hepatic microsomal enzyme system that metabolizes many other drugs. The interaction of ethanol with other drugs may lead to lethal overdoses or undermedication through effects on drug or alcohol metabolism, absorption, or action (see Table 11–5).

Progression of alcoholism leads to associated medical problems regarding the brain, the digestive tract, the heart, other muscles, blood, hormones, and pregnancy. Alcohol, heavy tobacco use, and deficiency of vitamins A and B all contribute to high cancer rates in the mouth, tongue, larynx, esophagus, stomach, liver, and pancreas (Fraumeni 1982). Alcohol dissolves mucus and irritates gastric lining, contributing to bleeding. Seventy-five percent of patients with chronic pancreatitis have alcoholism. Liver problems range from fatty liver to alcoholic hepatitis to

---

Table 11–5. Effects of some drug interactions with alcohol

Disulfiram (Antabuse)	Flushing, diaphoresis, vomiting, confusion
Anticoagulants (oral)	↑ Effect with acute; ↓ intoxication effect after chronic use
Antimicrobials	Minor Antabuse reactions
Tranquilizers, narcotics, antihistamines	Increased central nervous system depression
Diazepam	Increased absorption
Phenytoin	↑ Anticonvulsant effect with acute intoxication; alcohol intoxication or withdrawal may lower seizure threshold after chronic alcohol abuse
Salicylates	Gastrointestinal bleeding
Chlorpromazine	↑ Levels of alcohol
Monoamine oxidase inhibitor	Adverse reactions to tyramine in some alcoholic beverages

---

cirrhosis, which is life-threatening. Inflammation and later destruction of liver cells from this disease kill 10% to 30% of those persons who develop cirrhosis.

Alcoholic cardiomyopathy can develop after 10 or more years of drinking. Alcohol has chronic effects on other muscle tissue and reduces white blood cell count, which may affect the body's immune response. Infectious diseases have been common in this group. Alcohol interferes with male sexual functioning and fertility through direct effects on testosterone levels and testicular atrophy. In alcoholic females, severe gonadal failure, with inability to produce adequate amounts of female hormones, may also occur, affecting secondary sexual characteristics, reducing menstruation, and producing infertility.

Comorbidity

Depression, anxiety, personality disorders, and drug abuse have all been associated with alcohol abuse. Significant secondary depressions may occur in between one-quarter to two-thirds of alcoholic persons over a lifetime (Schuckit 1985). In a study of acute general hospital patients with a diagnosis of borderline personality disorder, 67% also had a substance abuse diagnosis (Dulit et al. 1990). Antisocial personality has been related to higher rates of alcohol abuse (Nestadt et al. 1992).

Kushner et al. (1990) reported that agoraphobia and social phobia appear to predate chronic alcohol use, and panic attacks and generalized anxiety disorder tend to follow pathological alcohol consumption. Evidence still suggests that heavy alcohol use causes and exacerbates general psychiatric distress, and baseline levels of high stress are predictive of poorer outcome (Dryman and Anthony 1989). Alcohol use is common in schizophrenia and may be related to poorer outcome (Drake et al. 1989). High rates of alcohol and other drug abuse occur in schizophrenic persons, and alcohol use may be related to subjective decreases in social anxiety, dysphoria, insomnia, and other nonpsychotic but unpleasant experiences (Noordsy et al. 1991).

Maternal alcohol misuse can lead to *fetal alcohol syndrome,* which consists of growth retardation before or after birth; abnormal features of the face and head, such as unusually small head circumference and/or flattening of facial features; and evidence of central nervous system (CNS) abnormalities (Rosett and Weiner 1984).

☐ Laboratory Testing in Alcoholism

Standard laboratory tests for alcoholism are listed in Table 11–6. Ancillary tests such as an electroencephalogram (EEG) and a computed tomography (CT) scan series may be ordered as indicated.

Table 11–6.   Standard laboratory tests for alcoholism

Complete blood count with differential	Calcium
Serum electrolytes	Magnesium
Liver function tests	Albumin with total protein
Bilirubin	Hepatitis B surface antigen
Blood urea nitrogen	B_{12} and folic acid levels
Creatinine	Stool guaiac
Fasting blood sugar	Urinalysis
Prothrombin time	Drug and alcohol urine screen
Cholesterol	Chest X ray
Triglycerides	Electrocardiogram

Serum gamma-glutamyltransferase (SGGT) is increased in more than 50% of patients with an alcohol problem and 80% of those with liver problems (Trell et al. 1984). Increased mean corpuscular volume, decreased white cell count, and increased levels of uric acid, triglyceride, aspartase aminotransferase, and urea are also common in alcoholism. A fingerprint of commonly available blood chemistry tests using quadratic discriminant analysis may be specific for recent heavy drinking; however, its usefulness in detecting alcoholism is limited by false negatives and false positives (Goodwin 1985a). EEGs show nonspecific slowing in intoxication and overdose of sedative-hypnotics. Additional testing is needed as indicated to diagnose the presence of complications of alcohol abuse.

As in other areas of psychiatry, the search for biological markers in alcoholism has not yet led to widely applicable clinically useful tests. Schuckit has found differences in the way corticosteroids and prolactin levels in sons of alcoholic persons change in response to an alcohol challenge (Schuckit 1984), as well as a P3-amplitude difference on alcohol challenge (Schuckit et al. 1988). Nonalcoholic men at high risk for alcoholism may have a relatively lower plasma gamma-aminobutyric acid (GABA) level than do control subjects (Moss et al. 1990).

☐ Causes of Alcoholism

Alcoholism is the final result of a complex interaction between biological vulnerability and environmental factors such as childhood experience, parental attitudes, social policies, and culture. Twin and adoption studies have found that genetic variables significantly influence causation, although the mechanism of genetic transmission is not known (Goodwin 1985b). Monozygotic twins have a two-times higher rate for the concordance of alcoholism compared with dizygotic twins, and the incidence of alcoholism is four times higher among male biological offspring of alcoholic fathers compared with offspring of nonalcoholic fathers, regardless of whether they are raised by foster parents or their biological parents. Hereditary factors among women are less clear. However, a very recent study has found genetic vulnerability in alcoholic women. In studies of familial alcoholism, those individuals with positive family history have earlier onset, more antisocial features, worse medical problems, and a poorer prognosis (Frances et al. 1984).

Several studies have subtyped alcoholic persons. The most prominent is the Type 1 versus Type 2 described by Bohman et al. (1987). The Type 1 milieu-limited prototype is characterized by onset of alcoholism after the age of 25; the presence of only isolated alcohol-related difficulties with health, marital relationships, or self-care; behavior inhibition; anticipatory worry; rigidity; reflectiveness; and sparse histories of arrests, violence, or abuse of other drugs. The Type 2 prototype is characterized by being a relative of an alcoholic man; onset of alcohol problems before the age of 25; antisocial traits, including histories of violence, arrests, and illegal drug abuse; and risk taking, impulsiveness, and quick temper.

In a prospective study, Vaillant (1984) found that there may not be any personality style predictive of alcoholism. McCord and McCord (1960) found aggressive and impulsive problems in adolescents with future drinking problems. Although Cloninger et al. (1979) reported that alcoholism, sociopathy, and depression are genetically distinct, other authors, such as Winokur et al. (1974), found that a broad-based genetic vulnerability may end up being expressed in either alcoholism or depression. Loranger and Tulis (1985) found a greater family history of alcoholism in borderline patients compared with bipolar or schizophrenic patients.

The search for a gene for alcoholism led to a report by Blum et al. (1990) of an A1 allele linkage of the dopamine D_2-receptor gene and alcoholism. This finding was not confirmed by Bolos et al. (1990). The effort to map the genes for addictive disorders using candidate probes is a high research priority. Tarter (1982) found that primary alcoholic persons reported a history of the prevalence of minimal brain disorder and had poorer performance on psychological tests.

☐ Pathophysiology

With increasing evidence that alcoholism is inherited, there has been growing attention to the question of exactly what is inherited. A number of hypotheses have been brought forward that are currently being studied:

1. Some factor such as serotonin or a prostaglandin may be at first increased and then decreased by alcohol.
2. Alcohol could lead to increased activity of endorphins or morphine-like substances such as tetrahydroisoquinoline (TIQ).
3. Alcohol may at first increase relaxation in susceptible individuals, such as sons of alcoholic fathers, as evidenced by slow-wave alpha activity on the EEG.
4. Sons of alcoholic fathers may be particularly prone to high tolerance in early stages of the problem.
5. Unpleasant physiological reactions to alcohol such as the "oriental flush" might be protective against alcoholism (Goodwin 1985a).

Changes in neuronal membranes may account for tolerance and physical dependence (Goldstein et al. 1982). Alcohol initially increases membrane fluidity and the sodium-potassium adenosine triphosphate activities. Behavioral tolerance and dependence are complex phenomena that may occur at a number of levels, including at the level of this membrane biological adaptation. Blass and Gibson (1977) reported a familial transketolase deficiency in humans that causes a vitamin B deficiency in a subgroup at risk for Korsakoff's syndrome. The question of whether alcohol has direct toxic effects on the liver, the cortex, and the fetus, or whether these effects are primarily due to malnutrition or other variables, has not been fully answered. Most likely, the combined effects of alcohol, diet, and heredity are important.

☐ Differential Diagnosis

It can be difficult to differentiate the effects of alcohol intoxication, overdose, and withdrawal; the effects of chronic use; and the complex interaction of alcoholism with other psychiatric disorders. Alcohol and alcoholism may mask or mimic a variety of other clinical syndromes. In any patient who presents intoxicated or in a coma it is important to consider the possibility of overdose. In any individual who is unconscious, signs of alcohol and drug abuse should be looked for: a red nose, red palms, skin tracks, scars, spider nevi, erythema, cigarette burns between the index and middle fingers, poor dental care, jaundice, enlarged liver, abdominal pain, reduced sensation, and muscle weakness. When patients present severely intoxicated, comatose, or semicomatose, other complications should be ruled out, including head and spinal cord injuries, hypoglycemia, diabetic coma, hepatic coma, cardiac arrhythmias, myasthenia, and other drug overdose.

☐ Alcohol-Induced Organic Mental Disorders

Alcohol Intoxication

Alcohol intoxication, the most frequently induced organic mental disorder, is time limited and, depending on individual variation and tolerance, may occur with varying amounts of alcohol use. Stages range from mild inebriation to anesthesia, coma, respiratory depression, and, rarely, death. A CNS depressant, alcohol may in low doses produce clinical excitement. In those who have not built up tolerance, BACs of 0.03 mg % can lead to euphoria, and those of 0.05 mg % can cause mild coordination problems.

Wernicke-Korsakoff Syndrome

The Wernicke-Korsakoff syndrome classically begins with abrupt-onset encephalopathy, with truncal ataxia, ophthalmoplegia, and mental confusion. Several authors (e.g., Brew 1986) have suggested that the diagnosis should not rely on the presence of all three criteria and that the presence of two of the three criteria is suggestive of limited forms of the disorder. The etiology of the syndrome involves thiamine deficiency due to dietary, genetic, or medical factors. Wernicke's encephalopathy may result in death or, more commonly, Korsakoff's psychosis, a chronic amnestic disorder. Approximately 80% of patients with Wernicke's encephalopathy who survive will develop Korsakoff's psychosis (Reuler et al. 1985).

Alcohol Withdrawal

Alcohol withdrawal symptoms relate to a relative drop in alcohol blood levels and therefore may occur during continuous alcohol consumption. Increased duration of drinking and binge patterns of alcohol ingestion are tied to an increase in withdrawal phenomena. A coarse, fast-frequency generalized tremor that is made worse by motor activity or stress is observed when the hand or the tongue is extended, with peak symptoms occurring 24 to 48 hours after the last drink and subsiding in 5 to 7 days, even without treatment, although irritability and insomnia may last 10 days or longer. Patients show signs of autonomic hyperactivity, including increased blood pressure, pulse rate greater than 100, sweating, malaise, nausea, vomiting, anxiety, tactile illusions or hallucinations, and disturbed sleep. These symptoms frequently lead to rapid return to drinking in order to reduce the withdrawal symptoms.

Alcohol Withdrawal Seizures

Withdrawal seizures may occur 7 to 38 hours after last alcohol use in chronic drinkers, peaking at approximately 24 hours (Adams and Victor 1981). In some series, 10% of patients with chronic alcoholism have recurrent seizures, and a considerably higher number have had solitary seizures (Espir and Rose 1987). Alcohol intoxication may also precipitate seizures by lowering seizure threshold. Hypomagnesemia, respiratory alkalosis, hypoglycemia, and increased intracellular sodium have been associated with alcohol seizures (Victor and Wolfe 1973).

Alcohol Withdrawal Delirium (Delirium Tremens)

Typical signs and symptoms are delusions, vivid hallucinations, agitation, insomnia, mild fever, and marked autonomic arousal, which may appear suddenly but can develop 2 to 3 days after cessation of heavy drinking, with peak intensity on the fourth or fifth day. Patients frequently report visual hallucinations of insects, small animals, or other perceptual distortions, along with terror and agitation. Patients may show similar patterns of behavior each time they withdraw from alcohol (Turner et al. 1989). Cause of death in delirium tremens is usually infections, fat emboli, and cardiac arrhythmias, which are usually associated with hyperkalemia, hyperpyrexia, and poor hydration. Delirium tremens occur more frequently and are most dangerous in those who have associated infection, subdural hematomas, trauma, liver disease, or metabolic disorder.

Chronic Alcohol Hallucinosis

Chronic alcohol hallucinosis is associated with vivid auditory hallucinations lasting at least 1 week and occurring shortly after the cessation or reduction of heavy ingestion of alcohol. The hallucinosis can develop in a clear sensorium with a lower amount of autonomic symptoms than is typical in delirium tremens. The hallucinations may include familiar noises or clear voices, which may be responded to with fear, anxiety, and agitation (Lishman 1978).

☐ Treatment of Alcohol-Induced Organic Disorders

Intoxication

Intoxication is managed supportively by decreasing external stimuli, interrupting alcohol ingestion, and protecting individuals from damaging themselves and others. In potentially fatal cases, hemodialysis has been attempted; otherwise, careful observation is all that is indicated.

Withdrawal Syndrome

The choice of inpatient versus outpatient treatment depends on the severity of symptoms, the stage of withdrawal, medical and psychiatric complications, polydrug abuse, patient cooperation, the patient's ability to follow instructions, social support systems, and past history. A good medical workup for alcohol withdrawal is essential. Nutritional deficiencies in B_{12}, thiamine, and folic acid can be corrected with multivitamins, oral thiamine (100 mg), folic acid, plus adequate nutrition. Thiamine may be necessary in cases of very poor nutrition and should be given prior to any situation in which glucose loading is required, because glucose infusion can affect stores of thiamine. Patients with a past history of alcohol withdrawal seizures should be given magnesium sulfate. Usually, intravenous fluid replacement is not needed, and overhydration may occur. However, in cases in which sweating, fever, or vomiting has caused severe dehydration, careful rehydration and attention to electrolyte replacement should be effected with medical supervision.

Generally, safe inpatient detoxification occurs with adequate sedation of the patient and gradual withdrawal of blood levels of any medication that is cross-tolerant with alcohol. Although a variety of agents have been used (including alcohol itself), benzodiazepines are preferred for withdrawal symptoms because of a relatively high therapeutic safety index, oral and intravenous routes of administration, anticonvulsant properties, and good prevention of delirium tremens. Patients with severe liver disease and elderly patients may be best detoxified with intermediate-acting benzodiazepines such as lorazepam or oxazepam, with their added advantage of renal versus liver excretion.

Outpatient detoxification with close follow-up, daily visits, and observation for complications is preferable for the majority of patients with mild withdrawal symptoms. Standard inpatient detoxification is accomplished with chlordiazepoxide, with nurses carefully watching for agitation, tremulousness, or change of vital signs. Patients who have had a history of epilepsy may require additional anticonvulsant medication such as phenytoin; however, in uncomplicated withdrawal seizures, adding anticonvulsants to benzodiazepines may not be needed.

☐ Rehabilitation and Treatment of Alcoholism

Once the diagnosis and treatment of intoxication and withdrawal syndromes have been accomplished, the greater challenge is tailoring the right longer-term treatment or the right combination of treatments to meet each patient's needs. Careful psychiatric diagnosis and sorting of primary and secondary conditions are of crucial importance. Differential therapeutics for the two-thirds of patients with alcoholism who have additional psychiatric diagnoses such as depression, anxiety disorders, and attention-deficit disorder utilized a wide range of advances in the field of alcoholism. Patients with both primary and secondary affective illness have an increased suicide rate, and recognition and appropriate treatment of the depression are important, even if no medication is indicated with secondary depression.

The search for pharmacological treatments for alcoholism has not led to breakthroughs; however, some promising drugs include serotonergic antidepressants, buspirone, and naltrexone. Fluoxetine was found to lower alcohol intake and craving during the first week of administration in a controlled pilot study. In a preliminary study by Volpicelli et al. (1992), naltrexone was found to reduce relapse in alcoholic patients.

Indications for inpatient treatment are described above in the subsection on treatment of the withdrawal syndrome. Most alcohol inpatient treatment services in the United States have emphasized a combination of psychoeducation, 12-step programs, disulfiram, and individual, group, and family counseling for 1–2 weeks to 1 month, modeled after Hazelton and the Naval Alcohol Treatment Centers. Some centers also emphasize psychiatric treatment with evaluation and with appropriate use of other modalities such as psychotherapy and pharmacotherapy, especially for the dual-diagnosis patient.

Evaluation and treatment of the families of patients with alcoholism are essential. A family system that has been altered to accommodate the patient's drinking may also reinforce it. Frequently it is a family crisis that brings the patient to treatment, and including the family in treatment planning increases the chances that the patient will engage in treatment. An emphasis on group and self-help aspects of treatment aids in a patient's resocialization.

Alcoholics Anonymous (AA) meetings provide members with acceptance, understanding, forgiveness, confrontation, and a means for positive identification. In a program of 12 steps, new members are asked to admit to a problem, give up a sense of personal control over the disease, do a personal assessment, make amends, and help others. Regular AA attendance is associated with favorable outcome (Vaillant 1984).

Individual supportive or dynamically oriented therapy may be especially needed in patients who refuse to accept Alcoholics Anonymous, group, or family treatment. The initial focus of treatment is on conflicts about acceptance of the diagnosis of dependency, the need for help, and the loss of loved ones and friends, jobs, health, and even alcohol. Gradually confronting other problems in self-care, self-esteem, assertiveness, the handling of aggression, and alcohol's role in allowing or distancing oneself from sexual life and issues around control may become important. Support is usually needed at first, with gradual increase in clarification, confrontation, and interpretation of denial, lying, splitting, and projective defenses. Professional treatment programs can work well in concert with self-help groups. A prospective study of employed alcoholic individuals found that treatment plus AA was more effective than AA alone in helping employed alcohol-abusing persons to attain and continue abstinence (Walsh et al. 1991).

Patients may enter treatment as a result of coercion by family, employer, physician, or probation officer. A thorough understanding of alcoholism and an empathic approach to the patient's resistances help the therapist form a working alliance with the patient who is initially hostile. Confrontation of lying and denial is important and may be aided by family meetings and the use of laboratory aids. Countertransference problems on the part of therapists most frequently occur either in response to patients' transferences of rebelliousness, dishonesty, or aggression; therapists' lack of knowledge about alcoholism or its treatment; or problems that the therapists have had with alcohol either themselves or in their close relationships.

In patients with alcoholism and psychiatric disorders, if the need for medication is not well explained and accepted, the abstinence emphasis of alcohol programs can work antithetically to prescribed psychotropic medication compliance. Many alcohol halfway houses will not accept patients on any medication. Confrontational methods found in some self-help groups may be detrimental to some psychologically ill patients. Facilities that treat dual-diagnosis patients with combined psychiatric treatment and substance disorder rehabilitation are expensive and have yet to demonstrate that tailoring treatment to the patient is cost-effective; however, at present, they provide state-of-the-art treatment in the field.

Treatment outcome studies in alcoholism indicate that a variety of treatment programs yield benefit and may be cost-effective; however, few studies exist that differentiate which treatments are best for which kinds of patients. In one well-designed outcome study, Woody et al. (1984) treated patients who had an additional psychiatric diagnosis along with a psychoactive substance use disorder(s) and found improved outcome of these poor-prognosis patients. So far, the outcome literature reflects that patient factors such as a stable family, stable job, less sociopathy, less psychopathology, and a negative family history for alcoholism are more powerful predictors of positive prognosis than is the type of treatment used (Frances et al. 1984).

■ SEDATIVE, HYPNOTIC, OR ANXIOLYTIC ABUSE AND DEPENDENCE

Benzodiazepines and barbiturates are useful medications with potential for abuse and dependence. In the early 1980s, 15% of the United States population used a benzodiazepine during a 1-year period. The ratios of female to male use and white to black use are approximately 3:1 (Gottschalk et al. 1979). Only a minority (16%) of users abuse sedatives (Rickels et al. 1983). Abuse may be iatrogenically caused or intentional. Emergency visits secondary to barbiturate overdoses have decreased because of the waning popularity of barbiturate use. Benzodiazepines have a higher index of therapeutic safety and produce less respiratory depression than barbiturates. However, they potentiate the CNS depression and euphoria of other sedatives and opioids.

Diagnosis of sedative abuse may be difficult. Such abuse may start in the context of treatment for anxiety, medical disorders, or insomnia. Individuals prone to polysubstance abuse may use sedatives for their calming effects or for their ability to potentiate euphoric effects of other drug classes such as opioids, or to self-medicate overwhelming affects including anxiety. Physical dependence can develop to low-dose use (10 to 40 mg per day) over several years or high-dose use over weeks to months (Dietch 1983). Individuals may develop tolerance to extremely high doses (up to 1,000 to 1,500 mg per day) of Valium. Tolerance to sedative-hypnotic effects can develop in 2 to 3 weeks; however, antianxiety effects may persist. Intoxication, withdrawal, withdrawal delirium, and amnestic disorder symptoms are similar to those found with alcohol. Benzodiazepines, however, have a much longer half-life. Valium withdrawal may not be evident until 7 to 10 days after cessation of use.

☐ Clinical Features

Indiscriminate use of benzodiazepines prescribed by physicians may contribute to abuse. A patient may become tolerant to considerable benzodiazepine dosages without showing behavioral pathology. In individuals with generalized anxiety, panic attacks, agitated depression, or personality disorders, in whom affect regulation is impaired, benzodiazepines may serve as self-medication, and alarmingly high doses of benzodiazepines may be used. These individuals may be prone to behavioral disinhibition, especially when alcohol, opioid, or cocaine abuse is also present. Social and legal consequences of abuse may present similarly to those of alcohol, opioid, and cocaine abuse.

Chronic sedative abuse may lead to neuropsychological impairment (Bergman et al. 1980). Deficits in memory (verbal and nonverbal), concentration, motor coordination, and speed have been described (O'Brien and Woody 1986). Overdose secondary to brain-stem depression is possible with little warning when benzodiazepines are used at extremely high dosages because of a patient's high tolerance to sedation. Enlargement of cerebrospinal fluid spaces in long-term abuse of benzodiazepines has been described (Schmauss and Krieg 1987).

It may be difficult to distinguish withdrawal symptoms and side effects from presumed underlying anxiety symptoms, and prognosis for benzodiazepine abuse is guarded. The primary sedative-hypnotic–abusing patient should be viewed with a high suspicion of underlying psychiatric symptoms. Alcohol and opioid CNS depression may interact with sedative-hypnotics with potentiation of depressive actions. Complex perceptual and motor tasks, such as driving, may be negatively affected because of acute neuropsychological impairment. Prescription-induced sedativism may become a lead-in to alcoholism, especially in women.

□ Treatment

The treatment of sedative, hypnotic, and anxiolytic withdrawal is similar to that of withdrawal from alcohol. A cross-tolerant sedative is given to prevent withdrawal symptoms and is gradually decreased. Long-acting barbiturates or benzodiazepines are preferred. Clonazepam has an extremely long half-life and has shown some promise in alprazolam withdrawal, which has proven to be a benzodiazepine that is particularly difficult to taper after long-term use or high-dose abuse. For inpatient detoxification, the most important factor in keeping complications to a minimum is to decrease dose by approximately 10% per day, with the terminal 10% dosage tapered slowly to zero over a 3- to 4-day period. Orders for as-needed dosages should be available for vital sign or marked subjective changes.

Generally, detoxification can be accomplished in a 10- to 14-day period, but longer detoxification may be required in certain individuals. For outpatient detoxification, a taper (25% a week) is generally well tolerated; however, more discomfort may be evident at the end of the taper. Factors such as neuroticism, female sex, and history of alcohol abuse may contribute to a patient's difficulty with withdrawal (Schweizer et al. 1990). Because of potential medical complications of detoxification, especially with high-dose abuse, initial inpatient treatment is preferred. Detoxification with shorter-acting benzodiazepines such as oxazepam or lorazepam is indicated in patients with liver or pulmonary disease. When indicated for dual-diagnosis patients with anxiety disorders and after other behavioral and pharmacological treatments have failed, use of benzodiazepines can be tried with patients who are abstinent and are not escalating doses and with close monitoring of the patient and family (Dupont and Saylor 1991).

■ OPIOID ABUSE AND DEPENDENCE

Consistent with that of other psychoactive substance dependence, the definition of diagnosis of opioid dependency in DSM-IV includes psychosocial factors, and the concept of abuse has been made more specific (Table 11–2). Frequently tolerance and withdrawal are present with dependence.

☐ Epidemiology

There were approximately 492,000 opioid-addicted individuals in the United States in 1980 (NIDA 1981). Recidivism rates as high as 90% contribute to this number's stability. Estimates of opioid use come from overdose reports, surveys, prevalence of medical complications, arrests, and admissions into treatment programs. The majority of opioid-dependent individuals are not in treatment, and recent attempts have been made to characterize this group. Availability of opioids is an important factor in the incidence. In 1977, narcotic addiction was estimated to be 1% to 2% among physicians, in contrast to 0.37% among the general population. Young teenagers tend to experiment with codeine or pentazocine before abusing heroin. Heroin abuse occurs more frequently in males than in females (3:1) in urban areas, and it is more common among the 18- to 25-year-old age group.

☐ Clinical Features

Intravenous heroin intoxication produces a subjective euphoric "rush" that can be highly reinforcing. Tolerance to this high develops with repeated use over time. Physical signs of intoxication include pupillary constriction, decreased gastrointestinal motility, marked sedation, slurred speech, and impairment in attention or memory. There is a clear association between heroin use and crime. Daily use of opioids over days to weeks, depending on dose and potency of the drug, will produce opioid withdrawal symptoms upon cessation of use. Rather intense but generally non–life-threatening withdrawal syndromes start approximately 10 hours after the last dose of short-acting opioids such as morphine and heroin. The onset of opioid withdrawal depends on the half-life of the opioid and the chronicity of use.

Mild opioid withdrawal presents a flu-like syndrome with symptoms of anxiety, dysphoria, yawning, sweating, rhinorrhea, lacrimation, pupillary dilation, piloerection, mild hypertension, tachycardia, and disrupted sleep. Severe symptoms include hot and cold flashes, deep muscle and joint pain, nausea, vomiting, diarrhea, abdominal pain, weight loss, fever, and waves of gooseflesh.

Contaminated needles and impure drugs can lead to endocarditis, septicemia, pulmonary emboli, and pulmonary hypertension. Contaminants can cause skin infections, hepatitis, and HIV spread. Opioid overdose should be suspected in any undiagnosed coma patient, especially when accompanied by respiratory depression, pupillary constriction, or the presence of needle marks. In any suspected opioid overdose, naloxone should be given immediately.

Addicted individuals frequently have a comorbid psychiatric disorder(s). In a diverse sample of 133 narcotic-addicted persons, there was a 93% rate of other diagnosable DSM-III psychiatric disorders, including depression in 60%, antisocial personality disorder in 35%, and other personality disorders in 30% (Khantzian and Treece 1985). It is often hard to separate out the influence of symptoms of chronic intoxication and withdrawal from other Axis I and Axis II pathology. Rounsaville et al. (1982) found that 80% of a sample of outpatients on methadone had lifetime histories of psychiatric disorders, with 74% meeting a lifetime diagnosis of affective disorder.

☐ Etiology

Pathophysiology

Basic research advances in the identification of distinct subtypes of opioid receptors have provided increased understanding of the mechanism of endogenous opioid neuroregulation and physiology. Cellular mechanisms of opioid neuroadaptation are being explored in relation to characteristics of opioid receptors and intracellular modulators of opioid action. Multiple subtypes of opioid receptors, designated mu, delta, kappa, sigma, and epsilon, have been described (Redmond and Krystal 1984).

Certain individuals may be more prone to opioid addiction because of a hypothesized lack of endogenous opioid peptide homeostasis. Other models have linked opioid tolerance and dependence to a disruption of balance between endogenous opioids and contraopioid ligands such as adrenocorticotropic hormone (ACTH). ACTH may interact with endogenous endorphins in a mutually antagonistic manner (Hendrie 1985). Neuroadaptation leads to tolerance of opioid effects, especially respiratory depression. Removal of opioid drug from receptors produces rebound withdrawal symptoms. Neuroadaptation appears to be a result of intracellular modulations that may affect the numbers or conformation of opioid receptors. Kosten (1990) reviewed the synaptic mechanisms of opiate action and opiate effects on second messenger systems, G-proteins, and regulatory phosphoroproteins. Alterations in the coupling of G-protein subunits may be involved in opioid dependency, tolerance, and withdrawal. "Resetting" of second messenger systems may aid in opioid detoxification.

Important clinical tools have resulted from basic research into opioid-norepinephrine interaction. The locus coeruleus is the primary source of noradrenergic interaction of the limbic system, cerebellar, and cerebral cortices. Endogenous opioid receptors have been found in the locus coeruleus, and the chronic administration of opioids inhibits the firing rates of the locus coeruleus noradrenergic system, probably through inhibitory action on common second messenger systems. Opioid withdrawal symptoms are mediated by noradrenergic activity in the locus coeruleus. 3-Methoxy-4-hydroxyphenylglycol (MHPG) levels in the CNS increase after naltrexone-precipitated withdrawal and correlate positively to the signs and symptoms of withdrawal (Charney et al. 1984). These findings have led to the use of clonidine to suppress and inhibit narcotic withdrawal symptoms.

Psychosocial Factors

Yamaguchi and Kandel (1984) have extensively studied patterns of psychoactive substance use in adolescence through young adulthood and found a progression from tobacco, alcohol, and marijuana to sedatives, cocaine, and finally opioids. Regular marijuana use, depressive symptoms, lack of closeness to parents, and dropping out of school may predispose the adolescent to later narcotic use. Low sensation-seeking scores have been found in opioid-dependent subjects, whereas highly sensation-seeking individuals have been found to use cocaine (Galizio and Stein 1983). Avoidance of excessive internal or external arousal may be a factor in opioid preference.

Khantzian (1985) found a strong interaction between dominant dysphoric feelings and drug preference. He emphasized an "anti-rage" property to opioids that provides a pharmacological solution to an overwhelming affect that is due to either deficient ego defenses or low frustration tolerance. Patients may seek mastery over pain through self-administered drug titration of withdrawal and dysphoria. Spotts and Shontz (1985) found that opioid-addicted persons had difficulty in maintaining intimate relationships, partly related to their social withdrawal and avoidance of sexual and aggressive conflict. Blatt et al. (1984) noted that, compared with normal subjects, addicted individuals experienced people to be less stable in affect; involved in less meaningful, purposeful, and constructive activity; and less well differentiated as persons.

☐ Treatment

Approaches to treatment of opioid addiction can be grouped into opioid substitution or maintenance versus abstinence approaches. New pharmacological tools such as clonidine and naltrexone allow a select minority of patients to be detoxified as outpatients. The course of heroin addiction typically involves a 2- to 6-year interval between regular heroin use and the seeking of treatment. Early experimentation with opioids may not lead to opioid addiction, but once addiction develops, a lifelong pattern of use and relapse frequently ensues. The need to secure the drug predisposes the addicted individual to participate in illegal activities or complicates an already existing tendency toward criminality. Attitudes toward one's self, society's attitudes toward addicted individuals, personality problems, unemployment, and empathic impairments are not responsive to psychopharmacological treatment alone; thus treatment almost always involves psychosocial rehabilitation. Family therapy, vocational training, and respect for indigenous community sensitivities and needs are factors that have received attention (Kosten and Kleber 1984).

Methadone Maintenance

Methadone is a relatively long-acting (half-life of 24 to 36 hours), cross-tolerant opioid that mutes extreme fluctuation in opioid blood level and blunts euphoric response to illicit heroin. Unlike heroin, which has a shorter half-life of 8 to 12 hours, methadone can be administered once daily without causing withdrawal and provides a treatment structure for rehabilitation without the need for illegal activities to support a costly habit.

A patient who gives a history of heroin use two or more times per day for several weeks and is unemployed has a moderate to severe degree of opioid dependence and warrants methadone maintenance. Methadone is administered orally and is most often reliably absorbed; it binds nonspecifically to body tissues and therefore maintains a fairly steady blood concentration. Subjectively, common side effects are sedation, mild euphoria, constipation, and reduced sweating if the dosage is too high. These symptoms usually remit after the first few weeks. Occasionally, transient ankle edema, skin problems, and reduced libido have been reported. Long-term euphoric effects persist in some patients, but many find methadone relatively dysphoric. Although a mainstay treatment, this therapy reaches only 20% to 25% of addicted individuals, with retention rates of 59% to 85% (Stimmel et al. 1977).

Dole and Nyswander (1965) advocated starting a methadone maintenance program at 20 to 40 mg the first day, with gradual increase up to a total of 120 mg a day in certain individuals, on a chronic basis to adequately suppress opioid hunger and block any response to illicit heroin. Other programs approach maintenance not as a lifelong substitution but as a transitional phase toward total abstinence. Large doses of heroin with this regimen may result in euphoria. Poor retention rate in low-dose programs is a critical factor in leading experts to favor higher doses (Brown et al. 1982). Some programs offer take-home medications for methadone patients who have had long-term success, and this is very appropriate for a subset of methadone maintenance clients; however, this can result in diversion to illegal methadone markets. Carefully selected patients may be able to have less frequent monitoring (Novick et al. 1988). Behavioral contingency contacting based on urine monitoring in methadone clients may play a role in reducing illicit drug use while the patient is on methadone and may improve compliance (Stine et al. 1991). Illicit use of drugs such as cocaine and alcohol continues to be a problem among individuals who use methadone. The optimal length of methadone maintenance treatment is difficult to predetermine. Advocates for long-term maintenance cite the benefits as a decrease in opioid drug use (if not total abstinence), less criminal behavior, less unemployment, and reduced sharing of needles with consequent lower risk of contracting HIV infection (Metzger et al. 1991).

Two new long-acting opioid agonists have some advantages over methadone. L-Alpha-acetyl-methadol (LAAM), an agonist similar to methadone, has a longer half-life, providing suppression of withdrawal symptoms for from 72 to 96 hours (Jaffe and Martin 1985). Therefore, LAAM can be given just 3 days per week, making take-home privileges unnecessary. Because of LAAM's slow induction, the potential for abuse is less. Generally LAAM compares favorably to methadone, but decreased retention rates and mood side effects may be drawbacks. Buprenorphine is a mixed mu-receptor agonist/antagonist. In experimental settings, patients who use heroin have sharply decreased their intake when started and maintained on subcutaneous buprenorphine.

Opioid Detoxification

Methadone.   Studies have suggested a 76% success rate of completion for methadone detoxification (Milby 1988). When attempted, detoxification should be very slow, because abstinence symptoms may be protracted. Some patients in methadone maintenance programs (15% to 34%) may not have a true opioid dependence when tested with antagonist challenge.

Conservative detoxification of methadone is achieved through decreasing doses by 10% per week until the 10-to-20 mg range is reached, and then decreasing by 3% per week (Table 11–7). This slow detoxification regimen is used to reduce relapse rates. This method is also appropriate for detoxification from equivalent dosages of heroin. Detoxification of weak opioids such as codeine conservatively can be achieved by starting methadone at 20 mg, and then decreasing this dosage by 1 mg per day over a 14- to 21-day period. Although it is frequently easy to decrease methadone level dose to 20 mg per day, it is hard to go lower because

Table 11–7. Opiate detoxification

Methadone

Outpatient: Decrease methadone 10% per week until 10–20 mg range, then decrease 3% per week

Inpatient: 1 mg/day over 20 days

Clonidine

After patient stabilized at 20 mg of methadone, can abruptly switch to clonidine 0.1–0.3 mg three times daily for 2 days, then third day 0.2–0.7 mg three times daily for 8 to 14 days, then discontinue.

subsequent mild withdrawal symptoms may be conditioned to fear of being off drugs in opioid-addicted individuals. Unless there are complications, deaths are not reported from opioid withdrawal, although patients may suffer extreme discomfort upon sudden withdrawal.

Methadone maintenance patients often have the added problem of polysubstance use. Cocaine and alcohol are frequently combined with or used instead of opioids. Alcoholism is a factor in 26% of terminations from methadone treatment and may be abused by 14% to 40% of all opioid patients (Joseph and Appel 1985). The majority of polysubstance-using individuals have had problems with alcohol prior to methadone treatment, and they frequently increase their alcohol use after methadone detoxification. The dual addiction of methadone and alcohol decreases survival rates, especially in black persons, and increases the chances of overdose and medical complications. Detoxification from multiple drug dependence is best achieved by beginning with sedative-hypnotic withdrawal while maintaining methadone. Combined use of methadone and benzodiazepines must be very carefully monitored because of the interaction of the two drugs and the greater danger of overdose. Methadone tends to potentiate the sedative effects of benzodiazepines.

Clonidine.   Clonidine has been found to be a nonopioid suppressor of opioid withdrawal symptoms. Clonidine generally provides good suppression of autonomic signs of withdrawal but may be less effective at relieving subjective discomfort (Jasinski et al. 1985). Withdrawal symptoms may be more prominent with clonidine in the early phase of withdrawal compared with methadone. Patients do better with an abrupt switch to clonidine if the methadone dose is first stabilized at 20 mg or less. Rounsaville et al. (1986) found outpatient detoxification failure in both clonidine- and methadone-assisted withdrawal. Sedation and hypotension are common side effects. Clonidine's main benefit may prove to be the period of 5 to 7 days in which the patient is opioid free, making it easier for the patient to be started on an opioid antagonist.

Naltrexone.   Naltrexone is an opioid antagonist that blocks opioid receptors, preventing the reinforcing euphoric effects of opioids. Its long-term use results in gradual extinction of drug-seeking behavior, and consequently it is a tool in abstinence-oriented treatment (Greenstein et al. 1984). Because of its antagonist properties, naltrexone can precipitate withdrawal symptoms if receptors are not clear of opioids. Dysphoria may result from naltrexone use in formerly opioid-addicted individuals long after use of opioids is stopped, and also occurs in normal subjects (Crowley et al. 1985).

   The clinical effectiveness of naltrexone has varied greatly according to the population studied and the degree of patient motivation for treatment (Kosten and Kleber 1984). High refusal rates of 70% and dropout rates of 90% in 9 months with naltrexone were found in urban outpatient clinic populations, indicating limited usefulness for most cases of hardcore addiction (Resnick et al. 1980). Washton and Resnick (1981) reported a 70% 1-year abstinence rate in an outpatient naltrexone program for highly motivated patients.

Clonidine and naltrexone.   Abrupt switch to clonidine may be started along with gradual low-dose naltrexone (antagonist) administration. The combination appears to shorten the withdrawal period to 3 to 4 days without increasing symptomatology, and can be used successfully on an outpatient basis (Kleber et al. 1987). The naltrexone may serve to "reset" the opioid homeostasis. Higher doses of naltrexone may speed withdrawal duration but require higher dose levels of clonidine to suppress symptoms.

☐ Psychosocial Treatment Outcome

Treatment outcome factors have included a variety of measures involving choice of drug of abuse, employment, psychosocial adjustment, degree of sociopathy, and severity of psychopathology. Total abstinence is often used as the only measure of success, but decreased opioid use and fewer episodes may have very positive effects on life quality.

   The prognosis of opioid-addicted patients is inversely related to severity of psychopathology; however, if psychotherapy is added, psychiatrically ill patients do better than they would otherwise have done (Woody et al. 1985). Antisocial personality alone is a negative predictor of psychotherapy outcome, but additional presence of depression improves therapy outcome considerably as measured by drug use and functioning (Woody et al. 1985). Rounsaville et al. (1986) found that a high psychiatric severity index scale rating in methadone patients best predicts poor functioning at 2.5-year follow-up. The ability to form a meaningful relationship in therapy is a positive prognostic factor. Good patient-therapist alliance and purity of technique may predict better therapy outcome (Luborsky et al. 1985).

Therapeutic communities remove the addicted individual from the drug environment, confront his or her attitudes with peer support, and emphasize assumption of personal responsibility. Only the highly motivated patients stay in treatment, with estimated dropout rates of 50% at 6 months and 90% at 12 months (Deleon et al. 1982). Select patients who do stay in treatment 3 to 6 months have a relatively good prognosis (Simpson 1981). These programs are generally drug free and highly structured. Overall success rates in therapeutic communities have not been impressive.

■ COCAINE

In DSM-IV, cocaine-related problems are discussed in relation to intoxication, cocaine intoxication paranoia, uncomplicated withdrawal, dependence, and abuse, and are similar to behavior found with amphetamine and other similarly acting stimulants. Diagnosis of intoxication requires recent use (within minutes to hours) and a "high" with euphoria, hyperalertness, grandiosity, and, often, impaired judgment. Chronic use may result in affective blunting, fatigue, and sadness. Individuals may be more gregarious or socially avoidant, and may have increased anxiety, restlessness and hypervigilance, and stereotypical behavior. Cocaine intoxication paranoia occurs with high-dose, chronic, or binge use and is usually of short duration. It is associated with aggression and violence, and distortion of perceived threat.

In DSM-IV, *dependence* is defined as compulsive self-administration of high doses of cocaine and the involvement with the drug to the exclusion of other important activities and responsibilities such as work, eating, and family, with adverse consequences to work, health, legal, and social relationships. Dependence may be episodic or continuous (daily). In DSM-IV, *abuse* is defined as repetitive self-administration of high doses of cocaine with consequent social or medical problems, without the compulsive quality that is present with dependence.

□ Epidemiology

The National Institute on Drug Abuse estimated that 5.4 million Americans had tried cocaine at least once by 1974, 21.6 million by 1982, and perhaps 25 to 40 million by 1986 (NIDA 1986). Emergency room visits and medical examiner deaths reportedly associated with cocaine use increased fourfold from 1976 to 1984 (Adams and Durell 1984). An estimated 79,398 emergency visits for cocaine use were made in 1990.

Bachman et al. (1990) traced lowering of cocaine and drug abuse in 3,000 high school seniors to perceived risk of physical and other harm and to disapproval. Cocaine use dropped dramatically after the deaths of a college basketball star and professional football player, and after the subsequent heavy media coverage dramatizing the dangers of drug use. Demand reduction programs have impacted cocaine and marijuana epidemics in youth but have not been as effective with poor, disadvantaged groups, who have maintained high levels of "crack" addiction.

Pope et al. (1990) found that seniors in college had reduced drug use in 1989 compared with seniors in 1969 and 1978. Cocaine use peaked in 1978 at 25% and was reduced to 20% in 1989. These trends indicate attitudinal changes in young Americans about drugs in the last decade. A PRIDE survey of junior high school students reported, however, a reversal in the 3-year trend in decrease of psychoactive substance use. Crack cocaine is used by a small subset of the general population; however, it is more popular among younger, more serious cocaine users (Smart 1991). There has been a decline in cocaine use, especially among middle-class and affluent populations and among students (Bachman et al. 1990; Perlstadt et al. 1991).

Cocaine use tends to decrease in social users as they assume adult responsibility. Kandel and Raveis's (1989) longitudinal study of nonclinical populations of teenagers found, however, a subset of users characterized by greater involvement with drug-using friends, more antisocial behavior, and increased dependence on marijuana. These teenagers were more likely to be involved with drugs at age 28 or 29.

☐ Clinical Features

Effects of intoxication depend on the dose and administration of the drug and include euphoria, hyperalertness, perceptual changes, disinhibition, enhanced sense of mastery, sexual arousal, and improved self-esteem (Kleber and Gawin 1986). This "rush" experience may be greatly intensified with intravenous or freebase use. Maladaptive behavioral changes include fighting, grandiosity, hypervigilance, psychomotor agitation, impaired judgment, and impaired social or occupational functioning. Tachycardia, pupillary dilation, elevated blood pressure, perspiration or chills, nausea or vomiting, and visual or tactile hallucinations are signs that may present within 1 hour of use.

With prolonged cocaine administration, a transient delusional psychosis, simulating paranoid schizophrenia, can be seen. Usually these symptoms remit, although heavy prolonged use or predisposing psychopathology may result in persistence of psychosis. Generally, higher doses distinguish overdose from simple intoxication. Cocaine abuse tends to occur in binge patterns. In humans, cocaine binges can last a few hours to several days, are highly reinforcing, and may lead to psychosis or death.

Pharmacology

Cocaine hydrochloride is a white crystal powder derived from coca leaves and coca paste. It is usually diluted, or "stepped on," to 20% pure by mixing it with other local anesthetics such as lidocaine, procaine, and various sugars. Cocaine freebase is a by-product in which the hydrochloride salt is removed by various substances. "Crack" or "rock" is a prepackaged freebased derivative ready for smoking. Intranasal cocaine's half-life is less than 90 minutes, with euphoric effects lasting 15 to 30 minutes. Most cocaine is hydrolyzed in the body to benzoylecgonine, which can be detected in the urine for up to 36 hours.

Cocaine blocks neuronal dopamine, serotonin, and norepinephrine reuptake. Dopaminergic pathways involving the ventral tegmental area, frontal lobe, septum, amygdala, and particularly the nucleus accumbens are important in reinforcing behavior (Roberts et al. 1977). The actions of cocaine on brain dopaminergic systems are essential to the drug's reinforcing properties, and cocaine-induced increase in dopamine neurotransmission appears prominent in its acute behavioral effects. Dopamine can increase psychomotor activity, induce stereotypical behavior, and decrease food consumption. Dopamine is involved in limbic pleasure centers, including those associated with food and sex. With repeated cocaine use, tolerance to cocaine's effect develops that may be due to hypothesized decreases in reuptake inhibition, decreased release of catecholamines, or catecholamine receptor sensitivity changes, either postsynaptic desensitization or presynaptic supersensitization. PET studies suggest that postsynaptic dopamine receptor availability decreases with chronic cocaine abuse (Volkow et al. 1990).

Abstinence Symptomatology

Using structural diagnostic interviews in a longitudinal fashion, Gawin and Kleber (1986) identified three phases of abstinence symptomatology, with possible implications for intervention and future biological research. Phase 1 consisted of the immediate postuse cocaine dysphoria known as "the crash." During prolonged intoxication, subjects reported receiving diminished euphoric effects from larger doses. Major depressive features and suicidal ideation can be prominent. Sedative agents such as benzodiazepines and alcohol were used as self-medication in attempts to sleep. Phase 1 lasted up to 3 days.

In Phase 2, low-level cocaine craving continued, with irritability, anxiety, and decreased capacity to experience pleasure. Frequently, this led to another binge cycle, which sometimes repeated itself every 3 to 10 days. If the first two phases were successfully completed, Phase 3, a period of milder episodic craving lasting several weeks, developed in a context of conditioned environmental stimuli. Many patients appeared to have a major depressive disorder shortly after cocaine cessation, but most of these symptoms eventually cleared.

Adverse Medical Sequelae

Cocaine has been associated with acute and chronic ailments. Chronic intranasal use can lead to septal necrosis due to vasoconstriction and subsequent dilation, producing nasal stuffiness and "the runs." The anesthetic properties of cocaine may lead to oral numbness and dental neglect. Malnutrition, severe weight loss, and dehydration often result from cocaine binges. Intravenous cocaine use complicated by impurities may produce endocarditis, septicemia, HIV spread, local vasculitis, hepatitis B, emphysema, pulmonary emboli, and granulomas. Freebase cocaine has been associated with decreased pulmonary exchange, and pulmonary dysfunction may persist (Itkomen et al. 1984). Intravenous cocaine injection sites are characterized by prominent ecchymosis, whereas those persons using opioids intravenously more frequently show needle scars.

Positive cocaine urine test results have been found increasingly in homicide victims, those arrested for murder, and those who die by overdose. In New York City, one out of every five persons who had completed suicide during a 1-year period had used cocaine immediately prior to committing suicide (Marzuk et al. 1992). Deaths among persons who use cocaine recreationally in low doses have been reported. Acute agitation, diaphoresis, tachycardia, metabolic and respiratory acidosis, cardiac dysrhythmia, and grand mal seizures can lead ultimately to respiratory arrest. Treatment of seizures and acidosis is essential, and intravenous propranolol and diazepam have been helpful adjuncts (Jonsson et al. 1983). Recurrent myocardial infarction in cocaine use associated with tachycardia and coronary vasoconstriction has been reported. Myocarditis and myocardial ischemia have all been reported to be associated with cocaine use (Nadamanee et al. 1989; Virmani et al. 1988).

☐ Interaction With Other Disorders

There may be a significant subset of patients with underlying affective mood disorder (cyclothymic or dysthymic); narcissistic, borderline, or antisocial personality disorder; other Axis I substance abuse; or attention-deficit disorder (Weiss and Mirin 1986). Weiss et al. (1988) reported lower levels of affective disorders. In cocaine-using subjects who sought treatment, 55% had a current psychiatric diagnosis other than substance abuse, and 73% had a lifetime diagnosis (Rounsaville et al. 1991). These subjects may differ from untreated cocaine-addicted individuals. Carroll and Rounsaville (1992) found that untreated cocaine-abusing subjects had higher levels of polysubstance abuse, fewer negative consequences of cocaine use, lower levels of participation in adult social roles, greater involvement with the legal system and with illegal activities, and a diminished sense of negative consequences of their use despite comparable severity of abuse and psychiatric symptomatology. Affective disorders and alcoholism usually followed the onset of drug abuse, whereas anxiety disorders, antisocial personality disorder, and attention-deficit disorder preceded drug abuse.

Depressed cocaine-addicted subjects in one study had started to use tobacco, marijuana, and cocaine at a significantly earlier age (Kleinman et al. 1990). Patients with attention-deficit disorder may, when not diagnosed or treated with methylphenidate, self-medicate with cocaine, which paradoxically sedates, decreases stimulation, and improves concentration. The majority of persons using cocaine do not have Axis I diagnoses other than those related to substance abuse. Several studies have highlighted the use of cocaine in schizophrenia (Salloum et al. 1991; Schneier and Siris 1987; Sevy et al. 1990). Compared with other psychiatric patients, schizophrenic patients seem to have higher rates of stimulant use and lower rates of alcohol abuse. This suggests that many schizophrenic individuals may be treating negative symptoms of their disease, despite the fact that stimulant abuse may worsen their prognosis (Brady et al. 1990). Persons using cocaine heavily who experience transient paranoia while intoxicated may be at higher risk for development of psychosis than those cocaine-using individuals who do not experience paranoia (Satel and Edell 1991).

☐ Treatment

The principles of cocaine rehabilitation are similar to treatment of alcoholism or sedativism, although new approaches have taken into account unique features of cocaine dependency. Patterns of use, administration, and psychopathological features are the main determinants of treatment choice.

Psychological Treatments

Kleber and Gawin (1986) recommend an initial trial of outpatient non-pharmacological treatment, especially for those who have passed the initial cocaine crash and craving. In uncomplicated cases, outpatient treatment has the advantage of keeping patients in their natural environment, allowing them to better master everyday temptations and conflicts. Inpatient hospitalization may be needed for severe crash symptoms, suicidal ideation, or psychotic symptoms. Washton (1990) recommends inpatient treatment for 1) chronic freebase or intravenous use, 2) concurrent dependency on other addictive drugs or alcohol, 3) serious medical or psychiatric problems, 4) severe impairment of psychosocial functioning, 5) insufficient motivation for outpatient treatment, 6) lack of family and supports, or 7) failure in outpatient treatment.

Initial treatment strategy focuses on confronting denial, teaching the disease concept of addictions, fostering in the patient an identification as a recovering person, rediscovering shades of affect, helping the patient to recognize the ambivalent relationship with cocaine, helping the patient to avoid situational and intrapsychic cues that stimulate craving, and formulating support plans. Carroll et al. (1991a) compared two purely psychotherapeutic treatments of cocaine abuse: relapse prevention and interpersonal psychotherapy. Those subjects with severe abuse who received relapse prevention treatment achieved abstinence significantly better than did those who received interpersonal therapy (59% versus 9%). Individuals with lower-severity abuse had no difference in outcome. Relapse prevention addresses ambivalence and strives to reduce cocaine availability, minimize high risk situations and develop coping strategies, recognize conditioned cues to craving, recognize decision patterns that can lead into actual use, and obtain a lifestyle modification with behavioral alternatives to cocaine use (Carroll et al. 1991b).

Behavior therapy contingency contracting can involve either positive or negative contingency contracting (Anker and Crowly 1982). One form of aversion conditioning is "Ulysses contracting," in which the patient thinks of the worst scenario of continued cocaine use. This adverse effect is then structured by written agreement with the therapist to occur after the next use of cocaine. This often takes a form of letters to employers or family members. Drug urine tests are given to ensure compliance. The constant reminder of the adverse consequences of cocaine is the most salient feature of this approach.

Alcohol and other mood-altering drugs should be avoided during treatment. Concurrent Axis I or II psychiatric disorders should be treated, with attention to the interaction with cocaine disorder. Treatment of clearly defined attention-deficit disorder or bipolar or unipolar depression should proceed along with attention to the addiction. Treatment of additional psychoactive disorders will be impossible if the addiction is not addressed.

Pharmacological Treatment

Cocaine intoxication, agitation, and anxiety can be treated with diazepam or, in persistent cases, propranolol. If cocaine psychosis persists, haloperidol or the more sedating chlorpromazine is effective. A schizophreniform picture may develop in some cocaine-using individuals, requiring continuing neuroleptic use.

Mirin and Weiss (1991) proposed four classes of pharmacological treatment for cocaine abuse: 1) antagonists, 2) aversive agents, 3) drugs that treat premorbid coexisting psychiatric disorders, and 4) drugs that treat cocaine-induced states such as intoxication, withdrawal, and craving. Kosten and Kosten (1991) reviewed blocking agents for cocaine and other stimulants. Mazindol, a competitor for the catecholamine reuptake carrier, and haloperidol, a D_2-receptor blocker, in theory could act as cocaine antagonists but have not been found to be clinically useful. Aversive agents have received scant attention. Experimental treatments of cocaine withdrawal, anhedonia, and craving have been based on neurobiological findings in cocaine use. More recently, dopamine autoreceptor supersensitivity has been related to the cocaine withdrawal syndrome. Flupentixol decanoate, a dopamine-blocking agent that is an antidepressant at low doses, in a preliminary study was found to have promise in decreasing craving in crack cocaine use (Gawin et al. 1989). Desipramine and nortriptyline are more potent norepinephrine reuptake blockers; however, Fischman et al. (1990) found that cocaine administration was not attenuated by desipramine and was associated with irritability and cardiovascular toxicity.

Until positive findings are well replicated and safety is well established, clinicians should be cautious about the use of antidepressants as an adjunct analogous to naltrexone in patients who are actively abusing cocaine and other substances. Low-dose desipramine has been found to be useful in the treatment of cocaine-related panic attacks (Bystritsky et al. 1991).

■ AMPHETAMINES

Amphetamines, or "speed," are compounds with stimulant and reinforcing effects similar to those of cocaine. Amphetamines block reuptake of dopamine, serotonin, and norepinephrine similarly to cocaine but produce more profound effects on dopamine storage release. Central stimulant drugs such as dextroamphetamine and methylphenidate are manufactured for the treatment of medical conditions such as narcolepsy and attention-deficit hyperactivity disorder. Illegal "black market" diversion and abuse peaked in the late 1960s.

The signs and symptoms of amphetamine use include tachycardia, elevated blood pressure, pupillary dilation, agitation, elation, loquacity, and hypervigilance. Adverse side effects may include insomnia, irritability, confusion, and hostility. Amphetamine psychosis can resemble acute paranoid schizophrenia, but visual hallucinations are common. As in cocaine use, binge episodes or runs may alternate with severe crash symptoms (Table 11–8). Patients who use amphetamines daily or intravenously may require a period of inpatient hospitalization for depression, suicidal ideation during withdrawal, psychosis, or violence during intoxication. Antipsychotic medication such as haloperidol may be needed to treat paranoid or delusional symptoms. Rehabilitation should include a comprehensive treatment approach, as described in the alcohol and cocaine sections earlier in this chapter.

■ PHENCYCLIDINE ("ANGEL DUST")

Phencyclidine (PCP) is an anesthetic that was initially manufactured for use in animal surgery. Street use of PCP first appeared in the 1960s and

---

Table 11–8. DSM-IV criteria for amphetamine (or a related substance) intoxication

A. Recent use of amphetamine or a related substance (e.g., methylphenidate).

B. Clinically significant maladaptive behavioral or psychological changes (e.g., euphoria or affective blunting; changes in sociability; hypervigilance; interpersonal sensitivity; anxiety, tension, or anger; stereotyped behaviors; impaired judgment; or impaired social or occupational functioning) that developed during, or shortly after, use of amphetamine or a related substance.

C. Two (or more) of the following, developing during, or shortly after, use of amphetamine or a related substance:
1. Tachycardia or bradycardia
2. Pupillary dilation
3. Elevated or lowered blood pressure
4. Perspiration or chills
5. Nausea or vomiting
6. Evidence of weight loss
7. Psychomotor agitation or retardation
8. Muscular weakness, respiratory depression, chest pain, or cardiac arrhythmias
9. Confusion, seizures, dyskinesias, dystonias, or coma

D. The symptoms are not due to a general medical condition and are not better accounted for by another mental disorder.

Specify if:
With perceptual disturbances

---

extended to widespread use in the 1970s. Street samples sold as PCP may vary greatly in dose and purity. Smoking marijuana cigarettes laced with PCP is the most common form of administration.

Phencyclidine has been reported to be reinforcing in animals (Grinspoon and Bakalar 1986). Although the mechanism of action is unclear, PCP has been known to affect several neurotransmitters and to affect the sigma opiate receptor. The DSM-IV definition of PCP abuse and dependence is defined as for other drugs (Tables 11–1 and 11–2). Phencyclidine abuse may occur in conjunction with multiple substance abuse and be associated with similar risk factors. Cases of pure PCP abuse have been reported. In our experience, these individuals appear to have significant psychopathology; however, it is difficult to distinguish drug effects from premorbid personality.

☐ Clinical Features

Psychoactive effects generally begin within 5 minutes and plateau at 30 minutes. Phencyclidine induces several organic mental disorders including intoxication, delirium, and delusional, mood, and flashback disorders. Volatile emotional affects are the predominant behavioral presentation, ranging from intense euphoria to anxiety, stereotypical repetitive behavior, and bizarre aggressive behavior. Violent murders have been attributed to complications of PCP abuse. Distorted perceptions, numbness, and confusion also are common. Physical signs include high blood pressure, muscle rigidity, ataxia, and, at higher dosages, hyperthermia, involuntary movements, and coma. Rhabdomyolysis in overdoses may lead to acute renal failure. Dilated pupils and nystagmus, particularly vertical nystagmus, may heighten suspicion of use. Chronic psychotic episodes are reported following use. Use of PCP may lead to long-term neuropsychological deficits (Davis 1982).

☐ Treatment

Acute adverse reactions generally require pharmacological adjuncts to control symptoms. Intravenous diazepam is the drug of first choice, but antipsychotics may occasionally be necessary as long as they are used with caution, because of the possibility of anticholinergic psychosis in unknown cases. When the diagnosis is unclear, other causes of delirium need to be considered. Because other supportive treatment may be necessary, treatment in a medical setting is preferred.

■ HALLUCINOGENS

Hallucinogens have not been reported to be reinforcing in animal studies. In humans, actual psychedelic use is infrequent, and psychedelic use greater than 20 times is considered chronic abuse. The DSM-IV definition of abuse and dependence is presented in Tables 11–1 and 11–2. Hallucinogen intoxication (DSM-IV) is defined in Table 11–9. Other disorders included in DSM-IV are hallucinogen persisting perception disorder (flashbacks); hallucinogen delirium; hallucinogen psychotic disorder, with delusions; hallucinogen psychotic disorder, with hallucinations; hallucinogen mood disorder; hallucinogen anxiety disorder; and hallucinogen use disorder not otherwise specified.

Lysergic acid diethylamide (LSD) and related drugs produce changes in perception that vary greatly with setting and user's personality. Rather intense perceptual changes in time, space, and body image can occur. Illusions and pseudohallucinations, primarily visual, can predominate in conjunction with intense emotional or mystical experiences. Generally, overall reality testing and orientation are preserved. "Flashbacks" are psychedelic drug experiences that occur spontaneously in the absence of concurrent use. These may occur in as many as 25% of users (Naditch and Fenwick 1977). Large numbers of prior psychedelic experiences, marijuana smoking, and emotional stress are common precipitating factors.

Chronic delusional and psychotic reactions, and rarely schizophreni-

---

Table 11–9.   DSM-IV criteria for hallucinogen intoxication

A.   Recent use of a hallucinogen.

B.   Clinically significant maladaptive behavioral or psychological changes (e.g., marked anxiety or depression, ideas of reference, fear of losing one's mind, paranoid ideation, impaired judgment, or impaired social or occupational functioning) that developed during, or shortly after, hallucinogen use.

C.   Perceptual changes occurring in a state of full wakefulness and alertness (e.g., subjective intensification of perceptions, depersonalization, derealization, illusions, hallucinations, synesthesias) that developed during, or shortly after, hallucinogen use.

D.   Two (or more) of the following signs, developing during, or shortly after, hallucinogen use:
      1.   Pupillary dilation
      2.   Tachycardia
      3.   Sweating
      4.   Palpitations
      5.   Blurring of vision
      6.   Tremors
      7.   Incoordination

E.   The symptoms are not due to a general medical condition and are not better accounted for by another mental disorder.

---

form states, have been reported in a minority of persons who use psyche-delics (Vardy and Kay 1983). In the vast majority of users, no characteristic personality is evident. Most use can be classified as experimental. Individuals who develop prolonged psychiatric syndromes tend to have schizophrenic susceptibility based on genetic or personality vulnerabilities. Generally, intoxicated patients can be "talked down" from frightening experiences in a quiet setting with minimal stimuli, stressing the time-limited extent of the drugs. Occasionally, diazepam is used as an adjunct, and rarely antipsychotics are needed in the case of marked disturbance.

■ CANNABIS

Three cannabis-related organic disorders are listed in the DSM-IV: 1) cannabis intoxication, 2) cannabis delirium, and 3) cannabis delusional disorder. Definitions of cannabis abuse and dependence follow definitions of other psychoactive substances (Tables 11–1 and 11–2). There is no cannabis withdrawal diagnosis in DSM-IV. Based on case reports, withdrawal symptoms in persons who chronically use high doses of cannabis have included anxiety, dysphoria, insomnia, anorexia, tremulousness, and sweating.

☐ Epidemiology

In 1979, more than 50 million people had used marijuana at least once. Alcohol, tobacco, and marijuana are the most frequent substances of abuse among adolescents. Adolescence and early adulthood are the peak ages of prevalence for marijuana abuse, and risk factors for this period have been most studied. A 1982 NIDA survey revealed that 21% of young teenagers, 40% of young adults ages 18 to 25, and only 10% of older adults had tried marijuana (Miller 1983). It is generally acknowledged that marijuana use among adolescents peaked in the late 1970s, and, possibly because of less peer approval, regular marijuana use dropped from 51% to 42% between 1979 and 1983. Daily users of marijuana dropped from 10.2% in 1978 to 5% in 1984. The regular use of marijuana had a disapproval rating among adolescents of 83% in 1983.

☐ Clinical Features

Peak intoxication with smoking generally occurs after 10 to 30 minutes, when delta-9-THC levels are maximal. Highly lipid soluble, delta-9-THC and metabolites tend to accumulate in fat cells and have a half-life of approximately 50 hours. Most marijuana cigarettes contain 5 to 20 mg of delta-9-THC (Jaffe 1980). Intoxication usually lasts from 2 to 4 hours depending on the dose used; however, behavioral and psychomotor impairment may continue several hours longer. Oral ingestion of marijuana produces a slower onset of intoxication (45 to 60 minutes) and more powerful psychoactive effects.

Intoxication can produce many subjective psychoactive effects that become the "high" experience repeatedly sought (Halikas et al. 1971). Persons who use marijuana experience slowed time; increased appetite; increased thirst; a keener sense of color, sound, pattern, textures, and tastes; euphoria; heightened introspection; ability to be absorbed in sensual experiences; feelings of relaxation and floating; and increased self-confidence. Other subjective symptoms include heightened sexual desire, transitory illusions, hallucinations, and increased interpersonal sensitivity. Conjunctivitis (i.e., red eyes), strong odor, dilated pupils, tachycardia, dry mouth, and coughing are physical signs of immediate use. Adverse effects such as mild anxiety, depression, and paranoia are infrequently treated in a medical setting and usually are not a deterrent to further use. Behavior may be marked by passivity and sedation or by hyperactivity and marked hilarity.

Numerous studies have outlined the neuropsychological changes and deficits related to marijuana intoxication, although effects can be highly variable. Decreases have been found in complex reaction time and digit code memory tasks, concept formation, memory, tactile form discrimination, motor function, time estimation, and the ability to track information over time (Klonoff et al. 1973). Psychosis, derealization, and aggression have been described to occur rarely. Weller and Halikas (1985) followed 97 persons who regularly used marijuana over a 5- to 6-year period. Continued use was associated with a decrease in pleasurable effects. Undesirable effects persisted, but decreases were found in tachycardia, dry mouth, and lightheadedness. Numerous studies have demonstrated that marijuana intoxication impairs automobile driving, airplane flying, and other complex skilled activities through impaired attention span, motor coordination, and depth perception for up to 10 hours or more after use.

Delta-9-THC–induced acute toxic psychosis has been described in first-time users and chronic users and may include organic features or persist in a clear consciousness (Spencer 1970; Weil 1970). Psychosis can present suddenly with first-rank Schneiderian symptoms, agitation, and amnesia for toxic events. Thacore and Shukla (1976) found that, compared with paranoid schizophrenia, cannabis psychosis is characterized by agitation, violence, flight of ideas, and less thought disorder. Prolonged psychotic episodes may herald residual psychopathology. Cannabis can precipitate "flashbacks" or psychotic experiences from past psychedelic or marijuana experiences.

Differential diagnosis of cannabis psychosis and schizophrenia can be difficult; however, assessment of past history, urine testing, and the short-lived nature of toxic symptoms usually help in making the diagnosis. Millman and Sbriglio (1986) suggested that by attributing their symptoms to marijuana abuse, some schizophrenic individuals may distance themselves from their underlying illness. In summary, marijuana use should be especially cautioned in individuals prone to psychotic illness.

☐ Etiology

Studies on the etiology of marijuana abuse have tended to focus on adolescent developmental issues and have not found simple generalizable factors. Kandel and Faust (1975) found that teenage use of liquor and cigarettes is associated with the highest rates of future marijuana abuse. The temporal order between alcohol and marijuana may be stronger than that between tobacco and marijuana. Marijuana use was found to be a key stepping-stone to other illicit drugs, and progression to harder drugs was directly related to the intensity of marijuana use. Recently, adolescents increasingly proceed to cocaine without extensive marijuana use. Marijuana introduces youth to drug subcultures and lowers inhibition to use of other drugs. Peer drug use, parents' substance use, and low parental monitoring are risk factors for marijuana abuse. Delinquency is a risk factor for abuse of marijuana and other substances; however, peer group choice is usually with other drug-using individuals more so than with delinquent persons. Kandel (1984) suggested that marijuana use in young adulthood is associated with a social context favorable to its use and with disaffection from social institutions. High-risk factors may operate independent of personality.

☐ Pathophysiology

In vitro studies have reported abnormal cell division and abnormal spermatogenesis, resulting in decreased sperm counts. High delta-9-THC exposure has been associated with birth and reproductive abnormalities in animals, and decreases in female sexual and reproductive hormones have been found in humans. However, marijuana's effect on human male or female fertility remains controversial.

Patients with underlying cardiovascular disease may not tolerate the increased heart rate and blood pressure that marijuana causes. Marijuana may have a mild immunosuppressant effect. Cannabis smoke contains carcinogens similar to those in tobacco smoke, and chronic heavy marijuana use may predispose to chronic obstructive lung disease or pulmonary neoplasm. A spectrum of cognitive and behaviorial difficulty may result secondarily to long-term cannabis abuse. Apathy and lack of motivation in these patients may represent one pole of the spectrum and may be the result of multiple factors (Millman and Sbriglio 1986).

☐ Treatment

Usually adverse effects of marijuana intoxication do not lead to professional attention. Support, reassurance, and reality testing by friends or family usually suffice. Physical symptoms such as tachycardia may contribute to a "fight or flight syndrome." Pointing out that marijuana can cause these symptoms and reassurance that they will pass usually helps these individuals. Anxiolytic agents occasionally are needed, and neuroleptics can be used in cases of protracted psychosis.

The treatment of marijuana abuse follows the general principles for that of other substance abuse, with special attention to developmental issues affecting adolescence. Marijuana abuse rarely requires inpatient treatment, and detoxification is not necessary. Occasionally with severe abuse or behavioral problems, especially in teenage populations, inpatient intervention is needed. Outpatient treatment consists of self-help 12-step groups, group and individual therapy, family therapy, and periodic urine testing to monitor abstinence. Adolescent drug programs may concentrate on promoting age-related behavior and increasing communication through various verbal and nonverbal modalities. Families need to become aware of how they can help or hurt the treatment process.

■ NICOTINE

Tobacco addiction is the number one preventable health problem in the United States. Awareness of the health risk factors associated with tobacco use has existed since the 1950s. Despite educational campaigns, self-help groups, self-help literature, treatment facilities, and governmental legislation, all attempting to decrease the numbers of smokers, tobacco addiction remains a significant but scientifically neglected area of research and treatment.

In DSM-IV, tobacco is listed under psychoactive substance use disorders. Tobacco's main psychoactive substance is nicotine. Nicotine is a psychoactive substance as evidenced by euphoric effects and by placebo and positive reinforcement properties similar to those of cocaine and opiates (Henningfield 1984). Tolerance develops to the effects of nicotine, and mild withdrawal syndromes have been described. Hughes and Hatsukami (1986) tested the signs and symptoms of tobacco withdrawal and found evidence of craving for tobacco, irritability, anxiety, difficulty concentrating, and restlessness. Decreased heart rate, increased eating, increased sleep disturbance, and decreased alcohol intake were also found.

☐ Etiology

Cigarette smoking generally begins in the teenage years and may be associated with peer tobacco use, parental tobacco use, and other substance abuse. Individuals may smoke for a period of time, attempt to quit, and then relapse. Tobacco addiction has many properties that are similar to those of opioid addiction. There is great similarity between cigarettes, alcoholism, and opioids in the temporal pattern of relapse, and circumstantial evidence suggests that tobacco use is usually an addictive form of behavior. High stress, poor social support, maladjustment, anxiety, and low self-confidence have been associated with poor treatment outcome, and these factors may play a part in promoting continued use. Psychological characteristics such as extraversion, anxiety, and anger have been proposed to be associated with tobacco use. There is a strong association between alcohol and smoking, especially in women and alcoholic persons.

☐ Clinical Features

Tobacco use can produce a calming, euphoric effect on chronic users, more characteristic after a period of tobacco deprivation. Acute nicotine poisoning consists of nausea, salivation, abdominal pain, vomiting and diarrhea, headaches, dizziness, and a cold sweat. Inability to concentrate, confusion, and tachycardia may also result. There are well-known associations between tobacco use and chronic obstructive lung disease, lung cancer, oral cancers, and hypertension. Tobacco use may complicate prescribed psychiatric medication by increasing liver drug metabolism and lowering neuroleptic and antidepressant levels. Low birth weight has been associated with smoking in pregnant mothers. This information has led to a decrease in smoking in pregnant women.

☐ Treatment

Various treatment approaches, including behavioral, cognitive, educational, self-help, and pharmacological, have been applied to tobacco addiction. Yet the vast majority (95%) of abstainers receive no formal intervention, and research is needed to clarify how and why these individuals ceased use. Environmental stress; poor social support, including having family members who continue to smoke; lack of exposure to educational information; being female; poor overall adjustment; low self-confidence; poor motivation; and high pretreatment cotinine (a metabolite of nicotine) levels were associated with poor long-term outcome (Tunstall et al. 1985).

Nicotine gum chewing is a pharmacological substitution approach in which smoking behavior is interrupted while blood levels of nicotine are maintained to minimize withdrawal (Raw 1985). Three-month success rates of 76% and 1-year success rates of 50% have been reported. Effectiveness is maximized with therapeutic contact. However, considerable relapse after gum use is terminated has been found (Hall et al. 1985). Hypnosis, rapid smoking, or aversive treatment and nicotine blockade with mecamylamine are other alternative treatments. The 1-year post-intervention effectiveness of most intensive smoking cessation programs is between 25% to 40%, which roughly parallels the postintervention effectiveness of programs for other substance abuse. Studies have demonstated successful outcomes using transdermal nicotine patches in combination with some form of behavioral smoking cessation intervention.

■ INHALANTS

Inhalants include substances with diverse chemical structures such as gasoline, airplane glue, aerosol (spray paints), lighter fluid, fingernail polish remover, typewriter fluid, a variety of cleaners, amyl and butyl nitrates, and nitrous oxide. Hydrocarbons are the most active ingredients. In 1980, 10% of 12- to 17-year-olds had reported using inhalants at least once, but the vast majority did not report abuse patterns (NIDA 1981).

A predominant number of persons who use inhalants are socio-economically deprived young males ages 13 to 15 years (Watson 1980). A high prevalence of abuse is found among Native American and Mexican Indians (Reed and May 1984). Amyl nitrate use was popular in the 1970s in a subset of the homosexual community, and nitrous oxide abuse may be predominant among health personnel with easy access, such as dentists. Typical signs and symptoms of intoxication may include grandiosity, a sense of invulnerability, immense strength, euphoria, slurred speech, and ataxia. Visual distortions and faulty space perception are also common.

■ REFERENCES

Adams EH, Durell J: Cocaine: a growing public health problem, in Cocaine: Pharmacology, Effects, and Treatment of Abuse (NIDA Res Monogr No 50; DHHS Publ No ADM 84-1326). Edited by Grabowski J. Rockville, MD, National Institute of Drug Abuse, 1984, pp 9–14

Adams RD, Victor M: Principles of Neurology. New York, McGraw-Hill, 1981

American Psychiatric Association: Diagnostic and Statistical Manual of Mental Disorders, 4th Edition. Washington, DC, American Psychiatric Association, 1994

Anker AL, Crowly TJ: Use of contingency contracting in specialty clinics for cocaine abuse, in Problems of Drug Dependence 1981 (NIDA Drug Res Monogr No 41). Edited by Harris LS. Rockville, MD, National Institute on Drug Abuse, 1982, pp 452–459

Bachman JG, Johnston LD, O'Malley PM: Explaining the recent decline in cocaine use among young adults: further evidence that perceived risks and disapproval lead to reduced drug use. J Health Soc Behav 31:173–184, 1990

Bergman H, Borg S, Holin L: Neuropsychological impairment and exclusive abuse of sedatives or hypnotics. Am J Psychiatry 137:215–217, 1980

Blass JP, Gibson GE: Abnormality of a thiamine-requiring enzyme in patients with Wernicke-Korsakoff syndrome. N Engl J Med 297:1367–1370, 1977

Blatt SJ, Berman W, Bloom-Feshbach S, et al: Psychological assessment of psychopathology in opiate addicts. J Nerv Ment Dis 172:156–165, 1984

Blum K, Noble EP, Sheridan PJ, et al: Allelic association of human dopamine D_2 receptor gene in alcoholism. JAMA 263:2055–2060, 1990

Bohman M, Cloninger CR, Sigvardsson S, et al: The genetics of alcoholism and related disorders. J Psychiatr Res 21:447–452, 1987

Bolos AM, Dean M, Lucas-Derse S, et al: Population and pedigree studies reveal a lack of association between the dopamine D_2 receptor gene and alcoholism. JAMA 264:3156–3160, 1990

Brady K, Anton R, Ballenger JC, et al: Cocaine abuse among schizophrenic patients. Am J Psychiatry 147:1164–1167, 1990

Brew BJ: Diagnosis of Wernicke's encephalopathy. Aust N Z J Med 16:676–678, 1986

Brown BS, Watters JK, Iglehart AS: Methadone maintenance dosage levels and program retention. Am J Drug Alcohol Abuse 9:129–139, 1982

Bystritsky A, Ackerman DL, Pasnau RO: Low dose desipramine treatment of cocaine-related panic attacks. J Nerv Ment Dis 179:755–758, 1991

Carroll KM, Rounsaville BJ: Contrast of treatment-seeking and untreated cocaine abusers. Arch Gen Psychiatry 49:464–471, 1992

Carroll KM, Rounsaville BJ, Gawin FH: A comparative trial of psychotherapies for ambulatory cocaine abusers: relapse prevention and interpersonal psychotherapy. Am J Drug Alcohol Abuse 17:229–247, 1991a

Carroll KM, Rounsaville FJ, Keller DS: Relapse prevention strategies for the treatment of cocaine abuse. Am J Drug Alcohol Abuse 17:249–265, 1991b

Charney DS, Redmond E, Galloway MP: Naltrexone precipitated opiate withdrawal in methadone addicted human subjects: evidence for noradrenergic hyperactivity. Life Sci 35:1263–1272, 1984

Cloninger RC, Reich T, Wetzel R: Alcoholism and affective disorders: familial associations and genetic models, in Alcoholism and Affective Disorders. Edited by Goodwin DW, Erickson CK. Jamaica, NY, Spectrum, 1979, pp 57–86

Crowley TJ, Wagner JE, Zerbe G, et al: Naltrexone-induced dysphoria in former opioid addicts. Am J Psychiatry 142:1081–1084, 1985

Davis BL: The PCP epidemic: a critical review. Int J Addict 17:1137–1155, 1982

Deleon D, Weiller HK, Jainchill N: The therapeutic community: success and improvement rates five years after treatment. Int J Addict 17:703–747, 1982

Dietch J: The nature and extent of benzodiazepine abuse: an overview of recent literature. Hosp Community Psychiatry 34:1139–1145, 1983

Dole VP, Nyswander ME: A medical treatment of heroin addiction. JAMA 193:646–650, 1965

Drake RE, Osher FC, Wallach MA: Alcohol use and abuse in schizophrenia: a prospective community study. J Nerv Ment Dis 177:408–414, 1989

Dryman A, Anthony JC: An epidemiologic study of alcohol use as a predictor of psychiatric distress over time. Acta Psychiatr Scand 80:315–321, 1989

Dulit RA, Fyer MR, Haas GL, et al: Substance use in borderline personality disorder. Am J Psychiatry 147:1002–1007, 1990

Dupont RL, Saylor KE: Sedatives/hypnotics and benzodiazepines, in Clinical Textbook of Addictive Disorders. Edited by Frances RJ, Miller SI. New York, Guilford, 1991, pp 69–102

Espir ML, Rose FC: Alcohol, seizures and epilepsy. J R Soc Med 9:542–543, 1987

Ewing JA: Detecting alcoholism: the CAGE questionnaire. JAMA 252:1905–1907, 1984

Fischman MW, Foltin RW, Nestadt G, et al: Effects of desipramine maintenance on cocaine self-administration by humans. J Pharmacol Exp Ther 253:760–770, 1990

Frances RJ, Franklin JE: Concise Guide to Treatment of Alcoholism and Addictions. Washington, DC, American Psychiatric Press, 1989

Frances RJ, Bucky S, Alexopoulos GS: Outcome study of familial and nonfamilial alcoholism. Am J Psychiatry 141:1469–1471, 1984

Fraumeni JF Jr: Epidemiology of cancer, in Cecil Textbook of Medicine, 16th Edition. Edited by Wyngaarden JB, Smith LH. Philadelphia, PA, W B Saunders, 1982

Galizio M, Stein FS: Sensation seeking and drug choice. Int J Addict 18:1039–1048, 1983

Gawin FH, Kleber HD: Abstinence symptomatology and psychiatric diagnosis in cocaine abusers. Arch Gen Psychiatry 43:107–113, 1986

Gawin FH, Allen D, Humblestone B: Outpatient treatment of "crack" cocaine smoking with flupenthixol decanoate: a preliminary report. Arch Gen Psychiatry 46:322–325, 1989

Goldstein DB, Chin JH, Lyon RC: Ethanol disordering of spin-labeled mouse brain membranes: correlation with genetically determined ethanol sensitivity of mice. Proc Natl Acad Sci U S A 79:4231–4233, 1982

Goodwin DW: Alcoholism and alcoholic psychoses, in Comprehensive Textbook of Psychiatry/IV, 4th Edition, Vol 1. Edited by Kaplan HI, Sadock BJ. Baltimore, MD, Williams & Wilkins, 1985a, pp 1016–1026

Goodwin DW: Alcoholism and genetics: the sins of the fathers. Arch Gen Psychiatry 42:171–174, 1985b

Gottschalk L, McGuire F, Haser F, et al: Drug abuse deaths in nine cities: a survey report (NIDA Res Monogr No 29). Rockville, MD, National Institute of Drug Abuse, 1979

Greenstein RA, Arndt IC, McLellan AT, et al: Naltrexone: a clinical perspective. J Clin Psychiatry 45 (No 9, Sec 2):25–28, 1984

Grinspoon L, Bakalar JB: Psychedelics and arylcyclohexylamines, in Psychiatry Update: American Psychiatric Association Annual Review, Vol 5. Edited by Frances AJ, Hales RE. Washington, DC, American Psychiatric Press, 1986, pp 212–225

Halikas JA, Goodwin DW, Guze SB: Marijuana effects. JAMA 217:692–694, 1971

Hall SM, Tunstall C, Rugg D, et al: Nicotine gum and behavioral treatment in smoking cessation. J Consult Clin Psychol 53:256–258, 1985

Helzer JE, Camino GJ, Hwu H, et al: Alcoholism: a cross-national comparison of population surveys with the DIS, in Alcoholism: A Medical Disorder. Edited by Rose RM, Barrett J. New York, Raven, 1986

Hendrie CA: Opiate dependence and withdrawal: a new synthesis. Pharmacol Biochem Behav 23:863–870, 1985

Henningfield JE: Pharmacologic basis and treatment of cigarette smoking. J Clin Psychiatry 45 (No 12, Sec 2):24–34, 1984

Hughes JR, Hatsukami D: Signs and symptoms of tobacco withdrawal. Arch Gen Psychiatry 43:289–294, 1986

Itkomen J, Schnoll S, Glassroth J: Pulmonary dysfunction in freebase cocaine users. Arch Intern Med 144:2195–2197, 1984

Jaffe JH: Drug addiction and drug abuse, in Goodman and Gilman's Pharmacological Basis of Therapeutics, 6th Edition. Edited by Gilman AG, et al. New York, Macmillan, 1980, pp 535–584

Jaffe JH, Martin WR: Opioid analysis and analgesics and antagonists, in Goodman and Gilman's The Pharmacological Basis of Therapeutics, 7th Edition. Edited by Gilman AG, Goodman LS, Rall TW, et al. New York, Macmillan, 1985, pp 491–531

Jasinski DR, Johnson RE, Kocher TR: Clonidine in morphine withdrawal: differential effects on signs and symptoms. Arch Gen Psychiatry 42:1063–1066, 1985

Jonsson S, O'Meara M, Young JB: Acute cocaine poisoning. Am J Med 75:1061–1064, 1983

Joseph H, Appel P: Alcoholism and methadone treatment: consequences for the patient and program. Am J Drug Alcohol Abuse 11:37–53, 1985

Kandel DB: Marijuana users in young adulthood. Arch Gen Psychiatry 41:200–209, 1984

Kandel D[B], Faust R: Sequence and stages in patterns of adolescent drug use. Arch Gen Psychiatry 32:923–932, 1975

Kandel DB, Raveis VH: Cessation of illicit drug use in young adulthood. Arch Gen Psychiatry 46:109–116, 1989

Khantzian EJ: The self-medication hypotheses of addictive disorders: focus on heroin and cocaine dependence. Am J Psychiatry 142:1259–1264, 1985

Khantzian EJ, Treece C: DSM-III psychiatric diagnosis of narcotic addicts: recent findings. Arch Gen Psychiatry 42:1067–1071, 1985

Kleber HD, Gawin FH: Cocaine, in Psychiatry Update: American Psychiatric Association Annual Review, Vol 5. Edited by Frances AJ, Hales RE. Washington, DC, American Psychiatric Press, 1986, pp 160–185

Kleber HD, Topazian M, Gaspari J, et al: Clonidine and naltrexone in outpatient treatment of opioid withdrawal. Am J Drug Alcohol Abuse 13:1–18, 1987

Kleinman PH, Miller AB, Millman RB, et al: Psychopathology among cocaine abusers entering treatment. J Nerv Ment Dis 178:442–447, 1990

Klonoff H, Low M, Marcus A: Neuropsychological effects of marijuana. Canadian Medical Association Journal 108:150–157, 1973

Kosten TR: Neurobiology of abused drugs: opioids and stimulants. J Nerv Ment Dis 178:217–227, 1990

Kosten TR, Kleber HD: Strategies to improve compliance with narcotic antagonists. Am J Drug Alcohol Abuse 10:249–266, 1984

Kosten TA, Kosten TR: Pharmacological blocking agents for treating substance abuse J Nerv Ment Dis 179:583–592, 1991

Kushner MG, Sher KJ, Beitman BD: The relation between alcohol problems and the anxiety disorders. Am J Psychiatry 147:685–695, 1990

Lishman WA: Organic Psychiatry. Philadelphia, PA, J B Lippincott, 1978

Loranger AW, Tulis EH: Family history of alcoholism in borderline personality disorder. Arch Gen Psychiatry 42:153–157, 1985

Luborsky L, McLellan AT, Woody GE, et al: Therapist success and its determinants. Arch Gen Psychiatry 42:602–611, 1985

Marzuk PM, Tardiff K, Leon AC, et al: Prevalence of cocaine use among residents of New York City who committed suicide during a one-year period. Am J Psychiatry 149:371–375, 1992

McCord W, McCord J: Origins of Alcoholism. Stanford, CA, Stanford University Press, 1960

Metzger D, Woody G, De Philippis D, et al: Risk factors for needle sharing among methadone-treated patients. Am J Psychiatry 148:636–640, 1991

Milby JB: Methadone maintenance to abstinence: how many make it? J Nerv Ment Dis 176:409–422, 1988

Miller JD: National Survey on Drug Abuse, Main Findings, 1982. Rockville, MD, National Institute on Drug Abuse, 1983

Millman RB, Sbriglio R: Patterns of use and psychopathology in chronic marijuana users. Psychiatr Clin North Am 9:533–545, 1986

Mirin SM, Weiss RD: Substance abuse and mental illness, in Clinical Textbook of Addictive Disorders. Edited by Frances RJ, Miller SI. New York, Guilford, 1991, pp 271–298

Moss HB, Yao JK, Burns M, et al: Plasma GABA-like activity in response to ethanol challenge in men at high risk for alcoholism. Biol Psychiatry 27:617–625, 1990

Myers JK, Weissman MM, Tischler GL, et al: Six-month prevalence of psychiatric disorders in three communities: 1980–1982. Arch Gen Psychiatry 41:959–967, 1984

Nadamanee K, Gorelick DA, Josephson MA: Myocardial ischemia during cocaine withdrawal. Ann Intern Med 111:876–880, 1989

Naditch MP, Fenwick S: LSD flashbacks and ego functioning. J Abnorm Psychol 86:352–359, 1977

National Institute on Drug Abuse: Client Oriented Data Acquisition Process (CODAP), Annual Data and Quarterly Reports, Statistical Series D and E. Rockville, MD, NIADA/MHA, 1981

National Institute on Drug Abuse: Drug use among American high school students and other young adults: national trends through 1985 (DHHS Publ No ADM 86-1450). Rockville, MD, National Institute on Drug Abuse, 1986

Nestadt G, Romanoski AJ, Samuels JF, et al: The relationship between personality and DSM-III Axis I disorders in the population: results from an epidemiological survey. Am J Psychiatry 149:1228–1233, 1992

Noordsy DL, Drake RE, Teague GB, et al: Subjective experiences related to alcohol use among schizophrenics. J Nerv Ment Dis 179:410–414, 1991

Novick DM, Pascarelli EF, Joseph H: Methadone maintenance patients in general medical practice: a preliminary report. JAMA 259:3299–3302, 1988

O'Brien CP, Woody GE: Sedative-hypnotics and antianxiety agents, in Psychiatry Update: American Psychiatric Association Annual Review, Vol 5. Edited by Frances AJ, Hales RE. Washington, DC, American Psychiatric Press, 1986, pp 186–199

Perlstadt H, Hembroff LA, Zonia SC: Changes in status, attitude and behavior toward alcohol and drugs on a university campus. Family and Community Health 14:44–62, 1991

Pope HG Jr, Ionescu-Pioggia M, Aizley HG, et al: Drug use and life-style among college undergraduates in 1989: a comparison with 1969 and 1978. Am J Psychiatry 147:998–1001, 1990

Raw M: Does nicotine chewing gum work? BMJ 290:1231–1232, 1985

Redmond DE, Krystal JH: Multiple mechanisms of withdrawal from opioid drugs. Annu Rev Neurosci 7:443–478, 1984

Reed BJ, May PA: Inhalant abuse and juvenile delinquency: a control study in Albuquerque, New Mexico. Int J Addict 19:789–803, 1984

Regier Da, Farmer ME, Rae DS, et al: Comorbidity of mental disorders with alcohol and other drug abuse: results from the Epidemiologic Catchment Area (ECA) study. JAMA 264:2511–2518, 1990

Resnick RB, Schuyten-Resnick E, Washton AM: Assessment of narcotic antagonists in the treatment of opiate dependence. Annu Rev Pharmacol Toxicol 20:463–474, 1980

Reuler JB, Girard DE, Cooney TG: Wernicke's encephalopathy. N Engl J Med 312:1035–1039, 1985

* Rickels K, Case WG, Downing RW, et al: Long-term diazepam therapy and clinical outcome. JAMA 251:767–771, 1983

Roberts DC, Corcoran ME, Fibiger HC: On the role of ascending catecholaminergic systems in intravenous self-administration of cocaine. Pharmacol Biochem Behav 6:615–620, 1977

Robins LN, Helzer JE, Weissman MM, et al: Lifetime prevalence of specific psychiatric disorders in three sites. Arch Gen Psychiatry 41:949–958, 1984

Rosett HL, Weiner L: Alcohol and the Fetus: A Clinical Perspective. New York, Oxford University Press, 1984

Rounsaville BJ, Weissman MM, Kleber H[D], et al: The heterogeneity of psychiatric diagnosis in treated opiate addicts. Arch Gen Psychiatry 39:161–166, 1982

Rounsaville BJ, Kosten TR, Weissman MM, et al: Prognostic significance of psychopathology in treated opiate addicts: a 2.5-year follow-up. Arch Gen Psychiatry 43:739–745, 1986

Rounsaville BJ, Anton SF, Carroll K, et al: Psychiatric diagnoses of treatment-seeking cocaine abusers. Arch Gen Psychiatry 48:43–51, 1991

Salloum IM, Moss HB, Daley DC: Substance abuse and schizophrenia: impediments to optimal care. Am J Drug Alcohol Abuse 3:321–336, 1991

Satel SL, Edell WS: Cocaine-induced paranoia and psychosis proneness. Am J Psychiatry 148:1708–1711, 1991

Schmauss C, Krieg JC: Enlargement of cerebrospinal fluid spaces in long-term benzodiazepine abusers. Psychol Med 17:869–873, 1987

Schneier FR, Siris SG: A review of psychoactive substance use and abuse in schizophrenia: patterns of drug choice. J Nerv Ment Dis 175:641–652, 1987

Schuckit MA: Differences in plasma cortisol after ingestion of ethanol in relatives of alcoholics and controls: preliminary results. J Clin Psychiatry 45:374–376, 1984

Schuckit MA: The clinical implications of primary diagnostic groups among alcoholics. Arch Gen Psychiatry 42:1043–1049, 1985

Schuckit MA, Gold EO, Croot K, et al: P300 latency after ethanol ingestion in sons of alcoholics and in controls. Biol Psychiatry 24:310–315, 1988

Schweizer E, Rickels K[V], Case WG, et al: Long-term therapeutic use of benzodiazepines. Arch Gen Psychiatry 47:908–915, 1990

Selzer ML: The Michigan Alcoholism Screening Test: the quest for a new diagnostic instrument. Am J Psychiatry 127:1653–1658, 1971

Sevy S, Kay SR, Opler LA, et al: Significance of cocaine history in schizophrenia. J Nerv Ment Dis 178:642–648, 1990

Simpson DD: Treatment for drug abuse: follow-up outcomes and length of time spent. Arch Gen Psychiatry 38:875–880, 1981

Smart RG: Crack cocaine use: a review of prevalence and adverse effects. Am J Drug Alcohol Abuse 17:13–26, 1991

Spencer DJ: Cannabis-induced psychosis. Br J Addict 65:369–372, 1970

Spotts JV, Shontz FC: A new perspective on intervention in heavy, chronic drug use. Int J Addict 20:1545–1565, 1985

Stine SM, Burns B, Kosten T: Methadone dose for cocaine abuse (letter). Am J Psychiatry 148:1268, 1991

Stimmel B, Goldberg J, Rotkopf E, et al: Ability to remain abstinent after methadone detoxification: a six-year study. JAMA 237:1216–1220, 1977

Tarter RE: Psychosocial history, minimal brain dysfunction and differential drinking patterns of male alcoholics. J Clin Psychol 38:867–873, 1982

Thacore VR, Shukla SRP: Cannabis psychosis and paranoid schizophrenia. Arch Gen Psychiatry 33:383–386, 1976

Trell E, Kristenson H, Fex G: Alcohol-related problems in middle-aged men with elevated serum gamma-glutamyltransferase: a preventive medical investigation. J Stud Alcohol 45:302–309, 1984

Tunstall CD, Ginsberg D, Hall SM: Quitting smoking. Int J Addict 20:1089–1112, 1985

Turner RG, Lichstein PR, Peden JG, et al: Alcohol withdrawal syndromes: a review of pathophysiology, clinical presentations and treatment. J Gen Intern Med 4:432–444, 1989

U.S. Department of Health and Human Services: Fifth special report to the United States Congress on alcohol and health from the Secretary of Health and Human Services (DHHS Publ No [ADM]-84-1291). Washington, DC, U.S. Department of Health and Human Services, 1984

Vaillant GE (preceptor): Alcohol abuse and dependence, in Psychiatry Update: American Psychiatric Association Annual Review, Vol 3. Edited by Grinspoon L. Washington, DC, American Psychiatric Press, 1984, pp 299–381

Vardy MM, Kay SR: LSD psychosis or LSD-induced schizophrenia? A multimethod inquiry. Arch Gen Psychiatry 40:877–883, 1983

Victor M, Wolfe SM: Causation and treatment of the alcohol withdrawal syndrome, in Alcoholism: Progress in Research and Treatment. Edited by Bourne G, Fox R. New York, Academic, 1973, pp 137–166

Virmani R, Robinowitz M, Smialek JE, et al: Cardiovascular effects of cocaine: an autopsy study of 40 patients. Am Heart J 115:1068–1076, 1988

Volkow ND, Fowler JS, Wolf AP, et al: Effects of chronic cocaine abuse on postsynaptic dopamine receptors. Am J Psychiatry 147:719–724, 1990

Volpicelli JR, Alterman AI, Hayashida M, et al: Naltrexone in the treatment of alcohol dependence. Arch Gen Psychiatry 49:876–880, 1992

Walsh DC, Ringson RW, Merrigan DM, et al: A randomized trial of treatment options for alcohol-abusing workers. N Engl J Med 325:775–782, 1991

Warheit GJ, Buhl Auth J: Epidemiology of alcohol abuse in adulthood (Chapter 18), in Psychiatry, Vol 3. Edited by Michels R, Cavenar JO Jr. Philadelphia, PA, JB Lippincott, 1985

Washton AM: Structured outpatient treatment of alcohol vs. drug dependencies. Recent Dev Alcohol 8:285–304, 1990

Washton AM, Resnick RG: Clonidine in opiate withdrawal: a review and appraisal of clinical findings. Pharmacotherapy 1:140–146, 1981

Watson JM: Solvent abuse by children and young adults: a review. Br J Addict 75:27–36, 1980

Weil AJ: Adverse reactions to marijuana. N Engl J Med 282:997–1000, 1970

Weiss RD, Mirin SM: Subtypes of cocaine abusers. Psychiatr Clin North Am 9:491–501, 1986

Weiss RD, Mirin SM, Griffin ML, et al: Psychopathology in cocaine abusers: changing trends. J Nerv Ment Dis 176:719–725, 1988

Weller RA, Halikas JA: Marijuana use and psychiatric illness: a follow-up study. Am J Psychiatry 142:848–850, 1985

Winokur GA, Cadoret R, Dorzab JA, et al: The division of depressive illness into depression spectrum disease and pure depressive illness. International Pharmacopsychiatry 9:5–13, 1974

Woody GE, McLellan AT, Luborsky L, et al: Severity of psychiatric symptoms as a predictor of benefits from psychotherapy: the Veterans Administration–Penn Study. Am J Psychiatry 141:1172–1177, 1984

Woody GE, McLellan AT, Luborsky L, et al: Sociopathy and psychotherapy outcome. Arch Gen Psychiatry 42:1081–1086, 1985

Yamaguchi K, Kandel DB: Patterns of drug use from adolescence to young adulthood, III: predictors of progression. Am J Public Health 74:673–680, 1984

CHAPTER

12

Schizophrenia, Schizophreniform Disorder, and Delusional Disorder

Donald W. Black, M.D.
Nancy C. Andreasen, M.D., Ph.D.

Schizophrenia is probably the most devastating illness that psychiatrists treat. An estimated 0.5% to 1% of the population suffer from schizophrenia. It strikes at a young age so that, unlike patients with cancer or heart disease, schizophrenic patients usually live many years after its onset and continue to suffer its effects, which prevents their full participation in society. Apart from its impact on individuals and families, schizophrenia creates an enormous economic burden for society. Despite its emotional and economic costs, schizophrenia has yet to receive sufficient recognition as a major health concern or the necessary research support to investigate its causes, treatments, and prevention.

Schizophrenia and related disorders have been recognized in almost all cultures and described throughout much of recorded time. Emil Kraepelin (1856–1926) is usually credited with delineating schizophrenia, principally on the basis of course and outcome. He observed that some of the seriously mentally ill persons whom he treated began to have symptoms such as delusions and emotional withdrawal at a relatively early age and that these patients were likely to have a chronic and deteriorating course. Kraepelin distinguished these patients from patients with the late-onset dementias by referring to the former as having "dementia praecox."

393

At the urging of Eugen Bleuler (1857–1939) (see Bleuler 1911/1950), dementia praecox was eventually renamed "schizophrenia." Bleuler was convinced that cross-sectional symptoms were more important defining features of schizophrenia than were course and outcome. He stressed that the fundamental and unifying abnormality in schizophrenia was cognitive impairment, which he conceptualized as a "splitting" or "loosening" in the "fabric of thought." He believed that "thought disorder" was the essential and pathognomonic symptom of schizophrenia. Bleuler also believed that affective blunting, peculiar and distorted thinking (i.e., autism), avolition, impaired attention, and conceptual indecisiveness (i.e., ambivalence) together were nearly equally important as thought disorder. He referred to this group of symptoms as "fundamental," whereas other symptoms such as delusions and hallucinations were regarded as "accessory," because they could occur in other disorders such as manic-depressive illness.

The influence of Bleuler led to an increasingly broad definition and conceptualization of schizophrenia as psychiatry gathered strength and momentum during the postwar years and through the 1950s and 1960s. This phenomenon was particularly apparent in the United States, where concepts such as "latent schizophrenia" became popular. By the late 1960s, however, a number of factors intervened to introduce a climate of change. The development of effective treatments such as antipsychotics, antidepressants, and, eventually, lithium carbonate made diagnosis an important clinical issue. In addition, studies of comparative diagnostic practices in the United States, England, and other nations alerted American psychiatrists to the fact that their diagnostic habits were out of step. For example Cooper et al. (1972) set out to learn why prevalence of schizophrenia was greater in New York than London, while the reverse was true for manic-depressive illness. The investigators found that the same patients were given different diagnoses in different countries because of conceptual and theoretical differences between different diagnostic systems.

In the context of these studies, an interest in reliable diagnosis emerged, leading to the development of structured interviews such as the Present State Examination (PSE; Wing et al. 1967). Structured interviews required the definition of a symptom in a way that would ensure close agreement among clinicians. The PSE helped to introduce the concepts of the German psychiatrist Kurt Schneider (1887–1967) and his emphasis on "first-rank symptoms" to the English-speaking world. These forces helped reshape the concept of schizophrenia into one of a relatively severe psychotic disorder, again bringing it closer to the original ideas of Kraepelin.

The DSM-III (American Psychiatric Association 1980) and DSM-III-R (American Psychiatric Association 1987) and now DSM-IV (American

Psychiatric Association 1994) represent a convergence of these various points of view with their Kraepelinian emphasis on course, through the requirement that the illness be present for at least 6 months; their emphasis on specific delusions and hallucinations thought important by Schneider; and their acknowledgment of the importance of fundamental Bleulerian symptoms (thought disorder in the form of associative loosening or incoherence and affective blunting).

■ DIAGNOSIS

According to DSM-IV, schizophrenia consists of characteristic positive or negative symptoms present for a significant portion of time during a 1-month period or less if successfully treated; deterioration in social, work, or interpersonal relations; and continuous signs of the disturbance for at least 6 months. In addition, schizoaffective disorder and mood disorder with psychotic features have been ruled out, and the disturbance is not due to the direct effects of a substance or a general medical condition. Schizophrenia is further classified according to course of illness, as shown in Table 12–1.

If an illness otherwise meets the criteria but has a duration of less than 6 months, it is termed a *schizophreniform disorder*. If it has lasted less than 4 weeks but more than 1 day, it may be classified as either a *brief psychotic disorder* or a *psychotic disorder not otherwise specified*, which is a residual category for psychotic disturbances that cannot be better classified.

The diagnosis of schizophrenia should be thought of as a diagnosis of exclusion because the consequences of the diagnosis are severe and limit therapeutic options. First, it is important that a thorough physical examination and medical history rule out psychoses due to the direct effects of a substance or to a general medical condition. Atypical presentations, such as a relatively recent onset, clouding of the sensorium, or onset occurring after age 30 years, should be carefully investigated. Psychotic symptoms have been found in a variety of other illnesses including substance abuse (e.g., hallucinogens, phencyclidine, amphetamines, cocaine, alcohol), intoxication due to commonly prescribed medications (e.g., corticosteroids, anticholinergics, levo-dopa), infections, metabolic and endocrine disorders, tumors and mass lesions, and temporal lobe epilepsy.

Routine laboratory tests may be helpful in ruling out possible organic etiologies. Testing may include a complete blood count (CBC), urinalysis, liver enzymes, serum creatinine, blood urea nitrogen (BUN), thyroid function tests, and serologic tests for evidence of an infection with syphilis or human immunodeficiency virus (HIV). Other tests will be indicated

Table 12–1. DSM-IV criteria for schizophrenia

A. *Characteristic symptoms:* Two (or more) of the following, each present for a significant portion of time during a 1-month period (or less if successfully treated):

1. Delusions
2. Hallucinations
3. Disorganized speech (e.g., frequent derailment or incoherence)
4. Grossly disorganized or catatonic behavior
5. Negative symptoms (i.e., affective flattening, alogia, or avolition)

Note: Only one criterion A symptom is required if delusions are bizarre or hallucinations consist of a voice keeping up a running commentary on the person's behavior or thoughts, or two or more voices conversing with each other.

B. *Social/occupational dysfunction:* For a significant portion of the time since the onset of the disturbance, one or more major areas of functioning such as work, interpersonal relations, or self-care are markedly below the level achieved prior to the onset (or when the onset is in childhood or adolescence, failure to achieve expected level of interpersonal, academic, or occupational achievement).

C. *Duration:* Continuous signs of the disturbance persist for at least 6 months. This 6-month period must include at least 1 month of symptoms (or less if successfully treated) that meet criterion A (i.e., active-phase symptoms) and may include periods of prodromal or residual symptoms. During these prodromal or residual periods, the signs of the disturbance may be manifested by only negative symptoms or two or more symptoms listed in criterion A present in an attenuated form (e.g., odd beliefs, unusual perceptual experiences).

D. *Schizoaffective and mood disorder exclusion:* Schizoaffective disorder and mood disorder with psychotic features have been ruled out because either 1) no major depressive, manic, or mixed episodes have occurred concurrently with the active-phase symptoms; or 2) if mood episodes have occurred during active-phase symptoms, their total duration has been brief relative to the duration of the active and residual periods.

E. *Substance/general medical condition exclusion:* The disturbance is not due to the direct physiological effects of a substance (e.g., a drug of abuse, a medication) or a general medical condition.

F. *Relationship to a pervasive developmental disorder:* If there is a history of autistic disorder or another pervasive developmental disorder, the additional diagnosis of schizophrenia is made only if prominent delusions or hallucinations are also present for at least 1 month (or less if successfully treated).

Classification of longitudinal course (can be applied only after at least 1 year has elapsed since the initial onset of active-phase symptoms):

Episodic with interepisode residual symptoms (episodes are defined by the re-emergence of prominent psychotic symptoms); *also specify if:* **With prominent negative symptoms**

Episodic with no interepisode residual symptoms   *(continued)*

Table 12–1.   DSM-IV criteria for schizophrenia *(continued)*

Continuous (prominent psychotic symptoms are present throughout the period of observation). *Also specify if:* **With prominent negative symptoms**

Single episode in partial remission. *Also specify if:* **With prominent negative symptoms**

Single episode in full remission

Other or unspecified pattern

in some patients, such as a serum ceruloplasmin to rule out Wilson's disease. Electroencephalography, computed tomography (CT), or magnetic resonance imaging (MRI) may be useful in selected cases to rule out alternate diagnoses, such as a tumor or mass lesion, or during the initial workup for new-onset cases.

The major differential diagnosis in psychiatric settings involves separating schizophrenia from schizoaffective disorder, mood disorder with psychotic features, delusional disorder, or a personality disorder. To rule out schizoaffective disorder and psychotic mood disorders, major depressive or manic episodes should have been absent during the active phase, or the mood episode should have been brief relative to the total duration of the psychotic episode. Unlike delusional disorder, schizophrenia is characterized by bizarre delusions, and hallucinations are common. Patients with personality disorders, particularly the "eccentric cluster" (e.g., schizoid, schizotypal, and paranoid personality), may be indifferent to social relationships and display restricted affect, have bizarre ideation and odd speech, or be suspicious and hypervigilant, but they do not have delusions, hallucinations, or grossly disorganized behavior. Furthermore, patients with schizophrenia may develop other symptoms, such as a profound thought disorder, behavioral disturbances, and enduring personality deterioration. These symptoms are uncharacteristic of the mood disorders, delusional disorder, or the personality disorders.

Other psychiatric disorders will also need to be ruled out, including schizophreniform disorder, brief psychotic disorder, factitious disorder with psychological symptoms, and malingering. If symptoms persist for more than 6 months, schizophreniform disorder will have been ruled out. The history of how the illness presents will help to rule out a brief psychotic disorder, because schizophrenia generally has an insidious onset and there are usually no precipitants. Factitious disorder may be difficult to separate from schizophrenia, especially when the person is knowledgeable about the disorder, but careful observation should enable the clinician to make the distinction. Furthermore, the disorganized speech of schizophrenia is very difficult to simulate. A malingering individual could attempt to feign schizophrenia, but as with factitious disorder, careful observation is essential. In malingering, there will be evidence of obvious secondary gain, such as avoiding military conscription, and the history will often suggest an antisocial personality disorder.

■ CLINICAL FINDINGS

☐ Perceptual and Cognitive Disturbances

Hallucinations have sometimes been considered the hallmark of schizophrenia. Although it is now widely known that hallucinations may occur in a variety of other disorders, including mood and organic disorders, they remain important symptoms of schizophrenia and schizophreniform disorder. *Hallucinations* are perceptions experienced without an external stimulus to the sense organs that have a quality similar to a true perception. Hallucinations are usually experienced as originating in the outside world, or within one's own body, but not within the mind as through imagination. They vary in complexity and in sensory modality. Schizophrenic patients commonly have auditory, visual, tactile, gustatory, or olfactory hallucinations, or a combination of several types. Auditory hallucinations are the type most frequently observed in schizophrenia and may be experienced as noises, music, or more typically "voices." Visual hallucinations, which may be simple or complex and include flashes of light, persons, animals, or objects, may be smaller or larger than a true perception. Olfactory and gustatory hallucinations are often experienced together, leading to unpleasant tastes and odors.

Delusions, which involve a disturbance in inferential thinking rather than in perception, are firmly held beliefs that are untrue. The judgment of "untrueness" must always be made within the context of the person's educational and cultural background. Delusions occurring in patients with schizophrenia may have somatic, grandiose, religious, nihilistic, or persecutory themes (Table 12–2). None is specific to schizophrenia, and, like hallucinations, delusions can differ by culture.

Certain types of auditory hallucinations and delusions were considered symptoms of the "first rank" by Schneider. He described these hallucinations as prolonged, clearly audible voices, often commenting upon a person's actions, arguing with each other about the patient, or repeating aloud the patient's thoughts. First-rank delusions were those of thought broadcasting, thought withdrawal, thought insertion, or delusions of passivity (i.e., of being controlled as if one were a puppet). Although found in up to three-quarters of schizophrenic patients, these delusions are also present in at least 10% of patients with psychotic mood disorders (Andreasen and Akiskal 1983).

Table 12–2. Varied content in delusions

Delusions	Foci of preoccupation
Grandiose	Possessing wealth, great beauty, or having a special ability (e.g., extrasensory perception); having influential friends; being an important figure (e.g., Napoleon, Hitler)
Nihilistic	Belief that one is dead or dying; belief that one does not exist or that the world does not exist
Persecutory	Being persecuted by friends, neighbors, or spouses; being followed, monitored, or spied on by the government (e.g., FBI, CIA) or other important organizations (e.g., the Catholic Church)
Somatic	Belief that one's organs have stopped functioning (e.g., that the heart is no longer beating) or are rotting away; belief that the nose or other body part is terribly misshapen or disfigured
Sexual	Belief that one's sexual behavior is commonly known; that one is a prostitute, a pedophile, or a rapist; that masturbation has led to illness or insanity
Religious	Belief that one has sinned against God; that one has a special relationship to God, or some other deity; that one has a special religious mission; that one is the Devil or is condemned to burn in Hell

Disorders of thinking and language are also characteristic of schizophrenia and schizophreniform disorder. *Thought disorder* was regarded as the most important symptom of schizophrenia by Bleuler. Historically, types of thought disorder have included associative loosening, illogical thinking, overinclusive thinking, and loss of ability to engage in abstract thinking. Other types of formal thought disorder have been identified, including perseveration, distractibility, clanging, neologisms, echolalia, and blocking; with the possible exception of clanging in mania, none appears to be specific to a particular disorder. Because these various forms of "thought disorder" are inferred from observing the speech of patients, the concept of "thought disorder" has evolved into the concept of "disorganized speech" and appears as such in the diagnostic criteria.

Lack of insight is a common symptom in schizophrenia. A patient may not believe he or she is ill or abnormal in any way. The hallucinations and delusions are real to him or her and not imagined. Poor insight is one of the most difficult symptoms to treat and may persist even when other symptoms (e.g., hallucinations) respond to treatment. Orientation and memory are usually normal, unless impaired by the patient's psychotic symptoms, inattention, or distractibility.

☐ Behavioral and Motor Disturbances

Many patients with schizophrenia develop diminished volition, various motor disturbances, and changes in social behavior. Abnormal behaviors range from catatonic stupor to excitement. In a catatonic stupor, the patient may become immobile, mute, and unresponsive, and yet remain fully conscious. In a state of catatonic excitement, a patient may exhibit uncontrolled and aimless motor activity. Some patients manifest waxy flexibility (*flexibilitas cerea*), in which they allow themselves to be placed in uncomfortable positions that are maintained without apparent distress. Occasionally patients assume bizarre or uncomfortable postures and maintain them for long periods. Patients may exhibit *stereotypy*, which is a repeated but non–goal-directed movement such as rocking; *mannerisms*, which are normal goal-directed activities that appear to have social significance but are either odd in appearance or out of context; and *mitgehen*, which is moving a limb in response to slight pressure on it despite being told to resist the pressure. Less common symptoms are *echopraxia*, which is imitating the movements and gestures of another person; *automatic obedience*, which is carrying out simple commands in a robot-like fashion, and *negativism*, which is refusing to cooperate with simple requests for no apparent reason.

Antipsychotic medications are often blamed for causing motor abnormalities and are clearly responsible for causing a variety of extrapyramidal side effects, as well as tardive dyskinesia. Schizophrenic patients are often unaware of their involuntary movements and, when these movements are pointed out, may be unconcerned about them (Caracci et al. 1990). Deterioration of social behavior often develops along with social withdrawal. Patients may neglect themselves and become messy or unkempt, and wear dirty, unmended, or inappropriate clothing. Patients may ignore their surroundings so that the latter become cluttered and untidy. Patients may develop other odd behaviors breaking most social conventions such as exhibiting crude table manners, masturbating in public, foraging through garbage bins, or shouting obscenities. Many of today's "homeless" persons are schizophrenic (Susser et al. 1989).

Psychoactive substance abuse, particularly alcohol abuse, is common in patients with schizophrenia at rates exceeding those found in the community (Dixon et al. 1991). Cigarette use is also very common, and in one study nearly three of every four schizophrenic patients was a smoker (Goff et al. 1992). Drug-taking schizophrenic patients tend to be younger and are more often male, and have more psychiatric symptoms, poor treatment compliance, and more frequent hospitalizations (Drake et al. 1989).

☐ Affective Disturbances

Schizophrenic patients may develop a reduced intensity of emotional expression and response that leaves them indifferent and apathetic. Many patients appear incapable of experiencing pleasure and may describe themselves as feeling emotionally empty. Expression of affect may be inappropriate, such as giggling when told of a relative's death. Up to 60% of schizophrenic patients develop significant depressive symptoms (Guze et al. 1983). Depression is often difficult to diagnose in schizophrenic patients, because the symptoms of schizophrenia and depression overlap. Further, antipsychotics can cause what appears to be a depression, but is actually a drug-induced akinesia. This "depression" may go away when the dosage of antipsychotic is reduced, or an anticholinergic medication is added (Johnson 1981). According to DSM-IV, a major depression occurring in a patient with well-established schizophrenia, is diagnosed as depressive disorder not otherwise specified.

☐ Positive and Negative Symptoms

Many clinicians have found it useful to describe typical schizophrenic symptoms as positive or negative. In practice, patients usually have a mixture of the two (Andreasen et al. 1990b). *Positive symptoms,* such as hallucinations, delusions, marked positive formal thought disorder (manifested by marked incoherence, derailment, tangentiality, or illogicality), and bizarre or disorganized behavior, reflect aberrant mental activity. *Negative symptoms* reflect a deficiency of a mental function that is normally present—for example, alogia (i.e., marked poverty of speech, or poverty of content of speech), affective flattening, anhedonia/asociality (i.e., inability to experience pleasure, few social contacts), avolition/apathy (i.e., anergia, lack of persistence at work or school), and attentional impairment.

☐ Other Symptoms

Nonlocalizing neurological soft signs occur in a substantial proportion of schizophrenic patients and include abnormalities in stereognosis, graphesthesia, balance, and proprioception (Heinrichs and Buchanan 1988). One hypothesis is that these abnormalities reflect defects in the integration of proprioceptive and other sensory information (Quitkin et al. 1976). Olfactory identification and acuity are reported to be poor in male schizophrenic patients (Kopala et al. 1989). Smooth pursuit eye movement (SPEM) is often impaired. Because abnormal SPEM has been observed in patients with remitted schizophrenia or schizotypal personality disorder, and is more frequently found in relatives of schizophrenic patients than in the general population (Holzman et al. 1984), it may represent a biological marker for schizophrenia. A similar abnormality in visual fixation has also been reported that may have greater familial specificity than SPEM (Amador et al. 1991). Other ocular abnormalities commonly include the absence and avoidance of eye contact, and staring for long periods; decreased or increased blink rates and paroxysmal bouts of rapid blinking may occur (Mackert et al. 1991).

Some patients display disturbances of sleep, sexual interest, or other bodily functions. A variety of disrupted sleep measures have been reported in schizophrenia. Decreased delta sleep with diminished Stage 4 is the most consistent finding (Neylan et al. 1992). Schizophrenic patients often have little interest in sexual activity and may derive little or no pleasure from sexual experiences (Lyketsos et al. 1983).

☐ Premorbid Personality

Several early writers, including Bleuler, noted that patients with schizophrenia often had odd personalities even before the onset of their illness. Research has since confirmed that as a group, chronic schizophrenic patients differ premorbidly from the rest of the population. In a study of chronic schizophrenic patients, 35% met the criteria for a DSM-III personality disorder premorbidly; 44% of these personality disorders were schizoid and the rest were a mixture of avoidant, paranoid, histrionic, compulsive, and other personality disorders (Pfohl and Winokur 1983). More recent studies suggest that poor premorbid adjustment may be an indication of a more severe form of schizophrenia characterized by negative symptoms, low educational achievement, poor social functioning, and structural brain abnormalities (Andreasen et al. 1990a).

☐ Cognitive Assessment

Schizophrenic patients score lower than expected on standardized measures of intelligence. Their premorbid IQ tends to be lower than scores of their siblings and peers of similar social class origin, but IQ does not characteristically decline premorbidly or after the onset of schizophrenia (Aylward et al. 1984). Although early studies focused on IQ, most researchers now use a variety of neuropsychological tests to provide a more thorough assessment of cognitive function. Saykin et al. (1991) studied 36 unmedicated schizophrenic patients and age-matched control subjects. Patients showed generalized impairment relative to the control subjects, and a selective deficit in memory and learning. Recently, Braff et al. (1991) showed that despite having average verbal intellectual abilities, a group of 40 patients with schizophrenia had clear neuropsychological deficits on tests of complex reasoning, psychomotor speed, new learning, incidental memory, and both motor and sensory perceptual abilities. Impairment was strongly associated with negative symptoms of schizophrenia.

Neuropsychological test abnormalities have been positively correlated with cerebral ventricular enlargement (Keilp et al. 1988). Although evidence of cognitive test abnormalities is consistent with the hypothesis that schizophrenia is a dementing illness, it may be that intellectual deterioration is characteristic of a subset of schizophrenic patients, particularly those exhibiting negative symptoms or having evidence of ventricular enlargement.

■ SUBTYPES OF SCHIZOPHRENIA AND SCHIZOPHRENIFORM DISORDER

The DSM-IV recognizes five subtypes of schizophrenia: paranoid, disorganized (i.e., hebephrenic), catatonic, undifferentiated, and residual. The main purpose of subtyping is to improve predictive validity, to help the clinician to select treatments and predict outcome, and to help the researcher to delineate homogeneous subtypes. Unfortunately, the validity of different schizophrenic subtypes has not been fully established. The DSM-IV subtypes are summarized in Table 12–3.

☐ Paranoid Schizophrenia

The paranoid subtype of schizophrenia is characterized by a preoccupation with one or more delusions or frequent auditory hallucinations; disorganized speech/behavior, catatonic behavior, and flat or inappropriate affect are not prominent. Kraepelin was the first to identify a paranoid subtype of schizophrenia, in which patients had bizarre and fragmented delusions and, ultimately, personality deterioration. Winokur et al. (1974) compared 62 paranoid patients with 115 hebephrenic patients. Paranoid patients had an older age at onset and were older at the time of admission than hebephrenic patients. They were also more likely to be married, to have children, and to be employed. The relatives of patients with paranoid schizophrenia also had a higher risk for schizophrenia than did the relatives of patients with hebephrenic schizophrenia. Fenton and McGlashan (1991) compared the course of 78 paranoid, 26 hebephrenic, and 83 undifferentiated schizophrenic patients. They, too, found that patients with paranoid schizophrenia had an older age at onset, and that this subtype often developed rapidly in individuals with good premorbid functioning and had a better outcome.

Table 12–3. DSM-IV subtypes of schizophrenia

Subtype	Criteria	Associated features
Paranoid	A. Preoccupation with one or more delusions or frequent auditory hallucinations. B. None of the following is prominent: disorganized speech, disorganized or catatonic behavior, flat or inappropriate affect.	Often associated with unfocused anger, anxiety, argumentativeness, or violence. Stilted, formal quality or extreme intensity of interpersonal interactions may be seen.
Disorganized	A. All of the following are prominent: 1. Disorganized speech 2. Disorganized behavior 3. Flat or inappropriate affect B. The criteria are not met for catatonic type.	Silly and childlike behavior is common. Associated with extreme social impairment, poor premorbid functioning, and poor long-term functioning.
Catatonic	The clinical picture is dominated by at least two of the following: 1. Motoric immobility as evidenced by catelepsy (including waxy flexibility) or stupor 2. Excessive motor activity (that is apparently purposeless and not influenced by extreme stimuli) 3. Extreme negativism (an apparently motiveless resistance to all instructions or maintenance of a rigid posture against attempts to be moved) or mutism 4. Peculiarities of voluntary movement as evidenced by posturing (voluntary assumption of inappropriate or bizarre postures), stereo-typed movements, prominent mannerisms or prominent grimacing 5. Echolalia or echopraxia	Marked psychomotor disturbance present (stupor or agitation), and unusual motor disturbances may be present. May need medical supervision due to malnutrition, exhaustion, hyperpyrexia, or self-injury. Amytal interview may be helpful diagnostically.

Undifferentiated	Symptoms that meet criterion A are present, but the criteria are not met for paranoid, disorganized, or catatonic types.	Probably the most common presentation in clinical practice.
Residual	The following criteria are met: A. Absence of prominent delusions, hallucinations, disorganized speech, and grossly disorganized or catatonic behavior B. Continuing evidence of the disturbance, as indicated by the presence of negative symptoms or two or more symptoms listed in criterion A for schizophrenia, present in an attenuated form (e.g., odd beliefs, unusual perceptual experiences)	Active-phase symptoms (i.e., psychotic symptoms) are not present, but patient still exhibits emotional blunting, eccentric behavior, illogical thinking, and mild loosening of associations.

☐ Disorganized Schizophrenia

Disorganized schizophrenia (i.e., hebephrenia) is characterized by disorganized speech and behavior, and flat or inappropriate affect; it does not meet the criteria for catatonic schizophrenia. Generally, delusions and hallucinations, if present, are fragmentary, unlike the well-systematized delusions of the paranoid schizophrenic patient. Hebephrenia typically has an early onset that begins with the insidious development of avolition, affective flattening, deterioration of habits, and cognitive impairment, as well as delusions and hallucinations (Winokur et al. 1974). Hebephrenic patients often seem silly and childlike. They may grimace or giggle inappropriately and often appear self-absorbed. Mirror gazing is frequently described.

☐ Catatonic Schizophrenia

In DSM-IV, catatonic schizophrenia is defined as a type of schizophrenia dominated by at least two of the following: motoric immobility as evidenced by catalepsy or stupor, excessive motor activity, extreme negativism or mutism, peculiarities of voluntary movement (e.g., stereotypies, mannerisms, grimacing) and echolalia or echopraxia. This subtype of schizophrenia is reported to be less common than in the past, possibly a benefit of the modern treatment era. Because these symptoms can be found in other subtypes of schizophrenia, in other psychiatric disorders (including mood and organic mental disorders), and in a variety of other conditions such as viral encephalitis, frontal lobe tumors, metabolic derangements (i.e., acute intermittent porphyria), and toxic reactions, a patient displaying catatonic features requires careful evaluation and differential diagnosis (Stoudemire 1982).

Intravenous sodium amobarbital may be helpful in the differential diagnosis of catatonia. Perry and Jacobs (1982) report that a catatonia of functional origin will clear temporarily during an "Amytal interview." A mute patient may begin to speak, for example. Patients in whom a catatonic syndrome has resulted from an organic disorder will become drowsy and less responsive.

☐ Undifferentiated and Residual Subtypes

The DSM-IV also includes the *undifferentiated* subtype, which is a residual category for patients meeting criteria for schizophrenia but not meeting criteria for the paranoid, disorganized, or catatonic subtypes. Although the term has been popular, many clinicians have used it indiscriminately. The *residual* subtype as described in DSM-IV is used for patients who no longer have prominent psychotic symptoms but who once met criteria for schizophrenia and have continuing evidence of illness. This may be indicated by the presence of negative symptoms, or two or more symptoms listed in Criterion A for schizophrenia, present in an attenuated form (e.g., odd beliefs, unusual perceptual experiences).

☐ Schizophreniform Disorder

The term *schizophreniform* was first used by Gabriel Langfeldt to describe psychoses that were acute and reactive and that occurred in persons with normal personalities (Langfeldt 1939). The DSM-IV provides a somewhat different conceptualization. The disorder requires active positive or negative symptoms, is not due to a schizoaffective disorder or a mood disorder with psychotic features, is not due to the direct effects of a substance or to a general medical condition and lasts more than 1 month but less than 6 months (Table 12–4). The diagnosis changes to schizophrenia once symptoms extend past 6 months, even if the symptoms are residual. The disorder can be further subdivided into cases with and without good prognostic features (e.g., acute onset).

This relatively new diagnosis has little empirical support, and the few relevant studies have yielded conflicting results. For example, Weinberger et al. (1982) found schizophreniform and schizophrenic patients to have similar CT scan abnormalities. Fogelson et al. (1982) concluded that at least a portion of schizophreniform patients have a mood disorder, based on family history, treatment response, and neuroendocrine testing. One long-term follow-up study (Coryell and Tsuang 1986) indi-

---

Table 12–4.   DSM-IV criteria for schizophreniform disorder

A.   Criteria A, D, and E of schizophrenia are met.

B.   An episode of the disorder (including prodromal, active, and residual phases) lasts at least 1 month but less than 6 months. (When the diagnosis must be made without waiting for recovery, it should be qualified as "provisional.")

Specify if:

Without good prognostic features

With good prognostic features as evidenced by two (or more) of the following:

1.   Onset of prominent psychotic symptoms within 4 weeks of the first noticeable change in usual behavior or functioning
2.   Confusion or perplexity at the height of the psychotic episode
3.   Good premorbid social and occupational functioning
4.   Absence of blunted or flat affect

---

cated that patients with schizophreniform disorder are heterogeneous. Outcome measures used in the study (e.g., marital status, living situation, occupational history, psychiatric symptoms) showed that schizophreniform patients were more similar in outcome to schizophrenic patients than to mood disorder patients. This finding implies that some patients with schizophreniform disorder actually have a mood disorder, and that the others, probably the majority, develop schizophrenia. The study also found that the morbidity risk for mood disorders among first-degree relatives of schizophreniform patients was no different from that observed among relatives of schizophrenic patients, but was significantly lower than that observed among the relatives of mood disorder patients. A more recent study (Pulver et al. 1991) did not confirm these results.

■ COURSE OF ILLNESS

Schizophrenia often begins with a *prodromal phase* that precedes the active phase of illness, sometimes by many years. This phase is characterized by social withdrawal and other subtle changes in behavior and emotional responsiveness. The prodromal phase is followed by an *active phase,* in which psychotic symptoms such as hallucinations and delusions predominate. This phase is florid and alarming to friends and relatives, and may lead to medical intervention, including hospitalization. A *residual phase* follows and is similar to the prodromal phase, although affective flattening and role impairment may be worse. Psychotic symptoms may persist during this phase, but at a lower level of intensity, and they may not be as troublesome to the patient. The residual phase may be interrupted by reoccurrences of the active phase, or "acute exacerbations." The frequency and timing of these exacerbations are unpredictable, although stressful situations may precede these relapses. Relapses may be preceded by changes in thought, feeling, or behavior noticed by the patient and family members.

The symptoms of schizophrenia tend to change over time. Patients may show a preponderance of positive symptoms early in their illness, but over time develop more negative or deficit symptoms. Pfohl and Winokur (1983) showed that 85% of patients with schizophrenia initially had persecutory delusions of some type at index admission, but after 10 years of illness only 50% had such delusions, and after 20 years of illness only 40% had them. This finding was true for hallucinations and motor symptoms as well. On the other hand, the authors found that negative symptoms, such as avolition, asociality, and affective flattening, increased in frequency with time.

■ OUTCOME

Studies of outcome in schizophrenia are difficult to compare directly, but according to a review of six outcome studies involving 3,137 patients (Cutting 1986), 13% had a good outcome, 45% had a bad outcome, and 42% had an intermediate outcome. Good outcome was defined as no hospital readmission during follow-up, and bad outcome, as continuous hospitalization during follow-up, or moderate to severe intellectual or social impairment.

Several long-term follow-up studies have been published using contemporary American definitions of schizophrenia. In the Iowa 500 Study, 20% of the schizophrenic patients were found to be psychiatrically well at follow-up, but 54% had incapacitating psychiatric symptoms; 21% were married or widowed, but 67% had never married; 34% lived in their own home or with a relative, but 18% were in mental institutions; 35% were economically productive, but 58% had never worked. The group experienced excess mortality from both natural and unnatural causes, and more than 10% committed suicide (Tsuang et al. 1979). This and other studies show that schizophrenia is a devastating illness that affects every aspect of a patient's life. Fortunately, as many as one in four or five patients with schizophrenia will have a relatively good outcome, and many will avoid the severe deterioration considered by some to be a hallmark of the disorder.

Although it is not easy to predict outcome in individual cases, many prognostic factors have been reported (Jonsson and Nyman 1984; McGlashan 1986). It appears that definitions of schizophrenia that exclude patients with mood symptoms or a duration of illness under 6 months, such as that in DSM-IV, predict a poor prognosis. This is, at least partly, because such definitions exclude patients with mood or schizophreniform disorders, who tend to have better outcomes. Perhaps the best evaluation of the predictive value of these factors was the IPSS (World Health Organization 1975). Regression analysis showed the five most powerful predictors of poor outcome to be social isolation, long duration of episode, history of past psychiatric treatment, being unmarried, and a history of behavioral problems in childhood such as truancy and tantrums.

For reasons that are not well understood, cross-cultural studies have shown that patients in less developed countries tend to have better outcomes than those in more developed countries. It may be that the schizophrenic patient is better accepted in less developed countries, has fewer external demands, and is more likely to be taken care of by family members. Women appear to have a more favorable course than do men on several outcome measures (Seeman 1986), including antipsychotic response, social functioning, and overall prognosis.

■ EPIDEMIOLOGY

☐ Incidence and Prevalence

Schizophrenia has presented a challenge to epidemiologists over the years because of disagreements about its definition. The development of operational criteria, such as those in DSM-IV, has led to a reassessment of earlier epidemiological studies that used older definitions.

Incidence and prevalence of schizophrenia are important measures of the distribution of schizophrenia in the community. The *incidence* of a disorder is the number of new cases arising in a given time per unit of population. *Prevalence* is the number of existing cases per unit of population present during a given time interval. A World Health Organization study (Sartorius et al. 1986) indicated that annual incidence rates for schizophrenia vary from 0.16 to 0.28 per 1,000 persons in industralized countries. The study also showed that incidence rates are remarkably stable across widely varying situations.

Estimates of prevalence from studies conducted over the past fifty years have varied widely. However, figures reported in the Epidemiologic Catchment Area survey (Robins et al. 1984) in the United States generated lifetime prevalence rates between 1.0% and 1.9%. The rate for schizophreniform disorder ranged from 0.1% to 0.3%. There was an approximate average prevalence for schizophrenia of 1.1% for men and 1.9% for women. The study found a preponderance of schizophrenia in women and in persons aged 18 to 44 years. If accurate, the United States has one of the highest reported prevalence rates for schizophrenia, affecting between 2.5 million and 4.75 million persons.

☐ Socioeconomic Status, Ethnicity, and Race

Research has confirmed the inverse relationship of social class status to risk for schizophrenia. Eaton (1985) reviewed 17 available studies of incidence of treated schizophrenia that included indicators of social class. The highest rate of schizophrenia was found in the lowest social class in 15 of the studies.

In a review of 22 studies in 14 countries, Jablensky and Sartorius (1975) concluded that except for a high rate in north Sweden (10.8 per 1,000) and a low rate reported for the Hutterite sect in the United States (1.1 per 1,000), the prevalence rates for schizophrenia appear to be very similar worldwide. High prevalence has also been reported in areas of Croatia, in Ireland, among Canadian Catholics, and among the Tamils of southern India. Low prevalence has been reported among American Old Order Amish, among aboriginal tribes in Taiwan, and among the black population in Ghana. Although early studies in the United States suggested a higher rate of schizophrenia in African-Americans than in whites, this finding may have been due to a systematic bias to overdiagnose schizophrenia in blacks (Mukherjee et al. 1983).

☐ Age at Onset and Sex Ratio

Schizophrenia typically has an onset in early adulthood, but can develop at any age, and, in fact, has been described in children as young as 5 years (Beitchman 1985). Both Bleuler and Kraepelin reported an earlier onset for men than women, a finding since confirmed by other investigators. Loranger (1984) examined age at onset in 100 men and 100 women meeting DSM-III criteria for schizophrenia. Mean age of first psychiatric episode for men was 21.4 years, and for women 26.8 years, but mean age at first treatment was 25.2 and 19.6 years in men and women, respectively. Nine of 10 men, but only two of three women, had developed the illness by age 30 years. Onset after age 35 occurred in 17% of women, but in only 2% of men. The reason that women develop schizophrenia later than men remains a mystery, but it is apparently not an artifact due to women leading a more sheltered existence that would thereby conceal their illness.

Early epidemiological studies showed approximately equal rates of schizophrenia for men and women, but the broad concept of schizophrenia used in the past may have led to the inclusion of a disproportionate number of women with mood disorders. Lewine et al. (1984) analyzed the effect of using six different diagnostic systems on the male-to-female ratio of schizophrenia among 387 inpatients. Diagnostic criteria that present a broad concept of schizophrenia, such as the New Haven Schizophrenia Index, yielded equal rates of schizophrenia among men and women. Diagnostic systems with more stringent criteria, such as the RDC, yielded a greater male-to-female ratio.

☐ Marital Status

Patients with schizophrenia are often unmarried and tend to be divorced more often if ever married. This pattern is especially characteristic of male patients (Eaton 1985). These findings are probably explained by the tendency of women to be younger than men when first married and therefore less likely to have experienced an initial psychotic episode. Furthermore, women have traditionally been less active in initiating and pursuing courtship. Early researchers tended to find low fertility rates and reproduction among schizophrenic patients (Kallman 1938), findings probably explained by several factors, including lack of interest in social relations, apathy, low sex drive, and lack of opportunity for sexual

relationships in institutions. Rates of reproduction in schizophrenic patients have probably increased since deinstitutionalization, although
they probably remain lower than those found in the general population
(Erlenmeyer-Kimling 1978).

☐ Mortality and Morbidity

Research over the past 50 years has continued to demonstrate increased
mortality in patients with schizophrenia (Black and Fisher 1992) due primarily to suicide and accidents. Data from the Oxford Case Register
(Herrman et al. 1983) show a twofold increase over expected mortality
for men and women. Those at risk for early death appear to be patients
younger than 55 years; in other words, the risk is greatest during the time
when the illness is most pronounced.

Schizophrenic patients have a high risk for committing suicidal acts.
About one-third will attempt suicide (Allebeck et al. 1987), and about 1 in
10 will complete suicide (Tsuang 1978). Between 2% and 3% of those persons who complete suicide have schizophrenia (Barraclough et al. 1974).
Risk factors for suicide include male gender, age less than 30 years, living
alone, unemployment, chronic relapsing course, prior depression, past
treatment for depression, depression during the last episode of illness,
history of substance abuse, and recent discharge (Allebeck et al. 1987;
Roy 1982). Unlike other psychiatric patients who commit suicide, schizophrenic patients may fail to communicate their suicidal intentions and
may act impulsively, making an attempt at intervention difficult. Methods used to commit suicide tend to be highly lethal among this population (Breier and Astrachan 1984). Although some investigators have
suggested that a high percentage of murderers are severely mentally ill
and are likely to have paranoid schizophrenia, the risk of homicide and
other serious crime is probably the same for patients with schizophrenia
as for members of the general population (Henn et al. 1976).

☐ Utilization of Health Services

Schizophrenic patients utilize a disproportionate share of general medical and psychiatric services. Data from the NIMH show schizophrenia to
be the first or second most frequent diagnosis for admissions to various
types of psychiatric inpatient services, ranging from 21% for private hospitals to 38% for state and county hospitals, with a length of stay averaging 18 to 42 days, respectively. There were over 1.6 million admissions for
patients with schizophrenia to inpatient facilities in 1980 (Taube and Barrett 1985). Data from the ECA study (Shapiro et al. 1984) show that nearly
78% of schizophrenic patients surveyed had had health care visits during

the previous 6 months; 45% of the visits had been for mental health care. Patients with schizophrenia tended to obtain mental health care from specialists rather than from general medical providers.

■ ETIOLOGY

Hypotheses about the etiology and pathophysiology of schizophrenia can be grouped into genetic, neurobiological, developmental, and sociocultural causes.

☐ Genetic Hypotheses

Evidence for a genetic contribution to schizophrenia is based on family studies, twin studies, and studies of adoptees. Summaries of individual family studies have shown siblings of schizophrenic patients to have a near 10% lifetime risk of developing schizophrenia, while children who have one parent with schizophrenia have a 5% to 6% lifetime expectancy (Gottesman and Shields 1982). The risk of a family member developing schizophrenia increases markedly when two or more family members have the illness, with a lifetime expectancy of schizophrenia of 17% for siblings with one sib and one parent with schizophrenia, and up to 46% in children of two schizophrenic parents. These findings strongly support the familial nature of schizophrenia, but do not confirm a genetic over a familial environmental cause.

Twin studies are based on the hypothesis that monozygotic twins are more likely to be concordant for genetic illness than dizygotic twins because of the greater genetic similarity. Despite varying methods, twin studies have been remarkably consistent in demonstrating high concordance rates for monozygotic twins (Farmer et al. 1987; Gottesman and Shields 1982). Rates have averaged 46% compared with 14% in dizygotic twins across multiple studies, with only one negative twin study (Tienari 1963). However, the failure of monozygotic twins to be 100% concordant suggests that a genetic role may be necessary but insufficient to cause schizophrenia, and that environmental factors are also important.

Adoption studies present another paradigm for evaluating genetic influences in familial illness. The best known adoption study was performed in Denmark using a national psychiatric case register and a register of adoptions. Kety et al. (1975) reported that schizophrenia and "schizophrenia spectrum" disorders were more common in the biological relatives of index adoptees who had schizophrenia than in the biological relatives of mentally healthy control adoptees. Schizophrenia spectrum disorders include personality disorders that share certain characteristics with schizophrenia, such as paranoid ideas or eccentric behavior, without meeting full syndromal criteria.

Molecular genetic techniques have recently been used in attempts to pin down the mode of inheritance and to locate a "schizophrenia gene." Sherrington et al. (1988) suggested that a schizophrenia gene may lie on chromosome 5, but subsequent investigators have failed to replicate this finding. The nonreplications, while not ruling out involvement of chromosome 5 in some families, may indicate only that schizophrenia is genetically heterogeneous.

☐ Neurobiological Hypotheses

Schizophrenia is widely believed to have a neurobiological basis. A variety of evidence indicates that the symptoms of schizophrenia may be due to neurochemical and/or structural brain abnormalities. This evidence derives from neurochemistry and neuropharmacology, neuroanatomy, and neurophysiology.

Neurochemistry and Neuropharmacology

The most popular pathophysiological explanation for the symptoms of schizophrenia is the "dopamine hypothesis," which suggests that the symptoms of schizophrenia are due primarily to hyperactivity in the dopaminergic system (Davis et al. 1991). If a functional hyperactivity in dopamine transmission does exist, it theoretically could occur in one of three ways: 1) transmitter neurons could produce excessive quantities of dopamine; 2) excessive quantities of dopamine could exist at the synaptic junction, due to failure of metabolic breakdown or reuptake; or 3) receptor neurons could be functionally hyperactive. Most of the available evidence appears to support the third explanation.

Evidence supporting this hypothesis includes the effectiveness of antipsychotic medications that block postsynaptic dopamine receptors (Seeman et al. 1976; Snyder 1976). The drugs that produce the strongest blockade in animals are also those that are most effective in reducing the symptoms of schizophrenia in humans (Creese et al. 1976). Other drugs that are powerful dopamine antagonists, such as reserpine, also reduce the symptoms of schizophrenia, although such drugs are rarely used clinically because their side effects are greater than those of antipsychotics. On the other hand, drugs that enhance dopamine transmission, such as the amphetamines, tend to exacerbate the symptoms of schizophrenia (Snyder 1972).

Direct support for the dopamine hypothesis has been provided through the study of postmortem brains and by the use of positron-emission tomography (PET). An increase in D_2 receptors in the caudate and nucleus accumbens has been documented in postmortem brains

(Clardy et al. 1993). This work indicates that patients with schizophrenia have a specific hyperactivity of D_2 receptors, but this finding may be an artifact of treatment with neuroleptics. Recently, PET has provided another direct line of evidence concerning neurochemical transmission in schizophrenia. This technique is sufficiently precise to permit direct measurement of the number of D_2 receptors. Farde et al. (1990) used PET to assess D_2 receptor density in schizophrenic patients who had never been medicated. The authors did not find an increase and so were unable to support the hypothesis of a general increase in central D_2 dopamine receptor density in schizophrenia. Other neurotransmitter systems are probably involved in the neurochemistry of schizophrenia as well. Norepinephrine, serotonin, glutamate, and GABA may also play some role in modulating the symptoms of schizophrenia (Meltzer 1987; Van Kammen et al. 1990).

Neuroanatomical and Neuroimaging Studies

Since the early work of Kraepelin, Alzheimer, and Nissl in the late 19th and early 20th centuries, many psychiatrists have been convinced that patients with schizophrenia have some type of functional or structural brain abnormality (Kraepelin 1919). Early pneumoencephalographic (PEG) and neuropathological studies provided partial support for this hypothesis, but in recent years new technology has been able to support it more fully. With the advent of new staining techniques, and brain-imaging techniques such as CT, MRI, and PET, there is now substantial evidence that some schizophrenic patients have structural brain abnormalities.

CT scan abnormalities in schizophrenia have perhaps become the most consistently replicated biological finding in this disorder. Cerebral ventricular enlargement is the most consistent finding, but sulcal enlargement or cerebellar atrophy is also reported. While these findings cannot be explained on the basis of such factors as treatment with medications, they may be explained in part by gender, because it may be predominantly a male effect (Flaum et al. 1990). There is substantial evidence to suggest that ventricular enlargement is associated with poor premorbid functioning, negative symptoms, poor response to treatment, and cognitive impairment. Computed tomographic scan abnormalities occur in up to 40% of schizophrenic patients. Although these findings are not diagnostically specific, structural abnormalities observed relatively early in the illness indicate that the brain may have suffered some type of injury or insult prior to the onset of symptoms, which could explain why some patients may be treatment refractory.

MRI offers many advantages over CT, including better resolution, absence of bony artifacts, the ability to image in multiple planes, and the absence of ionizing radiation. The first large MRI study in schizophrenia reported decreased cranial, cerebral, and frontal size in persons with this disorder (Andreasen et al. 1986); a subsequent study indicated that this finding was no longer present if control subjects were educationally and sociodemographically matched, suggesting that a common factor may influence both brain development and educational achievement or intelligence (Andreasen et al. 1990a). Several studies have indicated that temporal size may be decreased in schizophrenia and that there may even be a relatively specific abnormality in the superior temporal gyrus that is correlated with the presence of hallucinations (Barta et al. 1990; Suddath et al. 1990). Studies have also reported abnormalities in the basal ganglia (Jernigan et al. 1991; Swayze et al. 1992).

Neuropathology

A substantial amount of evidence suggests that structural abnormalities may also occur in schizophrenia at the cellular level, particularly in limbic and periventricular regions. Fisman (1975) described glial rosettes like those characteristic of viral encephalitis in the brains of psychotic patients, and Colon (1972) identified quantitative changes in the cortical cytoarchitectonics of patients suffering from schizophrenia. Stevens (1982) noted gliosis in the midbrain, diencephalic, and forebrain regions; these regions contain major tracts of the limbic system, thalamus, and basal ganglia. Bogerts et al. (1985) reported abnormalities in periventricular and limbic system regions in schizophrenia. Conrad et al. (1991) described neuronal loss and pyramidal cell disarray in the hippocampus, while Arnold et al. (1991) described cytoarchitectural abnormalities in the entorhinal cortex, which is part of the anterior parahippocampal gyrus. Benes et al. (1991) have also reported decreased density of interneurons in the prefontal cingulate and motor cortex, findings that are consistent with an accelerated process of neuronal dropout early in life, perhaps related to a perinatal insult.

Functional and Metabolic Studies

Beginning with the work of Ingvar and Franzen (1974), studies of regional cerebral blood flow (rCBF) have explored the possibility of functional or metabolic abnormalities in schizophrenia. Ingvar and Franzen's work suggested that schizophrenic patients had a relative hypofrontality and that blood flow to posterior brain regions may be increased. This finding has subsequently been confirmed by other investigators (Ariel et al. 1983; Buchsbaum et al. 1984). Research using PET has also consistently found evidence for a relative hypofrontality. Buchsbaum et al. (1992) confirmed lower metabolic rates in the inferior and medial frontal regions in neuroleptic-naive schizophrenic patients compared with control subjects. In general, research shows that hypofrontality is common in schizophrenic patients, is not due to prior medication or chronicity, and may be related to negative symptoms. Further, these studies suggest that there may be abnormalities in prefontal circuitry and function.

Electrophysiological Studies

Electrophysiological studies have shown that abnormal cerebral physiological events are associated with schizophrenia. Many schizophrenic patients have abnormal electroencephalographic tracings. The most consistent findings are of decreased alpha and increased delta activity. Research on evoked potentials appears more promising. One of the most consistent observations is the decrease in amplitudes of middle- and long-latency average event-related responses in schizophrenic subjects following auditory, visual, and somatosensory stimuli. Amplitude reduction may occur particularly in responses reflecting selective attention and stimulus evaluation. The most pronounced changes are in the P300 response, in which there is a reduced amplitude to surprising or unexpected stimuli using both auditory and visual paradigms. This research has supported the view that schizophrenic patients have an inability to properly filter or "gate" irrelevant information. Conceptually, this defect leads to information or sensory "overload" and an inability to screen out irrelevant stimuli (Braff and Geyer 1990).

Clinical Implications of Neurobiological Studies

Many of the symptoms of schizophrenia are consistent with frontal or temporolimbic disease. Lesion studies have indicated that injury to the prefrontal cortex leads to disorders of cognitive function (concreteness, impaired attention, difficulty abstracting or categorizing), diminished spontaneity of speech, a decrease in voluntary motor behavior, decreased will and energy, difficulty in shifting response set, and abnormalities of affect and emotion (Fuster 1980). These symptoms are strikingly similar to the negative symptoms observed in schizophrenia. Evidence from MRI, neuropathology, electrophysiology, and functional brain imaging techniques suggests that some patients with schizophrenia may have some type of frontal lobe abnormality.

Many of the symptoms of schizophrenia are also consistent with temporolimbic disease, including auditory hallucinations, disorganized speech, and abnormalities in verbal memory and other neuropsychological test abnormalities. Research on the dopamine hypothesis confirms the possibility that the temporolimbic region may be involved in schizophrenia. The dopaminergic system "drives" a substantial portion of the limbic system. Abnormalities in the limbic system in schizophrenia are also supported by some of the neuropathological studies cited above.

☐ Developmental Hypotheses

Family Environment

Clinicians working with families of schizophrenic patients became aware of frequent discord and social maladjustment within the family. Although these problems could have been the result of having a mentally ill family member, early work focused on family dysfunction itself as a cause of schizophrenia. The "schizophrenogenic mother" became a popular scapegoat (Fromm-Reichman 1948). According to this theory, schizophrenia results from an inadequate mother-child relationship; mothers of schizophrenic patients were described as rejecting, aloof, overly protective, or overtly hostile.

Parental influence and its effects on schizophrenia were amplified by communication theorists, most notably Bateson et al. (1956). They believed that schizophrenic patients were often subjected to vague, ambiguous, or confusing messages by their parents. This often resulted in the children being placed in a no-win response situation. Children exposed to this "double-bind" were vulnerable to develop schizophrenia because of the feelings of ambivalence and ambiguity. Bateson's hypothesis has stimulated research and discussion but has not been supported by more systematic clinical investigation (Leff 1978).

Although parental influences are no longer considered to cause schizophrenia, the influence of the family on the course of illness continues to be an active area of research and interest. Follow-up studies have examined families in which the schizophrenic member relapsed frequently (Brown et al. 1962). A family environment found to predispose to relapse was characterized by frequent, intense expression of emotion by the relatives to the schizophrenic patient, along with a pushy and critical attitude. This has been termed high "expressed emotion." Research in expressed emotion has continued and has included intervention trials to determine whether family therapy can lower expressed emotion and prevent schizophrenic patients from relapsing. These studies are discussed later in the chapter in the section on clinical management.

Neurodevelopmental Factors

Several lines of evidence support speculation that schizophrenia is a neurodevelopmental disorder resulting from brain injury occurring early in life that interferes with normal maturational events (Feinberg 1982; Weinberger 1987). The observation that perinatal complications often precede the development of severe neurological and psychological disorders, such as cerebral palsy and mental retardation, has led investigators to explore the role of perinatal and obstetrical complications in the etiology of schizophrenia. Schizophrenic patients are more likely than other psychiatric patients or normal control subjects to have a history of obstetrical complications (Lewis and Murray 1987). Prematurity, oxygen deprivation, and long labor are especially common.

A body of evidence suggests that obstetrical complications may have a relationship with cerebral ventricular size. Turner et al. (1986) reported that ventricular size was positively correlated with obstetrical complications in a small sample of first-episode schizophrenic patients, while Pearlson et al. (1985) similarly found that perinatal complications were associated with larger ventricles and earlier age at onset. DeLisi et al. (1986) noted that schizophrenic patients had larger ventricles than did their well siblings, and that 7 of 8 schizophrenic patients with ventricles more than one standard deviation larger than the control mean had a history of obstetrical complications or head injury.

The association of birth seasonality with schizophrenia also suggests a neurodevelopmental etiology. Throughout the temperate northern latitudes, the birth dates of schizophrenic patients tend to cluster in the winter months, although the excess is minor (Hare et al. 1973). This finding indicates that a seasonally varying influence, such as a viral infection, is acting in utero or in early life to cause brain injury. Thus, children born during the winter months would be more vulnerable because of the increased frequency of viral infections during the winter. Supporting a role for viral infection, Mednick et al. (1988) reported that individuals who were in their second trimester of fetal development during a 1957 A_2 influenza epidemic in Finland were at higher risk of hospitalization for schizophrenia than those born in the same months over the previous 6 years. The finding was replicated using data from influenza cases reported to the Ministry of Health in Denmark (Barr et al. 1990). Other attempts to link known influenza epidemics to an outbreak of schizophrenia have not been successful (Kendell and Kemp 1989).

Evidence from neuropathology and brain imaging also suggests the possibility of neurodevelopmental abnormalities in schizophrenia. In the early 1980s, Feinberg (1982) proposed that the peripubertal onset of the disorder may be due to the role of late brain maturation. According to this model, programmed synaptic elimination (or "pruning") in early adolescence could be delayed or decreased in at least some schizophrenic patients. This proposal has been supported by several subsequent neuroimaging studies and several neuropathology studies. Jernigan et al. (1991) and Swayze et al. (1992) have both observed increases in the size of basal ganglia structures, which could be attributed to a failure of pruning.

☐ Sociocultural Hypotheses

In a study of the geographic distribution of mental illness, Faris and Dunham (1939) found higher rates for mental hospital admissions, including admissions for schizophrenia, in central slums than in the suburbs. This finding was replicated in other cities in both the United States and Europe. The conclusion was drawn that schizophrenia was caused by the ill effect of the slum environment, where people are faced with enormous stress from social disorganization, poverty, and the general adversity imposed by poor living conditions. These conditions were believed to produce, or "breed," schizophrenia (Hare 1956).

Another explanation soon developed to explain the finding of geographic isolation of mentally ill persons. The "drift" hypothesis (Wender et al. 1973) stated that living in poor areas *resulted from* schizophrenia, and was not causal. Rather, schizophrenia leads to amotivation, cognitive impairment, poor hygiene, and other symptoms that make it impossible for the person with schizophrenia to maintain employment and survive in middle- and upper-class structures. Thus, persons with schizophrenia drift down in social class as their illness progresses. Subsequent research has supported this view (Silverton and Mednick 1984).

■ CLINICAL MANAGEMENT

☐ Pharmacological Approaches

Antipsychotic medication has been the mainstay of treatment for schizophrenia. All antipsychotics, with minor exceptions, have proven superior to placebo in the treatment of schizophrenia, reportedly due to their ability to block post-synaptic dopamine receptors in the limbic forebrain. Except for clozapine and risperidone, the first in a new generation of atypical antipsychotics, none has been shown to be superior to another. The choice of drug depends on the patient and his or her illness, as well as predicted side effects, prior treatment response, and perhaps family history of drug response. Both clozapine and risperidone are reported to be effective in many patients refractory to other antipsychotics, and have the advantage of few extrapyramidal side effects typical of most other antipsychotic medications. Therefore, patients who receive either of these drugs should be considered treatment refractory, or have severe extrapyramidal side effects from other agents. Since clozapine has the potential to induce agranulocytosis, blood counts need to be obtained weekly.

Acute Therapy

The acutely psychotic or agitated schizophrenic patient requires rapid control of symptoms. A daily dose of between 10 and 20 mg of haloperidol (or 500 to 600 mg of chlorpromazine) will produce improvement in many patients over several days or weeks; higher dosages may increase the likelihood of adverse side effects, and lower dosages may be ineffective (Baldessarini et al. 1988). Nearly 40 years after the introduction of these useful agents, a dose-response curve has not yet been defined and attempts to correlate plasma concentration of antipsychotics and their metabolites with therapeutic response have been disappointing. Plasma concentrations for many antipsychotics are available, but only haloperidol and clozapine levels have been positively correlated with clinical response (Perry et al. 1991); haloperidol may have a "therapeutic window" between 5 and 15 ng/ml, whereas clozapine blood levels greater than 500 ng/ml have been shown to have a 2.5-fold greater response rate than lower levels. More research is needed before the use of plasma levels becomes routine. Patients who smoke may require higher doses of antipsychotics because tobacco tends to stimulate hepatic enzymes, which increases drug metabolism (Goff et al. 1992).

Highly agitated patients who are out of control should be given frequent, equally spaced doses of an antipsychotic. A high-potency agent, such as haloperidol, can be given every 30 to 120 minutes until agitation is under control. Rarely is more than 20 to 30 mg of haloperidol required in a 24-hour period. It is likely that its effectiveness in subduing patients results from sedation rather than any specific antipsychotic effect. Because sedation is desired, a more rational approach may be to combine an antipsychotic with benzodiazepine for more rapid control of agitated psychotic patients.

Maintenance Therapy

Patients benefiting from short-term treatment with antipsychotics are candidates for long-term prophylactic treatment, which has as its goal the sustained control of psychotic symptoms. Because of the potential of these agents to cause tardive dyskinesia, continuing benefit to antipsychotic patients must be clearly established. A review of 38 studies (Baldessarini et al. 1988) showed that maintenance antipsychotics can reduce the chance of relapse by a factor of nearly fourfold within the first year (55% vs. 14%). However, it is clear that not all patients benefit equally; between 30% and 50% of patients on maintenance neuroleptics will eventually relapse, but up to 70% will relapse without medication (Crow et al. 1986).

Maintenance for one to two years is appropriate after an initial psychotic episode, usually at doses in the range of one-third to one-half of the original dose. After two such episodes, patients will probably benefit from longer prophylaxis (up to five years). At least five years of treatment are recommended for multi-episode patients since a high risk of relapse remains. Beyond this, data are incomplete, but indefinite and perhaps lifelong treatment is recommended for patients who pose a danger to themselves or others (Kissling 1991).

Over time, schizophrenic patients may develop an increase in negative symptoms and a decrease in positive symptoms, and, as a result, some may function well without medication. Positive symptoms, which may predominate early in the illness, tend to be more amenable to treatment. Therefore, the clinician should periodically reassess a patient to determine whether maintenance treatment is still required (Davis 1975). Research suggests that risk of relapse remains greater on oral rather than intramuscular antipsychotics, likely due to the problem of patient noncompliance (DeVito et al. 1978). Drug holidays, once recommended as a means of lowering the risk of tardive dyskinesia, lead only to more decompensation and rehospitalization, without lowering the risk for tardive dyskinesia (Carpenter et al. 1990).

Adjunctive Pharmacological Treatments

Adjunctive psychotropic medications are useful in the treatment of schizophrenia, although their role has not been clearly defined. Many patients benefit from anxiolytics (e.g., benzodiazepines) if anxiety is prominent. Other uses for these agents have been to help reduce psychotic agitation (Wolkowitz and Pickar 1991) or to relieve the akathisia associated with antipsychotic medications. Lithium carbonate may be useful to reduce impulsive and aggressive behaviors, hyperactivity, excitation, or to stabilize mood, although its effectiveness in this role has not been adequately determined. While early research suggested that antidepressants were not helpful in treating depressed schizophrenic patients and could cause a worsening of thought disorder, more recent research has shown that they may have a legitimate role in treating these patients (Siris et al. 1987, 1989). If used, antidepressants should be prescribed along with an antipsychotic to prevent worsening of psychosis, and should not be used routinely in floridly psychotic patients. A trial of an anti-parkinsonian agent to rule out an antipsychotic-induced akinesia should be tried initially. For patients who respond to adjunctive antidepressants, continuation treatment appears to be safe and effective. Other medications, including propranolol, carbamazepine, sodium valproate, clonidine, and verapamil, have been used experimentally, but have no current role in the treatment of schizophrenia.

☐ Physical Treatments

The primary usefulness of electroconvulsive therapy (ECT) is in the treatment of a few specific syndromes and in patients who do not respond to antipsychotic medication. Catatonia and depression secondary to schizophrenia have been recognized as indications for ECT. In both situations, ECT appears to be rapidly effective based on clinical reports, although neither its use in catatonia nor its use in depression secondary to schizophrenia has been subjected to careful study.

☐ Psychosocial Treatments

Psychosocial interventions play an important role in the management of patients with schizophrenia. Initially limited to traditional individual and group psychotherapies, interventions today may include assisting a patient to obtain access to governmental programs that provide the necessities for living, such as food and shelter. Clinicians must work actively to ensure that schizophrenic patients receive adequate mental health care and community benefits, and are encouraged to develop a close working relationship with local social service agencies. Optimal care necessitates the availability of a range of services to fit the needs of the patient, including social, vocational, and housing needs, but these services are inadequate in many communities (Lamb 1986).

Individual Psychotherapy

Although insight-oriented psychotherapy may not be helpful for most patients, and may be harmful to some (Mueser and Berenbaum 1990), this in no way diminishes the value that a long-term, supportive relationship with an interested clinician has for the schizophrenic patient. Supportive therapy that is reality oriented and pragmatic can be enormously helpful. For example, the clinician can help a patient to develop new coping strategies, to test reality, to resolve concrete problems, and to identify common stressors and prodromal symptoms of relapse. A strong "therapeutic alliance" may also help to boost medication compliance (Frank and Gunderson 1990).

Group Psychotherapy

Group therapy grew out of the observation that patients with similar problems could benefit from one another as well as from their physician. Although the primary goal in most traditional group therapies is facilitation of insight into personal and interpersonal problems, most work with schizophrenic patients is oriented toward providing support, an environment in which a patient can develop social skills, and a format that allows friendships to begin. Inpatient group therapy with schizophrenic patients is most successful when highly structured and when goals are limited to the capabilities of the individuals within the group (Yalom 1983). Patients who respond to group therapy while hospitalized may benefit from this approach on an outpatient basis.

Family Therapy

Family therapy has focused on families in which relatives of schizophrenic patients show high expressed emotion, a factor shown to increase risk of relapse (Falloon et al. 1985). Family therapy may be particularly valuable in preventing relapse when combined with antipsychotic medication. In a 2-year follow-up, Hogarty et al. (1991) found that family intervention along with maintenance medication forestalls relapse compared with medication only. Medication noncompliance was also less frequent in the group receiving family therapy. Thus, family therapy gains some of its impact through enhanced medication compliance. Family therapy also appears to enhance social adjustment and the ability to work.

Although our knowledge about the mechanism of improvement in family therapy may be limited, general recommendations can be made. First, families benefit from education about schizophrenia itself. This should include information about the chronic nature of the illness and the need for long-term management based on realistic expectations. Education will also improve the cooperation and compliance of both patient and family. Second, learning to minimize harsh criticism and emotional overinvolvement will decrease the schizophrenic patient's daily stress. This reduction may be helpful in preventing relapse.

Hospitalization

Long-term institutionalization is now rare, and most patients, when hospitalized, stay briefly in special psychiatric hospitals or in psychiatric units found in general hospitals. Reasons to hospitalize a schizophrenic patient include the patient being a danger to himself/herself or others; refusing to properly care for himself or herself; or the need for special medical observation, tests, or treatments. When the patient is a danger to himself/herself or others and refuses to enter the hospital, it is usually necessary to obtain a court order for hospitalization.

The design, structure, and organization of the ward can itself be therapeutic for patients with schizophrenia. The following characteristics are optimal: small units, short stays, high staff-to-patient ratio, low staff turnover, low percentage of psychotic patients, broad delegation of responsibility with clear lines of authority, low perceived levels of anger and aggression, high levels of support, and a practical problem-solving approach (Ellsworth 1983). Following hospital discharge, a similar milieu, such as that found in a residential treatment center (i.e., "halfway house"), can help the patient readjust to living in the community. A group residence in which clear limits and expectations are provided without intensive personal relationship is preferred. Unfortunately, such programs are expensive and may not be available (Lamb 1986).

Outpatient Treatment

During outpatient treatment, the patient should become an active participant in selecting medication and dose. This participation will reduce the sense of helplessness that many patients develop, thereby increasing the possibility of compliance. A depot neuroleptic will be the best choice for some patients; it will not only ensure that a patient receives needed medication, but will rid him or her of the need for oral dosing that serves as a daily reminder of disability. Although most of the antipsychotics are equally effective, some patients will respond better to certain agents for idiosyncratic reasons, or may subjectively "feel better" on a particular drug.

Alcohol/Drug Abuse

Psychoactive substance abuse aggravates the symptoms of schizophrenia, leads to medication noncompliance, and undermines other treatment interventions. Abstinence should be encouraged in all patients, and some will need referral for drug detoxification and rehabilitation. Although these services may not be helpful in acutely psychotic or agitated patients, they may be enormously beneficial once the patient has improved and the schizophrenic illness has stabilized.

Other Approaches

Once the acute symptoms of schizophrenia have subsided, other psychosocial interventions are possible. Social skills are usually deficient in schizophrenic patients (Cramer et al. 1992). There are a number of settings, including the living situation, individual or group therapies, or day hospital programs, where the patient may be helped to develop more appropriate social behaviors; many patients will benefit from specific programs in social skills training. Vocational training may benefit some patients. A simple, repetitive job environment with some opportunity for interpersonal distance may be the best initial work setting and is often found at a "sheltered workshop." Employment should be encouraged in able patients, but some patients will not be employable in any setting be-cause of apathy, amotivation, or chronic psychosis. For those patients who are unable to work, the clinician's role will be to assist them in ob-taining disability benefits.

■ DELUSIONAL DISORDER

Delusional disorder comprises a small but important group of distur-bances, characterized by the presence of well-systematized, nonbizarre delusions accompanied by affect appropriate to the delusion, and occur-ring in the presence of a relatively well-preserved personality. Kraepelin separated paranoia from dementia praecox and used the term to describe those patients with systematized delusions, an absence of hallucinations, and a prolonged course without recovery but not leading to mental dete-rioration (Kendler 1988). Bleuler also believed that paranoia was separate from dementia praecox, but he differed from Kraepelin in maintaining that hallucinations could occur in some patients. He was particularly in-terested in the psychological development of the disorder.

Recent American thought is represented in DSM-IV and is remark-ably similar to the definition put forth by Kraepelin. The term *paranoid disorder* has been discarded because the term paranoid is inherently am-biguous and is usually construed to mean "persecutory." The delusions observed in delusional disorder are not restricted to persecutory themes, but may include grandiose, erotomanic (i.e., delusions of being loved), and somatic themes as well (Winokur 1977).

☐ Diagnosis

According to DSM-IV (Table 12–5), delusional disorder is characterized by nonbizarre delusions lasting at least 1 month, behavior that is not ob-viously odd or bizarre apart from the delusion or its ramifications, rela-tive absence of active-phase symptoms that may occur in schizophrenia (e.g., hallucinations, disorganized speech, or negative symptoms), and the determination that the disorder is not due to a mood disorder with psychotic features or a substance-induced or secondary psychotic disor-der. The core feature, however, is the presence of a well-systematized, encapsulated, nonbizarre delusion. The term *systematized* is used to indi-cate that the delusion and its ramifications fit into an all-encompassing, complex scheme that makes sense to the patient. The term *encapsulated* indicates that apart from the delusion or its ramifications, the patient generally functions normally in most domains of life. The term *nonbizarre* implies that the delusion involves situations that can occur in real life, such as being followed, and not implausible or impossible situations.

Table 12–5. DSM-IV criteria for delusional disorder

A. Nonbizarre delusions (i.e., involving situations that occur in real life, such as being followed, poisoned, infected, loved at a distance, or deceived by spouse or lover, or having a disease) of at least 1 month's duration.

B. Criterion A for schizophrenia has never been met.

Note: Tactile and olfactory hallucinations may be present in delusional disorder if they are related to the delusional theme.

C. Apart from the impact of the delusion(s) or its ramifications, functioning is not markedly impaired and behavior is not obviously odd or bizarre.

D. If mood episodes have occurred concurrently with delusions, their total duration has been brief relative to the duration of the delusional periods.

E. The disturbance is not due to the direct physiological effects of a substance (e.g., a drug of abuse, a medication) or a general medical condition.

Specify type (the following types are assigned based on the predominant delusional theme):

Erotomanic type: delusions that another person, usually of higher status, is in love with the individual

Grandiose type: delusions of inflated worth, power, knowledge, identity, or special relationship to a deity or famous person

Jealous type: delusions that the individual's sexual partner is unfaithful

Persecutory type: delusions that the person (or someone to whom the person is close) is being malevolently treated in some way

Somatic type: delusions that the person has some physical defect or general medical condition

Mixed type: delusions characteristic of more than one of the above types but no one theme predominates

Unspecified type

A careful diagnostic assessment is necessary to rule out other functional or organic illnesses that could have caused the delusions. The workup must include physical examination to rule out alcoholism, amphetamine, cocaine, and other drug-induced states; dementia; infections; and metabolic and endocrine disorders (Manschreck and Petri 1978). Routine laboratory tests may be indicated depending on the results of the history and physical examination. CT or MRI may be useful in selected patients, especially when mass lesions are suspected.

The major differential diagnosis remains in separating delusional disorder from mood disorders, schizophrenia, and paranoid personality. The chief distinction is that in delusional disorder a full depressive or manic syndrome is absent, developed after the psychotic symptoms, or was brief in duration relative to the duration of the psychotic symptoms. Unlike schizophrenia, delusional disorder is characterized by *nonbizarre* delusions and generally either *no* hallucinations *or* hallucinations that are not prominent. Furthermore, patients with delusional disorder do not develop other schizophrenic symptoms such as incoherence or grossly disorganized behavior, and personality is generally preserved. Persons with paranoid personality are suspicious and hypervigilant, but are not delusional. Other features of delusional disorder may include anger, social isolation and seclusiveness, eccentric behavior, suspiciousness, hostility, and rarely violence, usually prompted by the delusion (Kennedy et al. 1992). Many patients become litigious and end up as lawyers' clients rather than as psychiatrists' patients.

☐ Epidemiology

Delusional disorder constitutes between 1% and 4% of psychiatric admissions, with a prevalence of between 24 to 30 per 100,000 population. Paranoia manifests predominantly in middle to late adult life with a peak frequency of first admissions in persons between 35 and 55 years of age. Patients are more likely to be female than male. Sixty to 75% of patients first admitted are married, but up to one-third are widowed, divorced, or separated at the time of admission. Patients with the disorder are judged to be relatively socially disadvantaged, both in economic and in educational terms, and are often immigrants (Kendler 1982).

☐ Etiology

Little is known about the etiology of delusional disorder. The weight of evidence suggests that it is not related to schizophrenia or the mood disorders. Kendler et al. (1985) reported no increase in the risk for mood disorders in families of paranoid probands. Kendler et al. (1981) found that cases of schizophrenia spectrum disorders (i.e., schizotypal personality and schizophrenia) were strongly concentrated in the biological relatives of schizophrenic adoptees, but not in adoptees with delusional disorder.

It is possible that psychosocial stressors have a role in the etiology of delusional disorder in some persons. Certain rare conditions illustrate this possibility. *Shared psychotic disorder* occurs when delusions are shared by two or more individuals. Usually the dominant person in the relationship develops a delusion, which is later adopted by the more passive individual. *Migration psychoses,* often persecutory in nature, are described in persons migrating from one country to another (although it is reasonable that persons in whom paranoia is prone to develop may be more likely to emigrate than others). *Prison psychosis* has been described in which isolation in prison, especially solitary confinement, has led to paranoia. *Querulent paranoia,* a special form of paranoia characterized by litigiousness, is believed by Scandinavian investigators to be a psychogenic disorder in which unlucky personal experiences precipitate paranoia in persons with deviant personalities (Astrup 1984).

☐ Course and Outcome

Delusional disorders have a relatively chronic, unremitting course. Studies evaluating outcome have not been entirely consistent, although delusional disorder appears to have a better outcome than does schizophrenia. Winokur (1977) reported that 79% of hospitalized patients with delusional disorder were discharged to the community compared with 26% of schizophrenic patients. At follow-up nearly 3 years later, 69% remained delusional, although 31% were considered "socially recovered." Retterstol (1970) found on long-term follow-up that 79% of his cohort were self-supporting and 74% had had no major periods without work; comparable figures for patients with schizophrenia were 31% and 30%, respectively. Only 39% of delusional disorder patients had been hospitalized since initial discharge and 27% were psychotic; comparable figures for schizophrenic patients were 90% and 80%, respectively.

☐ Clinical Management

There are no systematic data comparing treatments in delusional disorder; therefore any recommendations are based on clinical observation, not empirical evidence. Most patients have little insight about their illness and refuse to acknowledge that there may be a problem, so the initial obstacle is getting the patient to the physician. Most patients can be treated on an outpatient basis. Hospitalization is indicated if a potential for danger is present. In some cases, involuntary hospitalization will be necessary, especially when the threat of self-harm or harm to others is present.

Tact and skill are necessary to persuade a patient to accept treatment. It may help to first convince the patient that he or she should have treatment for depressive or anxiety symptoms and not his or her delusions. After establishing a therapeutic relationship, the physician may begin to gently challenge the delusional beliefs by showing how they interfere with the patient's life. The physician must neither condemn nor collude in the beliefs. The patient should be assured of confidentiality, and the physician should not discuss matters with the patient's family without the patient's approval. Insight-oriented psychotherapy and group therapy are generally not recommended, because suspiciousness and hypersensitivity may lead to misinterpretation.

The use of antipsychotic medications has never been properly evaluated in delusional disorder, although anecdotal evidence suggests that response is poor (Winokur 1977). These agents may help to diminish delusions and anxiety, but leave the core delusion untouched. Any of the standard antipsychotics may be used, but the selection of medication and dose will depend on age and anticipated side effects. If the patient responds to antipsychotics, depot forms may be helpful to ensure compliance. Some investigators suggest that specific forms of delusional disorder—for example, *monohypochondriacal paranoia* (i.e., delusional disorder, somatic type)—may have a good response to the antipsychotic pimozide (Munro 1978). Segal (1989) concluded that neuroleptics can help to reduce the intensity of the delusions in erotomania and the associated ideas of reference. Antidepressants and anxiolytics may be indicated for accompanying depressive or anxiety syndromes, but they have not been systematically evaluated in patients with delusional disorder.

■ REFERENCES

Allebeck P, Varla A, Kristjansson E, et al: Risk factors for suicide among patients with schizophrenia. Acta Psychiatr Scand 76:414–419, 1987

Amador XF, Sackheim HA, Mukerjee S, et al: Specificity of smooth pursuit eye movement and visual fixation abnormalities in schizophrenia: comparison to mania and normal controls. Schizophrenia Research 5:135–144, 1991

American Psychiatric Association: Diagnostic and Statistical Manual of Mental Disorders, 3rd Edition. Washington, DC, American Psychiatric Press, 1980

American Psychiatric Association: Diagnostic and Statistical Manual of Mental Disorders, 3rd Edition, Revised. Washington, DC, American Psychiatric Association, 1987

American Psychiatric Association: Diagnostic and Statistical Manual of Mental Disorders, 4th Edition. Washington, DC, American Psychiatric Association, 1994

Andreasen NC, Akiskal HS: The specificity of Bleulerian and Schneiderian symptoms: a critical reevaluation. Psychiatr Clin North Am 6:41–54, 1983

Andreasen NC, Nasrallah HA, Dunn V, et al: Structural abnormalities in the frontal system in schizophrenia: a magnetic resonance imaging study. Arch Gen Psychiatry 43:136–144, 1986

Andreasen NC, Ehrhardt JC, Swayze VW, et al: Magnetic resonance imaging of the brain in schizophrenia: the pathophysiologic significance of structural abnormalities. Arch Gen Psychiatry 47:35–44, 1990a

Andreasen NC, Flaum M, Swayze VW, et al: Positive and negative symptoms in schizophrenia: a critical reappraisal. Arch Gen Psychiatry 47:615–621, 1990b

Ariel RN, Golden CJ, Berg RA, et al: Regional cerebral blood flow in schizophrenics: tests using the xenon Xe 133 inhalation method. Arch Gen Psychiatry 40:258–263, 1983

Arnold SE, Hyman BT, Van Hoesen GW, et al: Some cytoarchitectural abnormalities of the entorhinal cortex in schizophrenia. Arch Gen Psychiatry 48:625–632, 1991

Astrup C: Querulent paranoia: a follow-up. Neuropsychobiology 11:149–154, 1984

Aylward E, Walker E, Bettes B: Intelligence in schizophrenia: meta-analysis of the research. Schizophr Bull 10:430–459, 1984

Baldessarini RJ, Cohen BM, Teicher MH: Significance of neuroleptic dose and plasma level in the pharmacologic treatment of psychoses. Arch Gen Psychiatry 45:79–91, 1988

Barr CE, Mednick SA, Munk-Jorgensen P: Exposure to influenza epidemics during gestation and adult schizophrenia: a 40-year study. Arch Gen Psychiatry 47:869–874, 1990

Barraclough B, Bunch J, Nelson B, et al: A hundred cases of suicide: clinical aspects. Br J Psychiatry 125:355–373, 1974

Barta PE, Pearlson GD, Powers RE, et al: Auditory hallucinations and smaller superior temporal gyral volume in schizophrenia. Am J Psychiatry 147:1457–1462, 1990

Bateson G, Jackson D, Haley J, et al: Towards a theory of schizophrenia. Behav Sci 1:251–264, 1956

Beitchman JH: Childhood schizophrenia—a review and comparison with adult onset schizophrenia. Pediatr Clin North Am 8:793–814, 1985

Benes FM, McSparren J, Bird ED, et al: Deficits in small interneurons in prefrontal and cingulate cortices of schizophrenic and schizoaffective patients. Arch Gen Psychiatry 48:996–1001, 1991

Black DW, Fisher R: Mortality in DSM-III-R schizophrenia. Schizophrenia Research 7:109–116, 1992

Bleuler E: Dementia Praecox, or the Group of Schizophrenias (1911). Translated by Zinken J. New York, International Universities Press, 1950

Bogerts B, Meertz E, Schönfeldt-Bausch R: Basal ganglia and limbic system pathology in schizophrenia: a morphometric study of brain volume and shrinkage. Arch Gen Psychiatry 42:784–791, 1985

Braff DL, Geyer MA: Sensorimotor gating and schizophrenia: human and animal model studies. Arch Gen Psychiatry 47:181–188, 1990

Braff DL, Heaton R, Kuck J, et al: The generalized pattern of neuropsychological deficits in outpatients with chronic schizophrenia with heterogeneous Wisconsin Card Sorting Test results. Arch Gen Psychiatry 48:891–898, 1991

Breier A, Astrachan BM: Characterization of schizophrenic patients who commit suicide. Am J Psychiatry 141:206–209, 1984

Brown GW, Monck EM, Carstairs GM, et al: Influence of family life on the course of schizophrenic illness. British Journal of Preventative and Social Medicine 16:55–68, 1962

Buchsbaum MS, DeLisi LE, Holcomb HH, et al: Antero-posterior gradients in cerebral glucose use in schizophrenia and affective disorders. Arch Gen Psychiatry 41:1159–1166, 1984

Buchsbaum MS, Haier RJ, Potkin SG, et al: Frontostriatal disorder of cerebral metabolism in never-medicated schizophrenics. Arch Gen Psychiatry 49:935–942, 1992

Caracci G, Mukherjee S, Roth SD, et al: Subjective awareness of abnormal involuntary movements in chronic schizophrenic patients. Am J Psychiatry 147:295–298, 1990

Carpenter WT Jr, Hanlon TE, Heinrichs DW, et al: Continuous versus targeted medication in schizophrenic outpatients: outcome results. Am J Psychiatry 147:1138–1148, 1990

Clardy JA, Hyde TM, Kleinman JE: Postmortem neurochemical and neuropathological studies in schizophrenia, in Schizophrenia: From Mind to Molecule. Edited by Andreasen NC. Washington, DC, American Psychiatric Press, 1993, pp 123–145

Colon EJ: Quantitative cytoarchitectonics in the lumen cerebral cortex in schizophrenic dementia. Acta Neuropathol (Berl) 20:1–10, 1972

Conrad AJ, Abebe T, Austin R, et al.: Hippocampal pyramidal cell disarray in schizophrenia as a bilateral phenomenon. Arch Gen Psychiatry 48:413–417, 1991

Cooper JE, Kendell RE, Gurland BJ, et al: Psychiatric Diagnosis in New York and London: A Comparative Study of Mental Hospital Admissions. Institute of Psychiatry Maudsley Monographs No 20. London, Oxford University Press, 1972

Coryell WH, Tsuang MT: Outcome after 40 years in DSM-III schizophreniform disorder. Arch Gen Psychiatry 43:324–328, 1986

Cramer P, Bowen J, O'Neill M: Schizophrenics and social judgement: why do schizophrenics get it wrong? Br J Psychiatry 160:481–487, 1992

Creese R, Burt BR, Snyder SH: Dopamine receptor binding predicts clinical and pharmacologic potencies of antipsychotic drugs. Science 192:81–84, 1976

Crow TJ, MacMillan JF, Johnson AL, et al: The Northwick Park Study of First Episodes of Schizophrenia, II: a randomised controlled study of prophylactic neuroleptic treatment. Br J Psychiatry 148:120–127, 1986

Cutting J: Outcome of schizophrenia: overview, in Contemporary Issues in Schizophrenia. Edited by Kerr TA, Snaith P. Washington, DC, American Psychiatric Press, 1986, pp 433–440

Davis JM: Overview: maintenance therapy in psychiatry, I: schizophrenia. Am J Psychiatry 132:1237–1245, 1975

Davis KL, Kahn RS, Ko G, et al: Dopamine in schizophrenia: a review and reconceptualization. Am J Psychiatry 148:1474–1486, 1991

DeLisi LE, Goldin LR, Hamovit JR, et al: A family study of the association of increased ventricular size with schizophrenia. Arch Gen Psychiatry 43:148–153, 1986

DeVito RA, Brink L, Sloan C, et al: Fluphenazine decanoate vs oral antipsychotics: a comparison of their effectiveness in the treatment of schizophrenia as measured by a reduction in hospital readmissions. J Clin Psychiatry 39:26–34, 1978

Dixon L, Haas G, Weiden PJ, et al: Drug abuse in schizophrenic patients: clinical correlates and reasons for use. Am J Psychiatry 148:224–230, 1991

Drake RE, Osher FC, Wallach MA: Alcohol use and abuse in schizophrenia: a prospective community study. J Nerv Ment Dis 177:408–414, 1989

Eaton WW: Epidemiology of schizophrenia. Epidemiol Rev 7:105–126, 1985

Ellsworth RB: Characteristics of effective treatment milieu, in Principles and Practice of Milieu Therapy. Edited by Gunderson JG, Will OA, Mosher LF. New York, Jason Aronson, 1983, pp 87–123

Erlenmeyer-Kimling L: Fertility in psychotics, in Annual Review of the Schizophrenic Syndrome, Vol 5. Edited by Cancro R. New York, Brunner/Mazel, 1978, pp 298–325

Falloon IRH, Boyd JL, McGill CW, et al: Family management in the prevention of morbidity of schizophrenia: clinical outcome of a two-year longitudinal study. Arch Gen Psychiatry 42:887–896, 1985

Farde L, Wiesel F-A, Stone-Elander S, et al: D_2 dopamine receptors in neuroleptic-naive schizophrenic patients: positron emission tomography study with [^{11}C]raclopride. Arch Gen Psychiatry 47:213–219, 1990

Faris REL, Dunham HL: Mental Disorder in Urban Areas. Chicago, IL, University of Chicago Press, 1939

Farmer AE, McGuffin P, Gottesman II: Twin concordance for DSM-III schizophrenia: scrutinizing the validity of the definition. Arch Gen Psychiatry 44:634–641, 1987

Feinberg I: Schizophrenia and late maturational brain changes in man. Psychopharmacol Bull 18(3):29–31, 1982

Fenton WS, McGlashan TH: Natural history of schizophrenia subtypes, I: longitudinal study of paranoid, hebephrenic, and undifferentiated schizophrenia. Arch Gen Psychiatry 48:969–977, 1991

Fisman M: The brain stem in psychosis. Br J Psychiatry 126:414–422, 1975

Flaum M, Arndt S, Andreasen NC: The role of gender in studies of ventrical enlargement in schizophrenia: a predominantly male effect. Am J Psychiatry 147:1327–1332, 1990

Fogelson DL, Cohen BM, Pope HG Jr: A study of DSM-III schizophreniform disorder. Am J Psychiatry 139:1281–1285, 1982

Frank AF, Gunderson JG: The role of the therapeutic alliance in the treatment of schizophrenia: relationship to course and outcome. Arch Gen Psychiatry 47:228–236, 1990

Fromm-Reichmann F: Notes on the development of treatment of schizophrenics by psychoanalytic psychotherapy. Psychiatry 11:263–273, 1948

Fuster JM: The Prefrontal Cortex. New York, Raven, 1980

Goff DC, Henderson DC, Amico E: Cigarette smoking in schizophrenia: relationship to psychopathology and medication side effects. Am J Psychiatry 149:1189–1194, 1992

Gottesman II, Shields J: Schizophrenia: The Epigenetic Puzzle. Cambridge, UK, Cambridge University Press, 1982

Guze SB, Cloninger CR, Martin RL, et al: A follow-up and family study of schizophrenia. Arch Gen Psychiatry 40:1273–1276, 1983

Hare EH: Mental illness and social conditions in Bristol. Journal of Mental Science 102:349–357, 1956

Hare EH, Price JS, Slater E: Mental disorder and season of birth. Nature 24:480, 1973

Heinrichs DW, Buchanan RW: Significance and meaning of neurological signs in schizophrenia. Am J Psychiatry 145:11–18, 1988

Henn FA, Herjanic M, Vanderpearl RH: Forensic psychiatry: diagnosis and criminal responsibility. J Nerv Ment Dis 162:423–429, 1976

Herrman HE, Baldwin JA, Christie D: A record linkage study of mortality and general hospital discharge in patients diagnosed as schizophrenic. Psychol Med 13:581–593, 1983

Hogarty GE, Anderson CM, Reiss DJ, et al: Family psychoeducation, social skills training, and maintenance chemotherapy in the aftercare treatment of schizophrenia, II: two-year effects of a controlled study on relapse and adjustment. Arch Gen Psychiatry 48:340–347, 1991

Holzman PS, Solomon CM, Levin S, et al: Pursuit eye movement dysfunctions in schizophrenia: family evidence for specificity. Arch Gen Psychiatry 41:136–139, 1984

Ingvar DH, Franzen G: Abnormalities of cerebral blood flow distribution in patients with chronic schizophrenia. Acta Psychiatr Scand 50:425–462, 1974

Jablensky A, Sartorius N: Culture and schizophrenia. Psychol Med 5:113–124, 1975

Jernigan TL, Zisook S, Heaton RK, et al: Magnetic resonance imaging abnormalities in lenticular nuclei and cerebral cortex in schizophrenia. Arch Gen Psychiatry 48:881–890, 1991

Johnson DAW: Studies of depressive symptoms in schizophrenia, III: a double-blind trial of orphenadrine against placebo. Br J Psychiatry 139:96–97, 1981

Jonsson H, Nyman AK: Prediction of outcome in schizophrenia. Acta Psychiatr Scand 69:274–291, 1984

Kallman FJ: The Genetics of Schizophrenia. New York, Augustin, 1938

Keilp JG, Sweeney JA, Jacobsen P, et al: Cognitive impairment in schizophrenia: specific relations to ventricular size and negative symptomatology. Biol Psychiatry 24:47–55, 1988

Kendell RE, Kemp IW: Maternal influenza in the etiology of schizophrenia. Arch Gen Psychiatry 46:878–882, 1989

Kendler KS: Demography of paranoid psychosis (delusional disorder): a review and comparison with schizophrenia and affective illness. Arch Gen Psychiatry 39:890–902, 1982

Kendler KS: Kraepelin and the diagnostic concept of paranoia. Compr Psychiatry 29:4–11, 1988

Kendler KS, Gruenberg AM, Strauss JS: An independent analysis of the Copenhagen sample of the Danish Adoption Study of Schizophrenia, III: the relationship between paranoid psychosis (delusional disorder) and the schizophrenia spectrum disorders. Arch Gen Psychiatry 38:985–987, 1981

Kendler KS, Masterson CC, Davis KL: Psychiatric illness in first-degree relatives of patients with paranoid psychosis, schizophrenia and medical illness. Br J Psychiatry 147:524–531, 1985

Kennedy HG, Kemp LI, Dyer DE: Fear and anger in delusional (paranoid) disorder: the association with violence. Br J Psychiatry 160:488–492, 1992

Kety SS, Rosenthal D, Wender PH, et al: Mental illness in the biologic and adoptive families of adopted individuals who have became schizophrenic: a preliminary report based on psychiatric interviews, in Genetic Research in Psychiatry. Edited by Fieve R, Rosenthal D, Brill H. Baltimore, MD, Johns Hopkins Press, 1975, pp 147–165

Kissling W (ed): Guidelines for Neuroleptic Relapse Prevention in Schizophrenia. Berlin, Springer-Verlag, 1991

Kopala L, Clark C, Hurwitz TA: Sex differences in olfactory function in schizophrenia. Am J Psychiatry 146:1320–1322, 1989

Kraepelin E: Dementia Praecox and Paraphrenia. Translated by Barkley RM. Edinburgh, E & S Livingstone, 1919

Lamb HR: Some reflections on treating schizophrenics. Arch Gen Psychiatry 43:1007–1011, 1986

Langfeldt G: Schizophreniform States. Copenhagen, E Munksguard, 1939

Leff J: Social and psychological causes of the acute attack, in Schizophrenia: Towards a New Synthesis. Edited by Wing JK. London, Academic, 1978, pp 139–165

Lewine R, Burbach D, Melzer HY: Effect of diagnostic criteria on the ratio of male to female schizophrenic patients. Am J Psychiatry 141:84–87, 1984

Lewis SW, Murray RM: Obstetric complications, neurodevelopmental deviance, and risk of schizophrenia. J Psychiatr Res 21:413–421, 1987

Loranger AW: Sex difference in age at onset of schizophrenia. Arch Gen Psychiatry 41:157–161, 1984

Lyketsos GC, Sakka P, Maïlis A: The sexual adjustment of chronic schizophrenics: a preliminary study. Br J Psychiatry 143:376–382, 1983

Mackert A, Flechtner KM, Woyth C, et al: Increased blink rates in schizophrenics: influences of neuroleptics and psychopathology. Schizophrenia Research 4:41–47, 1991

Manschreck TC, Petri M: The paranoid syndrome. Lancet 2:251–253, 1978

McGlashan TH: The prediction of outcome in chronic schizophrenia, IV: The Chestnut Lodge Follow-up Study. Arch Gen Psychiatry 43:167–176, 1986

Mednick SA, Machon RA, Huttunen MO, et al: Adult schizophrenia following prenatal exposure to an influenza epidemic. Arch Gen Psychiatry 45:189–192, 1988

Meltzer HY: Biological studies in schizophrenia. Schizophr Bull 13:77–111, 1987

Mueser KT, Berenbaum H: Psychodynamic treatment of schizophrenia: is there a future? Psychol Med 20:253–262, 1990

Mukherjee S, Shukla S, Woodle J, et al: Misdiagnosis of schizophrenia in bipolar patients: a multiethnic comparison. Am J Psychiatry 140:1571–1574, 1983

Munro A: Monosymptomatic hypochondriacal psychosis manifesting as delusions of parasitosis. Arch Dermatol 114:940–943, 1978

Neylan TC, van Kammen DP, Kelley ME, et al: Sleep in schizophrenic patients on and off haloperidol therapy: clinically stable vs relapsed patients. Arch Gen Psychiatry 49:643–649, 1992

Pearlson GD, Garbacz DJ, Moberg PJ, et al: Symptomatic, familial, perinatal, and social correlates of computerized axial tomography (CAT) changes in schizophrenics and bipolars. J Nerv Ment Dis 173:42–50, 1985

Perry JC, Jacobs D: Overview: clinical applications of the Amytal interview in psychiatric emergency settings. Am J Psychiatry 139:552–559, 1982

Perry PJ, Miller DD, Arndt SV, et al: Clozapine and norclozapine plasma concentrations and clinical response of treatment-refractory schizophrenic patients. Am J Psychiatry 148:231–235, 1991

Pfohl B, Winokur G: The micropsychopathology of hebephrenic/catatonic schizophrenia. J Nerv Ment Dis 171:296–300, 1983

Pulver AE, Brown CH, Wolyniec PS, et al: Psychiatric morbidity in the relatives of patients with DSM-III schizophreniform disorder: comparisons with the relatives of schizophrenic and bipolar patients. J Psychiatr Res 25:19–29, 1991

Quitkin F, Rifkin A, Klein DF: Neurologic soft signs in schizophrenia and character disorders: organicity in schizophrenia with premorbid asociality and emotionally unstable character disorders. Arch Gen Psychiatry 33:845–853, 1976

Retterstol N: Paranoid and Paranoiac Psychoses. Springfield, IL, Charles C Thomas, 1970

Robins LN, Helzer JE, Weissman MM, et al: Lifetime prevalence of specific psychiatric disorders in three sites. Arch Gen Psychiatry 41:949–958, 1984

Roy A: Suicide in chronic schizophrenia. Br J Psychiatry 141:171–177, 1982

Sartorius N, Jablensky A, Korten A: Early manifestations and first contact incidence of schizophrenia in different cultures: a preliminary report on the evaluation of the WHO Collaborative Study in Determinants of Outcome of Severe Mental Disorders. Psychol Med 16:909–928, 1986

Saykin AJ, Gur RC, Gur RE, et al: Neuropsychological function in schizophrenia: selective impairment in memory and learning. Arch Gen Psychiatry 48:618–624, 1991

Seeman MV: Current outcome in schizophrenia: women vs men. Acta Psychiatr Scand 73:609–617, 1986

Seeman P, Lee T, Chau-Wong M, et al: Antipsychotic drug doses and neuroleptic-dopamine receptors. Nature 261:717–719, 1976

Segal JH: Erotomania revisited: from Kraepelin to DSM-III-R. Am J Psychiatry 146:1261–1266, 1989

Shapiro S, Skinner EA, Kessler LG, et al: Utilization of health and mental health services: three Epidemiologic Catchment Area sites. Arch Gen Psychiatry 41:971–978, 1984

Sherrington R, Brynjolfsson J, Peturssen H, et al: Localization of a susceptibility locus for schizophrenia on chromosome 5. Nature 336:164–166, 1988

Silverton L, Mednick S: Class drift and schizophrenia. Acta Psychiatr Scand 70:304–309, 1984

Siris SG, Morgan V, Fagerstrom R, et al: Adjunctive imipramine in the treatment of postpsychotic depression: a controlled trial. Arch Gen Psychiatry 44:533–539, 1987

Siris SG, Cutler J, Owen K, et al: Adjunctive imipramine maintenance treatment in schizophrenic patients with remitted postpsychotic depression. Am J Psychiatry 146:1495–1497, 1989

Snyder SH: Catecholamines in the brain as mediators of amphetamine psychosis. Arch Gen Psychiatry 27:169–179, 1972

Snyder SH: The dopamine hypothesis of schizophrenia: focus on the dopamine receptor. Am J Psychiatry 133:197–202, 1976

Stevens JR: Neurology and neuropathology of schizophrenia, in Schizophrenia as a Brain Disease. Edited by Henn FA, Nasrallah HA. New York, Oxford University Press, 1982, pp 112–147

Stoudemire A: A differential diagnosis of catatonic states. Psychosomatics 23:245–251, 1982

Strauss JS, Carpenter WT Jr: Schizophrenia. New York, Plenum, 1981

Suddath RC, Christison GW, Torrey EF, et al: Anatomical abnormalities in the brains of monozygotic twins discordant for schizophrenia. N Engl J Med 322:789–794, 1990

Susser E, Struening EL, Conover S: Psychiatric problems in homeless men: lifetime psychosis, substance use, and current distress in new arrivals at New York City shelters. Arch Gen Psychiatry 46:845–850, 1989

Swayze VW, Andreasen NC, Alliger RJ, et al: Subcortical and temporal structures in affective disorder and schizophrenia: a magnetic resonance imaging study. Biol Psychiatry 31:221–240, 1992

Taube CA, Barrett SA (eds): Mental Health United States, 1985 (DHHS Publ No ADM 85-1378). Rockville, MD, National Institute of Mental Health, 1985

Tienari P: Psychiatric illness in identical twins. Acta Psychiatr Scand Suppl, No 171, 1963

Tsuang MT: Suicide in schizophrenics, manics, depressives, and surgical controls: a comparison with general population suicide mortality. Arch Gen Psychiatry 35:153–155, 1978

Tsuang MT, Woolson RF, Fleming JA: Long-term outcome of major psychoses, I: schizophrenia and affective disorders compared with psychiatrically symptom-free surgical conditions. Arch Gen Psychiatry 36:1295–1304, 1979

Turner SW, Toone BK, Brett-Jones JR: Computerized tomographic scan change in early schizophrenia. Psychol Med 16:209–225, 1986

Van Kammen DP, Peters J, Yao J, et al: Norepinephrine in acute exacerbations of chronic schizophrenia: negative symptoms revisted. Arch Gen Psychiatry 47:161–168, 1990

Weinberger DR: Implications of normal brain development for the pathogenesis of schizophrenia. Arch Gen Psychiatry 44:660–669, 1987

Weinberger DR, DeLisi LE, Perman GP, et al: Computed tomography and schizophreniform disorder and other acute psychiatric disorders. Arch Gen Psychiatry 39:778–783, 1982

Wender PH, Rosenthal D, Kety SS, et al: Social class and psychopathology in adoptees: a natural experimental method for separating the roles of genetic and experiential factors. Arch Gen Psychiatry 28:318–325, 1973

Wing JK, Birley JLT, Cooper JE, et al: Reliability of a procedure for measuring and classifying "present psychiatric state." Br J Psychiatry 113:499–515, 1967

Winokur G: Delusional disorder (paranoia). Compr Psychiatry 18:511–521, 1977

Winokur G, Morrison J, Clancy J, et al: Iowa 500: the clinical and genetic distinction of hebephrenic and paranoid schizophrenia. J Nerv Ment Dis 159:12–19, 1974

Wolkowitz OM, Pickar D: Benzodiazepines in the treatment of schizophrenia: a review and reappraisal. Am J Psychiatry 148:714–726, 1991

World Health Organization: Schizophrenia: The International Pilot Study of Schizophrenia, Vol 1. Geneva, World Health Organization, 1975

Yalom ID: Inpatient Group Psychotherapy, New York, Basic Books, 1983

Mood Disorders

James W. Jefferson, M.D.
John H. Greist, M.D.

In 1980, DSM-III (American Psychiatric Association 1980) divided the major affective disorders into *bipolar* (mixed, manic, and depressed) and *major depression* (single episode and recurrent). In DSM-III-R, the affective disorders of DSM-III were referred to as *mood disorders*. Mood was described as "a prolonged emotion that colors the whole psychic state" (American Psychiatric Association 1987, p. 213). Affect had been defined elsewhere as "the outward manifestation of a person's feeling, tone, or mood" (American Psychiatric Association 1984, p. 3). Semantics aside, mood disorders and affective disorders are one and the same, and, practically speaking, the terms are used interchangeably.

DSM-IV still refers to mood disorders, with some modifications from DSM-III-R (American Psychiatric Association 1994) (Table 13–1). Major depression is now known as *major depressive disorder*. Dysthymia has become *dysthymic disorder,* and its alternative appellation, *depressive neurosis,* has finally been put to rest. Depressive disorder NOS has incorporated conditions such as premenstrual dysphoria disorder, minor depressive disorder, and recurrent brief depressive disorder, all of which failed to achieve separate categoryhood, and postpsychotic depression of schizophrenia. In DSM-IV the bipolar disorders have been further refined to remove bipolar II disorder (i.e., recurrent major depressive episodes with hypomania) from the bipolar disorder NOS residual category and give it individual status.

Three new diagnostic categories have been established under mood disorders: mood disorder due to a general medical condition, substance-induced mood disorder, and mood disorder NOS. The first two are trans-

---

Table 13–1.   Mood disorders (DSM-IV)

Depressive disorders
    Major depressive disorder
        Single episode
        . Recurrent
    Dysthymic disorder
    Depressive disorder not otherwise specified (NOS)
        Examples:
            Premenstrual dysphoric disorder
            Minor depressive disorder
            Recurrent brief depressive disorder
            Postpsychotic depression of schizophrenia
Bipolar disorders
    Bipolar I disorder
        Single manic episode
        Most recent episode hypomanic
        Most recent episode manic
        Most recent episode mixed
        Most recent episode depressed
        Most recent episode unspecified
    Bipolar II disorder (recurrent major depressive episodes with hypomania)
Cyclothymic disorder
Bipolar disorder not otherwise specified (NOS)
    Examples:
        Recurrent hypomania without depression
        Manic episode superimposed on delusional disorder
Mood disorder due to a general medical condition
Substance-induced mood disorder
Mood disorder not otherwise specified (NOS)

---

fers from the organic mental disorders section in DSM-III-R, and the last may have been created for more ambivalent diagnosticians. Finally, that apparently large group of patients seen most commonly in primary care with a mixture of anxiety and depressive symptoms that does not meet diagnostic criteria for a mood disorder are addressed in DSM-IV in the category anxiety disorders NOS.

■ DEPRESSION: GENERAL CHARACTERISTICS

Depression is a term with meanings ranging from the transient dips in mood that are characteristic of life itself, to a clinical syndrome of substantial severity, duration, and associated signs and symptoms that is markedly different from normal. Grief, or bereavement, encompasses features of a depressive syndrome but is usually less pervasive and more limited in duration. The clinical features of depression fall into four broad categories:

1. **Mood (affect):** sad, blue, depressed, unhappy, down-in-the-dumps, empty, worried, irritable.
2. **Cognition:** loss of interest, difficulty concentrating, low self-esteem, negative thoughts, indecisiveness, guilt, suicidal ideation, hallucinations, delusions.
3. **Behavior:** psychomotor retardation or agitation, crying, social withdrawal, dependency, suicide.
4. **Somatic (physical):** sleep disturbance (insomnia or hypersomnia), fatigue, decreased or increased appetite, weight loss or gain, pain, gastrointestinal upset, decreased libido.

When many of the above-mentioned symptoms are prominent, depression is easily recognized. This is not always the case, however, because patients may present with prominent somatic manifestations while minimizing or denying the mood and cognitive components. Studies have found that over 50% of clinically important depression goes unrecognized in primary care. Diagnosis is further complicated in the presence of medical illnesses and medication side effects that may produce "pseudodepressive" manifestations (e.g., insomnia secondary to pain, weight loss from malignancy, lethargy caused by medication).

Depression is a potentially lethal disorder: about 15% of individuals with a primary affective disorder eventually kill themselves. Factors associated with an early (defined as within 1 year of interview) increased suicide risk in depressed patients include panic attacks, psychic anxiety, severe loss of interest and pleasure (i.e., anhedonia), difficulty concentrating, substance abuse, and marked insomnia (Fawcett et al. 1990). Long-term risk factors (i.e., 1 to 5 years after interview) include hopelessness, suicidal ideation, and prior suicide attempts. There is also evidence that comorbid depression increases the likelihood of death from other medical illnesses such as cardiovascular disease and cancer.

According to the Medical Outcomes Study, depression had a greater adverse impact on individuals than did other chronic conditions such as hypertension, diabetes, arthritis, and lung disease, as measured across the dimensions of physical functioning, role functioning, social functioning, number of days in bed due to poor health, perceived current health, and bodily pain (Wells et al. 1989).

The economic impact of depression includes the costs of treatment (i.e., direct costs) and the costs of lost productivity due to illness or death (i.e., indirect costs). Based on economic data from 1990, the annual financial cost of depression in the United States was estimated to be $43.7 billion ($12.4 billion in direct costs, $7.5 billion in mortality costs, and $23.8 billion in morbidity costs) (Greenberg et al. 1993).

■ MAJOR DEPRESSIVE EPISODE

Major depressive episodes occur in both major depression and bipolar disorder. They are subclassified according to *severity* (mild, moderate, severe without psychotic features or with psychotic features). The DSM-IV diagnostic criteria for a major depressive episode are listed in Table 13–2.

DSM-IV applies the term "with atypical features" to major depressive episodes that have mood reactivity (temporary mood improvement in response to positive events) and at least two of the following for at least 2 weeks:

1. Significant weight gain or increase in appetite
2. Hypersomnia
3. Leaden paralysis (i.e., heavy, leaden feelings in arms or legs)
4. Long-standing pattern of interpersonal rejection sensitivity (not limited to episodes of mood disturbance) resulting in significant social or occupational impairment

☐ Psychotic Depression

Psychotic depression is characterized by the presence of delusions and/or hallucinations that are usually mood-congruent. In other words, these features are consistent with the theme of depression (death, poverty, nihilism, disease, etc.). Although less common, mood-incongruent psychotic features may also occur (e.g., thought insertion, thought broadcasting, delusions of control).

☐ Melancholia

A major depressive episode with melancholic features is characterized in DSM-IV as shown in Table 13–3. Melancholic depression can occur in both major depression and bipolar disorder.

☐ Seasonal Pattern

Some mood disorders follow a regular seasonal pattern, with onset and remission of episodes usually occurring rather predictably at a particular time of year (Table 13–4). Seasonal pattern mood disorders are often referred to as seasonal affective disorders (SADs), a common form of which

---

Table 13–2. DSM-IV diagnostic criteria for major depressive episode

A. Five (or more) of the following symptoms have been present during the same 2-week period and represent a change from previous functioning; at least one of the symptoms is either (1) depressed mood or (2) loss of interest or pleasure. **Note:** Do not include symptoms that are clearly due to a general medical condition or mood-incongruent delusions or hallucinations.

    1. Depressed mood most of the day, nearly every day, as indicated either by subjective report (e.g., feels sad or empty) or observation made by others (e.g., appears tearful). **Note:** In children and adolescents, can be irritable mood.

    2. Markedly diminished interest or pleasure in all, or almost all, activities most of the day, nearly every day (as indicated either by subjective account or observation made by others).

    3. Significant weight loss when not dieting or weight gain (e.g., a change of more than 5% of body weight in a month), or decrease or increase in appetite nearly every day. **Note:** In children, consider failure to make expected weight gains.

    4. Insomnia or hypersomnia nearly every day.

    5. Psychomotor agitation or retardation nearly every day (observable by others, not merely subjective feelings of restlessness or being slowed down).

    6. Fatigue or loss of energy nearly every day.

    7. Feelings of worthlessness or excessive or inappropriate guilt (which may be delusional) nearly every day (not merely self-reproach or guilt about being sick).

    8. Diminished ability to think or concentrate, or indecisiveness, nearly every day (either by subjective account or as observed by others).

    9. Recurrent thoughts of death (not just fear of dying), recurrent suicidal ideation without a specific plan, or a suicide attempt or a specific plan for committing suicide.

B. The symptoms do not meet criteria for a mixed episode.

C. The symptoms cause clinically significant distress or impairment in social, occupational, or other important areas of functioning.

D. The symptoms are not due to the direct physiological effects of a substance (e.g., a drug of abuse, a medication) or a general medical condition (e.g., hypothyroidism).

E. The symptoms are not better accounted for by bereavement, i.e., after the loss of a loved one, the symptoms persist for longer than 2 months or are characterized by marked functional impairment, morbid preoccupation with worthlessness, suicidal ideation, psychotic symptoms, or psychomotor retardation.

---

is "winter" depression (late fall/winter onset) that is often linked to spring/summer hypomania. Depression in SAD is often characterized by hypersomnia, carbohydrate craving, overeating, weight gain, and fatigue, although there are many exceptions to this profile (Blehar and

---

Table 13–3.   DSM-IV diagnostic criteria for melancholic features specifier

Specify if: **With melancholic features** (can be applied to the current or most recent major depressive episode in major depressive disorder and to a major depressive episode in bipolar I or bipolar II disorder only if it is the most recent type of mood episode):

A.   Either of the following, occurring during the most severe period of the current episode:

   1.   Loss of pleasure in all, or almost all, activities

   2.   Lack of reactivity to usually pleasurable stimuli (does not feel much better, even temporarily, when something good happens)

B.   Three (or more) of the following:

   1.   Distinct quality of depressed mood (i.e., the depressed mood is experienced as distinctly different from the kind of feeling experienced after the death of a loved one)

   2.   Depression regularly worse in the morning

   3.   Early morning awakening (at least 2 hours before usual time of awakening)

   4.   Marked psychomotor retardation or agitation

   5.   Significant anorexia or weight loss

   6.   Excessive or inappropriate guilt

Lewy 1990). While winter depression responds to conventional antidepressant drug therapy, research has shown that it also responds well to bright artificial light.

☐ Postpartum Mood Disturbance

DSM-IV has included "with postpartum onset" as a course specifier that can be applied to either manic or major depressive episodes in bipolar disorder, major depressive disorder, or brief psychotic disorder. In addition to first-onset mood syndromes ranging from postpartum blues to postpartum psychosis (usually affective in nature), there is an increased risk of recurrence of preexisting mood disorders in the immediate postpartum period.

■ MAJOR DEPRESSIVE DISORDER

Major depressive disorder is identified by the presence of one or more major depressive episodes in the absence of a history of mania or hypomania.

Table 13–4.   DSM-IV diagnostic criteria for seasonal pattern specifier

---

A.   There has been a regular temporal relationship between the onset of major depressive episodes in bipolar I or bipolar II disorder or major depressive disorder, recurrent, and a particular time of the year (e.g., regular appearance of the major depressive episode in the fall or winter).
Note: Do not include cases in which there is an obvious effect of seasonal-related psychosocial stressors (e.g., regularly being unemployed every winter).

B.   Full remissions (or a change from depression to mania or hypomania) also occur at a characteristic time of the year (e.g., depression disappears in the spring).

C.   In the last 2 years, two major depressive episodes have occurred that demonstrate the temporal seasonal relationships defined in criteria A and B, and no nonseasonal major depressive episodes have occurred during that same period.

D.   Seasonal major depressive episodes (as described above) substantially outnumber the nonseasonal major depressive episodes that may have occurred over the individual's lifetime.

Note. This designation can be applied to the pattern of major depressive episodes in bipolar I disorder, bipolar II disorder, or major depressive disorder, recurrent.

☐ Epidemiology and Clinical Course

The National Institute of Mental Health (NIMH) Epidemiologic Catchment Area (ECA) study, based on a survey of over 18,000 adults in five United States communities, found a 1-month prevalence of 1.6% and a lifetime prevalence of 4.4% for major depressive disorder (Weissman et al. 1988a, 1988b). The mean age at onset was 27 years, with little difference according to sex. Studies have shown that individuals born in recent decades appear to have both an earlier age at onset and an increased rate of depression. The prevalence of depression in women is uniformly higher than in men, with most studies finding major depression to be twice as common (Weissman et al. 1988b).

According to DSM-IV, an episode of major depressive disorder must have a minimum duration of 2 weeks; an average untreated episode, however, lasts 6 or more months. The onset and termination of a major depressive episode may be gradual or abrupt. Although return to the premorbid state either spontaneously or with treatment is the rule, a chronic outcome is not rare. A 5-year follow-up of 431 depressive patients found that, although 50% had recovered within 6 months, 12% were still ill at 5 years (Keller et al. 1992). Risk factors for chronicity included long duration of illness prior to evaluation, history of alcoholism and other nonaffective psychiatric disorders, and low family income.

Major depressive disorder is usually a recurrent disorder. The likelihood of a single episode is well under 50%, and once recurrence is established, the risk of further episodes increases with subsequent episodes (Thase 1990). The pattern of recurrence is variable and generally unpredictable. Months, and even years, may separate episodes.

Major depressive disorder commonly coexists with other psychiatric conditions. Patients with dysthymic disorder usually have superimposed episodes of major depression (so-called double depression). Markowitz et al. (1992) found a 68% lifetime prevalence of major depression among their dysthymic patients. Anxiety disorders also coexist with major depressive disorder.

☐ Etiology

The causes of major depressive disorder and bipolar disorder are unknown, and a thoroughly satisfying explanation for the effectiveness of treatments is lacking. Nevertheless, elegant efforts have been made to integrate various etiologic perspectives.

Biological Models

Genetics.   Twin, adoption, and family studies have established a genetic predisposition toward major depressive disorder and bipolar disorder (Gershon 1990). There is a higher concordance for major mood disorders in identical (i.e., monozygotic) than in fraternal (i.e., dizygotic) twins. Concordance in monozygotic twinships is greater for bipolar disorder than for major depressive disorder, suggesting a stronger genetic basis for bipolar disorder. While co-twins tend to develop the same disorder, this is not always the case, and unipolar and bipolar disorders may coexist in a twinship. The few studies of identical twins reared apart have also supported a genetic basis for major mood disorder. Although fraught with design flaws, most adoption studies provide evidence that the biological parents of adoptees with major mood disorder have a higher incidence of mood disorder than do the adoptive parents.

The inheritable nature of major mood disorders indicates a need for genetic counseling. According to Gershon (1990), who reported on 300 adult offspring of one bipolar parent, the risk of major affective disorder was 29.5 percent; when two parents had affective illness, with one of them bipolar, the risk rose to 74 percent.

Biochemical (neurotransmitter) hypotheses.   A variety of biochemical hypotheses have been generated to explain the etiology of mood disorder. The observation that tricyclic antidepressants inhibit the neuronal uptake of norepinephrine and serotonin (5-hydroxytryptamine [5-HT]) suggested a role for these neurotransmitters in mood disorders. However, contrary evidence indicated that 1) uptake inhibition occurred within hours, whereas mood improvement lagged weeks behind; 2) uptake inhibitors such as amphetamine and cocaine were not particularly effective "antidepressants"; and 3) some effective antidepressants (e.g., trimipramine, bupropion, tianeptine) had negligible effects on uptake inhibition. Despite these inconsistencies, the recent influx of selective serotonin reuptake inhibitor (SSRI) antidepressants such as fluoxetine, fluvoxamine, paroxetine, and sertraline, has kept this theory alive.

With greater attention focused on receptors and receptor subtypes, more elegant theories have evolved to incorporate observed alterations in receptor sensitivity. The time necessary for antidepressant-induced beta-adrenergic receptor downregulation (i.e., decreased receptor density) closely parallels the course of clinical improvement. In addition, tricyclic and monoamine oxidase inhibitor (MAOI) antidepressants and electroconvulsive therapy (ECT) downregulate beta-receptors. Unfortunately for the theory, some antidepressants do not downregulate beta-receptors, and certain pharmacological maneuvers that shortened the time to downregulation do not speed up the time to clinical improvement. Interest shifted to the 5-HT$_2$ receptor that was found by some to be upregulated in depression and downregulated by antidepressants. This theory, too, is flawed by inconsistencies in that neuroleptics and lysergic acid diethylamide (LSD) also downregulate the receptor, whereas ECT upregulates it.

Single cell recordings of neuronal firing following microiontophoretically applied 5-HT suggest that the final common pathway of antidepressant efficacy may be through enhancement of 5-HT neurotransmission. Through a variety of mechanisms (sensitization of postsynaptic receptors, desensitization of presynaptic somatodendritic and terminal autoreceptors), tricyclics, tetracyclics, SSRIs, MAOIs, and ECT all facilitate 5-HT, but not norepinephrine, neurotransmission (Blier et al. 1987).

Neuroendocrine system.   Abnormalities of the *hypothalamic-pituitary-adrenal* (HPA) axis are commonly found in depression. The release of corticotropin-releasing factor (CRF) from the hypothalamus is partially regulated by neurotransmitters such as 5-HT, norepinephrine, acetylcholine, and gamma-aminobutyric acid (GABA). CRF, in turn, stimulates pituitary secretion of corticotropin (ACTH), leading to increased adrenocortical cortisol production. Cortisol hypersecretion has been noted in major depression, and, recently, increased levels of CRF have been found in the CSF of depressed patients. Anatomic support for an overactive HPA axis has been provided by small studies finding pituitary and adrenal gland enlargement in patients with major depression. These observations have been cited to support a role for "CRF overdrive" in the pathogenesis of depression.

Abnormalities in thyroid function have for years been linked to mood disorders, with hypothyroidism sometimes presenting as a depressive syndrome and hyperthyroidism occasionally the cause of secondary mania. A substantial minority of depressed patients show a blunted pituitary thyroid-stimulating hormone (TSH) response to the infusion of thyrotropin-releasing hormone (TRH). Similar findings have been noted in mania. Rapid-cycling bipolar disorder is often associated with abnormalities in thyroid function, and there is preliminary research evidence that this disorder can be treated effectively with hypermetabolic doses of L-thyroxine (T_4) (Bauer and Whybrow 1990). For years triiodothyronine (T_3) has been used by clinicians to augment antidepressants in treatment-resistant depression. Although research has not conclusively confirmed the efficacy of this approach, there is considerable clinical support for its continued use. Thyroid function testing has a well-established role in clinical psychiatry, but the meaning of minor perturbations of the *hypothalamic-pituitary-thyroid* (HPT) axis in the pathogenesis of major depression is far from established.

Sleep Studies

Disturbances of sleep are characteristic of mood disorders, with depression associated with insomnia or hypersomnia and mania with decreased sleep need. Sleep electroencephalographic studies of depression have found impaired sleep continuity, reduced total sleep time, shortened rapid eye movement (REM) latency (i.e., the time from falling asleep to the appearance of the first REM period), increased REM density, and reduced non-REM sleep. Shortened REM latency has been proposed as a biological marker for endogenous depression. Disturbances of sleep and other aspects of circadian rhythm continue to be promising areas of investigation. For example, sleep deprivation has a transient antidepressant effect and has been used to potentiate response to antidepressant drugs, to speed up their onset of action, to prevent recurrent mood episodes, and to predict response to treatment with antidepressant drugs or ECT (Leibenluft and Wehr 1992).

Psychological Models

Psychoanalytic.   In 1911, Abraham published the first psychoanalytic explanation of depression by relating it to repression of instincts (aggression turned inward). Freud suggested that early childhood loss results in introjection of the lost object. This theory influenced and misguided clinicians who generalized from it over the decades despite the fact that Freud stressed its limited applicability and later discounted it. Bemporad (1988) pointed out themes common to many of the psychodynamic models of depression: 1) ambivalent relationships, 2) narcissistic relationships, 3) helplessness and hopelessness, and 4) loss or threatened loss during childhood.

Cognitive/behavioral.   Beck proposed that the primary defect in depression involved cognition and that depressed mood is a consequence, rather than the cause, of cognitive impairment in depression (Beck et al. 1979). Beck's *cognitive triad* involves a depressed individual's negative views of self, environment, and future. The self is viewed as inadequate and defective and, hence, worthless. Depressed individuals also negatively interpret life experiences and view the future as offering nothing but failure and frustration. The cognitive model proposes that early adverse experiences establish negative concepts retained as "schemas" that are reactivated by adverse life experiences and result in depression.

Learned helplessness.   Seligman (1975) found that dogs exposed repeatedly to unavoidable electric shocks would eventually not escape the shocks even when they were free to do so. Being unable to control the painful situation led to a withdrawn helpless state. The *learned helplessness model of depression* postulates that past experiences of real helplessness imbue the individual with the conviction that future unpleasant situations will also be uncontrollable, and, therefore, such situations are responded to by passivity, resignation, and depressive acceptance.

Life events.   Most studies using healthy individuals, medical patients, and other psychiatric patients as controls found that depressed patients had a greater number of life events or more life stress over varying periods of time prior to the onset of depressive episodes. The increase of life events prior to the onset of illness was not confined to depression but was also present with other psychiatric disorders and with medical illnesses. Paykel (1982) estimated that life events play an important but not overwhelming role in the causation of depression. When an effort was made to identify event types that were particularly associated with depression, results were somewhat inconsistent but with a trend toward increases in "deaths and interpersonal separations," "failures and disappointments," and "arguments and discord with various key interpersonal figures."

Early childhood loss has been linked to increased vulnerability to depression. The role of early loss as a risk factor for later depression is less well-established than popular lore would suggest. In contrast to studies with humans, studies of nonhuman primates in controlled settings have found a consistent depression-like response in infants separated from their mothers. Characteristically, separation is followed initially by an agitated "protest" stage and later by a despair stage associated with social withdrawal, reduced activity level, and reduced food and water intake (McKinney 1988).

☐ Treatment

Most patients with major depressive disorder can be safely and effectively treated in an outpatient setting. Hospitalization may be required for suicidal or other severely disabled patients, and for crisis intervention, complex diagnostic evaluation, initiation of high-risk treatments, and ECT.

Before addressing the more specific treatments of major depressive disorder, certain terms, such as recovery, remission, relapse, and recurrence, require definition. *Full remission* refers to "a relatively brief . . . period during which an improvement of sufficient magnitude is observed that the individual is asymptomatic" (Frank et al. 1991, p. 853). *Partial remission* is a period during which the individual has more than minimal symptoms but these symptoms no longer meet the criteria for major depression. *Recovery* refers to a full remission of at least a minimum duration (not defined). A *relapse* represents "the return of the symptoms of a still ongoing but symptomatically suppressed episode" (Frank et al. 1991, p. 853), whereas a *recurrence* is a new episode of major depression. These concepts are important to clinicians who must treat an acute episode long enough to ensure that it remains in full remission when treatment is stopped (no relapse) and who must decide whether to initiate long-term maintenance to prevent new episodes (recurrences).

Psychotherapy for Major Depressive Disorder

Although many forms of psychotherapy have been used to treat major depression, most have not been subjected to the rigors of scientific scrutiny. *Supportive psychotherapy* lacks such a research foundation, although it is widely practiced and may be considered the background against which more specific therapies are conducted. Techniques include explaining and educating, reality testing, strengthening defenses, developing support systems, and providing empathy. In recent years, a number of *brief psychodynamic psychotherapies* have been developed. These include brief focal psychotherapy (Malan), short-term anxiety-provoking psychotherapy (Sifneos), time-limited psychotherapy (Mann), and broad-focus short-term dynamic psychotherapy (Davanloo).

Two forms of psychotherapy, interpersonal psychotherapy (IPT) and cognitive therapy (CT), have been found in research studies to be effective in the treatment of mild to moderate (and perhaps more severe) episodes of major depression. Karasu provides a thorough comparison of psychodynamic, cognitive, and interpersonal therapies for depression, pointing out the advantages and disadvantages of each approach (Karasu 1990). Both IPT and CT require specialized training, and although many clinicians have incorporated aspects of one or both into their practices, few of these individuals can be considered fully trained in these modalities.

The goal of IPT is to relieve depression through improving disturbed interpersonal relationships. It is a time-limited approach conducted over months rather than years. Typically, treatment is on a once-weekly basis over 3 to 4 months. It focuses on current rather than past interpersonal relationships, although the latter are not ignored. Likewise, IPT does not focus heavily on intrapsychic or personality issues other than to integrate them into the context of current interpersonal problems. The efficacy of IPT has been established in a number of research studies (Klerman and Weissman 1987). A 16-week comparison of IPT alone, amitriptyline alone, and combined IPT and amitriptyline found all to be more effective than supportive therapy received "on demand" in a control group of depressed outpatients. IPT and amitriptyline were equally effective, and the combination was even more effective (DiMascio et al. 1979).

Cognitive therapy and cognitive-behavior therapy (CBT) were developed by Beck et al. (1979) as treatments for nonpsychotic, nonbipolar depression. CT is a focused, directive, standardized, time-limited approach that attempts to correct the distorted cognitions or beliefs that are felt to cause depression. The goals of therapy are to both relieve depression and prevent recurrence. The therapist helps the patient identify negative thoughts and assumptions and replace them with more realistic and positive beliefs. Research studies have shown CT to compare favorably to antidepressant medication in the treatment of outpatient major depression (Wright and Thase 1992). Most studies have found CT to be effective even in the presence of endogenous or melancholic depression. For example, a study of depressed outpatients found that CT and pharmacotherapy (i.e., imipramine) were equally effective, even in the more seriously depressed subjects (Hollon et al. 1992).

Antidepressant Drug Therapy

Many clinicians consider medication the cornerstone of therapy with which other treatments must be compared. At the same time, it is widely believed that the combination of pharmacotherapy and psychotherapy provides the most comprehensively effective approach to treatment. All antidepressants marketed in the United States have established efficacy for major depression in placebo-controlled studies. When compared with each other, however, none has shown superiority. Outcome studies usually find that active drug is effective in 60% to 80% of patients compared with a placebo response rate of 30% to 40%. As the severity of depression increases, active drug/placebo differences become more robust, whereas with milder depressions there is less likely to be a drug/placebo difference. However, concluding that antidepressant drugs are appropriate only in more severe major depression may be premature in that there is evidence of drug efficacy in mild atypical depression (Stewart et al. 1992).

In the presence of psychotic (delusional) depression, antidepressant drug monotherapy has usually been found to be less effective than ECT or a combination of antidepressant and antipsychotic drug. The only exception appears to be amoxapine, which compared favorably to a combination of amitriptyline and perphenazine, probably because of its intrinsic dopamine receptor blocking properties. Atypical depression responds more favorably to MAOIs than to tricyclic antidepressants, although the latter are more effective than placebo.

Acute treatment.   As a result of their side-effect potential, some antidepressants (e.g., tricyclics and MAOIs) are started at low doses and increased gradually as tolerated until an antidepressant effect range is reached. The selective serotonin uptake inhibitors (e.g., fluoxetine, paroxetine, sertraline) are better tolerated and can be started at what will usually be an effective dose. These drugs appear to have a flat dose-response curve across their marketed range, and further increases are usually not necessary. Blood levels can be measured for all antidepressants, but only a few agents (e.g., nortriptyline, imipramine, desipramine) have ranges that have some correlation with therapeutic efficacy. In general, routine measurement of antidepressant blood levels is not necessary, although it can be helpful in evaluating compliance, side effects, toxicity, and the effects of interactions with other drugs.

The antidepressant effect of medications evolves slowly over many days or several weeks. Before concluding that a drug is ineffective, it should be used for at least 4 to 6 weeks at an appropriate dose. If there is inadequate or no response to single-drug therapy, treatment options include switching to a different drug (a washout period may be necessary) or augmenting with a medication such as lithium, thyroid hormone (i.e., triiodothyronine), buspirone, or another antidepressant. Research has shown that once a patient has entered a full remission, *continuation therapy* for at least 4 months will greatly reduce the risk of relapse (Kupfer 1991). If the decision is then made to discontinue treatment, the medication dose should be gradually reduced to avoid both withdrawal symptoms and possible reemergence depression if the decision turns out to be premature. (The long half-life of fluoxetine allows it to be abruptly stopped without withdrawal difficulty.)

Maintenance therapy.　Given the recurrent nature of major depressive disorder, long-term maintenance (i.e., preventive) therapy is often indicated. Both 3- and 5-year maintenance studies with imipramine have shown very significant prophylactic effects of active drug compared with placebo (Frank et al. 1990; Kupfer et al. 1992). Of great importance was the observation that compared with earlier lower-dose protocols, "full-dose" maintenance (i.e., the same amount that ended the acute episode) was considerably more protective against recurrence. Studies with other antidepressants (e.g., fluoxetine, paroxetine, phenelzine, sertraline) have also been positive, suggesting that whatever drug effectively resolves the acute episode can be used to prevent recurrences.

Other Somatic Therapies

Electroconvulsive therapy.　ECT is a well-established, effective treatment for depression. In conjunction with the use of general anesthesia and muscle relaxation, it is usually safe and well tolerated. A typical course of ECT involves a total of 9 to 12 treatments administered either unilaterally or bilaterally every 2 to 3 days. Maintenance treatments given at weekly to monthly intervals are felt by some experts to be useful in preventing recurrences, especially when long-term medication has failed or is not tolerated. Indications for ECT include treatment resistance, high suicide risk, psychotic depression, and a previous good response to ECT.

Light therapy.　The use of high-intensity artificial light to treat seasonal affective disorder (winter depression) appears to be quite beneficial. Exposure to 2,500 to 10,000 lux for 30 minutes to 2 hours is usually given in the morning. Response occurs over several days and is maintained for as long as treatment continues (Terman et al. 1989). Despite its wide acceptance, treatment with light is still investigational.

Exercise

Studies comparing running with psychotherapy found these modalities to be equally effective in treating mild to moderate depression (and both more effective than being on a waiting list). Exercise is simple, safe, and inexpensive and offers health benefits that extend beyond the treatment of depression (Greist et al. 1979).

■ DYSTHYMIC DISORDER

One can rather simplistically consider dysthymia to be a chronic low-grade depression that, according to Murphy (1991), is "an ill-defined and non-specific diagnostic 'catch-all', with limited useful clinical application" (p. 109). The full DSM-IV criteria for dysthymic disorder are listed in Table 13–5. If symptoms resembling dysthymic disorder evolve from an episode of major depressive disorder, the more appropriate diagnosis would be major depressive disorder, partial remission. If dysthymic disorder has been present for 2 years (1 year in children and adolescents) and major depressive disorder becomes superimposed, both diagnoses should be made (the term "double depression" is often used to describe this situation).

Dysthymic disorder seldom exists alone. The ECA study found that over 75% of persons with dysthymia had other conditions, the most common of which was major depressive disorder. Also overrepresented were panic disorder, any other anxiety disorder, and substance abuse, but not bipolar disorder. Other studies have found an increased comorbid incidence of attention-deficit disorder, conduct disorder, and personality disorder (Kocsis and Frances 1987).

The etiological theories of dysthymic disorder are usually extrapolations of those proposed for major depressive disorder.

☐ Epidemiology

In the ECA study a 3% lifetime prevalence of dysthymia was found in the adult population, with women being affected 1.5 to 3 times more often than men. Dysthymia was also "more common in women under age 65, unmarried persons, and young persons with low income and was associated with greater use of general health and psychiatric services and psychotropic drugs" (Weissman et al. 1988a, p. 815).

☐ Treatment

Because dysthymic disorder is a mild form of depression, it is often assumed to be nonbiological and, therefore, particularly amenable to treatment with psychotherapy. Contrary to the generally low regard in which antidepressant drugs have been held for treating mild chronic depression, there is considerable evidence to support their effectiveness (Howland 1991). Compared with research on major depressive disorder, however, the pharmacological research directed at dysthymic disorder has been rather limited, and conclusive recommendations cannot be made. The newer antidepressants, such as the selective serotonin uptake inhibitors and bupropion, have shown promise that awaits systematic confirmation.

Table 13–5. DSM-IV diagnostic criteria for dysthymic disorder

A. Depressed mood for most of the day, for more days than not, as indicated either by subjective account or observation by others, for at least 2 years. **Note:** In children and adolescents, mood can be irritable and duration must be at least 1 year.

B. Presence, while depressed, of two (or more) of the following:
   1. Poor appetite or overeating
   2. Insomnia or hypersomnia
   3. Low energy or fatigue
   4. Low self-esteem
   5. Poor concentration or difficulty making decisions
   6. Feelings of hopelessness

C. During the 2-year period (1 year for children or adolescents) of the disturbance, the person has never been without the symptoms in criteria A and B for more than 2 months at a time.

D. No major depressive episode has been present during the first 2 years of the disturbance (1 year for children and adolescents); i.e., the disturbance is not better accounted for by chronic major depressive disorder, or major depressive disorder in partial remission. **Note:** There may have been a previous major depressive episode provided there was a full remission (no significant signs or symptoms for 2 months) before development of the dysthymic disorder. In addition, after the initial 2 years (1 year in children or adolescents) of dysthymic disorder, there may be superimposed episodes of major depressive disorder, in which case both diagnoses may be given when the criteria are met for the major depressive episode.

E. There has never been a manic episode, a mixed episode, or a hypomanic episode, and criteria have never been met for cyclothymic disorder.

F. The disturbance does not occur exclusively during the course of a chronic psychotic disorder, such as schizophrenia or delusional disorder.

G. The symptoms are not due to the direct physiological effects of a substance (e.g., a drug of abuse, a medication) or a general medical condition (e.g., hypothyroidism).

H. The symptoms cause clinically significant distress or impairment in social, occupational, or other important areas of functioning.

Specify if:

Early onset: if onset is before age 21 years

Late onset: if onset is age 21 years or older

Specify (for most recent 2 years of dysthymic disorder):

With atypical features

■ MANIA AND HYPOMANIA

Mania is characterized by an elevated, expansive, or irritable mood. In its mildest form, hypomania may be difficult to distinguish from normalcy. Thus, the sense of well-being that often follows resolution of a depressive episode may be difficult to categorize. Similar problems exist at the other end of the manic spectrum, with psychotic or delirious mania impossible to distinguish in cross-section from other psychotic conditions. Diagnostic accuracy can be increased by obtaining a careful longitudinal history of current and previous episodes and a detailed family history from both patient and significant others.

The DSM-IV diagnostic criteria for a manic episode are listed in Table 13–6. Similar symptoms also occur in a hypomanic episode, but the hypomanic episode "is not severe enough to cause marked impairment in social or occupational functioning, or to necessitate hospitalization, and there are no psychotic features" (American Psychiatric Association 1994). At the same time, to qualify as hypomanic in DSM-IV, the episode must be "associated with an unequivocal change in functioning that is uncharacteristic of the person when not symptomatic." Thus, one can be happy without necessarily being hypomanic.

Manic episodes are subclassified according to severity (mild; moderate; severe, without psychotic features; severe, with psychotic symptoms) and the type of psychotic features (mood-congruent or mood-incongruent). The presence of a thought disorder during a manic episode may result in the misdiagnosis of schizophrenia. Studies have shown that the presence of a thought disorder during an acute episode carries no diagnostic specificity, although there may be qualitative differences between mania and schizophrenia that can aid in diagnosis (Goodwin and Jamison 1990). The prudent clinician will not attempt to reach diagnostic finality based solely on a cross-sectional view of the patient during an acute psychotic episode. Diagnostic clarity can be improved by obtaining a longitudinal history of both current and prior episodes. A manic syndrome caused by a specific medical condition such as multiple sclerosis would be categorized as a mood disorder due to a general medical condition. Mania caused by substance abuse (e.g., steroids) or substance withdrawal would be considered a substance-induced mood disorder. Like depression, mania has a clinical presentation that differs considerably from patient to patient.

☐ Mixed States

Not all major mood episodes can be neatly categorized as manic or depressed. In DSM-IV a mixed episode is defined as follows: "For every day during at least a one-week period, the criteria for a major depressive episode (except for duration) and a manic episode are both met." However, data-based criteria for mixed or dysphoric mania are less well established than is suggested in either DSM-III-R or DSM-IV. According to McElroy et al. (1992), "much of the ambiguity surrounding dysphoric mania is due to the lack of widely accepted, empirically based operational diagnostic

---

Table 13–6. DSM-IV diagnostic criteria for manic episode

A. A distinct period of abnormally and persistently elevated, expansive, or irritable mood, lasting at least 1 week (or any duration if hospitalization is necessary).

B. During the period of mood disturbance, three (or more) of the following symptoms have persisted (four if the mood is only irritable) and have been present to a significant degree:

1. Inflated self-esteem or grandiosity

2. Decreased need for sleep (e.g., feels rested after only 3 hours of sleep)

3. More talkative than usual or pressure to keep talking

4. Flight of ideas or subjective experience that thoughts are racing

5. Distractibility (i.e., attention too easily drawn to unimportant or irrelevant external stimuli)

6. Increase in goal-directed activity (either socially, at work or school, or sexually) or psychomotor agitation

7. Excessive involvement in pleasurable activities that have a high potential for painful consequences (e.g., engaging in unrestrained buying sprees, sexual indiscretions, or foolish business investments)

C. The symptoms do not meet criteria for a mixed episode.

D. The mood disturbance is sufficiently severe to cause marked impairment in occupational functioning or in usual social activities or relationships with others, or to necessitate hospitalization to prevent harm to self or others, or there are psychotic features.

E. The symptoms are not due to the direct physiological effects of a substance (e.g., a drug of abuse, a medication, or other treatment) or a general medical condition (e.g., hyperthyroidism).

Note. Manic-like episodes that are clearly caused by somatic antidepressant treatment (e.g., medication, electroconvulsive therapy, light therapy) should not count toward a diagnosis of bipolar I disorder.

---

criteria for the disorder" (p. 1633). It follows that the prevalence of dysphoric mania varies widely across studies (5% to 70%); nonetheless, a mean prevalence of 31% confirms that it is a common condition (McElroy et al. 1992). Dysphoric mania does appear to be more common in females, to be associated with a higher suicide risk, and to have a poorer prognosis (including a lessened responsiveness to lithium).

☐ Psychotic Mania

Psychotic symptoms (delusions and/or hallucinations) are common during manic episodes. The delusions of mania tend to be grandiose, expansive, religious, and sexual, but, less commonly, they are mood-incongruent. Manic hallucinations can be auditory and visual and are often of transient duration with ecstatic and religious content. An earlier age at onset of bipolar disorder is associated with more psychotic symptoms. The common occurrence of florid psychoses in adolescent bipolar patients has contributed to overdiagnosis of schizophrenia in this age group.

☐ Postpartum

The risk of recurrence of mania and depression is sufficiently high in the postpartum period that mood-stabilizing medications that were discontinued during pregnancy should usually be restarted shortly after delivery (Stewart et al. 1991).

■ BIPOLAR (MANIC-DEPRESSIVE) DISORDER

According to DSM-III-R, the essential feature of bipolar disorder is a history of at least one manic episode. Most individuals with the disorder have also experienced at least one major depressive episode, although this depends, in part, on the duration of the illness. Whether unipolar mania (i.e., recurrent manic episodes with no history of depression) is a bona fide variant of bipolar disorder is open to question. There is consensus that if unipolar mania exists, it is a variant of bipolar disorder, because of shared clinical features, family history, treatment response, and longitudinal course.

The most substantial modification of the bipolar disorder categories in DSM-IV was removing bipolar II (i.e., hypomania and recurrent major depressive episodes but no manic episodes) from the category of "Not Otherwise Specified" and placing it on the same classificatory level as bipolar I (i.e., at least one manic episode). This reordering has not fully resolved the controversy as to whether bipolar II is a distinct entity or a variant of bipolar I or of major depressive disorder (Keller 1987).

☐ Epidemiology and Comorbidity

The ECA study found a 1.2% lifetime prevalence of bipolar disorder with a 0.7% to 1.6% range across the five study sites (Weissman et al. 1988b). Other studies have shown a lifetime risk of between 0.6% and 0.9%. Although figures vary widely, bipolar disorder is estimated to represent about 20% of all cases of major mood disorder. An exception is the Old Order Amish study in which bipolar and unipolar disorder were equally represented. This may reflect, in part, the recognition of subtle bipolar II disorder in this relatively homogeneous population.

Bipolar disorder is uncommon in prepubertal children but does occur. As adolescence evolves, the condition begins to flourish as evidenced by ECA study findings of a median age at onset of 18 years in men and 20 years in women (Burke et al. 1990). Pooled data from a number of older studies showed median age at onset in the mid-20s. This cohort effect of earlier age at onset in those born more recently is similar to that observed with major depressive disorder. Mania appearing for the first time in the elderly is not rare but is commonly associated with an organic etiology.

Bipolar disorder is equally common in women and men, except in rapid cyclers, among whom women are overrepresented. The ECA study found a 1.2:1 female/male ratio. The underreporting of bipolar disorder in blacks may be an artifact of misdiagnosis and racial bias. More recent studies such as the ECA study found no significant black/white difference. Studies in industrialized Western countries found a similar incidence in bipolar prevalence. In the ECA study a lifetime prevalence of alcohol abuse or dependence was found in 46% of bipolar I patients. The overall lifetime prevalence for any substance abuse or dependence was 61% (compared with 27% for major depression) (Regier et al. 1990).

☐ Clinical Course

Bipolar disorder is an episodic, recurrent illness. The likelihood of having only a single episode is slim. As the number of episodes increases, the cycle length (i.e., the interval from the start of one episode to the start of the next) tends to decrease. The most pronounced changes occur over the first few episodes, until eventually a plateau is reached. There is also a tendency for later-onset bipolar disorder to be associated with shorter cycle lengths. The episodes themselves can be characterized as manic, hypomanic, major depressive, minor depressive, or mixed. The first episode has been reported to be manic in 34% to 79% of cases (Goodwin and Jamison 1990). Whereas men tend to have an equal number of manic and depressive episodes over the course of the illness, women are more susceptible to depression.

There is great variation in cycling patterns in bipolar disorder, with episodes occurring irregularly or linked together in a mania-depression-euthymia or a depression-mania-euthymia pattern. Continuous cycling indicates the absence of sustained periods of mood stability, while rapid cycling has been somewhat arbitrarily defined as at least four episodes per year. DSM-IV applies the term "rapid cycling" to bipolar I or bipolar II disorder if there have been "at least four episodes of a mood disturbance in the previous 12 months that meet criteria for a manic episode, a hypomanic episode, or a major depressive episode" (American Psychiatric Association 1994).

There are well-documented cases of ultrarapid cycling (more common in males), with episodes lasting 24 hours, and there is growing support for the existence of ultra-ultrarapid cycling (i.e., several to many episodes occurring daily). Rapid cycling and continuous cycling may coexist (i.e., continuous rapid cycling). Rapid cycling has been reported in 10% to 30% of bipolar patients (mostly women), with only 20% beginning to cycle rapidly at the onset of the illness. Later-onset rapid cycling has been linked by some to treatment with antidepressant medications.

☐ Etiology

Goodwin and Jamison (1990), who consider neurotransmitter, neuropeptide, neuroendocrine, and electrolyte hypotheses, suggest that "the genetic defect in manic-depressive illness involves the circadian pacemaker or systems that modulate it" (p. 589). Their hypothesis incorporates observations such as 1) the shortening of cycle length with successive episodes until a plateau is eventually reached, 2) increased sensitivity to light in manic-depressive disorder that appears to be trait- rather than state-dependent, 3) the seasonal pattern of illness seen in some bipolar patients, 4) the suggested commonality of serotonin and dopamine dysfunction in bipolar disorder and circadian rhythm disorders, and 5) the link between disturbed sleep and mood episodes.

The sensitization model of mood disorder considers both the role of *psychosocial stressor sensitization* in precipitating initial and early episodes and the role of *episode sensitization* in increasing the ease and frequency with which subsequent episodes occur. Post (1992) suggests that "the experience of an affective episode and its associated neurotransmitter and peptide alterations may leave behind memory traces that predispose to further episodes, i.e., it is possible that 'episodes beget episodes'" (p. 1004). If this is true, then initiating long-term maintenance treatment early in the course of the illness may reduce the likelihood of a catastrophic evolution.

☐ Treatment

Psychotherapy

Even more than with major depressive disorder, pharmacotherapy is central to the acute and long-term treatment of bipolar disorder. Nevertheless, psychotherapy plays a vitally important adjunctive role in all phases of the illness. Therapy issues range from the role of psychosocial stressors in precipitating and aggravating episodes, to the psychic, interpersonal, and social consequences of the disorder itself. Educating patients and significant others is essential, and having them participate in self-help groups such as the National Depressive and Manic-Depressive Association can be invaluable. Patients need to deal with the impact of having a chronic, recurrent illness, the need to take medication regularly and often indefinitely, and the risks of genetic transmission to children.

Pharmacotherapy

Acute mania. Severe manic episodes are usually treated in a hospital setting to ensure a safe environment in which to begin and stabilize medication. Lithium is currently the only drug with FDA labeling approval for the treatment of acute mania, although valproate was recently recommended for approval. Early placebo-controlled studies showed an overall response rate of 78% (Goodwin and Jamison 1990), but more recent observations suggest growing resistance to the antimanic effect of lithium. This increased resistance may reflect, in part, the observation that dysphoric or mixed mania is less responsive to lithium (McElroy et al. 1992). Because lithium has a relatively slow onset of action, adjunctive treatment with a neuroleptic and/or a benzodiazepine is often necessary. Both neuroleptics and benzodiazepines (especially clonazepam and lorazepam) may have intrinsic antimanic properties, although a nonspecific sedative effect is also likely.

The anticonvulsants carbamazepine and valproate are the most promising alternatives to lithium for treating mania. Both have been shown to be effective in placebo- and lithium-controlled studies, although they have not been compared with each other (Bowden et al. 1994; Keck et al. 1992). There is some suggestion that these agents may prove particularly useful for the rapid cycling and dysphoric states for which lithium has reduced efficacy. Combinations of lithium and an anticonvulsant are commonly used. ECT has been shown in anecdotal reports, in uncontrolled studies, and in a small number of controlled studies to be an effective treatment for mania.

Acute depression. The pharmacotherapy of bipolar depression resembles that of major depressive disorder. Lithium appears to be more effective for the former (79% response) than the latter (36% response), and it is considered by many to be the initial treatment of choice for bipolar depression (Goodwin and Jamison 1990). The use of conventional antidepressants for bipolar depression is complicated by the risk of inducing mania or rapid cycling. Consequently, these agents are often used in combination with lithium or another mood stabilizer. Tricyclic antidepressants appear to be less effective in bipolar than unipolar depression, while MAOIs are quite promising. The role for bupropion and selective serotonin uptake inhibitors such as fluoxetine, fluvoxamine, paroxetine, and sertraline requires further substantiation. If breakthrough depression occurs during the course of lithium maintenance, lithium-induced hypothyroidism should be ruled out. Otherwise, a temporary increase in serum lithium level may be effective. If an antidepressant drug must be added, it should be discontinued shortly after the episode remits to reduce the likelihood of drug-induced mania or rapid cycling.

Maintenance therapy.   Lithium has FDA labeling approval for long-term use in patients with a history of manic episodes. Its effectiveness is well established in placebo-controlled, double-blind studies (Goodwin and Jamison 1990). Lithium reduces the frequency, severity, and duration of both manic and depressive episodes, with a somewhat better outcome for mania. Gelenberg et al. (1989) showed that standard maintenance levels were more effective than low levels, although side effects and dropouts were greater in the former group over the 3 years of the study. Discontinuation of lithium after successful treatment is associated with a high recurrence rate. Even more disturbing, some long-term lithium responders who relapse after discontinuation fail to respond to retreatment with lithium (Post et al. 1992).

■ CYCLOTHYMIC DISORDER

Cyclothymic disorder is a chronic mood disturbance; the DSM-IV diagnostic criteria for cyclothymia are presented in Table 13–7. It is often difficult to distinguish between cyclothymic disorder and other conditions characterized by mood lability such as the cluster B personality disorders (i.e., antisocial, borderline, histrionic, and narcissistic).

☐ Epidemiology and Clinical Course

Cyclothymia has a prevalence of 0.4% to 1.1% and is equally distributed between men and women (American Psychiatric Association 1994). The age at onset of this disorder is similar to that of bipolar disorder (i.e., adolescence and early adulthood). Even after the prerequisite 2 years' duration, many individuals develop full-blown manic and/or depressive episodes. The clinical course of cyclothymic disorder may be one of predominant hypomania (hyperthymic temperament), of predominant depression, or of a similar number of hypomanic and depressive episodes. Although it lacks the severity of bipolar disorder, cyclothymic disorder can, nonetheless, cause substantial interpersonal, social, and occupational difficulties. Substance abuse may be a complicating factor.

Table 13–7.   DSM-IV diagnostic criteria for cyclothymic disorder

---

A. For at least 2 years, the presence of numerous periods with hypomanic symptoms (see American Psychiatric Association 1994, p. 338) and numerous periods with depressive symptoms that do not meet criteria for a major depressive episode.   **Note:** In children and adolescents, the duration must be at least 1 year.

B. During the above 2-year period (1 year in children and adolescents), the person has not been without the symptoms in criterion A for more than 2 months at a time.

C. No major depressive episode (see American Psychiatric Association 1994, p. 327), manic episode (see American Psychiatric Association 1994, p. 332), or mixed episode (see American Psychiatric Association 1994, p. 335) has been present during the first 2 years of the disturbance.

Note: After the initial 2 years (1 year in children and adolescents) of cyclothymic disorder, there may be superimposed manic or mixed episodes (in which case both bipolar I disorder and cyclothymic disorder may be diagnosed) or major depressive episodes (in which case both bipolar II disorder and cyclothymic disorder may be diagnosed).

D. The symptoms in criterion A are not better accounted for by schizoaffective disorder and are not superimposed on schizophrenia, schizophreniform disorder, delusional disorder, or psychotic disorder not otherwise specified.

E. The symptoms are not due to the direct physiological effects of a substance (e.g., a drug of abuse, a medication) or a general medical condition (e.g., hyperthyroidism).

F. The symptoms cause clinically significant distress or impairment in social, occupational, or other important areas of functioning.

☐ Treatment

Neither psychotherapy nor pharmacotherapy has been rigorously studied as a treatment for cyclothymic disorder. Because relationships often suffer, couples and family therapy as well as individual psychotherapy may be of value. The pharmacotherapy of cyclothymic disorder has focused predominantly on lithium, with a limited number of open clinical trials and case reports suggesting benefit (Jefferson et al. 1987). Guidelines for the use of lithium and other mood stabilizers in the treatment of cyclothymic disorder are similar to those followed for bipolar disorder.

■ DIFFERENTIAL DIAGNOSIS (Disorders of Mood Yet Not Mood Disorders)

The presence of depression or mania requires diagnostic considerations that extend beyond the primary mood disorders.

☐ Adjustment Disorder With Depressed Mood

The predominant features of adjustment disorder with depressed mood are symptoms such as low mood, hopelessness, and tearfulness. The distinction between this disorder and major depression is often not clear, especially since stressors may play an important role in both conditions. If the full criteria for a major depressive episode are met, that diagnosis should take precedence.

☐ Uncomplicated Bereavement

Uncomplicated bereavement is considered a normal reaction to the loss of a loved one and, as such, is not classified as a mental disorder. In general, uncomplicated bereavement is not associated with a pervasive sense of guilt and worthlessness, marked functional impairment, and suicidality. Bereavement usually begins shortly after the loss and improves over several months. If symptoms are sufficiently severe, pervasive, and long-lasting, bereavement should be considered complicated by a major depressive episode and managed accordingly.

☐ Organic and Psychoactive Substance– Induced Mood Disorders

Organic and psychoactive substance–induced mood disorders encompass both depressive and manic syndromes for which there are known or presumed specific organic etiologies. The search for organicity (and hopefully reversibility) is essential to the evaluation of all disorders of mood. Extensive lists of potential "organic" causes abound, but well-established criteria for causality tend to be lacking. These conditions are sometimes referred to as a form of secondary mood disorder.

☐ Schizoaffective Disorder

DSM-III-R acknowledges that schizoaffective disorder is an especially confusing and controversial concept, and suggests that the diagnosis "be considered for conditions that do not meet the criteria for either schizophrenia or a mood disorder, but that at one time have presented with both a schizophrenic and a mood disturbance and, at another time, with psychotic symptoms but without mood symptoms" (American Psychiatric Association 1987, p. 208). One criterion requires that during an episode there be "delusions or hallucinations for at least two weeks, but no prominent mood symptoms" (p. 210). If hallucinations and/or delusions were to occur only within the context of a prominent mood syndrome, the diagnosis would be either major depressive episode or manic episode with mood-congruent or mood-incongruent psychotic features. The DSM-IV criteria are similar.

Schizoaffective mania may benefit from lithium or other mood stabilizers, although an antipsychotic drug is often also necessary. Schizoaffective depression responds to both neuroleptics and antidepressants, or combinations thereof, although less well than does major depression. Lithium can be an effective long-term prophylactic treatment for schizoaffective disorder, but the adjunctive use of a neuroleptic is often necessary (Goodnick and Meltzer 1984).

☐ Dementia

There are many variations on the interactive themes of mood disorder and dementia. The two may coexist, for example, in an individual with a well-documented history of a recurrent mood disorder who later develops the insidious onset of Alzheimer's dementia. On the other hand, an individual may become depressed as a psychological reaction to an evolving dementia. Given the irreversible and untreatable nature of dementias such as Alzheimer's, the therapeutic implications of recognizing superimposed depression cannot be overstated. Although depression in the demented geriatric patient may be more difficult to treat because of reduced tolerance to antidepressant side effects and, perhaps, reduced therapeutic responsiveness, it is often a gratifyingly treatable condition.

☐ Secondary Depression

A distinction has been made between primary and secondary depression, with the latter defined as occurring in the context of a preexisting disorder such as schizophrenia or alcohol dependence. Classifying a depression as secondary is based solely on a chronological association and carries no etiological or causal implications. Depressions associated with other disorders encompass a broader mix, ranging from a psychological reaction to the coexisting illness, to the coexistence of two separate disorders, to disorders sharing a common biological substrate.

■ REFERENCES

American Psychiatric Association: Diagnostic and Statistical Manual of Mental Disorders, 3rd Edition. Washington, DC, American Psychiatric Association, 1980

American Psychiatric Association: American Psychiatric Glossary, 5th Edition. Washington, DC, American Psychiatric Association, 1984

American Psychiatric Association: Diagnostic and Statistical Manual of Mental Disorders, 3rd Edition, Revised. Washington, DC, American Psychiatric Association, 1987

American Psychiatric Association: Diagnostic and Statistical Manual of Mental Disorders, 4th Edition. Washington, DC, American Psychiatric Association, 1994

Bauer MS, Whybrow PC: Rapid cycling bipolar affective disorder, II: treatment of refractory rapid cycling with high-dose levothyroxine: a preliminary study. Arch Gen Psychiatry 47:435–440, 1990

Beck AT, Rush AJ, Shaw BF, et al: Cognitive Therapy of Depression. New York, Guilford, 1979

Bemporad JR: Psychodynamic models of depression and mania, in Depression and Mania. Edited by Georgotas A, Cancro R. New York, Elsevier, 1988, pp 167–180

Blehar MC, Lewy AJ: Seasonal mood disorders: consensus and controversy. Psychopharmacol Bull 26:465–494, 1990

Blier P, de Montigny C, Chaput Y: Modifications of the serotonin system by antidepressant treatments: implications for the therapeutic response in major depression. J Clin Psychopharmacol 7 (No 6, Suppl):24S–35S, 1987

Bowden CL, Brugger AM, Swann AC, et al: Efficacy of divalproate vs lithium and placebo with treatment of mania. JAMA 271:918–924, 1994

Burke KC, Burke JD Jr, Regier DA, et al: Age at onset of selected mental disorders in five community populations. Arch Gen Psychiatry 47:511–518, 1990

DiMascio A, Weissman MM, Prusoff BA, et al: Differential symptom reduction by drugs and psychotherapy in acute depression. Arch Gen Psychiatry 36:1450–1456, 1979

Fawcett J, Scheftner WA, Fogg L, et al: Time-related predictors of suicide in major affective disorder. Am J Psychiatry 147:1189–1194, 1990

Frank E, Kupfer DJ, Perel JM, et al: Three-year outcomes for maintenance therapies in recurrent depression. Arch Gen Psychiatry 47:1093–1099, 1990

Frank E, Prien RF, Jarrett RB, et al: Conceptualization and rationale for consensus definitions of terms in major depressive disorder: remission, recovery, relapse, and recurrence. Arch Gen Psychiatry 48:851–855, 1991

Gelenberg AJ, Kane JM, Keller MB, et al: Comparison of standard and low serum levels of lithium for maintenance treatment of bipolar disorder. N Engl J Med 321:1489–1493, 1989

Gershon ES: Genetics, in Manic-Depressive Illness. Edited by Goodwin FK, Jamison KR. New York, Oxford University Press, 1990, pp 373–401

Goodnick PJ, Meltzer HY: Treatment of schizoaffective disorders. Schizophr Bull 10:30–48, 1984

Goodwin FK, Jamison KR: Manic-Depressive Illness. New York, Oxford University Press, 1990

Greenberg PE, Stiglin LE, Finkelstein SN, et al: The economic burden of depression in 1990. J Clin Psychiatry 54:405–418, 1993

Greist JH, Klein MH, Eischens RR, et al: Running through your mind. J Psychosom Res 22:259–294, 1979

Hollon SD, DeRubeis RJ, Evans MD, et al: Cognitive therapy and pharmacotherapy for depression: singly and in combination. Arch Gen Psychiatry 49:774–781, 1992

Howland RH: Pharmacotherapy of dysthymia: a review. J Clin Psychopharmacol 11:83–92, 1991

Jefferson JW, Greist JH, Ackerman DL, et al: Lithium Encyclopedia for Clinical Practice, 2nd Edition, Revised. Washington, DC, American Psychiatric Press, 1987

Karasu TB: Toward a clinical model of psychotherapy for depression, I: systematic comparison of three psychotherapies. Am J Psychiatry 147:133–147, 1990

Keck PE Jr, McElroy SL, Nemeroff CB: Anticonvulsants in the treatment of bipolar disorder. J Neuropsychiatry Clin Neurosci 4:395–405, 1992

Keller MB: Differential diagnosis, natural course, and epidemiology of bipolar disorders, in Psychiatry Update: American Psychiatric Association Annual Review, Vol 6. Edited by Hales RE, Frances AJ. Washington, DC, American Psychiatric Press, 1987, pp 10–31

Keller MB, Lavori PW, Mueller TI, et al: Time to recovery, chronicity, and levels of psychopathology in major depression: a 5-year prospective follow-up of 431 subjects. Arch Gen Psychiatry 49:809–816, 1992

Klerman GL, Weissmann MM: Interpersonal psychotherapy (IPT) and drugs in the treatment of depression. Pharmacopsychiatry 20:3–7, 1987

Kocsis JH, Frances AJ: A critical discussion of DSM-III dysthymic disorder. Am J Psychiatry 144:1534–1542, 1987

Kupfer DJ: Long-term treatment of depression. J Clin Psychiatry 52 (No 5, Suppl):28–34, 1991

Kupfer DJ, Frank E, Perel JM, et al: Five-year outcome for maintenance therapies in recurrent depression. Arch Gen Psychiatry 49:769–773, 1992

Leibenluft E, Wehr TA: Is sleep deprivation useful in the treatment of depression? Am J Psychiatry 149:159–168, 1992

Markowitz JC, Moran ME, Kocsis JH, et al: Prevalence and comorbidity of dysthymic disorder among psychiatric outpatients. J Affect Disord 24:63–71, 1992

McElroy SL, Keck PE Jr, Pope HG Jr, et al: Clinical and research implications of the diagnosis of dysphoric or mixed mania or hypomania. Am J Psychiatry 149:1633–1644, 1992

McKinney WT: Animal models for depression and mania, in Depression and Mania. Edited by Georgotas A, Cancro R. New York, Elsevier, 1988, pp 181–196

Murphy DGM: The classification and treatment of dysthymia. Br J Psychiatry 158:106–109, 1991

Paykel ES: Life events and early environment, in Handbook of Affective Disorders. Edited by Paykel ES. New York, Guilford, 1982, pp 146–161

Post RM: Transduction of psychosocial stress into the neurobiology of recurrent affective disorder. Am J Psychiatry 149:999–1010, 1992

Post RM, Leverich GS, Altshuler L, et al: Lithium-discontinuation–induced refractoriness: preliminary observations. Am J Psychiatry 149:1727–1729, 1992

Regier DA, Farmer ME, Rae DS, et al: Comorbidity of mental disorders with alcohol and other drug abuse. JAMA 264:2511–2518, 1990

Seligman MEP: Helplessness: On Depression, Development, and Death. San Francisco, WH Freeman, 1975

Stewart DE, Klompenhouwer JL, Kendell RE, et al: Prophylactic lithium in puerperal psychosis: the experience of three centres. Br J Psychiatry 158:393–397, 1991

Stewart JW, McGrath PJ, Quitkin FM: Can mildly depressed outpatients with atypical depression benefit from antidepressants? Am J Psychiatry 149:615–619, 1992

Terman M, Terman JS, Quitkin FM, et al: Light therapy for seasonal affective disorder. Neuropsychopharmacology 2:1–22, 1989

Thase ME: Relapse and recurrence in unipolar major depression: short-term and long-term approaches. J Clin Psychiatry 51 (No 6, Suppl):51–57, 1990

Weissman MM, Leaf PJ, Bruce ML, et al: The epidemiology of dysthymia in five communities: rates, risks, comorbidity, and treatment. Am J Psychiatry 145:815–819, 1988a

Weissman MM, Leaf PJ, Tischler GL, et al: Affective disorders in five United States communities. Psychol Med 18:141–153, 1988b

Wells KB, Stewart A, Hays RD, et al: The functioning and well-being of depressed patients. JAMA 262:914–919, 1989

Wright JH, Thase ME: Cognitive and biological therapies: a synthesis. Psychiatric Annals 22:451–458, 1992

Anxiety Disorders

Eric Hollander, M.D.
Daphne Simeon, M.D.
Jack M. Gorman, M.D.

A nxiety disorders are the most common of all psychiatric illnesses and result in considerable functional impairment and distress. Recent research developments have had a broad impact on our understanding of the underlying mechanisms of illness and treatment response. In this chapter we have divided the anxiety disorders into four broad categories: panic and anxiety disorders (panic disorder and generalized anxiety disorder); phobic disorders (agoraphobia, social phobia, and specific phobia); obsessive-compulsive disorder; and posttraumatic stress disorder.

■ PANIC AND GENERALIZED ANXIETY DISORDERS

The DSM-IV (American Psychiatric Association 1994) definition of a panic attack is presented in Table 14–1. Panic disorder is subdivided into panic disorder with agoraphobia and without agoraphobia, depending on whether there is any secondary phobic avoidance (see Tables 14–2 and 14–3). The DSM-IV definition of generalized anxiety disorder (GAD) is presented in Table 14–4.

Panic attacks are known to occur not only in panic disorder but in other anxiety disorders as well (e.g., specific phobia, social phobia, and posttraumatic stress disorder). In these other disorders, panic attacks are situationally bound or cued—that is, they occur exclusively within the context of the feared situation. The DSM-IV presents the definition of a panic attack independently of panic disorder; it also specifies that a panic

---

Table 14–1.   DSM-IV definition of panic attack

A discrete period of intense fear or discomfort, in which four (or more) of the following symptoms developed abruptly and reached a peak within 10 minutes:
1. Palpitations, pounding heart, or accelerated heart rate
2. Sweating
3. Trembling or shaking
4. Sensations of shortness of breath or smothering
5. Feeling of choking
6. Chest pain or discomfort
7. Nausea or abdominal distress
8. Feeling dizzy, unsteady, lightheaded, or faint
9. Derealization (feelings of unreality) or depersonalization (being detached from oneself)
10. Fear of losing control or "going crazy"
11. Fear of dying
12. Paresthesias (numbness or tingling sensations)
13. Chills or hot flushes

The essential feature of a panic attack is a discrete period of intense fear or discomfort that is accompanied by at least 4 of 13 somatic or cognitive symptoms. The attack has a sudden onset and builds to a peak rapidly (usually in 10 minutes or less) and is often accompanied by a sense of imminent danger or impending doom and an urge to escape. The 13 somatic or cognitive symptoms are palpitations, sweating, trembling or shaking, sensations of shortness of breath or smothering, feeling of choking, chest pain or discomfort, nausea or abdominal distress, dizziness or lightheadedness, derealization or depersonalization, fear of losing control or "going crazy," fear of dying, paresthesias, and chills or hot flushes. Attacks that meet all other criteria but that have fewer than 4 somatic or cognitive symptoms are referred to as limited-symptom attacks.

Individuals seeking care for unexpected panic attacks will usually describe the fear as intense and report that they thought they were about to die, lose control, have a heart attack or stroke, or "go crazy." They also usually report an urgent desire to flee from wherever the attack is occurring. With recurrent attacks, some of the intense fearfulness may wane. Shortness of breath is a common symptom in panic attacks associated with panic disorder with and without agoraphobia. Blushing is common in situationally bound panic attacks related to social or performance anxiety. The anxiety that is characteristic of a panic attack can be differentiated from generalized anxiety by its intermittent, almost paroxysmal nature and its typically greater severity.

Panic attacks can occur in a variety of anxiety disorders (e.g., panic disorder, social phobia, specific phobia, posttraumatic stress disorder, acute stress disorder). In determining the differential diagnostic significance of a panic attack, it is important to consider the context in which the panic attack occurs. There are three characteristic types of panic attacks with different relationships between the onset of the attack and the presence or absence of situational triggers: **unexpected (uncued) panic attacks,** in which the onset of the panic attack is not associated with a situational trigger (i.e., occurring spontaneously "out of the blue"); **situationally bound (cued) panic attacks,** in which the

(continued)

Table 14–1.   DSM-IV definition of panic attack *(continued)*

panic attack almost invariably occurs immediately on exposure to, or in anticipation of, the situational cue or trigger (e.g., seeing a snake or dog always triggers an immediate panic attack); and **situationally predisposed panic attacks,**
which are more likely to occur on exposure to the situational cue or trigger,
but are not invariably associated with the cue and do not necessarily occur immediately after the exposure (e.g., attacks are more likely to occur while driving, but there are times when the individual drives and does not have a panic
attack or times when the panic attack occurs after driving for a half hour).

The occurrence of unexpected panic attacks is required for a diagnosis of panic
disorder (with or without agoraphobia). Situationally bound panic attacks are
most characteristic of social and specific phobias. Situationally predisposed
panic attacks are especially frequent in panic disorder but may at times occur
in specific phobia or social phobia. The differential diagnosis of panic attacks
is complicated by the fact that an exclusive relationship does not always exist
between the diagnosis and the type of panic attack. For instance, although
panic disorder definitionally requires that at least some of the panic attacks be
unexpected, individuals with panic disorder frequently report having situationally bound attacks, particularly later in the course of the disorder.

---

attack can be unexpected, situationally bound (i.e., cued), or situationally
predisposed. For a diagnosis of panic disorder to be made, the panic attacks must be unexpected (uncued). As with earlier versions, the DSM-IV
retains the diagnoses of panic disorder with agoraphobia, social phobia,
and specific phobia, but indicates that panic attacks can occur as part of
all three disorders.

The DSM-IV sharpened the distinction of GAD from "normal" anxiety by requiring that in the former the worry be excessive, pervasive, difficult to control, and associated with marked distress or impairment. The
DSM-IV also clarified when a diagnosis of GAD is excluded in the presence of other major Axis I disorders, with attention especially being
drawn to hypochondriasis and posttraumatic stress disorder.

A condition characterized by both anxiety *and* depressive symptoms
is often encountered but does not meet the criteria for either an anxiety
disorder or a depressive disorder. On one hand, the condition may cause
significant distress, and one would not want to miss or inconsistently
treat such individuals. On the other hand, there is a risk of overdiagnos-
ing psychiatric illness when it blends in with more universal human vi-
cissitudes, of encouraging nonspecific diagnoses made in nonpsychiatric
settings by nonexperts, and of overmedicating with drugs that may not
be effective or specific in their target symptoms. As a solution, the diagnosis of mixed anxiety-depressive disorder is included in an appendix to
DSM-IV. It is a diagnosis of exclusion and stipulates a 1-month duration
of symptoms.

Table 14–2.   DSM-IV diagnostic criteria for panic disorder with agoraphobia

---

A. Both (1) and (2):
  1. Recurrent unexpected panic attacks
  2. At least one of the attacks has been followed by 1 month of one
      (or more) of the following:
      a) persistent concern about having additional attacks;
      b) worry about the implications of the attack or its consequences
          (e.g., losing control, having a heart attack, "going crazy");
      c) a significant change in behavior related to the attacks

B. The presence of agoraphobia, i.e., anxiety about being in places or situations
    from which escape might be difficult (or embarrassing) or in which help
    may not be available in the event of having an unexpected or situationally
    predisposed panic attack or panic-like symptoms. Agoraphobic fears
    typically involve characteristic clusters of situations that include being
    outside the home alone; being in a crowd or standing in a line; being on
    a bridge; and traveling in a bus, train, or automobile. **Note:** Consider the
    diagnosis of specific phobia if limited to one or only a few specific situa-
    tions, or social phobia if the avoidance is limited to social situations.

C. The panic attacks are not due to the direct physiological effects of a sub-
    stance (e.g., a drug of abuse, a medication) or a general medical condition
    (e.g., hyperthyroidism).

D. The panic attacks are not better accounted for by another mental disorder,
    such as social phobia (e.g., occurring on exposure to feared social situations),
    specific phobia (e.g., on exposure to a specific phobic situation), obsessive-
    compulsive disorder (e.g., on exposure to dirt in someone with an obsession
    about contamination), posttraumatic stress disorder (e.g., in response to
    stimuli associated with a severe stressor), or separation anxiety disorder
    (e.g., in response to being away from home or close relatives).

If pathological anxiety is induced by either psychoactive substance
use or an Axis III physical illness, it is classified in the DSM-IV under the
anxiety disorders (substance-induced anxiety disorder or anxiety disorder due to a general medical condition, respectively). The DSM-IV specifies the subtype of organic anxiety as generalized anxiety, panic attacks,
or obsessive-compulsive symptoms.

☐ Clinical Descriptions

Panic Disorder

Onset.   In the typical onset of a case of panic disorder, subjects are engaged in some ordinary aspect of life when suddenly their heart begins
to pound and they cannot catch their breath. They feel dizzy, lightheaded, and faint, and are convinced they are about to die. Although the
first attack generally strikes during some routine activity, several events

Table 14–3. DSM-IV diagnostic criteria for panic disorder without agoraphobia

A. Both (1) and (2):
  1. Recurrent unexpected panic attacks
  2. At least one of the attacks has been followed by 1 month (or more) of one (or more) of the following:
     a) persistent concern about having additional attacks;
     b) worry about the implications of the attack or its consequences (e.g., losing control, having a heart attack, "going crazy");
     c) a significant change in behavior related to the attacks
B. Absence of agoraphobia [defined in Table 14–2(B)].
C. The panic attacks are not due to the direct physiological effects of a substance (e.g., a drug of abuse, a medication) or a general medical condition (e.g., hyperthyroidism).
D. The panic attacks are not better accounted for by another mental disorder, such as social phobia (e.g., occurring on exposure to feared social situations), specific phobia (e.g., on exposure to a specific phobic situation), obsessive-compulsive disorder (e.g., on exposure to dirt in someone with an obsession about contamination), posttraumatic stress disorder (e.g., in response to stimuli associated with a severe stressor), or separation anxiety disorder (e.g., in response to being away from home or close relatives).

are often associated with the early presentation of panic disorder. Not uncommonly, the first panic attack occurs in the context of a life-threatening illness or accident, the loss of a close interpersonal relationship, or during separation from family. Patients developing either hypo- or hyperthyroidism may get the first flurry of attacks at this time. Attacks also begin in the immediate postpartum period. Finally, many patients have reported experiencing their first attacks while taking mind-altering drugs.

Patients experiencing their first panic attack often rush to the nearest emergency room, where routine laboratory tests, electrocardiography, and physical examination are performed. All that is found is an occasional case of sinus tachycardia, and the patients are reassured and sent home. However, perhaps a few days or even weeks later they will again have the sudden onset of severe anxiety with all of the associated physical symptoms. Again, they seek emergency medical treatment. At this point, they may either be told the problem is "psychological," be given a prescription for a benzodiazepine tranquilizer, or be referred for extensive medical workup.

Symptoms. Typically, during a panic attack, a patient will experience the sudden onset of overwhelming fear, terror, apprehension, and a

---

Table 14–4.   DSM-IV diagnostic criteria for generalized anxiety disorder

---

A. Excessive anxiety and worry (apprehensive expectation), occurring more days than not for at least 6 months, about a number of events or activities (such as work or school performance).

B. The person finds it difficult to control the worry.

C. The anxiety and worry are associated with three (or more) of the following six symptoms (with at least some symptoms present for more days than not for the past 6 months). **Note:** Only one item is required in children.

1. Restlessness or feeling keyed up or on edge

2. Being easily fatigued

3. Difficulty concentrating or mind going blank

4. Irritability

5. Muscle tension

6. Sleep disturbance (difficulty falling or staying asleep, or restless, unsatisfying sleep)

D. The focus of the anxiety and worry is not confined to features of an Axis I disorder, e.g., the anxiety or worry is not about having a panic attack (as in panic disorder), being embarrassed in public (as in social phobia), being contaminated (as in obsessive-compulsive disorder), being away from home or close relatives (as in separation anxiety disorder), gaining weight (as in anorexia nervosa), having multiple physical complaints (as in somatization disorder), or having a serious illness (as in hypochondriasis), and the anxiety and worry do not exclusively during posttraumatic stress disorder.

E. The anxiety, worry, or physical symptoms cause clinically significant distress or impairment in social, occupational, or other important areas of functioning.

F. The disturbance is not due to the direct physiological effects of a substance (e.g., a drug of abuse, a medication) or a general medical condition (e.g., hyperthyroidism) and does not occur exclusively during a mood disorder, a psychotic disorder, or a pervasive developmental disorder.

---

sense of impending doom. Several of a group of associated symptoms, mostly physical, are also experienced: dyspnea, palpitations, chest pain or discomfort, choking or smothering sensations, dizziness or unsteady feelings, feelings of unreality (derealization and/or depersonalization), paresthesias, hot and cold flashes, sweating, faintness, trembling and shaking, and a fear of dying, going crazy, or losing control of oneself. Most of the physical sensations of a panic attack represent massive over-stimulation of the autonomic nervous system. Attacks usually last from 5 to 20 minutes, and rarely as long as an hour.

Most patients develop some degree of anticipatory anxiety consequent to the experience of repetitive panic attacks. The patient comes to dread experiencing an attack and starts worrying about doing so in the intervals between attacks. This can progress until the level of fearfulness and autonomic hyperactivity in the interval between panic attacks almost approximates the level during the actual attack itself. Such patients may be mistaken for GAD patients. *Hyperventilation* is a central feature in the pathophysiology of panic attacks and panic disorder. Patients with panic disorder have been shown to be chronic hyperventilators who also acutely hyperventilate during spontaneous and induced panic. This hyperventilation then induces hypocapnia and alkalosis, leading to decreased cerebral blood flow and to the dizziness, confusion, and derealization characteristic of panic attacks.

Generalized Anxiety Disorder

Generalized anxiety disorder is the main diagnostic category for prominent and chronic anxiety in the absence of panic disorder. The essential feature of this syndrome, according to the DSM-IV, is persistent anxiety lasting at least 6 months. The symptoms of this type of anxiety fall within two broad categories: apprehensive expectation and physical symptoms. Patients with GAD are constantly worried over trivial matters, fearful, and anticipating the worst. Muscle tension, inability to relax, difficulty concentrating, insomnia, irritability, and fatigue are typical signs of generalized anxiety.

☐ Epidemiology

The Epidemiologic Catchment Area (ECA) study examined the population prevalence of DSM-III–diagnosed panic disorder (Regier et al. 1988). The 1-month, 6-month, and lifetime prevalence rates for panic disorder were 0.5%, 0.8%, and 1.6%, respectively. Women had a significantly higher rate than men, and their attacks tended to continue longer into older age (Regier et al. 1988). Findings on GAD from the ECA revealed one-year prevalence rates of 3.8% versus 2.7% when concurrent panic or major depression was excluded. Lifetime prevalence when panic and major depression were excluded ranged from 4.1% to 6.6% (Blazer et al. 1991).

☐ Etiology

Biological Theories

Catecholamine theory.   Some investigators have found anxiety reactions associated with increases in levels of urinary catecholamines, especially epinephrine. Studies of normal subjects exposed to novel stress also demonstrate elevations in plasma catecholamine levels (Dimsdale and Moss 1980). Elevated plasma levels of epinephrine are not, however, a regular accompaniment of panic attacks induced in the laboratory (Liebowitz et al. 1985).

During a panic attack the patient complains of palpitations, tremulousness, and excessive sweating, all symptoms that are characteristic of massive stimulation of beta-adrenergic receptors. Frohlich et al. (1969) gave intravenous isoproterenol infusions to patients with a "hyperdynamic beta-adrenergic circulatory state" and produced "hysterical outbursts" that sound similar to panic attacks. Patients with spontaneous anxiety may be more sensitive to the effects of isoproterenol than are normal control subjects (Rainey et al. 1984). However, no study has ever shown that beta-adrenergic blockers are specifically effective in blocking spontaneous panic attacks.

Locus coeruleus theory.　　Another prominent hypothesis for the etiology of panic attacks involves the locus coeruleus. Support for this hypothesis comes from the fact that electrical stimulation of the animal locus coeruleus produces a marked fear and anxiety response, whereas ablation of the animal locus coeruleus renders an animal less susceptible to fear response in the face of threatening stimuli (Redmond 1979). Also, in humans, drugs capable of increasing locus coeruleus discharge in animals are anxiogenic, whereas many drugs that curtail locus coeruleus firing and decrease central noradrenergic turnover are antianxiety agents. Yohimbine, an alpha$_2$-adrenergic antagonist, is an example of a drug that increases locus coeruleus discharge and has been shown to provoke anxiety in humans. Examples of medications that curtail locus coeruleus firing are clonidine, propranolol, benzodiazepines, morphine, endorphin, and tricyclic antidepressants. The results from challenge tests with clonidine suggest noradrenergic dysregulation in panic, with hypersensitivity of some and subsensitivity of other brain alpha$_2$ adrenoreceptors (Charney et al. 1984). Similarly in patients with GAD, Abelson et al. (1991) reported a blunted growth hormone response to clonidine compared with responses in normal control subjects.

Lactate panicogenic metabolic theory.　　Lactate-provoked panic is specific to patients with prior spontaneous attacks, closely resembles such attacks, and can be blocked by the same drugs that block natural attacks (Liebowitz et al. 1984a). Pitts and McClure (1967) administered intravenous infusions of sodium lactate to patients with "anxiety" disorder and found that most of the patients suffered an anxiety attack during the infusion; normal control subjects did not experience panic attacks during the infusion. Having been replicated on numerous occasions, the finding that sodium lactate will provoke a panic attack in most patients with panic disorder is now a well-accepted fact. The mechanism, however, that may account for the observed biochemical and physiological changes (Liebowitz et al. 1985) has been subject to much controversy. Transient intracerebral hypercapnia is one theory that has received considerable interest and validation.

Carbon dioxide hypersensitivity theory. Controlled hyperventilation and respiratory alkalosis do not routinely provoke panic attacks in most patients with panic disorder. Surprisingly, however, giving these patients a mixture of 5% carbon dioxide in room air to breathe causes panic almost as often as does a sodium lactate infusion (Gorman et al. 1984). This finding has been consistently replicated. Similarly, sodium bicarbonate infusion provokes panic attacks in patients with panic disorder at a rate comparable to that induced by CO_2 inhalation (Gorman et al. 1989).

CO_2, when added to inspired air, causes a reliable dose-dependent increase in rat locus coeruleus firing (Elam et al. 1981). Alternatively, panic disorder patients may have hypersensitive brain-stem CO_2 chemoreceptors in their medulla. Indeed, during the CO_2 induction procedure, panic disorder patients who experience panic attacks while breathing 5% CO_2 demonstrate a much faster increase in inspiratory drive than do nonpanicking patients or normal control subjects; inspiratory drive is thought to reflect most directly the brain-stem component of respiratory regulation (Gorman et al. 1988). Such a model could account for the generally well-established fact that hyperventilation does not cause panic, whereas CO_2, lactate, and bicarbonate do. Infused lactate is metabolized to bicarbonate, which is then converted in the periphery to CO_2. This CO_2 then selectively crosses the blood-brain barrier and produces transient cerebral hypercapnia. The hypercapnia then sets off the brain-stem CO_2 chemoreceptors, leading to hyperventilation and panic.

GABA-benzodiazepine theory. Another area of inquiry that may relate to the biological etiology of GAD and panic is the study of the recently discovered brain benzodiazapine receptor. This receptor is linked to a receptor for the inhibitory neurotransmitter gamma-aminobutyric acid (GABA). Binding of a benzodiazepine to the benzodiazepine receptor facilitates the action of GABA, effectively slowing neural transmission. One series of compounds, the beta-carbolines, which are inverse agonists of this receptor complex, produce an acute anxiety syndrome when administered to laboratory animals or to normal human volunteers (Dorrow et al. 1983). Compared with normal control subjects, panic disorder patients demonstrate less reduced saccadic eye movement velocity in response to diazepam, suggesting hyposensitivity of the benzodiazepine receptor in panic (Roy-Byrne et al. 1990).

Genetic basis of anxiety and panic.   Family history studies of panic disorder have found a higher rate in relatives of probands with panic disorder than in relatives of normal subjects. Crowe et al. (1983) found a morbidity risk for panic disorder of 24.7% among relatives of patients with panic disorder compared with only 2.3% among normal control subjects. A 19.5% morbidity risk for GAD was found among relatives of GAD patients compared with 3.5% in normal control relatives (Noyes et al. 1987).

Early twin studies showed a higher concordance rate for anxiety disorder among monozygotic twins than among dizygotic twins. More recently, Torgersen (1983) found that panic attacks were five times more frequent in monozygotic than in dizygotic twins. However, the absolute concordance rate in monozygotic twins was 31%, suggesting that non-genetic factors play an important role in the development of the illness. Kendler et al. (1992a), studying GAD in female twins, determined that the familial component of the disorder was almost entirely genetic, with a modest heritability of about 30%.

Psychodynamic Theories

Freud's first theory of anxiety neurosis (id or impulse anxiety).   In his earliest concept of anxiety formation, Freud (1895a[1894]/1962) postulated that anxiety stems from the direct physiological transformation of libidinal energy into the somatic symptoms of anxiety, without the mediation of psychic mechanisms. Such anxiety would today be referred to as *id* or *impulse anxiety.* Freud subsequently modified his theory; although the basic tenet that anxiety stemmed from undischarged sexual energy remained the same, this was no longer posited to be due to external constraints such as sexual dysfunctions. In accordance with Freud's developing topographic theory of the mind, anxiety resulted from forbidden sexual drives in the unconscious being repressed by the preconscious.

Structural theory and intrapsychic conflict.   According to Freud's revised theory, anxiety is an affect belonging to the ego and acts as a signal alerting the ego to internal danger. The danger stems from intrapsychic conflict between instinctual drives from the id, superego prohibitions, and external reality demands. Anxiety acts as a signal to the ego for the mobilization of repression and other defenses to counteract the threat to intrapsychic equilibrium. This *intrapsychic conflict model of anxiety* continues to constitute a major tenet of contemporary psychoanalytic theory.

With the broadening of psychodynamic theory over the decades, different forms of anxiety have been elaborated and have received increased attention: annihilation (i.e., fusion or persecutory) anxiety, separation anxiety, anxiety over the loss of others' love, castration anxiety, superego anxiety, and id anxiety. In particular, greater emphasis on preoedipal dynamics and research in child development has brought to the forefront attachment theories, the importance of negotiating the ubiquitous fear of object loss, and the central role of separation anxiety in the genesis of psychopathology.

Separation anxiety. Klein (1964) advanced an etiological theory that agoraphobia with panic attacks represents an aberrant function of the biological substrate that underlies normal human separation anxiety. According to Klein (1981), the attachment of an infant animal or human to its mother is not simply a learned response, but is genetically programmed and biologically determined. Indeed, 20% to 50% of adults with panic disorder and agoraphobia recall manifesting symptoms of pathological separation anxiety, often taking the form of school phobia, when they were children. Gittelman-Klein and Klein (1971) conducted a study of imipramine treatment for children with school phobia. In these children, fear of separation from their mothers was usually the basis behind refusing to go to school. The drug proved successful in getting the children to return to school.

Learning Theories

Behavior or learning theorists hold that anxiety is conditioned by the fear of certain environmental stimuli. Anxiety attacks can be viewed as conditioned responses to fearful situations. For example, an infant learns that if his or her mother is not present (i.e., the conditioned stimulus) he or she will suffer hunger (i.e., the unconditioned stimulus), and learns to become anxious automatically whenever the mother is absent (i.e., the conditioned response). Several problems are posed by such a theory. First, although some traumatic situations seem paired with the onset of panic disorder, for many patients no such traumatic event can ever be located. For patients with GAD, attempting to find a precipitating event that makes sense as an unconditioned stimulus is even more difficult. It is also the case that most conditioned responses ultimately extinguish in laboratory animals if they are not at least intermittently reinforced. Clinical experience does not support that patients with panic disorder or GAD undergo repeat traumatic events, and therefore they should be able to "unlearn" their anxiety and panic.

☐ Diagnosis

The diagnosis of panic disorder is made when a patient experiences recurrent panic attacks that are discrete and unexpected and followed by a month of persistent anticipatory anxiety or behavioral change. These panic attacks are characterized by a sudden crescendo of anxiety and fearfulness, in addition to the presence of at least four physical symptoms. Finally, these attacks are not secondary to a known organic factor or due to another mental disorder.

The diagnosis of GAD is made when a patient experiences at least 6 months of chronic anxiety and excessive worry. At least three of six physical symptoms must also be present. Finally, this chronic anxiety must not be secondary to another Axis I disorder or a specific organic factor.

☐ Differential Diagnosis

Other Psychiatric Illnesses

Although the medical conditions that mimic anxiety disorder are usually easily ruled out, psychiatric conditions that involve pathological anxiety can make the differential diagnosis of panic disorder and GAD difficult. By far the most problematic is the differentiation of primary anxiety disorder from depression.

Patients with GAD or panic disorder generally do not demonstrate the full range of vegetative symptoms that are seen in depression. Thus, anxious patients usually have trouble falling asleep, not early morning awakening, and do not lose their appetite. Diurnal mood fluctuation is uncommon in anxiety disorder. Perhaps of greatest importance is the fact that most anxious patients do not lose the capacity to enjoy things or to be cheered up as endogenously depressed patients do.

The distinction between atypical depression and anxiety disorders is even more difficult. However, although patients with atypical depression can also be cheered up, they tend to slump faster than patients with anxiety disorder. Panic attacks and atypical depression frequently coexist, and coexisting panic attacks may increase the monoamine oxidase inhibitor (MAOI) responsivity of patients with atypical depression (Liebowitz et al. 1984b).

Patients with somatization disorder can present similarly to GAD patients because of their constant worry, but are distinguished from GAD patients by their almost exclusive preoccupation with physical complaints. Unlike panic disorder patients, somatizing patients present with physical problems that do not usually occur in episodic attacks, but are virtually constant. Patients with depersonalization disorder have episodes of derealization/depersonalization without the other symptoms of a panic attack. However, panic attacks not infrequently involve depersonalization and derealization as prominent symptoms.

Hyperthyroidism and Hypothyroidism

Both hyper- and hypothyroidism can present with anxiety unaccompanied by other signs or symptoms. For this reason, it is imperative that all patients complaining of anxiety undergo routine thyroid function tests, including the evaluation of the level of thyroid-stimulating hormone. It should be remembered, however, that thyroid disease can act as one of the predisposing triggers to panic disorder, so that even when the apparently primary thyroid disease is corrected, panic attacks may continue until specifically treated.

Cardiac Disease and Other Medical Illnesses

The relationship of mitral valve prolapse to panic disorder has attracted a great deal of attention over the years. This usually benign condition has been shown to occur more frequently in patients with panic disorder than in normal subjects. However, screening of patients known to have mitral valve prolapse reveals no greater frequency of panic disorder than is found in the overall population. Although patients with mitral valve prolapse occasionally complain of palpitations, chest pain, lightheadedness, and fatigue, symptoms of a full-blown panic attack are rare. Some have speculated that mitral valve prolapse and panic disorder may represent manifestations of the same underlying disorder of autonomic nervous system function (Gorman et al. 1981). Others have suggested that panic disorder, by creating intermittent states of high circulating catecholamine levels and tachycardia, actually causes mitral valve prolapse (Mattes 1981).

A variety of cardiac conditions can initially present as anxiety symptoms, although, in most cases, the patient complains prominently of chest pain, skipped beats, or palpitations. Ischemic heart disease and arrhythmias, especially paroxysmal atrial tachycardia, should be ruled out by electrocardiography.

Disease of the vestibular nerve can cause episodic bouts of vertigo, lightheadedness, nausea, and anxiety that mimic panic attacks. Rather than merely feeling dizzy, such patients often experience true vertigo in which the room seems to spin in one direction during each attack. Otolaryngology consultation is warranted when this condition is suspected.

Hyperparathyroidism occasionally presents with anxiety symptoms, warranting a serum calcium level before a definitive diagnosis is made.

Although many patients believe that their anxiety disorder is caused by reactive hypoglycemia, there is no scientific proof that this is a cause of psychiatric disturbance. The only convincing way to establish hypoglycemia as a cause of symptoms is to document a low blood-sugar level at the same time the patient is symptomatic. Studies with insulin tolerance tests in panic disorder have yielded negative results.

☐ Course and Prognosis

The course of illness without treatment is highly variable. The illness seems to have a waxing and waning course in which spontaneous recovery occurs, only to be followed months to years later by a new outburst. At the extreme, some patients become completely housebound for decades. Treatment aimed at blocking the occurrence of the spontaneous attack is appropriate at any point in the course of the illness when such attacks are occurring. Results are often dramatic. Pharmacological blockade of panic attacks early in the illness, before phobic avoidance has become an ingrained way of life, often leads to complete remission. Even years into the illness, effective disruption of the attacks with medication can lead to resolution of anticipatory anxiety and phobias without other treatment. However, a substantial number of patients with significant phobic avoidance remain anxious and frightened of confronting feared situations even after the attacks have been blocked.

The putative association between panic disorder and increased suicide risk was previously thought to have been due to the fact that patients with panic disorder are more prone than the normal population to major depressive disorder and to alcoholism at some point in their lives, and in part that probably remains valid. However, Allgulander and Lavori (1991) found an increased suicide risk in panic disorder in the absence of comorbid diagnoses. In the ECA study, the lifetime rate of suicide attempts in persons with uncomplicated panic disorder was found to be 7%, about the same as the 7.9% rate for persons with uncomplicated major depression (Johnson et al. 1990). How exactly panic disorder may lead to suicide remains unclear, although impaired quality of life, marred by a subjective sense of poor health, financial dependency, and occupational and social dysfunction, could lead to demoralization and hopelessness and pose a suicide risk.

☐ Treatment

Pharmacotherapy

Antidepressants. The central feature in the treatment of panic disorder is the pharmacological blockade of the spontaneous panic attacks. Several classes of medication have been shown to be effective in accomplishing this goal, and a summary of the pharmacological treatment of panic disorder is presented in Table 14–5. The most widely used and studied medications are the tricyclic antidepressants, especially imipramine. Other tricyclics, such as desipramine, have also been found effective, although they have not been studied as extensively as imipramine. Nortriptyline has not been systematically studied, but clinical experience

---

Table 14–5. Pharmacological treatment of panic disorder

Tricyclic antidepressants
General indication: Most established efficacy
Imipramine: Most studied
Desipramine: If low tolerance to anticholinergic side effects
Nortriptyline: If prone to orthostatic hypotension

Serotonin reuptake inhibitors
General indications: Inability to tolerate tricyclics; comorbid obsessive-compulsive symptoms
Clomipramine: Partial selectivity for serotonin and norepinephrine
Fluoxetine: Fewer anticholinergic side effects than tricyclics
Sertraline: Fewer anticholinergic side effects than tricyclics
Fluvoxamine: Established efficacy; fewer anticholinergic side effects than tricyclics

Monoamine oxidase inhibitors
General Indications: Poor response or tolerance of other antidepressants; comorbid atypical depression symptoms; comorbid social phobia symptoms
Phenelzine: Most studied
Tranylcypromine: Less sedation

High-potency benzodiazepines
General indications: Poor response or tolerance of antidepressants; prominent anticipatory anxiety or phobic avoidance
Alprazolam: Most studied
Clonazepam: Longer-acting, less frequent dosing, less withdrawal

---

tends to be that it is also efficacious. The presence of depressed mood is not a predictor or requirement for these drugs to be effective in blocking panic attacks.

When initiating a drug regimen for a patient with panic disorder, it is crucial for the patient to understand that the drug will block the panic attacks but may not necessarily decrease the amount of intervening anticipatory anxiety. For patients suffering from severe anxiety, in order to reduce the level of anticipatory anxiety, it may be helpful for them initially to take a concomitant benzodiazepine, which can be gradually tapered and discontinued after several weeks of antidepressant treatment. Some patients with panic disorder display an initial hypersensitivity to tricyclic antidepressants, during which they complain of jitteriness, agitation, a "speedy" feeling, and insomnia. Although this is usually transient, it is one of the main reasons why patients opt to discontinue medication early on. Therefore, it is recommended that patients with panic disorder be started on lower doses of tricyclics than would be given to depressed patients. Patients who experience excessive anticholinergic side effects to imipramine can be given desipramine instead. The elderly or patients who are otherwise very sensitive to orthostatic hypotension can be tried on nortriptyline.

Monoamine oxidase inhibitors are as equally effective as the tricyclics in treating panic. Both phenelzine and tranylcypromine successfully treat panic, although phenelzine has been studied more extensively. Tricyclics are typically preferred over MAOIs because they obviate the need for dietary restrictions and the risk of hypertensive crises. However, MAOIs are an option to consider for patients who fail to tolerate or to respond well to tricyclics. In patients with concomitant atypical depression or social phobia, MAOIs may be an appropriate first choice for treatment.

A number of open and controlled treatment trials have shown that serotonin reuptake blockers, such as clomipramine, fluoxetine, and fluvoxamine, are also highly effective in the treatment of panic. Given their higher safety and ease of administration compared with MAOIs, serotonin reuptake blockers may be preferable in patients who did not respond to or cannot tolerate tricyclics. In the presence of obsessive-compulsive symptoms, they would be indicated as first choice. Like the tricyclics, fluoxetine can cause uncomfortable overstimulation in panic patients if started at the usual dose.

Full remission of panic attacks with antidepressants usually requires 4 to 12 weeks of treatment. Subsequently, the duration of required treatment in order to prevent relapse is a function of the natural course of panic disorder. The disorder can probably best be characterized as chronic, with an exacerbating and remitting course. A reasonable recommendation in treating panic patients is to keep them on full-dose medication for at least 6 months to prevent early relapse. Afterward, patients can be tapered to half-dose medication and be followed to ensure that clinical improvement is maintained. Subsequently, the clinician may attempt gradual dose decreases every few months as long as the improvement is maintained, and reach a minimal dose on which the patient is relatively symptom-free. Some patients may eventually be able to discontinue medication. Other patients may require more chronic maintenance treatment, especially in light of the morbidity and mortality risk that may be associated with the disorder.

With regard to GAD, preliminary studies have indicated that tricyclic antidepressants may also be effective in treating chronically anxious patients independent of the presence of depressive symptoms. However, in all but one of these studies, the patients were not specifically diagnosed as having GAD. In one controlled study comparing imipramine and alprazolam specifically in the treatment of GAD, similar efficacy was found for the two medications, with imipramine acting more on negative affects and cognitions and alprazolam acting more on somatic symptoms (Hoehn-Saric et al. 1988).

Anxiolytics.   The high-potency benzodiazepine alprazolam appears to be an effective antipanic drug. In a large multicenter placebo-controlled study (Ballenger et al. 1988), 82% of patients treated acutely with alprazolam showed at least moderate improvement in panic, compared with 43% on placebo. There are fewer data about the efficacy of clonazepam and lorazepam, but what exists is also promising in the acute treatment of panic. Long-term efficacy and possible dependency are still under investigation, and little is known.

These medications have fewer initial side effects than tricyclics, serotonin reuptake inhibitors, and MAOIs. However, the general treatment principle is that anxiolytics should be reserved until the different classes of antidepressants have failed, because they pose some risk of tolerance, dependence, and withdrawal. For patients with severe acute distress and disability, who may require immediate relief, it may be indicated to start with a benzodiazepine and then replace it with an antidepressant. There is also some evidence that benzodiazepines may be more effective, at least initially, in ameliorating the associated anticipatory anxiety and phobic avoidance, and this may be another indication for their initial use.

The pharmacological treatment of GAD is less well established. Traditionally, chronically anxious patients have been placed on benzodiazepines. However, no study has yet shown benzodiazepines to be superior to other drugs or nonpharmacological treatment methods in patients specifically diagnosed with GAD. Although benzodiazepines are generally safe, with side effects limited mainly to sedation, there is a concern that some patients may become tolerant or even addicted to these agents.

A newer drug, buspirone, is a nonbenzodiazepine antianxiety agent that appears to have efficacy in treating GAD similar to that of the benzodiazepines. Its advantages are a better side-effect profile and the absence of tolerance and withdrawal. Its disadvantages are a slower rate of onset (Rickels et al. 1988), which can lead to early patient noncompliance. It has also been suggested that patients who have previously been treated with benzodiazepines may not respond as well to buspirone (Schweizer et al. 1986).

Other medications.   Beta-adrenergic blocking drugs, such as propranolol, are said by some to be useful in the treatment of a variety of anxiety disorders, but there is no scientific evidence that they are specifically effective in blocking spontaneous panic attacks. The same applies for GAD, in which propranolol may only be rarely indicated as an adjuvant in patients who experience significant palpitations or tremor.

Clonidine, which inhibits locus coeruleus discharge, would seem, for theoretical reasons, to be a good antipanic drug. Although in a small series two-thirds of patients responded initially, the therapeutic effect tends to be lost in a matter of weeks despite continuation of dose (Liebowitz et al. 1981).

Psychotherapy

Insight psychotherapy. Even after medication has blocked the actual panic attacks, a subgroup of panic patients remain wary of independence and assertiveness. In addition to supportive and behavioral treatment, traditional psychodynamic psychotherapy might be helpful for some of these patients. Significant unconscious conflict over separations during childhood sometimes appears to operate in patients with panic disorder, leading to a reemergence of anxiety symptoms in adult life each time a new separation is imagined or threatened. Furthermore, it has been found that comorbid personality disorder is the major predictor of continued social maladjustment in patients otherwise treated for panic disorder (Noyes et al. 1990), suggesting that psychodynamic therapy may be an important additional treatment for at least some patients with panic. However, in those patients with a predominant biological component to their illness, insistence on dynamic understanding and on responsibility for one's symptoms may be, in the long run, not only useless but potentially harmful, leading to further damage in self-esteem and strengthened masochistic defenses.

Psychodynamic psychotherapy may also be helpful in some patients with GAD, when unconscious conflict is believed by the clinician to be the cause of the patient's chronic anxiety. From a psychodynamic viewpoint, the more contained anxiety characteristic of GAD may be more akin to Freud's concept of signal anxiety and may thus be more amenable to psychodynamic exploration than is panic. Here, the emphasis is not on anxiety as an illness, but as a ubiquitous affect hinting at underlying conflict.

Supportive psychotherapy. Despite adequate treatment of panic attacks with medication, phobic avoidance may remain. Supportive psychotherapy and education about the illness are necessary to urge the patient to confront the phobic situation. Patients who fail to respond may then need additional psychotherapy, dynamic or behavioral. Encouragement from other patients with similar conditions often can be helpful.

Cognitive-behavior therapy. The major behavioral techniques for the treatment of panic attacks are breathing retraining, to control both acute and chronic hyperventilation; exposure to somatic cues, usually involving a hierarchy of exposure to feared sensations; and relaxation training. Cognitive treatment of panic involves cognitive restructuring so as to give the uncomfortable affects and physical sensations associated with panic a more benign interpretation. The extreme cognitive view is that panic attacks consist of normal physical sensations (e.g., palpitations, slight dizziness) to which panic disorder patients grossly overreact with catastrophic cognitions. A more middle-of-the-road view is that panic patients do have extreme physical sensations such as bursts of tachycardia, but still significantly help themselves by changing their interpretation of the event. Several studies have shown that cognitive-behavioral techniques can be successful in the treatment of panic attacks (Barlow et al. 1989; Beck et al. 1992; Michelson et al. 1990).

Relaxation may be a more useful technique for generalized anxiety. In anxiety management training for generalized anxiety, relaxation training is specifically applied to both imagined and real-life anxiety-provoking situations. Relaxation helps reduce tension and other physical manifestations of anxiety, and can be combined with cognitive restructuring to alleviate the cognitive component of negative anticipation and worrying. Although systematic evaluation and comparison of these techniques in GAD have been limited to date, they appear to hold some promise.

■ PHOBIC DISORDERS

A *phobia* is defined as a persistent and irrational fear of a specific object, activity, or situation that results in a compelling desire to avoid the dreaded object, activity, or situation (i.e., phobic stimulus). The fear is recognized by the individual as excessive or unreasonable in proportion to the actual dangerousness of the object, activity, or situation. Irrational fears and avoidance behavior are seen in a number of psychiatric disorders. However, in DSM-IV the diagnosis of phobic disorder is made only when single or multiple phobias are the predominant aspect of the clinical picture and a source of significant distress to the individual, and not the result of another mental disorder.

The major changes in the phobic disorders instituted in DSM-IV, in relation to DSM-III-R, were as follows. In agoraphobia without panic disorder, it is specified that the condition centers on the fear of developing incapacitating symptoms typically in characteristic situational clusters. It is also specified that agoraphobia related to embarrassment over a medical illness is a diagnosis that can be made subject to clinical judgment. The two major changes in social phobia and in specific phobia in DSM-IV are similar for the two disorders. First, it is made explicit that panic attacks can occur as a feature of these phobias, and therefore clinical judgment is required to make the differential diagnosis between panic disorder with agoraphobia versus social or specific phobia. Second, specific phobia is now divided into types, because new evidence has accumulated that phenomenology, natural history, and treatment response may differ according to type. The generalized type of social phobia was retained as in DSM-III-R. The DSM-IV diagnostic criteria for agoraphobia without history of panic disorder, social phobia, and specific phobia are presented in Tables 14–6, 14–7, and 14–8, respectively.

□ Clinical Descriptions

Agoraphobia

The clinical picture in agoraphobia consists of multiple and varied fears and avoidance behaviors that center around three main themes: 1) fear of leaving home, 2) fear of being alone, and 3) fear of being away from home in situations where one can feel trapped, embarassed, or helpless. According to DSM-IV, the fear is one of developing distressing symptoms in such situations where escape is difficult or help is unavailable. Typical agoraphobic fears are of using public transportation (buses, trains, subways, planes); being in crowds, theaters, elevators, restaurants, supermarkets, department stores; waiting in line; or traveling a distance from home. In severe cases patients may be completely housebound, fearful of leaving home without a companion or even of staying home alone.

Most cases of agoraphobia begin with a series of spontaneous panic

---

Table 14–6. DSM-IV diagnostic criteria for agoraphobia without history of panic disorder

A. The presence of agoraphobia related to fear of developing panic-like symptoms (e.g., dizziness or diarrhea). Agoraphobia: anxiety about being in places or situations from which escape might be difficult (or embarrassing) or in which help may not be available in the event of having an unexpected or situationally predisposed panic attack or panic-like symptoms. Agoraphobic fears typically involve characteristic clusters of situations that include being outside the home alone; being in a crowd or standing in a line; being on a bridge; and traveling in a bus, train, or automobile.

B. Criteria have never been met for panic disorder.

C. The disturbance is not due to the direct physiological effects of a substance (e.g., a drug of abuse, a medication) or a general medical condition.

D. If an associated general medical condition is present, the fear described in criterion A is clearly in excess of that usually associated with the condition.

Table 14–7.   DSM-IV diagnostic criteria for social phobia (social anxiety disorder)

A.   A marked and persistent fear of one or more social or performance situations in which the person is exposed to unfamiliar people or to possible scrutiny by others. The individual fears that he or she will act in a way (or show anxiety symptoms) that will be humiliating or embarrassing. **Note:** In children, there must be evidence of the capacity for age-appropriate social relationships with familiar people and the anxiety must occur in peer settings, not just in interactions with adults.

B.   Exposure to the feared situation almost invariably provokes anxiety, which may take the form of a situationally bound or situationally predisposed panic attack. **Note:** In children, the anxiety may be expressed by crying, tantrums, freezing, or shrinking from social situations with unfamiliar people.

C.   The person recognizes that the fear is excessive or unreasonable. **Note:** In children, this feature may be absent.

D.   The feared social or performance situations are avoided or else are endured with intense anxiety or distress.

E.   The avoidance, anxious anticipation, or distress in the feared social or performance situation(s) interferes significantly with the person's normal routine, occupational (academic) functioning, or social activities or relationships, or there is marked distress about having the phobia.

F.   In individuals under age 18 years, the duration is at least 6 months.

G.   The fear or avoidance is not due to the direct physiological effects of a substance (e.g., a drug of abuse, a medication) or a general medical condition and is not better accounted for by another mental disorder (e.g., panic disorder with or without agoraphobia, separation anxiety disorder, body dysmorphic disorder, a pervasive developmental disorder, or schizoid personality disorder).

H.   If a general medical condition or another mental disorder is present, the fear in criterion A is unrelated to it, e.g., the fear is not of stuttering, trembling in Parkinson's disease, or exhibiting abnormal eating behavior in anorexia nervosa or bulimia nervosa.

Specify if:

Generalized: if the fears include most social situations (also consider the additional diagnosis of avoidant personality disorder)

---

attacks. If the attacks continue, the patient usually develops a constant anticipatory anxiety characterized by continued apprehension about the possible occasion and consequences of the next attack. Agoraphobic symptoms represent a tertiary phase in the illness. Many patients will causally relate their panic attacks to the particular situation in which the attacks have occurred. They then avoid these situations in an attempt to prevent further panic attacks. Agoraphobic persons frequently fear situations in which they feel they cannot leave abruptly if an attack occurs, such as crowded rooms, bridges, and airplanes. One interesting aspect of

---

Table 14–8. DSM-IV diagnostic criteria for specific phobia

A. Marked and persistent fear that is excessive or unreasonable, cued by the presence or anticipation of a specific object or situation (e.g., flying, heights, animals, receiving an injection, seeing blood).

B. Exposure to the phobic stimulus almost invariably provokes an immediate anxiety response, which may take the form of a situationally bound or situationally predisposed panic attack. **Note:** In children, the anxiety may be expressed by crying, tantrums, freezing, or clinging.

C. The person recognizes that the fear is excessive or unreasonable. **Note:** In children, this feature may be absent.

D. The phobic situation(s) is avoided or else is endured with intense anxiety or distress.

E. The avoidance, anxious anticipation, or distress in the feared situation(s) interferes significantly with the person's normal routine, occupational (or academic) functioning, or social activities or relationships, or there is marked distress about having the phobia.

F. In individuals under age 18 years, the duration is at least 6 months.

G. The anxiety, panic attacks, or phobic avoidance associated with the specific object or situation are not better accounted for by another mental disorder, such as obsessive-compulsive disorder (e.g., fear of dirt in someone with an obsession about contamination), posttraumatic stress disorder (e.g., avoidance of stimuli associated with a severe stressor), separation anxiety disorder (e.g., avoidance of school), social phobia (e.g., avoidance of social situations because of fear of embarrassment), panic disorder with agoraphobia, or agoraphobia without history of panic disorder.

Specify type:
Animal type
Natural environment type (e.g., heights, storms, water)
Blood-injection-injury type
Situational type (e.g., airplanes, elevators, enclosed spaces)
Other type (e.g., phobic avoidance of situations that may lead to choking, vomiting, or contracting an illness; in children, avoidance of loud sounds or costumed characters)

---

agoraphobia is the effect of a trusted companion on phobic behavior. Many patients who are unable to leave the house alone can travel long distances and partake in most activities if accompanied by a spouse, family member, or close friend.

Social Phobia

In *social phobia,* the individuals' central fear is that they will act in such a way as to humiliate or embarrass themselves in front of others. Socially phobic individuals fear and/or avoid a variety of situations in which they would be required to interact with others or to perform a task in front of other people. Typical social phobias are of speaking, eating, or writing in public; using public lavatories; and attending parties or interviews. In addition, a common fear of socially phobic individuals is that other people will detect and ridicule their anxiety in social situations. An individual may have one, limited, or numerous social fears.

As in specific phobia, the anxiety in social phobia is stimulus-bound. When forced or surprised into the phobic situation, the individual experiences profound anxiety accompanied by a variety of somatic symptoms. Interestingly, different anxiety disorders tend to be characterized by their own constellation of most prominent somatic symptoms. Actual panic attacks may also occur in individuals with social phobia in response to feared social situations. Individuals who have only limited social fears may be functioning well overall and be relatively asymptomatic unless confronted with the necessity of entering their phobic situation. When faced with this necessity, they are often subject to intense anticipatory anxiety. Multiple social fears, on the other hand, can lead to chronic demoralization, social isolation, and disabling vocational and interpersonal impairment.

Specific Phobias

Specific phobias are circumscribed fears of specific objects, situations, or activities. This syndrome has three components: an anticipatory anxiety that is brought on by the possibility of confrontation with the phobic stimulus, the central fear itself, and the avoidance behavior by which the patient minimizes anxiety. In specific phobia, the fear is usually not of the object itself but of some dire outcome that the individuals believe may result from contact with that object. These fears are excessive, unreasonable, and enduring, so that although most individuals with specific phobias will readily acknowledge that they know "there is really nothing to be afraid of," reassuring them of this does not diminish their fear.

In DSM-IV, for the first time, types of specific phobias have been adopted: natural environment, animal, blood-injury-injection, situational, and other (e.g., choking, vomiting). The validity of such distinctions is supported by data showing that these types tend to differ with respect to age at onset, mode of onset, familial aggregation, and physiological responses to the phobic stimulus (Fyer et al. 1990; Himle et al. 1991; Ost 1987).

☐ Epidemiology

In the ECA study, phobias as a group were found to be the most common current psychiatric disorder, with 1-month and 6-month prevalence rates of 6.2% and 7.7%, respectively, and a lifetime rate of 12.5% (Regier et al. 1988). Specific phobias were the most common (11.3%), followed by agoraphobia (5.6%) and social phobia (2.7%). Specific phobias were more common in women than men (14.5% vs. 7.8%). Agoraphobia was also more common in women (7.9% vs. 3.2%). Social phobia was similar in the two sexes (2.9% in women vs. 2.5% in men) (Eaton et al. 1991).

☐ Etiology

Psychodynamic Theory

Early on, Freud (1895b[1894]/1962) did not consider phobias to be psychologically mediated. Rather he understood them, like anxiety neurosis, to be manifestations of a physiologically induced tension state. Undischarged libidinal energy was physiologically transformed into anxiety, which became attached to and partly discharged through objects that were, by their nature or in the patient's prior experience, dangerous. Freud later hypothesized that phobic symptoms occur as part of the resolution of intrapsychic conflict between instinctual impulses, superego prohibitions, and external reality constraints. Signal anxiety is experienced by the ego when such unconscious impulses threaten to break through. Such anxiety serves to mobilize not only further repression but, in the case of phobia formation, projection and displacement of the conflict onto a symbolic object, which can then be avoided as a neurotic solution to the original conflict.

Since Freud, the psychodynamic literature has to a degree shifted away from formulations that primarily emphasize libidinal wishes and castration fears in understanding phobias. For example, the significance of a trustworthy companion in individuals with agoraphobia could be understood as a simultaneous expression of aggressive impulses toward the companion and a magical wish to protect the companion from such impulses by always being together. Alternatively, excessive fear of object loss and its concomitant separation anxiety could explain both the fear of being away from home alone and the alleviation of this fear when a companion is present.

Conditioned Reflex Theories

In learning theory, phobic anxiety is thought to be a conditioned response acquired through association of the phobic object (i.e., the conditioned stimulus) with a noxious experience (i.e., the unconditioned stimulus). Avoidance of the phobic object prevents or reduces this conditioned anxiety and is therefore perpetuated through drive reduction. This classical learning theory model of phobias received much reinforcement from the relative success of behavioral (i.e., deconditioning) techniques in the treatment of many patients with simple phobia.

However, more recently the model has been criticized on the grounds that it is not consistent with a number of empirically observed aspects of phobic behavior in humans. Specifically, many cases of phobia do not appear to have begun with a traumatic incident in which the phobic object is associated with an unpleasant unconditioned stimulus. In addition, the range of phobic objects is actually relatively small and is neither random nor predominantly made up of those items that in a modern industrial society might be most likely to be frequently associated with noxious stimuli (e.g., electric switches, stoves, oncoming cars). Finally, learning theory does not account for the qualitative distinctions between panic and anticipatory anxiety delineated by pharmacological and sodium lactate infusion studies. Even though learning theory could account for the initial emergence of certain phobic symptoms, it does not fully account for their maintenance, as repeated exposure to the conditioned stimulus should extinguish the conditioned response.

Biological Theories

Seligman (1971) suggested that simple phobias are an example of evolutionarily prepared learning. The concept of "preparedness" refers to the observation that certain responses to stimuli are more easily learned than others and that the ease of learning in any one instance varies from species to species. Most specific phobias involve stimuli that over the course of evolution might have been dangerous to man, but are still reacted to as though intrinsically dangerous. In support of a biological component in specific phobias, Fyer et al. (1990) found high familial transmission for specific phobias, with a roughly threefold risk for first-degree relatives of affected subjects; interestingly, there was no increased risk for other phobic or anxiety disorders.

Social phobic symptoms are accompanied in perhaps 50% of cases by a surge of plasma epinephrine, distinguishing them from panic attacks, in which an adrenaline surge is not regularly seen. Cognitive features also play a role in social phobia, however, because rapid infusions of adrenaline in nonperformance situations do not fully reproduce the symptoms. Phenylethylamine or similar endogenous amines may be involved in our mood response to social approval and disapproval. This system could be poorly regulated in patients with social phobia and those with atypical depression (Liebowitz et al. 1984b). Both of these groups overreact to criticism or rejection, and greatly benefit from MAOIs, which reduce their sensitivity to rejection and also inhibit the metabolism of endogenous biogenic amines.

In a large study of phobias in twins, Kendler et al. (1992b) determined that the familial aggregation of phobias was mostly accounted for by genetic factors, with a modest heritability of 30% to 40% depending on the particular phobia.

☐ Diagnosis and Differential Diagnosis

Before the diagnosis of phobic disorder can be made, the presence of other disorders that may cause irrational fears and avoidance behaviors must be ruled out.

Agoraphobia

Widespread fears and avoidance of being alone or of leaving home can be seen in paranoid and psychotic states, posttraumatic disorders, and major depressive disorders. Psychotic states can be differentiated from agoraphobia by the presence of delusions, hallucinations, and thought process disorder. Although agoraphobic patients are frequently afraid that they are going crazy, they do not exhibit psychotic symptomatology. Patients with posttraumatic stress disorder have a typical history, such as a fear of being or traveling alone following an assault.

The distinction between depressive disorders and agoraphobia is more difficult. Both groups commonly experience spontaneous panic attacks. Patients with agoraphobia are frequently demoralized and will state that they feel depressed. Close questioning, however, usually does not reveal further vegetative symptoms or a loss of pleasure or interest in activities. Early morning awakening and pervasive anhedonia, which are common symptoms in endogenous depression, are rare in agoraphobia. Agoraphobic individuals will usually say they would love to leave home and engage in a variety of activities if only they could be sure of not panicking. In contrast, depressed individuals usually see no point in going out because nothing gives them any pleasure and they feel that people will be better off without them.

Social Phobia

Avoidance of social situations is seen as part of avoidant, schizoid, and paranoid personality disorders, agoraphobia, obsessive-compulsive disorder, depressive disorders, schizophrenia, and paranoid disorders. Persons with paranoid disorders fear that something unpleasant will be done to them by others. In contrast, social phobic individuals fear that they themselves will act inappropriately and cause their own embarrassment or humiliation. In avoidant personality disorder the central fear is also rejection, ridicule, or humiliation by others. The distinction between this and generalized social phobia is a subject of dispute.

Some agoraphobic patients say that they are afraid they will embarrass themselves by losing control if they panic while in a social situation.

These patients are distinguished from patients with social phobia by the presence of panic attacks that also occur in situations not involving evaluation by others. Interpersonal anxiety or fears of humiliation leading to social avoidance are not diagnosed as social phobia when occurring in the context of schizophrenia, schizophreniform or brief reactive psychoses, and major depressive disorder. Social withdrawal seen in depressive disorders is usually associated with a lack of interest or pleasure in the company of others rather than a fear of scrutiny. In contrast, individuals with social phobia generally express the wish to be able to interact appropriately with others and anticipate pleasure in this eventuality.

☐ Course and Prognosis

The usual age at onset of agoraphobia is between 18 and 35 years. Individuals whose "panic" episodes are characterized principally by feelings of unsteadiness and a fear of falling (leading to a fear of open spaces) typically have onset of the disorder in their 40s. Although in the case of those patients who eventually seek treatment the overall course of the illness is thought to be chronic, the general impression of experienced clinicians is that the illness waxes and wanes and that many patients have at least brief periods of improvement or even remission.

Social phobias are thought to have their onset mainly in adolescence and early adulthood, and the course of illness appears chronic. Mean age at onset is 19 years (Amies et al. 1983). Onset of symptoms is sometimes acute following a humiliating social experience, but is usually insidious over months or years and without a clear-cut precipitant. Men are equally or even more commonly affected than women, in distinction to other anxiety disorders, although in one large epidemiological survey of social phobia, Schneier et al. (1992) found that 70% of those afflicted were women.

Animal phobias usually begin in childhood, whereas situational phobias tend to start later in life. Marks (1969) found the mean age at onset for animal phobias to be 4.4 years, whereas patients with situational phobias had a mean age at onset of 22.7 years. It appears that specific phobias follow a chronic course unless treated.

☐ Treatment

Pharmacotherapy

Agoraphobia.   There continues to be disagreement regarding the best method of treatment of agoraphobia with panic attacks. Antipanic medication is given to block the occurrence of panic attacks, and its efficacy in this regard is well documented. However, medication alone is often not adequate treatment in patients with significant agoraphobic avoidance. It is generally accepted that some means of exposing agoraphobic patients to the feared situations is necessary for overall improvement. This may be achieved by various nonspecific methods, such as psychoeducation, reassurance, and supportive therapy. Cognitive-behavior therapy is, on the whole, more successful than nonspecific techniques in reducing agoraphobic avoidance. Consequently, the relative and combined efficacy of medications and cognitive-behavior therapy for panic with agoraphobia has been the focus of a number of investigations.

Some studies have not found imipramine to have a significant effect when given alone or with antiexposure instructions (Marks et al. 1983). Other studies found the combination of medication and behavioral treatment to be superior to behavioral treatment alone (Telch et al. 1985). Mavissakalian and Perel (1989) studied the impact of imipramine without any behavioral intervention and found that 83% of patients showed a marked improvement in panic and 67% of patients showed a marked improvement in phobia.

Social phobia.   In performance-type social phobia, studies suggest beta-blocker efficacy, particularly when these agents are used acutely prior to a performance. Many performing artists or public speakers find that propranolol reduces palpitations, tremor, and "the butterfly feeling."

The MAOI phenelzine has been found to be effective in mixed agoraphobic–social phobic samples. Liebowitz et al. (1992) conducted a controlled study comparing phenelzine, atenolol, and placebo in the treatment of patients with DSM-III social phobia. About two-thirds of patients had a marked response to phenelzine, whereas atenolol was not superior to placebo. Tranylcypromine was also associated with significant improvement in about 80% of patients with DSM-III social phobia treated openly for 1 year (Versiani et al. 1988). Gelernter et al. (1991) compared cognitive-behavioral group treatment with phenelzine, alprazolam, and placebo. Although all groups improved significantly with treatment, phenelzine tended to be superior in absolute clinical response and decreased impairment.

Specific phobias.   No medication has been shown to be effective in treating specific phobias.

Cognitive-Behavior Therapy

Agoraphobia.   The goal of psychotherapeutic intervention in agoraphobia is to encourage patients to reenter the phobic situation and demonstrate to themselves that they will no longer have panic attacks while on medication and therefore may give up both the avoidance and the worry, or anticipatory anxiety, about having attacks. At the start of treatment the therapist explains to the patient the three-stage development of the illness and the fact that the medication will block the spontaneous panics but may not alleviate anticipatory anxiety or the desire to avoid. Some patients, once the frequency of spontaneous panics has abated, will begin to try out previously avoided situations on their own; others need supportive psychotherapy. Focused behavioral therapies appear more effective for patients with more severe agoraphobia. A popular form of behavior therapy is group in vivo exposure, in which groups of agoraphobic patients (initially accompanied by the therapist) travel together to restaurants, shopping malls, etc. Self-help groups are also quite helpful for raising morale and sharing information among agoraphobic individuals.

Social phobia. A number of cognitive-behavioral techniques have been used in the treatment of social phobia: exposure (imaginal or in vivo; individual or group), cognitive restructuring, and social skills training. Exposure treatment involves imaginal or in vivo exposure to feared performance and social situations and has been linked to a traumatic (i.e., conditioned) etiology of social phobia. Social skills training employs modeling, rehearsal, role playing, and assigned practice (usually in groups) to help individuals learn appropriate behaviors and decrease anxiety in social situations. Cognitive restructuring focuses on poor self-concepts, the fear of negative evaluation by others, and the attribution of positive outcomes to chance or circumstance and negative outcomes to one's own shortcomings.

Heimberg et al. (1990) compared cognitive-behavioral group treatment to a credible psychoeducational-supportive control intervention in patients with DSM-III social phobia; both groups got better, but the cognitive-behavioral group showed more improvement, especially in patients' self-appraisal. It has been suggested that cognitive aspects may be of greater importance in social phobia than in other anxiety or phobic conditions, and therefore cognitive restructuring may be a necessary component to maximize treatment gains. Mattick et al. (1989) reported that combination treatment was superior to either exposure or cognitive restructuring alone in social phobia; cognitive restructuring was inferior to exposure in decreasing avoidant behavior, but exposure alone did not change self-perception and attitude.

Specific phobias. The treatment of choice for specific phobias is exposure. The problem is to persuade the patient that exposure is good for him or her. Exposure treatments may be divided into two groups depending on whether exposure to the phobic object is "in vivo" or "imaginal." In vivo exposure involves the patient in "real life" contact with the phobic stimulus. Imaginal techniques confront the phobic stimulus through the therapist's descriptions and the patient's imagination. Graded exposure uses a hierarchy of anxiety-provoking events, varying from least to most stressful. The patient begins at the least stressful level and gradually progresses up the hierarchy. Ungraded exposure begins with the patients confronting the most stressful items in the hierarchy.

◼ OBSESSIVE-COMPULSIVE DISORDER

The essential features of obsessive-compulsive disorder (OCD) are obsessions or compulsions. The definition and criteria of OCD in DSM-IV are presented in Table 14–9. Although some activities, such as eating, sexual behavior, gambling, or drinking, when engaged in excessively may be referred to as "compulsive," these activities are distinguished from true compulsions in that they are experienced as pleasurable, although their consequences may be unpleasant. Obsessive brooding, ruminations, or preoccupations may be unpleasant but are distinguished from true obsessions because they are not ego-dystonic, since the individual regards the ideation as meaningful, although possibly excessive. Patients with obsessions may be prone to obsessive broodings, and a common feature of both groups of patients is the inability to turn off a train of thought. However, most OCD patients have several different obsessions and compulsions over the course of their illness.

There are several presentations of OCD based on symptom clusters. One group includes patients with obsessions about dirt and contamination, whose rituals center around compulsive washing and avoidance of contaminated objects. A second group includes patients with pathological counting and compulsive checking. A third group includes "purely obsessional" patients with no compulsions. Primary obsessional slowness is evident in another group, in whom slowness is the predominant symptom. Patients may spend many hours every day getting washed, dressed, and eating breakfast, and life goes on at an extremely slow speed. Some OCD patients, called "hoarders," are unable to throw anything out for fear they might someday need something they discarded.

☐ Clinical Description

Onset

Obsessive-compulsive disorder usually begins in adolescence or early adulthood, but can begin prior to that time; 31% of first episodes occur between ages 10 and 15, with 75% developing by age 30 (Black 1974). In

Table 14–9. DSM-IV diagnostic criteria for obsessive-compulsive disorder

A.   Either obsessions or compulsions:

Obsessions as defined by (1), (2), (3), and (4):

1. Recurrent and persistent thoughts, impulses, or images that are experienced, at some time during the disturbance, as intrusive and inappropriate and that cause marked anxiety or distress.

2. The thoughts, impulses, or images are not simply excessive worries about real-life problems.

3. The person attempts to ignore or suppress such thoughts, impulses, or images or to neutralize them with some other thought or action.

4. The person recognizes that the obsessional thoughts, impulses, or images are a product of his or her own mind (not imposed from without as in thought insertion).

Compulsions as defined by (1) and (2):

1. Repetitive behaviors (e.g., handwashing, ordering, checking) or mental acts (e.g., praying, counting, repeating words silently) that the person feels driven to perform in response to an obsession or according to rules that must be applied rigidly.

2. The behaviors or mental acts are aimed at preventing or reducing distress or preventing some dreaded event or situation; however, these behaviors or mental acts either are not connected in a realistic way with what they are designed to neutralize or prevent or are clearly excessive.

B.   At some point during the course of the disorder, the person has recognized that the obsessions or compulsions are excessive or unreasonable. **Note:** This does not apply to children.

C.   The obsessions or compulsions cause marked distress, are time consuming (take more than 1 hour a day), or significantly interfere with the person's normal routine, occupational (or academic) functioning, or usual social activities or relationships.

D.   If another Axis I disorder is present, the content of the obsessions or compulsions is not restricted to it (e.g., preoccupation with food in the presence of an eating disorder; hair pulling in the presence of trichotillomania; concern with appearance in the presence of body dysmorphic disorder; preoccupation with drugs in the presence of a substance use disorder; preoccupation with having a serious illness in the presence of hypochondriasis; preoccupation with sexual urges or fantasies in the presence of a paraphilia; or guilty ruminations in the presence of major depressive disorder).

E.   The disturbance is not due to the direct physiological effects of a substance (e.g., a drug of abuse, a medication) or a general medical condition.

Specify if:
With poor insight: if, for most of the time during the current episode, the person does not recognize that the obsessions and compulsions are excessive or unreasonable

most cases, no particular stress or event precipitates the onset of OCD symptoms, and following an insidious onset there is a chronic and often progressive course.

Symptoms

Obsessions.   An obsession is an intrusive, unwanted mental event usually evoking anxiety or discomfort. Obsessions may be thoughts, ideas, images, ruminations, convictions, fears, or impulses, and are often of an aggressive, sexual, religious, disgusting, or nonsensical content. Obsessional ideas are repetitive thoughts that interrupt the normal train of thinking, while obsessional images are often vivid visual experiences. Much obsessive thinking involves horrific ideas. Obsessional convictions are based on magical ideas such as "step on the crack, break your mother's back." Obsessional fears often involve dirt or contamination, and differ from phobias because they are present in the absence of the phobic stimulus.

Attributing these obsessions to an internal source, the patient resists or controls them to a variable degree, and some impairment in functioning can result. *Resistance* is the struggle against an impulse or intrusive thought, and *control* is the patient's ability to divert his or her thinking. Obsessions are usually accompanied by compulsions but may also occur as the main or only symptom. Approximately 10% to 25% of OCD patients are purely obsessional or suffer predominantly from obsessions (Rachman and Hodgson 1980). In contrast to manic or psychotic patients, who manifest premature certainty, OCD patients are unable to achieve a sense of certainty between incoming sensory information and internal beliefs.

Compulsions.   A compulsive ritual is a behavior that usually reduces discomfort but is carried out in a pressured or rigid fashion. Such behavior may include rituals involving washing, checking, repeating, avoiding, striving for completeness, and being meticulous. "Washers" represent about 25% to 50% of most OCD samples (Rasmussen and Tsuang 1986). These individuals are concerned with dirt, contaminants, or germs, and may spend many hours a day washing their hands or showering. They may also attempt to avoid contaminating themselves with feces, urine, or vaginal secretions. "Checkers" have pathological doubt and thus compulsively check on things. Checking often fails to resolve the doubt and in some cases may actually exacerbate it. Mental compulsions are also quite common. Such patients, for example, may replay over and over in their minds past conversations with others to make sure they did not somehow incriminate themselves. Although distinct symptom clusters exist (washers, checkers, those who are purely obsessional, hoarders, and those with primary slowness), these symptoms may overlap or develop sequentially.

☐ Epidemiology and Comorbidity

Obsessive-compulsive disorder was previously considered one of the rarest mental disorders. OCD patients are often secretive about their symptoms, and on average wait 7.5 years before seeking psychiatric help (Rasmussen and Tsuang 1986). Data from the ECA study suggest that OCD is actually quite common, with a 1-month prevalence of 1.3%, a 6-month prevalence of 1.5%, and a lifetime rate of 2.5% (Regier et al. 1988).

In clinical samples of adult OCD, there is a roughly equal ratio of men to women (Black 1974). The ECA epidemiological sample found a slightly higher 1-month prevalence for women (1.5%) compared with men (1.1%), but this difference was not significant (Regier et al. 1988). However, in childhood-onset OCD, about 70% of patients are male (Swedo et al. 1989b).

There are reports demonstrating a comorbidity of OCD with schizophrenia; depression; other anxiety disorders such as panic disorder and simple and social phobia; eating disorders; autism; and Tourette's syndrome. Epidemiologically, the OCD comorbidity risk for other major psychiatric disorders was found to be fairly high but nondistinctive (Karno et al. 1988).

☐ Etiology

Biological Theories

Twin and family studies have found a greater degree of concordance for OCD among monozygotic twins compared with dizygotic twins (Carey and Gottesman 1981), suggesting that some predisposition to obsessional behavior is inherited. Studies of first-degree relatives of OCD patients show a higher-than-normal incidence of a variety of psychiatric disorders, including obsessionality and depression (Rapoport et al. 1981). Family studies suggest a genetic link between OCD and Tourette's syndrome (Nee et al. 1982).

Psychoanalytic Theory: Psychogenic Factors

Psychoanalytic theorists view OCD as residing on a continuum with obsessive-compulsive character pathology, and suggest that OCD develops when defense mechanisms fail to contain the obsessional character's anxiety. Obsessive-compulsive patients are thought to utilize the defense mechanisms of isolation, undoing, reaction formation, and displacement to control unacceptable sexual and aggressive impulses. *Isolation* is an attempt to separate the feelings from the thoughts, fantasies, or impulses that are associated with them. *Undoing* is an attempt to reverse a psychological event, such as a word, thought, or gesture, and involves magical thinking. An imagined act can be undone by a behaviorally opposite act. The defense of *reaction formation* emphasizes the opposite attitudes to the underlying impulses, giving rise to inappropriate behavior patterns.

In OCD, *regression* is theorized to take place from a genital oedipal phase to an earlier, never fully relinquished anal-sadistic phase. This regression helps the patient avoid genital conflicts and the anxiety associated with them. This anal phase, which involves a preoccupation with anger and dirt, consists of magical thinking, ambivalence, and a harsh and punitive superego and utilizes the defense mechanisms listed above.

In normal development, aggressive impulses are neutralized, and loving feelings predominate toward significant objects. In OCD, strong aggressive impulses are thought to reemerge toward love objects, resulting in displaced *ambivalence* and paralyzing doubts. In addition, magical thinking and lack of certainty may predominate, such that thoughts of harming someone may lead to uncertainty over actually having harmed someone.

Learning Theory

A prominent behavioral model of the acquisition and maintenance of obsessive-compulsive symptoms derives from the two-stage learning theory of Mowrer (1939). In Stage 1, anxiety is classically conditioned to a specific environmental event (i.e., classical conditioning). The person then engages in compulsive rituals (escape/avoidance responses) in order to decrease anxiety. If the individual is successful in reducing anxiety, the compulsive behavior is more likely to occur in the future (Stage 2: operant conditioning). Ritual behavior preserves the fear response, because the person avoids the eliciting stimulus and thus avoids extinction. Likewise, anxiety reduction following the ritual preserves the compulsive behavior.

Neurological Models

Although OCD has generally been viewed as having a psychological etiology, a number of findings now suggest a cerebral basis for OCD. Certain OCD comorbidity patterns, as well as sophisticated techniques better able to localize central nervous system dysfunction, have suggested that in OCD orbitofrontal–limbic–basal ganglia abnormalities are involved. OCD is closely associated with Tourette's syndrome, in which basal ganglia dysfunction results in abnormal involuntary movements. There is also an association between OCD and Sydenham's chorea, another disorder of the basal ganglia (Swedo et al. 1989a). Neuropsychiatric testing abnormalities in OCD, although not always consistent, have revealed frontal lobe dysfunction (Hollander et al. 1991c). After treatment of the OCD with serotonin reuptake blockers or behavior therapy, hyperactivity decreases in the caudate and orbitofrontal lobes in the patients with good treatment responses (Swedo et al. 1992b).

The role of the limbic system in OCD has also been highlighted. Animal models of bilateral hippocampal lesions (Pitman 1982) as well as chronic stimulant abuse in animals and humans have been reported to produce repetitive, stereotyped behavior bearing some similarity to compulsive rituals. Evidence from neurosurgical procedures shows improvement following surgical lesions of the cingulum (Jenike et al. 1991) and increased stereotypic movements after electrical stimulation of this region.

A neuroethological model of OCD has been proposed by Rapoport, Swedo, and their group (Swedo 1989; Wise and Rapoport 1989), based on the hypothesized orbitofrontal–limbic–basal ganglia dysfunction. The basal ganglia act as a gating station, which filters input from the orbitofrontal and the cingulate cortex and mediates the execution of motor patterns. Obsessions and compulsions are viewed as species-specific fixed action patterns that are normally adaptive but in OCD become inappropriately released, repetitive, and excessive. This could be due to a heightened internal drive state or increased responsivity to external releasers.

Biochemical Models

Serotonin (5-hydroxytryptamine) has been implicated in mediating impulsivity, suicidality, aggression, anxiety, social dominance, and learning. Dysregulation of this behaviorally inhibitory neurotransmitter could possibly contribute to the repetitive obsessions and ritualistic behaviors seen in OCD patients. Despite some conflicting and nonreplicated data, extensive research has now implicated the serotonergic system in the pathogenesis of OCD.

Considerable indirect evidence supporting the role of serotonin in OCD stems from the anti-obsessional effects of serotonin reuptake inhibitors such as clomipramine, fluoxetine, and fluvoxamine. Noradrenergic antidepressants such as desipramine have not been found to be effective in treating OCD. Furthermore, reduction of OCD symptoms during clomipramine treatment was shown to correlate with a decrease in platelet serotonin level (Flament et al. 1987) and cerebrospinal fluid (CSF) 5-hydroxyindoleacetic acid (5-HIAA) (Swedo et al. 1992a). The reduction in these serotonergic measures appeared to be due to the higher baseline platelet serotonin and CSF 5-HIAA in those patients who responded to clomipramine compared with those who did not respond.

The use of challenge agents to stimulate or block serotonin receptors has been more fruitful in elucidating the neurochemistry of OCD. Oral *m*-chlorophenylpiperazine (m-CPP), a partial serotonin agonist, has been found to transiently exacerbate obsessive-compulsive symptoms in a subgroup of OCD patients (Hollander et al. 1992). After treatment with serotonin reuptake blockers such as clomipramine or fluoxetine, m-CPP challenge no longer induced symptom exacerbation (Hollander et al. 1991a). Other serotonin agonists, such as tryptophan, fenfluramine, and ipsapirone, or antagonists, such as metergoline, have not been shown to induce consistent behavioral or neuroendocrine response abnormalities in patients with OCD.

The serotonergic system may, in part, be modulating or compensating for dysfunction in other neurotransmitter systems or dysfunctional neuromodulators. Decreased CSF arginine vasopressin was found to be significantly associated with OCD symptom severity, possibly implicating attention and memory difficulties in children with checking rituals (Swedo et al. 1992a). The noradrenergic alpha$_2$ agonist clonidine has been reported to induce a transient improvement in OCD symptoms (Hollander et al. 1991b). Dopaminergic dysregulation has been variously implicated in OCD (Goodman et al. 1990; Swedo et al. 1992a; McDougle et al. 1990).

☐ Course and Prognosis

Studies of the natural course of the illness suggest that 24% to 33% of patients have a fluctuating course, 11% to 14% have a phasic course with periods of complete remission, and 54% to 61% have a constant or progressive course (Black 1974). The disorder usually has a major impact on daily functioning; patients are often socially isolated, marry at an older age, and have high celibacy rates (particularly in males) and a low fertility rate. Depression and anxiety are common complications.

With developments in behavioral and pharmacological treatments, the prognosis has somewhat improved. Predictors of favorable outcome include mild or atypical symptoms, absence of compulsions, short duration of symptoms, and good premorbid personality (Goodwin et al. 1969). Early age at onset is predictive of poor prognosis and multiple obsessions and compulsions.

☐ Diagnosis and Differential Diagnosis

Psychoanalytic theorists have suggested that there is a continuum between compulsive personality and OCD. However, phenomenological and epidemiological evidence suggests that OCD is qualitatively distinct from obsessive-compulsive personality disorder. OCD symptoms are ego-dystonic, whereas obsessive-compulsive personality traits are ego-systonic and do not involve a sense of compulsion that must be resisted against. When patients with obsessional traits develop severe psychopathology, they often develop depression, paranoia, or somatic symptoms rather than OCD.

Depression

Patients with OCD and complicating depressions may be difficult to distinguish from depressed patients who have complicating obsessive symptoms. Patients with psychotic depression, agitated depression, or premorbid obsessional features prior to depression are particularly likely to develop obsessions (Gittleson 1966). These "secondary" obsessions often involve aggressive themes. Patients with OCD tend to develop agitation when they become depressed. Depressive ruminations, in contrast to obsessions, are often focused on a past incident and are rarely resisted.

Schizophrenia

The course of OCD may more closely resemble that of schizophrenia than that of "neurotic" disorders, with chronic debilitation and impairment in social and occupational functioning occurring. Sometimes it is difficult to distinguish between an obsession (i.e., contamination) and a delusion (i.e., being poisoned). An obsession is ego-dystonic, resisted, and recognized as having an internal origin. A delusion is not resisted and is believed to be external.

Phobic Disorders

Compulsive cleaners are very similar to phobic individuals and are often mislabeled "germ phobics." Both have avoidant behavior, both show intense subjective and autonomic responses to focal stimuli, and both are said to respond to similar behavioral interventions (Rachman and Hodgson 1980). Both have excessive fear, although disgust is prominent in OCD patients and not in phobic patients. Also, OCD patients can never entirely avoid the obsession, whereas phobic patients have more focal, external stimuli that they can successfully avoid.

Patients with OCD who experience high levels of anxiety may describe panic-like episodes, but these are secondary to obsessions and do not arise spontaneously.

☐ Treatment

Pharmacotherapy

The pharmacological treatment approach to OCD is summarized in Table 14–10. The most extensively studied medication for the treatment of OCD is clomipramine, a potent serotonin reuptake blocker. A series of well-controlled double-blind studies have undisputedly documented the efficacy of clomipramine in reducing OCD symptoms (Flament et al. 1985; Insel et al. 1983). Improvement with clomipramine is relatively slow, with maximal response occurring after 5 to 12 weeks of treatment. Some of the more common side effects reported by patients are dry mouth, tremor, sedation, nausea, and ejaculatory failure in men. Clomipramine is equally effective for OCD patients with pure obsessions and those with rituals, in contrast to behavioral treatments, which are less useful for patients suffering predominantly from obsessions. Controlled studies have also demonstrated that clomipramine is effective in treating OCD when other antidepressants have no therapeutic effect (Leonard et al. 1989; Zohar and Insel 1987), suggesting that improvement in OCD symptoms is mediated through the blockade of serotonin reuptake.

Studies with more selective serotonin reuptake blockers such as fluoxetine and fluvoxamine further support this hypothesis. Jenike et al. (1989) found an average improvement with fluoxetine in obsessive-compulsive symptoms of 38%, and Liebowitz et al. (1989) reported that half of the patients in their sample improved by at least 50%. Fluvoxamine has also been found to have a significant antiobsessional effect in controlled studies (Jenike et al. 1990).

Behavior Therapy

Behavioral treatments of OCD involve two separate components: 1) exposure procedures that aim to decrease the anxiety associated with obsessions, and 2) response prevention techniques that aim to decrease the frequency of rituals or obsessive thoughts. Exposure techniques range from systematic desensitization with brief imaginal exposure, to flooding, in which prolonged exposure to the real-life ritual-evoking stimuli causes profound discomfort. Exposure techniques aim to ultimately decrease the discomfort associated with the eliciting stimuli through habituation.

It is generally agreed that combined behavioral techniques yield the greatest improvement. Using the combined techniques of in vivo exposure and response prevention, up to 75% of ritualizing patients willing and able to undergo the arduous treatment were reported to show significant improvement (Marks et al. 1975). Marks et al. (1988) reported

Table 14–10.   Pharmacological treament of obsessive-compulsive disorder

Serotonin reuptake inhibitors
General indication: First treatment of choice
Clomipramine: Most studied in efficacy
Fluvoxamine: Superior to desipramine and to placebo, well studied
Fluoxetine: Effective
Sertraline: Effective, less well studied
Paroxetine: Effective, less well studied

Augmentation strategies
General indications: Partial response to serotonin reuptake inhibitors; presence of other target symptoms
Buspirone: Anxiety
Clonazepam: Anxiety, insomnia, panic attacks
Fenfluramine: Depression
Trazodone: Insomnia, depression
Lithium: Affective lability, bipolar features
Pimozide: Tics, schizotypal features, delusional symptoms
Haloperidol: Tics, schizotypal features, delusional symptoms

Combination treatments
General indications: Poor tolerance of clomipramine or selective serotonin reuptake inhibitor alone; partial response to clomipramine or selective serotonin reuptake inhibitor alone
Precautions: Use low doses of each medication. Follow clomipramine levels.
Clomipramine + a selective serotonin reuptake inhibitor (i.e. fluoxetine, sertraline, fluvoxamine)

that self-exposure constitutes the most powerful treatment component; however, clomipramine doses in this study were low and therapist-aided exposure was instituted late in the treatment and briefly. The addition of imaginal exposure to in vivo exposure/response prevention is reported to help maintain treatment gains, perhaps by moderating obsessive fears of future catastrophes (Steketee et al. 1982).

Other Psychotherapy

Patients with OCD frequently present with symptoms that appear laden with unconscious symbolism and dynamic meaning. However, OCD has generally proven refractory to psychoanalytically oriented, as well as loosely structured, nondirective psychotherapies. OCD patients need supportive treatment even while pharmacotherapy or behavior therapy is being applied. In contrast with its lack of efficacy in treating chronic OCD, psychotherapy may be helpful for acute cases and for dealing with obsessive character traits of perfectionism, doubting, procrastination, and indecisiveness (Salzman 1985).

■ POSTTRAUMATIC STRESS DISORDER

Posttraumatic stress disorder (PTSD) was first introduced in DSM-III, spurred in part by the increasing recognition of posttraumatic conditions in veterans of the Vietnam war. The current DSM-IV criteria for posttraumatic stress disorder (PTSD) are presented in Table 14–11. The disorder is classified with the anxiety disorders, and the major criteria involve an extreme precipitating stressor, intrusive recollections, emotional numbing, and hyperarousal.

Beyond the symptoms of PTSD per se, increasing attention has been drawn to an enduring constellation of traits that frequently develop in individuals subjected to chronic trauma as children or adults. Some investigators have suggested that a discrete entity of complicated posttraumatic syndromes be recognized, otherwise designated as "DESNOS" (disorders of extreme stress not otherwise specified)—one that is characterized by lasting changes in identity, interpersonal relationships, and the sense of life's meaning (Herman et al. 1989; van der Kolk and Saporta 1991).

☐ Clinical Description

The characteristic features that may develop following a traumatic event include psychic numbing, reexperiencing of the trauma, and increased autonomic arousal. The trauma is reexperienced in recurrent painful, intrusive recollections, daydreams, or nightmares. Dissociative states may occur, lasting from minutes to days, in which there is an actual reliving of the event. Psychic numbing or emotional anesthesia is manifest by diminished responsiveness to the external world, with feelings of being detached from other people, loss of interest in usual activities, and inability to feel emotions such as intimacy, tenderness, or sexual interest. Symptoms of excessive autonomic arousal may include hyperactivity and irritability, an exaggerated startle response, difficulty concentrating, and sleep abnormalities.

Other symptoms may include guilt about having survived, guilt about not having prevented the traumatic experience, depression, anxiety, panic attacks, shame, and rage. There may be prolonged episodes of intense affect; increased irritability; explosive, hostile behavior; and impulsive behavior. Other accompanying symptoms associated with PTSD

Table 14–11. DSM-IV diagnostic criteria for posttraumatic stress disorder

---

A. The person has been exposed to a traumatic event in which both of the following were present:
  1. The person experienced, witnessed, or was confronted with an event or events that involved actual or threatened death or serious injury or a threat to the physical integrity of self or others.
  2. The person's response involved intense fear, helplessness, or horror. **Note:** In children, this may be expressed instead by disorganized or agitated behavior.
B. The traumatic event is persistently reexperienced in one (or more) of the following ways:
  1. Recurrent and intrusive distressing recollections of the event, including images, thoughts, or perceptions. **Note:** In young children, repetitive play may occur in which themes or aspects of the trauma are expressed.
  2. Recurrent distressing dreams of the event. **Note:** In children, there may be frightening dreams without recognizable content.
  3. Acting or feeling as if the traumatic event were recurring (includes a sense of reliving the experience, illusions, hallucinations, and dissociative flashback episodes, including those that occur on awakening or when intoxicated). **Note:** In young children, trauma-specific reenactment may occur.
  4. Intense psychological distress at exposure to internal and external cues that symbolize or resemble an aspect of the traumatic event.
  5. Physiologic reactivity on exposure to internal or external cues that symbolize or resemble an aspect of the traumatic event.
C. Persistent avoidance of stimuli associated with the trauma and numbing of general responsiveness (not present before the trauma), as indicated by three (or more) of the following:
  1. Efforts to avoid thoughts, feelings, or conversations associated with the trauma
  2. Efforts to avoid activities, places, or people that arouse recollections of the trauma
  3. Inability to recall an important aspect of the trauma
  4. Markedly diminished interest or participation in significant activities
  5. Feeling of detachment or estrangement from others
  6. Restricted range of affect (e.g., unable to have loving feelings)
  7. Sense of a foreshortened future (e.g., does not expect to have a career, marriage, children, or a normal life span)
D. Persistent symptoms of increased arousal (not present before the trauma), as indicated by two (or more) of the following:
  1. Difficulty falling or staying asleep
  2. Irritability or outbursts of anger
  3. Difficulty concentrating
  4. Hypervigilance
  5. Exaggerated startle response

(continued)

Table 14–11.   DSM-IV diagnostic criteria for posttraumatic stress disorder *(continued)*

E.   Duration of the disturbance (symptoms in criteria B, C, and D) is more than 1 month.

F.   The disturbance causes clinically significant distress or impairment in social, occupational, or other important areas of functioning.

Specify if:
Acute: if duration of symptoms is less than 3 months
Chronic: if duration of symptoms is 3 months or more

Specify if:
With delayed onset: if onset of symptoms is at least 6 months after the stressor

---

may include substance abuse, self-injurious behavior and suicide attempts, occupational impairment, and interference with interpersonal relationships.

☐ Epidemiology and Comorbidity

Although there are marked individual differences in how people react to stress, when stressors become extreme the rate of morbidity rapidly increases (Eitinger 1971). Posttraumatic syndromes may be found in up to 30% of victims of disasters (Chapman 1962). Long-term physical health effects have been noted in persons 30 years after their having survived concentration camps (Eitinger 1971).

With respect to PTSD in the general population lifetime prevalence has been found to range from 1% to 9.2%. Prevalence was higher in women (1.3% to 11.3%) than in men (0.5% to 6%) (Breslau et al. 1991; Helzer et al. 1987). The nature of the precipitating trauma differed in the two sexes. Combat and witnessing someone's injury or death were the two traumas identified in men, whereas physical attack or threat accounted for almost half of the traumas in women. The highest comorbidity was with affective disorders and OCD. Men with PTSD had no increased risk for panic disorder or phobias, whereas women with PTSD had a three- to fourfold risk of these disorders (Helzer et al. 1987).

☐ Etiology

The severity of the stressor in PTSD differs in magnitude from that found in adjustment disorder, which is usually less severe and within the range of common life experience. A definite dose-response relationship exists between the impact of the trauma and PTSD. Still, it is rare even for overwhelming trauma to lead to PTSD in more than half of the exposed populations, suggesting that other etiological factors also play a role (McFarlane 1990).

Psychological Predictors

Although PTSD can develop in people without significant preexisting psychopathology, some studies suggest that predisposing psychological factors may render individuals more vulnerable to the development of PTSD. It has been suggested that the greater the amount of previous trauma experienced by an individual, the more likely he or she is to develop symptoms after a stressful life event (Horowitz et al. 1980). In addition, individuals with prior traumatic experiences may be more likely to become exposed to future traumas, as they can be prone to behaviorally reenact the original trauma (van der Kolk 1989). McFarlane (1989) found that, while the severity of exposure to disaster was the major determinant of early posttraumatic morbidity, preexisting psychological disorders better predicted the persistence of posttraumatic symptoms after 29 months. Patients with anxious premorbid states and family histories of anxiety may also respond to a trauma with pathological anxiety and develop PTSD (Scrignar 1984).

Risk factors for exposure to trauma identified in one epidemiological survey were male sex, childhood conduct problems, extraversion, and family history of substance abuse or psychiatric problems. Risk factors for developing PTSD after traumatic exposure were disrupted parental attachments, anxiety, depression, and family history of anxiety. Compared with nonchronic PTSD, chronic PTSD of greater than 1 year's duration has been specifically associated with female sex, higher rates of comorbid anxiety and depressive disorders, and a family history of antisocial behavior (Breslau and Davis 1992; Breslau et al. 1991).

Biological Theories

Freud (1919/1955) implicated a biological basis to posttraumatic symptoms, in the form of a physical fixation to the trauma. Kardiner (1959) comprehensively described the phenomenology of war "traumatic neurosis," identifying five cardinal features: 1) persistence of startle response, 2) fixation on the trauma, 3) atypical dream life, 4) explosive outbursts, and 5) overall constriction of the personality. He labeled this condition as a "physioneurosis," implying an interaction of psychological and biological processes, which serves as a forerunner of current psychobiological models of PTSD.

Hyperarousal.   The neurobiogical response to acute stress and trauma involves the release of various stress hormones that allow the organism to respond adaptively to stress. These releases include heightened secretion of catecholamines and cortisol. When PTSD develops under severe or repeated trauma, the stress response becomes dysregulated and chronic autonomic hyperactivity sets in. This manifests itself in the "positive symptoms of PTSD," that is, the hyperarousal and intrusive recollections.

The noradrenergic system, originating in the locus coeruleus, regulates arousal. In patients with PTSD, heightened physiological responses to stressful stimuli, such as blood pressure, heart rate, respiration, galvanic skin response, and electromyographic activity, have been consistently documented (Pitman et al. 1987). Long-standing increases in the urinary catecholamines norepinephrine and epinephrine have been found in PTSD patients (Kosten et al. 1987). Agents that stimulate the arousal system, such as lactate (Rainey et al. 1987) and yohimbine (Southwick et al. 1991), induce flashbacks in patients with PTSD. Clinical improvement in intrusive recollections and hyperarousal during open treatment with adrenergic blocking agents, such as clonidine or propranolol, also suggests adrenergic hyperactivity (Kolb et al. 1984).

A decrease in the number and sensitivity of alpha$_2$-adrenergic (α_2) receptors, possibly as a consequence of chronic noradrenergic hyperactivity, has been reported in PTSD (Perry et al. 1987). In addition, there is evidence that chronic hyperarousal blunts the adaptive steroid response to stress.

A kindling model has also been proposed to understand the positive symptoms of PTSD (Lipper 1990). It posits that intrusive recollections, such as flashbacks or nightmares, are actual reexperiences of stored memories, triggered by oversensitization of the limbic system. Presumably, such kindling is a result of the repeated traumatic experiences and associated hyperarousal, which progressively sensitize the limbic neurons and lower their firing threshold. Another neurophysiological model posits that the intrusive and hyperactive symptoms in PTSD are secondary symptoms of release that result from inadequate cortical inhibition of lower brain-stem structures, such as the hypothalamus and the locus coeruleus (Kolb 1987).

Numbing.   While, in the past, affective numbing was understood primarily as a psychological defense against overwhelming emotional pain, recent research has suggested a biological component to the "negative symptoms" of PTSD. It has been suggested that in persons who have sustained prolonged or repeated trauma, endogenous opiates are readily released with any stimulus that is reminiscent of the original trauma, leading to analgesia and psychic numbing (van der Kolk et al. 1984). After a transient opioid burst upon reexposure to traumatic stimuli, accompanied by a subjective sense of calm and control, opiate withdrawal may set in. This withdrawal may then contribute to the hyperarousal symptoms of PTSD, leading the individual to a vicious cycle of traumatic reexposures in order to gain transient symptomatic relief.

Clonidine, an alpha$_2$-adrenergic agonist, has been shown to suppress opiate withdrawal symptoms in opiate addiction (Gold et al. 1980). Open treatment with clonidine in Vietnam veterans with PTSD demonstrated substantial decreases in hyperreactivity (Kolb et al. 1984). Clonidine's opiate-enhancing effects may be mediated either through suppression of the noradrenergic system or by a direct morphine-like agonist effect.

Serotonergic system. The serotonergic system has also been implicated in the symptomatology of PTSD (van der Kolk and Saporta 1991). The septohippocampal brain system contains serotonergic pathways and mediates behavioral inhibition and constraint. The role of serotonergic deficit in impulsive aggression has been studied extensively. The irritability and outbursts seen in patients with PTSD may be related to serotonergic dysfunction. Recent open clinical trials have suggested that selective serotonin reuptake blockers may be the most effective medications for both the positive and negative symptoms of PTSD (Shay 1992).

☐ Course and Prognosis

Scrignar (1984) divides the clinical course of PTSD into three stages. Stage I involves the response to trauma. Nonsusceptible persons may experience an adrenergic surge of symptoms immediately after the trauma but do not dwell on the incident. Predisposed persons have higher levels of anxiety at baseline, an exaggerated response to the trauma, and an obsessive preoccupation with it following the trauma. If symptoms persist beyond 4 to 6 weeks, the patient enters Stage II, or acute PTSD. Feelings of helplessness and loss of control, symptoms of increased autonomic arousal, reliving of the trauma, and somatic symptoms may occur. The patient's life becomes centered around the trauma, with subsequent changes in life-style, personality, and social functioning. Phobic avoidance, startle responses, and angry outbursts may occur. In Stage III, chronic PTSD develops, with disability, demoralization, and despondency. The patient's emphasis changes from preoccupation with the actual trauma, to preoccupation with the physical disability resulting from the trauma. Somatic symptoms, chronic anxiety, and depression are common complications at this time, as well as substance abuse, disturbed family relations, and unemployment. Some patients may focus on compensation and lawsuits.

The DSM-IV states that delayed PTSD occurs when symptoms do not begin until 6 months after the trauma. Survivors of major catastrophes rather than ordinary accidents are more likely to have delayed-onset PTSD.

☐ Diagnosis and Differential Diagnosis

The diagnosis of PTSD is usually not difficult if there is a clear history of exposure to a traumatic event, followed by symptoms of intense anxiety lasting at least 1 month, with arousal and stimulation of the autonomic nervous system, numbing of responsiveness, and avoidance or reexperiencing of the traumatic event. However, a wide variety of anxiety, depressive, somatic, and behavioral symptoms for which the relationship between their onset and the traumatic event is less clear-cut may easily lead to misdiagnosis.

Organic Mental Disorders

Following acute physical traumas, head trauma, or concussion, an organic mental disorder must be ruled out. Organic mental disorders that could mimic PTSD include organic personality syndrome, delirium, amnestic syndrome, organic hallucinosis, or organic intoxication and withdrawal states. Mild concussions may leave no immediate apparent neurological signs but may have residual long-term effects on mood and concentration. Malnutrition may occur during prolonged stressful periods and may also lead to organic brain syndromes. Survivors of death camps may have symptoms of an organic mental disorder such as failing memory, difficulty concentrating, emotional lability, headaches, and vertigo.

Mood and Anxiety Disorders

There is much overlap between PTSD and major mood disorders. Symptoms such as psychic numbing, irritability, sleep disturbance, fatigue, anhedonia, impairments in family and social relationships, anger, concern with physical health, and pessimistic outlook may occur in both disorders. Major depression is a frequent complication of PTSD; dysthymic symptoms are also frequently secondary to PTSD.

Following a traumatic event, patients may be aversively conditioned to the surroundings of the trauma and develop a phobia of objects, surroundings, or situations that remind them of the trauma itself. In PTSD, the phobia may be symptomatically similar to specific phobia, but the nature of the precipitant and the symptom cluster of PTSD distinguish this condition from simple phobia.

The symptoms of GAD, such as motor tension, autonomic hyperactivity, apprehensive expectation, and vigilance and scanning, are also present in PTSD. However, the onset and course of the illness differ: GAD has an insidious or gradual onset and a course that fluctuates with environmental stressors, whereas PTSD has an acute onset often followed by a chronic course. Phobic symptoms, which are absent in GAD, are often present in PTSD. Patients with PTSD may also experience panic attacks. In some patients, panic attacks predate the PTSD, or do not occur exclusively in the context of stimuli reminiscent of the traumatic event. In some patients, however, panic attacks develop after the PTSD and are cued solely by traumatic stimuli. Adjustment disorder differs from PTSD, because the stressor is usually less severe and within the range of common experience, and the characteristic symptoms of PTSD, such as reexperiencing the trauma, are absent.

☐ Treatment

Pharmacotherapy

A variety of different agents have been used in the treatment of PTSD. Most reports, on the pharmacotherapy of PTSD involve the use of antidepressants. A retrospective study by Bleich et al. (1986) of PTSD patients treated with a variety of different antidepressants, including tricyclics and MAOIs, reported good or moderate results in 67% of cases treated. Antidepressants appeared to be more useful than major tranquilizers. While antidepressants improved intrusion-type symptoms, the most prominent overall effects were in alleviation of insomnia and in overall sedation. Antidepressants also were found to have a positive impact on psychotherapy in 70% of cases.

Burstein (1984), in administering imipramine to patients with PTSD of recent onset, observed significant improvement in intrusive recollections, sleep and dream disturbance, and flashbacks. Similar improvement in intrusive symptomatology was reported with an open trial of desipramine (Kauffman et al. 1987) A positive effect of imipramine on posttraumatic night terrors was reported by Marshall (1975).

Clinical findings support the role of noradrenergic hyperactivity in the maintenance of autonomic arousal symptoms in PTSD. In a retrospective treatment review of Cambodian patients with PTSD, Kinzie and Leung (1989) found that the majority of patients benefited from the combination of clonidine and a tricyclic, as opposed to either medication taken alone.

A study of monoamine oxidase inhibitors compared phenelzine, imipramine, and placebo in veterans with PTSD (Frank et al. 1988). Both antidepressants resulted in some overall improvement in patients' posttraumatic symptoms, and phenelzine tended to be superior to imipramine. The most marked improvement was the decrease in intrusive symptoms in patients on phenelzine, with 60% average reduction on the intrusion scale measure.

In an open trial of the anticonvulsant carbamazepine in 10 patients with PTSD, Lipper et al. (1986) reported moderate to great improvement in intrusive symptoms in 7 patients. Wolf et al. (1988) reported decreased impulsivity and angry outbursts in 10 veterans who were also treated with carbamazepine; all patients had normal EEGs.

Open trials with selective serotonin reuptake inhibitors suggest that these medications may hold promise for the treatment of PTSD. In patients with PTSD related to life-threatening accidents or sexual abuse, therapy with fluoxetine resulted in marked improvement of both intrusive and avoidant symptoms (Davidson et al. 1991). Shay (1992) reported that two-thirds of patients experienced decreased anger, reduced explosive outbursts, and better mood with fluoxetine.

Silver et al. (1990) concluded that the positive PTSD symptoms of hyperarousal and intrusive reexperiencing are responsive to more medications than are the negative symptoms of avoidance and withdrawal. The negative symptoms may be more amenable to psychotherapy, especially once the severity of the positive symptoms is alleviated with medication. Selective serotonin reuptake inhibitors may also hold some promise for negative symptoms.

Psychotherapy

It is generally agreed on that some form of psychotherapy is necessary in the treatment of posttraumatic pathology. Crisis intervention shortly after the traumatic event is effective in reducing immediate distress, possibly preventing chronic or delayed responses, and, if the pathological response is still tentative, may allow for briefer intervention. Brief dynamic psychotherapy has been advocated both as an immediate treatment procedure and as a way of preventing chronic disorder.

Attempting to modify preexisting conflicts, developmental difficulties, and defensive styles that render the person especially vulnerable to traumatization by particular experiences is central to the treatment of traumatic syndromes. The "phase oriented" treatment model suggested by Horowitz (1976) strikes a balance between initial supportive interventions to minimize the traumatic state, and increasingly aggressive "working through" at later stages of treatment. Establishment of a safe and communicative relationship, reappraisal of the traumatic event, revision of the patient's inner model of self and world, and planning for termination with a reexperiencing of loss are all important therapeutic issues in the treatmentof PTSD. Herman et al (1989) emphasized the importance of validating the patient's traumatic experiences as a precondition for reparation of damaged self-identity.

Embry (1990) outlined seven major parameters for effective psychotherapy in war veterans with chronic PTSD: 1) initial rapport building, 2) limit setting and supportive confrontation, 3) affective modeling,

4) defocusing on stress and focusing on current life events, 5) sensitivity to transference-countertransference issues, 6) understanding of secondary gain, and 7) therapist's maintenance of a positive treatment attitude.

Group psychotherapy can also serve as an important adjunctive treatment, or as the central treatment mode, in traumatized patients (van der Kolk 1987). Because of past experiences, such patients are often mistrustful and reluctant to depend on authority figures, whereas the identification, support, and hopefulness of peer settings can facilitate therapeutic change.

Behavior Therapy

A variety of behavioral techniques have been applied to the treatment of PTSD. People involved in traumatic events such as accidents frequently develop phobias or phobic anxiety related to or associated with these situations. When a phobia or phobic anxiety is associated with PTSD, systematic desensitization or graded exposure has been found to be effective. This is based on the principle that when patients are gradually exposed to a phobic or anxiety-provoking stimulus, they will become habituated or deconditioned to the stimulus. Variations of this treatment include using imaginal techniques (i.e., imaginal desensitization) and exposure to real-life situations (i.e., in vivo desensitization). Prolonged exposure (i.e., flooding), if tolerated by patients, can be useful and has been reported to be successful in the treatment of Vietnam veterans (Fairbank and Keane 1982).

Relaxation techniques produce the beneficial physiological result of reducing motor tension and lowering the activity of the autonomic nervous system—effects that may be particularly efficacious in PTSD. Progressive muscle relaxation involves contracting and relaxing various muscle groups to induce the relaxation response. This is useful for symptoms of autonomic arousal such as somatic symptoms, anxiety, and insomnia. Hypnosis has also been used to induce the relaxation response with success in PTSD.

Cognitive therapy and thought stopping, in which a phrase and momentary pain are paired with thoughts or images of the trauma, have been used to treat unwanted mental activity in PTSD.

■ REFERENCES

Abelson JL, Glitz D, Cameron OG, et al: Blunted growth hormone response to clonidine in patients with generalized anxiety disorder. Arch Gen Psychiatry 48:157–162, 1991

Allgulander C, Lavori PW: Excess mortality among 3302 patients with "pure" anxiety neurosis. Arch Gen Psychiatry 48:599–602, 1991

American Psychiatric Association: Diagnostic and Statistical Manual of Mental Disorders, 4th Edition. Washington, DC, American Psychiatric Association, 1994

Amies PL, Gelder MG, Shaw PM: Social phobia: a comparative clinical study. Br J Psychiatry 142:174–179, 1983

Ballenger JC, Burrows GD, DuPont RL Jr, et al: Alprazolam in panic disorder and agoraphobia: results from a multicenter trial, I: efficacy in short-term treatment. Arch Gen Psychiatry 45:413–422, 1988

Barlow DH, Craske MG, Cerny JA, et al: Behavioral treatment of panic disorder. Behavior Therapy 20:261–282, 1989

Beck AT, Sokol L, Clark DA, et al: A crossover study of focused cognitive therapy for panic disorder. Am J Psychiatry 149:778–783, 1992

Black A: The natural history of obsessional neurosis, in Obsessional States. Edited by Beech HK. London, Methuen Press, 1974

Blazer DG, Hughes D, George LK: Generalized anxiety disorder, in Psychiatric Disorders in America. Edited by Robins LN, Regier DA. New York, Free Press, 1991, pp 180–203

Bleich A, Siegel B, Garb R, et al: Post-traumatic stress disorder following combat exposure: clinical features and psychopharmacological treatment. Br J Psychiatry 149:365–369, 1986

Breslau N, Davis GC: Posttraumatic stress disorder in an urban population of young adults: risk factors for chronicity. Am J Psychiatry 149:671–675, 1992

Breslau N, Davis GC, Andreski P, et al: Traumatic events and posttraumatic stress disorder in an urban population of young adults. Arch Gen Psychiatry 48:216–222, 1991

Burstein A: Treatment of post-traumatic stress disorder with imipramine. Psychosomatics 25:681–687, 1984

Carey G, Gottesman II: Twin and family studies of anxiety, phobic, and obsessive disorders, in Anxiety: New Research and Changing Concepts. Edited by Klein DF, Rabkin J. New York, Raven Press, 1981, pp 117–136

Chapman D: A brief introduction to contemporary disaster research, in Man and Society in Disaster. Edited by Boher G, Chapman D. New York, Basic Books, 1962

Charney DS, Heninger GR, Breier A: Noradrenergic function in panic anxiety: effects of yohimbine in healthy subjects and patients with agoraphobia and panic disorder. Arch Gen Psychiatry 41:751–763, 1984

Crowe RR, Noyes R, Pauls DL, et al: A family study of panic disorder. Arch Gen Psychiatry 40:1065–1069, 1983

Davidson J, Roth S, Newman E: Fluoxetine in post-traumatic stress disorder. Journal of Traumatic Stress 4:419–423, 1991

Dimsdale JE, Moss J: Plasma catecholamines in stress and exercise. JAMA 243:340–342, 1980

Dorrow R, Horowski R, Paschelke G, et al: Severe anxiety induced by FG-7142, a beta-carboline ligand for benzodiazepine receptors. Lancet 1:98–99, 1983

Eaton WW, Dryman A, Weissman MM: Panic and phobia, in Psychiatric Disorders in America. Edited by Robins LN, Regier DA. New York, Free Press, 1991, pp 155–179

Eitinger L: Organic and psychosomatic after effects of concentration camp imprisonment. International Psychiatry Clinics 8:205–215, 1971

Elam M, Yoat TP, Svensson TH: Hypercapnia and hypoxia: chemoreceptor-mediated control of locus ceruleus neurons and splanchnic, sympathetic nerves. Brain Res 222:373–381, 1981

Embry CK: Psychotherapeutic interventions in chronic posttraumatic stress disorder, in Posttraumatic Stress Disorder: Etiology, Phenomenology, and Treatment. Edited by Wolf ME, Mosnaim AD. Washington, DC, American Psychiatric Press, 1990, pp 226–236

Fairbank TA, Keane TM: Flooding for combat-related stress disorders: assessment of anxiety reduction across traumatic memories. Behavior Therapy 13:499–510, 1982

Flament MF, Rapoport JL, Berg CJ, et al: Clomipramine treatment of childhood obsessive-compulsive disorder: a double-blind controlled study. Arch Gen Psychiatry 42:977–983, 1985

Flament MF, Rapoport JL, Murphy DL, et al: Biochemical changes during clomipramine treatment of childhood obsessive-compulsive disorder. Arch Gen Psychiatry 44:219–225, 1987

Frank JB, Kosten TR, Giller EL Jr, et al: A randomized clinical trial of phenelzine and imipramine for posttraumatic stress disorder. Am J Psychiatry 145:1289–1291, 1988

Freud S: On the grounds for detaching a particular syndrome from neurasthenia under the description "anxiety neurosis" (1895a[1894]), in The Standard Edition of the Complete Psychological Works of Sigmund Freud, Vol 3. Translated and edited by Strachey J. London, Hogarth Press, 1962, pp 85–117

Freud S: Obsessions and phobias (1895b[1894]), in The Standard Edition of the Complete Psychological Works of Sigmund Freud, Vol 3. Translated and edited by Strachey J. London, Hogarth Press, 1962, pp 69–84

Freud S: Introduction to Psychoanalysis and the War Neuroses (1919), in The Standard Edition of the Complete Psychological Works of Sigmund Freud, Vol 17. Translated and edited by Stratchey J. London, Hogarth Press, 1955, pp 205–215

Frohlich ED, Tarazi KC, Duston HP: Hyperdynamic beta-adrenergic circulatory state. Arch Intern Med 123:1–7, 1969

Fyer AJ, Mannuzza S, Gallops MS, et al: Familial transmission of simple phobias and fears: a preliminary report. Arch Gen Psychiatry 47:252–256, 1990

Gelernter CS, Uhde TW, Cimbolic P, et al: Cognitive-behavioral and pharmacological treatments of social phobia: a controlled study. Arch Gen Psychiatry 48:938–945, 1991

Gittelman-Klein R, Klein DF: Controlled imipramine treatment of school phobia. Arch Gen Psychiatry 25:204–207, 1971

Gittleson NL: The effect of obsessions on depressive psychosis. Br J Psychiatry 112:253–259, 1966

Gold M, Pottash AC, Sweeney DR, et al: Opiate withdrawal using clonidine. JAMA 243:343–346, 1980

Goodman WK, McDougle CJ, Price LH, et al: Beyond the serotonin hypothesis: a role for dopamine in some forms of obsessive compulsive disorder? J Clin Psychiatry 51 (No 8, Suppl):36–43, 1990

Goodwin DW, Guze SB, Robins E: Follow-up studies of obsessional neurosis. Arch Gen Psychiatry 20:182–187, 1969

Gorman JM, Fyer AF, Gliklich J, et al: Effect of imipramine on prolapsed mitral valves of patients with panic disorder. Am J Psychiatry 138:977–978, 1981

Gorman JM, Askanazi J, Liebowitz MR, et al: Response to hyperventilation in a group of patients with panic disorder. Am J Psychiatry 141:857–861, 1984

Gorman JM, Fyer MR, Goetz R, et al: Ventilatory physiology of patients with panic disorder. Arch Gen Psychiatry 45:31–39, 1988

Gorman JM, Battista D, Goetz RR, et al: A comparison of sodium bicarbonate and sodium lactate infusion in the induction of panic attacks. Arch Gen Psychiatry 46:145–150, 1989

Heimberg RG, Dodge CS, Hope DA, et al: Cognitive behavioral group treatment for social phobia: comparison with a credible placebo control. Cognitive Therapy and Research 14:1–23, 1990

Helzer JE, Robins LN, McEvoy L: Post-traumatic stress disorder in the general population: findings of the Epidemiologic Catchment Area survey. N Engl J Med 317:1630–1634, 1987

Herman JL, Perry JC, van der Kolk BA: Childhood trauma in borderline personality disorder. Am J Psychiatry 146:490–495, 1989

Himle JA, Crystal D, Curtis GC, et al: Mode of onset of simple phobia subtypes: further evidence of heterogeneity. Psychiatry Res 36:37–43, 1991

Hoehn-Saric R, McLeod DR, Zimmerli WD: Differential effects of alprazolam and imipramine in generalized anxiety disorder: somatic versus psychic symptoms. J Clin Psychiatry 49:293–301, 1988

Hollander E, DeCaria C, Gully R, et al: Effects of chronic fluoxetine treatment on behavioral and neuroendocrine responses to meta-chlorophenylpiperazine in obsessive-compulsive disorder. Psychiatry Res 36:1–17, 1991a

Hollander E, DeCaria C, Nitescu A, et al: Noradrenergic function in obsessive-compulsive disorder: behavioral and neuroendocrine responses to clonidine and comparison to healthy controls. Psychiatry Res 37:161–177, 1991b

Hollander E, Liebowitz MR, Rosen WG: Neuropsychiatric and neuropsychological studies in obsessive-compulsive disorder, in The Psychobiology of Obsessive-Compulsive Disorder. Edited by Zohar J, Insel T, Rasmussen S. New York, Springer, 1991c, pp 126–145

Hollander E, DeCaria CM, Nitescu A, et al: Serotonergic function in obsessive-compulsive disorder: behavioral and neuroendocrine responses to oral m-chlorophenylpiperazine and fenfluramine in patients and healthy volunteers. Arch Gen Psychiatry 49:21–28, 1992

Horowitz MJ: Stress-Response Syndromes. New York, Jason Aronson, 1976

Horowitz MJ, Wilner N, Kaltreider N, et al: Signs and symptoms of posttraumatic stress disorders. Arch Gen Psychiatry 37:88–92, 1980

Insel TR, Murphy DL, Cohen RM, et al: Obsessive-compulsive disorder: a double-blind trial of clomipramine and clorgyline. Arch Gen Psychiatry 40:605–612, 1983

Jenike MA, Buttolph L, Baer L, et al: Open trial of fluoxetine in obsessive-compulsive disorder. Am J Psychiatry 146:909–911, 1989

Jenike MA, Hyman S, Baer L, et al: A controlled trial of fluvoxamine in obsessive-compulsive disorder: implications for a serotonergic theory. Am J Psychiatry 147:1209–1215, 1990

Jenike MA, Baer L, Ballantine HT, et al: Cingulotomy for refractory obsessive-compulsive disorder: a long-term follow-up of 33 patients. Arch Gen Psychiatry 48:548–555, 1991

Johnson J, Weissman MM, Klerman GL: Panic disorder, comorbidity, and suicide attempts. Arch Gen Psychiatry 47:805–808, 1990

Kardiner A: Traumatic neurosis of war, in American Handbook of Psychiatry, Vol 1. Edited by Arieti S. New York, Basic Books, 1959, pp 245–257

Karno M, Golding JM, Sorenson SB, et al: The epidemiology of obsessive-compulsive disorder in five US communities. Arch Gen Psychiatry 45:1094–1099, 1988

Kauffman CD, Reist C, Djenderedjian A, et al: Biological markers of affective disorders and posttraumatic stress disorder: a pilot study with desipramine. J Clin Psychiatry 48:366–367, 1987

Kendler KS, Neale MC, Kessler RC, et al: Generalized anxiety disorder in women: a population-based twin study. Arch Gen Psychiatry 49:267–272, 1992a

Kendler KS, Neale MC, Kessler RC, et al: The genetic epidemiology of phobias in women: the interrelationship of agoraphobia, social phobia, situational phobia, and simple phobia. Arch Gen Psychiatry 49:273–281, 1992b

Kinzie JD, Leung P: Clonidine in Cambodian patients with posttraumatic stress disorder. J Nerv Ment Dis 177:546–550, 1989

Klein DF: Delineation of two drug responsive anxiety syndromes. Psychopharmacologia 5:397–408, 1964

Klein DF: Anxiety reconceptualized, in Anxiety: New Research and Changing Concepts. Edited by Klein DF, Rabkin JG. New York, Raven Press, 1981, pp 235–263

Kolb LC: A neuropsychological hypothesis explaining posttraumatic stress disorders. Am J Psychiatry 144:989–995, 1987

Kolb LC, Burris BC, Griffiths S: Propranolol and clonidine in treatment of the chronic post-traumatic stress disorders of war, in Post-Traumatic Stress Disorder: Psychological and Biological Sequelae. Edited by van der Kolk BA. Washington, DC, American Psychiatric Press, 1984, pp 97–105

Kosten TR, Mason JW, Giller EL, et al: Sustained urine norepinephrine and epinephrine elevation in PTSD. Psychoneuroendocrinology 12:13–20, 1987

Leonard HL, Swedo SE, Rapoport JL, et al: Treatment of obsessive-compulsive disorder with clomipramine and desipramine in children and adolescents: a double-blind crossover comparison. Arch Gen Psychiatry 46:1088–1092, 1989

Liebowitz MR, Fyer AJ, McGrath P, et al: Clonidine treatment of panic disorder. Psychopharmcol Bull 17(3):122–123, 1981

Liebowitz MR, Fyer AJ, Gorman JM, et al: Lactate provocation of panic attacks, I: clinical and behavioral findings. Arch Gen Psychiatry 41:764–770, 1984a

Liebowitz MR, Quitkin FM, Stewart JW, et al: Phenelzine v imipramine in atypical depression: a preliminary report. Arch Gen Psychiatry 41:669–677, 1984b

Liebowitz MR, Gorman JM, Fyer AJ, et al: Lactate provocation of panic attacks, II: biochemical and physiological findings. Arch Gen Psychiatry 42:709–719, 1985

Liebowitz MR, Hollander E, Schneier F, et al: Fluoxetine treatment of obsessive-compulsive disorder: an open clinical trial. J Clin Psychopharmacol 9:423–427, 1989

Liebowitz MR, Schneier F, Campeas R, et al: Phenelzine vs atenolol in social phobia: a placebo-controlled comparison. Arch Gen Psychiatry 49:290–300, 1992

Lipper S: Carbamazepine in the treatment of posttraumatic stress disorder: implications for the kindling hypothesis, in Posttraumatic Stress Disorder: Etiology, Phenomenology, and Treatment. Edited by Wolf ME, Mosnaim AD. Washington, DC, American Psychiatric Press, 1990, pp 184–203

Lipper S, Davidson JRT, Grady TA, et al: Preliminary study of carbamazepine in post-traumatic stress disorder. Psychosomatics 27:849–854, 1986

Marks IM: Fears and Phobias. New York, Academic, 1969

Marks IM, Hodgson R, Rachman S: Treatment of chronic obsessive-compulsive neurosis by in vivo exposure: a two-year follow-up and issues in treatment. Br J Psychiatry 127:349–364, 1975

Marks IM, Gray S, Cohen D, et al: Imipramine and brief therapist-aided exposure in agoraphobics having self-exposure homework. Arch Gen Psychiatry 40:153–162, 1983

Marks IM, Lelliott P, Basoglu M, et al: Clomipramine, self-exposure and therapist-aided exposure for obsessive-compulsive rituals. Br J Psychiatry 152:522–534, 1988

Marshall JR: The treatment of night terrors associated with posttraumatic syndrome. Am J Psychiatry 132:293–295, 1975

Mattes J: More on panic disorder and mitral valve prolapse (letter). Am J Psychiatry 138:1130, 1981

Mattick RP, Peters L, Clarke JC: Exposure and cognitive restructuring for social phobia: a controlled study. Behavior Therapy 20:3–23, 1989

Mavissakalian M, Perel JM: Imipramine dose-response relationship in panic disorder with agoraphobia: preliminary findings. Arch Gen Psychiatry 46:127–131, 1989

McDougle CJ, Goodman WK, Price LH, et al: Neuroleptic addition in fluvoxamine-refractory obsessive-compulsive disorder. Am J Psychiatry 147:652–654, 1990

McFarlane AC: The aetiology of post-traumatic morbidity: predisposing, precipitating and perpetuating factors. Br J Psychiatry 154:221–228, 1989

McFarlane AC: Vulnerability to posttraumatic stress disorder, in Posttraumatic Stress Disorder: Etiology, Phenomenology, and Treatment. Edited by Wolf ME, Mosnaim AD. Washington, DC, American Psychiatric Press, 1990, pp 2–20

Michelson L, Marchione K, Greenwald M, et al: Panic disorder: cognitive-behavioral treatment. Behav Res Ther 28:141–151, 1990

Mowrer O: A stimulus response analysis of anxiety and its role as a reinforcing agent. Psychological Review 46:553–565, 1939

Nee LE, Caine ED, Polinsky RJ, et al: Gilles de la Tourette syndrome: clinical and family study of 50 cases. Ann Neurol 7:41–49, 1982

Noyes R Jr, Clarkson C, Crow RR, et al: A family study of generalized anxiety disorder. Am J Psychiatry 144:1019–1024, 1987

Noyes R Jr, Reich JH, Christiansen J, et al: Outcome of panic disorder: relationship to diagnostic subtypes and comorbidity. Arch Gen Psychiatry 47:809–818, 1990

Ost LG: Age of onset of different phobias. J Abnorm Psychol 96:223–229, 1987

Perry BD, Giller EL Jr, Southwick SM: Altered plasma α_2-adrenergic binding sites in posttraumatic stress disorder (letter). Am J Psychiatry 144:1511–1512, 1987

Pitman RK: Neurological etiology of obsessive-compulsive disorders? (letter). Am J Psychiatry 139:139–140, 1982

Pitman RK, Orr SP, Forgue DF, et al: Psychophysiologic assessment of post-traumatic stress disorder imagery in Vietnam combat veterans. Arch Gen Psychiatry 44:970–975, 1987

Pitts FN, McClure JN: Lactate metabolism in anxiety neurosis. N Engl J Med 277:1329–1336, 1967

Rachman SJ, Hodgson RJ: Obsessions and Compulsions. Englewood Cliffs, NJ, Prentice-Hall, 1980

Rainey JM Jr, Pohl RB, Williams M, et al: A comparison of lactate and isoproterenol anxiety states. Psychopathology 17 (suppl 1):74–82, 1984

Rainey JM Jr, Aleem A, Ortiz A, et al: Laboratory procedure for the inducement of flashbacks. Am J Psychiatry 144:1317–1319, 1987

Rapoport J[L], Elkins R, Langer DH, et al: Childhood obsessive-compulsive disorder. Am J Psychiatry 138:1545–1554, 1981

Rasmussen SA, Tsuang MT: Clinical characteristics and family history in DSM-III obsessive compulsive disorder. Am J Psychiatry 143:317–322, 1986

Redmond DE Jr: New and old evidence for the involvement of a brain norepinephrine system in anxiety, in Phenomenology and Treatment of Anxiety. Edited by Fann WE, Karacan I, Pokorny AD, et al. New York, Spectrum, 1979, pp 153–203

Regier DA, Boyd JH, Burke JD Jr, et al: One-month prevalence of mental disorders in the United States, based on five Epidemiologic Catchment Area sites. Arch Gen Psychiatry 45:977–986, 1988

Rickels K, Schweizer E, Csanalosi I, et al: Long-term treatment of anxiety and risk of withdrawal: prospective comparison of clorazepate and buspirone. Arch Gen Psychiatry 45:444–450, 1988

Roy-Byrne PP, Cowley DS, Greenblatt DJ, et al: Reduced benzodiazepine sensitivity in panic disorder. Arch Gen Psychiatry 47:534–538, 1990

Salzman L: Comments on the psychological treatment of obsessive-compulsive patients, in Obsessive-Compulsive Disorder: Psychological and Pharmacological Treatment. Edited by Mavissakalian M, Turner SM, Michelson L. New York, Plenum, 1985, pp 155–165

Schneier FR, Johnson J, Hornig CD, et al: Social phobia: comorbidity and morbidity in an epidemiologic sample. Arch Gen Psychiatry 49:282–288, 1992

Schweizer E, Rickels K, Lucki I: Resistance to the anti-anxiety effect of buspirone in patients with a history of benzodiazepine use. N Engl J Med 314:719–720, 1986

Scrignar CB: Post-Traumatic Stress Disorder: Diagnosis, Treatment, and Legal Issues. New York, Praeger, 1984

Seligman ME: Phobias and preparedness. Behavior Therapy 2:307–320, 1971

Shay J: Fluoxetine reduces explosiveness and elevates mood of Vietnam combat vets with PTSD. Journal of Traumatic Stress 5:97–101, 1992

Silver JM, Sandberg DP, Hales RE, et al: New approaches in the pharmacotherapy of posttraumatic stress disorder. J Clin Psychiatry 51 (suppl 10):33–38, 1990

Southwick SM, Krystal JH, Charney DS: Yohimbine and m-chloro-phenyl-piperazine in PTSD, in New Research Program and Abstracts, 144th annual meeting of the American Psychiatric Association, NR348, 1991, pp 131–132

Steketee GS, Foa EB, Grayson JB: Recent advances in the behavioral treatment of obsessive-compulsives. Arch Gen Psychiatry 39:1365–1371, 1982

Swedo SE: Rituals and releasers: an ethological model of obsessive-compulsive disorder, in Obsessive-Compulsive Disorder in Children and Adolescents. Edited by Rapoport JL. Washington, DC, American Psychiatric Press, 1989, pp 269–288

Swedo SE, Rapoport JL, Cheslow DL, et al: Increased incidence of obsessive-compulsive symptoms in patients with Sydenham's chorea. Am J Psychiatry 146:246–249, 1989a

Swedo SE, Rapoport JL, Leonard H, et al: Obsessive-compulsive disorder in children and adolescents: clinical phenomenology of 70 consecutive cases. Arch Gen Psychiatry 46:335–341, 1989b

Swedo SE, Leonard HL, Kruesi MJP, et al: Cerebrospinal fluid neurochemistry in children and adolescents with obsessive-compulsive disorder. Arch Gen Psychiatry 49:29–36, 1992a

Swedo SE, Pietrini P, Leonard HL, et al: Cerebral glucose metabolism in childhood-onset obsessive-compulsive disorder: revisualization during pharmacotherapy. Arch Gen Psychiatry 49:690–694, 1992b

Telch MJ, Agras WG, Taylor CM, et al: Combined pharmacological and behavioral treatment for agoraphobia. Behav Res Ther 23:325–335, 1985

Torgersen S: Genetic factors in anxiety disorders. Arch Gen Psychiatry 40:1085–1089, 1983

van der Kolk BA: The role of the group in the origin and resolution of the trauma response, in Psychological Trauma. Edited by van der Kolk BA. Washington, DC, American Psychiatric Press, 1987, pp 153–171

van der Kolk BA: The compulsion to repeat the trauma: reenactment, revictimization, and masochism. Psychiatr Clin North Am 12:389–411, 1989

van der Kolk BA, Saporta J: The biological response to psychic trauma: mechanisms and treatment of intrusion and numbing. Anxiety Research 4:199–212, 1991

van der Kolk BA, Boyd H, Krystal J, et al: Post-traumatic stress disorder as a biologically based disorder: implications of the animal model of inescapable shock, in Post-Traumatic Stress Disorder: Psychological and Biological Sequelae. Edited by van der Kolk BA. Washington, DC, American Psychiatric Press, 1984, pp 123–134

Versiani M, Mundim FD, Nardi AE, et al: Tranylcypromine in social phobia. J Clin Psychopharmacol 8:279–283, 1988

Wise SP, Rapoport JL: Obsessive-compulsive disorder: is it a basal ganglia dysfunction?, in Obsessive-Compulsive Disorder in Children and Adolescents. Edited by Rapoport JL. Washington, DC, American Psychiatric Press, 1989, pp 327–344

Wolf ME, Alavi A, Mosnaim AD: Posttraumatic stress disorder in Vietnam veterans, clinical and EEG findings: possible therapeutic effects of carbamazepine. Biol Psychiatry 23:642–644, 1988

Zohar J, Insel TR: Obsessive-compulsive disorder: psychobiological approaches to diagnosis, treatment, and pathophysiology. Biol Psychiatry 22:667–687, 1987

CHAPTER 15

Psychological Factors Affecting Medical Conditions

J. Stephen McDaniel, M.D.
Michael G. Moran, M.D.
James L. Levenson, M.D.
Alan Stoudemire, M.D.

The fact that psychological factors and psychiatric disorders may affect the clinical course of medical illness is incontrovertible and is no longer the topic of serious debate. For example, psychiatric disorders may adversely affect outcome and length of stay in general hospital patients (Saravay et al. 1991), and the presence of major depression increases morbidity rates in patients with coronary artery disease (Carney et al. 1988). In some situations, timely psychiatric intervention in medical patients can improve psychosocial adjustment (Evans et al. 1988) and even survival (Spiegel et al. 1989). Behavioral factors such as cigarette smoking, obesity, alcohol and substance dependency, and hazardous sexual practices are major causes of premature death and medical morbidity (Stoudemire et al. 1987). A scheme to describe areas of investi-

The authors would like to thank other members of the Work Group involved in revising the diagnostic criteria for this category in DSM-IV, whose background literature research contributed substantially to the information contained in this chapter. These individuals include Gale Beardsley, M.D., Claudia Bemis, M.D., Susan Glocheski, M.D., Michael Goldstein, M.D., F. Cleveland Kinney, M.D., David G. Folks, M.D., Robert E. Hales, M.D., M. Eileen McNamara, M.D., and Raymond Niaura, Ph.D.

gation (Lipowski 1986) for classifying the areas in which psychological, behavioral, and social factors may affect physical health is presented in Table 15–1.

The revised diagnostic criteria for the DSM-IV (American Psychiatric Association 1994) category "Psychological Factors Affecting Medical Conditions" are presented in Table 15–2. These criteria emphasize the clinician's noting of relationships between psychological factors and medical conditions in regard to not only the onset but also the course and outcome of illness.

■ THE ROLE OF PSYCHOLOGICAL FACTORS IN CANCER ONSET AND PROGRESSION

The relationship between psychological factors and the onset and course of neoplastic disease serves as a prototype in examining the literature in this area, because many health care professionals and lay people believe

---

Table 15–1. **Psychological and behavioral factors affecting medical conditions**

I. Psychophysiology
    A. Physiological reactions to psychological and behavioral variables
    B. Biological regulatory mechanisms associated with behavioral and psychological variables
        1. Psychoneurophysiology
        2. Psychoneuroendocrinology
        3. Psychoneuroimmunology
        4. Psychocardiology
II. Effects of concurrent psychiatric illness on the course and outcome of medical disorders
III. Behavioral risk factors for disease and injury
    A. Personality variables
    B. Cigarette smoking
    C. Dietary habits
    D. Alcohol and substance abuse
    E. Hazardous sexual behavior
    F. Risk-taking behaviors (accidents, injury)
    G. Noncompliance with medical treatment
    H. Violence, suicide, homicide
    I. Stressful or disruptive life change

Source. Reprinted from Stoudemire A, Hales RE: "Psychological and Behavioral Factors Affecting Medical Conditions and DSM-IV: An Overview." *Psychosomatics* 32:5–13, 1991. Copyright 1991, American Psychiatric Association. Used with permission.

that psychological factors play a major role in cancer onset and progression. This belief has been strengthened, in part, by a rapidly growing literature, both scientific and popular, examining the role of psychological factors in cancer.

☐ Affective States and Cancer

The relationship between depression and cancer has been the focus of extensive study, with early research indicating that depression was associated with an increased risk of cancer (Shekelle et al. 1981). More recent epidemiological studies, however, have demonstrated negative findings (Hahn and Petitti 1988). Dattore et al. (1980) found significantly *lower* depression scores in men who subsequently developed any type of cancer.

Table 15–2.   DSM-IV diagnostic criteria for psychological factor affecting [general] medical condition

---

A. A general medical condition (coded on Axis III) is present.

B. Psychological factors adversely affect the general medical condition in one of the following ways:

  1. The factors have influenced the course of the general medical condition as shown by a close temporal association between the psychological factors and the development or exacerbation of, or delayed recovery from, the general medical condition.

  2. The factors interfere with treatment of the general medical condition.

  3. The factors constitute additional health risks for the individual.

  4. Stress-related physiological responses precipitate or exacerbate symptoms of the general medical condition.

Choose name based on the nature of the psychological factors (if more than one factor is present, indicate the most prominent):

Mental disorder affecting general medical condition (e.g., Axis I disorder such as major depressive disorder delaying recovery from a myocardial infarction)

Psychological symptoms affecting general medical condition (e.g., depressive symptoms delaying recovery from surgery; anxiety exacerbating asthma)

Personality traits or coping style affecting general medical condition (e.g., pathological denial of the need for surgery in a patient with cancer; hostile, pressured behavior contributing to cardiovascular disease)

Maladaptive health behaviors affecting general medical condition (e.g., overeating; lack of exercise; unsafe sex)

Stress-related physiological response affecting general medical condition (e.g., stress-related exacerbations of ulcer, hypertension, arrhythmia, or tension headache)

Other or unspecified psychological factors affecting general medical condition (e.g., interpersonal, cultural, or religious factors)

A more recent study (Zonderman et al. 1989) found no significant depressive symptoms that could be seen as predictors of cancer morbidity or mortality.

Breast cancer patients who demonstrated a "fighting spirit" or who used denial had a higher survival rate than those with stoic acceptance or expressed hopelessness and helplessness (Greer et al. 1979). Although clinical studies have not found a relationship between depression and cancer outcome (Cassileth et al. 1985), one study involving radiation therapy patients actually found high anxiety or depression to be predictive of lower mortality 3 years later (Leigh et al. 1987).

☐ Coping Styles, Personality Traits, and Cancer

Cassileth et al. (1988) found that none of the multiple psychosocial factors thought to be predictive of health predicted cancer survival. Other studies have demonstrated no differences in coping styles between breast cancer patients and control subjects (Buddeberg et al. 1991), or head and neck cancer patients and control subjects (Yamagiwa et al. 1991), and no relationship between coping style and breast cancer course (Edwards et al. 1990). Epidemiological studies have not supported a relationship between "emotional repression" and cancer incidence or mortality (Shekelle et al. 1981).

Some other work has linked stressful life events to cancer progression or recurrence (Funch and Marshall 1983; Ramirez et al. 1989). Many other studies, however, have failed to find an association between preceding stressful life events and cancer onset (Edwards et al. 1990). In a review of human and animal studies, Fox (1983) concluded that if stressful events and/or other psychological factors do have an effect on cancer incidence, it is small.

☐ Psychosocial Intervention and Cancer Outcome

In contrast with lack of convincing support of an etiological relationship between psychological factors and cancer, studies have shown improvement in the quality of life in cancer patients receiving group therapy (Fawzy et al. 1990a; Spiegel et al. 1989). Relaxation training (Bindemann et al. 1991; Holland et al. 1991) and cognitive-behavior therapy (Greer et al. 1991) have also reduced anxiety and depression in cancer patients.

Spiegel et al. (1989) performed a small randomized, controlled trial of supportive group therapy with training in self-hypnosis for pain control in women with metastatic breast cancer. At 1 year, the psychotherapy treatment group had less mood disturbance and fewer phobic responses and complained of less pain. The treatment group also had increased survival compared with the control group (34.8 vs. 18.9 months). Greater longevity was associated with less mood disturbance and higher vigor. Fawzy et al. (1990a) evaluated the immediate and prolonged effects of a 6-week structured psychiatric group intervention for postsurgical patients with malignant melanoma. Patients who received the intervention had higher vigor than did control subjects at 6 weeks and less depression, fatigue, and total mood disturbance at 6-month follow-up. Experimental subjects demonstrated more active coping than control subjects both at the conclusion of the intervention and at follow-up. The investigators also reported that patients who received group therapy had statistically significant increases in immunological function at 6-month follow-up (Fawzy et al. 1990b).

In controlled comparisons of women with metastatic breast cancer who did or did not receive psychotherapy, Grossarth-Maticek et al. also found psychotherapy to be associated with increased survival and higher lymphocyte counts (Grossarth-Maticek and Eysenck 1989). Although psychotherapeutic interventions may be of great benefit to cancer patients, if it is suggested in an overly optimistically manner that such therapy will deliver cure or remission, there is a risk of deeply disappointing patients and their families and distracting from the direct benefits of psychiatric treatment for quality of life. Psychiatrists should keep in mind that psychosocial interventions are more likely to contribute to quality than to quantity of life in cancer patients. Despite enthusiasm among many professional and laypersons for treatments promising to overcome cancer through "mind over body," current scientific evidence supports a more cautious view. Psychiatric interventions are primarily justified if they reduce distress and dysfunction, such as when depressive or anxiety disorders are diagnosed in the context of oncological illness.

■ PSYCHONEUROIMMUNOLOGY

The observation that psychosocial variables may affect outcome in cancer has focused attention on the immune sytem as a mediating mechanism, since the interrelationship of the brain and the immune system has now been well documented. This evidence ranges from anatomical confirmation of central nervous system (CNS) innervation of immune organs to reports documenting behavioral effects on immune response and tumor acquisition in experimental animals.

The natural progression of study in psychoneuroimmunology has led investigators to focus on how psychological and psychosocial factors operate to influence physical health. There is a consistent literature describing the association of bereavement and immune function. Researchers have documented decreased mitogen stimulation in vitro in recently bereaved subjects, as well as decreased natural killer cell activity in vitro in individuals with anticipatory bereavement. The largest research focus has examined a possible relationship between depression and the immune system. However, the studies have led to considerable confusion regarding conceptualizations, methods, experimental designs, and results. Stein et al. (1991) concluded that "alterations in the immune system in MD [major depression] and MDD [major depressive disorder] do not appear to be a specific biological correlate of this disorder, but, rather, may occur in association with other variables that characterize depressed patients, including age and symptom severity" (p. 175). These conclusions were drawn as a result of their study in which significant age-related differences between depressed subjects and control subjects were found. Specifically, the depressed patients did *not* show increases in lymphocyte function or number of CD_4 lymphocytes with advancing age as did the control subjects.

The possible role of psychological interventions affecting immune parameters has recently been studied in a group of postsurgical patients with malignant melanoma (Fawzy et al. 1990a). Those individuals randomized to the group intervention showed reduced psychological distress and enhanced longer-term effective coping. At 6-month follow-up, these patients also showed increases in the percentage of large granular lymphocytes and natural killer cells, as well as increased natural killer cytotoxic activity. Clinical implications of psychonneuroimmunology research indicates that particularly in those patients experiencing bereavement and other significant psychosocial stress, as well as the spectrum of mood disorders, the possibility of coexisting immune changes should be considered.

■ PSYCHOLOGICAL FACTORS AND ENDOCRINE DISEASE

Although there is a considerable literature base examining the field of psychoneuroendocrinology, particularly in relation to the biology of mood disorders, there is a paucity of methodologically sound research regarding the clinical aspects of psychological factors and how these factors potentially influence endocrine diseases. An extensive review of this area was recently published by Beardsley and Goldstein (1993). Of the existing literature, most research is focused on diabetes mellitus and Graves' disease.

□ Diabetes Mellitus

Investigators have speculated on the role of psychological factors in affecting the course of diabetes mellitus. Although early studies were flawed primarily due to difficulties in accurately measuring glucose control, more recent measures of glycosylated hemoglobin have proven more reliable. One group of investigators studied 15 patients with insulin-dependent diabetes mellitus who self-monitored psychological stress, diet, exercise, insulin dose, and blood glucose levels over 8 weeks (Halford et al. 1990). Seven of the 15 subjects had statistically significant associations between measures of daily psychological stress and blood glucose levels. Another study monitored continuous blood glucose in patients with insulin-dependent diabetes mellitus who were undergoing brief standardized stressors during two laboratory sessions (Gonder-Frederick et al. 1990). The authors found significant changes in the glucose levels of 8 of 14 subjects when the subjects were exposed to the active stressor during their first session. Significant changes were not found during the second session, which occurred 12 weeks after the original session, perhaps suggesting development of habituation in this population (Gonder-Frederick et al. 1990). Although based on small numbers of subjects, these studies show some support for the hypothesis that psychological stress is associated with changes in glucose control in at least a subset of insulin-dependent diabetes mellitus patients.

Rovet and Ehrlich (1988) examined the effect of temperament on metabolic control in children with insulin-dependent diabetes mellitus. Diabetic children who were more active, were better at following routines, displayed milder responses to external stimuli, were less attentive, and were more prone to negative moods had improved metabolic control compared with the other diabetic children. No cause-effect relationship was implied from this study. Another investigation examined the relationship between specific personality traits and glucose regulation in diabetic children. Children with Type A behavior as identified by their responses to video games were found to have a hyperglycemic response to stress that was not exhibited by children with a Type B behavior pattern (Stabler et al. 1987). Other investigators have examined such measures as social competence and the relation of low social competence to worsening of metabolic control (Hanson et al. 1987).

☐ Graves' Disease

Minimal evidence to date suggests that psychological characteristics of patients predispose them to develop Graves' disease, or for that matter any thyroid disorder (Weiner 1977). However, one study suggested that negative life events may be risk factors for Graves' disease (Winsa et al. 1991). These investigators studied 219 eligible patients with newly diagnosed Graves' disease and 372 matched control subjects over a 2-year period. Patients and control subjects responded to a mailed questionnaire assessing demographic variables, life events, social support, and personality. Compared with control subjects, patients with Graves' disease had more negative life events in the 12 months preceding the diagnosis, and negative life events scores were significantly higher. These findings are of interest with regard to their psychosomatic implication; however, prospective studies are needed to confirm these results.

■ PSYCHOCARDIOLOGY

The effects of psychosocial and behavioral factors in cardiovascular disease have garnered considerable research attention. This research has looked both at hypertension and at more general aspects of coronary artery disease, including myocardial infarction and sudden cardiac death. Because approximately 85% of hypertension cases are classified as primary, or essential, hypertension in which the exact regulatory disruption leading to elevated blood pressure cannot be specified, psychological factors have been closely studied as part of the pathogenesis. These factors have been categorized as, on the one hand, "pressure reactivity" and, on the other, personality/behavioral factors. Relatively strong evidence indicates that subsets of individuals have greater blood pressure reactivity to a variety of stressors than do others. However, the evidence linking reactivity in normotensive individuals with the eventual development of hypertension is equivocal. Perhaps most importantly, pressure reactivity in patients who have already developed hypertension may exacerbate and even accelerate their disease process.

Research examining personality traits in hypertension has been criticized because of the lack of prospective, longitudinal design. The most positive correlates have specifically involved anger coping styles, but a positive relationship has been found between inhibited anger expression and excessive anger expression.

Some treatment interventions have been specifically aimed at affecting psychological factors related to hypertension. Various behavioral procedures (including biofeedback and relaxation training), as well as psychotherapy, have been used to treat hypertension. A number of investigators have reported clinically significant success in controlled studies, whereas other investigators have not found significant treatment effects when compared with the effects of interventions designed to act as a placebo or as attention control conditions.

The role of stress as a behavioral risk factor in coronary artery disease is another major area of research focus in psychocardiology. Stress has been shown to cause a sympatheticoadrenomedullary alarm reaction characterized by excess catecholamine secretion. It is felt that catecholamine-mediated cardiac effects such as increased heart rate, contractility, and conduction velocity, as well as a shorter atrioventricular refractory period, may be pathogenically related to adverse cardiac events.

Another method of examining behavioral risks factors has resulted from Friedman's investigation of psychosocial variables in coronary artery disease (Friedman and Rosenman 1959). These investigations led to the Type A versus Type B categorization first proposed in the 1950s. A review of these studies suggests that the Type A behavior pattern is a risk factor for developing coronary artery disease; however, once coronary artery disease is present, the presence of a Type A behavior pattern does not appear to increase the risk of subsequent cardiac morbidity. Therefore, further studies have examined possible aspects of the Type A behavior pattern that are themselves more strongly associated with coronary artery disease. A multidimensional item analysis from the Cook-Medley Hostility Scale derived from the Minnesota Multiphasic Personality Inventory (MMPI) has shown a significant relationship to mortality when specifically focusing on the items of cynicism, hostile affect, and aggressive responding in patients with a Type A behavior pattern (Goldstein and Niaura 1992).

The role of mood states and cardiovascular morbidity and mortality has also been an important focus in cardiovascular research. One study showed that a major depression was the best predictor of major cardiac events during the 12 months after cardiac catheterization (Carney et al. 1988). Subsequent events were independent of such variables as severity of cardiac disease, left ventricular function, and smoking. Mood states associated with acute situational disturbances have been linked to sudden cardiac death. Reich et al. (1981) found that the onset of malignant ventricular arrhythmias was associated with identifiable psychologically stressful events in 21% of their patients referred for antiarrhythmic management.

Such sociological factors as work overload and life stress in the face of lack of social support have been shown to enhance coronary risk. A reduced level of socioeconomic resources enhances risk for cardiovascular death with coronary artery disease after all other risk factors are controlled (Williams et al. 1992). Nonmarried individuals with coronary artery disease are also at higher risk for death when compared with married individuals (Chandra et al. 1983). The role of social connections in the onset and course of coronary disease is an important focus of psychosomatic research, particularly as data continue to support the hypothesis that more socially isolated and/or less socially integrated individuals are overall less healthy psychologically and physically.

Because of the role of pressure reactivity in patients with hypertension and its association with Type A behavior patterns, those patients who exhibit manifestations of Type A behavior should be strongly considered for psychological interventions. Particularly in view of existing evidence that Type A behavior patterns may be a risk factor for developing coronary artery disease, and new evidence that mental stress is associated with decreased myocardial perfusion, patients who are at risk of developing, or those who currently have a diagnosis of, coronary artery disease are potentially excellent candidates for such interventions as stress management, biofeedback, and relaxation training. The recent study by Carney et al. (1988) that showed major depression as the best predictor for significant cardiac events following catheterization suggests that all cardiac patients should be screened for depressive disorders.

■ LIFE–STYLE RISK FACTORS

It is now well established that life-style behaviors are risk factors that significantly contribute to the mortality rate in the United States. The most widely studied risk factors are cigarette smoking and obesity, both of which affect the development, perpetuation, and exacerbation of medical illnesses. Cigarette smoking is a powerful independent contributor to the occurrence of myocardial infarction, sudden death, peripheral vascular disease, and stroke (Figure 15–1).

After cigarette smoking, obesity is the second most widely studied risk factor associated with increased morbidity and mortality. There is a strong association between obesity and hypertension, hypercholesterolemia, and diabetes mellitus as risk factors for cardiovascular disease. Obesity may also increase the risk of prostate, colon, and rectal cancer in men and endometrial, cervical, ovarian, breast, and gall bladder cancer in women.

Other life-style factors that have been associated with negative health outcomes are as follows: 1) a sedentary life-style and diet high in cholesterol and fats and low in fiber; 2) sexual practices known to increase the risk of infection with the human immunodeficiency virus (HIV); 3) exposure to sun and other ultraviolet light; 4) lack of use of safety restraints when riding in motor vehicles; and 5) psychoactive substance use and abuse (Stoudemire et al. 1993).

With the currently established evidence of the morbidity and mortality associated with life-style risk factors, psychiatrists, perhaps more so than other clinicians, have an active role to play in assisting patients with behavioral changes. With cigarette smoking being the single most important modifiable risk factor for illness in this country, treatment of nicotine dependence should play a central role in the treatment plans of those patients who continue to abuse tobacco. Unfortunately, smoking cessation is a difficult intervention. The difficulty is compounded by the physical dependence on nicotine in chronic smokers, which has led to a separate category for nicotine dependence in DSM-IV. Such dependence

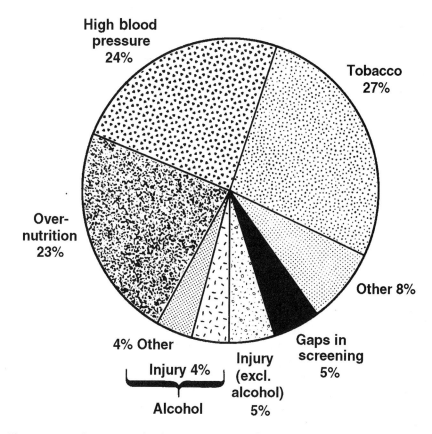

Figure 15–1. Premature deaths. Three precursors—tobacco, high blood pressure, and overnutrition—account for 73.5% of premature deaths in the United States. Reprinted from Amler RW, Eddins DL: "Cross-Sectional Analysis: Precursors of Premature Death in the United States." *American Journal of Preventive Medicine* 3 (No 5, Suppl):181–187, 1987. Copyright 1987, Society for Neuroscience. Used with permission.

can now be treated effectively, especially when behavioral and pharmacological approaches are combined.

Similarly, interventions for modifying obesity are paramount in preventing and treating such conditions as heart disease, diabetes mellitus, pulmonary disease, and certain cancers. Although weight reduction for obese individuals has become an important medical intervention, evidence has shown that individuals who repeatedly diet are more likely to increase their weight over time when compared with obese individuals who do not repeatedly attempt to lose weight. This finding has led to speculation that repeated dieting may be associated with increases in morbidity. At the very least, psychoeducation into the above risk behaviors, as well as into risk behaviors that include unsafe sexual practices, exposure to sun, psychoactive substance use and abuse, use of safety restraints in motor vehicles, and certain dietary risks, should be addressed with patients when considering their overall psychosomatic-psychophysiological profile (Brown et al. 1993; Clark et al. 1993).

■ PULMONARY DISEASES

Asthma historically was considered to be a classic "psychosomatic" illness. Most practitioners now embrace a multifactorial model in which a range of childhood trauma and predispositions (including genetic ones) set the stage for vulnerability to asthma in childhood or later in life (Knapp and Mathe 1985). Confirmation of these models, which emphasize that optimal psychophysiological regulatory functions occur within a successful infant-mother attachment, is derived in part from observations that derangement or disruption of this attachment in monkeys may cause dysregulation of affect and physiological processes such as sleepwake cycle, body temperature, and heart rate, among others (Reite and Short 1986). Some authors have proposed that adult asthma patients with a poor ability to manage loss and others stressors through verbal expression may be at increased risk for asthma attacks (Gaddini 1978).

From a more purely biological perspective, the usefulness of sympathomimetic agents in the treatment of asthma led to the formulation of asthma as a state of relative parasympathetic dominance (or β_2-receptor blockade). Beta$_2$-receptor blockade can produce bronchoconstriction in susceptible individuals, including most asthmatic persons. Stress and anxiety should produce functionally increased sympathetic outflow and should at least theoretically not worsen or provoke an attack. Asthmatic patients, however, may respond to stressful events with abnormally low epinephrine secretion (Mathe and Knapp 1969).

Studies of chronic obstructive pulmonary disease (COPD) have centered on personality types, ability to interpret symptoms such as dyspnea, and patient and family factors in ventilator dependence. Although there is agreement that major personality disorders and mood disorders contribute to functional disability in COPD patients (Weiner 1985), no studies clearly designate these factors as predisposing traits or maladaptive consequences of COPD. COPD itself, through adverse effects on arterial oxygen concentrations, can cause neuropsychiatric disturbances that impair compliance.

A clear-cut connection between stressful events and aggravation of asthmatic symptoms should lead to psychiatric consultation. A specific aim of the consultation would include helping the patient develop heightened awareness of the typical stressors that appear to trigger breathing-related symptoms so that the patient can develop coping strategies for dealing with them. Some asthmatic patients also have panic disorder that is at times indistinguishable from the expectable physiological reaction to severe dyspnea, and they may inappropriately use bronchodilatory medications for the treatment of such episodes.

If anxiety or depressive affect is severe enough, pulmonary outcome is eroded in at least two ways: through the patient's inability to adhere to the treatment regimen and, possibly, through autonomic pathways (Yellowlees and Kalucy 1990). In addition, nonspecific induction of stress may worsen the course of the asthma (Gorman 1990). Certain pathological family dynamics, especially the presence of severe avoidance and denial of intense affect, suggest a poor prognosis for ventilator-dependent patients with COPD, and require early and firm intervention by the psychiatrist. Family sessions focused on the family members' helplessness and anger are crucial in the overall approach.

■ RHEUMATOLOGICAL DISEASE

Among patients and physicians there is widespread anecdotal agreement that emotional factors affect the clinical course of rheumatoid arthritis (RA). The presence of certain psychological factors appear to be predictive of a poor course with RA, including poor motivation, low intelligence, depressed mood unassociated with pain, poor impulse control, and deficits in ego strength (Molodofsky and Chester 1970). These factors operate through such mechanisms as diminished energy for rehabilitation, decreased understanding of the treatment regimen, and impulsive, maladaptive acting out of anger and depressed mood as reactions to the chronic illness. Psychological strengths that affect the course of RA in a constructive sense include a positive attitude toward rehabilitation personnel and a flexible and adjustable view of the goals of the rehabilitation process (Vogel and Rosillo 1971).

Psychiatrists treating patients with rheumatological diseases should be especially alert to the development of anxiety and depression (Meenan 1981). Both can erode the patient's capacity and will for long-term adherence to medical treatment plans, essential components of therapeutic success in these patients. The frustration and self-criticism associated with depression undermine the patient's willingness and ability to continue physical therapy. Aggressive attempts should be made to maintain the involvement of the patient's family and friends. Family involvement and support, frequent rheumatology office visits, home visits by physician-assistants or nurse-specialists, and psychotherapy and pharmacotherapy directed at the depressed mood all play a role in ensuring maintenance of function and early detection of relapse.

■ GASTROINTESTINAL DISORDERS

Personality factors can contribute to the active disregard of known risk factors for peptic ulcer disease (PUD, such as smoking or use of alcohol and salicylates) (Folks and Kinney 1992b). Depressive affect and anxiety may discriminate ulcer from nonulcer patients. Type A characteristics of aggression, sense of time urgency, and competitiveness have been linked to PUD (Magni et al. 1987). Limited capacity for emotional expression may be more common in dyspepsia and ulcer patients (Talley et al. 1988). Serum pepsinogen, a precursor in the secretory pathway for gastric acid, correlates positively with increasing personality scores for hostility, irritability, and hypersensitivity (Walker et al. 1988).

In irritable bowel syndrome (IBS), as in asthma, target organ hypersensitivity to mechanical and chemical stimuli plays a major pathophysiological role. Increased vagal activity appears to have a mediating function in both disorders (Read 1987). The clinical picture of IBS resembles that of lactose malabsorption. Symptoms include abdominal pain and alterations in bowel habits, either constipation or diarrhea, in the absence of abnormalities on physical examination or traditional laboratory and radiologic tests. Underlying motility disturbances appear to be responsive to psychological symptoms (Folks and Kinney 1992b) and produce a relapsing-remitting course. Morphology of the intestine does not appear to be altered in IBS, but electrical and motor activities are increased compared with such activities in control subjects (Latimer et al. 1981).

Up to 70% of IBS patients meet criteria for a psychiatric disorder (Latimer et al. 1981). Compared with ulcerative colitis patients, persons with IBS appear to have more premorbid psychopathology. From the perspective of psychological testing, IBS patients are a heterogeneous group, differing from normal control subjects but not PUD patients (Sjodin and Svedlund 1985). Developmental histories reveal that control subjects had many *fewer* childhood doctor visits and less discomfort with bowel symptoms than did individuals with IBS (Lowman et al. 1987). Loss and separation are recurrent early developmental themes in IBS. The early patienthood may reflect an attempt by the child to find a regulatory relationship outside the family unit. Persistent or neurotic pursuit of such regulation by others may account for the frequently reported histories of conflicted, dependent marriages in IBS patients (Lowman et al. 1987).

Patients with PUD whose condition is refractory to treatment should be screened for high state and trait anxiety characteristics. Psychotherapy focused on intellectualizing and problem-solving techniques can help patients feel a greater sense of mastery over feared calamities. Careful psychotherapeutic assessment and treatment of mood disorder and also the propensity for conflicted adult relationships may help the IBS patient avoid destructive repetitions of those losses.

■ DERMATOLOGICAL DISORDERS

The range of normal emotions affect skin appearance: flushing, sweating, and blanching. Psychopathological processes come into play—through neglect of normal skin care and reduced adherence to prescribed treatment of skin diseases; through overt self-inflicted lesions such as scratches and cuts; and through "stress" and anxiety—to produce a number of dermatoses by way of incompletely understood mechanisms. Because of the central social and psychological role played by the skin and its appearance, skin diseases in turn can produce a host of psychological reactions, including depressive affect, shame, social withdrawal, rage, and paradoxical aggravation of a primary skin condition (Folks and Kinney 1992a). Psychiatric consultation is thus an important part of the treatment approach with many dermatological patients.

The anxiety and shame associated with psoriasis combine to exact a tremendous psychological toll on patients, with intense anticipation of rejection, a sense of defectiveness, and social withdrawal. Despair and stigmatization have maladaptive effects, being highly associated with noncompliance with prescribed treatment (Gupta et al. 1989).

Many psychological studies of patients with acne show a high prevalence of emotional symptoms, with poor self-esteem and negative self-image being the most common (Rubinow et al. 1987). Successful treatment of severe acne tends to reverse symptoms such as depressive affect and anxiety, but produces little change in personality structure (Van der Meeren et al. 1985).

Self-induced dermatoses occur frequently among psychiatric patients. Representing the effects of rage and narcissistic injury (borderline personality disorder), psychosis (schizophrenia), malingering, and agitation and poor impulse control (mental retardation), the lesions can be wide ranging in their appearance and course. Serious lesions may result in tendon and nerve injury, as well as infection.

For many patients with chronic dermatitis, psychosocial stressors have a direct exacerbating effect, and supportive psychotherapy, with or without careful use of anxiolytics, may help immensely in mitigating the adverse effects of such stressors. Patients with idiopathic urticaria commonly experience flares due to anxiety. Assessment of the severity of the attacks and their correlation with emotional triggers can direct the psychiatrist toward supportive psychotherapy in the less severe cases, and to use of prophylactic antidepressants in those more affected patients with panic disorder.

■ END-STAGE RENAL DISEASE

As treatment for end-stage renal disease (ESRD) has evolved, there has been extensive interest in the psychiatric and psychosocial aspects of dialysis and transplantation. A number of studies have compared psychosocial quality of life with dialysis versus renal transplantation. Most have found better psychosocial functioning in transplant patients (Petrie 1989; Simmons and Abress 1990). Similar results have been demonstrated in children with renal failure (Brownbridge and Fielding 1991). Investigators have also compared the quality of life between patients receiving different dialysis modalities. Some have found continuous ambulatory peritoneal dialysis (CAPD) to be associated with better psychological outcome (Brownbridge and Fielding 1991; Rydholm and Pauling 1991).

A Canadian research group found that *depression* was a better predictor of shorter survival than was age or a composite physiological index of clinical variables (Burton et al. 1986). Several other investigators have noted that depression in ESRD patients is associated with higher mortality and morbidity (Numan et al. 1981; Shulman et al. 1989). Other studies have found no effects of depression on survival (Devins et al. 1990; Husebye et al. 1987). A fundamental weakness of most of these studies is that no attempt was made to measure and/or to control for disease severity, a major confounding factor in studies relating psychopathology to outcome in the medically ill (Levenson et al. 1990).

From a clinical standpoint, compliance is an important factor in the management of dialysis patients, but formal definition and measurement have been problematic. Psychosocial factors with demonstrated effects on compliance in ESRD include patients' beliefs about their health behaviors (Cummings et al. 1982), "locus of control" and self-efficacy (Schneider et al. 1991), family problems (Cummings et al. 1982), and social support (O'Brien 1990). Small studies in kidney transplant patients have shown that pretransplant noncompliance predicts posttransplant noncompliance and graft failure. Noncompliant kidney transplant patients are more likely to be depressed and have other psychosocial problems than are compliant patients (Rodriguez et al. 1991).

Psychiatric consultation may be requested when long-term dialysis patients wish to discontinue treatment, raising clinical (Greene 1983), liaison (Slevin 1983), and ethical (Holley et al. 1989) issues. In a large study of dialysis patients (Neu and Kjellstrand 1986), dialysis was discontinued in 9%, accounting for 22% of all deaths. Half of the patients withdrawn were incompetent and required surrogate decision making. Early studies that had pointed to a very high rate of suicide in dialysis patients overestimated suicide prevalence by not distinguishing rational treatment withdrawal from suicide.

The current state of research allows for informed speculation on how psychological factors such as depression might influence outcome in ESRD. Depression may adversely affect immune function (Stein et al. 1991). Clinical experience is that depressed ESRD patients are more likely to evidence poor self-care, noncompliance, and poor medical follow-up. Depression has been associated in other populations with increased use of analgesics, which in turn have been demonstrated to have a role in the etiology and exacerbation of chronic renal failure (Sandler et al. 1989; Schwarz et al. 1989). Depression may adversely impact outcome in ESRD by serving as a risk factor for other medical comorbidity—for example, myocardial infarction (Booth-Kewley and Friedman 1987) or reduced aerobic capacity (Carney et al. 1986).

Depression is the most common psychiatric disorder in ESRD patients, and the symptoms may be difficult to distinguish from uremia or other comorbid medical conditions (Levenson and Glocheski 1991). Careful differential diagnosis will identify those patients who should be treated for depression, with subsequent expectable improvement in quality of life and functional capacity.

Noncompliance remains the reason psychiatrists are most often consulted by nephrologists. The psychiatrist should help the ESRD treatment team avoid simplistic thinking about noncompliance and be aware of the risk of scapegoating the patient. The most extreme form of noncompliance is refusal to accept, or withdrawal from, treatment for ESRD. Some clinicians err in regarding such patients as always depressed and suicidal, while others err in the opposite direction. Psychiatrists have a crucial role in what can be a difficult distinction between autonomous rational decision making versus irrational suicidal giving up, symptomatic of a treatable depression.

■ REFERENCES

American Psychiatric Association: Diagnostic and Statistical Manual of Mental Disorders, 4th Edition. Washington, DC, American Psychiatric Association, 1994

Amler RW, Eddins DL: Cross-sectional analysis: precursors of premature death in the United States. Am J Prev Med 3 (No 5, suppl):181–187, 1987

Beardsley G, Goldstein MG: Psychological factors affecting physical condition: endocrine disease literature review. Psychosomatics 34:12–19, 1993

Bindemann S, Soukop M, Kaye SB: Randomized controlled study of relaxation training. European Journal of Cancer 27:170–174, 1991

Booth-Kewley S, Friedman HS: Psychological predictors of heart disease: a quantitative review. Psychol Bull 101:343–362, 1987

Brown RA, Goldstein MG, Niarua R, et al: Nicotine dependence: assessment and management, in Psychiatric Care of the Medical Patient. Edited by Stoudemire A, Fogel BS. New York, Oxford University Press, 1993, pp 877–901

Brownbridge G, Fielding DM: Psychosocial adjustment to end-stage renal failure: comparing hemodialysis, continuous ambulatory peritoneal dialysis and transplantation. Pediatr Nephrol 5:612–616, 1991

Buddeberg C, Wolf C, Sieber M, et al: Coping strategies and course of disease of breast cancer patients: results of a 3-year longitudinal study. Psychother Psychosom 55:151–157, 1991

Burton JJ, Kline SA, Lindsay RM, et al: Relationship of depression to survival in chronic renal failure. Psychosom Med 48:261–269, 1986

Carney RM, Wetzel RD, Hagberg J, et al: The relationship between depression and aerobic capacity in hemodialysis patients. Psychosom Med 48:143–147, 1986

Carney RM, Rich MW, Freedland KE, et al: Major depressive disorder predicts cardiac events in patients with coronary artery disease. Psychosom Med 50:627–633, 1988

Cassileth BR, Lusk EJ, Miller DS, et al: Psychological correlates of survival in advanced malignant disease? N Engl J Med 312:1551–1555, 1985

Cassileth BR, Walsh WP, Lusk EJ: Psychosocial correlates of cancer survival: a subsequent report 3 to 8 years after cancer diagnosis. J Clin Oncol 6:1753–1759, 1988

Chandra V, Szklo M, Goldberg R, et al: The impact of marital status on survival after an acute myocardial infarction: a population-based study. Am J Epidemiol 117:320–325, 1983

Clark MM, Ruggiero L, Pera V, et al: Assessment, classification, and treatment of obesity: a psychobiobehavioral perspective, in Psychiatric Care of the Medical Patient. Edited by Stoudemire A, Fogel BS. New York, Oxford University Press, 1993, pp 903–926

Cummings K, Becker M, Kirscht J, et al: Psychosocial factors affecting adherence to medical regimens in a group of hemodialysis patients. Med Care 20:567–580, 1982

Dattore PJ, Shontz FC, Coyne L: Premorbid personality differentiation of cancer and noncancer groups: a test of the hypothesis of cancer proneness. J Consult Clin Psychol 48:388–394, 1980

Devins GM, Mann J, Mandin H, et al: Psychosocial predictors of survival in end-stage renal disease. J Nerv Ment Dis 178:127–133, 1990

Edwards JR, Cooper CL, Pearl SS, et al: The relationship between psychosocial factors and breast cancer: some unexpected results. Behav Med 16:5–14, 1990

Evans DL, McCartney CF, Haggerty JJ, et al: Treatment of depression in cancer patients is associated with better life adaptation: a pilot study. Psychosom Med 50:72–76, 1988

Fawzy FI, Cousins N, Fawzy NW, et al: A structured psychiatric intervention for cancer patients, I: changes over time in methods of coping and affective disturbance. Arch Gen Psychiatry 47:720–725, 1990a

Fawzy FI, Kemeny ME, Fawzy NW, et al: A structured psychiatric intervention for cancer patients, II: changes over time in immunological measures. Arch Gen Psychiatry 47:729–735, 1990b

Folks DG, Kinney FC: The role of psychological factors in dermatologic conditions. Psychosomatics 33:45–54, 1992a

Folks DG, Kinney FC: The role of psychological factors in gastrointestinal conditions: a review pertinent to DSM-IV. Psychosomatics 33:257–270, 1992b

Fox BH: Current theory of psychogenic effects on cancer incidence and prognosis. Journal of Psychosocial Oncology 1:17–31, 1983

Friedman M, Rosenman RH: Association of specific overt behavior pattern with blood and cardiovascular findings. JAMA 169:1085–1096, 1959

Funch DP, Marshall J: The role of stress, social support and age in survival from breast cancer. J Psychosom Res 27:77–83, 1983

Gaddini R: Transitional object origins and the psychosomatic symptom, in Between Fantasy and Reality: Transitional Objects and Phenomena. Edited by Grolnick A, Barkin L. New York, Jason Aronson, 1978, pp 17–21

Goldstein MG, Niaura R: Psychological factors affecting physical condition: cardiovascular disease literature review, Part I: coronary artery disease and sudden death. Psychosomatics 33:134–145, 1992

Gonder-Frederick LA, Carter WR, Cox DJ, et al: Environmental stress and blood glucose change in IDDM. Health Psychol 9:503–515, 1990

Gorman JM: Psychobiological aspects of asthma and the consequent research implications (editorial). Chest 97:514–515, 1990

Greene WA: Problems in discontinuation of hemodialysis, in Psychonephrology 2: Psychological Problems in Kidney Failure and Their Treatment. Edited by Levy NB. New York, Plenum, 1983, pp 131–144

Greer S, Morris T, Pettingale KW: Psychological response to breast cancer: effect on outcome. Lancet 2:785–787, 1979

Greer S, Moorey S, Baruch J: Evaluation of adjuvant psychological therapy for clinically referred cancer patients. Br J Cancer 63:257–260, 1991

Grossarth-Maticek R, Eysenck HJ: Length of survival and lymphocyte percentage in women with mammary cancer as a function of psychotherapy. Psychol Rep 65:315–321, 1989

Gupta MA, Gupta AK, Kirkby S, et al: A psychocutaneous profile of psoriasis patients who are stress reactors: a study of 127 patients. Gen Hosp Psychiatry 11:166–173, 1989

Hahn RC, Petitti DB: Minnesota Multiphasic Personality Inventory–rated depression and the incidence of breast cancer. Cancer 61:845–848, 1988

Halford WK, Cuddily S, Mortimer RH: Psychological stress and blood glucose regulation in type 1 diabetic patients. Health Psychol 9:516–528, 1990

Hanson CL, Henggeler SW, Burghen GA: Social competence and parental support as mediators of the link between stress and metabolic control in adolescents with insulin-dependent diabetes mellitus. J Consult Clin Psychol 55:529–533, 1987

Holland JC, Morrow GR, Schmale A, et al: A randomized clinical trial of alprazolam versus progressive muscle relaxation in cancer patients with anxiety and depressive symptoms. J Clin Oncol 9:1004–1011, 1991

Holley JL, Finucane TE, Moss AH: Dialysis patients' attitudes about cardiopulmonary resuscitation and stopping dialysis. Am J Nephrol 9:245–251, 1989

Husebye DG, Westlie L, Styrovoky TJ, et al: Psychological, social, and somatic prognostic indicators in old patients undergoing long-term dialysis. Arch Intern Med 147:1921–1924, 1987

Knapp PH, Mathe AA: Psychophysiologic aspects of bronchial asthma: a review, in Bronchial Asthma: Mechanisms and Therapeutics. Edited by Weiss EB, Segal MS, Stein M. Boston, Little, Brown, 1985, pp 914–931

Latimer P, Sarna S, Campbell D, et al: Colonic motor and myoelectrical activity: a comparative study of normal subjects, psychoneurotic patients, and patients with irritable bowel syndrome. Gastroenterology 80:893–901, 1981

Leigh H, Percarpio B, Opsahl C, et al: Psychological predictors of survival in cancer patients undergoing radiation therapy. Psychother Psychosom 47:65–73, 1987

Levenson JL, Glocheski S: Psychological factors affecting end-stage renal disease: a review. Psychosomatics 32:382–389, 1991

Levenson JL, Colenda C, Larson DB, et al: Methodology in consultation-liaison research: a classification of biases. Psychosomatics 31:367–376, 1990

Lipowski ZJ: Psychosomatic medicine: past and present, Part III: current research. Can J Psychiatry 31:14–21, 1986

Lowman BC, Drossman DA, Cramer EM, et al: Recollection of childhood events in adults with irritable bowel syndrome. J Clin Gastroenterol 9:324–330, 1987

Magni G, DiMario F, Borgherini G, et al: Personality and duodenal ulcer response to antisecretory treatment. Digestion 38(3):152–155, 1987

Mathe AA, Knapp PH: Decreased plasma free fatty acids and urinary epinephrine in bronchial asthma. N Engl J Med 281:234–238, 1969

Meenan RF: The impact of chronic disease: a sociomedical profile of rheumatoid arthritis. Arthritis Rheum 24:544–549, 1981

Molodofsky H, Chester WJ: Pain and mood patterns in patients with rheumatoid arthritis. Psychosom Med 32:309–317, 1970

Neu S, Kjellstrand CM: Stopping long-term dialysis: an empirical study of withdrawal of life-supporting treatment. N Engl J Med 314:14–20, 1986

Numan IM, Barklind KS, Lubin B: Correlates of depression in chronic dialysis patients: morbidity and mortality. Res Nurs Health 4:295–297, 1981

O'Brien ME: Compliance behavior and long-term maintenance dialysis. Am J Kidney Dis 15:209–214, 1990

Petrie K: Psychological well-being and psychiatric disturbance in dialysis and renal transplant patients. Br J Med Psychol 62:91–96, 1989

Ramirez AJ, Craig TKJ, Watson JP, et al: Stress and relapse of breast cancer. BMJ 298:291–293, 1989

Read NW: Irritable bowel syndrome (IBS)—definition and pathophysiology. Scand J Gastroenterol Suppl 130:7–13, 1987

Reich P, DeSilva RA, Lown B, et al: Acute psychological disturbance preceding life-threatening ventricular arrhythmias. JAMA 246:233–235, 1981

Reite M, Short R: Behavior and physiology in young bonnet monkeys. Dev Psychobiol 19:567–579, 1986

Rodriguez A, Diaz M, Colon A, et al: Psychosocial profile of noncompliant transplant patients. Transplantation Proceedings 23:1807–1809, 1991

Rovet J, Ehrlich RM: Effect of temperament on metabolic control in children with diabetes mellitus. Diabetes Care 11:77–82, 1988

Rubinow DR, Peck GL, Squillace KM, et al: Reduced anxiety and depression in cystic acne patients after successful treatment with oral isotretinoin. J Am Acad Dermatol 17:25–32, 1987

Rydholm L, Pauling J: Contrasting feelings of helplessness in peritoneal and hemodialysis patients: a pilot study. American Nephrological Nurses Association Journal 18:183–186, 187, 200, 1991

Sandler DP, Smith JC, Weinberg CR, et al: Analgesic use and chronic renal disease. N Engl J Med 320:1238–1243, 1989

Saravay SM, Steinberg MD, Weinschel B, et al: Psychological comorbidity and length of stay in the general hospital. Am J Psychiatry 148:324–329, 1991

Schneider MS, Friend R, Whitaker P, et al: Fluid noncompliance and symptomatology in end-stage renal disease: cognitive and emotional variables. Health Psychol 10:209–215, 1991

Schwarz A, Kunzendorf U, Keller F, et al: Progression of renal failure in analgesic-associated nephropath. Nephron 53:244–249, 1989

Shekelle RB, Raynor WJ Jr, Ostfeld AM: Psychological depression and 17-year risk of death from cancer. Psychosom Med 43:117–125, 1981

Shulman R, Price JD, Spinelli J: Biopsychosocial aspects of long-term survival on end-stage renal failure therapy. Psychol Med 19:945–954, 1989

Simmons RG, Abress L: Quality of life issues for end-stage renal disease patients. Am J Kidney Dis 15:201–208, 1990

Sjodin I, Svedlund J: Psychological aspects of non-ulcer dyspepsia: a psychosomatic view focusing on a comparison between the irritable bowel syndrome and peptic ulcer disease. Scand J Gastroenterol Suppl 109:51–58, 1985

Slevin SE: Termination of hemodialysis treatment: staff reactions, in Psychonephrology 2: Psychological Problems in Kidney Failure and Their Treatment. Edited by Levy NB. New York, Plenum, 1983, pp 117–130

Spiegel D, Bloom JR, Kraemer HC, et al: Effect of psychosocial treatment on survival of patients with metastatic breast cancer. Lancet 2:888–891, 1989

Stabler B, Surwit RS, Lane JD, et al: Type A behavior pattern and blood glucose control in diabetic children. Psychosom Med 49:313–316, 1987

Stein M, Miller AH, Trestman RL: Depression, the immune system, and health and illness: findings in search of meaning. Arch Gen Psychiatry 48:171–177, 1991

Stoudemire A, Hales RE: Psychological and behavioral factors affecting medical conditions and DSM-IV: an overview. Psychosomatics 32:5–13, 1991

Stoudemire A, Wallack L, Hedemark N: Alcohol dependence and abuse. Am J Prev Med 3 (No 5, suppl):9–18, 1987

Stoudemire A, Beardsley G, Folks DG, et al: Psychological Factors Affecting Physical Condition (PFAPC) 316.00: proposals for revisions in DSM-IV, in DSM-IV Sourcebook: Literature Reviews. Edited by Widiger TA, Frances A, Pincus H, et al. Washington DC, American Psychiatric Press, 1993

Talley NJ, Ellard K, Jones M, et al: Suppression of emotions in essential dyspepsia and chronic duodenal ulcer: a case-control study. Scand J Gastroenterol 23:337–340, 1988

Van der Meeren HLM, Van der Schaar WW, Van den Hurk CMAM: The psychological impact of severe acne. Cutis 36:84–86, 1985

Vogel ML, Rosillo RH: Correlation of psychological variables and progress in physical rehabilitation, III: ego functions and defensive and adaptive mechanisms. Arch Phys Med Rehabil 52:15–21, 1971

Walker P, Luther J, Samloff IM, et al: Life events stress and psychosocial factors in men with peptic ulcer disease, II: relationships with serum pepsinogen concentrations and behavioral risk factors. Gastroenterology 94:323–330, 1988

Weiner H: Psychobiology and Human Disease. New York, Elsevier, 1977

Weiner H: Respiratory disorders, in Comprehensive Textbook of Psychiatry/IV, 4th Edition, Vol . Edited by Kaplan HI, Sadock BJ. Baltimore, MD, Williams & Wilkins, 1985, pp 1159–1167

Williams RB, Barefoot JC, Califf RM, et al: Prognostic importance of social and economic resources among medically treated patients with angiographically documented coronary artery disease. JAMA 267:520–524, 1992

Winsa B, Adami HO, Bergstrom R, et al: Stressful life events and Graves' disease. Lancet 338:1475–1479, 1991

Yamagiwa M, Harada T, Kubo M, et al: Psychological states and personality as factors in the morbidity of head and neck malignant tumors. Nippon Jibiinkoka Gakkai Kaiho 94:67–73, 1991

Yellowlees PM, Kalucy RS: Psychobiological aspects of asthma and the consequent research implications. Chest 97:628–634, 1990

Zonderman AB, Costa PT Jr, McCrae RR: Depression as a risk for cancer morbidity and mortality in a nationally representative sample. JAMA 262:1191–1195, 1989

CHAPTER 16

Somatoform Disorders

Ronald L. Martin, M.D.
Sean H. Yutzy, M.D.

Somatoform disorders were first delineated as a class of psychiatric disorders in DSM-III (American Psychiatric Association, 1980) to facilitate the differential diagnosis of psychiatric disorders characterized primarily by physical symptoms (hence, "somatoform") for which there are no demonstrable organic findings. With minor modifications, this grouping has been retained in DSM-IV (American Psychiatric Association 1994). In contrast to factitious disorders and malingering, somatoform disorder symptoms are *not* under voluntary control. The stipulation in DSM-IV that symptoms are *not* fully accounted for by known physiological mechanisms distinguishes somatoform disorders from certain disorders formerly designated as psychophysiological disorders. The disorders included under the somatoform rubric in DSM-IV are listed in Table 16–1.

Although the validity of the somatoform disorders category has been questioned by some (as summarized by Murphy 1990), others maintain that the somatoform grouping represents a major advance over previous systems (Cloninger 1987). The specific disorders in the somatoform grouping are heterogeneous. In somatization, undifferentiated somatoform, conversion, and pain disorders, the focus is on symptoms themselves. In hypochondriasis and body dysmorphic disorder, the emphasis is on preoccupations derived from symptoms. In hypochodriasis the preoccupation is with interpretation and implications of bodily symptoms, and in body dysmorphic disorder, with an imagined or exaggerated defect in appearance. In several ways hypochondriasis and body dysmorphic disorder more closely resemble obsessive-compulsive or even psychotic disorders than they do the symptom-centered somatoform disorders.

Table 16–1. DSM-IV somatoform disorders: a comparison

DSM-IV somatoform disorder	General description	Temporal and other requirements	Exclusions by other psychiatric illness	Other exclusions
Somatization disorder	History of many physical complaints: pain in at least four different sites or functions, two non-pain gastrointestinal, one sexual or reproductive, one pseudoneurological (conversion or dissociative).	Onset before age 30. Occurs over a period of several years. Treatment sought or significant impairment in social, occupational, or other important areas of functioning.	Not specified.	Not fully explained by a known general medical condition or the direct effect of a substance.
Undifferentiated somatoform disorder	One or more physical complaints.	Duration of at least 6 months. Clinically significant distress or impairment in social, occupational, or other important areas of functioning.	Not better accounted for by another mental disorder.	Not fully explained by a known general medical condition or pathophysiological mechanism (i.e., the effects of injury, medication, drugs, alcohol).

Conversion disorder	Symptoms or deficits affecting voluntary motor or sensory function suggesting a neurological or other general medical condition.	Psychological factors associated. Clinically significant distress or impairment in social, occupational, or other important areas of functioning; or warrants medical evaluation.	Not limited to pain or sexual dysfunction. Not exclusively during course of somatization disorder. Not better accounted for by another mental disorder.	Not intentionally produced or feigned. Not fully explained by a neurological or other general medical condition, or by the direct effect of a substance, or as a culturally sanctioned behavior or experience.
Pain disorder	Pain as predominant focus of clinical presentation. Of sufficient severity to warrant clinical attention.	Clinically significant distress or impairment in social, occupational, or other important areas of functioning. Psychological factors have an important role.	Not better accounted for by a mood, anxiety, or psychotic disorder, and does not meet criteria for dyspareunia.	Not specified.
Hypochondriasis	Preoccupation with fears of having, or the idea that one has, a serious disease based on the misinterpretation of bodily symptoms. Persists despite appropriate medical evaluation and reassurance.	Duration of at least 6 months. Clinically significant distress or impairment in social, occupational, or other important areas of functioning.	Not exclusively during course of a generalized anxiety, obsessive-compulsive, or panic disorder; a major depressive episode; separation anxiety; or another somatoform disorder.	Not of delusional intensity. Not restricted to circumscribed concern about appearance.

(continued)

Table 16–1. DSM-IV somatoform disorders: a comparison (*continued*)

DSM-IV somatoform disorder	General description	Temporal and other requirements	Exclusions by other psychiatric illness	Other exclusions
Body dysmorphic disorder	Preoccupation (may be of delusional intensity) with imagined defect in appearance or markedly excessive concern with slight physical anomaly.	Clinically significant distress or impairment in social, occupational, or other important areas of functioning.	Not better accounted for by another mental disorder (e.g., dis-satisfaction with body shape or size in anorexia nervosa).	Not specified.
Somatoform disorder not otherwise specified	Disorders with somatoform symptoms. Examples: pseudo-cyesis; disorders of less than 6 months with fatigue or body weakness, nonpsychotic hypochondriacal symptoms, or other physical complaints.	Can be of less than 6 months' duration.	Does not meet criteria for any specific somatoform disorder.	Not specified.

Source. Adapted from "Somatoform Disorders in the General Hospital Setting," in *Handbook of Studies on General Psychiatry.* Edited by Judd FK, Burrows GD, Lipsitt DR. Amsterdam, Elsevier, 1991. Copyright 1991, Elsevier Science Publishers. Used with permission.

■ SOMATIZATION DISORDER

The core features of somatization disorder are recurrent multiple physical complaints that are not fully explained by physical factors and that result in medical attention or significant impairment. Somatization disorder is the most pervasive somatoform disorder. By definition it is a polysymptomatic disorder affecting multiple body systems. Two specific somatoform disorders, *pain disorder* and *conversion disorder,* are subsumed within it. Undifferentiated somatoform disorder, in essence, represents a syndrome similar to somatization disorder but with a less extensive manifestation. From a hierarchial perspective, none of these three disorders is diagnosed if symptoms occur exclusively during the course of somatization disorder. Diagnostic preemption also applies to hypochondriasis, although the validity of this has been questioned.

□ Diagnosis and Differential Diagnosis

The DSM-IV diagnostic criteria for somatization disorder are listed in Table 16–2. The symptom picture encountered in somatization disorder is frequently nonspecific and can overlap with a multitude of medical disorders. According to Cloninger (1986), there are three features that are useful in discriminating between somatization disorder and physical illness: 1) involvement of multiple organ systems, 2) early onset and chronic course without development of physical signs of structural abnormalities, and 3) absence of characteristic laboratory abnormalities of the suggested physical disorder. Several medical disorders may be confused with somatization disorder. Multiple sclerosis (MS) and systemic lupus erythematosus (SLE) can both present with vague functional and sensory disturbances with unclear physical signs. Acute intermittent porphyria (AIP) may present with a history of episodic pain and various neurological disturbances that lead to its being confused with somatization disorder.

In addition to somatic symptoms, patients with somatization disorder often have complaints of a psychological or interpersonal nature. Wetzel et al. (1994) summarized these as "psychoform symptoms," and reported that the Minnesota Multiphasic Personality Inventory (MMPI) profiles of somatization disorder patients mimicked multiple psychiatric disorders. According to Cloninger (1986), three psychiatric disorders should be carefully considered in the differential diagnosis of somatization disorder: anxiety disorders (in particular, panic disorder), mood disorders, and schizophrenia. Individuals with generalized anxiety disorder may have a multitude of physical complaints that are also frequently found in patients with somatization disorder. Similarly, patients with somatization disorder often report panic attacks. Although the usual

---

Table 16–2.   DSM-IV diagnostic criteria for somatization disorder

A.   A history of many physical complaints beginning before age 30 years that occur over a period of several years and result in treatment being sought or significant impairment in social, occupational, or other important areas of functioning.

B.   Each of the following criteria must have been met, with individual symptoms occurring at any time during the course of the disturbance.

    1.   *Four pain symptoms:* a history of pain related to at least four different sites or functions (e.g., head, abdomen, back, joints, extremities, chest, rectum, during menstruation, during sexual intercourse, or during urination)

    2.   *Two gastrointestinal symptoms:* a history of at least two gastrointestinal symptoms other than pain (e.g., nausea, bloating, vomiting other than during pregnancy, diarrhea, or intolerance of several different foods)

    3.   *One sexual symptom:* a history of at least one sexual or reproductive symptom other than pain (e.g., sexual indifference, erectile or ejaculatory dysfunction, irregular menses, excessive menstrual bleeding, vomiting throughout pregnancy)

    4.   *One pseudoneurological symptom:* a history of at least one symptom or deficit suggesting a neurological disorder not limited to pain (conversion symptoms such as impaired coordination or balance, paralysis or localized weakness, difficulty swallowing or lump in throat, aphonia, urinary retention, hallucinations, loss of touch or pain sensation, double vision, blindness, deafness, seizures, dissociative symptoms such as amnesia, or loss of consciousness other than fainting)

C.   Either (1) or (2):

    1.   After appropriate investigation, each of the symptoms in criterion B cannot be fully explained by a known general medical condition or the direct effects of a substance (e.g., a drug of abuse, a medication).

    2.   When there is a related general medical condition, the physical complaints or resulting social or occupational impairment is in excess of what would be expected from the history, physical examination, or laboratory findings.

D.   The symptoms are not intentionally produced or feigned (as in factitious disorder or malingering).

---

parameters of age at onset and course may not be helpful in differentiating between an anxiety disorder and somatization disorder, the presence of histrionic personality traits, conversion and dissociative symptoms, sexual and menstrual problems, and social impairment supports a diagnosis of somatization disorder. In addition, men are more likely to suffer from anxiety disorders than from somatization disorder.

Persons with mood disorders (depression or mania but especially depression) may present with somatic complaints, primarily headaches, gastrointestinal disturbances, or unexplained pains. These symptoms resolve with treatment of the mood disorder, whereas in somatization disorder the physical complaints continue. From the other perspective, persons with somatization disorder often present with depressive complaints (Wetzel et al. 1994). In fact, as described by DeSouza et al. (1988), patients with somatization disorder who fulfilled criteria for major depression had more depressive complaints than did patients with major depression and some somatic complaints, but did not fulfill criteria for somatization disorder. In this study, somatization disorder patients were more likely to report guilt, decreased concentration, confused thinking, decreased self-esteem, self-deprecation, death wish, suicide plan, suicide attempt, and increased appetite, and to have a history of drug abuse and antisocial symptoms.

Individuals with schizophrenia may present with unexplained somatic complaints. Careful evaluation will reveal delusions, hallucinations, and/or a formal thought disorder. Rarely will the somatic symptoms be extensive enough to meet the criteria for somatization disorder. If so, however, both diagnoses can be made. Occasionally a patient with extensive somatization symptomatology and no evidence of psychosis will subsequently develop the clinical picture of schizophrenia (Goodwin and Guze 1989).

☐ Course

Somatization disorder is unusual in children younger than age 9. In the majority of cases, characteristic symptoms begin during adolescence, and the criteria are satisfied by the mid-20s (Guze and Perley 1963). Somatization disorder is a chronic illness with fluctuations in the frequency and diversity of symptoms, but it rarely, if ever, remits (Guze et al. 1986). The most active symptomatic phase is usually early adulthood, but aging does not lead to total remission. Pribor et al. (1994) found that somatization disorder patients 55 years of age and older did not differ from younger patients in terms of the number of somatization symptoms or the utilization of health care services.

The most frequent and important complications of somatization disorder are repeated surgical operations, drug dependence, marital separation or divorce, and suicide attempts (Goodwin and Guze 1989). Because of awareness that somatization disorder is an explanation for various pains and other symptoms, invasive techniques can be withheld or postponed when objective indications are equivocal. Avoidance of prescribing habit-forming or addictive substances for recurrent or persistent complaints of pain should be paramount in the mind of the treating physician.

☐ Epidemiology

The lifetime risk for somatization disorder is estimated at about 2–3% in women when age at onset and method of assessment are taken into account (Cloninger et al. 1984). However the ECA study (Robins et al. 1984) found a lifetime risk of somatization disorder of only 0.2% to 0.3% of women. It is thought that the prevalence of somatization disorder is underestimated in studies, such as ECA, relying on interviews by non-physicians.

Somatization disorder is diagnosed predominantly in women, rarely in men. Some have suggested that this may be artifactual since the somatization disorder criteria are biased against making the diagnosis in men because some of the symptoms are inapplicable (e.g., pregnancy and menstrual complaints). Also, noting that men tend to report fewer symptoms than do women, some investigators have suggested that a mechanism be developed to adjust for this discrepancy (Temoshok and Attkisson 1977). However, when criteria to equalize men and women were applied, men had a mixed picture of anxiety and personality disorders and a syndrome that did not cluster in families with somatization disorder subjects of either gender (Cloninger 1986).

☐ Etiology

The etiology of somatization disorder is unknown, but it is clearly a familial disorder. From a number of studies, it appears that approximately 20% of the female first-degree relatives of patients with somatization disorder also meet criteria for this disorder (Guze et al. 1986). Several studies have suggested that male relatives of female patients with somatization disorder have an increased risk of antisocial personality disorder and alcoholism (Cloninger 1986). Somatization in women appears to share a common etiology with antisocial personality; somatization in men may be more related to anxiety disorders (Cloninger et al. 1986).

Bohman et al. (1984) found that women adopted prior to age 3 years had a fivefold increase in"high frequency somatization," (characterized by frequent headaches, backaches, gastrointestinal disturbances, and gynecological complaints) if their biological parents were alcoholic or antisocial. It was also noted that risk of somatization disorder in the adopted children varied according to the social status of the adoptive parents. These findings indicate that both biological and environmental factors contribute to the development of this disorder.

Experimental neuropsychological testing indicates that individuals with somatization disorder demonstrate difficulty with information processing related to problems with attention and memory (Almgren et al. 1978). Flor-Henry et al. (1981) found that, in comparison with normal controls, subjects with somatization disorder had bilateral, symmetrical patterns of frontal lobe dysfunction. The authors also noted increased nondominant hemisphere dysfunction in the anterior as opposed to the posterior regions as well as dominant hemisphere impairment. This latter finding is consistent with findings in antisocial personality disorder.

☐ Treatment

Somatization disorder is difficult to treat, and there appears to be no single superior treatment approach (Murphy 1982). Although primary care physicians can generally manage patients with somatization disorder adequately, the expertise of a psychiatrist is often useful. In a prospective, randomized, controlled study, Smith et al. (1986) found a reduction in health care costs in patients with somatization disorder receiving a psychiatric consultation relative to the time prior to the consultation, as well as in comparison to costs in those who did not receive such consultation.

The general principles of treatment for somatization disorder (Cloninger 1986; Smith et al. 1986) include the following goals: 1) to establish a firm therapeutic alliance with the patient; 2) to educate the patient regarding the manifestations of somatization disorder; and 3) to provide consistent reassurance. Implementation of these principles may prevent potentially serious complications, including the effects of unnecessary diagnostic and therapeutic procedures. A review of relevant literature did not reveal the superiority of any more specific treatment approaches (Kellner 1989).

Establishing a firm "therapeutic alliance" is often difficult with somatization disorder patients. Generally, these patients have already visited multiple physicians; they often have been advised that no explanation could be identified for their disorder, and have received the message that their difficulty is "mental," "psychological," or "psychiatric" in origin. To circumvent this, a therapeutic alliance is necessary. The first step in establishing such an alliance is to acknowledge the patient's pain and to convey an interest in providing help. Conducting an exhaustive review of the patient's medical history can then strengthen the therapeutic bond by demonstrating the physician's willingness to take the time and effort to understand the patient.

With respect to the principle of "education," Cloninger (1986) favors informing the patient of the diagnosis and describing the various facets of somatization disorder in a positive light. Advising the patient that he or she is not "crazy" but is suffering from a medically recognized illness, and that the condition will not lead to chronic mental or physical deterioration or death, may bring some comfort.

Patients with somatization disorder often become concerned that the physician is not performing a sufficiently thorough evaluation and may threaten to seek care from a different physician. Such challenges should be directly addressed with reassurance that the possiblity of an undiscovered physical illness is being appropriately assessed on a continuing basis and that changing physicians would place decisions in the hands of someone unaware of the complexities of their case. The patient should be reassured that there is no evidence of physical cause for the complaint but that there may be a link with "stress." A thorough review of complaints often identifies a temporal association with interpersonal, social, or occupational problems. Discussion may help the patient gain insight into such linkages. In patients for whom introspection is difficult, simple behavioral management techniques may be useful.

Use of prescription medications for patients with somatization disorder who complain of anxiety or depression should be held to a minimum and carefully monitored. Wheatley (1965) found that low doses of anxiolytic drugs provided some symptom improvement in a series of double-blind clinical trials. The use of pharmacotherapy must be tempered with the knowledge that these patients may take medicines inconsistently and unpredictably, develop drug dependence, and overdose in suicide attempts or gestures.

The clinician should develop a relationship with the patient's family. This facilitates attaining a better appreciation of the patient's social structure, which may be crucial to the understanding and management of the somatization disorder patient's often chaotic personal life-style. When appropriate, the clinician must place firm limits on excessive demands, manipulations, and attention seeking (Murphy 1982).

■ UNDIFFERENTIATED SOMATOFORM DISORDER

The essential aspect of undifferentiated somatoform disorder is the presence of one or more clinically significant medically unexplained somatic symptoms with a duration of 6 months or more that are not better accounted for by another mental disorder, such as multiple sclerosis (MS), systemic lupus erythematosus (SLE) or acute intermittent porphyria. In effect, this category serves to capture syndromes that resemble somatization disorder but do not meet the full criteria. Symptoms that may be seen include the same as those that are considered for somatization disorder.

☐ Diagnosis and Differential Diagnosis

Principal diagnostic considerations include the question of whether or not, with follow-up, criteria for somatization disorder will be met. Patients with somatization disorder are typically inconsistent historians, such that at one evaluation they may report a large number of symptoms and fulfill criteria for the full syndrome, while at another time they may report many fewer symptoms, perhaps only fulfilling criteria for an abridged syndrome (Martin et al. 1979). Another consideration is whether the somatic symptoms qualifying a patient for a diagnosis of undifferentiated somatoform disorder are the manifestation of a depressive or an anxiety disorder. Indeed, high rates of major depression and anxiety disorders have been found in somatizing patients attending family medicine clinics (Kirmayer et al. 1993).

☐ Epidemiology

Some investigators have argued that undifferentiated somatoform disorder is the most common somatoform disorder. Escobar et al. (1991), using a construct requiring six somatic symptoms for women and four for men, reported that in the United States 11% of non-Hispanic whites and Hispanics, and 15% of blacks, and in Puerto Rico 20% of Puerto Ricans fulfilled the criteria. A preponderance of women was evident in all groups except the Puerto Rican sample.

☐ Etiology

If undifferentiated somatoform disorder is an abridged form of somatization disorder, etiological theories reviewed under that diagnosis should apply here also. Of theoretical interest would be the question of why the syndrome is fully expressed in some and only partially in others. Some investigators have postulated that somatization can be viewed as a pattern of illness behavior by which bodily idioms of distress serve as symbolic means of social regulation as well as protest (Kirmayer and Robbins 1991).

☐ Treatment

A number of studies suggest that psychotherapy of a supportive, rather than a nondirective, type promotes improvement. However, a substantial proportion of patients improve or recover with no formal psychotherapy. Judicious use of pharmacotherapy may be of benefit: antidepressant medications for patients with depressive syndromes, and benzodiazepines and propranolol for patients with anxiety symptoms.

■ CONVERSION DISORDER

The essential features of conversion disorder are nonintentional symptoms or deficits affecting voluntary motor or sensory function that suggest yet are not fully explained by a neurological or other general medical condition, the direct effects of a substance, or as a culturally sanctioned behavior or experience. Specific conversion symptoms mentioned in DSM-IV include motor symptoms such as impaired coordination or balance, paralysis or localized weakness, tremor, difficulty swallowing or lump in throat (e.g., "globus hystericus"), aphonia, and urinary retention; sensory symptoms including hallucinations, loss of touch or pain sensation, double vision, blindness, and deafness; and seizures or convulsions with voluntary motor or sensory components. Single episodes usually involve one symptom, but, longitudinally, other conversion symptoms will be evident as well. Psychological factors may be involved in that symptoms often occur in the context of a conflictual situation that is resolved, at least in part, with the development of the symptom.

☐ Diagnosis and Differential Diagnosis

As defined in DSM-IV (Table 16–3), nonintentional "symptoms or deficits affecting voluntary motor or sensory function" (American Psychiatric Association 1994) are central to conversion disorder. The majority of such symptoms will suggest a neurological condition (i.e., are "pseudoneurological"), but other general medical conditions may be suggested as well. By definition, symptoms limited to pain or disturbance in sexual functioning are not included.

As in the other somatoform disorders, symptoms cannot be fully explained by a known physical disorder, and are not fully explained as a "culturally sanctioned behavior or experience." Symptoms occurring in conjunction with certain religious ceremonies such as "seizure-like episodes," and culturally expected responses such as women "swooning" in certain cultures and eras, would qualify as examples.

DSM-IV specifies that the symptoms in conversion disorder are not intentionally produced, thus distinguishing conversion symptoms from those of malingering or a factitious disorder. While this judgment is often difficult, it is important because the management and prognosis of these conditions are markedly different. Clinical judgment is also required in determining whether psychological factors are etiologically related to the symptom. Inclusion of this criterion is perhaps a holdover from the initial conceptualization of conversion symptoms as representing the "conversion" of unconscious psychic conflict into a physical symptom. As reviewed by Cloninger (1987), such determination is virtually impossible except in cases in which there is a temporal relationship between a psychosocial stressor and the symptom, or in cases in which similar situations led to conversion symptoms in the past.

A major diagnostic problem is that symptoms of neurological or general medical conditions are misdiagnosed as conversion. A number of studies have found that significant proportions of patients with diag-

---

Table 16–3.   DSM-IV diagnostic criteria for conversion disorder

A.   One or more symptoms or deficits affecting voluntary motor or sensory function that suggest a neurological or other general medical condition.

B.   Psychological factors are judged to be associated with the symptom or deficit because the initiation or exacerbation of the symptom or deficit is preceded by conflicts or other stressors.

C.   The symptom or deficit is not intentionally produced or feigned (as in factitious disorder or malingering).

D.   The symptom or deficit cannot, after appropriate investigation, be fully explained by a general medical condition, or by the direct effects of a substance, or as a culturally sanctioned behavior or experience.

E.   The symptom or deficit causes clinically significant distress or impairment in social, occupational, or other important areas of functioning or warrants medical evaluation.

F.   The symptom or deficit is not limited to pain or sexual dysfunction, does not occur exclusively during the course of somatization disorder, and is not better accounted for by another mental disorder.

Specify type of symptom or deficit:

With motor symptom or deficit
With sensory symptom or deficit
With seizures or convulsions
With mixed presentation

---

nosed conversion symptoms have neurological illness on follow-up. Slater and Glithero (1965) found a rate of 50% during a 7- to 11-year follow-up, while Gatfield and Guze (1962) reported 21%. These studies underscore the need to remain tentative in making a diagnosis of conversion disorder.

Symptoms of many neurological illnesses may appear inconsistent with known neurophysiology or neuropathology, and suggest conversion. Such diseases include MS (consider blindness secondary to optic neuritis with initially normal fundi), myasthenia gravis, periodic paralysis, myoglobinuric myopathy, polymyositis, other acquired myopathies (all of which may present with marked weakness in the presence of normal deep tendon reflexes), and Guillain-Barré syndrome, in which early weakness of the arms and legs may be inconsistent (Cloninger 1986). As reviewed by Ford and Folks (1985), over 13% of actual neurological cases are diagnosed as "functional" before the elucidation of a neurological illness.

Further complicating diagnosis is the fact that physical illness and conversion (or other apparent psychiatric overlay) are not mutually exclusive. Patients with physical illnesses that are incapacitating and frightening may appear to be exaggerating symptoms. Also, patients with actual neurological illness may have "pseudosymptoms" as well.

The most reliable predictor that a patient with apparent conversion symptoms will not later be shown to have a physical disorder is a history of previous conversion or other unexplained symptoms (Cloninger 1986). When apparent conversion symptoms occur in the context of somatization disorder, an underlying physical disorder is unlikely. Conversion symptoms first occurring in middle age or later should increase suspicion of an occult physical illness.

DSM-IV text lists "hallucinations" among the sensory nervous system conversion symptoms. Generally, conversion disorder hallucinations differ in several ways from hallucinations in psychotic conditions and are referred to by some as "pseudohallucinations." Conversion disorder hallucinations typically occur in the absence of other psychotic symptoms. Insight that the hallucinations are not "real" is generally retained. Whereas hallucinations in psychoses generally involve a single sensory modality (especially auditory, secondarily tactile), conversion hallucinations often involve more than one modality. They may have a naive, fantastic, or childish content as in a fairy tale, are described eagerly as an interesting story, and are often psychologically meaningful. Because hallucinations as part of psychoses may also share some of these features, vigilance must be maintained for the emergence of other signs of psychosis. A diagnosis of conversion disorder should not be made if the hallucinations are better accounted for by posttraumatic stress disorder or dissociative identity disorder (i.e., multiple personality disorder).

By definition, conversion symptoms affect voluntary motor and sensory functioning, and dissociative symptoms affect memory and identity. Traditionally, such symptoms have been attributed to similar psychological mechanisms and often occur in the same individual, sometimes during the same episode of illness. Thus, patients with conversion disorder should be screened for dissociative symptoms, and patients with a dissociative disorder should be evaluated for conversion symptoms.

□ Course

Onset is generally from late childhood to early adulthood. Conversion disorder is rare before the age of 10 (Maloney 1980) and seldom first presents after age 35, but has been reported to begin as late as the ninth decade (Weddington 1979). When onset is in middle or late age, the possibility of a neurological or other medical condition is increased. Onset is generally acute but may be characterized by gradually increasing symptomatology. The course of individual conversion symptoms is generally short, with from half (Folks et al. 1984) to nearly all (Carter 1949) patients showing disappearance of symptoms by the time of hospital discharge. However, from 20% to 25% will relapse within 1 year.

Factors associated with good prognosis include acute onset, presence of clearly identifiable stress at the time of onset, a short interval between onset and institution of treatment, and good intelligence (Toone 1990). Conversion blindness, aphonia, and paralysis are associated with relatively good prognosis, whereas conversion seizures and tremor are associated with poorer prognosis (Toone 1990). Generally, individual conversion symptoms are self-limited and do not lead to physical changes or disabilities. Risk of marital and occupational impairment is less than that in somatization disorder (Tomasson et al. 1991). In a long-term follow-up study of persons with conversion disorder, excess mortality by unnatural causes (but not suicide) was observed (Coryell and House 1984).

☐ Epidemiology

Lifetime prevalence rates of treated conversion symptoms in general populations have ranged from 11/100,000 to 300/100,000 (Ford and Folks 1985; Toone 1990). Conversion disorder appears to be more often diagnosed in women than in men, with ratios varying from 2:1 (Stefansson et al. 1976) to 10:1 (Raskin et al. 1966). In part, this may relate to referral patterns, but it also appears that indeed a predominance of women relative to men develop conversion symptoms.

From under 5% to 24% of psychiatric outpatients, 5% to 14% of general hospital patients, and 1% to 3% of outpatient psychiatric referrals have a history of conversion symptoms (Cloninger 1986; Toone 1990). There is an association with lower socioeconomic status, with less educated and less psychologically sophisticated and/or rural populations overrepresented (Martin and Yutzy 1994). Consistent with this finding, much higher rates (nearly 10%) of outpatient psychiatric referrals in developing countries are for conversion symptoms. As countries develop there may be a declining incidence over time, which may relate to increasing levels of education and sophistication (Stefanis et al. 1976).

☐ Etiology

The term "conversion" derives from the hypothesized "conversion" of psychological conflict into a somatic symptom. A number of psychological factors have been implicated in the pathogenesis, or at least pathophysiology, of conversion disorder.

Theoretically, conversion symptoms involve a "primary gain," whereby anxiety is reduced by keeping an internal conflict or need out of awareness by its symbolic expression. However, individuals with active conversion symptoms often continue to show marked anxiety, especially on psychological tests (Cloninger 1987). Symbolism is infrequently evident, and its evaluation involves highly inferential and unreliable judgments (Raskin et al. 1966). "Secondary gain," whereby conversion symptoms allow avoidance of noxious activities or the obtaining support, may also occur in persons with medical conditions taking advantage of such benefits (Watson and Buranen 1979).

Individuals with conversion disorder may show a lack of concern out of keeping with the nature or implications of the symptom (the so-called *la belle indifference*). However, indifference to symptoms is not invariably present in conversion disorder (Lewis and Berman 1965), and is also seen in individuals with general medical conditions, sometimes on the basis of denial or stoicism (Pincus 1982). Many persons with conversion disorder have a history of disturbed sexuality (Lewis 1974), with one-third reporting a history of sexual abuse, especially incestuous. Individuals with conversion disorder are reported to often be the youngest, or else the youngest of a sex, in sibling order, but these are not consistent findings (Stephens and Kamp 1962).

Accumulated data from twin studies show 9 concordant and 33 discordant monozygotic pairs, and no concordant and 43 discordant dizygotic pairs (Inouye 1972). Nongenetic familial factors, particularly incestuous childhood sexual abuse, may also be frequent. Nearly one-third of individuals with medically unexplained seizures reported childhood sexual abuse, as compared with less than 10% of those with complex partial epilepsy (Alper et al. 1993).

Many factors have been suggested as predisposing to conversion disorder, including preexisting personality disorders, rural backgrounds, and lack of psychological and medical sophistication. A tendency to conversion symptoms has been attributed to "modeling"—that is, patients with neurological disorders are likely to observe in others, as well as in themselves, various neurological symptoms that they at other times simulate as conversion symptoms.

☐ Treatment

Generally, the initial aim in treatment is the removal of the symptom(s). The urgency behind this depends on the degree of distress and disability (Merskey 1989). If the patient is not in particular discomfort, and the need to regain function is not great, decisive action may not be necessary. Direct confrontation is not recommended since this may cause intensified feelings of isolation. A conservative approach of reassurance and relaxation is effective, whether from a psychiatrist or the primary physician. Short-term prognosis is good; Folks et al. (1984) found that half of 50 general hospital patients with conversion symptoms showed complete remission by the time of discharge.

If symptoms do not resolve promptly, treatment is important since the duration of conversion symptoms is associated with greater risk of recurrence and chronic disability (Cloninger 1986). A number of techniques, including narcoanalysis, hypnotherapy, and behavior therapy, may be tried (Merskey 1989). In narcoanalysis, amobarbital or another sedative-hypnotic medication such as lorazepam is given to the patient intravenously to the point of drowsiness. This may be followed by administration of a stimulant medication such as methylamphetamine. The patient is then encouraged to discuss stressors and conflicts. This technique may be effective acutely, leading to at least temporary symptom relief and expansion of the information known about the patient but has not been shown to be effective with more chronic symptoms. In hypnotherapy, symptoms may be removed during a hypnotic state, with the suggestion that the symptoms will gradually improve posthypnotically. Behavior therapy, including relaxation training and even aversion therapy, has been proposed and reported to be effective.

■ HYPOCHONDRIASIS

The essential feature in hypochondriasis is the fear or idea of having a serious disease, based on the misinterpretation of bodily signs and sensations. The preoccupation persists despite evidence to the contrary and reassurance from physicians that the fears are groundless. As reviewed by Kellner (1987), 10% to 20% of "normal" and 45% of "neurotic" persons have intermittent, unfounded worries about illness, with 9% of patients doubting reassurances given by physicians. Kellner (1985) estimates that 50% of all patients attending physicians' offices have some degree of hypochondriacal symptomology.

☐ Diagnosis and Differential Diagnosis

Specific criteria for the diagnosis of hypochondriasis are presented in Table 16–4. "Bodily symptoms" may be interpreted broadly to include misinterpretation of normal bodily functions. The requirement that the preoccupation persist despite medical evaluation and reassurance emphasizes the disease conviction of the syndrome. The exclusionary criterion of delusion distinguishes hypochondriasis from delusional disorders, somatic type. To distinquish hypochondriasis from clinically insignificant states, the requirement for distress or impairment is as in the other somatoform disorders. A requirement of 6 months' duration distinguishes hypochondriasis from transient syndromes, the longitudinal course of which has been shown to be more variable, suggesting heterogeneity (Barsky et al. 1993).

The first step is to assess the possibility of physical disease. The list of serious diseases that may lead to the sort of complaints with which hypochondriacal patients present is extensive, yet certain general categories should be considered (Kellner 1987). These include neurological diseases such as myasthenia gravis and MS, endocrine diseases, systemic diseases such as SLE that affect several organ systems, and occult malignancies. One differentiating feature of patients with such diseases is that they may actually accept medical assurances (even though erroneuous) better than do patients with hypochondriasis.

Next, whether the hypochondriacal symptoms represent a primary disorder of hypochondriasis or are secondary to another psychiatric illness must be considered. Somatic delusions of serious illness are seen in some cases of major depressive disorder and with schizophrenia. Patients with hypochondriasis are generally able to acknowledge the possibility that their concerns are unfounded; delusional patients, on the other hand, are not. Generally, schizophrenic patients with delusions of the presence of a serious illness would also show other signs of schizophrenia such as looseness of associations, peculiarities of thought and behavior, hallucinations, and other delusions. A patient with hypochondriasis secondary to depression should show other symptoms of depression such as dysphoric mood, sleep and appetite disturbances, feelings of worthlessness, self-reproach, and so forth, although particularly elderly patients may deny sadness or other expressions of depressed mood. Patients with obsessive-compulsive disorder may also have preoccupations

---

Table 16–4.   DSM-IV diagnostic criteria for hypochondriasis

A.   Preoccupation with fears of having, or the idea that one has, a serious disease based on the person's misinterpretation of bodily symptoms.

B.   The preoccupation persists despite appropriate medical evaluation and reassurance.

C.   The belief in criterion A is not of delusional intensity (as in delusional disorder, somatic type) and is not restricted to a circumscribed concern about appearance (as in body dysmorphic disorder).

D.   The preoccupation causes clinically significant distress or impairment in social, occupational, or other important areas of functioning.

E.   The duration of the disturbance is at least 6 months.

F.   The preoccupation is not better accounted for by generalized anxiety disorder, obsessive-compulsive disorder, panic disorder, a major depressive episode, separation anxiety, or another somatoform disorder.

Specify if:
With poor insight: if, for most of the time during the current episode, the person does not recognize that the concern about having a serious illness is excessive or unreasonable

with illness. The presence of other nonhealth-related preoccupations distinguishes such patients.

☐ Course

Limited data suggest that approximately one-quarter of patients with a diagnosis of hypochondriasis do poorly, two-thirds show a chronic but fluctuating course, and one-tenth recover. A much more variable course is seen in patients with just some hypochondriacal concerns.

☐ Etiology

Hypochondriasis has been discussed extensively in the psychoanalytic literature, with a number of explanatory theories suggested. Freud hypothesized that hypochondriasis represented "the return of object libido onto the ego with cathexis to the body" (Viederman 1985). This theory has formed the basis for a number of psychoanalytic interpretations, including disturbed object relations, and repressed hostility displaced to the body so that anger can be communicated indirectly to others, as well as dynamics involving masochism, guilt, conflicted dependency needs, and a need to suffer and be loved at the same time (Stoudemire 1988). Such a "narcissistic" mechanism has been thought to make such patients unanalyzable. Other psychological theories involve defenses against feelings of low self-esteem and inadequacy, perceptual and cognitive abnormalities, and reinforcement for assuming the "sick role."

☐ Treatment

Depressive and even anxiety symptoms secondary to hypochondriasis may improve with appropriate pharmacological intervention. Hypochondriasis as a primary condition does not seem to be responsive to psychopharmacological drugs, although recently selective serotonin reuptake inhibitors such as fluoxetine, sertraline and paroxetine, have shown promise.

Overall, hypochondriacal patients benefit from psychiatric intervention. Patients referred early for psychiatric evaluation and treatment have a better prognosis than those continuing with only medical evaluations and treatments. A large number of psychotherapeutic approaches have been tried, including supportive, rational, ventilative, and educative approaches (Kellner 1987). Hospitalization, unnecessary medical tests, and medications with addictive potential are to be avoided. Focus should gradually be shifted from symptoms to social or interpersonal problems. Such a plan may be too time-consuming for a busy primary care physician and may require the involvement of other professionals.

■ BODY DYSMORPHIC DISORDER

The essential feature of body dysmorphic disorder is a preoccupation with some imagined defect in appearance, or a markedly excessive concern with a minor physical anomaly (Table 16–5). Such preoccupation persists even after medical reassurances. Complaints include a diversity of imagined flaws of the face or head, including various defects in the hair (too much or too little), skin, shape of the face, or facial features. However, other body parts may be the focus, including genitals, breasts, buttocks, the extremities, and shoulders, and even overall body size. De Leon et al. (1989) stated that the nose, ears, face, or sexual organs are most often involved. Patients with body dysmorphic disorder are often found among persons seeking cosmetic surgery.

☐ Diagnosis and Differential Diagnosis

In DSM-IV, the essential feature of body dysmorphic disorder is preoccupation with an imagined defect in appearance, or markedly excessive concern for a slight anomaly. In DSM-IV, diagnosis requires that the preoccupation causes clinically significant distress or impairment to exclude trivial symptoms. Body dysmorphic disorder is not diagnosed when the body preoccupation is better accounted for by another mental disorder. Anorexia nervosa, in which there is dissatisfaction with body shape and size, is specifically mentioned in the criteria as an example of such a situation. If preoccupation is limited to discomfort or a sense of inappropriateness of one's primary and secondary sex characteristics, coupled with a strong and persistent cross-gender identification, body dysmorphic disorder would not be diagnosed.

Mood-congruent ruminations of major depression sometimes involve concern with an unattractive appearance in association with poor self-esteem, but such preoccupations generally lack the focus on a particular body part that is seen in body dysmorphic disorder. The preoccupations of body dysmorphic disorder may resemble obsessions and ruminations as seen in obsessive-compulsive disorder. In body dysmorphic disorder the preoccupations are limited to concerns with appear-

---

Table 16–5.   DSM-IV diagnostic criteria for body dysmorphic disorder

A.   Preoccupation with an imagined defect in appearance. If a slight physical anomaly is present, the person's concern is markedly excessive.

B.   The preoccupation causes clinically significant distress or impairment in social, occupational, or other important areas of functioning.

C.   The preoccupation is not better accounted for by another mental disorder (e.g., dissatisfaction with body shape and size in anorexia nervosa).

---

ance. Preoccupations in body dysmorphic disorder may reach delusional proportions, and patients with this disorder may show ideas of reference in regard to defects in their appearance, which may lead to the consideration of schizophrenia. However, other bizarre delusions and hallucinations are not seen in body dysmorphic disorder. Unlike in hypochondriasis, if the preoccupation is of psychotic proportions, a diagnosis of body dysmorphic disorder can still be made.

In body dysmorphic disorder, it appears that a continuum exists between preoccupations and delusions and individual patients seem to move along this continuum. Some investigators suggest that any boundary between the two would be artificial. Both body dysmorphic disorder and delusional disorder, somatic type diagnoses can be made if a dysmorphic preoccupation is delusional.

Because patients with body dysmorphic disorder often become isolative, social phobia may be suspected. Indeed, the two conditions may coexist. In social phobia alone, however, the person may feel self-conscious but will not focus on a specific imagined defect. Persons with histrionic personality disorder may be vain and excessively concerned with appearance. However, in this disorder, the focus is on maintaining a good or even exceptional appearance, rather than preoccupation with a defect.

☐ Course

Onset may have two peaks: one in adolescence or early adulthood, and the other, at least for women, at menopause (De Leon et al. 1989). It is thought that the late-onset cases are generally associated with mood disorders. Body dysmorphic disorder is generally a chronic condition, with a waxing and waning of intensity, but rarely full remission. In some persons, the same preoccupation remains unchanged, but over a lifetime, multiple preoccupations are typical; one study found an average of four preoccupations (Phillips et al. 1993). In others, preoccupations with newly perceived defects are added to the original ones. In others still, symptoms remit, only to be replaced by others.

Body dysmorphic disorder is highly incapacitating. Almost all persons with this disorder show marked impairment in social and occupational activities. Perhaps a third become housebound. Most attribute their limitations to embarrassment concerning their "defect." Superimposed depressive episodes are common, as are suicidal ideation and suicide attempts.

☐ Epidemiology

Andreasen and Bardach (1977) estimated that 2% of patients seeking corrective cosmetic surgery suffer from this disorder. Generally, patients with body dysmorphic disorder are seen psychiatrically only after referral from plastic surgery, dermatology, and otorhinolaryngology clinics (De Leon et al. 1989).

☐ Treatment

Simply recognizing that a complaint derives from body dysmorphic disorder may have therapeutic benefit by interrupting an unending procession of repeated evaluations by additional physicians, and the possiblity of needless surgery. Surgery has actually been recommended as a treatment for this disorder, but there is no clear evidence that this is effective. There are anecdotal reports of benefit from a diversity of treatments, including behavior therapy, dynamic psychotherapy, and pharmacotherapy, the last involving neuroleptics and antidepressants, particularly monoamine oxidase inhibitors (De Leon et al. 1989) and, more recently, selective serotonin reuptake inhibitors (Phillips et al. 1993).

The delusional syndromes often respond to neuroleptics, whereas body dysmorphic disorder, even when the bodily preoccupations are psychotic, does not. Pimozide has been singled out as a neuroleptic having specific effectiveness for somatic delusions, but this drug does not appear to be any more effective than other neuroleptics in treating body dysmorphic disorder. Some reports of positive response to antidepressant drugs may be due to improvement in depressive symptoms rather than direct effects on dysmorphic body disorder. Exceptions may be treatment with clomipramine or selective serotonin reuptake inhibitors, such as fluoxetine, with which over 50% of patients with body dysmorphic disorder showed a partial or complete remission, a response not predicted on the basis of coexisting major depression or obsessive-compulsive disorder (Phillips et al. 1993).

■ SOMATOFORM DISORDER NOT OTHERWISE SPECIFIED

Somatoform disorder not otherwise specified (NOS) is the true residual category for the somatoform disorders. Disorders considered under this category are characterized by somatic symptoms but do not meet criteria for any of the "specified" somatoform disorders or for undifferentiated somatoform disorder, which requires a 6-month duration. In fact, some disorders may be relegated to "NOS" on the basis that they do not meet the time requirements for a specified somatoform disorder.

☐ Diagnosis and Differential Diagnosis

The basic requirement is for a disorder with somatoform symptoms that does not meet the criteria for a "specified" somatoform disorder. With the restriction of conversion to voluntary motor and sensory function, pseudocyesis was relegated to the NOS category (Table 16–6); however, given its rarity, it is not listed as a "specified" somatoform disorder. Unlike delusional pregnancies, pseudocyesis is associated with objective signs of pregnancy (Small 1986). While, in most, if not all, cases a neuroendocrine change accompanies, or at times antedates, the false belief of pregnancy, in pseudocyesis a discrete general medical conditon (such as a hormone-secreting tumor) cannot be identified.

☐ Epidemiology, Etiology, and Treatment

A syndrome that would warrant a "specified" somatoform disorder diagnosis except for insufficient duration (less than 6 months) is probably best considered to be in the "spectrum" of the resembled disorder. Thus, the epidemiological, etiological, and treatment considerations pertaining to the "specified" disorder should be reviewed, for these may apply, at least in part, to the briefer syndromes. As to treatment, Whelan and Stewart (1990) emphasize two principles. First, the patient is to be clearly, yet "empathically" advised that she (or the rare he) is not pregnant. If this fails, objective procedures such as ultrasound are recommended to demonstrate to the patient that there is no visible evidence of a fetus. Alternatively, menses are to be induced. Such straightforward approaches are often effective (Cohen 1982). The second principle is that the patient's expectations, fears, and fantasies be explored to discover the "reason" that the false pregnancy was "needed." It is also advised to provide a

---

Table 16–6. DSM-IV diagnostic criteria for somatoform disorder not otherwise specified

This category includes disorders with somatoform symptoms that do not meet the criteria for any specific somatoform disorder. Examples include

1. *Pseudocyesis:* a false belief of being pregnant that is associated with objective signs of pregnancy, which may include abdominal enlargement (although the umbilicus does not become everted), reduced menstrual flow, amenorrhea, subjective sensation of fetal movement, nausea, breast engorgement and secretions, and labor pains at the expected date of delivery. Endocrine changes may be present, but the syndrome cannot be explained by a general medical condition that causes endocrine changes (e.g., a hormone-secreting tumor).

2. A disorder involving nonpsychotic hypochondriacal symptoms of less than 6 months' duration.

3. A disorder involving unexplained physical complaints (e.g., fatigue or body weakness) of less than 6 months' duration that are not due to another mental disorder.

"face-saving" resolution to the patient's lack of pregnancy such as allowing the patient to take the position that a "miscarriage" has occurred. Whatever the therapy, relapses are common. Concomitant disorders such as major depression should be treated in the usual manner.

■ REFERENCES

Almgren P-E, Nordgren L, Skantze H: A retrospective study of operationally defined hysterics. Br J Psychiatry 132:67–73, 1978

Alper K, Devinsky O, Vasquez B, et al: Nonepileptic seizures and childhood sexual and physical abuse. Neurology 43:1950–1953, 1993

American Psychiatric Association: Diagnostic and Statistical Manual of Mental Disorders, 3rd Edition. Washington, DC, American Psychiatric Association, 1980

American Psychiatric Association: Diagnostic and Statistical Manual of Mental Disorders, 4th Edition. Washington, DC, American Psychiatric Association, 1994

Andreasen NC, Bardach J: Dysmorphophobia: symptom or disease? Am J Psychiatry 134:673–676, 1977

Barsky AJ, Cleary PD, Sarnie MK, et al: The course of transient hypochondriasis. Am J Psychiatry 150:484–488, 1993

Bohman M, Cloninger CR, von Knorring A-L, et al: An adoption study of somatoform disorders, III: cross-fostering analysis and genetic relationship to alcoholism and criminality. Arch Gen Psychiatry 41:872–878, 1984

Carter AB: The prognosis of certain hysterical symptoms. BMJ 1:1076–1079, 1949

Cloninger CR: Somatoform and dissociative disorders, in The Medical Basis of Psychiatry. Edited by Winokur G, Clayton P[J]. Philadelphia, PA, WB Saunders, 1986, pp 123–151

Cloninger CR: Diagnosis of somatoform disorders: a critique of DSM-III, in Diagnosis and Classification in Psychiatry: A Critical Appraisal of DSM-III. Edited by Tischler GL. New York, Cambridge University Press, 1987, pp 243–259

Cloninger CR, Sigvardsson S, von Knorring A-L, et al: An adoption study of somatoform disorders, II: identification of two discrete somatoform disorders. Arch Gen Psychiatry 41:863–871, 1984

Cloninger CR, Martin RL, Guze SB, et al: A prospective follow-up and family study of somatization in men and women. Am J Psychiatry 143:873–878, 1986

Cohen LM: A current perspective of pseudocyesis. Am J Psychiatry 139:1140–1144, 1982

Coryell W, House D: The validity of broadly defined hysteria and DSM-III conversion disorder: outcome, family history, and mortality. J Clin Psychiatry 45:252–256, 1984

De Leon J, Bott A, Simpson GM: Dysmorphophobia: body dysmorphic disorder or delusional disorder, somatic subtype? Compr Psychiatry 30:457–472, 1989

DeSouza C, Othmer E, Gabrielli W Jr, et al: Major depression and somatization disorder: the overlooked differential diagnosis. Psychiatric Annals 18:340–348, 1988

Escobar JI, Swartz M, Rubio-Stipec M, et al: Medically unexplained symptoms: distribution, risk factors, and comorbidity, in Current Concepts of Somatization: Research and Clinical Perspectives. Edited by Kirmayer LJ, Robbins JM. Washington, DC, American Psychiatric Press, 1991, pp 63–78

Flor-Henry P, Fromm-Auch D, Tapper M, et al: A neuropsychological study of the stable syndrome of hysteria. Biol Psychiatry 16:601–626, 1981

Folks DG, Ford CV, Regan WM: Conversion symptoms in a general hospital. Psychosomatics 25:285–295, 1984

Ford CV, Folks DG: Conversion disorders: an overview. Psychosomatics 26:371–383, 1985

Gatfield PD, Guze SB: Prognosis and differential diagnosis of conversion reactions (a follow-up study). Diseases of the Nervous System 23:623–631, 1962

Goodwin DW, Guze SB: Psychiatric Diagnosis, 4th Edition. New York, Oxford University Press, 1989

Guze SB, Perley MJ: Observations on the natural history of hysteria. Am J Psychiatry 119:960–965, 1963

Guze SB, Cloninger CR, Martin RL, et al: A follow-up and family study of Briquet's syndrome. Br J Psychiatry 149:17–23, 1986

Inouye E: Genetic aspects of neurosis. International Journal of Mental Health 1:176–189, 1972

Kellner R: Functional somatic symptoms and hypochondriasis: a survey of empirical studies. Arch Gen Psychiatry 42:821–833, 1985

Kellner R: Hypochondriasis and somatization. JAMA 258:2718–2722, 1987

Kellner R: Somatization disorder, in Treatments of Psychiatric Disorders: A Task Force Report of the American Psychiatric Association, Vol 3. Washington, DC, American Psychiatric Association, 1989, pp 2166–2171

Kirmayer LJ, Robbins JM: Introduction: concepts of somatization, in Current Concepts of Somatization: Research and Clinical Perspectives. Edited by Kirmayer LJ, Robbins JM. Washington, DC, American Psychiatric Press, 1991, pp 1–19

Kirmayer LJ, Robbins JM, Dworkind M, et al: Somatization and the recognition of depression and anxiety in primary care. Am J Psychiatry 150:734–741, 1993

Lewis WC: Hysteria: the consultant's dilemma: twentieth century demonology, pejorative epithet, or useful diagnosis? Arch Gen Psychiatry 30:145–151, 1974

Lewis WC, Berman M: Studies of conversion hysteria, I: operational study of diagnosis. Arch Gen Psychiatry 13:275–282, 1965

Maloney MJ: Diagnosing hysterical conversion disorders in children. J Pediatr 97:1016–1020, 1980

Martin RL, Yutzy SH: Somatoform disorders, in American Psychiatric Press Textbook of Psychiatry, Second edition. Edited by Hales RE, Yudofsky SC, Talbott JA. Washington, DC, American Psychiatric Press, 1994, pp 591–622

Martin RL, Cloninger CR, Guze SB: The evaluation of diagnostic concordance in follow-up studies, II: a blind prospective follow-up of female criminals. J Psychiatr Res 15:107–125, 1979

Merskey H: Conversion disorder, in Treatments of Psychiatric Disorders: A Task Force Report of the American Psychiatric Association, Vol 3. Washington, DC, American Psychiatric Association, 1989, pp 2152–2159

Murphy GE: The clinical management of hysteria. JAMA 247:2559–2564, 1982

Murphy MR: Classification of the somatoform disorders, in Somatization: Physical Symptoms and Psychological Illness. Edited by Bass C. Oxford, UK, Blackwell Scientific, 1990, pp 10–39

Phillips KA, McElroy SL, Keck PE Jr, et al: Body dysmorphic disorder: 30 cases of imagined ugliness. Am J Psychiatry 150:302–308, 1993

Pincus J: Hysteria presenting to a neurologist, in Hysteria. Edited by Roy A. London, Wiley, 1982, pp 131–144

Pribor EF, Smith DS, Yutzy SH: Somatization disorder in the elderly. Am J Geriatric Psychiatry 2:109–117, 1994

Raskin M, Talbott JA, Meyerson AT: Diagnosis of conversion reactions: predictive value of psychiatric criteria. JAMA 197:530–534, 1966

Robins LN, Helzer JE, Weissman MM, et al: Lifetime prevalence of specific psychiatric disorders in three sites. Arch Gen Psychiatry 41:949–958, 1984

Slater ETO, Glithero C: A follow-up of patients diagnosed as suffering from "hysteria." J Psychosom Res 9:9–13, 1965

Small GW: Pseudocyesis: an overview. Can J Psychiatry 31:452–457, 1986

Smith GR Jr, Monson RA, Ray DC: Psychiatric consultation in somatization disorder: a randomized controlled study. N Engl J Med 314:1407–1413, 1986

Stefanis C, Markidis M, Christodoulou G: Observations on the evolution of the hysterical symptomatology. Br J Psychiatry 128:269–275, 1976

Stefansson JH, Messina JA, Meyerowitz S: Hysterical neurosis, conversion type: clinical and epidemiological considerations. Acta Psychiatr Scand 59:119–138, 1976

Stephens JH, Kamp M: On some aspects of hysteria: a clinical study. J Nerv Ment Dis 134:305–315, 1962

Stoudemire GA: Somatoform disorders, factitious disorders, and malingering, in American Psychiatric Press Textbook of Psychiatry. Edited by Talbott JA, Hales RE, Yudofsky SC. Washington, DC, American Psychiatric Press, 1988, pp 533–556

Temoshok L, Attkisson CC: Epidemiology of hysterical phenomena: evidence for a psychosocial theory, in Hysterical Personality. Edited by Horowitz MJ. New York, Jason Aronson, 1977, pp 143–222

Tomasson K, Kent D, Coryell W: Somatization and conversion disorders: comorbidity and demographics at presentation. Acta Psychiatr Scand 84:288–293, 1991

Toone BK: Disorders of hysterical conversion, in Physical Symptoms and Psychological Illness. Edited by Bass C. London, Blackwell Scientific, 1990, pp 207–234

Viederman M: Somatoform and factitious disorders, in Psychiatry, Vol 1. Edited by Cavenar JO. Philadelphia, PA, JB Lippincott, 1985

Watson CG, Buranen C: The frequency and identification of false positive conversion reactions. J Nerv Ment Dis 167:243–247, 1979

Weddington WW: Conversion reaction in an 82-year-old man. J Nerv Ment Dis 167:368–369, 1979

Wetzel RD, Guze SB, Cloninger CR, et al: Briquet's syndrome (hysteria) is both a somatoform and a "psychoform" illness: an MMPI study. Psychosom Med 56:554–569, 1994

Wheatley D: General practitioner clinical trials: chlordiazepoxide in anxiety states, II: long-term study. Practitioner 195:692–695, 1965

Whelan CI, Stewart DE: Pseudocyesis—a review and report of six cases. Int J Psychiatry 20:97–108, 1990

CHAPTER

17

Factitious Disorders and Malingering

John M. Plewes, M.D.
Joe G. Fagan, M.D.

■ FACTITIOUS DISORDERS

Factitious disorders have long been a medical enigma and are character-ized by the intentional production or feigning of physical or psychologi-cal signs or symptoms. Patients having this disorder frequently are misunderstood by clinicians and may receive innappropriate diagnostic and therapeutic interventions, often to the patients' detriment. Unlike malingerers, who may attempt to gain financial advantage, disability, or relief from onerous or dangerous duties (as in the military), persons with factitious disorder "seem to gain nothing except the discomfiture of un-necessary investigations or operations" (Asher 1951, p. 339). They appear to have only one goal: to take on the sick role (Tables 17–1 and 17–2).

The most notorious of the factitious disorders in DSM-IV (American Psychiatric Association 1994) is *Munchausen's syndrome*. In this special type of factitious disorder, pathological lying (*pseudologia fantastica*) is prominent. The patient shows a pattern of feigning illness at numerous hospital emergency rooms, often in different cities, gaining admission and sometimes receiving invasive procedures, becoming quarrelsome with the staff, and being discharged against medical advice when the ruse is discovered. In 1951, Asher initiated the use of the term Mun-chausen's syndrome to describe these patients. He drew the term from Rudolf Erich Raspe's book *Baron Münchausen's Narrative of His Marvelous Travels and Campaigns in Russia* (1784), which detailed the exaggerated

---

Table 17–1.   DSM-IV diagnostic criteria for factitious disorder

A.   Intentional production or feigning of physical or psychological signs or symptoms.

B.   The motivation for the behavior is to assume the sick role.

C.   External incentives for the behavior (such as economic gain, avoiding legal responsibility, or improving physical well-being, as in malingering) are absent.

Code based on type:

300.16   With predominantly psychological signs and symptoms: if psychological signs and symptoms predominate in the clinical presentation

300.19   With predominantly physical signs and symptoms: if physical signs and symptoms predominate in the clinical presentation

300.19   With combined psychological and physical signs and symptoms: if both psychological and physical signs and symptoms are present, but neither predominates in the clinical presentation

---

Table 17–2.   DSM-IV description of factitious disorder not otherwise specified

300.19 This category includes disorders with factitious symptoms that do not meet the criteria for factitious disorder. An example is factitious disorder by proxy: the intentional production or feigning of physical or psychological signs or symptoms in another person who is under the individual's care for the purpose of indirectly assuming the sick role.

---

accounts of the sporting and military adventures, as well as the peregrinations, of Baron Karl Friedrich Hieronymous von Münchausen. A former cavalry officer in the Russian army, Münchausen was widely known for his outrageous stories and his habit of wandering from town to town to find a new audience for them, and, as one might surmise, new admirers and benefactors.

Asher (1951) described three major patterns of the disorder. The first was the "acute abdominal type" in which the patient had a history of multiple abdominal surgeries leaving him or her with a "gridiron" pattern of surgical scars on the abdomen. The second type was characterized by simulated hemotysis or hematemesis and was called the "hemorrhagic type." The third type, the "neurological type," included presentations of feigned neurological symptoms such as headaches, seizures, or loss of consciousness.

Asher's description of the Munchausen syndrome has remained generally accepted by most clinicians and has been used for the majority of clinical presentations falling within the rubric of factitious disorder, including presentations with symptoms in the dermatological and cardiac systems, as well as for factitious fevers. Spiro in 1968 recommended that the term "chronic factitious illness" be substituted for Munchausen syndrome. Spiro's concern was that the Munchausen syndrome was too closely associated with lying, swindling, and the negative connotations of these behaviors. He suggested using the term chronic factitious illness because it was not pejorative and was more accurate and objective. In 1980, Spiro's term received formal recognition in DSM-III as *chronic factitious disorder with physical symptoms.* Munchausen syndrome remained, however, the preferred term, possibly because, as Nadelson (1979) noted, "the Baron's name is a more charming, evocative, antique, and noble reference and makes a more mouth-filling phrase" (p. 11).

Factitious disorders have been and continue to be controversial, because the establishment of the diagnosis requires the physician to deviate significantly from the traditional physician-patient relationship in order to determine whether the patient is or is not fabricating the signs and/or symptoms of an illness. The physician must then determine if the patient has consciously and willfully fabricated the illness. Finally the physician must conclude that the patient will not profit from the fabrication of the illness. The diagnostic process often creates an adversarial relationship between physician and patient that exacerbates the existing tendency within the factitious disorder patient to be truculent and frequently leads to premature disruption in the medical care. The diagnostic process also raises questions concerning ethics and patients' right to confidentiality.

Data on incidence and prevalence rates, etiology, natural course, diagnostic reliability and validity, and appropriateness of treatment for the factiticious disorders are difficult to gather and are accordingly suspect, because individuals with factitious disorder are unreliable historians and most of the reporting clinicians have not verified their data. Additionally, many of the case histories are abbreviated. Unfortunately, case reports give primarily a single cross-sectional look at a chronic disorder, and series of cases are hard to gather because of the deceptive and wandering nature of many of the patients. These patients are opportunistic in seeking medical attention and frequently change the nature and type of symptoms and signs with which they present in order to facilitate the desired medical attention or hospitalization. In fact, they often will shift their symptom complex during a single hospital stay.

In DSM-IV, factitious disorder is described by the general criteria for the disorder followed by codes used to differentiate between the types of signs and symptoms that predominate (Tables 17–1 and 17–2). The three codes are for predominantly physical, psychological, or combined physical and psychological symptoms and signs. The key word in the description of the disorder that defines the code is the word "predominantly"; the clinician should decide which of the signs or symptoms are the most important, and assign an appropriate code accordingly. Many patients will have both physical and psychological signs and symptoms, in which case the code for the combined type should be used. The code for factitious disorder NOS should be used for disorders with factitious symptoms that do not meet criteria for a specific factitious disorder.

☐ Differential Diagnosis

The most important differential diagnosis in a patient thought to have a factitious disorder is a "real" disorder—that is, a verifiable medical or surgical illness requiring intervention. Factitious patients are at first pleased to receive the care and attention of a physician who is attempting to unravel their history, signs, and symptoms and place these into a schema for investigation. The challenge to the physician is to distinguish between actual and feigned illness. Even if the patient is clumsy enough to be discovered in the deception, the fact that he or she may have had numerous abdominal surgical procedures, for example, may predispose him or her to actual intestinal obstruction, and the patient may be a candidate for yet another exploratory surgery. Also, patients may become seriously ill while carrying out their plan to be evaluated and treated. An example is the former nurse who repeatedly injected herself subcutaneously with saline contaminated with fecal material; she developed a true septicemia and an infection of her heart valves, and congestive heart failure resulted. The clinician must walk a delicate line: he or she must be alert to potential problems and pursue them vigorously, while minimizing, whenever possible, procedures or tests that are unneccessary or dangerous.

Pope et al. (1982), observing difficulties in distinguishing between factitious, malingering, and somatizing patient presentations, proposed that these disorders are closely related and should be studied as a group. Some of the diagnostic difficulties with these patients may be related to the differences in clinical presentations by males and females. Reference is made to the possibility that somatization disorder or conversion disorder in a female with an underlying histrionic personality disorder is equivalent to Munchausen syndrome or malingering in a male with an underlying antisocial personality disorder. In this model, the factitious symptoms and signs seen in the various diagnostic categories may simply represent gender-specific or culture-specific manifestations of a single disorder. Malingering should only be diagnosed in the absence of other psychiatric illness and in the presence of sociopathic behavior adaptive to a long-term goal (Spiro 1968).

Pope et al. further proposed that to distinguish factitious disorders from somatization disorder, conversion disorder, or malingering, the diagnostic focus should be on more objective factors such as demographics, associated phenomenology, biological findings (if any), family history, treatment response, and long-term outcome rather than on evaluating a patient's motivation in conscious or unconscious terms. In contrast, one should be aware that there is a commonly held view that somatization disorder, conversion disorder, and malingering are quite distinct, in terms of motivation for the behaviors, from the factitious disorders. Conversion disorder is felt to have unconscious causation and unconscious motivation; in DSM-IV, no mention is made of motivation, conscious or unconscious, for somatization disorder. Malingering is thought to have willful causation and the conscious motivation of secondary gain.

Other disorders that should be considered in the differential for factitious disorders are true psychoses (such as schizophrenia), mood disorders, and antisocial personality disorder. It may initially be difficult to distinguish feigned from true psychosis; however, with continued observation of behaviors and of the response to test doses of antipsychotic medications in a ward setting, inconsistencies in the presentation are revealed. The antisocial patient may also exhibit pseudologia fantastica, few close relationships, and a history of criminal activity and substance abuse, but these behaviors usually have an earlier onset than is the case in factitious disorder. Also, most antisocial patients do not seek a life of chronic hospitalization.

☐ Factitious Disorder by Proxy

Another type of factitious illness, described by Meadow (1977, 1982), is called *Munchausen syndrome by proxy* (although at least one attempt was made to call the disorder Meadow's syndrome, after its describer [O'Shea 1987]). In DSM-IV, this entity is termed *factitious disorder by proxy* and appears in the appendix as a diagnosis warranting further study. It is anticipated that with the aging of the population, clinicians should be alert to cases of factitious disorder by proxy in the elderly population, as well as in children.

In Meadow's original description, one person persistently fabricates symptoms or signs in another person for the purpose of indirectly assuming the sick role. In most cases, the situation includes a caretaker/victim (e.g., parent/child) dyad. In this type of factitious disorder, the gain to the caretaker is still to assume the sick role, but in an indirect fashion through the "victim." The psychiatric disorder is given to the person who induces the symptoms (e.g., the parent who feeds his child ground glass and presents the child as having "bloody stools"). However, if there is evidence that the individual with the symptoms colluded in their production, he or she receives the diagnosis of factitious disorder and the perpetrator receives the diagnosis of factitious disorder by proxy (e.g., a caretaker assisting the patient in draining blood from a subclavian catheter, producing a dramatic factitious anemia that results in hospitalization).

☐ Etiology

There is no evidence that factitious disorders have a direct genetic or biological basis. Psychodynamic explanations of these parodoxical disorders have been provided by Nadelson (1985), Viederman (1985), and Folks and Freeman (1985). Nadelson conceptualized factitious disorder as a manifestation of borderline character pathology rather than as an isolated clinical syndrome. The patient becomes both the "victim and victimizer" by garnering medical attention from physicians and other health care workers while defying and devaluing them. Projection of hostility and worthlessness onto the caretaker occurs as he or she is both desired and rejected.

Folks and Freeman (1985) pointed out that secondary gain, such as receiving attention, support, sympathy, and relief from responsibility, may underlie the need to assume the sick role in these patients. Viederman (1985) noted that early life experiences such as a history of abuse, emotional deprivation, childhood illness and hospitalization, abandonment in childhood, or a lack of nurturance may contribute to the development of a personality structure that lends itself to factitious behaviors. In this model, relatedness to parental or authority figures is marked by abuse, leading to masochistic tendencies whereby caring is associated with submissiveness and pain.

☐ Treatment

Foremost in the treatment of factitious disorders is making the correct diagnosis. It is imperative that true medical illness not be overlooked and that it be pursued as vigorously as good medical judgment allows. There is an art to crafting an evaluation scheme that enables the clinician to be comfortable that the criteria for the disorder are met and still allows him or her not to miss essential medical problems. Once the diagnosis is made, close collaboration between the psychiatrist and the primary clinician must be effected. A joint confrontation is preferable, and the psychiatrist should ensure that the encounter itself proceeds as therapeutically as possible. The patient may expect (and hope) that the clinicians will be angry at being duped; every attempt should be made to approach the patient in a matter-of-fact way. The clinician should recognize that no matter how carefully the intervention is carried out, the patient may become upset and attempt to leave the hospital against medical advice, especially if the patient is on a medical or surgical ward when the intervention is initiated. Establishing good rapport with the patient, which may require "a significant period" of time, "may partially prevent abrupt termination of treatment" (Stoudemire 1988, p. 552).

Once the confrontation is made, the patient should be transferred to an inpatient psychiatry setting where 24-hour observation and psychiatric intervention are possible. There are a number of reports documenting the potential beneficial effects of psychotherapy in this group of patients (Mayo and Haggerty 1984; Yassa 1978). However, it is the essence of this disorder that the patient opposes attempts to uncover the ruse and to eliminate the core causation of the disorder, so considerable resistance should be expected. The goal of treatment should be to prevent further unnecessary or dangerous evaluations and treatments. Future hospitalizations should be expected and anticipated, and it may prove beneficial to plan "prophylactic" psychiatric or even medical hospitalizations with the primary medical caregiver as a partner in treatment to contain some of the patient's tendency to seek care inappropriately.

■ MALINGERING

Malingering is usually considered to occur rarely. However, examples abound. Almost everyone has malingered an illness at some time in his or her life: as a child, most have feigned a headache or stomachache to avoid going to school. In DSM-IV, malingering is defined as "the intentional production of grossly exaggerated physical or psychological symptoms, motivated by external incentives such as avoiding military duty, avoiding work, obtaining financial compensation, evading criminal prosecution, or obtaining drugs" (American Psychiatric Association 1994). In some circumstances, malingering may represent adaptive behavior.

In malingering, as differentiated from factitious disorders, the motivation for the symptom production is an external incentive (i.e., the identifiable goal is something besides achieving the "sick" role). In contrast to somatoform disorders and conversion disorder, malingering involves the intentional production of symptoms in the face of obvious external incentives. The malingering individual is much less likely to present his or her symptoms in the context of emotional conflict, and the presenting symptoms are much less likely to be related to an underlying emotional conflict. When compared with symptoms in conversion disorder, malingered symptoms are less likely to be relieved by suggestion, hypnosis, or an amobarbital interview. However, even experienced clinicians may find it difficult to distinguish malingering from true illness or from somatoform, factitious, or conversion disorders.

According to Yudofsky (1985), any combination of the following should alert the physician to the possibility of malingering:

1. *Staged events:* Events may be carefully planned that embellish an "injury," such as arranging to be "hit" by a slow-moving automobile on a city street, or staging a "fall" at the workplace.
2. *Data tampering:* Medical tests or results may be changed or contaminated to simulate abnormal or perplexing findings.
3. *Opportunistic malingering:* Individuals may intentionally take advantage of an accident or injury to maximize the financial compensation by exaggerating the symptoms.
4. *Symptom intervention:* Symptoms are created without previous evidence of disease or injury. Malingering of this kind can take any one of a number of presentations and includes neurological (seizures, headache, weakness, visual disturbances, syncope), psychiatric (feigned psychosis, psychogenic amnesia and fugue states, and posttraumatic stress disorder), and surgical-orthopedic injuries.

Stoudemire (1988) added a fifth form of malingering to the above:

5. *Self-destructive behavior:* Behavior may occur that is actively self-destructive or mutilative, the goal of which is the avoidance of duties or obligations. An example would be a person's shooting oneself in the leg to avoid performing dangerous military duties such as combat.

In DSM-IV it is advised that malingering should be strongly suspected if the patient displays any of the following presentations:

1. Medicolegal presentation (e.g., the person is referred to the physician by his or her attorney for evaluation).
2. Marked discrepancy between the person's claimed stress or disability and the objective findings.
3. Lack of cooperation during the diagnostic evaluation and in complying with the treatment regimen.
4. Presence of antisocial personality disorder.

Yudofsky (1985) listed a number of clinical indicators that should raise the index of suspicion for malingering. These indicators encompass both of the above lists and add the following suggested criteria: symptoms are vague or ill-defined; announcement of a favorable prognosis is met with resistance; unsuspected drugs or toxins appear in drug screens; there is a history of multiple accidents or injuries; and the patient has made requests for addictive drugs.

The majority of the literature concerning malingering is focused on the medical-legal issues engendered by the patient's reaction to the diagnosis. A high index of suspicion is required, and the physician should use tests and procedures judiciously. Because many malingering individuals are also seeking narcotics or other drugs of abuse, caution should be exercised in the prescription of these medications for patients with questionable medical histories or signs and symptoms. As in factitious disorder, the first task of the physician is to ensure that a true medical cause for the symptoms is not overlooked. A thorough and well-planned evaluation, noting objectively the presence or absence of clinical findings and relating these findings to known patterns or disease syndromes, will allow the physician to decide more reasonably whether malingering is a diagnostic consideration. The sagacious physician should keep in mind that the malingering person may use threats of litigation in an attempt to coerce the clinician; careful documentation is absolutely necessary in assessing these patients. Obtaining a second opinion is usually indicated and helpful.

■ REFERENCES

American Psychiatric Association: Diagnostic and Statistical Manual of Mental Disorders, 4th Edition. Washington, DC, American Psychiatric Association, 1994

Asher R: Munchausen's syndrome. Lancet 1:339–341, 1951

Clinical Case Conference. N Engl J Med 311:108–115, 1984

Folks DG, Freeman AM: Munchausen's syndrome and other factitious illness. Psychiatr Clin North Am 8:263–278, 1985

Mayo JP Jr, Haggerty J Jr: Long-term psychotherapy of Munchausen syndrome. Am J Psychother 38:571–578, 1984

Meadow R: Munchausen by proxy: the hinterland of child abuse. Lancet 2:343–345, 1977

Meadow R: Munchausen syndrome by proxy. Arch Dis Child 57:92–98, 1982

Nadelson T: The Munchausen spectrum: borderline character features. Gen Hosp Psychiatry 1:11–17, 1979

Nadelson T: The false patient: chronic factitious disease, Munchausen syndrome, and malingering (Chapter 101), in Psychiatry, Vol 2. Edited by Cavenar JO Jr. Philadelphia, PA, JB Lippincott, 1985

O'Shea B: Meadow's syndrome. Irish Journal of Psychotherapy and Psychosomatic Medicine 4:6–8, 1987

Pope HG Jr, Jonas JM, Jones B: Factitious psychosis: phenomenology, family history, and long-term outcome of nine patients. Am J Psychiatry 139:1480–1483, 1982

Spiro HR: Chronic factitious illness: Munchausen's syndrome. Arch Gen Psychiatry 18:569–579, 1968

Stoudemire GA: Somatoform disorders, factitious disorders, and malingering, in The American Psychiatric Press Textbook of Psychiatry. Edited by Talbott JA, Hales RE, Yudofsky SC. Washington, DC, American Psychiatric Press, 1988, pp 533–556

Viederman M: Somatoform and factitious disorders (Chapter 35), in Psychiatry, Vol 1. Edited by Cavenar JO Jr. Philadelphia, PA, JB Lippincott, 1985

Yassa R: Munchausen's syndrome: a successfully treated case. Psychosomatics 19:242–243, 1978

Yudofsky SC: Conditions not attributable to a mental disorder, in Comprehensive Textbook of Psychiatry/IV, 4th Edition. Edited by Kaplan HI, Sadock BJ. Baltimore, MD, Williams & Wilkins, 1985, pp 1862–1865

CHAPTER 18

Dissociative Disorders

David Spiegel, M.D.

The dissociative disorders involve a disturbance in the integrated organization of identity, memory, perception, or consciousness. Events normally experienced on a smooth continuum are isolated from the other mental processes with which they would ordinarily be associated. When it is memories that are poorly integrated, the resulting disorder is *dissociative amnesia.* Fragmentation of identity results in *dissociative fugue* or *dissociative identity disorder.* Disordered perception yields *depersonalization disorder.* Dissociation of aspects of consciousness produces *acute stress disorder* and various dissociative trance and possession states.

These dissociative disorders are more a disturbance in the organization or structure of mental contents than in the contents themselves. Memories in dissociative amnesia are not so much distorted or bizarre as they are segregated one from another. The identities lost in dissociative fugue, or those fragmented in dissociative identity disorder, are two-dimensional aspects of an overall personality structure. In this sense, it has been said that patients with dissociative identity disorder suffer not from having more than one personality, but rather from having less than one personality. The problem is the failure of integration rather than the contents of the fragments.

Repression as a general model for keeping information out of conscious awareness differs from dissociation in four important ways:

1. Dissociated information is stored in a discrete and untransformed manner, whereas repressed information is usually disguised and fragmented. Even when repressed information becomes available to consciousness, its meaning is hidden (e.g., in dreams, slips of the tongue, etc.).

2. Retrieval of dissociated information can often be direct. Techniques such as hypnosis can be used to access warded-off memories. In contrast, uncovering of repressed information often requires repeated recall trials through intense questioning, psychotherapy, or psychoanalysis with subsequent interpretation (i.e., of dreams).

3. The information kept out of awareness in dissociation is often for a discrete and sharply delimited period of time, whereas repressed information may be for a type of encounter or experience scattered across times.

4. Dissociation seems to be elicited as a defense especially after episodes of physical trauma, whereas repression is a response to warded-off fears and wishes, or in response to other dynamic conflicts.

There is debate about whether dissociation is a subtype of repression or vice versa. Such a dispute is probably not resolvable, but what has become clear in recent years is that given the complexity of human information processing, the accomplishment of a sense of mental unity is an achievement, not a given (Kihlstrom and Hoyt 1990; Spiegel D 1990a). What is remarkable is not that dissociative disorders occur, but rather that they do not occur more often, given the fact that information processing comprises a variety of reasonably autonomous subsystems involving perception, memory storage and retrieval, intention, and action (Cohen and Servan-Schreiber 1992).

■ MODELS AND MECHANISMS OF DISSOCIATION

☐ Dissociation and Memory Systems

Modern research on memory demonstrates that there are at least two broad categories of memory, variously described as explicit and implicit (Schacter 1992; Squire 1992) or episodic and semantic (Tulving 1983). These two memory systems serve different functions. *Explicit (or episodic) memory* involves recall of personal experience identified with the self (e.g., "I was at the ball game last week"). The other type, *implicit* (or *semantic) memory,* involves the execution of routine operations, such as riding a bicycle or typing. Such operations may be carried out with a high degree of proficiency with little conscious awareness of either their current execution or the learning episodes upon which the skill is based. Indeed, these two types of memory may well have different anatomic localizations: the limbic system, especially the hippocampal formation, and mammillary bodies for episodic memory, and the basal ganglia and cortex for procedural memory (Mishkin 1991; Squire 1992).

Indeed, the distinction between these two types of memory may account for certain dissociative phenomena (Spiegel D et al. 1993). The automaticity observed in certain dissociative disorders may be a reflection of the separation of self-identification in certain kinds of explicit memory from routine activity in implicit or semantic memory. It is thus not at all foreign to our mental processing to act in an automatic way devoid of explicit self-identification. Were it necessary for us to retrieve explicit memories of how and when we learned all of the activities we are required to perform, it is highly unlikely that we would be able to function with anything like the degree of efficiency we have. There is thus a fundamental model in memory research for the dissociation between identity and performance that may well find its pathological reflection in such disorders as dissociative amnesia, fugue, and identity disorder.

☐ Dissociation and Trauma

An important development in the modern understanding of dissociative disorders is the exploration of the link between trauma and dissociation (Spiegel D and Cardeña 1991). Trauma can be understood as the experience of being made into an object or thing, the victim of someone else's rage or of nature's indifference. It is the ultimate experience of helplessness and loss of control over one's own body. There is growing clinical and some empirical evidence that dissociation may occur especially as a defense during trauma—an attempt to maintain mental control at the very moment when physical control has been lost (Kluft 1984; Putnam 1985; Spiegel D et al. 1988). Such individuals often report seeking comfort from imaginary playmates or imagined protectors, or absorbing themselves in some perceptual distraction, such as the pattern of the wallpaper. There is recent evidence (Terr 1991) that children exposed to multiple traumas are more likely to use dissociative defense mechanisms, which include spontaneous trance episodes and amnesia.

An accumulating literature suggests a connection between a history of physical and sexual abuse in childhood and the development of dissociative symptoms (Coons and Milstein 1986; Kluft 1984). Similarly, evidence is accumulating that dissociative symptoms are more prevalent in patients with Axis II disorders such as borderline personality disorder when there has been a history of childhood abuse (Chu and Dill 1990). However, another way to examine the connection between dissociation and trauma is to look at the link between recent trauma and dissociative symptoms (Spiegel D 1991; Spiegel D and Cardeña 1991). If it is indeed the case that trauma seems to elicit dissociative symptoms, this should be observable in the immediate aftermath of natural disasters, combat, and physical assault.

Several researchers have observed that numbing (i.e., loss of responsiveness in the wake of trauma) is a predictor of later posttraumatic stress disorder (PTSD) symptomatology. For example, Solomon et al. (1989) observed that psychic numbing accounted for 20% of the variance in later PTSD among Israeli combat soldiers, and, similarly, McFarlane (1986) found that numbing in response to the Ash Wednesday Bush Fires in Australia was a strong predictor of later posttraumatic symptomatology.

Similarly, research on hostages and survivors of other life-threatening events indicates that more than half have experienced feelings of unreality, automatic movements, lack of emotion, and a sense of detachment (Madakasira and O'Brien 1987; Sloan 1988). Symptoms of depersonalization and hyperalertness also frequently occur (Noyes and Slymen 1978–1979). Numbing, loss of interest, and an inability to feel deeply about anything were reported in about a third of the survivors of the Hyatt Regency skywalk collapse (Wilkinson 1983) and in a similar proportion of survivors of the North Sea oil rig collapse (Holen 1993). This is consistent with our studies of survivors of the Loma Prieta earthquake (Cardeña and Spiegel D 1993), in which a quarter of a sample of normal students reported marked depersonalization during and immediately afterward.

Such dissociative experiences, especially numbing, have been found to be rather strong predictors of later PTSD (Solomon et al. 1989; Koopman et al. 1994). Indeed, more extreme dissociative disorders, such as dissociative identity disorder, have been conceptualized as chronic posttraumatic stress disorders (Kluft 1984, 1991). Recollection of trauma tends to have an off-on quality involving either intrusion or avoidance (Horowitz 1976), in which victims either intensively relive the trauma as though it were recurring, or have difficulty remembering it (Cardeña and Spiegel 1993; Christianson and Loftus 1987; Madakasira and O'Brien 1987). Thus, physical trauma seems to elicit dissociative responses.

■ ACUTE STRESS DISORDER

Although acute stress disorder is classified among the anxiety disorders in DSM-IV (American Psychiatric Association 1994), mention is made of it in this chapter because half of the symptoms of this disorder are dissociative in nature (Table 18–1). The diagnostic criteria for this disorder would designate as symptomatic approximately one-third of individuals exposed to serious trauma. These symptoms are strongly predictive of later development of PTSD (Koopman et al. 1994). Similarly, the occurrence of PTSD is predicted by intrusion, avoidance, and hyperarousal symptoms in the immediate aftermath of rape (Rothbaum and Foa 1993) and combat trauma (Blank 1993). Although most individuals experiencing serious trauma are initially symptomatic, the majority will recover without developing PTSD. Most studies demonstrate that 25% or less of those who

---

Table 18–1. DSM-IV diagnostic criteria for acute stress disorder

---

A. The person has been exposed to a traumatic event in which both of the following were present:

   1. The person experienced, witnessed, or was confronted with an event or events that involved actual or threatened death or serious injury, or a threat to the physical integrity of self or others.

   2. The person's response involved intense fear, helplessness, or horror.

B. Either while experiencing or immediately after experiencing the distressing event, the individual has three (or more) of the following dissociative symptoms:

   1. A subjective sense of numbing, detachment, or absence of emotional responsiveness

   2. A reduction in awareness of his or her surroundings (e.g., "being in a daze")

   3. Derealization

   4. Depersonalization

   5. Dissociative amnesia (i.e., inability to recall an important aspect of the trauma)

C. The traumatic event is persistently reexperienced in at least one of the following ways: recurrent images, thoughts, dreams, illusions, flashback episodes, or a sense of reliving the experience; or distress on exposure to reminders of the traumatic event.

D. Marked avoidance of stimuli that arouse recollections of the trauma (e.g., thoughts, feelings, conversations, activities, places, people).

E. Marked symptoms of anxiety or increased arousal (e.g., difficulty sleeping, irritability, poor concentration, hypervigilance, exaggerated startle response, and motor restlessness).

F. The disturbance causes clinically significant distress or impairment in social, occupational, or other important areas of functioning or impairs the individual's ability to pursue some necessary task, such as obtaining necessary assistance or mobilizing personal resources by telling family members about the traumatic experience.

G. The disturbance lasts for a minimum of 2 days and a maximum of 4 weeks and occurs within 4 weeks of the traumatic event.

H. The disturbance is not due to the direct physiological effects of a substance (e.g., a drug of abuse, a medication) or a general medical condition, is not better accounted for by brief psychotic disorder, and is not merely an exacerbation of a preexisting Axis I or Axis II disorder.

---

experience serious trauma later become symptomatic.

This new diagnostic category should be useful not only for research on the normal and abnormal processes of adjusting to trauma, but also as a means of providing an important opportunity for early preventive intervention. It may be that dissociation works well at the time of trauma, but that if the defense persists too long, it interferes with the work necessary to put traumatic experience into perspective and reduce the likelihood of later symptomatology. Therefore, psychotherapy aimed at helping individuals acknowledge, bear, and put into perspective traumatic experience shortly after the trauma should be helpful in reducing the incidence of later PTSD.

■ DISSOCIATIVE AMNESIA

Dissociative amnesia is the classical functional disorder of memory and involves difficulty in retrieving discrete components of episodic memory (Table 18–2). It has three primary characteristics:

1. The memory loss is episodic. The first-person recollection of certain events is lost, rather than knowledge of procedures.
2. The memory loss is for a discrete period of time, ranging from minutes to years. It is not vagueness or inefficient retrieval of memories, but rather a dense unavailability of memories that had been clearly available. Unlike in the amnestic disorders, for example, from damage to the medial temporal lobe in surgery (Squire and Zola-Morgan 1991), or in Wernicke-Korsakoff syndrome, there is usually no difficulty in learning *new* episodic information. Thus the amnesia is typically retrograde rather than anterograde (Loewenstein 1991), with one or more discrete periods of past information becoming unavailable.
3. The memory loss is generally for events of a traumatic or stressful nature. In one study (Coons and Milstein 1986), the majority of cases involved child abuse (60%), but disavowed behaviors such as marital problems, sexual activity, suicide attempts, criminal behavior, and the death of a relative were also precipitants.

Table 18–2.   DSM-IV diagnostic criteria for dissociative amnesia

A. The predominant disturbance is one or more episodes of inability to recall important personal information, usually of a traumatic or stressful nature, that is too extensive to be explained by ordinary forgetfulness.

B. The disturbance does not occur exclusively during the course of dissociative identity disorder, dissociative fugue, posttraumatic stress disorder, acute stress disorder, or somatization disorder and is not due to the direct physiological effects of a substance (e.g., a drug of abuse, a medication) or a neurological or other general medical condition (e.g., amnestic disorder due to head trauma).

C. The symptoms cause clinically significant distress or impairment in social, occupational, or other important areas of functioning.

Dissociative amnesia is most frequent in the third and fourth decades of life. It usually involves one episode, but multiple periods of lost memory are not uncommon (Coons and Milstein 1986). Comorbidity with conversion disorder, bulimia, alcohol abuse, and depression is common, and Axis II diagnoses of histrionic, dependent, and borderline personality disorders occur in a substantial minority of such patients (Coons and Milstein 1986). Legal difficulties, such as driving under the influence of alcohol, also accompany dissociative amnesia in a minority of cases.

Dissociative amnesia usually involves discrete boundaries around the period of time unavailable to consciousness. Individuals with such a disorder lose the ability to recall what happened during a specific period of time. They demonstrate not vagueness or spotty memory, but rather a loss of any episodic memory for a finite period of time. Such individuals may not initially be aware of the memory loss—that is, they may not remember that they do not remember. However, they may find new purchases in their homes but have no memory of having obtained them. They report being told that they have done or said things that they cannot remember.

Dissociative amnesia most frequently occurs after an episode of trauma, and the onset may be sudden or gradual. Some individuals do suffer from episodes of selective amnesia, usually for specific traumatic incidents, which may be more interwoven with periods of intact memory. In these cases, the amnesia is for a type of material remembered rather than for a discrete period of time.

Despite the fact that certain information is kept out of consciousness in dissociative amnesia, such information may well exert an influence on consciousness. For example, a rape victim with no conscious recollection of the assault will nonetheless behave like someone who has been sexually victimized. Such individuals often suffer detachment and demoralization, are unable to enjoy intimate relationships, and show hyperarousal to stimuli reminiscent of the trauma. Individuals with dissociative amnesia generally do not suffer disturbances of identity, except to the extent that their identity is influenced by the warded-off memory. It is not uncommon for such individuals to develop depressive symptoms as well, especially when the amnesia is in the wake of a traumatic episode.

☐ Treatment

Some cases of dissociative amnesia revert spontaneously. In most cases, the amnesia can be breached using techniques such as hypnosis. Most dissociative disorder patients are highly hypnotizable on formal testing and therefore are easily able to make use of hypnotic techniques such as age regression (Spiegel H and Spiegel D 1978[1987]). Such a patient is hypnotized and instructed to experience a time prior to the onset of the amnesia as though it were the present. Then the patient is reoriented in hypnosis to experience events during the amnestic time period. Hypnosis can enable such patients to reorient temporally and therefore to achieve access to otherwise dissociated memories.

If there is traumatic content to the warded-off memory, patients may abreact (i.e., express strong emotion) as these memories are elicited, and they will need psychotherapeutic help in integrating these memories and the associated affect into consciousness. The psychotherapy of dissociative amnesia involves accessing the dissociated memories, working through affectively loaded aspects of these memories, and supporting the patient through the process of integrating these memories into consciousness.

One technique that can help bring such memories into consciousness while modulating the affective response to them is the screen technique (Spiegel D 1981). In this approach, such patients are taught, using hypnosis, to relive the traumatic event as if they were watching it on an imaginary movie or television screen. This technique is often helpful for individuals who are unable to relive the event as if it were occurring in the present tense, either because that process is too emotionally taxing, or because they are not sufficiently hypnotizable to be able to engage in hypnotic age regression. The screen technique can also be used to provide dissociation between the psychological and somatic aspects of the memory retrieval. Individuals can be put into self-hypnosis as above and instructed to get their body into a state of floating comfort and safety. They are reminded that no matter what they see on the screen their bodies will be safe and comfortable.

■ DISSOCIATIVE FUGUE

Dissociative fugue combines failure of integration of certain aspects of personal memory with loss of customary identity and automatisms of motor behavior (Table 18–3). It involves one or more episodes of sudden, unexpected, purposeful travel away from home, coupled with an inability to recall portions or all of one's past, and a loss of identity or the assumption of a new identity. The onset is usually sudden, and it frequently occurs after a traumatic experience or bereavement. A single episode is not uncommon, and spontaneous remission of symptoms can occur without treatment.

It used to be thought that the assumption of a new identity was typical of dissociative fugue. However, Reither and Stoudemire (1988), in a recent review of the literature, document that in the majority of cases there is loss of personal identity but no clear assumption of a new iden-

Table 18–3. DSM-IV diagnostic criteria for dissociative fugue

A. The predominant disturbance is sudden, unexpected travel away from home or one's customary place of work, with inability to recall one's past.

B. Confusion about personal identity or assumption of a new identity (partial or complete).

C. The disturbance does not occur exclusively during the course of dissociative identity disorder and is not due to the direct physiological effects of a substance (e.g., a drug of abuse, a medication) or a general medical condition (e.g., temporal lobe epilepsy).

D. The symptoms cause clinically significant distress or impairment in social, occupational, or other important areas of functioning.

tity. Many cases of dissociative fugue remit spontaneously. But again, hypnosis can be useful in accessing dissociated material.

Hypnosis can be helpful in accessing otherwise unavailable components of memory and identity. The approach used is similar to that for dissociative amnesia. Hypnotic age regression can be used as the framework for accessing information available at a previous time. Demonstrating to such patients that such information can be made available to consciousness enhances their sense of control over this material and facilitates the therapeutic working through of emotionally laden aspects of it.

Once reorientation is established and the overt aspects of the fugue have been resolved, it is important to work through interpersonal or intrapsychic issues that underlie the dissociative defenses. Individuals with dissociative fugue are often relatively unaware of their reactions to stress because they can so effectively dissociate them (Spiegel H 1974). Thus, effective psychotherapy is also anticipatory, helping patients to recognize and modify their tendency to set aside their own feelings in favor of those of others.

Patients with dissociative fugue may be helped with a psychotherapeutic approach that facilitates conscious integration of dissociated memories and motivations for behavior previously experienced as automatic and unwilled. It is often helpful to address current psychosocial stressors, such as marital conflict, with the involved individuals. To the extent that current psychosocial stress triggers fugue, resolution of that stress can help resolve the fugue state and reduce the likelihood of reoccurrence. Highly hypnotizable individuals prone to these extreme dissociative symptoms (Spiegel D et al. 1988) often have great difficulty in asserting their own point of view in a personal relationship. Rather, they interact with others as though they were undergoing a spontaneous trance experience. Psychotherapy can be effective in helping such individuals recognize and modify their tendency toward unthinking compliance with others and extreme sensitivity to rejection and disapproval.

In the past, sodium amobarbital or other short-acting sedatives were used to reverse dissociative amnesia or fugue. However, such techniques offer no advantage over hypnosis and are not especially effective (Perry and Jacobs 1982). Not infrequently, the ceremony of injecting the drug elicits spontaneous hypnotic phenomena before the pharmacological effect is felt, and sedation and other side effects can be troublesome.

■ DEPERSONALIZATION DISORDER

The essential feature of depersonalization disorder is the occurrence of persistent feelings of unreality, detachment, or estrangement from oneself, or one's body, usually with the feeling that one is an outside observer of one's own mental processes (Steinberg 1991). Thus, depersonalization disorder is primarily a disturbance in the integration of perceptual experience (Table 18–4). Individuals suffering depersonalization are distressed by it. They are aware of some distortion in their perceptual experience and therefore are not delusional. The symptom is not infrequently transient and may co-occur with a variety of other symptoms, especially anxiety, panic, or phobic symptoms. Indeed, the content of the anxiety may involve fears of "going crazy."

Derealization frequently co-occurs, in which affected individuals notice an altered perception of their surroundings, resulting in the world seeming unreal or dreamlike. Affected individuals will often ruminate about this alteration and be preoccupied with their own somatic and mental functioning.

Unlike other dissociative disorders, the presence of which excludes other mental disorders such as schizophrenia and substance abuse, depersonalization frequently co-occurs with such disorders. It is often a symptom of anxiety and PTSD, and also occurs as a symptom of alcohol

---

Table 18–4.   DSM-IV diagnostic criteria for depersonalization disorder

A.   Persistent or recurrent experiences of feeling detached from, and as if one is an outside observer of, one's mental processes or body (e.g., feeling like one is in a dream).

B.   During the depersonalization experience, reality testing remains intact.

C.   The depersonalization causes clinically significant distress or impairment in social, occupational, or other important areas of functioning.

D.   The depersonalization experience does not occur exclusively during the course of another mental disorder, such as schizophrenia, panic disorder, acute stress disorder, or another dissociative disorder and is not due to the direct physiological effects of a substance (e.g., a drug of abuse, a medication) or a general medical condition (e.g., temporal lobe epilepsy).

and drug abuse, as a side-effect of prescription medication, and during stress and sensory deprivation. Depersonalization is considered a disorder when it is a persistent and predominant symptom. The phenomenology of the disorder involves both the initial symptoms themselves and the reactive anxiety caused by them.

☐ Treatment

Depersonalization is most often transient and may remit without formal treatment. Recurrent or persistent depersonalization should be thought of both as a symptom in and of itself and as a component of other syndromes requiring treatment, such as anxiety disorders and schizophrenia.

The symptom itself may respond to training in self-hypnosis. The symptoms are presented as a spontaneous form of hypnotic dissociation that can be modified. Individuals for whom this approach is effective can be taught to induce a pleasant sense of floating lightness or heaviness in place of the anxiety-related somatic detachment. Often the use of an imaginary screen to picture problems in a way that detaches them from the typical somatic response is also helpful (Spiegel H and Spiegel D 1978[1987]). Other relaxation techniques such as systematic desensitization, progressive muscle relaxation, and biofeedback may also help. Psychotherapy aimed at working through emotional responses to any traumatic or other stressors eliciting the depersonalization is also helpful.

Pharmacological approaches involve balancing therapeutic benefit and risk. Antianxiety medications are most commonly used, and they may be helpful in reducing the amplification of depersonalization caused by anxiety. However, depersonalization and derealization may also be side effects of antianxiety drugs, so their use should be carefully monitored. Increasing dosage, a standard technique when there is lack of therapeutic response, may also increase symptoms in this manner. Appropriate pharmacological treatment for comorbid disorders is an important part of treatment. Use of antianxiety medications for generalized anxiety or phobic disorders, and antipsychotic medications for schizophrenia, should help in these conditions.

■ DISSOCIATIVE IDENTITY DISORDER (MULTIPLE PERSONALITY DISORDER)

☐ Prevalence

There are no convincing studies of the absolute prevalence of dissociative identity disorder. The estimated prevalence is approximately 3% of psychiatric inpatients (Ross et al. 1991). There has been an enormous rise in the number of reported cases in recent years. Factors that account for this increase include a more general awareness of the diagnosis among mental health professionals; the availability of specific diagnostic criteria (Table 18–5); and reduced misdiagnosis of dissociative identity disorder as schizophrenia or borderline personality disorder. While the increase in reported cases is best documented in North America, a recent study shows similar phenomenology and trauma history in Europe (Boon and Draijer 1993).

Other authors have attributed the increase in reported cases to hypnotic suggestion and misdiagnosis (Frankel 1990). Proponents of this point of view argued that individuals with dissociative identity disorder are as a group highly hypnotizable and therefore quite suggestible, and that not infrequently a few specialist clinicians make the vast majority of diagnoses. However, it has been observed that the symptomatology of patients diagnosed by specialists in dissociation does not differ from that assessed by psychiatrists, psychologists, and physicians in more general practice who diagnose one or two cases a year. Furthermore, were such patients so suggestible and subject to directive influence by diagnosticians, it is surprising that they persist in presenting symptoms for an average of 6.5 years before attaining the diagnosis (Putnam et al. 1986). Rather, it would seem likely that such patients would accept a suggestion that they have another disorder(s), such as schizophrenia or borderline personality disorder, because they encounter many clinicians who are unaware of or not familiar with the disorder, especially if it is suggested that the patients have something else. Because these patients are indeed highly hypnotizable and therefore suggestible, care must be taken in the manner in which the illness is presented to them. However, it is unlikely that the increased number of cases currently reported is accounted for by suggestion alone. Rather, reduction in previous misdiagnosis, and in-

---

Table 18–5.   DSM-IV diagnostic criteria for dissociative identity disorder (multiple personality disorder)

A.   The presence of two or more distinct identities or personality states (each with its own relatively enduring pattern of perceiving, relating to, and thinking about the environment and self).

B.   At least two of these identities or personality states recurrently take control of the person's behavior.

C.   Inability to recall important personal information that is too extensive to be explained by ordinary forgetfulness.

D.   The disturbance is not due to the direct physiological effects of a substance (e.g., blackouts or chaotic behavior during alcohol intoxication) or a general medical condition (e.g., complex partial seizures). **Note:** In children, the symptoms are not attributable to imaginary playmates or other fantasy play.

creased recognition of the prevalence and sequelae of physical and sexual abuse in childhood (Kluft 1991; Terr 1991), are also likely explanations.

☐ Course

Dissociative identity disorder is diagnosed in childhood with increasing frequency (Kluft 1984) but typically emerges between adolescence and the third decade of life; it rarely presents as a new disorder after age 40, but there is often considerable delay between initial symptom presentation and diagnosis (Putnam et al. 1986). Untreated, it is a chronic and recurrent disorder. It rarely remits spontaneously, but the symptoms may not be evident for a period of time.

☐ Comorbidity

The major comorbid psychiatric illnesses of dissociative identity disorder are the depressive disorders, substance use disorders, and borderline personality disorder. Sexual, eating, and sleep disorders occur less commonly. Approximately a third of dissociative identity disorder patients fit the criteria for borderline personality disorder as well. Such individuals also show higher levels of depression (Horevitz and Braun 1984). Conversely, recent research shows dissociative symptoms in many patients with borderline personality disorder, especially those who report histories of physical and sexual abuse (Chu and Dill 1990; Ogata et al. 1990).

Comorbidity is complex in that patients with concurrent diagnoses of dissociative identity disorder and borderline personality disorder (approximately one-third) are also more likely to meet the criteria for major depressive disorder. In addition, they frequently meet the criteria for PTSD, with intrusive flashbacks to recurring dreams of physical and sexual abuse, avoidance and loss of pleasure of usually pleasurable activities, and symptoms of hyperarousal, especially when exposed to reminders of childhood trauma (Kluft 1991; Spiegel D 1990b).

These patients are not infrequently misdiagnosed as having schizophrenia. This diagnostic confusion is understandable given that the first-rank criterion for schizophrenia is that the patient has an apparent delusion (i.e., that his or her body is occupied by more than one person). These patients frequently have auditory hallucinations in which one personality state speaks to or comments on the activities of another (Kluft 1987). When misdiagnosed as having schizophrenia, these patients are frequently put on neuroleptics, with poor therapeutic response.

Individuals with dissociative identity disorder frequently report an average of 15 somatic or conversion symptoms (Ross et al. 1990), and other psychosomatic symptoms such as migraine headaches (Spiegel D

1987). Studies show that approximately one-third of these patients have complex partial seizures (Schenk and Bear 1981).

☐ Psychological Testing

Unlike individuals with schizophrenia, those with dissociative identity disorder score far higher than normal individuals on standard measures of hypnotizability, whereas schizophrenic patients tend to show lower than normal or the absence of high hypnotizability (Lavoie and Sabourin 1980; Pettinati et al. 1990; Spiegel D et al. 1982; Van der Hart and Spiegel 1993). More recently, scales of trait dissociation have been developed (Bernstein and Putnam 1986; Ross 1989), and patients with dissociative identity disorder score extremely high on these scales in contrast to normal populations and other patient groups (Ross et al. 1990; Steinberg et al. 1990).

☐ Treatment

Psychotherapy

It is possible to help dissociative identity disorder patients gain control in several ways over the dissociative process underlying their symptoms. The fundamental psychotherapeutic stance should involve meeting patients halfway in the sense of acknowledging that they experience themselves as fragmented, yet the reality is that the fundamental problem is a failure of integration of disparate memories and aspects of the self. In this sense, these patients suffer from having less than one personality, rather than more than one. Therefore, the goal in therapy is to facilitate integration of disparate elements. This can be done in a variety of ways.

Hypnosis. Hypnosis can be helpful in therapy as well as in diagnosis (Braun 1984; Kluft 1982; Spiegel H and Spiegel D 1978[1987]). First, the simple structure of hypnotic induction may elicit dissociative phenomena. Most of these patients have the experience of being unable to stop dissociative symptoms, but are often intrigued by the possibility of starting them. This carries with it the potential for changing or stopping the symptoms as well.

Hypnosis can be helpful in facilitating access to dissociated personalities. The personalities may simply occur spontaneously during hypnotic induction. An alternative strategy is to hypnotize the patient and use age regression to help the patient reorient to a time when a different personality state was manifest. An instruction later to change times back to the present tense usually elicits a return to the other personality state. This then becomes an alternative means of teaching the patient control over the dissociations.

Alternatively, entering the state of hypnosis may make it possible to simply call up different personalities. Patients can be taught a simple self-hypnosis exercise, after which it is often possible to simply ask to speak with a given alter personality, without the formal use of hypnosis.

Memory retrieval.   Because loss of memory in dissociative identity disorder is complex and chronic, its retrieval is likewise a more extended and integral part of the psychotherapeutic process. The therapy becomes an integrating experience of information-sharing among disparate personality elements. Conceptualizing dissociative identity disorder as a chronic posttraumatic stress disorder, the psychotherapeutic strategy involves a focus on working through traumatic memories in addition to controlling the dissociation.

Controlled access to memories greatly facilitates psychotherapy. As with dissociative amnesia, a variety of strategies can be employed to help dissociative identity disorder patients break down amnesic barriers. Techniques employing hypnosis can be quite helpful, because such patients are as a group extremely hypnotizable. They can be taught age regression to a time when a seemingly unaccessible alter personality was "out." Usually this alter will then provide memories previously unaccessible to consciousness.

A second strategy involves hypnotizing the patient and asking to speak with one or more of the other personality states. Often such a patient has an imagined inner "place" where various aspects of his or her inner structure gather. Using hypnosis to go to that place in imagination and ask one or more such parts of the self to interact can be helpful. Once these memories of earlier traumatic experience have been brought into consciousness, it is crucial to help the patient work through the painful affect, inappropriate self-blame, and other reactions to these memories. A model of grief work is helpful, enabling the patient to acknowledge and bear the import of such memories (Spiegel D 1981). It may be useful to have the patient visualize the memories rather than relive them as a way of making their intensity more manageable. It can also be useful to have the patient divide the memories from one side of an imaginary screen—for example, picturing something an abuser did to him or her, and on the other side, how the patient tried to protect himself or herself from the abuse.

The "rule of thirds."   Psychotherapy with a dissociative identity disorder patient can be a time-consuming and emotionally taxing process. The "rule of thirds" (Kluft 1991) is a helpful guideline. Spend the first third of the psychotherapy session assessing the patient's current mental state and life problems and defining a problem area that might benefit from retrieval into conscious memory and working through. Spend the second third of the session accessing and working through this memory. Allow a final third for helping the patient assimilate the information, regulate and modulate emotional responses, and discuss any responses to the therapist and plans for the immediate future.

Given the intensity of the material that often emerges involving memories of sexual and physical abuse, and the sudden shifts in mental state accompanied by amnesia, the therapist is called upon to take a clear and structured role in managing the psychotherapy. Appropriate limits must be set about self-destructive or threatening behavior, and agreements made regarding physical safety, and treatment compliance, and other matters must be presented to the patient in such a way that dissociative ignorance is not an acceptable explanation for failure to live up to agreements.

Traumatic transference.   Transference applies with special meaning in patients who have been physically and sexually abused. These patients have experienced individuals who were presumed to be caretakers who acted instead in an exploitative and sometimes sadistic fashion. The patients thus expect this from therapists. Attention to these issues can diffuse, but not eliminate, such traumatic transference distortions of the therapeutic relationship (Spiegel D 1988).

Integration.   The ultimate goal of psychotherapy for dissociative identity disorder is integration of the disparate states. There can be considerable resistance to this process. Early in therapy, the patient views the dissociation as tremendous protection. Indeed, he or she may experience efforts of integration as an attempt on the part of the therapist to "kill" personalities. These fears must be worked through and the patient shown how to control the degree of integration. This gives the patient a sense of gradually being able to control his or her dissociative processes in the service of working through traumatic memories. The process of the psychotherapy, in emphasizing control, must alter rather than reinforce the content, which involves reexperiencing of helplessness, a symbolic reenactment of trauma (Spiegel D 1986).

Setting aside the defense also means acknowledging and bearing the discomfort of helplessness at having been victimized, and working through the irrational self-blame that gave the patient a fantasy of control over events that he or she was in fact helpless to control. Yet difficult as it is, ultimately, the goal of psychotherapy is mastery over the dissociative process, controlled access to dissociative states, integration of warded-off painful memories and material, and a more integrated continuum of identity, memory, and consciousness.

Psychopharmacology

As with other dissociative disorders, there is little evidence that psychoactive drugs are of great help in reversing functional amnesias. While in the past short-acting barbiturates such as sodium amobarbital were used intravenously to reverse functional amnesias, this technique is no longer employed, largely because of poor results (Perry and Jacobs 1982).

Benzodiazepines have at times been employed to facilitate recall through controlling secondary anxiety associated with retrieval of traumatic memories. However, these effects may be nonspecific at best.

Antidepressants are the most useful class of psychotropic agents for patients with dissociative identity disorder. Such patients frequently have dysthymic disorder or major depression, and when these disorders are present, especially with somatic signs and suicidal ideation, antidepressant medication can be helpful. The newer selective serotonin reuptake inhibitors are useful because of their lower danger in overdose compared with tricyclics and monoamine oxidase inhibitors (MAOIs).

Anticonvulsants have been used to treat both seizure disorders, which have a high rate of comorbidity with dissociative identity disorder, and the impulsiveness associated with personality disorders. These agents are rarely definitively helpful, but may add to control of symptoms such as impulsiveness.

■ DISSOCIATIVE TRANCE DISORDER

Dissociative phenomena are ubiquitous around the world, occurring in virtually every culture (Lewis-Fernandez 1993). These phenomena seem to be more prevalent in the less heavily industrialized second- and third-world countries, although they can be found everywhere. Furthermore, the trance and possession categories of dissociative trance disorder constitute by far the most common kind of dissociative disorder around the world. Several studies of dissociative disorders in India, for example, demonstrate that dissociative trance and possession is far and away the most prevalent dissociative disorder (i.e., approximately 3.5% of psychiatric admissions; Adityanjee et al. 1989; Saxena and Prasad 1989). On the other hand, dissociative identity disorder, which is relatively more common in the United States, is virtually never diagnosed in India. Cultural as well as biological factors may account for the different content and form of dissociative symptoms.

☐ Classification

Dissociative trance disorder has been divided into two broad categories: dissociative trance and possession trance (Table 18–6).

Table 18–6.   DSM-IV (appendix) diagnostic criteria for dissociative trance disorder

---

A. Either (1) or (2):
 1. Trance, i.e., temporary marked alteration in the state of consciousness or loss of customary sense of personal identity without replacement by an alternate identity, associated with at least one of the following:
   a. Narrowing of awareness of immediate surroundings or unusually narrow and selective focusing on environmental stimuli
   b. Stereotyped behaviors or movements that are experienced as being beyond one's control
 2. Possession trance, i.e., a single or episodic alteration in the state of consciousness characterized by the replacement of customary sense of personal identity by a new identity. This is attributed to the influence of a spirit, power, deity, or other person, as evidenced by one (or more) of the following:
   a. Stereotyped and culturally determined behaviors or movements that are experienced as being controlled by the possessing agent
   b. Full or partial amnesia for the event
B. The trance or possession trance state is not accepted as a normal part of a collective cultural or religious practice.
C. The trance or possession trance state causes clinically significant distress or impairment in social, occupational, or other important areas of functioning.
D. The trance or possession trance state does not occur exclusively during the course of a psychotic disorder (including mood disorder with psychotic features and brief psychotic disorder) or dissociative identity disorder and is not due to the direct physiological effects of a substance or a general medical condition.

Note.   The diagnostic criteria for DSM-IV dissociative trance disorder appear in Appendix B: "Criteria Sets and Axes Provided for Further Study."

Dissociative Trance

Dissociative trance phenomena are characterized by a sudden alteration in consciousness not accompanied by distinct alternative identities. In this form the dissociative symptom involves consciousness rather than identity. Also, in dissociative trance the activities performed are rather simple, usually involving sudden collapse, immobilization, dizziness, shrieking, screaming, or crying. Memory is rarely affected, and amnesia, if any, is fragmented.

Dissociative trance phenomena frequently involve sudden, extreme changes in sensory and motor control. Classic examples include *ataque de nervios*, which is prevalent throughout Latin America. This condition is estimated, for example, to have a 12% lifetime prevalence rate in Puerto Rico (Lewis-Fernandez 1993). Typically, the individual suddenly starts to shake convulsively, hyperventilate, scream, and exhibit agitation and aggressive movements. These behaviors may be followed by collapse and loss of consciousness. Afterward, such individuals report being exhausted and may have some amnesia for the event (Lewis-Fernandez 1993).

Falling-out occurs frequently among African Americans in the southern United States. Affected individuals may collapse suddenly, unable to see or speak even though they are conscious. These persons may be confused afterward, but usually are not amnesic to the episode (Lewis-Fernandez 1993).

In the Malay version of trance disorder, *latah,* affected individuals may have a sudden vision of a spirit that is threatening them. These persons scream or cry, strike out physically, and may need restraints. They may report amnesia, but they do not clearly take on the identity of the offending spirit (Lewis-Fernandez 1993).

Possession Trance

In contrast to dissociative trance, possession trance involves the assumption of a distinct alternate identity, usually that of a deity, ancestor, or spirit. The person in this trance often engages in rather complex activities, which may take the form of expressing otherwise forbidden thoughts or needs, negotiating for change in family or social status, or engaging in aggressive behavior. Possession usually involves amnesia for a large portion of the episode during which the alternate identity was in control of the person's behavior.

In Indian possession syndrome, the affected individual suddenly begins speaking in an altered voice with an altered identity, usually that of a deity recognizable to others. Through this voice, a person may refer to herself or himself in the third person. The affected person's "spirit" may negotiate for changes in the family environment or become agitated or aggressive. Possession syndrome typically occurs in a recently married woman who finds herself uncomfortable or unwelcome in her mother-in-law's home. Such individuals are usually unable to directly express their discomfort.

☐ Treatment

Treatment of these disorders varies from culture to culture. Rubbing the body with special potions, negotiating to change the affected person's social circumstances, and physical restraint are often used. Ceremonies to remove or appease the invading spirit are also used.

■ REFERENCES

Adityanjee, Raju GSP, Khandelwal SK: Current status of multiple personality disorder in India. Am J Psychiatry 146:1607–1610, 1989

American Psychiatric Association: Diagnostic and Statistical Manual of Mental Disorders, 4th Edition. Washington, DC, American Psychiatric Association, 1994

Bernstein EM, Putnam FW: Development, reliability, and validity of a dissociation scale. J Nerv Ment Dis 174:727–735, 1986

Blank AS Jr: The longitudinal course of posttraumatic stress disorder, in Posttraumatic Stress Disorder: DSM-IV and Beyond. Edited by Davidson JRT, Foa EB. Washington, DC, American Psychiatric Press, 1993, pp 3–22

Boon S, Draijer N: Multiple personality disorder in The Netherlands: a clinical investigation of 71 patients. Am J Psychiatry 150:489–494, 1993

Braun BG: Uses of hypnosis with multiple personality. Psychiatric Annals 14:34–36, 39–40, 1984

Cardeña E, Spiegel D: Dissociative reactions to the San Francisco Bay Area earthquake of 1989. Am J Psychiatry 150:474–478, 1993

Christianson SA, Loftus EF: Memory for traumatic events. Applied Cognitive Psychology 1:225–239, 1987

Chu JA, Dill DL: Dissociative symptoms in relation to childhood physical and sexual abuse. Am J Psychiatry 147:887–892, 1990

Cohen JD, Servan-Schreiber D: Introduction to neural network models in psychiatry. Psychiatric Annals 22:113–118, 1992

Coons PM, Milstein V: Psychosexual disturbances in multiple personality: characteristics, etiology, and treatment. J Clin Psychiatry 47:106–110, 1986

Frankel FH: Hypnotizability and dissociation. Am J Psychiatry 147:823–829, 1990

Holen A: Normal and pathological grief: recent views. Tidsskrift for den Norske Laegeforening 113:2089–2091, 1993

Horevitz RP, Braun BG: Are multiple personalities borderline? An analysis of 33 cases. Psychiatr Clin North Am 7:69–87, 1984

Horowitz MJ: Stress Response Syndromes. New York, Jason Aronson, 1976

Kihlstrom JF, Hoyt IP: Repression, dissociation, and hypnosis, in Repression and Dissociation: Implications for Personality Theory, Psychopathology, and Health. Edited by Singer JL. Chicago, IL, University of Chicago Press, 1990, pp 181–208

Kluft RP: Varieties of hypnotic intervention in the treatment of multiple personality. Am J Clin Hypn 24:230–240, 1982

Kluft RP: Multiple personality in childhood. Psychiatr Clin North Am 7:121–134, 1984

Kluft RP: First-rank symptoms as a diagnostic clue to multiple personality disorder. Am J Psychiatry 144:293–298, 1987

Kluft RP: Multiple personality disorder, in American Psychiatric Press Review of Psychiatry, Vol 10. Edited by Tasman A, Goldfinger SM. Washington, DC, American Psychiatric Press, 1991, pp 161–188

Koopman C, Classer C, Spiegel D: Predictors of post-traumatic stress symptoms among Oakland/Berkeley firestorm survivors. Am J Psychiatry 151:888–894, 1994

Lavoie G, Sabourin M: Hypnosis and schizophrenia: a review of experimental and clinical studies, in Handbook of Hypnosis and Psychosomatic Medicine. Edited by Burrows GD, Dennerstein L. New York, Elsevier, 1980

Lewis-Fernandez: Culture and dissociation: a comparison of ataque de nervios among Puerto Ricans and "possession syndrome" in India, in Dissociation: Culture, Mind, and Body. Edited by Spiegel D. Washington, DC, American Psychiatric Press, 1993

Loewenstein RJ: An official mental status examination for complex chronic dissociative symptoms and multiple personality disorder. Psychiatr Clin North Am 14:567–604, 1991

McFarlane AC: Posttraumatic morbidity of a disaster: a study of cases presenting for psychiatric treatment. J Nerv Ment Dis 174:4–14, 1986

Madakasira S, O'Brien KF: Acute posttraumatic stress disorder in victims of a natural disaster. J Nerv Ment Dis 175:286–290, 1987

Mishkin M: Cerebral memory circuits, in 1990 Yakult International Symposium: Perception, Cognition and Brain. Tokyo, Yakult Honsha Co, 1991

Noyes R Jr, Slymen DJ: The subjective response to life-threatening danger. Omega 9:313–321, 1978–1979

Ogata SN, Silk KR, Goodrich S, et al: Childhood sexual and physical abuse in adult patients with borderline personality disorder. Am J Psychiatry 147:1008–1013, 1990

Perry JC, Jacobs D: Overview: clinical applications of the Amytal interview in psychiatric emergency settings. Am J Psychiatry 139:552–559, 1982

Pettinati HM, Kogan LG, Evans FJ, et al: Hypnotizability of psychiatric inpatients according to two different scales. Am J Psychiatry 147:69–75, 1990

Putnam FW Jr: Dissociation as a response to extreme trauma, in Childhood Antecedents of Multiple Personality. Edited by Kluft RP. Washington, DC, American Psychiatric Press, 1985, pp 65–97

Putnam FW, Guroff JJ, Silberman EK, et al: The clinical phenomenology of multiple personality disorder: review of 100 recent cases. J Clin Psychiatry 47:285–293, 1986

Reither AM, Stoudemire A: Psychogenic fugue states: a review. South Med J 81:568–571, 1988

Ross CA: Multiple Personality Disorder: Diagnosis, Clinical Features, and Treatment. New York, Wiley, 1989

Ross CA, Miller SD, Reagor P, et al: Structured interview data on 102 cases of multiple personality disorder from four centers. Am J Psychiatry 147:596–601, 1990

Ross CA, Anderson G, Fleisher WP, et al: The frequency of multiple personality disorder among psychiatric inpatients. Am J Psychiatry 148:1717–1720, 1991

Rothbaum BO, Foa EB: Subtypes of posttraumatic stress disorder and duration of symptoms, in Posttraumatic Stress Disorder: DSM-IV and Beyond. Edited by Davidson JRT, Foa EB. Washington, DC, American Psychiatric Press, 1993

Saxena S, Prasad KVSR: DSM-III subclassification of dissociative disorders applied to psychiatric outpatients in India. Am J Psychiatry 146:261–262, 1989

Schacter DL: Understanding implicit memory: a cognitive neuroscience approach. Am Psychol 47:559–569, 1992

Schenk L, Bear D: Multiple personality and related dissociative phenomena in patients with temporal lobe epilepsy. Am J Psychiatry 138:1311–1316, 1981

Sloan P: Posttraumatic stress in survivors of an airplane crash landing: a clinical and exploratory research intervention. Journal of Traumatic Stress 1:211–229, 1988

Solomon Z, Mikulincer M, Benbenisty R: Combat stress reaction—clinical manifestations and correlates. Military Psychology 1:17–33, 1989

Spiegel D: Vietnam grief work using hypnosis. Am J Clin Hypn 24:33–40, 1981

Spiegel D: Dissociation, double binds, and posttraumatic stress in multiple personality disorder, in Treatment of Multiple Personality Disorder. Edited by Braun BG. Washington, DC, American Psychiatric Press, 1986, pp 61–77

Spiegel D: Chronic pain masks depression, multiple personality disorder. Hosp Community Psychiatry 38:933–935, 1987

Spiegel D: Dissociation and hypnosis in posttraumatic stress disorders. Journal of Traumatic Stress 1:17–33, 1988

Spiegel D: Hypnosis, dissociation, and trauma: hidden and overt observers, in Repression and Dissociation: Implications for Personality Theory, Psychopathology, and Health. Edited by Singer JL. Chicago, IL, University of Chicago Press, 1990a, pp 121–142

Spiegel D: Trauma, dissociation, and hypnosis, in Incest-Related Syndromes of Adult Psychopathology. Edited by Kluft RL. Washington, DC, American Psychiatric Press, 1990b, pp 247–261

Spiegel D: Dissociation and trauma, in American Psychiatric Press Review of Psychiatry, Vol 10. Edited by Tasman A, Goldfinger SM. Washington, DC, American Psychiatric Press, 1991, pp 261–275

Spiegel D, Cardeña E: Disintegrated experience: the dissociative disorders revisited. J Abnorm Psychol 100:366–378, 1991

Spiegel D, Detrick D, Frischholz E[J]: Hypnotizability and psychopathology. Am J Psychiatry 139:431–437, 1982

Spiegel D, Hunt T, Dondershine HE: Dissociation and hypnotizability in posttraumatic stress disorder. Am J Psychiatry 145:301–305, 1988

Spiegel D, Frischholz EJ, Spira J: Functional disorders of memory, in American Psychiatric Press Review of Psychiatry, Vol 12. Edited by Oldham JM, Riba MB, Tasman A. Washington, DC, American Psychiatric Press, 1993, pp 747–782

Spiegel H: The grade 5 syndrome: the highly hypnotizable person. Int J Clin Exp Hypn 22:303–319, 1974

Spiegel H, Spiegel D: Trance and Treatment: Clinical Uses of Hypnosis. New York, Basic Books, 1978 [Reprinted by American Psychiatric Press, Washington, DC, 1987]

Squire LR: Memory and the hippocampus: a synthesis from findings with rats, monkeys, and humans. Psychol Rev 99:195–231, 1992

Squire LR, Zola-Morgan S: The medial temporal lobe memory system. Science 253:1380–1386, 1991

Steinberg M: The spectrum of depersonalization: assessment and treatment, in American Psychiatric Press Review of Psychiatry, Vol 10. Edited by Tasman A, Goldfinger SM. Washington, DC, American Psychiatric Press, 1991, pp 223–247

Steinberg M, Rounsaville B, Cicchetti DV: The Structured Clinical Interview for DSM-III-R Dissociative Disorders: preliminary report on a new diagnostic instrument. Am J Psychiatry 147:76–82, 1990

Terr LC: Childhood traumas: an outline and overview. Am J Psychiatry 148:10–20, 1991

Tulving E: Elements of Episodic Memory. Oxford, UK, Clarendon Press, 1983

Van der Hart O, Spiegel D: Hypnotic assessment and treatment of trauma-induced psychoses: the early psychotherapy of Breukink and modern views. Int J Clin Exp Hypn 41:191–209, 1993

Wilkinson CB: Aftermath of a disaster: the collapse of the Hyatt Regency hotel skywalks. Am J Psychiatry 140:1134–1139, 1983

CHAPTER

19

Sexual and Gender Identity Disorders

Judith V. Becker, Ph.D.
Richard J. Kavoussi, M.D.

■ GENDER IDENTITY DISORDERS

□ Gender and Sexual Differentiation

The genetic sex of an individual is determined at conception, but development from that point on is influenced by many factors. For the first few weeks of gestation, the gonads are undifferentiated. If the Y chromosome is present in the embryo, the gonads will differentiate into testes. A substance referred to as the H-Y antigen is responsible for this transformation. If the Y chromosome or H-Y antigen is not present in the developing embryo, the gonads will develop into ovaries.

Like the gonads, the internal and external genital structures are initially undifferentiated in the fetus. If the gonads differentiate into testes, fetal androgen (i.e., testosterone) is secreted, and these structures develop into male genitalia (epididymis, vas deferens, ejaculatory ducts, penis, and scrotum). In the absence of fetal androgen, these structures develop into female genitalia (fallopian tubes, uterus, clitoris, and vagina). It is important to note that the development of genitalia in utero depends on the presence or absence of fetal androgen, from whatever source.

Psychosexual development is also thought to be influenced by a complex interaction of factors, both pre- and postnatal. Before discussing these factors, however, it is important to break down psychosexual be-

605

havior into several components. *Gender identity* is an individual's perception and self-awareness of being male or female. *Gender role* is the behavior that an individual engages in that identifies him or her to others as being male or female (e.g., wearing dresses/makeup). *Sexual orientation* is the erotic attraction that an individual feels (e.g., arousal to men, women, children, nonsexual objects, and so on).

Gender identity appears to develop in the early years of life and is generally established by age 3 years. Gender identity seems to depend on the sex in which an individual is reared, regardless of biological factors. The evidence for this comes from studies of children born with genitalia that are ambiguous or opposite from their genetic sex (Money and Ehrhardt 1974). Gender identity, once firmly established, is extremely resistant to change. For example, if a genetic female is reared as a boy (e.g., due to exposure to fetal androgens) but suddenly develops breasts and other female secondary sex characteristics during puberty, his gender identity will remain male, and he will want to correct the changes.

If gender identity develops between birth and age 3 and depends on sex of rearing, what are the factors that contribute to its development? Several theories attempt to answer this question. There may be biological factors that influence the development of gender identity that have not yet been discovered, and there are instances in which it has been suggested that biological factors may override sex assignment at birth (Ehrhardt and Meyer-Bahlburg 1981). According to a learning theory model, gender identity begins to develop when the child imitates or identifies with same-sexed models. The child is then reinforced for this identification and for engaging in "appropriate" sex-role behaviors. In psychoanalytic theory, gender identity develops as part of overall identity formation in the phase of separation and individuation and is very much dependent on the quality of the mother-infant dyad. Later, during the oedipal phase, gender role and sexual orientation are shaped.

☐ Criteria for Diagnosing Gender Identity Disorders

Gender identity disorders are characterized by strong and persistent cross-gender identification (not merely a desire for any perceived cultural advantages of being the other sex). In children the disorder is manifested by at least four of the criteria shown in Table 19–1. In adolescents or adults, the symptoms include:

- A stated desire to be the opposite sex
- Frequently "passing" as the opposite sex
- A desire to live or be treated as a member of the opposite sex
- Having the conviction that one experiences the typical feelings and reactions of the opposite sex

---

Table 19–1.   DSM-IV diagnostic criteria for gender identity disorder

---

A.   A strong and persistent cross-gender identification (not merely a desire for any perceived cultural advantages of being the other sex).

In children, the disturbance is manifested by four (or more) of the following:

1.   Repeatedly stated desire to be, or insistence that he or she is, the other sex
2.   In boys, preference for cross-dressing or simulating female attire; in girls, insistence on wearing only stereotypical masculine clothing
3.   Strong and persistent preferences for cross-sex roles in make-believe play or persistent fantasies of being the other sex
4.   Intense desire to participate in the stereotypical games and pastimes of the other sex
5.   Strong preference for playmates of the other sex

In adolescents and adults, the disturbance is manifested by symptoms such as a stated desire to be the other sex, frequent passing as the other sex, desire to live or be treated as the other sex, or the conviction that he or she has the typical feelings and reactions of the other sex.

B.   Persistent discomfort with his or her sex or sense of inappropriateness in the gender role of that sex.

In children, the disturbance is manifested by any of the following: in boys, assertion that his penis or testes are disgusting or will disappear or assertion that it would be better not to have a penis, or aversion toward rough-and-tumble play and rejection of male stereotypical toys, games, and activities; in girls, rejection of urinating in a sitting position, assertion that she has or will grow a penis, or assertion that she does not want to grow breasts or menstruate, or marked aversion toward normative feminine clothing.

In adolescents and adults, the disturbance is manifested by symptoms such as preoccupation with getting rid of primary and secondary sex characteristics (e.g., request for hormones, surgery, or other procedures to physically alter sexual characteristics to simulate the other sex) or belief that he or she was born the wrong sex.

C.   The disturbance is not concurrent with a physical intersex condition.

D.   The disturbance causes clinically significant distress or impairment in social, occupational, or other important areas of functioning.

Code based on current age: **Gender identity disorder in children**
Gender identity disorder in adolescents or adults

Specify if (for sexually mature individuals): **Sexually attracted to males**
Sexually attracted to females
Sexually attracted to both
Sexually attracted to neither

Gender identity disorder not otherwise specified

This category is included for coding disorders in gender identity that are not classifiable as a specific gender identity disorder. Examples include

1.   Intersex conditions (e.g., androgen insensitivity syndrome or congenital adrenal hyperplasia) and accompanying gender dysphoria
2.   Transient, stress-related cross-dressing behavior
3.   Persistent preoccupation with castration or penectomy without a desire to acquire the sex characteristics of the other sex

---

- Persistent discomfort with one's sex or sense of inappropriateness in the gender role of that sex

☐ Gender Identity Disorder of Adulthood (Transsexualism)

Gender identity disorder of adulthood (transsexualism) is rare, with estimates of 30,000 cases worldwide (Lothstein 1980). There have been cases described throughout history, but it is only in the past 25 years that scientific and media attention has focused on this phenomenon and specialized gender identity clinics have been developed. Transsexual individuals most commonly present by requesting *sex reassignment*—that is, change in their physical appearance (usually by hormonal and surgical means) to correspond with their self-perceived gender. However, it is important to remember that not all those who seek sex reassignment are transsexual; cross-gender wishes may occur in transvestism (i.e., wearing opposite gender clothes for erotic purposes) or effeminate homosexuality. Therefore it is important to conduct a thorough evaluation before recommending sex reassignment.

Gender dysphoria has been classified as primary or secondary (Person and Ovesey 1974). *Primary transsexuals* have a lifelong, profound disturbance of core gender identity. They have histories of cross-dressing as children, but never were aroused by wearing opposite-sex clothes. They usually have a clear history of engaging in opposite-sex gender-role behaviors. *Secondary transsexuals* can also have a long history of gender identity confusion; however, in this case the identity disturbance follows other cross-gender behavior such as transvestism or effeminate homosexuality.

Etiology

There are no well-established or exhaustive explanations for the development of gender identity disorder. As noted earlier, gender identity appears to be established and influenced by psychosocial factors during the first few years of life. However, many authors have argued that biological factors, if not causative, may predispose an individual to disordered gender identity. Although no correlation has been made with specific temporal lobe abnormalities, there have been case reports of individuals who became transsexual following onset of temporal lobe seizures and who improved with anticonvulsant medication. Some researchers have found decreased levels of testosterone in male transsexuals and abnormally high levels of testosterone in female transsexuals, but the findings have been inconsistent and the studies from which they were obtained were not well controlled.

Learning theory models suggest that gender dysphoria arises from absent or inconsistent reinforcement for identification with same-sexed models. Psychoanalytic theory argues that early deprivation of the male child by his mother leads to a symbiotic merger with the mother and lack of full individuation as a separate person. In the case of borderline personality disorder, this process leads to general identity confusion and loss of ego boundaries when the individual is under stress. In gender dysphoria, the defect is isolated to gender.

Diagnosis and Evaluation

Individuals who request sex reassignment require careful and patient evaluation by a psychiatrist or psychologist with experience in the management of gender identity disorders. As noted earlier, patients with other primary psychiatric diagnoses may present as transsexuals. Psychotic patients may have delusions centered around their genitalia. When the psychosis is treated, the cross-gender wishes usually resolve. Individuals with severe personality disorders, especially borderline, can have transient wishes to change gender as part of their overall identity diffusion during times of stress. Effeminate homosexuals may present with a desire to change sex in order to be more attractive to men; usually this desire fluctuates with time.

Treatment

Because most gender dysphoric individuals present with adamant requests for sex reassignment, it is extremely difficult to engage these patients in treatment with anything other than surgical sex reassignment as the goal. These patients see psychotherapy as a means of discouraging them from surgery. However, because surgery is irreversible, it is important to engage these patients in psychotherapy, even if surgery is indicated.

Supportive psychotherapy can serve various purposes in the transsexual individual. First, there have been reports of reversal of patients' disordered gender identity, albeit few in number. Second, a trial of psychotherapy is often useful in cases in which the diagnosis is not clear. Third, dealing with patients' fears of homosexuality can alleviate the wish for surgical reassignment. Fourth, psychotherapy plays an important role in the patient's adjustment to the process of sex reassignment. Finally, therapy is often helpful in the postsurgical adjustment of patients with gender identity disorder. Psychoanalysis is generally not indicated in the treatment of transsexuals because of their poor ego functioning.

Behavior therapy has been used with success in male transsexuals (Barlow et al. 1979). The treatment involves identifying female patterns of behavior, which are then changed using videotapes and modeling of masculine behavior that the patient is trained to engage in. Attempts are also made to change the patient's arousal pattern from homosexual to heterosexual; however, this was successful in only one of three cases.

Sexual reassignment to the opposite gender has been the most widely used and studied treatment modality for adults with gender identity disorder. Early reports of outcome were extremely positive, with dramatic changes in social functioning and satisfaction. Hormonal treatment and surgery became more readily available for adults with gender identity disorder, often with little preparation other than a brief consultation with a psychiatrist. This led to an increase in the reports of poor results and realization that sex reassignment was not a panacea.

☐ Gender Identity Disorder of Childhood

Because of the difficulty and turmoil involved in treating late adolescent and adult patients who have gender disorder, researchers and clinicians began to evaluate and treat children with gender identity problems. Strictly speaking, this disorder is seen in a child who perceives himself or herself as being of the opposite sex. However, it is often difficult to separate gender identity from gender role behavior in children. Boys with normal gender identity may play with "girl" dolls. Many girls in our culture are "tomboys" and like rough and contact games. However, in this gender identity syndrome there is a repeated pattern of opposite gender role behavior accompanied by a disturbance in the child's perception of "being" a boy or a girl. The exact incidence of gender identity disorder in children is not known, but, like adult gender dysphoria, it is a rare disorder.

Etiology

As with adult gender dysphoria, the etiology of childhood gender identity disorder is unclear. The theories outlined above with adults have also been applied to these children. Additional factors that have been suggested are parents' indifference to or encouragement of opposite-sex behavior; regular cross-dressing as a young boy by a female; lack of male playmates during a boy's first years of socialization; excessive maternal protection, with inhibition of rough-and-tumble play; or absence of or rejection by an older male early in life (Green 1974).

Course

Retrospective studies of transsexuals (Green 1974) have shown a high incidence of childhood cross-gender behavior. Follow-up of children with gender disorder has found a high incidence of continued manifestations in adulthood, with a higher incidence of homosexual or bisexual behavior and fantasies than in a control group (Green 1985).

Treatment

Treatment of the child with gender identity disorder is offered in an attempt to help the child avoid peer ostracism and humiliation, be comfortable with his or her own sex, and avoid the possible development of adult gender dysphoria. Behavior therapy has been used to modify specific cross-gender behaviors in a manner similar to that described above for adults and also through the use of contingency management (e.g., reinforcing appropriate behaviors with tokens). An eclectic approach to treatment has been advocated that involves the development of a close, trusting relationship between a male therapist and the boy, stopping parental encouragement of feminine behaviors, interrupting the excessively close relationship between mother and son, enhancing the role of father and son, and reinforcing male behaviors (Green 1974).

■ SEXUAL DYSFUNCTIONS

□ Male and Female Physiology

Human sexual functioning requires a complex interaction of the nervous, vascular, and endocrine systems to produce arousal and orgasm. Sexual arousal in men occurs in the presence of visual stimuli, fantasies, or physical stimulation of the genitals or other areas of the body. This leads to involuntary discharge in the parasympathetic nerves that control the diameter and valves of the penile blood vessels. There is then increased blood flow into the corpora cavernosa, two cylinders of specialized tissue that distend with blood to produce an erection. Continued stimulation leads to emission of semen and ejaculation, which are controlled through sympathetic fibers and the pudendal nerve. Dopaminergic systems in the central nervous system facilitate arousal and ejaculation, while serotonergic systems inhibit these functions. In addition, androgens must be present to expedite sexual arousal (and to some extent erection and ejaculation as well).

In women, as in men, arousal depends on fantasies, visual stimuli, and physical stimulation; in general, the latter is more important for women, whereas visual cues are more important for men. Again this leads to parasympathetic nervous discharge that increases blood flow to the female genitalia, resulting in lubrication of the vagina and some enlargement of the clitoris. Continued stimulation of the clitoris either directly or through intercourse results in orgasm. Estrogens and progestins play a role in female sexual functioning; however, androgens are important in the maintenance of sexual arousal in women. As in men, dopaminergic systems facilitate female sexual arousal and orgasm, while serotonergic systems inhibit these functions.

It is readily apparent that these sexual processes require intact neural and vascular connections to the genitals along with normal endocrine functioning. Any illness that interferes with these systems can lead to sexual dysfunction: neurological diseases (e.g., multiple sclerosis, lumbar or sacral spinal cord trauma, herniated disks), thrombosis of the arteries or veins of the penis, diabetes mellitus (which causes both neurological and vascular damage), endocrine disorders (e.g., hyperprolactinemia), liver disease (which leads to a buildup of estrogens), and so forth. Similarly, drugs that affect any part of this system can also impair sexual functioning. Thus, antihypertensives, because their antiadrenergic effects, can impair erectile function in men and lubrication in women. Antipsychotics, tricyclic antidepressants, and monoamine oxidase inhibitors can inhibit these same functions through their anticholinergic effects. Antipsychotics can impair arousal and orgasm because of their dopamine-blocking effects, while serotonin reuptake blockers (e.g., fluoxetine, sertraline, and paroxetine) can inhibit arousal and orgasm through their serotonergic effects. Spironolactone, steroids, and estrogens can decrease sexual desire through their antiandrogenic effects.

The sexual response cycle of men and women consists of four stages: appetitive, excitement, orgasm, and resolution (Masters and Johnson 1970). The *appetitive stage* is characterized by sexual fantasies or a desire to be sexual. The *excitement stage* in both men and women is characterized by erotic feelings that lead to vaginal lubrication in women and penile erection in men. There also is an increase in both heart rate and blood pressure. During the male *orgasmic phase*, semen is ejaculated from the penis in spurts. Orgasm for women consists of reflex rhythmic contractions of the circumvaginal muscles. During *resolution*, the final stage, the sex-specific physiological responses return to a resting state. In men, there is a refractory period after orgasm during which it is not possible to have another erection (the length of this period varies between individuals and increases with age). Women are variable: some have a refractory period after orgasm, whereas others do not and can have multiple sequential orgasms.

☐ Sexual Dysfunctions

Sexual dysfunctions (Table 19–2) occur when there are disruptions of any of the four stages of sexual response because of anatomic, physiological, or psychological factors. Sexual orientation is not a determining factor;

Table 19–2.   Sexual dysfunctions

Hypoactive sexual desire disorder	Dyspareunia (not due to a general medical condition)
Sexual aversion disorder	
Female sexual arousal disorder	Vaginismus (not due to a general medical condition)
Male erectile disorder	
Female orgasmic disorder (i.e., inhibited female orgasm)	Sexual dysfunction due to a general medical condition
Male orgasmic disorder (i.e., inhibited male orgasm)	Substance-induced sexual dysfunction
Premature ejaculation	Sexual dysfunction not otherwise specified

consequently, heterosexual, homosexual, or bisexual individuals may experience a sexual dysfunction at some point in their lives. Sexual dysfunctions may be lifelong or may develop after a period of normal sexual functioning. For example, a woman who has never achieved an orgasm would be classified as having a primary female orgasmic disorder, whereas a woman who has been orgasmic at one point in her life but is presently unable to orgasm is experiencing a secondary orgasmic disorder. Sexual dysfunctions may be further characterized as to whether they are present in all sexual activities or are situational in nature. For example, a man who has an erection during masturbation but not during sexual interaction with a partner has a situational erectile disorder. When making the diagnosis of a sexual dysfunction, the following types should be specified: dysfunction due to psychological factors, or dysfunction due to combined psychological factors and a general medical condition. The dysfunction may be recent or lifelong.

Epidemiology

The exact prevalence of sexual dysfunctions is difficult to determine. Nathan (1986) analyzed the findings of 22 general population sex surveys to estimate prevalence rates for various sexual dysfunctions; Spector and Carey (1990) evaluated 23 community samples to estimate prevalence rates. These studies found a wide range in prevalence estimates; 5%–30% of women and 4%–10% of men reported orgasmic disorders. The most frequent disorder, premature ejaculation, was reported by 35%–38% of men in these studies.

Etiology

Kaplan (1974) argued for a multicausal theory of sexual dysfunctions on several levels—intrapsychic, interpersonal, and behavioral—and lists four factors as playing a role in the development of these disorders:

1. Misinformation or ignorance regarding sexual and social interaction
2. Unconscious guilt and anxiety concerning sex
3. Performance anxiety, as the most common cause of erectile and orgasmic dysfunctions
4. Partners' failure to communicate to each other their sexual feelings and those behaviors in which they want to engage

Differential Diagnosis

Patients presenting with a sexual dysfunction should be medically evaluated by a gynecologist or urologist to rule out treatable organic etiologies. As noted earlier, these organic factors may be local diseases of the genitals, vascular illnesses, neurological disease, endocrine disorders, or systemic illness. The patient should always be asked about medications, including over-the-counter medicines as well as illegal drugs.

■ DESCRIPTION AND TREATMENT OF SPECIFIC SEXUAL DYSFUNCTIONS

☐ Sexual Desire Disorders

Hypoactive Sexual Desire Disorder

Hypoactive sexual desire disorder (also known as inhibited sexual desire, or ISD) is characterized by persistent or recurrently deficient sexual fantasies and desire for sexual activity. The disturbance also causes marked distress or interpersonal difficulty. The diagnosis is made if the dysfunction does not occur exclusively during the course of another Axis I disorder (e.g., major depression) and is not due to the direct effects of a substance (alcohol or illegal drugs or prescription drugs) or a general medical condition.

Hypoactive sexual desire disorder has been the most difficult of all the dysfunctions to treat. Testosterone has been used (in both men and women) to treat ISD; however, masculinizing side effects make its use problematic in women. There is no consistent evidence that it is useful in raising sexual interest in men, even when serum testosterone levels are low (O'Carroll and Bancroft 1984). In addition, a placebo-controlled study in women found no advantage of testosterone over therapy (Dow and Gallagher 1989). The most effective treatments involve a combination of cognitive therapy to deal with maladaptive beliefs, behavioral treatment, and marital therapy.

Sexual Aversion Disorder

Sexual aversion disorder is characterized by a persistent or recurrent extreme aversion to and avoidance of all (or almost all) genital sexual contact with a partner. The disturbance causes marked distress or interpersonal difficulties and does not occur exclusively during the course of another Axis II disorder. It is important to differentiate this disorder from hypoactive sexual desire disorder (Ponticas 1992). The major goal of treatment is to reduce the patient's fear and avoidance of sex. This can be accomplished via systematic desensitization in which the patient is gradually exposed in imagination and then in vivo to the actual sexual situations that generate anxiety. Kaplan et al. (1982) reported the successful treatment of sexual phobias using tricyclic medications and sex therapy.

☐ Sexual Arousal Disorders

Male Erectile Disorder

Male erectile disorder is characterized by persistent or recurrent inability to attain or maintain an adequate erection until completion of the sexual activity. Another criterion is that the disturbance causes marked distress or interpersonal difficulty.

The treatment of erectile problems is generally easier if the patient has a willing sexual partner to participate in therapy. However, treatment is possible without a partner's attendance. Initially, the clinician should inform the patient with male erectile dysfunction that he is not alone in this problem and that, in fact, most men are unable to generate an erection at some time in their lives. The most successful treatment for arousal and erectile disorders in patients with partners has been the use of behavioral assignments to gradually decrease performance anxiety. Sensate focus exercises (Masters and Johnson 1970) are one such technique in which the patient engages in nongenital, nondemand caressing with a partner and concentrates on pleasurable feelings. Gradually, the patient engages in pleasurable, genital sexual activities (e.g., touch, oral contact) with no penetration permitted until anxiety has been decreased sufficiently to permit full erectile function. Group therapy, hypnotherapy, and systematic desensitization have also been used successfully in cases of erectile difficulties. Again, these treatments act to reduce anxiety associated with being sexual. Various somatic treatments can also be used to treat erectile disorders, even when these disorders are primarily due to nonorganic factors.

Oral medications such as yohimbine, an alpha-adrenergic antagonist, have also been used to treat erectile dysfunction. Full or partial improvement has been reported in about 34% to 38% of patients when compared with placebo, although these benefits can take several weeks to develop (Sonda et al. 1990). Dopamine agonists such as bromocriptine have also been found to be effective in preliminary trials (Lal et al. 1991).

A major noninvasive, nonpharmacological treatment for erectile dysfunction is the use of an external vacuum device. These devices consist of a plastic cylinder with one open end and the other end connected to a vacuum pump. A vacuum is created that draws blood into the penis. A tension ring is then slipped from the cylinder to the base of the penis for up to 30 minutes. This treatment has a high success rate (about 85%) and a low drop-out rate (about 20% per year) (Turner et al. 1991). These devices have the advantages of being noninvasive, relatively inexpensive, and having few side effects (bruising, physical discomfort, and blocked ejaculation are the most common). Disadvantages are that erections last only 30 minutes and the patient must interrupt sexual activity to use the device (Turner et al. 1992).

Female Sexual Arousal Disorder

Female sexual arousal disorder is characterized by persistent or recurrent inability to attain or maintain an adequate lubrication-swelling response of sexual excitement until completion of the sexual activity. Diagnosis is made if the disorder does not occur exclusively during the course of another Axis I disorder and is not due to the direct effects of a substance (illegal or prescription drugs) or a general medical condition. Treatment of impairment of sexual arousal in women often involves the reduction of anxiety associated with sexual activity. Thus, behavioral techniques such as those involving sensate focus are most often effective (Kaplan 1974).

☐ Orgasm Disorders

Female Orgasmic Disorder

Female orgasmic disorder (also known as inhibited female orgasm) is characterized by persistent or recurrent delay in, or absence of, orgasm following a normal sexual excitement phase. Clinicians should take into consideration that females exhibit great variability in both the type and the intensity of stimulation required to trigger an orgasm. Other factors to be evaluated include the woman's age and sexual experience and the adequacy of sexual stimulation she receives. As with the other dysfunctions the diagnosis is made if the disorder causes marked distress or interpersonal difficulty, if it does not occur exclusively during the course of another Axis I disorder, and if it is not due to the direct effects of a substance or a general medical condition.

The most likely way for a woman with general anorgasmia (i.e., never having had an orgasm) to become orgasmic is through a program of directed masturbation (LoPiccolo and Stock 1986). Any discomfort the patient may feel about exploring her own body should be discussed. Next, the patient should be instructed in a systematic program for exercising the pubococcygeus muscle, a muscle involved in orgasms. Once the patient has mastered these exercises, she is placed on a masturbatory program that begins with a gradual visual and tactile exploration of her body and moves toward focused genital touching.

The most frequent complaint of women experiencing an orgasmic problem is that they are not orgasmic through penile-vaginal intercourse. When becoming orgasmic through intercourse is a patient's treatment goal, the clinician should ensure that she and her partner are aware that adequate stimulation both prior to and during intercourse is necessary. In addition, the clinician may suggest various sexual positions that allow stimulation of the clitoris by the patient or her partner during intercourse.

Male Orgasmic Disorder

Male orgasmic disorder (also known as inhibited male orgasm or retarded ejaculation) is characterized by persistent or recurrent delay in or absence of orgasm following a normal sexual excitement phase during sexual activity. The patient's age, as well as the focus, intensity, and duration of sexual stimulation, must be considered. As with the other disorders, the disturbance must cause marked distress. The treatment for this disorder is similar to that used for inhibited orgasm in females. The patient should be told that when he masturbates, he should masturbate as quickly as possible to ejaculation while fantasizing that his penis is inside his partner's vagina and ejaculating. A second technique is to teach the patient and his partner sensate focus exercises.

Premature Ejaculation

Premature ejaculation is characterized by persistent or recurrent ejaculation with minimal sexual stimulation before, upon, or shortly after penetration and before the person wishes. The patient's age, novelty of situation, sexual partner, and frequency of sexual activity must be taken into consideration in making this diagnosis.

The treatment of premature ejaculation involves training the individual to tolerate high levels of excitement without ejaculating, and reducing anxiety associated with sexual arousal. One successful intervention is the start-stop technique (Semans 1956). This procedure involves having the patient lie on his back while his partner strokes his penis. The patient focuses on the pleasurable feelings resulting from the penile stimulation and the sensations that precede his urge to ejaculate.

When he feels that he is about to ejaculate, he signals his partner to stop stimulation. The patient should start and stop at least four times before he allows himself to ejaculate. A second procedure, the "squeeze" technique (Masters and Johnson 1970), can be done in conjunction with the start-stop technique. In the squeeze technique, the patient's partner is taught to place her thumb on the frenulum of the penis and her first and second fingers on the opposite sides of the head of the penis. When the patient feels that he is going to ejaculate, the partner squeezes for up to 5 seconds and then releases the penis for up to 30 seconds. This is continued until the individual is no longer on the verge of ejaculating; then the patient's partner resumes penile stimulation.

☐ Sexual Pain Disorders

Dyspareunia

Dyspareunia is characterized by recurrent or persistent genital pain in either a male or female before, during, or after sexual intercourse. A substance-induced disorder and other Axis I disorders or general medical conditions should be ruled out. It is imperative that a comprehensive physical and gynecological examination be conducted. In the absence of organic pathology, the patient's fear and anxiety underlying sexual functioning should be investigated. Systematic desensitization has been found to be successful in the treatment of this disorder in some women.

Vaginismus

Vaginismus is characterized by recurrent or persistent involuntary spasm of the musculature of the outer one-third of the vagina that interferes with sexual intercourse. This problem can only be diagnosed with certainty by a gynecological examination. Some women who are anxious about sex may experience muscular tightening and some pain during penetration, but these women do not have vaginismus. It is important to rule out other Axis I disorders (e.g. somatization disorder), substance-induced disorders, or a general medical condition. Systematic desensitization has been the most effective treatment method for vaginismus. A useful procedure involves the systematic insertion of dilators of graduated sizes, either in the doctor's office or in the privacy of the patient's home. Some clinicians have the patient or her partner gradually insert a tampon or fingers until penile penetration can be effected (Kaplan 1974).

Sexual Dysfunction Due to a General Medical Condition

The diagnosis of sexual dysfunction due to a general medical condition is made if there is evidence from the history, physical examination, or laboratory findings of a general medical condition judged to be etiologically related to the sexual dysfunction (e.g., male erectile disorder due to a general medical condition, dyspareunia due to a general medical condition).

Substance-Induced Sexual Dysfunction

The diagnosis of substance-induced sexual dysfunction is made if the patient has been using either medications or drugs that result in the impairment of sexual functioning, and the symptoms of the dysfunction are manifested either during use of the substance or within 6 weeks of cessation of the substance. Individuals who abuse drugs have a high rate (up to 60%) of sexual dysfunctions (Schiavi 1990).

■ PARAPHILIAS

The paraphilia disorders (Table 19–3) are characterized by experiencing, over a period of at least 6 months, recurrent intense sexual urges and sexually arousing fantasies that involve nonhuman objects or nonconsenting partners. Examples are fetishism (i.e., sexual arousal to nonliving objects, female undergarments, etc.), transvestic fetishism (i.e., sexual urges and fantasies involving cross-dressing), and pedophilia (i.e., sexual urges and fantasies involving prepubescent children). Sexual sadism involves urges toward and sexually arousing fantasies of acts (real, not simulated) in which the psychological and/or physical suffering (including humiliation) of the victim is sexually exciting to the perpetrator. In sexual masochism an individual derives sexual excitement from being humiliated, beaten, bound, or otherwise made to suffer. In diagnosing all of the paraphilias a further criterion is that the person has acted on the urges or is markedly distressed by them.

☐ Epidemiology

The paraphilias rarely cause personal distress, and individuals with these disorders usually come for treatment because of pressure from their part-

Table 19–3.   Paraphilias

Exhibitionism	Sexual sadism
Fetishism	Transvestic fetishism
Frotteurism	Voyeurism
Pedophilia	Paraphilia not otherwise specified
Sexual masochism	Sexual disorder not otherwise specified

ners or the authorities. Thus there are few data on the prevalence or course of many of these disorders. The vast majority of individuals with these disorders are men. For example, among reported cases of sexual abuse, over 90% of offenders are men (Finkelhor 1986).

☐ Etiology

Various theories have been put forth to explain the development of paraphilias. As with the gender identity disorders, biological factors have been postulated. Destruction of parts of the limbic system in animals causes hypersexual behavior (Klüver-Bucy syndrome), and temporal lobe diseases such as psychomotor seizures or temporal lobe tumors have been implicated in some persons with paraphilias. It has also been suggested that abnormal levels of androgens may contribute to inappropriate sexual arousal. The majority of studies, however, have dealt only with violent sex offenders and have yielded inconclusive results (Bradford and McLean 1984).

Psychoanalytic theories have postulated that severe castration anxiety during the oedipal phase of development leads to the substitution of a symbolic object (inanimate or an anatomic part) for the mother, as in fetishism and transvestism. Some psychoanalytic theories have suggested that a paraphilia represents an attempt by an individual to recreate and master early childhood punishment or humiliation (Stoller 1975).

☐ Diagnosis

It is important to distinguish paraphilias such as fetishism and transvestism from normal variations of sexual behavior. Some couples occasionally augment their usual sexual activities with activities such as bondage or cross-dressing. Transvestism, however, would only be diagnosed if a heterosexual male, over a period of at least 6 months, had recurrent intense sexual urges and sexually arousing fantasies involving cross-dressing, and if the person is distressed by the urges, or has acted on them. It is only when these activities are the exclusive or preferred means of achieving sexual excitement and orgasm, or when the sexual behavior is not consensual, that the diagnosis of paraphilia is made. Obviously, nonconsensual sexual activities such as sexual contact with children or exhibitionism can never be appropriate—children can never give consent for sexual activity with an adult.

In evaluating an individual for paraphilic behavior, a careful psychiatric evaluation must be done to exclude the above-noted possible causes of this behavior. A detailed sexual history should be taken, noting the onset and course of paraphilic and appropriate sexual fantasies and behavior, and the present degree of control over the deviant behavior. In addition, the individual should be evaluated for faulty beliefs about his or her sexual behavior (i.e., cognitive distortions), social and assertive skills with appropriate adult partners, sexual dysfunctions, and sexual knowledge.

Phallometric assessments (i.e., measurements of penile erection) have been used to objectively assess sexual arousal in individuals who have engaged in paraphilic behavior. This is important because persons with paraphilias, especially those in trouble with the law, are reluctant to disclose the full extent of their deviant behavior and fantasies. A transducer (either a thin metal ring or mercury-in-rubber strain gauge) is placed around the penis, and the degree of erection is recorded while the individual is exposed to various sexual stimuli (audiotapes, slides, videotapes) depicting paraphilic and appropriate sexual scenes. This information is then recorded on a polygraph or computer, and the degree of arousal to deviant sexual scenes is compared with arousal to nonparaphilic scenes.

☐ Treatment

Biological treatments have traditionally been reserved for individuals with pedophilia or exhibitionism, although occasionally individuals with other paraphilias present for treatment with medications. In view of the important role androgens play in the maintenance of sexual arousal, treatments have focused on blocking or decreasing the level of circulating androgens. Surgical castration has been widely used in Europe with incarcerated sex offenders. However, studies have suggested this is not an effective means of eliminating deviant sexual behavior and that almost one-third of castrated men can still engage in intercourse (Heim 1981).

Stein and colleagues (1992) reported on the use of serotonergic medications (i.e., fluoxetine, clomipramine, fluvoxamine, or flufluramine) in the treatment of patients who presented with sexual obsessions, addictions, and paraphilias. In contrast to the studies cited above, these authors found that these medications were ineffective in treating the paraphilias. The authors hypothesized that compulsivity and impulsivity may be on a neurobiological spectrum in which obsessions and compulsions are at the compulsive end of the spectrum and paraphilias at the impulsive end.

Psychoanalysis and psychodynamic therapy have been used in treating paraphilias. Identification and resolution of early conflicts, trauma, and humiliation are thought to remove the individual's anxiety toward appropriate partners and enable him or her to give up the paraphilic fantasies. Although useful in some individuals, there has been disappointment with the results of psychodynamic psychotherapy as the sole form of treatment in cases of deviant sexual arousal (Crawford 1981).

A variety of behavior therapies have been used to treat paraphilias. Various aversive conditioning methods (e.g., noxious odors) and covert sensitization have been used to decrease deviant sexual behavior. (In the latter, the individual pairs his or her inappropriate sexual fantasies with aversive, anxiety-provoking scenes, under the guidance of a therapist.) Satiation is a technique in which the individual uses his or her deviant fantasies postorgasm in a repetitive manner to the point of satiating himself or herself with the deviant stimuli, in essence making the fantasies and behavior boring (Marshall and Barbaree 1978).

☐ Sexual Disorder Not Otherwise Specified

There are several sexual disturbances that are neither dysfunctions nor paraphilias but yet are still considered sexual disturbances. These include marked feelings of inadequacy concerning sexual performance or other traits related to self-imposed standards of masculinity of femininity, distress about a pattern of repeated sexual relationships involving a succession of lovers who are experienced by the person only as things to be used, or persistent and marked distress about one's sexual orientation.

■ REFERENCES

Barlow DH, Abel GG, Blanchard EB: Gender identity change in transsexuals: follow-up and replications. Arch Gen Psychiatry 36:1001–1007, 1979

Bradford JMW, McLean D: Sexual offenders, violence, and testosterone: a clinical study. Can J Psychiatry 29:335–343, 1984

Crawford D: Treatment approaches with pedophiles, in Adult Sexual Interest in Children. Edited by Cook M, Howells K. New York, Academic, 1981, pp 181–217

Dow MGT, Gallagher J: A controlled study of combined hormonal and psychological treatment for sexual unresponsiveness in women. Br J Clin Psychol 28:201–212, 1989

Ehrhardt AA, Meyer-Bahlburg HFL: Effects of prenatal sex hormones on gender-related behavior. Science 211:1312–1318, 1981

Finkelhor D: Source Book on Child Sex Abuse. Beverly Hills, CA, Sage, 1986

Green R: Sexual Identity Conflict in Children and Adults. New York, Basic Books, 1974

Green R: Gender identity in childhood and later sexual orientation: follow-up of 78 males. Am J Psychiatry 142:339–341, 1985

Heim N: Sexual behavior of castrated sex offenders. Arch Sex Behav 10:11–19, 1981

Kaplan HS: The New Sex Therapy: Active Treatment of Sexual Dysfunctions. New York, Brunner/Mazel, 1974

Kaplan HS, Fyer AJ, Novick A: Sexual phobia. J Sex Marital Ther 8:3–28, 1982

Lal S, Kiely ME, Thavundayil JX, et al: Effect of bromocriptine in patients with apomorphine-responsive erectile impotence: an open study. J Psychiatry Neurosci 16:262–266, 1991

LoPiccolo J, Stock WE: Treatment of sexual dysfunction. J Consult Clin Psychol 54:158–167, 1986

Lothstein L: The postsurgical transsexual: empirical and theoretical considerations. Arch Sex Behav 9:547–564, 1980

Marshall WL, Barbaree HE: The reduction of deviant arousal: satiation treatment for sexual aggressors. Criminal Justice and Behavior 5:294–303, 1978

Masters WH, Johnson VE: Human Sexual Inadequacy. Boston, MA, Little, Brown, 1970

Money J, Ehrhardt AA: Man and Woman, Boy and Girl: The Differentiation and Dimorphism of Gender Identity From Conception to Maturity. Baltimore, MD, Johns Hopkins Press, 1974

Nathan SG: The epidemiology of the DSM-III psychosexual dysfunctions. J Sex Marital Ther 12:267–281, 1986

O'Carroll R, Bancroft J: Testosterone therapy for low sexual interest and erectile dysfunctions in men: a controlled study. Br J Psychiatry 145:146–151, 1984

Person E, Ovesey L: The transsexual syndrome in males, II: secondary transsexualism. Am J Psychother 28:174–193, 1974

Ponticas Y: Sexual aversion versus hypoactive sexual desire: a diagnostic challenge. Psychiatr Med 10:273–281, 1992

Schiavi RC: Chronic alcoholism and male sexual dysfunction. J Sex Marital Ther 16:23–33, 1990

Semans JH: Premature ejaculation: a new approach. South Med J 9:353–357, 1956

Sonda LP, Mazo R, Chancellor MB: The role of yohimbine for the treatment of erectile impotence. J Sex Marital Ther 16:15–21, 1990

Spector IP, Carey MP: Incidence and prevalence of the sexual dysfunctions: a critical review of the empirical literature. Arch Sex Behav 19:389–408, 1990

Stein DJ, Hollander E, Anthony DT, et al: Serotonergic medications for sexual obsessions, sexual addictions and paraphilias. J Clin Psychiatry 53:267–271, 1992

Stoller RJ: Perversion: the Erotic Form of Hatred. New York, Pantheon, 1975

Turner LA, Althof SE, Levine SB, et al: External vacuum devices in the treatment of erectile dysfunction: a one-year study of sexual and psychosocial impact. J Sex Marital Ther 17:81–93, 1991

Turner LA, Althof SE, Levine SB, et al: Twelve-month comparison of two treatments for erectile dysfunction: self-injection versus external vacuum devices. Urology 39:139–144, 1992

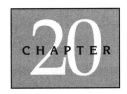

CHAPTER 20

Adjustment Disorder

James J. Strain, M.D.
Jeffrey Newcorn, M.D.
Dennis Wolf, M.D.
George Fulop, M.D.

Adjustment disorder is a subthreshold diagnosis that, as with all subthreshold diagnoses, presents major taxonomical and diagnostic dilemmas. In the gray area of diagnoses that lie between normal behavior on the one hand and major disorders on the other, reside the subthreshold disorders, which are often poorly defined, overlap with other diagnostic groupings, have indefinite symptomatology, and present problems of reliability and validity. These disorders are also juxtaposed between problem-level diagnoses and more clearly defined disorders.

At the same time, the indefiniteness of these subthreshold disorders permits the classification of early or temporary states when the clinical picture is vague and indiscrete, and yet the morbid state is more than that expected in a normal reaction. Therefore, adjustment disorder occupies an important place in the psychiatric lexicon spectrum: normal, problem-level diagnoses (V Codes), adjustment disorder, disorders not otherwise specified (NOS), and major disorders. As such, adjustment disorder would "trump" problem-level disorders, but be "trumped" by a specific diagnosis, even if it were in the NOS category.

Adjustment disorder is a stress-related phenomenon in which the stressor has resulted in maladaptation and symptoms that are time-limited until the stressor is removed or a new state of adaptation has occurred. The stress disorders are unique in the psychiatric DSM lexicon in that they are diagnoses with a known etiology and in which the etiological agent is central to the diagnosis. The DSM by design was intended to have an atheoretical and phenomenological base as the cornerstone of its conceptual framework for diagnostic assignment. The deviance of the stress-induced disorders requires the diagnostician to impute etiological significance to a life event—a stressor—and relate its effect in clinical terms to the patient. The diagnosis of adjustment disorder also requires a careful titration of the timing of the stressor to the adverse psychological sequelae that ensue.

■ DEFINITION AND DIAGNOSIS

Historically, the concept of adjustment disorder included the notion of a "transient situational disturbance," initially codified by developmental epochs, and then evolved to embody a disorder of adjustment characterized by mood, behavior, or work (or academic) inhibition (DSM-III [American Psychiatric Association 1980]), and finally to include physical complaints as well (DSM-III-R [American Psychiatric Association 1987]).

With the opportunity to develop another evolutionary step of the *Diagnostic and Statistical Manual of Mental Disorders* (i.e., DSM-IV), the authors were asked to reexamine the subthreshold diagnostic category of adjustment disorder. From a review of the literature, reanalysis of existing data sets, and observations of the other pertinent diagnoses (e.g., minor depression, PTSD, minor anxiety), suggested modifications for DSM-IV and their rationale were formulated.

As a result of the review of the literature and the Western Psychiatric Institute and Clinic data reanalysis, the American Psychiatric Association (APA) Task Force on Psychological System Interface Disorders recommended that the following changes be included in DSM-IV:

1. Enhance the language.
2. Describe the time of the reaction to reflect duration: acute (less than 6 months) or chronic (6 months or greater).
3. Allow for the continuation of the stressor for an indefinite period.
4. Eliminate the subtypes of mixed emotional features, work (or academic) inhibition, withdrawal, and physical complaints.

In reviewing the diagnosis of adjustment disorder for DSM-IV, two issues emerge as fundamental. First, the effect of the imprecision of this diagnosis on reliability and validity, because of the lack of behavioral or operational criteria, must be determined. Second, the classification of syndromes that do not fulfill the criteria for a major mental illness but present with serious (or incipient) symptomatology that requires intervention and/or treatment, by default, may be viewed as "subthreshold" and afforded a subthreshold interest by health care workers and third-party payers. Thus, the construct of adjustment disorder is designed as a means for classifying psychiatric conditions having a symptom profile that is as yet insufficient to meet the more specifically operationalized criteria for the major syndromes but that is 1) clinically significant and deemed to be in excess of a normal reaction to the stressor in question; 2) associated with impaired vocational or interpersonal functioning; and 3) not solely the result of a psychosocial problem (V code) requiring medical attention (e.g., noncompliance, phase of life problem, etc.).

The issue of boundaries between the major syndromes depression NOS, anxiety NOS, and adjustment disorder also remains problematic. How often are the major syndromes associated with a stressor? How different are the symptom profiles of depression and anxiety NOS from those of adjustment disorder?

Although the diagnosis of adjustment disorder is not scientifically rigorous, it is just this imprecision that makes the diagnosis so useful to psychiatry. It is difficult to identify an emerging illness in its early stages, and in such instances the diagnosis of adjustment disorder serves as a "temporary" diagnosis that can be modified with information from longitudinal evaluation and treatment. It is a way to "tag" an individual for possible difficulty.

Even serious symptomatology (e.g., suicidal behavior) that is not regarded as part of a major mental disorder needs treatment and a "diagnosis" under which it can be placed. De Leo et al. (1986a, 1986b) reported on adjustment disorder and suicidality. It had been suggested by the Adjustment Disorder DSM-IV Work Group that suicide could be a subtype of adjustment disorder, but the problem of suicidal symptomotology without another psychiatric diagnosis will now be placed in the F-code section for other problems "that may be a focus of clinical attention" (American Psychiatric Association 1994). Clearly, what is regarded as a subthreshold diagnosis—adjustment disorder—does not necessarily imply the presence of subthreshold symptomatology within its domain (Table 20–1).

The issues of diagnostic rigor and clinical utility seem at odds for adjustment disorder, and field studies that would employ reliable and valid instruments (e.g., depression or anxiety rating scales, stress assessments, length of disability, treatment outcome, family patterns, etc.) would allow more exact specification of the parameters of the diagnosis. Identification of the time course, remission or evolution to another diagnosis, and the evaluation of stressors (characteristics, duration, and the nature of adaptation to stress) would enhance understanding of the concept of a stress-response illness.

Regardless of their position on the diagnostic tree, subthreshold syndromes can encompass significant psychopathology that must be not only recognized but treated (e.g., suicidal ideation/behavior). Cross-

---

Table 20–1.   DSM-IV diagnostic criteria for adjustment disorders

---

A.   The development of emotional or behavioral symptoms in response to an identifiable stressor(s) occurring within 3 months of the onset of the stressor(s).

B.   These symptoms or behaviors are clinically significant as evidenced by either of the following:

   1.   Marked distress that is in excess of what would be expected from exposure to the stressor

   2.   Significant impairment in social or occupational (academic) functioning

C.   The stress-related disturbance does not meet the criteria for another specific Axis I disorder and is not merely an exacerbation of a preexisting Axis I or Axis II disorder.

D.   The symptoms do not represent bereavement.

E.   Once the stressor (or its consequences) has terminated, the symptoms do not persist for more than an additional 6 months.

Specify if:

Acute: if the disturbance lasts less than 6 months

Chronic: if the disturbance lasts for 6 months or longer

Adjustment disorders are coded based on the subtype, which is selected according to the predominant symptoms. The specific stressor(s) can be specified on Axis IV.

309.0	**With depressed mood**
309.24	**With anxiety**
309.28	**With mixed anxiety and depressed mood**
309.3	**With disturbance of conduct**
309.4	**With mixed disturbance of emotions and conduct**
309.9	**Unspecified**

---

sectionally, adjustment disorder may appear to be the incipient phase of an emerging major syndrome. Consequently, adjustment disorder, despite the problems of reliability and validity associated with such a category, could serve an important diagnostic function in the practice of psychiatry, especially when the typology is more fully developed. Problem- and subthreshold-level diagnoses are critical to the function of any medical discipline. Because this may be the initial phase, or a mild form, of a dysfunction that is not yet fully developed, there is a need to describe the relationship of the incipient to the developed, and the subthreshold to the defined. This apparent chaos, lack of specificity, and questionable reliability and validity are the hallmark of interface disorders and subthreshold phenomena, whether they be in diabetes mellitus, hypertension, or depression.

The characteristics of a mental disorder vary over the life cycle, and this is clearly illustrated by adjustment disorder. Certain developmental epochs may be associated with a particular symptom profile. The effect of the stressor may vary, and the assessment of functioning must be "measured" according to the demands of the developmental stage. The symptom characteristics and functional assessment of other diagnoses may also vary along the developmental schema from birth to senescence; illnesses such as major depressive disorders, organic mental disorders, sexual dysfunctions, and eating disorders need to be "recast" in another hierarchy to incorporate the stage of the life cycle extant at the time of the assessment. Such considerations as the normal variations across developmental epochs would make adjustment disorder and the other DSM disorders much more applicable and less vulnerable to their being characterized as "unfair" in regard to the "aged," the "child/youth," or the "medically ill" (Strain 1981).

■ EPIDEMIOLOGY

Andreasen and Wasek (1980) reported that 5% of an inpatient and outpatient sample were labeled as having adjustment disorder. Fabrega et al. (1987) observed that 2.3% of a sample of patients presenting to a walk-in clinic met criteria for adjustment disorder, with no other diagnoses on Axis I or Axis II; 20% had the diagnosis of adjustment disorder when patients with other Axis I diagnoses were also included. In general hospital psychiatric consultation populations, adjustment disorder was diagnosed as 21.5% and 11.5% (Popkin et al. 1990; Snyder and Strain 1989). Andreasen and Wasek (1980), utilizing a chart review, reported that more adolescents than adults experienced acting out and behavioral symptoms, but adults had significantly more depressive symptomatology (87.2% vs. 63.8%). Anxiety symptoms were frequent at all ages.

Fabrega et al. 1987 evaluated 64 symptoms currently present in three cohorts: subjects with specific diagnoses, those with adjustment disorder, and those who were not ill. Vegetative, substance use, and characterological symptoms were greatest in the specific-diagnosis group, intermediate in the adjustment disorder group, and least in the group with no illness. The symptoms of mood and affect, general appearance, behavior, disturbance in speech and thought pattern, and cognitive functioning had a similar distribution. The adjustment disorder group was significantly different from the no-illness group with regard to more "depressed mood" and "low self-esteem." The adjustment disorder and no-illness groups both had minimal pathology of thought content and perception. Twenty-nine percent of adjustment disorder versus 9% of the no-illness group had a positive response on the suicide indicators. The three cohorts did not differ on the frequency of Axis III disorders.

■ ETIOLOGY

Stress has been described as the etiological agent for adjustment disorder. However, diverse variables and modifiers are involved regarding who will experience an adjustment disorder following a stress. Cohen (1981) argues that 1) acute stresses are different from chronic ones in both psychological and physiological terms; 2) the meaning of the stress is affected by "modifiers" (i.e., ego strengths, support systems, prior mastery); and 3) one must differentiate the manifest and latent meanings of the stressor(s) (e.g., loss of job may be a relief or a catastrophe). An objectively overwhelming stress may have little impact on one individual, whereas a minor one could be regarded as cataclysmic by another. A recent minor stress superimposed on a previous underlying (major) stress that has no observable effect on its own may have a significant additive impact (i.e., concatenation of events) (B. Hamburg, personal communication, 1990).

The chronological relationship of the stressor and symptoms has been examined less extensively. Depue and Monroe (1986) and Rahe (1990) stated that the model of a single stressor impinging on an undisturbed individual to cause symptoms at a single point in time is insufficient to account for the many presentations of stress and illness in the clinical situation. Limitations of the current construct of stress for research have been described (Cohen 1981). Holmes and Rahe (1967) assigned relative values to specific stressors, but there has been much concern about the methodology used and the results obtained (Cohen 1981). Other life event scales (Paykel and Tanner 1976; Paykel et al. 1971; Tennant 1983) have also been shown to be inconsistent in their ability to link stress and illness. Many authors have cautioned that the vulnerability of the individual (e.g., ego strengths, support system, underlying personality disorders, the timing and concatenation of the stress(es), the issue of control over the stressor, and the desirability of the event, etc.) needs to be assessed to ascertain the import of the situation on the individual.

Hirschfeld (1981) and Winokur (1985) discussed both sides of the controversy regarding "neurotic" (i.e., related to a stressor) and "endogenous" (i.e., not related to a stressor) depression. From the examination of several studies, it has been difficult to demonstrate a significant temporal link between the onset of an identified stressor and the occurrence of depressive illness (Andreasen and Winokur 1979; Garvey et al. 1984; Hirschfeld 1981; Paykel and Tanner 1976; Winokur 1985).

Andreasen and Wasek (1980) described the differences between the types of stressors found in adolescents versus those in adults: respectively, 59% and 35% of the precipitants had been present for a year or more, and 9% and 39% for 3 months or less. Fabrega et al. (1987) reported that their adjustment disorder group had greater registration of stressors compared with the specific diagnosis and the non-illness cohorts. There was a significant difference in the amount of stressors reported relevant to the clinical request for evaluation: the group with adjustment disorder, compared with the specific diagnosis and the non-illness patients, was overrepresented in the "higher stress" category. Popkin et al. (1990) reported that in 68.6% of the cases in their consultation cohort, the medical illness itself was judged to be the primary psychosocial stressor. Snyder and Strain (1989) observed that stressors as assessed on Axis IV were significantly higher for consultation patients with adjustment disorder than for patients with other diagnostic disorders.

■ CLINICAL FEATURES

In DSM-IV, adjustment disorder has been reduced to six types that are classified according to their clinical features: adjustment disorder with depressed mood; adjustment disorder with anxious mood; adjustment disorder with mixed anxiety and depressed mood; adjustment disorder with disturbance of conduct; adjustment disorder with mixed disturbance of emotions and conduct; adjustment disorder not otherwise specified (NOS) (Table 20–2).

■ TREATMENT

Treatment of adjustment disorder rests primarily upon psychotherapeutic measures that enable the reduction of the stressor, enhanced coping with the stressor that cannot be reduced or removed, and the establishment of a support system to maximize adaptation. The first goal is to note significant dysfunction secondary to a stressor and help the patient to moderate this imbalance. Many stressors may be avoided or minimized—for example, taking on more responsibility than can be managed by the individual, or putting oneself at risk (e.g., unprotected sex with an unknown partner). Other stressors may elicit an overreaction on the part of the patient (e.g., abandonment by a lover). The patient may attempt suicide or become reclusive, damaging his or her source of income. In this situation, the therapist would attempt to help the patient put his or her feelings and rage into words rather than into destructive actions, and assist more optimal adaptation and mastery of the trauma-stressor.

The role of verbalization cannot be overestimated in an attempt to reduce the pressure of the stressor and enhance coping. The therapist also needs to clarify and interpret the meaning of the stressor for the patient. For example, a mastectomy may have devastated a patient's feel-

---

Table 20–2. Types of DSM-IV adjustment disorder

Adjustment disorder with depressed mood: The predominant symptoms are those of a minor depression. For example, the symptoms might be depressed mood, tearfulness, and hopelessness.

Adjustment disorder with anxious mood: This type of adjustment disorder is diagnosed when anxiety symptoms are predominant, such as nervousness, worry, and jitteriness. The differential diagnosis would include anxiety disorders.

Adjustment disorder with mixed anxiety and depressed mood: This category should be used when the predominant symptoms are a combination of depression and anxiety or other emotions. An example would be an adolescent who, after moving away from home and parental supervision, reacts with ambivalence, depression, anger, and signs of increased dependence.

Adjustment disorder with disturbance of conduct: The symptomatic manifestations are those of behavioral misconduct that violated societal norms or the rights of others. Examples are fighting, truancy, vandalism, and reckless driving.

Adjustment disorder with mixed disturbance of emotions and conduct: This diagnosis is made when the disturbance combines affective and behavioral features of adjustment disorder with mixed emotional features and adjustment disorder with disturbance of conduct.

Adjustment disorder not otherwise specified (NOS): This is a residual diagnosis within the diagnostic category. This diagnosis can be used when a maladaptive reaction that is not classified under other adjustment disorders occurs in response to stress. An example would be a patient who, when diagnosed as having cancer, denies the diagnosis of malignancy and is noncompliant with treatment recommendations.

Source. Adapted from American Psychiatric Association: *Diagnostic and Statistical Manual of Mental Disorders,* 4th Edition. Washington, DC, American Psychiatric Association, 1994. Copyright 1994, American Psychiatric Association. Used with permission.

---

ings about her body and herself. It is necessary to clarify that the patient is still a woman, capable of having a fulfilling relationship, including a sexual one, and that patients can have their cancer removed/treated and not have a recurrence. Otherwise the patient's pernicious fantasies—"all is lost"—may take over in response to the stressor (i.e., the mastectomy) and make her dysfunctional in work and/or sex, and precipitate a painful dysphoria or disturbance of mood that is incapacitating.

Counseling, psychotherapy, crisis intervention, family therapy, and group treatment may be employed to encourage the verbalization of fears, anxiety, rage, helplessness, and hopelessness to the stressors imposed upon a patient. The goal of treatment in each case is to expose the concerns and conflicts that the patient is experiencing, identify means to reduce the stressor(s), enhance the patient's coping skills, and help the patient gain perspective on the adversity and establish relationships (i.e., a support network) to assist in the management of the stressor and the self. The primary treatment for adjustment disorder is talking. However, in some patients small doses of antidepressants and anxiolytics may be appropriate.

■ COURSE AND PROGNOSIS

With regard to the long-term outcome of adjustment disorder, Andreasen and Hoenk (1982) suggested that the prognosis is good for adults, but that in adolescents many major psychiatric illnesses eventually occur. At 5-year follow-up, 71% of adults were completely well, 8% had an intervening problem, and 21% developed a major depressive disorder or alcoholism. In adolescents at 5-year follow-up, only 44% were without a psychiatric diagnosis, 13% had an intervening psychiatric illness, and 43% went on to develop major psychiatric morbidity (i.e., schizophrenia, schizoaffective disorders, major depression, bipolar disorder, substance abuse, and personality disorders). In contrast to the adults, the chronicity of the illness and the presence of behavioral symptoms in the adolescents were the strongest predictors for major pathology at the 5-year follow-up. The number and type of symptoms were less useful than the length of treatment and chronicity of symptoms as predictors of future outcome. Strain et al. (1981) found that many of the subtypes of adjustment disorder were infrequently used (e.g., "with mixed emotional features"), while "with physical complaints," a DSM-III-R category, has had insufficient time to be observed.

■ REFERENCES

American Psychiatric Association: Diagnostic and Statistical Manual of Mental Disorders, 3rd Edition. Washington, DC, American Psychiatric Association, 1980

American Psychiatric Association: Diagnostic and Statistical Manual of Mental Disorders, 3rd Edition, Revised. Washington, DC, American, 1987

American Psychiatric Association: Diagnostic and Statistical Manual of Mental Disorders, 4th Edition. Washington, DC, American Psychiatric Association, 1994

Andreasen NC, Hoenk PR: The predictive value of adjustment disorders: a follow-up study. Am J Psychiatry 139:584–590, 1982

Andreasen NC, Wasek P: Adjustment disorders in adolescents and adults. Arch Gen Psychiatry 37:1166–1170, 1980

Andreasen NC, Winokur G: Secondary depression: familial, clinical, and research perspectives. Am J Psychiatry 136:62–66, 1979

Cohen F: Stress and bodily illness. Psychiatr Clin North Am 4:269–286, 1981

De Leo D, Pellegrini C, Serraiotto L: Adjustment disorders and suicidality. Psychol Rep 59:355–358, 1986a

De Leo D, Pellegrini C, Serraiotto L, et al: Assessment of severity of suicide attempts: a trial with the dexamethasone suppression test and two rating scales. Psychopathology 19:186–191, 1986b

Depue RA, Monroe SM: Conceptualization and measurement of human disorder in life stress research: the problem of chronic disturbance. Psychol Bull 99:36–51, 1986

Fabrega H Jr, Mezzich JE, Mezzich AC: Adjustment disorder as a marginal or transitional illness category in DSM-III. Arch Gen Psychiatry 44:567–572, 1987

Garvey MJ, Tollefson GD, Mungas D, et al: Is the distinction between situational and nonsituational primary depression valid? Compr Psychiatry 25:372–375, 1984

Hirschfeld RMA: Situational depression: validity of the concept. Br J Psychiatry 139:297–305, 1981

Holmes TH, Rahe RH: The Social Readjustment Rating Scale. J Psychosom Res 11:213–218, 1967

Paykel ES, Tanner J: Life events, depressive relapse and maintenance treatment. Psychol Med 6:481–485, 1976

Paykel ES, Prusoff BA, Uhlenhuth EH: Scaling of life events. Arch Gen Psychiatry 25:340–347, 1971

Popkin MK, Callies AL, Colón EA, et al: Adjustment disorders in medically ill patients referred for consultation in a university hospital. Psychosomatics 31:410–414, 1990

Rahe RH: Psychosocial stressors and adjustment disorder: Van Gogh's life chart illustrates stress and disease. J Clin Psychiatry 51 (No 11, suppl):13–19, 1990

Snyder S, Strain JJ: Differentiation of major depression and adjustment disorder with depressed mood in the medical setting. Gen Hosp Psychiatry 12:159–165, 1989

Strain JJ: Diagnostic considerations in the medical setting. Psychiatr Clin North Am 4:287–300, 1981

Tennant C: Life events and psychological morbidity: the evidence from prospective studies (editorial). Psychol Med 13:483–486, 1983

Winokur G: The validity of neurotic-reactive depression: new data and reappraisal. Arch Gen Psychiatry 42:1116–1122, 1985

CHAPTER 21

Impulse Control Disorders Not Elsewhere Classified

Michael G. Wise, M.D.
John G. Tierney, M.D.

The DSM-IV (American Psychiatric Association 1994a) diagnostic category called "Impulse Control Disorders Not Elsewhere Classified" is a "residual" diagnostic category, even though there is no other distinct group of disorders in DSM-IV classified as impulse disorders. The diagnoses found in this category are intermittent explosive disorder, kleptomania, pyromania, pathological gambling, trichotillomania, and impulse control disorder not otherwise specified (NOS). The features common to all of these impulse disorders are as follows:

1. Failure to resist an impulse, drive, or temptation to perform some act that is harmful to the person or others.
2. An increasing sense of tension or arousal before commiting the act.
3. A sense of pleasure, gratification, or release at the time of committing the act, or shortly thereafter.

Recent research has stimulated discussion as to whether the impulse control disorders are "affective spectrum disorders" (McElroy et al. 1992), are related to obsessive-compulsive disorder (OCD) (Swedo et al. 1989), or are a convergence of mood, impulse, and compulsive disorders (Kafka and Coleman 1991).

■ INTERMITTENT EXPLOSIVE DISORDER

☐ Definition and Diagnostic Criteria

The DSM-IV diagnostic criteria for intermittent explosive disorder (Table 21–1) eliminate the requirement that impulsivity be absent between episodes, and add additional exclusionary diagnoses. Two DSM-IV diagnoses are currently available to the clinician who wishes to diagnose a patient who primarily manifests episodic violent behavior: *intermittent explosive disorder* and *personality change due to a general medical condition, aggressive type*. Intermittent explosive disorder has numerous exclusion criteria, whereas personality change due to a general medical condition requires the presence of a specific organic factor that is judged to be causally related to the violence. The majority of individuals with episodic violent behavior will not meet the diagnostic criteria for either disorder, but will have another psychiatric disorder such as schizophrenia, paranoid disorder, mania, substance abuse, drug withdrawal, delirium, a personality disorder (especially borderline or antisocial), mental retardation, a conduct disorder, or organic brain disease (Tardiff 1992).

☐ Epidemiology

Monopolis and Lion (1983) called attention to the tendency of clinicians to diagnose intermittent explosive disorder without using any diagnostic criteria. A literature review prepared for the sourcebook for DSM-IV (American Psychiatric Association 1994b) reaffirmed this impression and notes that authors typically use the occurrence of one or more explosive outbursts as sufficient for the diagnosis. Males account for 80% of persons who display episodic violence (American Psychiatric Association 1994b).

Table 21–1. DSM-IV diagnostic criteria for intermittent explosive disorder

A. Several discrete episodes of failure to resist aggressive impulses that result in serious assaultive acts or destruction of property.

B. The degree of aggressiveness expressed during the episodes is grossly out of proportion to any precipitating psychosocial stressors.

C. The aggressive episodes are not better accounted for by another mental disorder (e.g., antisocial personality disorder, borderline personality disorder, a psychotic disorder, a manic episode, conduct disorder, or attention-deficit/hyperactivity disorder) and are not due to the direct physiological effects of a substance (e.g., a drug of abuse, a medication) or a general medical condition (e.g., head trauma, Alzheimer's disease).

☐ Etiology

Despite the knowledge that individuals who exhibit episodic violence often have personality disorders, no investigator of intermittent explosive disorder has evaluated personality in a systematic fashion. This is a critical factor, because antisocial personality disorder and borderline personality disorder are part of the exclusion criteria for the intermittent explosive disorder diagnosis.

The characteristics of 842 individuals who were reported to display episodic violent behavior are summarized in Table 21–2 (American Psychiatric Association 1994b). When all 842 cases were carefully reviewed and compared to DSM-III-R criteria for intermittent explosive disorder, only 17 patients who might have intermittent explosive disorder were found. Patients with episodic violent behavior frequently have neurological abnormalities. When examined, a significant percentage have abnormal neurological exams (65%), abnormal neuropsychological tests (58%), abnormal electroencephalograms (EEGs) (55%), a history of attention-deficit hyperactivity disorder (45%), or a history of learning disability

Table 21–2.   Characteristics of 842 patients with episodic violent behavior

	Percentage of patients examined out of total sample (N = 842)	Number positive/total examined (%)
History of seizures	87	215/733 (29%)
Legal problems	74	216/621 (35%)
Head trauma	73	182/617 (30%)
History of attention deficit	69	262/582 (45%)
Drugs involved	65	82/547 (15%)
Neurological abnormality	64	350/539 (65%)
History of psychosis	62	33/527 (6%)
Antisocial personality	53	15/445 (3%)
Alcohol abuse/pathological intoxication	50	238/417 (57%)
Electroencephalogram (EEG)	44	202/368 (55%)
Family history of violence	31	109/264 (41%)
Prodromal symptoms	24	77/202 (38%)
Other personality disorder	20	39/168 (23%)
Neuropsychological tests	20	97/167 (58%)
Presence of remorse	18	96/153 (63%)
Genetic abnormality	18	4/151 (3%)
Learning disability	12	38/99 (38%)
Computed tomography scan	12	16/98 (16%)

Source.   Reprinted from literature review on intermittent explosive disorder authored by Michael Wise et al. in American Psychiatric Association 1994b. Used with permission.

(38%). Despite evidence of CNS dysfunction, it is often impossible to establish a clear cause-and-effect relationship between the CNS dysfunction and episodic violent behavior.

Research has implicated abnormalities in noradrenergic and serotonergic function in individuals who display episodic violence (Eichelman 1992; Tardiff 1992). This research is promising, and further investigation into the relationship between biological factors and behavioral disorders is warranted.

☐ Treatment and Prognosis

According to a review of the literature published between 1937 and 1991, episodic violent behavior is quite common in the general population, but strictly diagnosed intermittent explosive disorder is quite rare (American Psychiatric Association 1994b). Consequently, although information on the management and treatment of aggressive behavior is available, no information exists on the treatment, course, or prognosis of rigorously diagnosed intermittent explosive disorder.

Presently, there is no drug specifically approved by the Food and Drug Administration (FDA) for the treatment of aggression. However, numerous pharmacological agents, including neuroleptics, benzodiazepines, lithium, beta-blockers (especially propranolol), anticonvulsants (especially carbamazepine), serotonin-modulating drugs (tryptophan, trazodone, buspirone, clomipramine, fluoxetine), polycyclic antidepressants, monoamine oxidase inhibitors, and psychostimulants, and long-term psychotherapy are effective in diminishing violent behavior in some individuals (Eichelman 1992; Tardiff 1992).

The management of a patient who becomes acutely violent, regardless of the underlying etiology, commonly involves physical restraint, seclusion, and sedation. Neuroleptics and benzodiazepines, such as haloperidol and lorazepam (or a combination of the two), are often appropriate and effective interventions to control an acutely violent individual. Because there are no universally effective "antiaggression" medications, selection of a pharmacological agent is based on the clinical diagnosis of the patient. In the absence of a treatable psychiatric condition, lithium, carbamazepine, propranolol, and more recently serotonin-selective agents are increasingly being used in the management of chronic aggressive behavior.

■ KLEPTOMANIA

There is no systematic research on kleptomania to establish or refute the validity of the existing DSM criteria (American Psychiatric Association 1994b). The DSM-IV diagnostic criteria for kleptomania are given in Table 21–3. The only modification in these criteria from those in DSM-III-R is the addition of mania as an exclusionary diagnosis.

The reader must exercise caution when reading literature about "kleptomania." Much of the literature presents information about shoplifters and thiefs, and does not discuss the rare subgroup of those individuals who meet the diagnostic criteria for kleptomania. Shoplifters and thieves are different from kleptomanic persons in that thieves steal for financial gain or to use the stolen object for personal use (and are excluded by criterion A of the DSM-IV diagnostic criteria for kleptomania).

☐ Epidemiology

Little is known about the epidemiology of kleptomania, because it is a relatively rare disorder and is seldom the subject of research. According to McElroy et al. (1991), most of the information on kleptomania is derived from three sources: studies of "legally referred" shoplifters, case reports or small series of psychiatric patients, and cases of kleptomania patients with eating disorders. Consequently, estimates on the incidence and sex ratios of kleptomania vary widely. Among shoplifters, the incidence of kleptomania has been estimated as "no clear entity exists" (Gibbens and Prince 1962), 3.8% (Arieff and Bowie 1947), 8% (Medlicott 1968), and less than 5% (American Psychiatric Association 1994b).

In a study by Bradford and Balmaceda (1983), a 1:1 male-to-female ratio among shoplifters was found; however, more females (62%) than males (38%) were sent for pretrial psychiatric evaluation, which would skew the data. In a study by McElroy et al. (1991), 15 of 20 (75%) individuals who met DSM-III-R criteria for kleptomania were female. The peak frequency of stealing was 27 episodes per month; the mean age was 36 years; and the mean duration of illness was 16 years.

☐ Etiology

Hypotheses about the cause of kleptomania are legion and little agreement exists. Hypotheses to explain stealing behavior in kleptomania in-

---

Table 21–3.   DSM-IV diagnostic criteria for kleptomania

A.   Recurrent failure to resist impulses to steal objects that are not needed for personal use or for their monetary value.

B.   Increasing sense of tension immediately before committing the theft.

C.   Pleasure, gratification, or relief at the time of committing the theft.

D.   The stealing is not committed to express anger or vengeance and is not in response to a delusion or a hallucination.

E.   The stealing is not better accounted for by conduct disorder, a manic episode, or antisocial personality disorder.

clude that such behavior is an antidepressant, compensation for an actual or anticipated loss, an act for intrapsychic profit, a fetishistic behavior, a sexual act, a symptom of an underlying conflict, a behavior related to depression, a defense, a neurotic conflict, a form of psychopathy, or an OCD-related disorder (Goldman 1991). Stealing is also occasionally a presenting feature of brain disease (Wood and Garralda 1990) or a response to medications.

Bradford and Balmaceda (1983) in their study found an association between shoplifting and psychosocial stress: 78% of shoplifters had a mild to moderate psychosocial stressor on DSM-III Axis IV, and an additional 14% had a severe level of stress. McElroy et al. (1991) found that none of the 20 persons with kleptomania whom they studied developed stealing as a result of stressful or traumatic events.

McElroy et al. (1991) found that all 20 of her patients who met the DSM-III-R diagnostic criteria for kleptomania had either a current diagnosis (65%) or a lifetime history (100%) of depression. Also, a particularly high association with bipolar disorder was noted (35%). In addition, 17 (85%) met criteria during their lifetime for at least four or more other psychiatric disorders, including psychoactive substance use disorders (50%), anxiety disorders (80%), eating disorders (60%), and other impulse control disorders (60%).

☐ Treatment and Prognosis

Recent literature reviews of kleptomania report no systematic studies of rigorously diagnosed kleptomanic individuals (American Psychiatric Association 1994b; Goldman 1991; McElroy et al. 1991). The secretive nature of the disorder also complicates systematic study. In addition, as noted in the foregoing discussion, many case reports and studies fail to adequately distinguish between shoplifting and kleptomania. Without systematic studies and careful differentiation of kleptomania from shoplifting, little useful information exists about treatment, course, or prognosis of kleptomanic individuals. Available information on treatment is limited to a number of case reports that use a broad range of therapeutic interventions.

Somatic therapies are credited with partial or full remission in kleptomanic symptoms. For example, McElroy et al. (1991) cite several reports of electroconvulsive therapy (ECT) alone, or ECT in combination with antidepressants, decreasing kleptomanic behavior. Burstein (1992) reports remission of kleptomanic behavior in one patient treated with a combination of fluoxetine and lithium. McElroy et al. (1991) suggest that kleptomania is part of a group of disorders called affective spectrum disorders. Included in this category are OCD, eating disorders, and major mood disorders. These disorders are hypothesized to represent a spectrum of behaviors that occur secondary to abnormalities in the serotonergic system. Consequently, much of their research focuses on treatment using antidepressants that modulate serotonergic activity.

■ PYROMANIA

Pyromania has been described as "motiveless arson" (Koson and Dvoskin 1982). This description would imply that if no motivation can be determined, pyromania exists. The problem with this diagnostic approach is that arsonists often do not admit motivation, or even the crime for that matter. To do so would admit guilt. This has led to misclassification of arsonists as pyromaniacs and contaminates much of the data on pyromania. Geller (1987) cautions that "pathologic fire setting needs to be viewed not as pathognomonic of pyromania but as a symptom, present in a range of psychiatric disorders, that must be addressed clinically" (p. 501). Geller notes that the pyromanic individual may make considerable advanced preparation before setting the fire, be an avid fire watcher, set off false fire alarms, be interested in fire-fighting paraphernalia, and even seek work as a firefighter.

In a literature review on pyromania (American Psychiatric Association 1994b), there was found to be "a small frequency of pyromania in reported cases of fire setting since 1970 and *no* cases reported in the literature from the United States since 1970." Because there is little new literature on pyromania, DSM-IV made few changes to the DSM-III-R diagnostic criteria for pyromania. The additions to DSM-IV state that pyromania is not diagnosed if fire setting occurs only during a manic episode or if fire setting is better accounted for by a conduct disorder or an antisocial personality disorder (Table 21–4).

☐ Epidemiology

The diagnosis of pyromania is rarely made when DSM-III or DSM-III-R criteria are applied; the diagnosis is much more readily given in studies of arsonists in which no clear diagnostic criteria are used. Therefore, one cannot be sure whether pyromanic individuals are adequately differentiated in the literature from persons who exhibit other types of fire setting or arson. This flaw brings into question the characteristics often associated with pyromania.

Lewis and Yarnell (1951) conducted the largest study of this topic, making a detailed survey of 1,145 adult male cases. (Even with intense efforts, these authors were able to find only 201 records of adult female fire setters.) The peak incidence of fire setting occurred at age 17. Of the males, 48% were classified as "morons" or "imbeciles"; 22% as having borderline to dull normal intelligence; and 13% as having dull to low av-

---

Table 21–4.   DSM-IV diagnostic criteria for pyromania

A. Deliberate and purposeful fire setting on more than one occasion.

B. Tension or affective arousal before the act.

C. Fascination with, interest in, curiosity about, or attraction to fire and its situational contexts (e.g., paraphernalia, uses, consequences).

D. Pleasure, gratification, or relief when setting fires or when witnessing or participating in their aftermath.

E. The fire setting is not done for monetary gain, as an expression of socio-political ideology, to conceal criminal activity, to express anger or vengeance, to improve one's living circumstances, in response to a delusion or hallucination, or as a resault of impaired judgment (e.g., in dementia, mental retardation, substance intoxication).

F. The fire setting is not better accounted for by *conduct disorder*, a *manic episode*, or *antisocial personality disorder*.

Note.   Italics indicate changes to DSM-III-R criteria.

---

erage intelligence. Only 17% of the entire group were rated as having average to superior intelligence. More recent studies indicate that the clinical phenomenon of pyromania is more rare than found in Lewis and Yarnell's samples.

Whereas pyromania is a rare disorder, fire-setting behavior among adults and children with other psychiatric disorders is not (Kolko and Kazdin 1992). In a study of psychiatric patients in a state hospital, 26% had a history of fire-setting behaviors and 16% had actually set fires (Geller and Bertsch 1985). Preliminary data on another chronic mentally ill population showed a lifetime prevalence rate of 30% in fire-setting behaviors.

☐ Etiology

Fire symbolizes many things, from the "fires of Hell" to "fiery passion." The diverse symbolism of fire is represented in the psychoanalytic interpretations of pyromania. Sigmund Freud (1932[1931]/1964) considered fire setting a masturbatory equivalent with homosexual features. Fenichel (1945) discussed pyromania as a specific form of urethral-erotic fixation and emphasized the sadistic and destructive symbolism of fire. Later writers, such as Lewis and Yarnell (1951), stressed that revenge is an important underlying motive for pyromania. Geller (1987) suggests that fire setting as a symptom can best be understood as a communication from an individual with few social skills.

Research (Virkkunen et al. 1987) has raised questions about whether the behavior of arson is associated with reactive hypoglycemia and/or lower concentration of 3-methoxy-4-hydroxyphenylglycol (MHPG) and 5-HIAA in CSF. A small subgroup of pyromanic subjects in this study

(3 of 20 arsonists) had the lowest blood glucose nadirs among the arsonists. In addition, impulse fire setters who are violent offenders are often alcoholics and have a father who is an alcoholic (Linnoila et al. 1989).

□ Treatment and Prognosis

Most writers on the treatment of pyromania approach the patients from a psychoanalytic perspective (Macht and Mack 1968; Stekel 1924). Mavromatis and Lion (1977) pointed out that "treatment for fire setters has been traditionally problematic due to the frequent refusal to take responsibility for the act, the use of denial, the existence of alcoholism, and the lack of insight" (p. 955). Most behavioral researchers have used aversive therapy to treat fire setters (McGrath and Marshall 1979), although others have used positive reinforcement with threats of punishment, stimulus satiation, and operant structured fantasies with positive reinforcement (Bumpass et al. 1983).

The pyromanic impulse to set fires is episodic and often self-limited, and frequently appears during a developmental or situational crisis. Fire setting associated with mental retardation, alcoholism, or a ritualistic pattern indicates a poor prognosis. A better prognosis exists if the patient can verbalize and work through frustrations in therapy. Studies indicate that the recidivism rate for fire setters ranges from 4.5% (Mavromatis and Lion 1977) to 28% (Lewis and Yarnell 1951).

■ PATHOLOGICAL GAMBLING

Gambling is now legal in some form in 48 out of 50 states and in more than 90 countries, and consequently increases the likelihood that clinicians will encounter individuals who have this disorder (Lesieur and Rosenthal 1990).

The diagnostic criteria for pathological gambling in DSM-IV incorporate features from the criteria found in DSM-III and DSM-III-R (Table 21–5). The reader will note that the criteria for pathological gambling are similar to the criteria for psychoactive substance abuse disorders. Freud was one of the first to recognize this similarity, which prompted him to categorize pathological gambling as an addiction along with alcoholism and drug dependence (Lesieur and Rosenthal 1990).

□ Clinical Features

The compulsive gambler is a risk taker who fails to profit from his gambling misadventures. The compulsive gambler is often described as fiercely competitive, highly independent, individualistic, overconfident, and profoundly optimistic. He resents the intrusion of authority figures

---

Table 21–5.   DSM-IV diagnostic criteria for pathological gambling

A.   Persistent and recurrent maladaptive gambling behavior as indicated by
      five (or more) of the following:
   1. Is preoccupied with gambling (e.g., preoccupied with reliving past
      gambling experiences, handicapping or planning the next venture, or
      thinking of ways to get money with which to gamble).
   2. Needs to gamble with increasing amounts of money in order to achieve
      the desired excitement.
   3. Has repeated unsuccessful efforts to control, cut back, or stop gambling.
   4. Is restless or irritable when attempting to cut down or stop gambling.
   5. Gambles as a way of escaping from problems or of relieving a dysphoric
      mood (e.g., feelings of helplessness, guilt, anxiety, depression).
   6. After losing money gambling, often returns another day to get even
      ("chasing" one's losses).
   7. Lies to family members, therapist, or others to conceal the extent of
      involvement with gambling.
   8. Has committed illegal acts such as forgery, fraud, theft, or embezzle-
      ment to finance gambling.
   9. Has jeopardized or lost a significant relationship, job, or educational or
      career opportunity because of gambling.
  10. Relies on others to provide money to relieve a desperate financial
      situation caused by gambling.
B.   The gambling behavior is not better accounted for by a manic episode.

---

into his life, just as he resented his parents' intrusions during his childhood. The compulsive gambler is likely to marry and provide reasonably
well for his family before his gambling losses precipitate a financial crisis.
Contrary to what one might suspect, the compulsive gambler is extremely knowledgeable about the technical aspects of gambling and his
skills are impressive, particularly when winning. It is when he is "chas-
ing" his losses by larger and larger wagers that he disregards his technical knowledge. The compulsive gambler rarely seeks psychiatric help on
his own, but is generally forced into consultation.

The pathological gambler is progressively preoccupied with gambling; spends more time gambling and needs higher bets to experience
excitement; experiences withdrawal symptoms if gambling is abruptly
discontinued; may use gambling to forget or avoid dysphoric mood
states; wagers larger and larger amounts to win back losses (called "chas-
ing"); creates family and job disruption by telling lies to sustain gambling
and performing illegal acts to pay debts; will request and often receive
financial help (a "bailout") from family and/or friends to pay off debts
and to sustain gambling; and attempts unsuccessfully to cut back or stop
gambling.

☐ Epidemiology

Dickerson (1984) estimated that 1% of adult males are pathological gamblers, an estimate that is consistent with Volberg and Steadman's (1988) data; in DSM-IV (American Psychiatric Association 1994a) the prevalence is estimated as being 2% to 3% of the adult population. The rate among psychiatric inpatients is higher and goes largely unrecognized. Lesieur and Blume (1990) found that 6.7% of patients admitted to an adult general psychiatry ward were pathological gamblers. Prevalence rates among alcohol- and substance-abusing individuals are estimated from 8% to 25% (Lesieur and Rosenthal 1990). It is likely that equal numbers of men and women gamble, but the vast majority of compulsive gamblers are men.

☐ Etiology

Numerous theories have been invoked to explain the origin of pathological gambling, including unconscious motivations, behavioral anomalies, the presence of an affective disorder, addiction, and biological abnormalities. Hollander et al. (1992) reiterated the idea that pathological gambling might be an OCD-related disorder. Any one explanation seems a gross oversimplification given the heterogeneous nature of the patient population.

Gambling is an activity that is reinforced by both the cash that one may win and the many exciting stimuli associated with the process. The validity of this hypothesis to explain pathological gambling is challenged by the observation that individuals have losing streaks that last for months. The compulsive gambler will continue gambling regardless of the losses.

Many studies (Lesieur and Rosenthal 1990; Linden et al. 1986; McCormick et al. 1984) have reported an extremely high incidence of affective disorders among pathological gamblers. Gambling may also be an antidepressant, protecting the gambler from dysphoria and depression. The analogy can be drawn between the manic and depressive cycles of a bipolar patient, and the frenetic, high-energy mood of a winning gambler versus the desperate low of the losing gambler.

There are many similarities between substance abuse, particularly alcoholism, and compulsive gambling. In both disorders dependencies are developed that exclude basic human needs such as sleep, food, and sex. The insidious downward trajectory of both disorders leads to loss of family, friends, and position. Custer (1982) noted that compulsive gamblers who abruptly stop gambling during a hospital admission are frequently tremulous and experience headaches, abdominal pain, diarrhea, nightmares, and cold sweats. The course of a recovering substance abuser and that of a compulsive gambler are very much alike in that relapses are common and occur at times of increased stress.

☐ Treatment and Prognosis

A number of diverse treatments for compulsive gambling have been reported (Legg England and Götestam 1991). These include psychoanalysis, behavior therapy, cognitive therapy, medications, and ECT. There are no controlled studies that compare these treatment modalities. Regardless of the choice of therapy, the pathway to recovery is likely to be fraught with difficulties. Relapses are common, as are missed sessions. During treatment, financial crises may occur and legal sequelae of gambling may arise.

The high incidence of major affective disorders among pathological gamblers leads one to question the relationship between these disorders. In some gamblers the affective disorder may promote the gambling, whereas in other gamblers it seems likely that the depletion of resources (e.g., emotional, family, friends, financial) is responsible for the affective state of the gambler when he enters treatment. There may be a subgroup of compulsive gamblers who remain depressed in spite of abstinence.

Behavioral treatments, particularly aversive therapy, have been used to treat compulsive gamblers. However, review of the literature on aversive treatments reveals disappointing results. Greenberg and Rankin (1982) reported on the behavioral treatment of 25 compulsive gamblers. Following treatment, 5 (20%) had their gambling "well under control," 7 (28%) alternated between periods of control and periods of gambling, and 14 (56%) were gambling when last followed up.

Custer (1982) recommends that the compulsive gambler be admitted to an inpatient psychiatric treatment center, particularly when there is a risk of suicide, emotional decompensation, or exhaustion. The initial assessment must include the compulsive gambler's areas of "high risk": marital problems, large debts, demands or threats from creditors, loss of employment, legal problems, and isolation from friends and relatives. The treatment plan is then designed to treat problems identified during the intake process.

The clinical course of pathological gambling is outlined in Figure 21-1. Once the gambler falls behind, he is unable to cut his losses, which leads to a tightening spiral of involvement and fewer options. In a study of 50 compulsive gamblers, Lesieur (1979) noted that all 50 participated in some activity such as pool, golf, and bowling hustling; bookmaking; obtaining loans from friends, loan sharks, or loan companies; "borrowing" from personal checking accounts and from work; and committing petty larceny. Seventeen (34%) participated in check forgery, burglary, fencing stolen goods, stealing company checks, or swindling. The prognosis of

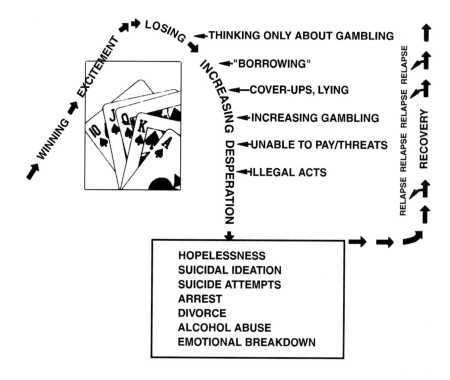

Figure 21–1.   Clinical course of pathological gambling.

the untreated compulsive gambler is unknown. Few creditable data exist about the prognosis of the treated pathological gambler. Taber et al.'s (1987) follow-up study of 66 male veterans 6 months after the completion of a 28-day inpatient program indicates that 56% were totally abstinent. Outcome in this study was found to correlate with attendance at Gamblers Anonymous meetings.

■ TRICHOTILLOMANIA

Trichotillomania is a term created by Hallopeau in 1889 (Krishnan et al. 1985) to describe a compulsion to pull out one's own hair. Although there has been more recent research on trichotillomania than on most of the other disorders in this chapter, insufficient information was available at the time DSM-IV was developed to warrant significant changes to the DSM-III-R diagnostic criteria.

Trichotillomania produces irregular, nonscarring focal patches of hair loss that are linear, rectangular, or oval. Hair loss usually occurs in the scalp region but can involve eyebrows, eyelashes, or pubic hair. These areas of hair loss are more likely found on the opposite side of the body from the dominant hand. Within the area of hair loss, broken hairs of varying lengths are found, and the scalp may have a slight brownish discoloration secondary to rubbing the area. Two clinical findings can help with the diagnosis. In trichotillomania, the patient should not have changes in fingernails or toenails (except possibly signs of nail biting) usually associated with dermatologic conditions. Second, the application of collodion to the area of hair loss for 1 week permits regrowth of the hair.

☐ Epidemiology

The frequency of trichotillomania in the adult population is unknown, but most literature suggests that it is rare. The literature also suggests that females have the disorder much more frequently than do males. However, Christenson et al. (1991c) concluded that trichotillomania may not be as rare as previously suspected and that males may be affected as frequently as females. Prevalence for males ranged between 0.6% and 1.5%, and for females between 0.6% and 3.4%.

Christenson et al. (1991a) reported on the characteristics of 60 adult hair pullers. The mean age at onset was 13 years, and 93% of the subjects were female. Hair was pulled primarily from the scalp (67%); however, other locations were involved, such as eyelashes (22%), eyebrows (8%), facial hair (2%), and pubic hair (2%). Subjects in this study were just as likely to use the nondominant as the dominant hand for hair pulling. All subjects felt that their hair pulling was an excessive or unusual behavior, and 95% reported a diurnal variation, with the worst hair pulling in the evening. The comorbidity with other psychiatric disorders was striking.

☐ Etiology

Oguchi and Miura (1977) believed that when trichotillomania occurs in a child, the hair pulling is a manifestation of mild frustration and is analogous to nail biting. In children, the syndrome usually develops at a time of psychosocial stress (Oranje et al. 1986), such as when there is a disturbed mother-child relationship, hospitalization, or when there is family stress associated with raising a mentally retarded child. These authors believe that the hair pulling can develop into a habit even though the stressor(s) is no longer present.

Krishnan et al. (1985) noted that trichotillomania can be present as a major symptom in OCD, mental retardation, schizophrenia, borderline personality disorder, and depression. Some authors have even questioned the validity of trichotillomania as a unique diagnostic entity (Dean et al. 1992; Werry 1990). It has been suggested that trichotillomania might be a type of OCD (Jenike 1989; Swedo et al. 1989).

☐ Treatment and Prognosis

There is no specific treatment for trichotillomania; rather psychoanalytic, behavioral, or pharmacological treatment may each potentially decrease hair pulling. Swedo et al. (1989) found that clomipramine was significantly more effective than desipramine in a double-blind crossover treatment of trichotillomania. This study has been criticized for selection bias toward OCD patients, because 9 of 20 subjects were self-referred to the study after a television advertisement on OCD (Dean et al. 1992). Christenson et al. (1991b), in another placebo-controlled, double-blind crossover study, reported the response of 21 patients with chronic hair pulling to fluoxetine. Stein and Hollander (1992) found that augmentation of serotonergic agents with pimozide (a dopamine blocker) led to improvement in 6 of 7 patients. Isolated case reports of successful treatment of trichotillomania have been published discussing the use of medications (chlorpromazine [in a schizophrenic individual]; amitriptyline; a monoamine oxidase inhibitor), hypnosis (with and without other treatments), and numerous behavior modification techniques (Krishnan et al. 1985).

According to Stroud (1983), most cases of trichotillomania in young children resolve spontaneously. In younger children, trichotillomania usually represents a transient behavior in response to a psychosocial stressor, or it may represent a habit, without the presence of an obvious precipitant. However, if hair loss persists, psychiatric consultation is indicated, and inquiry into areas of parent-child relationships or other areas of potential conflict may illuminate the problem.

■ IMPULSE CONTROL DISORDER NOT OTHERWISE SPECIFIED

The diagnosis of impulse control disorder not otherwise specified (ICDNOS) remains a residual category for impulse control disorders that do not meet the criteria for other impulse control disorders discussed in this chapter.

■ REFERENCES

American Psychiatric Association: Diagnostic and Statistical Manual of Mental Disorders. 4th Edition. Washington, DC, American Psychiatric Association, 1994a

American Psychiatric Association: DSM-IV Sourcebook. Washington, DC, American Psychiatric Association, 1994b

Arieff AJ, Bowie CG: Some psychiatric aspects of shoplifting. J Clin Psychopathology 8:565–576, 1947

Bradford J, Balmaceda R: Shoplifting: is there a specific psychiatric syndrome? Can J Psychiatry 28:248–254, 1983

Bumpass ER, Fagelman FD, Brix RJ: Intervention with children who set fires. Am J Psychother 37:328–345, 1983

Burstein A: Fluoxetine-lithium treatment for kleptomania (letter). J Clin Psychiatry 53:28–29, 1992

Christenson GA, Mackenzie TB, Mitchell JE: Characteristics of 60 adult chronic hair pullers. Am J Psychiatry 148:365–370, 1991a

Christenson GA, Mackenzie TB, Mitchell JE, et al: A placebo-controlled, double-blind crossover study of fluoxetine in trichotillomania. Am J Psychiatry 148:1566–1571, 1991b

Christenson GA, Pyle RL, Mitchell JE: Estimated lifetime prevalence of trichotillomania in college students. J Clin Psychiatry 52:415–417, 1991c

Custer RL: An overview of compulsive gambling, in Addictive Disorders Update: Alcoholism, Drug Abuse, Gambling. Edited by Carone PA, Yolles SF, Kieffer SN, et al. New York, Human Sciences Press, 1982, pp 107–124

Dean JT, Nelson E, Moss L: Pathologic hair-pulling: a review of the literature and case reports. Compr Psychiatry 33:84–91, 1992

Dickerson MG: Compulsive Gambling. New York, Longman Group Ltd, 1984

Eichelman B: Aggressive behavior: from laboratory to clinic. Quo vadit? Arch Gen Psychiatry 49:488–492, 1992

Fenichel O: The Psychoanalytic Theory of Neurosis. New York, WW Norton, 1945

Freud S: The acquisition and control of fire (1932[1931]), in Standard Edition of the Complete Psychological Works of Sigmund Freud, Vol 22. Translated and edited by Strachey J. London, Hogarth Press, 1964, pp 181–193

Geller JL: Firesetting in the adult psychiatric population. Hosp Community Psychiatry 38:501–506, 1987

Geller JL, Bertsch G: Fire-setting behavior in the histories of a state hospital population. Am J Psychiatry 142:464–468, 1985

Gibbens TCN, Prince J: Shoplifting. London, Institute for the Study and Treatment of Delinquency, 1962

Goldman MJ: Kleptomania: making sense of the nonsensical. Am J Psychiatry 148:986–996, 1991

Greenberg D, Rankin H: Compulsive gamblers in treatment. Br J Psychiatry 140:364–366, 1982

Hollander E, Frenkel M, DeCaria C, et al: Treatment of pathological gambling with clomipramine (letter). Am J Psychiatry 149:710–711, 1992

Jenike MA: Obsessive-compulsive and related disorders (editorial). N Engl J Med 321:539–541, 1989

Kafka MP, Coleman E: Serotonin and paraphilias: the convergence of mood, impulse, and compulsive disorders (editorial). J Clin Psychopharmacol 11:223–224, 1991

Kolko DJ, Kazdin AE: The emergence and recurrence of child firesetting: a one-year prospective study. J Abnorm Child Psychol 20:17–37, 1992

Koson DF, Dvoskin J: Arson: a diagnostic study. Bull Am Acad Psychiatry Law 10:39–49, 1982

Krishnan KRR, Davidson JRT, Guajardo C: Trichotillomania—a review. Compr Psychiatry 26:123–128, 1985

Legg England S, Götestam KG: The nature and treatment of excessive gambling. Acta Psychiatr Scand 84:113–120, 1991

Lesieur HR: The compulsive gambler's spiral of options and involvement. Psychiatry 42:79–87, 1979

Lesieur HR, Blume SB: Characteristics of pathological gamblers identified among patients on a psychiatric admissions service. Hosp Community Psychiatry 41:1009–1012, 1990

Lesieur HR, Rosenthal RJ: Pathological gambling, a review of the literature prepared for DSM-IV Work Group on Disorders of Impulse Control Not Elsewhere Classified. Washington, DC, American Psychiatric Association, 1990

Lewis NDC, Yarnell H: Pathological Firesetting (Pyromania) (Nervous and Mental Disease Monogr 82). New York, Coolidge Foundation, 1951

Linden RD, Pope HG Jr, Jonas JM: Pathological gambling and major affective disorder: preliminary findings. J Clin Psychiatry 47:201–203, 1986

Linnoila M, De Jong J, Virkkunen M: Family history of alcoholism in violent offenders and impulsive fire setters. Arch Gen Psychiatry 46:613–616, 1989

Macht LB, Mack JE: The firesetter syndrome. Psychiatry 31:277–288, 1968

Mavromatis M, Lion JR: A primer on pyromania. Diseases of the Nervous System 38:954–955, 1977

McCormick RA, Russo AM, Ramirez LF, et al: Affective disorders among pathological gamblers seeking treatment. Am J Psychiatry 141:215–218, 1984

McElroy SL, Pope HG Jr, Hudson JI, et al: Kleptomania: a report of 20 cases. Am J Psychiatry 148:652–657, 1991

McElroy SL, Hudson JI, Pope HG Jr, et al: The DSM-III-R impulse control disorders not elsewhere classified: clinical characteristics and relationship to other psychiatric disorders. Am J Psychiatry 149:318–327, 1992

McGrath P, Marshall PG: A comprehensive treatment program for a fire setting child. J Behav Ther Exp Psychiatry 10:69–72, 1979

Medlicott RW: Fifty thieves. N Z Med J 67:183–188, 1968

Monopolis S, Lion JR: Problems in the diagnosis of intermittent explosive disorder. Am J Psychiatry 140:1200–1202, 1983

Oguchi T, Miura S: Trichotillomania: its psychopathological aspect. Compr Psychiatry 18:177–182, 1977

Oranje AP, Pureboom-Wynia JDR, De Raeymaechec CMJ: Trichotillomania in childhood. J Am Acad Dermatol 16:614–619, 1986

Stein DJ, Hollander E: Low-dose pimozide augmentation of serotonin reuptake blockers in the treatment of trichotillomania. J Clin Psychiatry 53:123–126, 1992

Stekel W: Peculiarities of Behavior: Wandering Mania, Dipsomania, Cleptomania, Pyromania and Allied Impulsive Acts, Vol 2. New York, Liveright, 1924

Stroud JD: Hair loss in children. Pediatr Clin North Am 30:641–657, 1983

Swedo SE, Leonard HL, Rapoport JL, et al: A double-blind comparison of clomipramine and desipramine in the treatment of trichotillomania (hair pulling). N Engl J Med 321:497–501, 1989

Taber JI, McCormick RA, Russo AM, et al: Follow-up of pathological gamblers after treatment. Am J Psychiatry 144:757–761, 1987

Tardiff K: The current state of psychiatry in the treatment of violent patients. Arch Gen Psychiatry 49:493–499, 1992

Virkkunen M, Nuutila A, Goodwin FK, et al: Cerebrospinal fluid monoamine metabolite levels in male arsonists. Arch Gen Psychiatry 44:241–247, 1987

Volberg RA, Steadman HJ: Refining prevalence estimates of pathological gambling. Am J Psychiatry 145:502–505, 1988

Werry JS: Trichotillomania—taxonomic issues. Literature review prepared for the DSM-IV Task Force Childhood Disorders Committee. Washington, DC. American Psychiatric Association, 1990

Wood A, Garralda ME: Kleptomania in a 13-year old boy: a sequel of a 'lethargic' encephalitic/depressive process? Br J Psychiatry 157:770–772, 1990

CHAPTER 22

Personality Disorders

Katharine A. Phillips, M.D.
John G. Gunderson, M.D.

All clinicians encounter patients with personality disorders. These patients are commonly seen in a variety of treatment settings, both inpatient and outpatient. Personality disorders are relatively common in the general population, with a prevalence of 10% to 18% (Weissman 1993). Patients with personality disorders present with problems that are among the most complex and challenging that clinicians encounter. This complexity is amplified by the fact that these and other personality disorder characteristics are not simply a problem the patient has, but are in fact central to who the patient is.

Personality disorders, according to DSM-IV (American Psychiatric Association 1994), are patterns of inflexible and maladaptive personality traits that cause subjective distress, significant impairment in social or occupational functioning, or both. These traits must also "deviate markedly" from the culturally expected and accepted range (or "norm"), with this deviation being manifested in more than one of the following areas: cognition, affectivity, control over impulses and need gratification, and ways of relating to others. The deviation must have been stably present and enduring since adolescence or early adulthood, and it must be pervasive—that is, it must manifest itself across a broad range of situations, rather than in only one specific "triggering" situation or in response to a particular stimulus.

Personality disorders cause significant problems for those who have them. Persons with these disorders often suffer, and their relationships with others are problematic. They have difficulty responding flexibly and adaptively to the environment and to the changes and demands of life, and they lack resilience under stress. Instead, their usual ways of responding tend to perpetuate and intensify their difficulties. However, these individuals are often oblivious to the fact that their personality causes them problems, and they may instead blame others for their difficulties or even deny that they have any problems at all.

Personality disorders also often cause problems for others and are costly to society. Individuals with personality disorders often have considerable difficulty in their family, academic, occupational, and other roles. They have elevated rates of separation, divorce, and child-custody proceedings as well as increased rates of accidents, emergency room visits, suicide attempts, and completed suicide. It has also been found that 70% to 85% of criminals, 60% to 70% of alcoholic individuals, and 70% to 90% of persons who abuse drugs have a personality disorder.

Finally, personality disorders need to be identified because of their treatment implications. These disorders often need to be a focus of treatment or, at the very least, should be taken into account when comorbid Axis I disorders are treated, because their presence often affects an Axis I disorder's prognosis and treatment response. In addition, the characteristics of patients with a personality disorder are likely to be manifested in the treatment relationship, whether or not the personality disorder is the focus of treatment.

■ GENERAL CONSIDERATIONS

Since DSM-III (American Psychiatric Association 1987), the personality disorders have been grouped into three clusters: the *odd or eccentric cluster* (schizotypal, schizoid, and paranoid); the *anxious or fearful cluster* (avoidant, dependent, and obsessive-compulsive); and the *dramatic, emotional, or erratic cluster* (borderline, histrionic, narcissistic, and antisocial) (Table 22–1). Although these clusters were originally based on face validity alone, they have since received some empirical support (Kass et al. 1985; Zimmerman and Coryell 1989). Nonetheless, these clusters are limited because they are based on descriptive similarities rather than on similarities in etiology or external validators such as family history or treatment response.

Another classification issue is whether the personality disorders are best classified as dimensions or categories (Frances 1982; Gunderson et al. 1991). Do personality disorders exist along dimensions that reflect extreme variants of normal personality, or are they distinct categories that are qualitatively different, and clearly demarcated, from normal personality traits and one another? Although DSM-IV is based primarily on the categorical model, it to some extent also incorporates a dimensional approach in that it encourages clinicians to identify problematic personality

Table 22–1. Summary of personality disorder features

Cluster	Model	Key clinical features	Treatment	Course/ Prognosis
A **Odd, eccentric**	Spectrum disorders	Social deficits, absence of close relationships	Structure, rehabilitation, support, medication	Stable/poor
B **Dramatic, emotional, erratic**	Self disorders	Social and interpersonal instability	Support, exploration, sociotherapy, individual therapy, medication	Unstable/some remission with age
C **Anxious, fearful**	Dimensional disorders	Interpersonal and intrapsychic conflicts	Exploration, individual therapy, group therapy	Modifiable/ good

traits that are subthreshold for any particular diagnosis. Classification models that incorporate both a dimensional and a categorical approach may ultimately prove most useful to clinicians, and several such models have been proposed (Gunderson 1992).

☐ Assessment Issues and Methods

The assessment of Axis II disorders is in some ways more complex than that of Axis I disorders. It can be difficult to assess multiple domains of experience and behavior (i.e., cognition, affects, intrapsychic experience, and interpersonal interactions) and to determine that traits are not only distressing, impairing, and of early onset, but also pervasive and enduring. Nonetheless, a personality disorder assessment is essential to the comprehensive evaluation and adequate treatment of all patients.

Comprehensiveness of Evaluation

A skilled, psychodynamically informed clinical interview is the mainstay of personality disorder diagnosis and is particularly useful if the clinician is familiar with DSM criteria, takes a longitudinal view, and uses multiple sources of information. However, because an open-ended approach may inadequately cover all Axis II disorders, the additional use of a self-report or semistructured (i.e., interviewer administered) personality disorder assessment instrument can be useful (Table 22–2). Although self-report instruments have the advantage of saving interviewer time, they often give false positive diagnoses and allow contamination of Axis II traits by Axis I states. Semistructured interviews facilitate accurate diagnosis in several ways by allowing the interviewer to attempt to differentiate Axis II traits from Axis I states, clarify contradictions or ambiguities in the patient's response, and determine that traits are pervasive rather than limited to a specific situation.

Syntonicity of Traits

Because personality disorders to some extent reflect who the person is—and not simply what he or she has—some patients are unaware of the traits that reflect their disorder or may not perceive them as problematic. This limited self-awareness can interfere with personality disorder assessment. This problem can be minimized by the use of a skilled psychodynamic interview, comprehensive coverage of all personality disorder criteria with a semistructured assessment instrument, and the use of multiple sources of information.

State Versus Trait

Another potential problem in personality disorder assessment is that the presence of an Axis I state can complicate the assessment of Axis II traits. In some cases, assessment of Axis II disorders may need to wait until the Axis I condition, such as florid psychosis or mania, has subsided. However, personality traits can often be successfully differentiated from Axis I states during an Axis I episode by asking the patient to describe his or her usual personality outside of Axis I episodes; the use of informants who have observed the patient over time and without an Axis I disorder can help with this task. In addition, a prior systematic assessment of Axis I conditions is invaluable in terms of alerting the clinician to which Axis II traits will need particularly careful assessment.

Medical Illness Versus Trait

Similarly, it is important that the interviewer ascertain that what appear to be personality traits are not symptoms of a medical illness. For example, aggressive outbursts caused by a seizure disorder should not be attributed to borderline or antisocial personality disorder. A medical and neurological evaluation should be included in a thorough patient assessment.

Table 22–2. Features of interviews and self-report instruments for the assessment of personality disorders

Interview or instrument	Author	Type	Special features
Structured Interview for DSM-III-R Personality Disorders (SIDP)	Pfohl et al. 1989	Interview	Patient and informant questions
Personality Disorder Examination (PDE)	Loranger 1988	Interview	Detailed instruction manual
Structured Clinical Interview for DSM-III-R Personality Disorders (SCID-II)	Spitzer et al. 1990	Interview	Axis I section; Axis II screening questionnaire
Diagnostic Interview for Personality Disorders (DIPD)	Zanarini et al. 1987	Interview	Best test-retest reliability
Personality Interview Questions–II (PIQ-II)	Widiger 1987	Interview	Nine-point scale for traits and behaviors
Personality Diagnostic Questionnaire—Revised (PDQ-R)	Hyler et al. 1987	Self-report	Face-valid items
Millon Clinical Multiaxial Inventory–II (MCMI-II)	Millon 1987	Self-report	Dimensions of Axis I and Axis II psychopathology
Wisconsin Personality Inventory (Revised) (WPI-R)	M. Klein 1990	Self-report	Integrates structural analysis of social behavior model[a]
Schedule for Normal and Abnormal Personality (SNAP)	Clark 1990	Self-report	Normal and abnormal personality measures
Minnesota Multiphasic Personality Inventory (MMPI) scales for DSM-III personality disorders	Morey et al. 1985	Self-report	Constructed from MMPI item pool

Note. All of the instruments listed assess the full range of personality disorders. Other instruments are available to assess certain individual personality disorders.
[a]See Benjamin 1974.
Source. Modified from Skodol and Oldham 1991.

Situation Versus Trait

The interviewer should also ascertain that personality disorder features are pervasive—that is, not limited to only one situation or occurring in response to only one specific trigger. Similarly, these features should be enduring rather than transient. Asking the patient for behavioral examples of traits can help clarify whether the characteristic is indeed present in a wide variety of situations and is expressed in many relationships.

Sex and Cultural Bias

Although most research suggests that personality disorder criteria are relatively free of sex bias, interviewers can unknowingly allow such bias to affect their assessments. Interviewers should also be careful to avoid cultural bias when diagnosing personality disorders, especially when evaluating such traits as promiscuity, suspiciousness, or recklessness, which may have different norms in different cultures.

Diagnosing Children and Adolescents

Because the personality of children and adolescents is still developing, personality disorders should be diagnosed with care in this age group. It is in fact often preferable to defer these diagnoses until late adolescence or early adulthood, at which time a personality disorder diagnosis may be appropriate if its features appear to be pervasive, stable, and likely to be enduring.

☐ Treatment

Personality disorders consist of deeply ingrained attitudes and behavior patterns that cannot be readily changed. Treatment efforts are further confounded by the degree to which patients view their personality disorder traits as constituting who they are and not as what they have.

The original conception of neurosis as a discrete set of symptoms related to a discrete developmental phase or to discrete conflicts was gradually replaced by the idea that more enduring defensive styles and identification processes were the building blocks of character traits. From this perspective, Wilhelm Reich (1949) and others developed the concept of character analysis and defense analysis. A parallel development in technique evolved from group therapy experience. Maxwell Jones (1953) identified the value of confrontations delivered within group settings in which peer pressure made it difficult for patients to ignore feedback or to leave the group. Here, too, a primary goal of treatment was to render the ego-syntonic but maladaptive aspects of the patient's interpersonal and behavioral style more dystonic. This general principle was subsequently adopted by other forms of sociotherapies, notably those within hospital milieus and family therapies.

Families or couples may present other complications insofar as the designated patient's disordered interpersonal and behavioral patterns may serve functions for, or be complementary to, those of persons with whom the patient is closely associated. Under these circumstances, treatment is primarily directed not at confronting the maladaptive aspects of one person's character traits but rather at identifying the way in which these aspects may be welcomed and reinforced in one setting but maladaptive and impairing in others.

Cognitive-behavioral strategies generally are more focused and structured than psychodynamic therapies and offer the hope of more discrete, time-limited forms of intervention. Behavioral strategies typically involve efforts to diminish impulsivity or increase assertiveness by using relaxation techniques or role-playing exercises. Cognitive strategies involve identifying specific internal mental schemes by which patients typically misunderstand certain situations or misrepresent themselves, and then learning how to modify those internal schemes.

The use of pharmacotherapy for personality disorders has begun to be explored. To the prospect of using specific medications for specific disorders has been added that of identifying biological dimensions of personality psychopathology that may respond to different medication classes (Cloninger 1987; Siever and Davis 1991). Research has increasingly suggested that impulsivity and aggression may respond to serotonergic medications, mood instability and lability may respond to serotonergic medications and to other antidepressants, and psychoticlike experiences may respond to neuroleptics.

■ SPECIFIC PERSONALITY DISORDERS

□ Paranoid Personality Disorder

Persons with paranoid personality disorder have a pervasive, persistent, and inappropriate mistrust of others (Table 22–3). They are suspicious of others' motives and assume that others intend to harm, exploit, or trick them. Thus, they may question, without justification, the loyalty or trustworthiness of friends or sexual partners, and they are reluctant to confide in others for fear the information will be used against them. Persons with paranoid personality disorder appear guarded, tense, and hypervigilant. They often find "evidence" of malevolence by misinterpreting benign events as demeaning or threatening. In response to perceived

---

Table 22–3.   DSM-IV diagnostic criteria for paranoid personality disorder

---

A.   A pervasive distrust and suspiciousness of others such that their motives are interpreted as malevolent, beginning by early adulthood and present in a variety of contexts, as indicated by four (or more) of the following:

1.   Suspects, without sufficient basis, that others are exploiting, harming, or deceiving him or her.

2.   Is preoccupied with unjustified doubts about the loyalty or trustworthiness of friends or associates.

3.   Is reluctant to confide in others because of unwarranted fear that the information will be used maliciously against him or her.

4.   Reads hidden demeaning or threatening meanings into benign remarks or events.

5.   Persistently bears grudges, i.e., is unforgiving of insults, injuries, or slights.

6.   Perceives attacks on his or her character or reputation that are not apparent to others and is quick to react angrily or to counterattack.

7.   Has recurrent suspicions, without justification, regarding fidelity of spouse or sexual partner.

B.   Does not occur exclusively during the course of schizophrenia, a mood disorder with psychotic features, or another psychotic disorder and is not due to the direct physiological effects of a general medical condition.

Note: If criteria are met prior to the onset of schizophrenia, add "premorbid," e.g., "paranoid personality disorder (premorbid)."

---

or actual insults or betrayals, these individuals overreact, quickly becoming excessively angry and responding with counterattacking behavior. They are unable to forgive or forget such incidents and instead bear long-term grudges against their supposed betrayers.

Differential Diagnosis

Unlike paranoid personality disorder, paranoid schizophrenia and delusional disorder, paranoid type, are both characterized by prominent and persistent paranoid delusions of psychotic proportions; paranoid schizophrenia is also accompanied by hallucinations or other core symptoms of schizophrenia. Although paranoid and schizotypal personality disorders both involve suspiciousness, paranoid personality disorder does not entail perceptual distortions and eccentric behavior.

Etiology

The defense mechanism of projection is still generally believed to be involved in the expression of this disorder's features (Vaillant 1992). Some theories suggest that persons with this disorder have been the object of excessive parental rage, whereas others suggest that these persons have been humiliated by others.

It seems likely that paranoid personality disorder has biogenetic contributions. An association between this disorder and Axis I delusional disorder, persecutory type, has received some support from family history studies that found a greater morbid risk of paranoid personality disorder in the first-degree relatives of delusional disorder probands than in the relatives of probands with schizophrenia or medical illness (Kendler and Gruenberg 1982). Such a link implicates the likely involvement of both environmental and constitutional factors in the etiology of paranoid personality disorder.

Treatment

Because they mistrust others, persons with paranoid personality disorder usually avoid psychiatric treatment. Engaging them and keeping them in treatment can best be accomplished by maintaining an unusually respectful, straightforward, noncontrolling, and unintrusive style aimed at building trust. It is best to avoid an overly warm style, which might exacerbate the patient's paranoid tendencies. A supportive psychotherapy may be the best treatment for these patients.

Although group treatment or cognitive-behavioral treatment (Turkat and Maisto 1985) aimed at anxiety management and the development of social skills might be of benefit, these patients tend to resist such approaches. Antipsychotic medications are sometimes useful and are particularly indicated in the treatment of the overtly psychotic decompensations that these patients sometimes experience.

☐ Schizoid Personality Disorder

Schizoid personality disorder is characterized by a profound defect in the ability to relate to others in a meaningful way (Table 22–4). Persons with this disorder have little or no desire for relationships with others and are extremely socially isolated. They prefer to pursue solitary activities and often create an elaborate fantasy world into which they retreat. As a result of their lack of interest in relationships, they have few or no close friends. They date infrequently and seldom marry, and they often work at jobs requiring little interpersonal interaction. These individuals are also notable for their lack of affect. They usually appear cold, detached, and aloof; few, if any, activities or experiences give them pleasure.

Table 22–4.   DSM-IV diagnostic criteria for schizoid personality disorder

---

A.   A pervasive pattern of detachment from social relationships and a restricted range of expression of emotions in interpersonal settings, beginning by early adulthood and present in a variety of contexts, as indicated by four (or more) of the following:

1.   Neither desires nor enjoys close relationships, including being part of a family.
2.   Almost always chooses solitary activities.
3.   Has little, if any, interest in having sexual experiences with another person.
4.   Takes pleasure in few, if any, activities.
5.   Lacks close friends or confidants other than first-degree relatives.
6.   Appears indifferent to the praise or criticism of others.
7.   Shows emotional coldness, detachment, or flattened affectivity.

B.   Does not occur exclusively during the course of schizophrenia, a mood disorder with psychotic features, another psychotic disorder, or a pervasive developmental disorder and is not due to the direct physiological effects of a general medical condition.

Note: If criteria are met prior to the onset of schizophrenia, add "premorbid," e.g., "schizoid personality disorder (premorbid)."

Differential Diagnosis

Schizoid personality disorder shares social isolation and restricted emotional expression with schizotypal personality disorder, but it lacks the latter disorder's cognitive and perceptual distortions. Unlike individuals with avoidant personality disorder, who intensely desire relationships but avoid them because of exaggerated fears of rejection, persons with schizoid personality disorder have little or no interest in developing relationships with others.

Etiology

Clinicians have noted that schizoid personality disorder occurs in adults who experienced cold, neglectful, and ungratifying relationships in early childhood. Constitutional factors may also contribute to the disorder. Although family history studies give stronger support to a link between schizophrenia and schizotypal personality disorder, some studies suggest an association of schizophrenia with schizoid personality disorder, which would implicate the importance of genetic factors in the latter disorder's etiology.

Treatment

Persons with schizoid personality disorder rarely seek treatment. They do not perceive the formation of any relationship—including a therapeutic relationship—as potentially valuable or beneficial. Whereas some patients can tolerate only a supportive therapy or treatment aimed at the resolution of a crisis or an associated Axis I disorder, others do well with psychodynamic psychotherapy aimed at effecting a basic shift in their comfort with intimacy and affects.

Development of an alliance may be difficult and can be facilitated by an interested and caring attitude and an avoidance of early interpretation or confrontation. So-called inanimate bridges, such as writing and artistic productions, can ease the patient into the therapy relationship. Cognitive-behavioral approaches that encourage gradually increasing social involvement may be of value (Liebowitz et al. 1986). Group therapy may also facilitate the development of social skills and relationships.

☐ Schizotypal Personality Disorder

Persons with schizotypal personality disorder experience cognitive or perceptual distortions, behave in an eccentric manner, and are socially inept and anxious (Table 22–5). Their cognitive and perceptual distortions include ideas of reference, bodily illusions, and unusual telepathic and clairvoyant experiences. These distortions occur frequently and are an important and pervasive component of the person's experience. They are in keeping with the odd and eccentric behavior characteristic of this disorder. These individuals may talk to themselves in public, gesture for no apparent reason, or dress in a peculiar or unkempt fashion. Their speech is often odd and idiosyncratic and their affect is constricted or inappropriate. Persons with schizotypal personality disorder are also socially uncomfortable and isolated, and they have few friends. If they develop a relationship they tend to remain distant or may terminate it because of their persistent social anxiety and paranoia.

Differential Diagnosis

Schizotypal personality disorder shares the feature of suspiciousness with paranoid personality disorder and social isolation with schizoid personality disorder, but these latter two disorders lack markedly peculiar behavior and significant cognitive and perceptual distortions. Schizotypal personality disorder, although on a spectrum with Axis I schizophrenia, lacks enduring overt psychosis.

Table 22–5. DSM-IV diagnostic criteria for schizotypal personality disorder

A. A pervasive pattern of social and interpersonal deficits marked by acute discomfort with, and reduced capacity for, close relationships as well as by cognitive or perceptual distortions and eccentricities of behavior, beginning by early adulthood and present in a variety of contexts, as indicated by five (or more) of the following:

1. Ideas of reference (excluding delusions of reference)
2. Odd beliefs or magical thinking that influences behavior and is inconsistent with subcultural norms (e.g., superstitiousness, belief in clairvoyance, telepathy, or "sixth sense"; in children and adolescents, bizarre fantasies or preoccupations)
3. Unusual perceptual experiences, including bodily illusions
4. Odd thinking and speech (e.g., vague, circumstantial, metaphorical, overelaborate, or stereotyped)
5. Suspiciousness or paranoid ideation
6. Inappropriate or constricted affect
7. Behavior or appearance that is odd, eccentric, or peculiar
8. Lack of close friends or confidants other than first-degree relatives
9. Excessive social anxiety that does not diminish with familiarity and tends to be associated with paranoid fears rather than negative judgments about self

B. Does not occur exclusively during the course of schizophrenia, a mood disorder with psychotic features, another psychotic disorder, or a pervasive developmental disorder.

Note: If criteria are met prior to the onset of schizophrenia, add "premorbid," e.g., "schizotypal personality disorder (premorbid)."

Etiology

Schizotypal personality disorder is a schizophrenia-spectrum disorder—that is, it is related to Axis I schizophrenia. Phenomenological, biological, genetic, treatment response, and outcome data support this link. However, it may be that certain subtypes of this personality disorder are not related to schizophrenia. For those variants of schizotypal personality disorder that are related to schizophrenia, it is not clear whether they represent a milder, traitlike, nonpsychotic variant of schizophrenia or in fact constitute schizophrenia's core features, upon which the more florid psychotic episodes of schizophrenia can be superimposed.

Treatment

Persons with schizotypal personality disorder usually avoid psychiatric treatment. It is difficult to establish an alliance with schizotypal patients, and they are unlikely to tolerate exploratory techniques that emphasize interpretation or confrontation. A supportive relationship that counters cognitive distortions and ego-boundary problems may be useful (Stone 1985). This may involve an educational approach that fosters the development of social skills, encourages risk-taking behavior in social situations, or, if these approaches fail, encourages the development of activities with less social involvement. Cognitive-behavior therapy and highly structured educational groups with a social skills focus may also be helpful. Low-dose antipsychotic medications may be useful (Goldberg et al. 1986; Serban and Siegel 1984).

□ Antisocial Personality Disorder

The central characteristic of antisocial personality disorder is a long-standing pattern of socially irresponsible behaviors that reflects a disregard for the rights of others (Table 22–6). Many persons with this disorder engage in repetitive unlawful acts. The more prevailing personality characteristics include a lack of interest in or concern for the feelings of others and, most notably, a lack of remorse over the harm they may cause others. These characteristics generally make these individuals fail in roles requiring fidelity (e.g., as a spouse or a parent) or honesty (e.g., as an employee). A subgroup of these persons take sadistic pleasure in their ability to outwit, harm, and exploit others.

Table 22–6.   DSM-IV diagnostic criteria for antisocial personality disorder

A. There is a pervasive pattern of disregard for and violation of the rights of others occurring since age 15 years, as indicated by three (or more) of the following:
  1. Failure to conform to social norms with respect to lawful behaviors as indicated by repeatedly performing acts that are grounds for arrest
  2. Deceitfulness, as indicated by repeated lying, use of aliases, or conning others for personal profit or pleasure
  3. Impulsivity or failure to plan ahead
  4. Irritability and aggressiveness, as indicated by repeated physical fights or assaults
  5. Reckless disregard for safety of self or others
  6. Consistent irresponsibility, as indicated by repeated failure to sustain consistent work behavior or honor financial obligations
  7. Lack of remorse, as indicated by being indifferent to or rationalizing having hurt, mistreated, or stolen from another
B. The individual is at least age 18 years.
C. There is evidence of conduct disorder with onset before age 15 years.
D. The occurrence of antisocial behavior is not exclusively during the course of schizophrenia or a manic episode.

Differential Diagnosis

The primary differential diagnostic issue involves narcissistic personality disorder. Indeed, these two disorders may be variants of the same basic type of psychopathology (Hare et al. 1991). However, the antisocial person, unlike the narcissistic person, is likely to be reckless and impulsive. In addition, narcissistic persons' exploitativeness and disregard for others are attributable to their sense of uniqueness and superiority rather than to a desire for materialistic gains.

Etiology

Twin and adoptive studies indicate that genetic factors predispose to the development of antisocial personality disorder (Grove et al. 1990; Mednick et al. 1984). In addition, the early family life of these persons often poses severe environmental handicaps in the form of absent, assaultive, or inconsistent parenting. Indeed, many family members also have significant action-oriented psychopathology such as substance abuse or antisocial personality disorder itself.

Treatment

It is important to recognize antisocial personality disorder because an uncritical acceptance of these individuals' glib or shallow statements of good intention and collaboration can permit them to have a disruptive influence on treatment teams and other patients. In confined settings, such as the military or prisons, depressive and introspective concerns may surface (Vaillant 1975). Under these circumstances, confrontation by peers may bring about changes in the antisocial person's social behaviors. Some antisocial patients demonstrate an ability to form a therapeutic alliance with psychotherapists, which augurs well for these patients' future course (Woody et al. 1985). The prevalence of this disorder diminishes with age as these individuals become more aware of the social and interpersonal maladaptiveness of their most noxious social behaviors.

☐ Borderline Personality Disorder

The borderline personality disorder construct originated from the observations of psychoanalytic psychotherapists who were impressed by these patients' demanding search for nurturance, their disregard for the usual boundaries of therapy, and their tendency to regress in unstructured situations. Borderline personality disorder is the most widely studied personality disorder. It is also common, occurring in about 2% to 3% of the population and in every culture.

Central to this disorder's psychopathology are a severely impaired capacity for attachment and predictably maladaptive behavior patterns related to separation (Gunderson 1984). When borderline patients feel cared for, held on to, and supported, depressive features (notably loneliness and emptiness) are most evident (Table 22–7). When the loss of such a sustaining relationship is threatened, the lovingly idealized image of a beneficent caregiver is replaced by a hatefully devalued image of a cruel persecutor—a shift called *splitting*. An impending separation also evokes intense abandonment fears. To minimize these fears and to prevent the separation, rageful accusations of mistreatment and cruelty and angry self-destructive behaviors often occur. These behaviors often elicit a guilty or fearful protective response from others. When patients experience an absence of a sustaining, holding, or caring relationship, dissociative experiences, ideas of reference, or desperate impulsive acts predictably occur.

Differential Diagnosis

Borderline patients' intense feelings of being bad or evil are different from the idealized self-image of narcissistic persons. Although borderline patients, like persons with antisocial personality disorder, may be reckless and impulsive, their behaviors are primarily interpersonally oriented and aimed toward obtaining support rather than materialistic gains.

Table 22–7.   DSM-IV diagnostic criteria for borderline personality disorder

A pervasive pattern of instability of interpersonal relationships, self-image and affects, and marked impulsivity beginning by early adulthood and present in a variety of contexts, as indicated by five (or more) of the following:

1. Frantic efforts to avoid real or imagined abandonment. **Note:** Do not include suicidal or self-mutilating behavior covered in criterion 5.
2. A pattern of unstable and intense interpersonal relationships characterized by alternating between extremes of idealization and devaluation.
3. Identity disturbance: markedly and persistently unstable self-image or sense of self.
4. Impulsivity in at least two areas that are potentially self-damaging (e.g., spending, sex, substance abuse, reckless driving, binge eating). **Note:** Do not include suicidal or self-mutilating behavior covered in criterion 5.
5. Recurrent suicidal behavior, gestures, or threats, or self-mutilating behavior.
6. Affective instability due to a marked reactivity of mood (e.g., intense episodic dysphoria, irritability, or anxiety usually lasting a few hours and only rarely more than a few days).
7. Chronic feelings of emptiness.
8. Inappropriate, intense anger or difficulty controlling anger (e.g., frequent displays of temper, constant anger, recurrent physical fights).
9. Transient, stress-related paranoid ideation or severe dissociative symptoms.

Etiology

Psychoanalytic theories have emphasized the importance of early parent-child relationships in the etiology of borderline personality disorder. Such reports have emphasized maternal mismanagement of the 2- to 3-year-old child's efforts to become autonomous (Masterson 1972), exaggerated maternal frustration that aggravates the child's anger (Kernberg 1975), and inattention to the child's emotions and attitudes (Adler 1985). These traumatic experiences occur within a context of sustained neglect from which the preborderline child develops an enduring rage and self-hatred. The lack of stably involved attachment during development is a source of their inability to maintain a stable sense of themselves or of others without ongoing contact. Efforts to identify inherited temperamental predispositions to borderline personality disorder have yielded support for the presence of nonspecific problems with regulation of affects and impulses. The existing data, however, indicate that borderline personality disorder is only weakly heritable (Torgersen 1984).

Treatment

Clinicians encounter extreme difficulties with these patients, problems that derive from the patients' appeal to their treaters' nurturing qualities and their rageful accusations in response to their treaters' perceived failures. Often therapists develop intense countertransference reactions that lead them to attempt to re-parent or reject borderline patients. The treatment literature has focused on the value of intensive exploratory psychotherapies directed at modifying borderline patients' basic character structure. However, improvement may be related not to the acquisition of insight but to the corrective experience of developing a stable, trusting relationship with a therapist who fails to retaliate in response to these patients' angry and disruptive behaviors. Supportive psychotherapies or group therapies may bring about similar changes.

Studies indicate that many medications may diminish specific problems such as impulsivity, affective lability, or intermittent cognitive and perceptual disturbances (Cowdry and Gardner 1988; Soloff 1989). Behavioral treatment consisting of a fairly intensive individual and group regimen can effectively diminish the self-destructive behaviors of borderline patients (Linehan et al. 1991).

☐ Histrionic Personality Disorder

Central to histrionic personality disorder is an overconcern with attention and appearance (Table 22–8). Persons with this disorder spend excessive time seeking attention and making themselves attractive. The desire to be found attractive may lead to inappropriately seductive or

Table 22–8. DSM-IV diagnostic criteria for histrionic personality disorder

A pervasive pattern of excessive emotionality and attention seeking, beginning by early adulthood and present in a variety of contexts, as indicated by five (or more) of the following:

1. Is uncomfortable in situations in which he or she is not the center of attention.
2. Interaction with others is often characterized by inappropriate sexually seductive or provocative behavior.
3. Displays rapidly shifting and shallow expression of emotions.
4. Consistently uses physical appearance to draw attention to self.
5. Has a style of speech that is excessively impressionistic and lacking in detail.
6. Shows self-dramatization, theatricality, and exaggerated expression of emotion.
7. Is suggestible, i.e., easily influenced by others or circumstances.
8. Considers relationships to be more intimate than they actually are.

provocative dress and flirtatious behavior, while the desire for attention may lead to other flamboyant acts or self-dramatizing behavior. Persons with histrionic personality disorder also display an effusive but labile and shallow range of feelings. They are often overly impressionistic and given to hyperbolic descriptions of others. These persons do not attend to detail or facts, and they are reluctant or unable to make reasoned critical analyses of problems or situations.

Differential Diagnosis

Histrionic individuals are often willing, even eager, to have others make decisions and organize their activities for them. However, unlike persons with dependent personality disorder, histrionic persons are uninhibited and lively companions who willfully forgo appearing autonomous because they believe this is desired by others. Unlike persons with borderline personality disorder, they do not perceive themselves as bad, and they lack ongoing problems with rage or willful self-destructiveness. Persons with narcissistic personality disorder also seek attention to sustain their self-esteem but differ in that their self-esteem is characterized by grandiosity, and the attention they crave must be admiring.

Etiology

Psychoanalytic theory proposes that histrionic personality disorder originates in the oedipal phase of development. More recent research suggests that qualities like emotional expressiveness and attention-seeking may be characteristics of biogenetically determined temperament.

Treatment

Individual psychodynamic psychotherapy, including psychoanalysis, re-mains the cornerstone of most treatment. This treatment is directed at increasing patients' awareness of 1) how their self-esteem is maladap-tively tied to their ability to attract attention at the expense of developing other skills, and 2) how their shallow relationships and emotional ex-perience reflect unconscious fears of real commitments. Most of this increase in awareness occurs through analysis of the here-and-now doctor-patient relationship rather than via the reconstruction of child-hood experiences.

☐ Narcissistic Personality Disorder

Because persons with narcissistic personality disorder have grandiose self-esteem, they are vulnerable to intense reactions when their self-image is damaged (Table 22–9). They respond with strong feelings of hurt or anger to even small slights, rejections, defeats, or criticisms. As a result, they usually go to great lengths to avoid exposure to such experi-ences and, when that fails, react by becoming devaluative or rageful. In relationships, narcissistic persons are often quite distant, try to sustain "an illusion of self-sufficiency" (Modell 1975), and may exploit others for

---

Table 22–9. DSM-IV diagnostic criteria for narcissistic personality disorder

A pervasive pattern of grandiosity (in fantasy or behavior), need for admiration, and lack of empathy, beginning by early adulthood and present in a variety of contexts, as indicated by five (or more) of the following:

1. Has a grandiose sense of self-importance (e.g., exaggerates achievements and talents, expects to be recognized as superior without commensurate achievements).
2. Is preoccupied with fantasies of unlimited success, power, brilliance, beauty, or ideal love.
3. Believes that he or she is "special" and unique and can only be understood by, or should associate with, other special or high-status people (or institutions).
4. Requires excessive admiration.
5. Has a sense of entitlement, i.e., unreasonable expectations of especially favorable treatment or automatic compliance with his or her expectations.
6. Is interpersonally exploitative, i.e., takes advantage of others to achieve his or her own ends.
7. Lacks empathy: is unwilling to recognize or identify with the feelings and needs of others.
8. Is often envious of others or believes that others are envious of him or her.
9. Shows arrogant, haughty behaviors or attitudes.

---

self-serving ends. They are likely to feel that those with whom they associate need to be special and unique because they see themselves in these terms.

Differential Diagnosis

Like persons with antisocial personality disorder, those with narcissistic personality disorder are capable of exploiting others but usually rationalize their behavior on the basis of the specialness of their goals or their personal virtue. In contrast, antisocial persons' goals are materialistic, and their rationalizations are based on a view that others would do the same to them. The narcissistic person's excessive pride in achievements, relative constraint in expression of feelings, and disregard for other people's rights and sensitivities help distinguish him or her from persons with histrionic personality disorder.

Etiology

This disorder appears to develop in persons who have had their fears, failures, or dependency responded to with criticism, disdain, or neglect during their childhood years. They develop a veneer of invulnerability and self-sufficiency that masks their underlying emptiness and constricts their capacity to feel deeply.

Treatment

Individual psychodynamic psychotherapy, including psychoanalysis, is the cornerstone of treatment. Some therapists believe that the vulnerability to narcissistic injury indicates that intervention should be directed at conveying empathy for the patient's sensitivities and disappointments. This approach, in theory, allows a positive idealized transference to develop that will then be gradually disillusioned by the inevitable frustrations encountered in therapy—disillusionment that will clarify the excessive nature of the patient's reactions to frustrations and disappointments. An alternative view holds that the vulnerability should be addressed earlier and more directly by interpretations and confrontations. With either approach, the psychotherapeutic process usually requires a relatively intensive schedule over a period of years in which a recognition of the narcissistic patient's hypersensitivity to slights is foremost in the therapist's mind and interventions.

☐ Avoidant Personality Disorder

Persons with avoidant personality disorder experience excessive and pervasive anxiety and discomfort in social situations and in intimate relationships (Table 22–10). Although strongly desiring relationships, they avoid them because they fear being ridiculed, criticized, rejected, or humiliated. These fears reflect their low self-esteem and their hypersensitivity to negative evaluation by others. When these persons do enter into social situations or relationships, they feel inept and are self-conscious, shy, awkward, and preoccupied with being criticized or rejected.

Differential Diagnosis

Persons with schizoid personality disorder are socially isolated, but do not desire relationships, whereas the avoidant person desires them but avoids them because of anxiety and fears of humiliation and rejection. Whereas avoidant personality disorder is characterized by pervasive fears of all situations and relationships involving possible rejection or disappointment, Axis I social phobia usually consists of specific fears related to social performance.

Etiology

Millon (1981) suggests that the disorder develops from parental rejection and censure, which may be reinforced by rejecting peers. Psychodynamic theory suggests that avoidant behavior may derive from early life experiences that lead to an exaggerated desire for acceptance or an intolerance of criticism. Work in the biological sphere implicates the importance of inborn temperament in the development of avoidant behavior (Kagan 1989).

Table 22–10.   DSM-IV diagnostic criteria for avoidant personality disorder

---

A pervasive pattern of social inhibition, feelings of inadequacy, and hypersensitivity to negative evaluation, beginning by early adulthood and present in a variety of contexts, as indicated by four (or more) of the following:

1. Avoids occupational activities that involve significant interpersonal contact, because of fears of criticism, disapproval, or rejection.
2. Is unwilling to get involved with people unless certain of being liked.
3. Shows restraint within intimate relationships because of the fear of being shamed or ridiculed.
4. Is preoccupied with being criticized or rejected in social situations.
5. Is inhibited in new interpersonal situations because of feelings of inadequacy.
6. Views self as socially inept, personally unappealing, or inferior to others.
7. Is unusually reluctant to take personal risks or to engage in any new activities because they may prove embarrassing.

Treatment

Engagement in psychotherapy may be facilitated by the therapist's use of supportive techniques, sensitivity to the patient's hypersensitivity, and gentle interpretation of the defensive use of avoidance. Although early in treatment these patients may tolerate only supportive techniques, they may eventually respond well to all kinds of psychotherapy, including short-term, long-term, and psychoanalytic approaches. Assertiveness and social skills training may increase patients' confidence and willingness to take risks in social situations. Cognitive techniques that gently challenge patients' pathological assumptions about their sense of ineptness may also be helpful. Group experiences may also prove useful. Anxiolytics sometimes help patients better manage the associated anxiety.

☐ Dependent Personality Disorder

Dependent personality disorder is characterized by an excessive need to be cared for by others, which leads to submissive and clinging behavior and excessive fears of separation from others (Table 22–11). These persons rely excessively on "powerful" others to initiate and do things for them, make their decisions, assume responsibility for their actions, and guide them through life. Low self-esteem and doubt about their effectiveness lead them to avoid positions of responsibility. Because they feel unable to function without excessive guidance, they go to great lengths to maintain the dependent relationship. If the dependent relationship ends, these individuals feel helpless and fearful because they feel incapable of caring for themselves, and they often indiscriminately find another relationship to provide them with direction or nurturance.

Differential Diagnosis

Although persons with borderline personality disorder also dread being alone and need ongoing support, dependent persons want others to assume a controlling function that would frighten the borderline patient. Moreover, persons with dependent personality disorder become appeasing rather than rageful or self-destructive when threatened with separation. Although both avoidant and dependent personality disorders are characterized by low self-esteem, rejection sensitivity, and an excessive need for reassurance, those persons with dependent personality disorder seek out rather than avoid relationships, and they quickly and indiscriminately replace ended relationships instead of further withdrawing from others.

Table 22–11. DSM-IV diagnostic criteria for dependent personality disorder

A pervasive and excessive need to be taken care of that leads to submissive and clinging behavior and fears of separation, beginning by early adulthood and present in a variety of contexts, as indicated by five (or more) of the following:

1. Has difficulty making everyday decisions without an excessive amount of advice and reassurance from others.
2. Needs others to assume responsibility for most major areas of his or her life.
3. Has difficulty expressing disagreement with others because of fear of loss of support or approval. **Note:** Do not include realistic fears of retribution.
4. Has difficulty initiating projects or doing things on his or her own (because of a lack of self-confidence in judgment or abilities rather than a lack of motivation or energy).
5. Goes to excessive lengths to obtain nurturance and support from others, to the point of volunteering to do things that are unpleasant.
6. Feels uncomfortable or helpless when alone because of exaggerated fears of being unable to care for himself or herself.
7. Urgently seeks another relationship as a source of care and support when a close relationship ends.
8. Is unrealistically preoccupied with fears of being left to take care of himself or herself.

Etiology

Abraham (1923) suggested that the dependent character derives from either overindulgence or underindulgence during the oral phase of development. Subsequent empirical data have given more support to the underindulgence hypothesis. However, studies of adults have not supported a specific association between feeding or other oral habits in childhood and dependency in adulthood. It may be that ongoing patterns unrelated to the oral phase per se are more important to this disorder's development. Genetic/constitutional factors, such as innate submissiveness, may also contribute to the etiology of this disorder, as may cultural and social factors. Dependent personality disorder may represent an exaggerated and maladaptive variant of normal dependency.

Treatment

Patients with dependent personality disorder often enter therapy with complaints of depression or anxiety that may be precipitated by the threatened or actual loss of a dependent relationship. They often respond well to various types of individual psychotherapy. Treatment may be particularly helpful if it explores patients' fears of independence; uses the transference to explore their dependency; and is directed toward increasing patients' self-esteem, sense of effectiveness, assertiveness, and independent functioning. These patients often seek an excessively dependent relationship with the therapist, which can lead to countertransference problems that may actually reinforce their dependence. Group therapy and cognitive-behavior therapy aimed at increasing independent functioning, including assertiveness and social skills training, may be useful. If the patient is in a relationship that is maintaining and reinforcing his or her excessive dependence, couples or family therapy may be helpful.

☐ Obsessive-Compulsive Personality Disorder

Persons with obsessive-compulsive personality disorder are excessively orderly (Table 22–12). They are neat, punctual, overly organized, and overconscientious. These traits must be so extreme as to cause significant distress or impairment in functioning. As Abraham (1923) noted, these individuals' perseverance is unproductive. Although these individuals tend to work extremely hard, they do so at the expense of leisure activities and relationships. These individuals also tend to be overly concerned with control—not only over the details of their own lives but over their emotions and other people. They have difficulty expressing warm and tender feelings. And they may be obstinate and reluctant to delegate tasks or to work with others unless others submit exactly to their way of doing things, which reflects their need for interpersonal control as well as their fear of making mistakes. Their tendency to doubt and worry also manifests itself in their inability to discard worn-out or worthless objects that might be needed for future catastrophes. And persons with an obsessive-compulsive personality are miserly toward themselves and others.

Differential Diagnosis

Obsessive-compulsive personality disorder differs from Axis I obsessive-compulsive disorder in that the latter disorder consists of specific repetitive thoughts and ritualistic behaviors rather than personality traits. In addition, obsessive-compulsive disorder has traditionally been considered ego-dystonic and obsessive-compulsive personality disorder ego-syntonic.

Etiology

Freud's (1908/1924) view that obsessive-compulsive personality disorder derives from difficulties occurring during the anal stage of psychosexual development (i.e., age 2 to 4) was echoed and elaborated upon by sub-

---

Table 22–12. DSM-IV diagnostic criteria for obsessive-compulsive
personality disorder

A pervasive pattern of preoccupation with orderliness, perfectionism, and
mental and interpersonal control, at the expense of flexibility, openness, and
efficiency, beginning by early adulthood and present in a variety of contexts,
as indicated by four (or more) of the following:

1. Is preoccupied with details, rules, lists, order, organization, or schedules to
    the extent that the major point of the activity is lost.
2. Shows perfectionism that interferes with task completion (e.g., is unable
    to complete a project because his or her own overly strict standards are
    not met).
3. Is excessively devoted to work and productivity to the exclusion of leisure
    activities and friendships (not accounted for by obvious economic necessity).
4. Is overconscientious, scrupulous, and inflexible about matters of morality,
    ethics, or values (not accounted for by cultural or religious identification).
5. Is unable to discard worn-out or worthless objects even when they have
    no sentimental value.
6. Is reluctant to delegate tasks or to work with others unless they submit to
    exactly his or her way of doing things.
7. Adopts a miserly spending style toward both self and others; money is
    viewed as something to be hoarded for future catastrophes.
8. Shows rigidity and stubbornness.

---

sequent psychoanalytic thinkers. According to this theory, children's infantile anal-erotic libidinal impulses conflict with parental attempts to so-
cialize them—in particular, to toilet train them. Although these theories
emphasize the importance of children's perception of parental disapproval during toilet training, and of ensuing parent-child control struggles, these factors are not currently considered central to this disorder's
etiology. It may be, however, that conflicts that arise during toilet training and that continue during other developmental stages, do play a role
in this disorder's etiology (Perry and Vaillant 1989). In particular, excessive parental control, criticism, and shaming may result in an insecurity
that is defended against with perfectionism, orderliness, and an attempt
to maintain excessive control. Freud believed that constitutional factors
also play an important role in the formation of this personality type.

Treatment

These patients often respond well to psychoanalytic psychotherapy or
psychoanalysis. Therapists usually need to be relatively active in treatment. Rather than intellectualizing with the patient, therapists should focus on the feelings these patients usually avoid. Other defenses common

in this disorder, such as rationalization, isolation, undoing, and reaction formation, should be identified and clarified. Power struggles that may occur in treatment offer opportunities to address the patient's excessive need for control. Cognitive techniques may be used to diminish the patient's excessive need for control and perfection. Dynamically oriented groups that focus on feelings may provide insight and increase their comfort with exploring and expressing new affects.

■ OTHER PERSONALITY DISORDERS

The following personality disorders were considered for inclusion on DSM-IV Axis II on the basis of their historical tradition, clinical utility, and/or empirical support. However, for various reasons they were thought to require further study. Both disorders involve chronically morose people who have problems with direct expression of their aggression.

☐ Depressive Personality Disorder

Of all the personality disorders, depressive personality disorder may have the longest clinical tradition, having been recognized 2,000 years ago by Hippocrates (Phillips et al. 1990). Kraepelin (1921) also described this temperament and considered it a depressive-spectrum disorder—a constitutional traitlike variant of the more severe depressive disorders and one predisposing to their occurrence. Kernberg (1988) emphasized this personality type's psychodynamic features, which include a severe superego, the inhibited expression of aggression, and an excessive dependence that is defended against with counterdependence. Because of the strength of this disorder's historical tradition, depressive personality disorder was added to the appendix in DSM-IV.

Persons with depressive personality disorder are persistently gloomy, burdened, worried, serious, pessimistic, and incapable of enjoyment or relaxation. They also tend to feel guilty and be moralistic, self-denying, passive, nonassertive, and introverted. They have low self-esteem and are excessively sensitive to criticism and rejection. Although they may be critical of others, they have difficulty directing criticism or any form of aggression toward others and find it easier to criticize themselves. They are also overly dependent on the love and acceptance of others, but they inhibit the expression of this dependency and may instead appear counterdependent.

Available data suggest that this disorder's overlap with dysthymia, major depression, and other personality disorders is far from complete. Depressive personality disorder appears to be a distinct construct, although family history and other data suggest that it may be related to other disorders (Klein 1990). This disorder should not be diagnosed if it occurs only during major depressive episodes.

Depressive personality disorder has been noted to respond well to psychoanalytic psychotherapy and psychoanalysis. It has been proposed that the major depressive episodes that can co-occur with this personality type may be particularly responsive to antidepressant medications (Akiskal 1983).

☐ Passive-Aggressive (Negativistic) Personality Disorder

This appendix category is a replacement for the excessively narrow DSM-III-R category of passive aggressive personality disorder, which was more representative of a single defense mechanism than a personality disorder. Another limitation of the DSM-III-R category was its limited empirical support. Negativistic personality disorder is a broader construct that has some historical precedents, including Schneider's (1923) "ill-tempered depressives."

This disorder describes a pervasive pattern of passive resistance to demands for social and occupational performance. It also encompasses a wide range of negativistic attitudes and behaviors, such as anger, pessimism, and cynicism; whining and grumbling; feelings of being luckless and jinxed; and envy of those who are perceived as more fortunate. In addition, these individuals tend to alternate between hostile self-assertion and contrite submission. The clinical features of this disorder and its differentiation from other personality disorders remain to be empirically confirmed.

■ REFERENCES

Abraham K: Contributions to the theory of the anal character. Int J Psychoanal 4:400–418, 1923

Adler G: Borderline Psychopathology and Its Treatment. New York, Jason Aronson, 1985

Akiskal HS: Dysthymic disorder: psychopathology of proposed chronic depressive subtypes. Am J Psychiatry 140:11–20, 1983

American Psychiatric Association: Diagnostic and Statistical Manual of Mental Disorders, 3rd Edition, Revised. Washington, DC, American Psychiatric Association, 1987

American Psychiatric Association: Diagnostic and Statistical Manual of Mental Disorders, 4th Edition. Washington, DC, American Psychiatric Association, 1994

Benjamin LS: Structural analysis of social behavior. Psychol Rev 81:392–425, 1974

Cloninger CR: A systematic method for clinical description and classification of personality variants. Arch Gen Psychiatry 44:573–588, 1987

Cowdry RW, Gardner DL: Pharmacotherapy of borderline personality disorder: alprazolam, carbamazepine, trifluoperazine, and tranylcypromine. Arch Gen Psychiatry 45:111–119, 1988

Frances A: Categorical and dimensional systems of personality diagnosis: a comparison. Compr Psychiatry 23:516–527, 1982

Freud S: Character and anal erotism (1908), in Collected Papers, Vol 2. London, Hogarth, 1924, pp 45–50

Goldberg SC, Schulz C, Schulz PM, et al: Borderline and schizotypal personality disorders treated with low-dose thiothixene vs placebo. Arch Gen Psychiatry 43:680–686, 1986

Grove WM, Eckert ED, Heston L, et al: Heritability of substance abuse and antisocial behavior: a study of monozygotic twins reared apart. Biol Psychiatry 27:1293–1304, 1990

Gunderson JG: Borderline Personality Disorder. Washington, DC, American Psychiatric Press, 1984

Gunderson JG: Diagnostic controversies, in American Psychiatric Press Review of Psychiatry, Vol 11. Edited by Tasman A, Riba M. Washington, DC, American Psychiatric Press, 1992, pp 9–24

Gunderson JG, Links PS, Reich JH: Competing models of personality disorders. Journal of Personality Disorders 5:60–68, 1991

Hare RD, Hart SD, Harpur TJ: Psychopathy and the DSM-IV criteria for antisocial personality disorder. J Abnorm Psychol 100:391–398, 1991

Jones M: The Therapeutic Community—A New Treatment in Psychiatry. New York, Basic Books, 1953

Kagan J: Temperamental influences on the preservation of styles of social behavior. McLean Hosp J 14:23–34, 1989

Kass F, Skodol AE, Charles E, et al: Scaled ratings of DSM-III personality disorders. Am J Psychiatry 142:627–630, 1985

Kendler KS, Gruenberg AM: Genetic relationship between paranoid personality disorder and the "schizophrenic spectrum" disorders. Am J Psychiatry 139:1185–1186, 1982

Kernberg OF: Borderline Conditions and Pathological Narcissism. New York, Jason Aronson, 1975

Kernberg OF: Clinical dimensions of masochism. J Am Psychoanal Assoc 36:1005–1029, 1988

Klein DN: Depressive personality: reliability, validity, and relation to dysthymia. J Abnorm Psychol 99:412–421, 1990

Kraepelin E: Manic-Depressive Insanity and Paranoia. Translated by Barclay RM. Edited by Robertson GM. Edinburgh, E & S Livingstone, 1921

Liebowitz MR, Stone MH, Turkat ID: Treatment of personality disorders, in Psychiatry Update: American Psychiatric Association Annual Review, Vol 5. Edited by Frances AJ, Hales RE. Washington, DC, American Psychiatric Press, 1986, pp 356–393

Linehan MM, Armstrong HE, Suarez A, et al: Cognitive-behavioral treatment of chronically parasuicidal borderline patients. Arch Gen Psychiatry 48:1060–1064, 1991

Masterson JF: Treatment of the Borderline Adolescent: A Developmental Approach. New York, Wiley-Interscience, 1972

Mednick S, Gabrielli W, Hutchings B: Genetic factors in criminal behavior: evidence from an adoption cohort. Science 224:891–893, 1984

Millon T: Disorders of Personality—DSM-III: Axis II. New York, Wiley, 1981

Modell AH: A narcissistic defense against affects and the illusion of self-sufficiency. Int J Psychoanal 56:275–282, 1975

Perry JC, Vaillant GE: Personality disorders, in Comprehensive Textbook of Psychiatry/V, 5th Edition, Vol 2. Edited by Kaplan HI, Sadock BJ. Baltimore, MD, Williams & Wilkins, 1989, pp 1352–1387

Phillips KA, Gunderson JG, Hirschfeld RMA, et al: A review of the depressive personality. Am J Psychiatry 147:830–837, 1990

Reich W: On the technique of character analysis, in Character Analysis, 3rd Edition. New York, Simon & Schuster, 1949, pp 39–113

Schneider K: Die psychopathischen Personlichkeiten. Vienna, Deuticke, 1923

Serban G, Siegel S: Response of borderline and schizotypal patients to small doses of thiothixene and haloperidol. Am J Psychiatry 141:1455–1458, 1984

Siever LJ, Davis KL: A psychobiological perspective on the personality disorders. Am J Psychiatry 148:1647–1658, 1991

Skodol AE, Oldham JM: Assessment and diagnosis of borderline personality disorder. Hosp Community Psychiatry 42:1021–1028, 1991

Soloff PH: Psychopharmacologic therapies in borderline personality disorder, in American Psychiatric Press Review of Psychiatry, Vol 8. Edited by Tasman A, Hales RE, Frances AJ. Washington, DC, American Psychiatric Press, 1989, pp 65–83

Stone M: Schizotypal personality: psychotherapeutic aspects. Schizophr Bull 11:576–589, 1985

Torgersen S: Genetic and nosological aspects of schizotypal and borderline personality disorders: a twin study. Arch Gen Psychiatry 41:546–554, 1984

Turkat I, Maisto S: Application of the experimental method to the formulation and modification of personality disorders, in Clinical Handbook of Psychological Disorders. Edited by Barlow D. New York, Guilford, 1985, pp 502–570

Vaillant GE: Sociopathy as a human process: a viewpoint. Arch Gen Psychiatry 32:178–183, 1975

Vaillant GE: Ego Mechanisms of Defense: A Guide for Clinicians and Researchers. Washington, DC, American Psychiatric Press, 1992

Weissman MM: The epidemiology of personality disorders: a 1990 update. Journal of Personality Disorders 7:44–62, 1993

Woody GE, McLellan AT, Luborsky L, et al: Sociopathy and psychotherapy outcome. Arch Gen Psychiatry 42:1081–1086, 1985

Zimmerman M, Coryell W: DSM-III personality disorder diagnoses in a nonpatient sample: demographic correlates and comorbidity. Arch Gen Psychiatry 46:682–689, 1989

CHAPTER 23

Disorders Usually First Diagnosed in Infancy, Childhood, or Adolescence

Charles W. Popper, M.D.
Ronald J. Steingard, M.D.

Childhood is recognized in psychiatry as a period of vulnerability and progressive development toward adult personality and character. More recently, the psychiatric disorders of children are coming into focus as serious, treatable conditions and as precursors of adult psychopathology. These disorders often emerge in combinations, interact with each other over time, change in presentation during maturation, and can be obscured or amplified by intervening developmental events.

Multiple psychiatric disorders are typical in a single child psychiatric patient. A primary psychiatric disorder in childhood can lead to secondary developmental complications such as conduct disorder or school failure, or more persistently to low self-esteem and disorders of social assertiveness. Primary syndromes quickly expand with secondary complications during development and blur the boundaries of the "original" psychopathology. Certain disorders move in clusters through families

The authors wish to thank Margaret Beuman, M.D., Dennis Cantwell, M.D., David Carter, Alan Crocker, M.D., Martin Drell, M.D., Barry Garfinkel, M.D., Jeffrey Newcorn, M.D., Jean Pallone, Leland Perry, David Urion, M.D., Fred Volkmar, M.D., and Charles Zeanah, M.D. for their wisdom, support, and vision.

and individuals, and interact with each other to produce more virulent forms of the disorders. These interactive effects of multiple concurrent disorders are particularly evident in children and adolescents. Even though personality diagnoses are usually withheld prior to age 18, the average child psychiatric outpatient carries two separate DSM-IV (American Psychiatric Association 1994) diagnoses, and the average inpatient carries four.

Where were adult psychiatric patients during their childhoods? Part of the answer rests in our ability to see disease in children. Just a few years ago, it was believed that mood disorders did not begin until mid or late adolescence. Now we know that all "adult" psychiatric disorders in DSM-IV can begin during childhood. Any diagnosis can be used as a primary diagnostic label in a child. Even personality disorders (all except antisocial personality disorder) may be used in the diagnosis of children if the characteristics of such disorders appear pervasive and unusually persistent. We also now know that all childhood-onset disorders can have major sequelae in adults or develop into adult disorders.

Medical conditions in children are crucial in evaluating behavior, because even mild or transient Axis III medical problems can cause flagrant behavioral symptoms, especially in young children (Cantwell and Baker 1988). There is a doubling of the prevalence of psychiatric disorders in children with non-central nervous system (CNS) physical handicaps and diseases (Rutter and Yule 1970). On Axis IV, DSM-IV provides a modified version of Severity of Psychosocial Stressors Scale for children and adolescents. Parental absence or neglect, physical and sexual abuse, psychiatric disorders among caregivers, and puberty exert age-specific effects. The Axis V Global Assessment of Functioning Scale incorporates features of the Children's Global Assessment Scale (Shaffer et al. 1983).

Developmental stage can influence the presentation and significance of symptoms and alter the course of a psychiatric disorder. Coping functions and adaptive strengths can change with development and are not related in a simple way to chronological age. Under the current DSM system, such developmental characteristics are not classified, and the clinician is left to personal judgment to assess the developmental stage of the individual and the developmental significance of the presenting symptoms. The DSM-IV category "Disorders Usually First Diagnosed in Infancy, Childhood, or Adolescence" includes conditions that not only begin in childhood but also are typically diagnosed during childhood (Table 23–1). Some behavior patterns can be normal at certain developmental stages but become pathological beyond their developmental stage (e.g., separation anxiety disorder, enuresis, encopresis, and oppositional defiant disorder). The majority of these disorders, however, are not "normal" at any age. Just as psychopathological influences can undergo developmental expansion during early life, so can early therapeu-

Table 23–1.   DSM-IV disorders usually first diagnosed in infancy, childhood, or adolescence

Mental retardation
Mild mental retardation
Moderate mental retardation
Severe mental retardation
Profound mental retardation
Mental retardation, severity unspecified

Learning disorders (academic skills disorders)
Reading disorder
Mathematics disorder
Disorder of written expression
Learning disorder not otherwise specified

Motor skills disorder (developmental coordination disorder)

Pervasive developmental disorders
Autistic disorder
Rett's disorder
Childhood disintegrative disorder
Asperger's disorder
Pervasive developmental disorder not otherwise specified

Attention-deficit and disruptive behavior disorders
Attention-deficit/hyperactivity disorder
Predominantly inattentive type
Predominantly hyperactive-impulsive type
Combined type
Not otherwise specified
Conduct disorder
Oppositional defiant disorder
Disruptive behavior disorder not otherwise specified

Feeding and eating disorders of infancy or early childhood
Pica
Rumination disorder of infancy
Feeding disorder of infancy or early childhood

Tic disorders
Tourette's disorder
Chronic motor or vocal tic disorder
Transient tic disorder
Tic disorder not otherwise specified

Communication disorders
Expressive language disorder
Mixed receptive-expressive language disorder
Phonological disorder
Stuttering
Communication disorder not otherwise specified

Elimination disorders
Encopresis
Enuresis

Other disorders of infancy, childhood, or adolescence
Separation anxiety disorder
Selective mutism
Reactive attachment disorder of infancy or early childhood
Stereotypic movement disorder
Disorder of infancy, childhood, or adolescence not otherwise specified

tic interventions. In knowing and treating childhood psychopathology, we serve children and the adults they become as well as adults (i.e., parents and caregivers) and the children they once were.

■ DISRUPTIVE BEHAVIOR AND ATTENTION–DEFICIT DISORDERS

Behavior disorders are highly prevalent in "normal" schoolchildren and in child psychiatric patients. For this large class of child psychiatric disorders, parents generally appear more distressed than the child and typically bring a reluctant child for help. The child often sees no personal problems or else views the parents as "the problem." These conditions are called *externalizing* disorders, emphasizing that children and adolescents with these disorders "act out" their conflicts, feelings, and impulses.

Disruptive behavior and attention-deficit disorders is a DSM-IV umbrella term that encompasses attention-deficit/hyperactivity disorder, conduct disorder, and oppositional defiant disorder in children. These disorders are often present concurrently in the same child and are identified with different components of behavioral unmanageability.

□ Attention-Deficit/Hyperactivity Disorder

Children or adults with attention-deficit/hyperactivity disorder (ADHD) show the behavioral characteristics of motor hyperactivity (or impulsivity), the cognitive characteristics of inattention (such as short attention span and distractibility), or both. The DSM-IV criteria (Table 23–2) no longer suggest that ADHD is a child's disorder, a loose mix of annoying behaviors and scattered attention, or a problem that may be seen in just one setting. Although ADHD is now understood to afflict people of all ages, most of the available research has concentrated on children and adolescents. Many documented findings about ADHD in children and adolescents have led to working hypotheses and speculations about ADHD in adults. So far, most findings on ADHD in adults have been consistent with prior findings in youths with ADHD.

Psychostimulant therapy of behavior disorder is one of the oldest and most established psychopharmacological treatments, with more than 170 double-blind demonstrations of its clinical effectiveness in children. In clinical practice, the disorder is often claimed to be "diagnosed" after a therapeutic response to an empirical trial of psychostimulant medication. However, drug-responsiveness cannot be taken as a biological marker of a single disorder. Because many behavioral conditions respond to psychostimulants, this diagnostic procedure is invalid. Fur-

Table 23–2.   DSM-IV diagnostic criteria for attention-deficit/hyperactivity disorder

A. Either (1) or (2):

1. Six (or more) of the following symptoms of *inattention* have persisted for at least 6 months to a degree that is maladaptive and inconsistent with developmental level:

Inattention

⟋a. Often fails to give close attention to details or makes careless mistakes in schoolwork, work, or other activities.

b. Often has difficulty sustaining attention in tasks or play activities.

c. Often does not seem to listen when spoken to directly.

d. Often does not follow through on instructions and fails to finish schoolwork, chores, or duties in the workplace (not due to oppositional behavior or failure to understand instructions).

e. Often has difficulties organizing tasks and activities.

f. Often avoids, dislikes, or is reluctant to engage in tasks that require sustained mental effort (such as schoolwork or homework).

g. Often loses things necessary for tasks or activities (e.g., toys, school assignments, pencils, books, or tools).

h. Is often easily distracted by extraneous stimuli.

i. Is often forgetful in daily activities.

2. Six (or more) of the following symptoms of *hyperactivity-impulsivity* have persisted for at least 6 months to a degree that is maladaptive and inconsistent with developmental level:

Hyperactivity

a. Often fidgets with hands or feet or squirms in seat.

b. Often leaves seat in classroom or in other situations in which remaining seated is expected.

c. Often runs about or climbs excessively in situations in which it is inappropriate (in adolescents or adults, may be limited to subjective feelings of restlessness).

d. Often has difficulty playing or engaging in leisure activities quietly.

e. Is often "on the go" or often acts as if "driven by a motor."

f. Often talks excessively.

Impulsivity

g. Often blurts out answers before questions have been completed.

h. Often has difficulty awaiting turn.

i. Often interrupts or intrudes on others (e.g., butts into conversations or games).

B. Some hyperactive-impulsive or inattentive symptoms that caused impairment were present before age 7 years.

C. Some impairment from the symptoms is present in two or more settings (e.g., at school [or work] and at home).

(continued)

Table 23–2.   DSM-IV diagnostic criteria for attention-deficit/hyperactivity disorder *(continued)*

D.   There must be clear evidence of clinically significant impairment in social, academic, or occupational functioning.

E.   The symptoms do not occur exclusively during the course of a pervasive developmental disorder, schizophrenia, or other psychotic disorder and are not better accounted for by another mental disorder (e.g., mood disorder, anxiety disorder, dissociative disorder, or a personality disorder).

Code based on type:

314.01   **Attention-deficit/hyperactivity disorder, combined type:** if both criteria A1 and A2 are met for the past 6 months.

314.00   **Attention-deficit/hyperactivity disorder, predominantly inattentive type:** if criterion A1 is met but criterion A2 is not met for the past 6 months.

314.01   **Attention-deficit/hyperactivity disorder, predominantly hyperactive-impulsive type:** if criterion A2 is met but criterion A1 is not met for the past 6 months.

Coding note: For individuals (especially adolescents and adults) who currently have symptoms that no longer meet full criteria, "in partial remission" should be specified.

---

thermore, despite 50 years of identification and treatment, behavioral predictors of psychostimulant response are quite nonspecific. In children, particularly, it is unsatisfying that this drug-treatable disorder is defined purely by the co-occurrence of common childhood behaviors. Unfortunately, in adults and children, the clinical use of this diagnostic label is often functionally equivalent to "stimulant-responsive impulsivity."

Clinical Description

Major symptoms of ADHD include motoric hyperactivity, impulsivity, inattention, and emotional lability. Generally, measures of activity and attention in ADHD are only weakly correlated, and these symptoms reflect independent dimensions of psychopathology. Factor-analytic studies of behavior yield two separate factors for "inattention" and "hyperactivity/impulsivity" both in children with ADHD and in nonreferred samples. The subtyping of ADHD into "predominantly inattentive," "predominantly hyperactive-impulsive," and "combined" types allows the diagnostic label of ADHD to designate persons with or without prominent hyperactivity (as well as with or without prominent inattention). The separate assessment of inattention and hyperactivity/impulsivity becomes clinically necessary, because each may have at least a partially distinct prognosis and response to treatment.

Persons with ADHD tend to be symptomatic in many if not all settings, but the intensity of symptoms varies across settings. Symptoms can vary with environmental structure, sensory stimulation, and emotional state, as well as with physiological factors such as general alertness, hunger, and sleep deprivation. Most children experience more environmental and affective "pressure" at school than at home, and the "overflow" into hyperactivity and impulsivity is particularly clear in the classroom. Hyperactivity/impulsivity and inattention are also increased in noisy places or group settings, such as hallways or crowded waiting rooms. Depending on whether the home or the hospital unit is more stimulating or disruptive, an ADHD child can become more symptomatic or can "improve" when hospitalized. The child may appear quite different to observers in different environments. Symptoms are often more apparent to the teacher in noisy or crowded settings than to the physician in a quiet office.

Although the DSM-IV label emphasizes cognitive and motoric characteristics, pathological impulsivity is also seen in motivation, emotionality, behavioral control, and aggressivity. Motivational variability, noncompliance with instructions or plans, difficulty in completing projects, and other symptoms of "disorganization" are common in ADHD. Emotional impulsivity, seen in anger and fighting, can be readily triggered in response to minor provocation. Once anger is felt, it can stimulate a further increase in impulsivity.

Exploratory behavior can seem "aggressive," involving an energetic foraging into new places and things. On entering a room, the child may immediately begin to touch and climb. These "exploratory" inclinations can lead to rough handling of objects, accidental breakage, intrusive entry into unsafe areas, physical injuries including bone fractures, and accidental ingestions. Property damage may result without intent (i.e., destructiveness can occur without anger).

Epidemiology

Approximately 10% of boys and 2% of girls have ADHD, so general prevalence is estimated at 6% (range 3% to 10%) of the school-age population in the United States. There is a strong male predominance (3:1 to 10:1 ratio of boys to girls). ADHD often appears in combination with other psychiatric disorders and is present in 30% to 50% of childhood psychiatric outpatients and 40% to 70% of child psychiatric inpatients. About 17% of ADHD children are extrafamilial adoptees, compared with 4% of child psychiatric patients and 1% of the general population (Deutsch et al. 1982). Accurate figures concerning the prevalence of ADHD in the adult population are not yet available.

Girls are generally believed to constitute 10% to 25% of ADHD children, although this may be an underestimate resulting from diagnostic expectations. There are suggestions that women may constitute a higher proportion of the adult ADHD population and may present for treatment more frequently than do men (Wender 1987). Data on ADHD in girls and women are sparse, for nearly all ADHD research has been conducted on boys.

Etiology

There is no evidence that only one attention deficit or that a single brain mechanism is responsible for all manifestations of ADHD. Different etiologies and different sites of psychostimulant action may be relevant for different individuals with ADHD. Family studies indicate a genetic etiological component (Pauls 1991). ADHD runs in families, particularly in male relatives of ADHD children. The prevalence of psychopathology is two to three times higher in relatives of ADHD children. In adopted ADHD children, biological parents have more psychopathology than do adopting parents.

Familial transmission can be explained by genetic or psychosocial mechanisms. There is no evidence of a single gene defect or of a specific mechanism of genetic transmission in ADHD, and the hereditary component will probably be explained as polygenic (Vandenberg et al. 1986). Although ADHD is diagnosed less commonly in girls, ADHD girls have a stronger family history for ADHD (in effect, a higher genetic loading for ADHD) than do ADHD boys (Vandenberg et al. 1986). A variety of biological, psychodynamic, and cultural factors can be postulated to account for this "gender threshold effect": reduced penetrance for the expression of the genetic form of ADHD in girls, a gender-related difference in profiles of ADHD etiologies or symptoms, or cultural differences in the frequency or recognition of aggressivity in boys and girls. In any case, it seems that genetic loading can interact with gender-related factors in modulating the appearance of ADHD.

There are a variety of other presumed neuromedical etiologies of ADHD, including brain damage, neurological disorder, low birth weight, and neurotoxin exposure. Obstetrical problems during pregnancy or delivery (such as bleeding or perinatal hypoxia) can cause neurological trauma. However, contrary to early belief, obstetrical difficulties and perinatal asphyxia are not tightly correlated with the appearance of neurological disorders such as cerebral palsy (Nelson and Ellenberg 1986) and probably do not account for more than a small percentage of cases of ADHD (Nichols and Chen 1981). Prenatal factors are probably more important than birth complications in the etiology of these neuropsychiatric disorders; that is, prenatal predisposing factors appear to produce both the birth complications and the ADHD. For example, low birth weight is partially predictive of subsequent ADHD, with or without obstetrical complications. Intrauterine exposure to toxic substances, including alcohol or lead, can produce teratogenic effects on behavior.

Overt neurological disorders, most commonly seizures and cerebral palsy, are diagnosable in 5% of children with ADHD. Findings on the electroencephalogram (EEG) are abnormal in 20% of ADHD children (vs. 15% generally), and computed tomography (CT) scans are typically normal. Nonlocalizing neurological "soft signs" (such as clumsiness, left-right confusion, perceptual-motor dyscoordination, and dysgraphia) are commonly seen in ADHD children, but 15% of normal children show up to five soft signs.

Cerebral imaging and numerous neuropsychological studies are consistent with the hypothesis that functioning of the frontal cortex is impaired in certain ADHD children. ADHD-like symptoms are typically observed in humans with lesions and disorders of the relevant regions of the frontal cortex. These frontal regions are believed to inhibit subcortically guided automatic (i.e., "impulsive") responses to sensory stimulation from external sources, and to prepare the brain for voluntary movements based on external stimuli. Brain localization is probably crucial to specific ADHD symptoms and might be related to variations in clinical presentation of ADHD. Among children with right hemisphere syndrome (i.e., cortical dysfunctions of the right hemisphere), 93% were found to have ADHD-like symptoms (Voeller 1986).

Attention-deficit/hyperactivity disorder is commonly seen in association with other psychiatric disorders, particularly conduct disorder (Table 23–3). Concomitant disorders can appear fully coincidentally

---

Table 23–3.   Psychiatric disorders often associated with attention-deficit/hyperactivity disorder (ADHD)

Disruptive behavior disorders	Posttraumatic stress disorder
Conduct disorder	Obsessive-compulsive disorder
Oppositional defiant disorder	Tic disorder: Tourette's disorder
Learning disorders	Schizophrenia
Motor skills disorder	Substance abuse
Communication disorders	Mental retardation
Mood disorders	Pervasive developmental disorders,
Major depression	including autistic disorder
Bipolar disorder	

Note.   Various psychiatric states should be assessed clinically in individuals with ADHD, even though strong statistical associations have not been demonstrated for each of these conditions.

(i.e., independently), but usually operate as exacerbating (i.e., interactive), mechanistically related (i.e., having common or shared cause), or etiological (i.e., causal) factors. For example, ADHD is often seen comorbidly with mood and anxiety disorders (typically with each disorder exacerbating the course of the other disorder), but ADHD-like symptoms can also be due to the mood and anxiety disorders. ADHD look-alikes can include conduct disorder, oppositional defiant disorder, major depressive disorder, bipolar disorder, posttraumatic stress disorder, abuse or neglect, and Tourette's disorder. Thus, for many reasons, various conditions need to be considered in the context of ADHD.

There is also a high prevalence of ADHD in all learning, motor skills, and communication disorders. ADHD occurs so commonly in association with psychotic disorders (including schizophrenia) and pervasive developmental disorders (including autistic disorder) that these disorders are considered relative exclusion criteria for ADHD. ADHD often presents comorbidly with mental retardation, but it is then considered a separate diagnosis. Conduct problems or conduct disorder is seen in 40% to 70% of children with ADHD, so a large portion of the ADHD literature is actually about the combination of ADHD and conduct disorder. Aggressivity, behavioral disorders, and subsequent antisocial personality disorder are commonly seen in association with ADHD.

There is an overrepresentation of ADHD in Tourette's disorder (at least 25% of males with Tourette's disorder) and probably obsessive-compulsive disorder (OCD) in children. ADHD boys have a high score for obsessive-compulsive features on the Achenbach and Edelbrock Child Behavior Checklist (Achenbach and Edelbrock 1983).

There is also an overrepresentation of ADHD in children who have major depressive disorder (both disorders are associated with decreased rapid eye movement [REM] latency, tricyclic-responsiveness, and genetic interrelationships), bipolar disorder (approximately 50% of lithium-responsive children are hyperactive), and anxiety disorders. Also, certain children of mothers with schizophrenia have motor and attentional deficits and, in follow-up studies, appear at high risk to grow up to become adults with schizophrenia; their non-ADHD siblings have a low incidence of adult schizophrenia (Marcus et al. 1985). Thus, certain children with ADHD may have "precursor conditions" of adult mood or psychotic disorders.

Other medical causes of ADHD or ADHD-like symptoms include generalized resistance to thyroid hormone (Hauser et al. 1993), hyperthyroidism, and, perhaps, chronic constipation and chronic hunger. Both dietary and immunological etiologies have been proposed but have not been established. Drug-induced ADHD can result from treatment with carbamazepine, benzodiazepines, or phenobarbital, as well as other medications such as caffeine or theophylline.

Clinical research has yielded a wide variety of biological findings on ADHD (and ADHD look-alikes) that potentially contribute to the descriptive and etiological understanding of this disorder (Table 23–4). These biological findings partially reflect both the diversity of etiologies

---

Table 23–4.   Physical and laboratory findings in attention-deficit/ hyperactivity disorder (ADHD)

Note.   Some findings appear only in certain subgroups or individuals rather than throughout the entire ADHD population.

Motor activity meters
Increased locomotion during daytime (especially during quiet activities) and sleep.

Clinical laboratory
Lead levels increased.
Thyroid abnormalities.

Neuromedical examination
Multiple minor physical anomalies, including neurological "soft signs."
Seizure disorders, with slight increased occurrence of abnormalities on the EEG.

Psychological testing
Various signs of distractibility and attentional pathology, variable motivational state, and various localized cortical deficits (associated with comorbid learning disorders).

Autonomic responsiveness
Mixed findings of increased or decreased autonomic and central "tone."

Sleep physiology
Decreased REM latency.
Increased sleep latency (initial insomnia).
Increased motor activity (restlessness during sleep).

Neurotransmitter metabolites
Mixed findings on neurochemical assays of biogenic amines in cerebrospinal fluid, but tendency to low levels of dopamine, norepinephrine, and phenylethylamine, and elevation of serotonin.

Regional metabolism in brain
High blood flow in primary sensory regions of temporal and occipital cortex, and low blood flow in frontal cortex (and usually caudate nuclei).
Cerebral glucose metabolism reduced by 8%, with decrease in many brain regions, with the largest reductions in the premotor cortex and superior prefrontal cortex.

---

that lead to ADHD and the shared characteristics of ADHD that are common across the numerous etiological and phenomenologically similar subgroups.

Neurochemical studies of ADHD have been largely organized around the catecholamine hypothesis, particularly regarding the role of dopamine (in the limbic or caudate regions) and norepinephrine (in the reticular formation). Laboratory studies have yielded contradictory findings.

The dopamine hypothesis is supported by findings that 1) the stimulants have strong (though not exclusively) dopaminergic effects, and their therapeutic effects are reduced when dopamine receptors are blocked; 2) experimental rats with neonatal lesions of their dopamine neuronal systems have motoric hyperactivity and learning deficits, which are reversed by psychostimulants; 3) children with von Economo's encephalitis had an ADHD-like clinical picture (and adults had parkinsonism); and 4) low levels of the dopamine metabolite homovanillic acid appear in the cerebrospinal fluid (CSF) of children with ADHD. However, dopamine receptor blockers also exert therapeutic effects, and not all dopamine agonists are therapeutic.

The norepinephrine hypothesis is supported by 1) therapeutic efficacy of tricyclic antidepressants and monoamine oxidase (MAO) inhibitors (though both also modify serotonin transmission) as well as clonidine, and 2) reports of low levels of 3-methoxy-4-hydroxyphenylglycol (MHPG).

In an imaging study of cerebral blood flow, ADHD children showed high blood flow in primary sensory regions of the occipital and temporal cortex. All 11 ADHD children had hypoperfusion of the frontal lobes (especially white matter), and 7 out of 11 had hypoperfusion of the caudate nuclei. Psychostimulant medication increased blood flow in the basal ganglia (consistent with activation of dopamine neurons) and decreased flow in primary sensory and motor cortex (Lou et al. 1989).

In cognitive studies, ADHD children show distractibility (especially when bored) and other abnormalities in attention regulation (including attention span), stimulus seeking, and motivational variability. Sustained focus on a specific task in continuous performance tests is impaired in children with ADHD, but also in children with learning disorders or mental retardation. State-dependent learning on psychostimulants (i.e., learning on medication that is not maintained after medication is stopped) is reported in laboratory studies of ADHD children, but not clinically.

Neurophysiological studies show that ADHD children differ in autonomic responsiveness from other children (exhibiting either more or less reactivity), both in the tonic resting state and in response to novel situations. However, these findings are also observed in children with learning disorders or mental retardation. In sleep studies, ADHD children show decreased REM latency (similar to that seen in adults with major depressive disorder), increased motoric activity during sleep (i.e., restlessness), and increased sleep latency (i.e., time required to fall asleep), but no other consistent EEG architectural changes.

This diversity of medical, neurological, psychiatric, biological, and neuropsychological findings and disorders associated with ADHD might eventually be systematically subdivided into a nosological classification. At present, clinicians are using the simple diagnostic label of ADHD to refer in a general way to this rich field of mechanistic happenings.

Course and Prognosis

The most frequent outcome of childhood ADHD is clinical normalcy, but features of impulsivity persist into adolescence in 70% of ADHD children and into adulthood in 30% to 50% (Barkley 1990; Gittelman et al. 1985; Weiss and Hechtman 1986). Motoric hyperactivity commonly improves in childhood and early adolescence. Mild but clear residual ADHD symptoms (such as restlessness or fidgeting) can be seen in some adults, with good adjustment and outcome.

ADHD is not, however, a benign or self-limited childhood disorder. In young adulthood, there is a significant compromise in social skills and low self-esteem. There are fewer completed years of schooling, more car accidents, more moves, more alcohol use (at age 14 but not subsequently), more marijuana use (at age 19 but not subsequently), more court appearances, and more felony convictions. These individuals have more suicide attempts, phobic anxiety, somatization, and psychosexual traumas, but no general excess of alcohol abuse, drug abuse, or schizophrenia (Weiss and Hechtman 1986).

A major finding on children with ADHD, confirmed in several follow-up studies, is the 25% to 30% prevalence of antisocial personality disorder in adulthood, especially concentrated in individuals who also had prior conduct disorder. Children with ADHD are at increased risk for the development of criminality, but this risk appears to operate through the mediating variables of comorbid conduct disorder and antisocial personality (Mannuzza et al. 1989). Although 40% to 70% of children with ADHD have associated conduct problems, ADHD without aggressiveness does not appear to lead to conduct disorder, aggressivity, or antisocial behavior in adulthood (August et al. 1983).

Many adults continue to show inattention, impulsivity, and emotional changeability long after the motoric hyperactivity is no longer clinically prominent. The diagnosis of ADHD is valid in adults with a history of ADHD during childhood. The residual symptoms remain stimulant-responsive (Wender 1987). One specific area of potential complication concerns family functioning, potentially influencing parental satisfaction, marital harmony, and sibling development. Parent and sibling responses to the behavior of ADHD children can aggravate or improve the course of the child's illness.

Evaluation

Clinical evaluation entails assessing etiologies of ADHD, delineating concomitant neurological and psychiatric disorders, and considering similarly presenting diagnoses (Table 23–5).

Psychodynamic, psychosocial, and developmental evaluation of the individual and family is standard. Special emphasis is placed on school reports of grades and behavior (including behavior in bus and cafeteria) or work history, obstetrical history (maternal alcohol use, fetal overactivity, prenatal or perinatal injury), family residence (lead exposure in paints and exhaust fumes), family psychiatric history (including ADHD in males), family medical history (thyroid disorder), medication usage (barbiturates, benzodiazepines, stimulants), history of child neglect or abuse, concomitant learning (plus motor skills and communication) dis-

---

Table 23–5. Differential diagnosis of attention-deficit/hyperactivity disorder (ADHD)

Psychiatric	Neurological
Conduct disorder	Neurological damage (posttrauma, postinfection)
Oppositional defiant disorder	
Major depression	Lead poisoning
Anxiety (situational, developmental)	**Medical**
Separation anxiety disorder	Thyroid disorders
Posttraumatic stress disorder	Drug-induced agitation
Panic disorder	Recreational stimulants
Phobic disorder	Medical stimulants: pseudo-ephedrine
Dissociative disorders	
Psychotic, prepsychotic, or intermittent psychotic disorders (bipolar, schizophrenic, borderline)	Barbiturates, benzodiazepines
	Carbamazepine
	Theophylline
Attention-seeking or manipulative behavior	**Dietary**
Psychosocial	Excessive caffeine
Physical or sexual abuse	**Hunger**
Neglect	**Constipation**
Boredom	**Minor persistent pain**
Overstimulation	**Normal behavior**
Sociocultural deprivation	

orders and major psychiatric disorders, and potential risks of medication abuse by the patient or family members.

Physical examination is routine for physical anomalies, thyroid disorder, and premedication clearance. Neurological examination documents possible neurological trauma, neuromaturational signs (choreiform movements, overflow and mirror movements, tremor, gross and fine motor function, laterality), and (prior to starting medication) tics and dystonias. Laboratory screening includes thyroid battery; blood levels of zinc protoporphyrin (ZPP) and, possibly, lead; and a premedication electrocardiogram (ECG).

Educational and possibly neuropsychological evaluations are useful to assess attention, academic achievement, intelligence, neurocortical functioning, learning, motor skills, and communication disorders. Differential diagnosis is particularly challenging in certain cases. ADHD can be difficult to distinguish from many other child psychiatric disorders, and it may present concurrently with many psychiatric diagnoses. The identification of specific and sensitive criteria for ADHD can aid in differential diagnosis. Certain previous criteria for ADHD were discarded after the field trials for DSM-IV because they lacked the power to differentiate ADHD from other psychiatric disorders; excessive talking, intruding and interrupting, and thoughtless self-endangering behavior were found to be too nonspecific to warrant their continued use.

Treatment

A variety of treatment modalities are useful, and multimodal approaches are generally needed. Some interventions are specific to particular etiologies, but certain treatments are helpful regardless of etiology.

Environmental management of sensory stimulation involves arranging the patient's home and school (or job) setting to reduce stimuli and distractions. For children at home, parents are advised to establish quiet spaces, decorate with simple furniture and subdued colors, keep toys away in the closet, permit one friend visiting at a time, avoid supermarkets and parties, and encourage fine motor exercises (e.g., jigsaw puzzles). These recommendations have not been supported by controlled studies but are commonly offered.

Special education is generally required, because children with ADHD are typically below achievement levels expected for school grade, even after accounting for IQ (Cantwell and Baker 1988). At school, a small and perhaps self-contained classroom, small group activities, thoughtful selection of seating location, high teacher-to-student ratio, routine and predictable structure, one-to-one tutoring, or use of a resource room can be beneficial. Supervised or modified recess, gym, bus, and cafeteria arrangements are sometimes helpful.

Psychopharmacological treatment is useful for many of these children and adolescents (Green 1991). The same treatments seem largely successful for adults, although studies in this population are much less plentiful. Even dose ranges in adults and children are approximately comparable because of the faster hepatic biotransformation of drugs in youths.

Approximately 75% of ADHD children respond therapeutically to psychostimulants or tricyclic antidepressants. It is common practice to treat with a short-acting psychostimulant (D-amphetamine or methylphenidate); if one psychostimulant fails, there is a 25% chance that the other will be helpful. These psychostimulants have therapeutic effects that last about 4 to 6 hours; a "rebound" period can then ensue, during which behavioral symptoms may become more severe than at baseline and tics may emerge. Methamphetamine is a commercially available alternative that has a longer duration of action. Long-acting formulations of stimulants do not generally live up to their name and often are less effective than standard formulations. Low doses of antidepressants provide therapeutic effects that last more than 24 hours, so daily use avoids rebound symptoms. Controversy about cardiovascular toxicity of tricyclic antidepressants, especially the poorly understood cases of sudden death during the course of desipramine treatment in children (Riddle et al. 1991) and adolescents, has led to doubts about the use of tricyclic antidepresssants for treatment of nonlethal conditions such as ADHD.

Monoamine oxidase inhibitor antidepressants are also clinically effective but are not typically used for treating ADHD because of the dietary restrictions and potential risks. Clonidine appears to be a very useful and underused treatment for ADHD (Hunt et al. 1990), but more extensive documentation is needed. If these medications fail, magnesium pemoline might be considered, but it carries a 1% to 3% risk of hepatotoxic metabolite formation. Bupropion has been effective in several early trials. Carbamazepine is commonly used in England, but formal demonstration of its efficacy is unavailable. Major tranquilizers in low-dose range can also be considered, but their effects are nonspecific and their side effects make them unsuitable for long-term treatment. Lithium is generally not effective and is reported to worsen the symptoms of typical ADHD; however, it can be helpful if the "ADHD" is bipolar disorder presenting with impulsivity, inattention, and hyperactivity. It is also necessary to avoid benzodiazepines and barbiturates, which can cause excitation and agitation. Diphenhydramine and chloral hydrate are less likely to cause paradoxical excitation and can be used to induce sleep in ADHD children.

Drug treatment may continue for several years, with periodic dose adjustments needed for changes in body weight, varying environmental or developmental stress, or metabolic (and drug-induced autometabolic) changes of drug biotransformation rate. In some cases, treatment is no longer required by adolescence, but many individuals show a continuing need for treatment into adulthood.

Psychostimulant effects in ADHD include a clinical improvement in impulsivity, hyperactivity, inattention, and emotional lability. This quieting is distinct from the caffeine-induced focusing of attention, the anti-anxiety effect of benzodiazepines, or the tranquilization of antipsychotic agents. These agents act by different neurochemical and neurophysiological mechanisms, and produce different chemical forms of "sedation." Children with ADHD can show a calming response to other medical stimulants (pseudoephedrine) and behavioral excitation to sedatives (benzodiazepines and barbiturates). Such "paradoxical" clinical effects may not be specific to hyperactive children.

Behavior therapy is employed for treatment of defiance and aggressivity. Behavioral treatment, including contingent rewards, response-cost management, and time-outs, can help impulse control, although generalization beyond the treatment setting may be limited. Cognitive-behavior therapy is used for the teaching of problem-solving strategies, self-monitoring, verbal mediation (using internal speech) for self-praise and self-instruction, and seeing rather than glossing over errors.

Education and support for parents and family members are crucial and can be provided through programmed group training sessions (Barkley 1990). In addition, national organizations for parents, such as CHADD (Children and Adults With Attention Deficits Disorders), have local chapters which may be particularly helpful in providing support, education, and advocacy for families.

Certain treatments are unestablished. Studies on the Feingold diet (which involves omitting salicylates and food dyes) have yielded contradictory findings, but food dye restriction might be helpful for a subgroup (5% to 10%) of ADHD children. Claims that sugar toxicity, sugar withdrawal, or reactive hypoglycemia produces ADHD symptoms do not appear to be valid, except perhaps if there are prior nutritional deficiencies. Dietary treatments based on trace mineral content in hair analysis (particularly zinc deficiency and cadmium excess) are unevaluated. Megavitamin treatments appear ineffective and can cause toxic effects. Food allergies have been proposed as a possible mechanism, but there is little documentation to support the notion that features of ADHD are primary presenting symptoms of immunological reactions.

To monitor treatment effects in children, it is useful to receive behavioral reports from teachers. The Child Attention/Activity Profile (CAP), developed by Edelbrock (1987), is sensitive to both inattention and hyperactivity/impulsivity factors and can yield a score that is sensitive to the effects of stimulant medications.

Multimodal treatment of ADHD is currently the standard of care for ADHD children with major behavioral problems, aggressivity, ego developmental difficulties, concomitant biopsychiatric or neurological disorders, or learning disorders. Satterfield et al.'s study of multimodal treatment is generally encouraging: a combination of medication, special education, and psychotherapy resulted in improved education, attentional functioning, reduced antisocial activity, and better psychosocial adjustment (Satterfield et al. 1981). However, the 50% drop-out rate at 3 years limits its generalizability to the full ADHD population. Despite current limitations of available treatment outcome data, multimodal therapies are commonly used to treat children at high risk for multiple developmental and adult disorders.

Treatment outcome studies of ADHD have led to some striking findings. Psychostimulants appear to help inattention, impulsivity, and hyperactivity during the period of drug treatment only and can lead to enduring improvement in social skills and attitudes toward self. However, psychostimulant treatment alone has not routinely led to improved academic performance or school grades, even in children whose attention and classroom behavior improved (Barkley and Cunningham 1978). Stimulants do not produce lasting improvement in aggressivity, conduct disorder, criminality, education achievement, job functioning, marital relationships, or long-term adjustment.

The clear value of psychostimulants in treating the defining behavioral and cognitive symptoms of ADHD contrasts with their ineffectiveness—when used alone—for more complex integrated aspects of psychological functioning and for future development. The experience with psychostimulants may serve as a reminder that the value of an effective treatment can be easily overestimated, and that empirical studies are required to define the use and scope of medical interventions.

☐ Conduct Disorder

Conduct disorder is the most common diagnosis of child and adolescent patients in both clinic and hospital settings. Conduct disorder entails repeated violations of personal rights or societal rules, including violent and nonviolent behaviors. The syndrome is not a single medical entity, but a final common pathway for a variety of forms of "misbehavior," ranging from frequent lying, cheating, running away, and truancy, to vandalism, arson, rape, and armed robbery (Table 23–6). The validity of a single categorical grouping has been questioned by proponents of a more symptomatic or dimensional approach to conduct problems. Conduct disorder can derive from biopsychiatric disease (mood disorders, psychosis), organic impairment (and mental retardation), or psychodevelopmental (or personality) disorders; however, socioeconomic and environmental factors contribute heavily in many individuals.

Table 23–6.   DSM-IV diagnostic criteria for conduct disorder

A. A repetitive and persistent pattern of behavior in which the basic rights of others or major age-appropriate societal norms or rules are violated, as manifested by the presence of three (or more) of the following criteria in the past 12 months, with at least one criterion present in the past 6 months:

Aggression to people and animals

1. Often bullies, threatens, or intimidates others.
2. Often initiates physical fights.
3. Has used a weapon that can cause serious physical harm to others (e.g., a bat, brick, broken bottle, knife, gun).
4. Has been physically cruel to people.
5. Has been physically cruel to animals.
6. Has stolen while confronting a victim (e.g., mugging, purse snatching, extortion, armed robbery).
7. Has forced someone into sexual activity.

Destruction of property

8. Has deliberately engaged in fire setting with the intention of causing serious damage.
9. Has deliberately destroyed others' property (other than by fire setting).

Deceitfulness or theft

10. Has broken into someone else's house, building, or car.
11. Often lies to obtain goods or favors or to avoid obligations (i.e., "cons" others).
12. Has stolen items of nontrivial value without confronting a victim (e.g., shoplifting, but without breaking and entering; forgery).

Serious violations of rules

13. Often stays out at night despite parental prohibitions, beginning before age 13 years.
14. Has run away from home overnight at least twice while living in parental or parental surrogate home (or once without returning for a lengthy period).
15. Is often truant from school, beginning before age 13 years.

B. The disturbance in behavior causes clinically significant impairment in social, academic, or occupational functioning.

C. If the individual is age 18 years or older, criteria are not met for antisocial personality disorder.

Specify type based on age at onset:

Childhood-onset type: Onset of at least one criterion characteristic of conduct disorder prior to age 10 years.

Adolescent-onset type: Absence of any criteria characteristic of conduct disorder prior to age 10 years.

(continued)

Table 23–6.   DSM-IV diagnostic criteria for conduct disorder *(continued)*

Specify severity:

Mild: Few if any conduct problems in excess of those required to make the diagnosis **and** conduct problems cause only minor harm to others.

Moderate: Number of conduct problems and effect on others intermediate between "mild" and "severe."

Severe: Many conduct problems in excess of those required to make the diagnosis **or** conduct problems cause considerable harm to others.

Clinical Description

Conduct disorder accounts for 50% of convicted juvenile delinquents and a higher proportion of incarcerated youths. These youths often come from low socioeconomic status, broken homes with family discord, maternal rejection, and absent or alcoholic fathers. They have measurably lower cognitive and moral development, more behavioral impulsivity, greater susceptibility to boredom and stimulus-seeking behavior, and often lower nutritional status. There is an overrepresentation of homicidal behavior in these youths, often directed against their parents. Outcome and course depend upon the nature of the delinquency group and the availability of alternative social supports.

Not all delinquent behavior is considered to be the result of conduct disorder. Youths with "subcultural delinquency" or "adaptive delinquency" are conceptualized to have made an "adaptive" response to social and cultural disadvantage, parental neglect, and delinquent peers. Viewed as social victims rather than as having a mental illness, these youths were commonly seen in juvenile delinquency centers and inner city clinics, and less commonly in prisons. Such delinquency may be seen in a wide range of severities, sometimes merging into the inapparent. The diagnosis of conduct disorder was developed to identify more serious cases that may have psychiatric dimensions.

Across a diversity of presentations, children and adolescents with conduct disorder may show alterations of attention (and learning disorders), mood (sullenness, impulsive anger), cognition (distortions of size and time awareness; lack of sense of prior events and consequences; disrupted view of causal connections, particularly regarding their own behavior; weak logical thinking; impaired moral reasoning; reduced problem-solving ability), pathological defenses (minimizing, avoiding, lying, externalizing, unconscious manipulation, denial), and interpersonal impairments (suspiciousness or paranoia, with cognitive distortions sometimes triggering fights and resentments; lack of guilt and empathy; difficulty in relating to professionals). Although some adolescents with conduct disorder are involved in driving recklessly, carrying weapons, or demonstrating impulsive violence, wanton dangerousness to the public is not typical of all youths with conduct disorder.

Epidemiology

The prevalence of the conduct disorder in the general child and adolescent population in the United States is approximately 10% (range 5% to 15%). There is a male predominance for property crimes (4:1) and violent crimes (8:1). In recent years, the prevalence of conduct disorder has been increasing in females, so consequently the male predominance is decreasing over time. The epidemiology of conduct disorder will continue to vary, depending on changes in population size and distribution, family and community structure, and socioeconomic conditions.

Etiology

A wide variety of etiological factors have been described, reflecting the full range of explanatory models of behavioral causation and the importance of delinquency as a central societal problem. Early speculation centered on intrapsychic structures such as "superego defects" (Aichhorn 1925/1955), and on parental influences on unconscious motivation (Johnson et al. 1941) such as "superego lacunae" and the "acting out" of parents' unverbalized antisocial wishes or impulses. These psychoanalytic speculations were never subjected to large-scale or epidemiological studies in children or adults.

Sociological theories focused on the effects of social deprivation (poverty and cultural disadvantage), local variations in behavioral norms (street corner gangs), status seeking, escape from social entrapment, early rejection by peers, and school failure. Current sociological research is using sophisticated mathematical modeling to determine the role of socialization experiences in the path that leads to delinquent behavior and drug use (Elliott et al. 1985).

Family history studies show an overrepresentation of antisocial personality, substance abuse and addictive behavior, mood disorders, ADHD, schizophrenia, learning disorders, and other behavioral problems. There is a higher incidence of antisocial behavior and conduct disorder in fathers and male relatives of children with conduct disorder. These effects can be explained by familial or genetic transmission.

Genetic studies suggest some inheritable predisposing factors. There are elevated rates of conduct disorder in adopted-away children (complicating the use of adoption studies), but twin studies suggest that both genetic and environmental factors are operational.

Neurological factors appear to be significant for certain individuals with conduct disorder, especially for more aggressive and violent children. There is an increased incidence in conduct disorder of both "hard" and "nonlocalizing" neurological symptoms, neuropsychological deficits (especially inattention), and seizures. Degree of aggressivity correlates with a history of physical abuse, head and face injuries, neurological findings, ADHD, and possibly perinatal problems.

Biological markers of conduct disorder might be interpreted as suggesting biological etiologies. Decreased resting heart rate has been reported in numerous studies. The combination of decreased heart rate, lowered skin conductance, and increased slow wave activity on the EEG at age 15 were found to correlate to the presence of criminality at age 24 (independently of some demographic and academic factors), suggesting that autonomic underarousal (perhaps associated with low levels of anxiety) may be a biological mediator of the tendency toward the development of conduct disorder (Raine et al. 1990).

Concomitant psychopathology can operate as a pathogenic factor: ADHD, mood disorders, learning and communication disorders, and individual psychodynamic features such as counterphobic behavior and avoidance, identification with the aggressor, and stimulus seeking may predispose to conduct disorder. The pathogenic relationships among conduct disorder, ADHD, and oppositional defiant disorder are believed to be quite complex.

Parent, caregiver, and home "microenvironment" characteristics have also been linked to the appearance of conduct disorder. Large family, absent or alcoholic father, proximity of a delinquent peer group, parental rejection, harsh discipline, shifting caregivers, parental abandonment, institutional care, parental overstimulation or understimulation, parental manipulative behavior, parental role-modeling of impulsive or injurious behaviors, inadequate limit setting, and inconsistent or unpredictable discipline are proposed mechanisms. Empirical evidence for these factors varies in strength. Speculatively, each factor probably contributes significantly in individual cases.

Course and Prognosis

The major outcome risk of conduct disorder in childhood is the occurrence of antisocial personality disorder in adulthood. In a 30-year follow-up study of 500 child guidance clinic patients (Robins 1966), antisocial behavior in childhood was found to predict maladjustment and high prevalence (37%) of severe psychopathology in adulthood, as evidenced by antisocial behavior, alcohol abuse, psychiatric hospitalization, child neglect, nonsupport, financial dependency, and poor employment and military records. The next generation of children showed a high prevalence of truancy, running away, theft, and dropping out of high school. The natural course did not appear to be influenced by psychiatric treatment, lengthy incarceration, job or military experiences, or religion.

However, there was evidence of help associated with marriage to a stable spouse, support from siblings and parents, and brief incarceration.

Factors that are associated with the chronicity of conduct disorder include early onset, attentional problems, family discord and deviance, and arson. Family risk factors have been proposed to be more prognostically significant for the development of conduct disorder than for any other child psychiatric diagnosis (Fendrich et al. 1990; Wolfgang et al. 1972).

Greater socialization skills and experiences are useful in predicting a better long-term outcome (Rutter and Giller 1984). The nature of involvement with peers is also a predictor of course and severity. Peer ratings of misbehavior and low popularity in first grade were found to predict delinquent behavior during adolescence (Tremblay et al. 1988). Furthermore, ratings of aggressivity made by a child's peers at age 8 years may predict certain features of the psychiatric, marital, and legal status at ages 28 to 30 (Huesmann et al. 1984). Intelligence and small family size have been repeatedly found to be protective factors in the development or persistence of conduct disorder.

Complications of conduct disorder are numerous: school failure, school suspension, legal problems, injuries due to fighting or retaliation, accidents, sexually transmitted disease, teenage pregnancy, prostitution, being raped or murdered, fugitive status, abandonment of family, drug addiction, suicide, and homicide. Consequences of comorbid attention deficits and learning disorders can include educational failure, low frustration tolerance, loss of interest in school, underdevelopment of verbal skills, dropping out of school, and subsequent unemployment. Children with conduct disorder have a high occurrence of physical injuries, accidents, and illnesses, as well as a large number of emergency room visits and hospitalizations. The most common causes of death at follow-up are suicide, motor vehicle accidents, and death from uncertain causes (Rydelius 1988).

Despite the extremely high incidence of major psychopathology, maladjustment, and incarceration, about 50% of children with conduct disorder are able to achieve a favorable adult adjustment (Rutter and Giller 1984). There is a tendency toward a reduction in antisocial symptoms after age 40 (Hare et al. 1988). Although later onset and good socialization skills are partial predictors of a better course and adult outcome, it is unknown to what extent good outcome is associated with the natural course of illness, life experiences, therapeutic intervention, comorbidity, or preexisting characteristics.

Evaluation

For youths with conduct disorder who have impaired verbal skills, use manipulative defenses, or become uncomfortable in talking with professionals, interactive diagnostic interviews can be difficult. Specific verbal inquiries or repetitive questioning can elicit inconsistent or hostile responses. For these individuals, standard interviews can be ineffective or even counterproductive. Assessments based on such verbal and structured interviews may overestimate psychopathology and underestimate the interpersonal or mechanical strengths of these individuals.

Child self-reports of conduct symptoms are not fully reliable. Although parents' reports are often viewed by clinicians as more trustworthy, there are good reasons to question the accuracy of their data. Because the behaviors may have a low rate of occurrence, historical rather than observational data are often preferred. Yet the secrecy of the behaviors, the fears or wishes for punishment, and the amplifying or diminishing influences of extraneous feelings and biases confound the reliability of all reporters (child, parents, teachers, police). Correlations between the behavioral reports of different types of reporters are quite low (Achenbach and McConaughty 1987), leading to unresolved clinical dilemmas concerning how to combine the data derived from different informants.

A search for comorbid psychiatric diagnoses is critical, especially depressive disorders in boys (McGee and Williams 1988). Approximately one-third of prepubertal children with major depressive disorder present with concomitant conduct disorder (Puig-Antich 1982), which may persist after the resolution of the mood disorder (Kovacs et al. 1988). Childhood bipolar disorder may be associated with an even higher prevalence of conduct disorder. Prepsychotic and intermittently psychotic children may fulfill the criteria for conduct disorder. Substance use is often present and commonly underdiagnosed. ADHD involves a concomitant diagnosis of conduct disorder in 40% to 70% of cases.

Treatment

Given the diversity of presentations and severities of conduct disorder, it is not surprising that treatment can move in several directions: legal sanctions, family interventions, social support, psychotherapeutic treatment of individual or family psychopathology, or neuromedical treatment (Kazdin 1987). The treatment site can be a home, school, hospital, residential school, or specialized delinquency program.

From the very start and to the end of treatment, the quick establishment of a containment structure and of an expectation of effective limit setting—to provide both safety and a holding environment for treatment—is essential. Creating or reinforcing limits can involve parent counseling, psychiatric treatment of parents, increased supervision at home, surveillance at school, or use of legal mechanisms. Guardianship, hearings before judges, counseling by parole officers, and brief incarceration may be essential for effective limit setting and for communicating the significance of behavioral violations.

Psychiatric treatment depends more on individual variables than on diagnostic variables. Pharmacotherapy can involve virtually any psychotropic drug, depending on the concomitant neuropsychiatric findings in the individual: psychostimulants for ADHD, antidepressants or lithium for mood disorders or aggressivity, neuroleptics for psychotic features (or, in low doses, for impulsivity), beta-adrenergic blocking agents for aggressivity, or anticonvulsants (Green 1991). Cognitive-behavior therapy can help develop skills for managing anger, controlling impulsivity, and communicating (Faulstich et al. 1988). Training in problem-solving skills may be more effective than individual psychotherapy (Kazdin et al. 1989). Parent guidance can help decision making concerning management of difficult behaviors, and promote effective setting of limits on impulsive behavior. Family therapy can be useful in certain cases for reducing interpersonal manipulativeness (Patterson 1982) and for limiting projective identification between family members (Tolan et al. 1986). Group therapy often permits the "gang orientation" to promote positive change and to improve socialization skills. School interventions can include special attention to behavioral control, individualized educational programming, vocational training, and remediation of language and learning disorders. There is evidence that the early treatment of learning disorders may help prevent the development of conduct disorder.

☐ Oppositional Defiant Disorder

Children with oppositional defiant disorder show argumentative and disobedient behavior, but, unlike children with conduct disorder, they respect the personal "rights" of other people. Similar provocative and antiauthority behavior is common in children with conduct disorder as well as those with mood and psychotic disorders, and can be seen in combination with a variety of other childhood psychiatric disorders. However, this disruptive behavior disorder is meant to describe children whose provocative, antiauthority, or angry behavior occurs apart from conduct disorder, symptomatic periods of mood disorders, or psychosis. Oppositional defiant disorder can be diagnosed in association with ADHD or other psychiatric diagnoses (Table 23–7).

Clinical Description

Oppositional and defiant features can be normal for young children (at 18 to 36 months) and for adolescents, but the 6-month duration criterion for oppositional defiant disorder is used to exclude ordinary develop-

---

Table 23–7.   DSM-IV diagnostic criteria for oppositional defiant disorder

A.   A pattern of negativistic, hostile, and defiant behavior lasting at least 6 months, during which four (or more) of the following are present:

1.   Often loses temper.
2.   Often argues with adults.
3.   Often actively defies or refuses to comply with adults' requests or rules.
4.   Often deliberately annoys people.
5.   Often blames others for his or her mistakes or misbehavior.
6.   Is often touchy or easily annoyed by others.
7.   Is often angry and resentful.
8.   Is often spiteful or vindictive.

Note: Consider a criterion met only if the behavior occurs more frequently than is typically observed in individuals of comparable age and developmental level.

B.   The disturbance in behavior causes clinically significant impairment in social, academic, or occupational functioning.

C.   The behaviors do not occur exclusively during the course of a psychotic or mood disorder.

D.   Criteria are not met for conduct disorder, and, if the individual is age 18 years or older, criteria are not met for antisocial personality disorder.

---

mental phenomena. Anger-related symptoms are the presenting behavioral problems, but management of anger appears to be a circumscribed problem. Unlike children with ADHD, the oppositional and angry behavior demonstrated by these children does not lead to impulsivity throughout their behavior, affect, and cognition. The anger is typically directed at parents and teachers, and a lesser degree of anger dyscontrol may be seen in peer relationships. Temper tantrums subside typically in minutes, at most in 30 minutes. Children with mood disorders can require considerably longer to reorganize after an angry outburst.

A crucial feature of oppositional struggling is the self-defeating stand that these children take in arguments. They may be willing to lose something they want (a privilege or toy) rather than lose a struggle. The oppositional struggle takes on a life of its own in the child's mind and becomes more important than the reality of the situation. This "holding onto" or "winning" the struggle may feel paramount to the child. "Rational" objections voiced to the child become counterproductive, and the child may experience these interventions as the adult's continuing of the argument.

Children may show oppositional or defiant behavior during major affective episodes (depression or hypomania) or for long periods in chronic mood disorder. The oppositional and defiant symptoms are generally reported by parents and caregivers, and the children are typically not able to provide reliable information pertaining to this diagnosis. In addition, intentional defiance is a hallmark of this disorder. Behavioral problems may include verbal fighting and bullying.

Epidemiology

Approximately 6% of children are estimated to have oppositional defiant disorder. A male predominance of 2:1 to 3:1 was reported in a non-referred epidemiological sample (Anderson et al. 1987). Oppositional defiant disorder is commonly seen in classrooms for children who are emotionally disturbed or have a learning disability.

Etiology

In the absence of direct studies of the etiology of oppositional defiant disorder, several psychosocial mechanisms have been hypothesized:

1. Parental problems in disciplining, structuring, and limit setting
2. Identification by the child with an impulse-disordered parent who sets a role model for oppositional and defiant interactions with other people
3. Parental unavailability

However, neurobiological influences and temperamental factors may also contribute. Preliminary studies suggest a familial aggregation of oppositional defiant disorder, but mechanisms of transmission are undetermined.

Course and Prognosis

Oppositional defiant disorder can be diagnosed after age 3 years, but usually appears in late childhood. Follow-up studies suggest that 40% of children with oppositional defiant disorder will retain the diagnosis for at least 4 years, and 93% will retain psychiatric symptoms (Cantwell and Baker 1989). Certain individuals undergo a developmental progression from oppositional defiant disorder to ADHD or conduct disorder, as well as to other psychiatric disorders.

Evaluation and Treatment

Psychiatric evaluation of the child and family is needed to rule out possible conduct disorder, ADHD, and mood disorders, and to investigate family and psychosocial factors. It is also worthwhile to evaluate for a learning or language disorder, or low IQ, which can contribute to the child's oppositionality.

There are virtually no psychiatric studies of the treatment of children with oppositional defiant disorder. The few available studies appear in the psychology literature and show that behavioral techniques can modify oppositionality.

■ LEARNING, MOTORS SKILLS, AND COMMUNICATION DISORDERS

Developmental impairments in the acquisition or performance of specific skills are usually first evident in childhood but often have major consequences for lifetime functioning. Three major domains of skills are addressed in DSM-IV. The *learning disorders* involve a series of impairments in the learning of academic skills, particularly reading, arithmetic, and expressive writing. *Motor skills disorder* entails difficulty with physical coordination. The *communication disorders* involve developmental problems with speech and language, specifically expressive language, receptive (plus expressive) language, stuttering, and articulation.

These disorders commonly occur in combination, and often with other psychiatric comorbidity in the individual and in the families. In practice, children with these disorders often present with psychiatric or behavioral problems, and it is only secondarily that the learning and communication disorders are uncovered. Most of these disorders are defined by a particular area of functioning that is impaired relative to general intelligence. DSM-IV criteria specify that the diagnosis should be based on more than clinical observation: whenever possible, standardized test protocols are essential to document the presence of a specific deficit. Depending on the disorder, formal measurements of both IQ and specific skills may be required for diagnosis.

As a group, these disorders are widespread and involve 10% to 15% of the school-age population. All of these disorders run in families. There is a male predominance of 3:1 to 4:1 for these disorders, with the notable exception of mixed receptive/expressive language disorder.

The etiology of the learning, motor skills, and communication disorders, although unknown, is generally believed to be related to slow maturation, dysfunction, or damage of the cerebral cortex or other brain areas related to these specific processing functions. However, the strength of the direct evidence for genetic or biological abnormalities varies with each disorder, and nonbiological factors are clearly also involved. There is no reason to assume that each disorder is due to a single pathological mechanism, and subtyping may become possible as the brain mechanisms involved become better understood. The clustering of these disorders in the same individuals suggests that these developmental neuropsychological impairments may reflect wide-ranging cerebral dysfunctions, requiring multimodal educational remediation.

Learning disorders, language disorders, and coordination disorder are commonly associated with high rates of comorbid psychiatric disorders as well as a variety of psychological complications, including low self-esteem, poor frustration tolerance, passivity, rigidity in new learning situations, truancy, and dropping out of school. Disruptive behavior disorder can be a complication, but may appear prior to school failure and even in the preschool years. Although there has been considerable emphasis on the "emotional overlay" resulting from learning and communication disorders, there is an increasing awareness of the neuropsychiatric and sociofamilial antecedents of these disorders.

Over time, mild cases may "resolve" by persistent education and practice. Certain individuals may compensate by "overlearning," but others retain specific deficits in adulthood. Often, the associated behavioral symptoms and intrapsychic complications persist beyond the duration of the developmental deficits and may remain problematic during adult life (Cohen J 1985).

Evaluation includes intelligence testing, a battery of specific achievement tests (full range of academic skills, language, speech, and motor coordination), and observation of the child's behavior in the classroom. A general determination of the quality of teaching available at the school is needed prior to diagnosis. It is also essential to evaluate the patient for possible mental retardation, ADHD, mood disorder (low motivation), and other psychiatric and neurological disorders. Sensory perception tests are obtained to assess possible impairments of vision or hearing that can aggravate or mimic features of these disorders.

Treatment for these disorders in public schools is guaranteed (in principle) by law. The Education for Handicapped Children Act of 1978 (Public Law PL 94-142) mandates "special education" of all children with learning disabilities in the "least restrictive environment." PL 94-142 is usually interpreted to include, at most, the learning disorders, communication disorders, and ADHD, although some other psychiatric disorders that entail symptoms of inattention are sometimes considered. Multidisciplinary communication is essential, because many specialists and teachers may be involved in the education of a single child.

Learning, motor skills, and communication disorders are widespread and can be lifelong. Since the enactment of PL 94-142, these underdiagnosed and undertreated disorders have come into focus and now receive rehabilitation in childhood. Despite the national use of many types of psychoeducational and educational techniques, these methods are rarely evaluated in comparative studies. Psychopharmacological therapy is not helpful in treating learning, motor skills, or communication disorders.

☐ Learning Disorders

The learning disorders involve deficits in the acquisition and performance of reading, writing (not handwriting but expressive writing), or arithmetic. These conditions are meant to designate individuals who are qualitatively different from other slow learners and demonstrate specific deficits in acquiring skills and neurointegrative processing. Persons with learning disorders commonly also have a communication or motor skills disorder, and perhaps other symptoms of cortical dysfunction, anxiety, motivational problems, or associated psychiatric disorders. These disorders are defined to exclude individuals whose slow learning is explainable by weak educational opportunities, low intelligence, motor or sensory (visual or auditory) handicaps, or neurological problems. It is helpful to keep a broad psychiatric and neurological view on development in childhood and functioning in adulthood, because the estimated 5% to 10% of the population with a learning disorder is at increased risk for other psychiatric disorders.

Diagnosis is often made initially during grade school. During the early school years, basic skills, attention, and motivation are building blocks for subsequent learning. Major impairments in these functions are identified as requiring remediation. In later school years, organizational skills become significant: problems with note taking, time management, and book and paper arrangements may be signs of cortical deficits, even if basic skills are well remedied. In high school and college, individuals may have difficulty in learning foreign languages, writing efficiently, or reading for fun (Cohen J 1985).

Depending on the type of disorder, a child might be encouraged to make use of a calculator, typewriter, or word processor; be permitted to take "time-extended" tests; be tutored individually or in a small group; or use self-paced programmed texts or computerized self-instruction. Behavioral techniques are often employed to emphasize success, develop pride, foster enjoyment of mastering a skill, and enhance general learning by reducing rigidity and promoting interests in new situations and new experiences.

Reading Disorder

Common *dyslexia* is characterized by a slow acquisition of reading skills. Slow reading speed, impaired comprehension, word omissions and distortions, and letter reversals are outside of the expected performance levels based on age and IQ (Table 23–8). Although learning to read can be

Table 23–8.   DSM-IV diagnostic criteria for reading disorder

A. Reading achievement, as measured by individually administered standardized tests of reading accuracy or comprehension, is substantially below that expected given the person's chronological age, measured intelligence, and age-appropriate education.
B. The disturbance in criterion A significantly interferes with academic achievement or activities of daily living that require reading skills.
C. If a sensory deficit is present, the reading difficulties are in excess of those usually associated with it.

Coding note: If a general medical (e.g., neurological) condition or sensory deficit is present, code the condition on Axis III.

compromised in a variety of ways, reading disorder is a specific neuropsychiatric cause of reading disability that is seen even in the presence of normal intelligence, education, motivation, and emotional control.

For reading acquisition to develop in the normal way, numerous neurological and psychiatric functions must be intact. Eye control (not slipping off letters or lines), spatial orientation (attacking letters and words from the left, retaining a memory trace of letter forms), verbal sequencing, grasping the structural sense of a sentence, and abstraction and categorization require intact eye and brain functions as well as cortical integration. There is a simultaneous use of visual-spatial perception (shape discrimination), sequencing (spatial and temporal), cross-modal visual-auditory processing, phonemic processing (linguistic sound units), syntactic (grammar) and semantic (meaning) analysis, as well as the pursuit of understanding. Attention, motivation, and effort must be intact. In addition, "reading readiness" skills are necessary, including the ability to take instruction and to avoid disrupting other individuals in the classroom. In general, reading ability correlates with IQ (especially verbal coding and sequencing). A general reading acquisition slowness or the specific reading disorder might result from problems affecting any of these functions. Difficulty in reading may result from mental retardation, brain damage, psychiatric disturbance (especially influences on attention and anxiety), sensory deficits, cultural deprivation, and inadequate schooling.

Clinical description.   Commonly, individuals with reading disorder show difficulty in the "paired-associate task" of translating verbal symbols (letters) into auditory-based sounded words. In addition, left-right orientation, sound discrimination, and perceptual-motor skills are often impaired. Signs of visual and perceptual motor skill impairment include letter reversals, word transposition, omissions, and substitution. Virtually all individuals with reading disorder have spelling problems, which may be more severe and long-lasting than the reading problem. About 80% have other verbal language deficits. Many have disorder of written expression, phonological disorder, motor skills disorder, or poor handwriting. Some have seizures or symptoms of nondominant hemisphere injury. Attentional difficulties are common, including for tasks unrelated to reading and language. About 25% have conduct disorder, usually beginning before adolescence or even before school years. About one-third of children with conduct disorder have reading disorder.

Epidemiology.   Prevalence estimates for reading disorder vary widely, but usually are about 3% to 10% of the general population. There is a 3:1 to 4:1 male predominance. Prevalence varies highly with geographic region. Also, increased prevalence is associated with low socioeconomic class, large family size, and social disadvantage.

Etiology.   The main etiological factors appear to be neurological, but symptom severity and duration are subject to learning and experience. When neuropsychological testing identifies patterns similar to individuals with localizable brain disorders, brain defects in similar cortical regions are postulated.

Neuropathological studies (Galaburda et al. 1985) have demonstrated neuroanatomic anomalies that imply developmental abnormalities of the cerebral cortex. These neuronal ectopias and dysplasias are widespread throughout the cortex, but are primarily concentrated in the left hemisphere, especially in the perisylvian region. In the inferior frontal and superior temporal regions, these neuronal anomalies include micropolygyria, neuronal ectopias in layer l, nodules (brain warts), and architectonic dysplasias.

There is also an absence of the usual cerebral pattern of a larger language-dominant region (Broca's area) in the left hemisphere (Haslam et al. 1981). Instead, the planum temporale is symmetrical in these brains, so the normal development of a differentiated language center is not seen. The usual asymmetry in this part of the brain is absent. Cerebral blood flow was found to be more left-asymmetric during a semantics task in individuals with reading disorder (Rumsey et al. 1985a).

In addition to the evidence of a relatively underdeveloped Broca's area (left planum temporale), more widespread cortical anomalies are seen. The neuronal ectopias and anomalous symmetry imply a relative failure in brain development that is not restricted to language-dominant regions. These anomalous brain structures are associated with a broad range of cerebral functions, including spatial and verbal abilities, motor dominance (i.e., handedness), and left-right sense.

Family psychiatric histories show an overrepresentation of reading, speech, and language disorders in the siblings and parents. A concordance rate approaching 100% in identical twins has been found in several studies (Vandenburg et al. 1986). The lower concordance in fraternal twins supports a clear genetic factor. Family pedigrees are not consistent with a single mode of transmission, suggesting that the disorder is genetically heterogeneous. Gene linkage analysis has implicated chromosome 15 in the autosomal dominant transmission of certain cases of reading disorder (Smith et al. 1983).

Despite the neurogenetic factors that can lead to reading disorder, its expression is influenced by educational opportunities, family support, individual personality, and drive and ambition. Maternal smoking, low birth weight, prenatal and perinatal mishaps, overt neurological disorders, and abnormalities on the EEG appear to be associated with the development of reading disorder.

Course and prognosis.   Delayed acquisition of reading skills is usually identified in grade school. Typically, by third grade the child with reading disorder is 1 to 2 years behind expectations. Adequate reading skills may eventually be acquired with sufficient time and effort. However, in adolescence, the individual may still show a slow learning of foreign languages, little ease in reading, and little reading for pleasure. Complications include frustration and loss of interest in school, dropping out of school, and the exacerbation of concomitant psychiatric disorders, especially disruptive behavior disorders. Over time, the reading usually improves, but spelling problems and delinquency may persist. In adulthood, unemployment and unskilled job placements are more likely.

Evaluation.   Neurological and psychiatric assessment (especially regarding disruptive behavior and attention-deficit disorders, other learning and communication disorders, and social deprivation), hearing and vision tests, and IQ, psychological, neuropsychological, and educational measurements are useful. The new imaging techniques are expected to contribute significantly to diagnostic assessment in the future.

Treatment.   Early educational intervention may use one of the many remedial systems, but comparative studies of the different educational approaches to reading disorder are lacking. There is little evidence supporting the use of any particular teaching method, including the usual perceptual training based on an individual's "strong" learning modality (e.g., auditory vs. visual). Self-esteem may need to be bolstered to help the child (or adult) tolerate the remedial efforts. Treatment should be directed at the reading disorder and the possibly associated learning and communication disorders, conduct disorder, and ADHD. Parental involvement is crucial in providing support for the educational program and for the child's persistent efforts in a criticism-free learning environment. There is evidence that parents can help by listening to their children read at home daily (Tizard et al. 1982). There is no evidence, however, that medications, vitamins, or diet is helpful.

Mathematics Disorder

The capacity for making simple mathematical calculations is critical in a consumer economy and high-technology culture. Arithmetic, calculation (fractions, decimals, percentages), measurement (space, time, weight), and logical reasoning are basic skills.

Individuals with mathematics disorder (Table 23–9) have difficulty in learning to count, in doing simple mathematical calculations, in conceptualizing sets of objects, and in thinking spatially (right-left, up-down, east-west). Deficits may be seen in copying shapes, mathematical memory, number and procedure sequencing, and the naming of mathematical concepts and operations. Typically, some reading and spelling problems are seen in association with mathematics disorder.

Factors that produce slow academic development of mathematical abilities include neurological, genetic, psychological, and socioeconomic conditions, and learning experiences. Typically, arithmetic ability correlates with IQ and classroom training; however, mathematics disorder is defined to designate not individuals who are merely slow learners or who have poor educational opportunities, but individuals with a specific neurocortical or psychiatric abnormality. However, there is little available psychiatric description of this disorder.

Approximately 6% of the population is affected by mathematics disorder, and the gender ratio is undetermined. Lower socioeconomic classes show an overrepresentation of mathematics disorder as well as other learning disorders. Etiological factors are not well defined. Language-dominant hemispheric damage is not typically demonstrable in

---

Table 23–9.   DSM-IV diagnostic criteria for mathematics disorder (developmental arithmetic disorder)

A.   Mathematical ability, as measured by individually administered standardized tests, is substantially below that expected given the person's chronological age, measured intelligence, and age-appropriate education.

B.   The disturbance in criterion A significantly interferes with academic achievement or activities of daily living that require mathematical ability.

C.   If a sensory deficit is present, the difficulties in mathematical ability are in excess of those usually associated with it.

Coding note: If a general medical (e.g., neurological) condition or sensory deficit is present, code the condition on Axis III.

---

mathematics disorder, but neuropsychological deficits may be demonstrated in number manipulations, spatial relationships, and mathematical reasoning. Both verbal (sequencing) and visuospatial deficits can contribute, so bilateral hemisphere dysfunction may be involved (Rourke and Strang 1983). Subcortical mechanisms have also been proposed.

Evaluation for mathematics disorder includes psychiatric (i.e., disruptive behavior disorders, mental retardation, and other learning disorders), neurological, cognitive (i.e., IQ, psychological tests, neuropsychological tests, and educational achievement tests), and social assessments. The standardized tests of arithmetic skills may need adjustment for the child's educational experience with an old (rote calculation) or new (logical concept) mathematics curriculum.

Treatment of mathematics disorder involves special education, with initial evaluation and subsequent monitoring of need for psychiatric and neurological intervention.

Disorder of Written Expression

The disorder of written expression is not well characterized in the psychiatric literature, and assessment and treatment are not well developed. Difficulties in spelling, grammar, sentence and paragraph formation, organizational structure, and punctuation are characteristic (Table 23–10). Symptoms include slow writing speed and low volume output, illegibility, letter reversals, word-finding and syntax errors, erasures, rewritings, spacing errors, and punctuation and spelling problems. Low productivity, refusal to complete work or submit assignments, and chronic underachievement may be suggestive of a more generalized "developmental output failure" (Levine et al. 1981). Ideational content and intellectual

---

Table 23–10.   DSM-IV diagnostic criteria for disorder of written expression

A. Writing skills, as measured by individually administered standardized tests (or functional assessments of writing skills), are substantially below those expected given the person's chronological age, measured intelligence, and age-appropriate education.

B. The disturbance in criterion A significantly interferes with academic achievement or activities of daily living that require the composition of written texts (e.g., writing grammatically correct sentences and organized paragraphs).

C. If a sensory deficit is present, the difficulties in writing skills are in excess of those usually associated with it.

Coding note: If a general medical (e.g., neurological) condition or sensory deficit is present, code the condition on Axis III.

abstraction may be limited, but not necessarily. A "sense of audience," involving social cognition of the interests and needs of the reader, may be impaired (Gregg and McAlexander 1989).

These deficits in written expression may result from underlying problems with graphomotor (hand and pencil control), fine motor, and visuomotor function; attention; memory; concept formation and organization (prioritizing and flow); and expressive language function. Like other learning disorders, disorder of written expression is presumed to result from neurocortical characteristics as modified by environmental experiences.

The prevalence of disorder of written expression has not yet been determined, but there appears to be the standard 3:1 to 4:1 male predominance seen in most learning disorders.

Formal methods for assessment and measurement of expressive writing have been developed, but adequate clinical screening can be obtained from samples of copied, dictated, and spontaneous writing.

Genuine remedial therapy is possible. Educational interventions have typically consisted of alternative writing formats and skill building. The availability of commercial word processors can contribute to remediation of some individuals. Pending additional psychiatric research, psychiatric evaluation and intervention follow general guidelines for the learning disorders.

☐ Motor Skills Disorder (Developmental Coordination Disorder)

Developmental coordination disorder involves impaired learning and performance of motor skills (Table 23–11). Memory of motor tasks and integration of motor functions are also impaired. None of the motor impairments can be explained by fixed or localizable neurological abnormalities or mechanical interference. Although this disorder is rarely a primary complaint leading to psychiatric evaluation, it is commonly found in association with many psychiatric disorders, especially learning disorders.

About 5% of children have significant impairments of gross or fine motor functions, which are manifest in running, throwing a ball, buttoning, holding a pencil, moving with grace, or in generalized physical awkwardness.

Three main areas of motor deficits have been defined: clumsiness, adventitious movements, and dyspraxia. *Clumsiness,* which is technically defined as a slowness or awkwardness in the movement of single joints, involves disruption of the integration of agonist and antagonist muscle groups. Although clumsiness is defined in terms of effects at the basic level of single-joint movements, it may reduce the capacity to perform

---

Table 23–11.   DSM-IV diagnostic criteria for motor skills disorder (developmental coordination disorder)

A.   Performance in daily activities that require motor coordination is substantially below that expected given the person's chronological age and measured intelligence. This may be manifested by marked delays in achieving motor milestones (e.g., walking, crawling, sitting), dropping things, "clumsiness," poor performance in sports, or poor handwriting.

B.   The disturbance in criterion A significantly interferes with academic achievement or activities of daily living.

C.   The disturbance is not due to a general medical condition (e.g., cerebral palsy, hemiplegia, or muscular dystrophy) and does not meet criteria for a pervasive developmental disorder.

D.   If mental retardation is present, the motor difficulties are in excess of those usually associated with it.

Coding note: If a general medical (e.g., neurological) condition or sensory deficit is present, code the condition on Axis III.

---

more complex motor tasks, such as riding a bike or drawing. Clumsiness may be seen alone or in association with ADHD, learning disorders, or mental retardation, and sometimes is aggravated by anticonvulsants. It is easily observed in finger tapping or in picking up very small objects.

Adventitious movements may include involuntary movements that occur during voluntary movements. Overflow movements (i.e., synkinesias) may include mirror movements (which occur in symmetrically active muscles) or motions seen in unrelated muscle groups. Other adventitious movements include tics, tremor, or chorea. Clinically, adventitious movements can be observed while the child is performing specific tasks that emphasize voluntary control.

Dyspraxia, the impaired learning or performance of sequential voluntary movements (relative to age or verbal intelligence) that cannot be attributed to sensory or mechanical limitations, does not improve when specific tasks are executed without time limits or hurry. Its expression may involve a range of muscle movements, from localized to global, and may depend partially on cerebral dominance (both in spatial vs. linguistic functions and in left- vs. right-sided tasks). Dyspraxia may also be seen in mental retardation, especially fragile X syndrome. Dyspraxia may be screened clinically by asking the child to imitate some unusual hand or finger positions and by pantomiming some sequential tasks.

Common concomitants of developmental coordination disorder include ADHD, and common complications include scapegoating, impaired self-esteem, and sports avoidance.

Recommendations of treatment may seem debatable in clinical settings, especially for mild presentations. However, remediation is warranted to promote general development. It is unclear whether developmental coordination disorder, apart from identifiable neurological disorders or more focal findings, has prognostic significance in psychiatry beyond those factors related to its comorbidity (Deuel and Robinson 1987).

☐ Communication Disorders

Speech problems (regarding sound production) are seen in about 15% of the general school-age population, and language problems (involving the communicative use of speech as well as other communicative modalities) are seen in about 6%. The frequent association of communication disorders, including disorders of speech or language, with learning disorders highlights the general cerebral dysfunctions that characterize both groups of disorders. There is some evidence to suggest that language disorders may be developmental precursors of learning disorders rather than being merely comorbid disorders of independent etiology (Tallal 1988). Early language disorders in young children may not become clinically evident until the appearance of learning disorders during the school years.

About 50% of children with communication disorders have concomitant psychiatric diagnoses, and an additional 20% show an eventual appearance of learning disorders (Beitchman 1986 et al.; Cantwell and Baker 1987). Among child psychiatric patients, about 25% to 50% have communication disorders.

Research in communication disorders is moving from an emphasis on deficits in audio-perceptual processing toward a conceptualization based on language and symbolic functions. There is a close connection between sensory, perceptual, motor, and cognitive processsses in cerebral development. During the course of early development of the cerebral cortex, there is a progressive leftward lateralization of language functions, including speech (sound production), phonetic and syntactic analysis, and verbal (as well as nonverbal) sequence analysis. The right hemisphere is involved in sound recognition. Gender differences in cortical maturation may relate to girls' developmental advantage in verbal skills (which lasts until adolescence), comparable to boys' advantage in spatial processing.

Deficits in articulation (diction or speech sound production), expression (oral language production and use), and reception (comprehension) may be notable by age 2 to 3 years. Early speech and language problems frequently improve during development, and these early delays are not strongly predictive of subsequent learning disorders. However, children with early genuine speech and language problems are at high risk for later learning disorders as well as persistent communication disorders.

Most preschool children with communication disorders (70%) will be placed in special education or will repeat a grade within 10 years (Aram et al. 1984).

Hearing loss plays a significant role in the etiology of the communication disorders. Hearing is crucial in the development of speech and language, and impairments of hearing operate etiologically alongside genetic, neurological, environmental, and educational factors. Deafness is associated with clear reduction in communication skills, but more mild hearing decrements may also be developmentally significant. A mild hearing loss (25 to 40 decibels) resulting from chronic otitis media or perforation of the tympanic membrane may delay development of articulation, expressive and receptive language, reading, and spelling. During the formative period for language development, fluctuating hearing capacity can diminish verbal intelligence and academic performance in a persistent way (Howie 1980).

Early middle-ear pathology may cause language or speech symptoms, particularly if the hearing impairment is chronic. Otitis media, a common infectious disease in children, may leave a residual hearing decrement in 20% of the American population. The degree of language and speech delay may correlate to the number of otitis episodes.

Evaluation includes a medical, psychiatric, social, and developmental workup as well as language and speech assessment (Cantwell and Baker 1987). Because 20% of children have hearing deficits due to otitis media, it is helpful to test for hearing acuity, using methods such as audiometry or auditory evoked response. Parents may give a history of few startle reactions, lack of sound imitation (at 6 months) or reactiveness (at 12 months), unintelligibility (at 2.5 years), loud speech, frequent misunderstandings, speech avoidance, or communication-associated embarrassment or tension (e.g., blinking). Assessing family characteristics, as well as observing free speech between parents and child, may be useful.

Treatment of communication disorders includes educational and behavioral interventions, as well as treatment of concomitant medical, neurological, and psychiatric problems. Aggressive treatment of otitis media is particularly indicated in these children, despite the uncertainty about the relation of this disease to language and speech development. It is particularly helpful to encourage social involvement, imitation, and imaginative play as a means of increasing verbal, communicative, and symbolic exercise.

Expressive Language Disorder

In this linguistic "encoding" problem, the symbolic production and communicative use of language are impaired. The individual cannot put the idea into words and also has problems in nonverbal expression. There are similar difficulties with repeating, imitating, pointing to named objects, or acting on commands. Unlike autistic and pervasive developmental disorders, there is typically normal comprehension in verbal and nonverbal communication. In verbal languages, both semantic and syntactic errors occur so that word selection and sentence construction may be impaired; paraphrasing, narrating, and explaining are unintelligible or incoherent. The child with expressive language disorder may use developmentally earlier forms of language expression and may rely more on nonverbal communication for requests and comments. Short sentences and simple verbal structures may be employed, even with nonverbal communications such as sign language (Paul et al. 1983) (Table 23–12).

Individuals with expressive language disorder may learn language in a normal sequence, but slowly. These children can adjust their speech to talk appropriately to young children (Fey et al. 1981), suggesting some facility and flexibility in the use of their language skills. There may be associated learning disorders, phonological disorder, impulsivity, inattentiveness, or aggressivity. When frustrated, the child may have tantrums during early years, or briefly refuse to speak when older. Problems in social interactions may lead to peer problems and overdependence on family members.

Approximately 1 out of 1,000 children have a severe form of expressive language disorder, but mild forms may be 10-fold more common.

Table 23–12.   DSM-IV diagnostic criteria for expressive language disorder

A. The scores obtained from standardized individually administered measures of expressive language development are substantially below those obtained from standardized measures of both nonverbal intellectual capacity and receptive language development. The disturbance may be manifest clinically by symptoms that include having a markedly limited vocabulary, making errors in tense, or having difficulty recalling words or producing sentences with developmentally appropriate length or complexity.

B. The difficulties with expressive language interfere with academic or occupational achievement or with social communication.

C. Criteria are not met for mixed receptive-expressive language disorder or a pervasive developmental disorder.

D. If mental retardation, a speech-motor or sensory deficit, or environmental deprivation is present, the language difficulties are in excess of those usually associated with these problems.

Coding note: If a speech-motor or sensory deficit or a neurological condition is present, code the condition on Axis III.

The standard 3:1 to 4:1 male predominance of other developmental disorders is seen in this disorder.

Diverse etiologies involving neurological, genetic, environmental, and familial factors have been described. Teratogenic, perinatal, toxic, and metabolic influences are linked to certain cases. When hearing loss is present, the degree to which hearing is lost strongly correlates to the amount of language impairment (Martin 1980). Children with expressive language disorder are reported to have low cerebral blood flow to the left hemisphere (Raynaud et al. 1989).

Expressive language disorder is often associated with seemingly secondary behavioral and attentional problems. However, a high incidence of various psychiatric problems is also observed in the relatives, suggesting that concomitant psychiatric disorders may be present in children with difficulties in expressive language.

Evaluation includes psychiatric (attention and behavior problems), neurological, cognitive, and educational assessments. Intelligence is determined by a nonverbal measure of IQ. A test of hearing acuity is sensible, and workup for concomitant learning disorders is essential.

Mixed Receptive-Expressive Language Disorder

Mixed receptive-expressive language disorder is the impaired development of language comprehension that entails impairments in both decoding (i.e., comprehension) and encoding (i.e., expression). Multiple cortical deficits are usually observed, including sensory, integrative, recall, and sequencing functions (Table 23–13). Because it involves both receptive and expressive language deficits, mixed receptive-expressive language disorder is considerably more severe and socially disruptive than expressive language disorder (Cohen D et al. 1976).

In mild cases, there may be slow comprehension of complicated sentences or slow "processing" of certain linguistic forms (e.g., unusual, uncommon, or abstract words; spatial or visual language). There may also be difficulty in understanding humor and idioms, and in "reading" situational cues. In severe cases, these difficulties may extend to more simple phrases or words, reflecting slow "auditory processing." Muteness, echolalia, or neologisms may be observed. During the developmental period, the learning of expressive language skills becomes impaired by the slowness of the receptive language processing.

About 3% to 10% of school-age children have mixed receptive-expressive language disorder, but severe cases have a prevalence of 1 out of 2,000. Unlike the male predominance of expressive language disorder and the learning disorders, there is an equal gender ratio in mixed receptive/expressive language disorder.

Table 23–13.   DSM-IV diagnostic criteria for mixed receptive-expressive language disorder

---

A. The scores obtained from a battery of standardized individually administered measures of both receptive and expressive language development are substantially below those obtained from standardized measures of nonverbal intellectual capacity. Symptoms include those for expressive language disorder as well as difficulty understanding words, sentences, or specific types of words, such as spatial terms.

B. The difficulties with receptive and expressive language significantly interfere with academic or occupational achievement or with social communication.

C. Criteria are not met for a pervasive developmental disorder.

D. If mental retardation, a speech-motor or sensory deficit, or environmental deprivation is present, the language difficulties are in excess of those usually associated with these problems.

Coding note: If a speech-motor or sensory deficit or a neurological condition is present, code the condition on Axis III.

The main etiology of mixed receptive-expressive language disorder appears to be neurobiological, usually genetic factors or cortical damage. Neurological examination reveals abnormalities in about two-thirds of cases. Electroencephalographic findings include a slight increase in nondiagnostic abnormalities, especially in the language-dominant hemisphere. CT scans may show abnormalities, but these are not uniform or diagnostic. Similarly, dichotic listening may be abnormal, but without specific or lateralizing findings.

Evaluation includes assessment of nonverbal IQ, social skills, hearing acuity, articulation, receptive skills (understanding single words, word combinations, and sentences), nonverbal communication (vocalizations, gestures, and gazes), and expressive language skills. Expressive language skills can be measured by the mean length of utterances (MLU), which is compared with developmental norms. Syntactic structures should be assessed and also compared with developmental norms. There are standardized instruments to assess comprehension, with norms starting at 18 months. Concomitant medical, neurological, and psychiatric diagnoses should be considered.

For treatment of expressive and receptive language problems, special education should be maintained until symptoms improve. Once a child is "mainstreamed," supplemental academic and language supports may still be helpful. Psychiatric treatment for attention and behavior problems, and speech therapy for phonological disorder, may be needed.

Phonological Disorder

Diction problems, especially for late-acquired sounds, may be seen with normal vocabulary and grammar. This impairment in articulation and in learning sound production for speech includes substitutions, omissions, additions, and distortions (Table 23–14). Speech may be slightly or largely unintelligible, or sound like "baby talk." The understandability of speech may be further compromised by problems that are not part of phonological disorder: accent, intonation (e.g., neurologically induced), stuttering, cluttering, physical conditions (orofacial disorders such as cleft palate), neurological disease, or psychotropic medication (especially neuroleptics).

The etiology of phonological disorder is often unknown, but contributing factors may include faulty speech models within the family, mild hearing impairment, or neurocortical deficits.

In addition to evaluation of intelligence, these children should receive a full language assessment, because many have an associated disorder of grammatical (syntactic) expression.

Spontaneous recovery usually occurs by age 8, but individual or group speech therapy may help the speed and completeness of speech development. The risk of "communicative low self-esteem" is a potential complication.

Stuttering

Stuttering, the disruption of normal speech flow, is characterized by involuntary and irregular hesitations, prolongations, repetitions, or blocks on sounds, syllables, or words (Table 23–15). Unlike in cluttering and other dysfluencies in children, in stuttering anxiety produces a notice-

---

Table 23–14.   DSM-IV diagnostic criteria for phonological disorder

A. Failure to use developmentally expected speech sounds that are appropriate for age and dialect (e.g., errors in sound production, use, representation or organization such as, but not limited to, substitutions of one sound for another [use of /t/ for target /k/ sound] or omissions of sounds such as final consonants).

B. The difficulties in speech sound production interfere with academic or occupational achievement or with social communication.

C. If mental retardation, a speech-motor or sensory deficit, or environmental deprivation is present, the speech difficulties are in excess of those usually associated with these problems.

Coding note: If a speech-motor or sensory deficit or a neurological condition is present, code the condition on Axis III.

Table 23–15.   DSM-IV diagnostic criteria for stuttering

A.   Disturbance in the normal fluency and time patterning of speech (inappropriate for the individual's age), characterized by frequent occurrences of one or more of the following:

1.   Sound and syllable repetitions
2.   Sound prolongations
3.   Interjections
4.   Broken words (e.g., pauses within a word)
5.   Audible or silent blocking (filled or unfilled pauses in speech)
6.   Circumlocutions (word substitutions to avoid problematic words)
7.   Words produced with an excess of physical tension
8.   Monosyllabic whole-word repetitions (e.g., "I-I-I-I see him")

B.   The disturbance in fluency interferes with academic or occupational achievement or with social communication.

C.   If a speech-motor or sensory deficit is present, the speech difficulties are in excess of those usually associated with these problems.

Coding note: If a speech-motor or sensory deficit or a neurological condition is present, code the condition on Axis III.

---

able aggravation in speech rhythm and rate. There may be a transient worsening during periods of performance anxiety or "communicative stress" (e.g., during public speaking or a job interview). In laboratory studies, abnormalities of speech behavior and body movement are seen even during periods of apparently fluent speech.

Approximately 2% to 4% of children have this speech disorder. Spontaneous improvement occurs in 50% to 80% of cases, and 1% of adolescents and adults continue to fulfill criteria for the disorder. There is a male predominance of 3:1 to 4:1.

Etiological theories of stuttering include genetic, neurological, psychodynamic, and behavioral concepts. There may be several etiological subgroups of stuttering. A strikingly higher concordance in monozygotic than dizygotic twins suggests a large genetic etiological factor (Vandenberg et al. 1986). For 60% of persons who stutter, the disorder runs in families, appearing in about 20% to 40% of first-degree relatives (especially males). Because the prevalence is lower in females but the familial prevalence is higher in the relatives of female stutterers, a gender threshold effect on penetrance is apparent.

Certain forms of acquired stuttering are clearly neurological—for example, after stroke or secondary to degenerative brain disease. These acquired forms may be transient but can persist particularly if there is bilateral and multifocal brain disease. Several studies found that non-right-handedness (mixed or left handedness) is overrepresented in persons who stutter (and in their first- and second-degree relatives), suggesting that stuttering may be associated with anomalous cortical organization (Geschwind and Galaburda 1985).

Psychodynamic theory has focused on the role of anal-sadistic impulses, partially defended anger, and inappropriate maternal speech patterns. Behavioral theories have emphasized the role of reinforcement in maintaining dysfluencies and secondary aggravation by frustration.

Evaluation of stuttering includes a workup for possible neurological causes (cortical, basal ganglial, cerebellar). A full developmental history and general evaluation of speech, language, and hearing are needed. Behavioral assessment includes delineating possible restrictions in social interactions and activities. Referral for evaluation to a speech and language pathologist is indicated in all cases of stuttering. Children who stutter are extremely aware of their symptoms, find that anxiety worsens their dysfluency, and cannot readily improve their speech by slowing their speech rate or by focusing attention on their speech.

Speech therapy involves some elements of behavior therapy, including modifying environmental and conversational factors that trigger stuttering, relaxation, rhythm control, feedback, and dealing with accessory body movements, as well as fostering self-esteem and social assertiveness. Methods can include imitation, role-playing, practice in speaking, talking in different settings, and talking with different people.

■ MENTAL RETARDATION

Intelligence (e.g., as measured by IQ) might be considered an independent dimension that deserves its own separate DSM-IV axis. However, the diagnosis of mental retardation encompasses more than low intelligence and also includes deficits in adaptive functioning. The diagnostic concept of mental retardation as constituting low IQ plus adaptive deficits was developed by the American Association on Mental Retardation (1992) and essentially adopted as the DSM-IV alternative. This concept emphasizes that mental retardation is not an innate characteristic of an individual, but a changeable result of an interaction between personal intellectual capacities and the environment.

At least 90% of individuals with low intelligence are identified by age 18, but the diagnosis of mental retardation requires its onset during the developmental period. Further, developmental understanding is basic to the treatment of mental retardation, though psychiatric treatment of persons with mental retardation is typically provided by adult as well as child psychiatrists.

The definition of mental retardation encompasses three features: 1) subaverage intelligence (e.g., IQ of 70 or below), 2) impaired adaptive functioning, and 3) childhood onset (Table 23–16). DSM-IV subclassifies the severity of mental retardation based on IQ scores, but the American Association on Mental Retardation (1992) instead subclassifies based on the required "intensity and pattern of support systems" (i.e., intermittent, limited, extensive, and pervasive).

Intelligence is routinely measured by standardized tests, such as the Wechsler Adult Intelligence Scale (WAIS), the Wechsler Intelligence Scales for Children—Revised (WISC-R) for 6- to 16-year-olds, the Stanford-Binet IQ—Revised for 2- to 18-year-olds, or sections of the Bayley Scales of Mental Development for 2-month-olds to 2.5-year-olds. Specialized test protocols are being developed for infants. Major limitations of these standardized methods include cultural variations in question meaning and test performance, language and communication differences between individuals, the unresponsiveness of standardized tests to "creative" responses, the dangers of employing a rigid construct of intelligence that masks individual strengths, and overreliance on test findings in planning education and forming self-esteem.

Adaptive capacities may be judged by many means, including standardized instruments for assessing social maturity and adaptive skills. For example, the Vineland Adaptive Behavior Scales (Sparrow et al. 1984) constitute a multidimensional measure of adaptive behaviors in five "domains": communication, daily living skills, socialization, motor skills, and maladaptive behaviors. Data are provided by a semistructured inter-

---

Table 23–16. DSM-IV diagnostic criteria for mental retardation

A. Significantly subaverage intellectual functioning: an IQ of approximately 70 or below on an individually administered IQ test (for infants, a clinical judgment of significantly subaverage intellectual functioning).

B. Concurrent deficits or impairments in present adaptive functioning (i.e., the person's effectiveness in meeting the standards expected for his or her age by his or her cultural group) in at least two of the following areas: communication, self-care, home living, social/interpersonal skills, use of community resources, self-direction, functional academic skills, work, leisure, health, and safety.

C. The onset is before age 18 years.

Code based on degree of severity reflecting level of intellectual impairment:

317 **Mild mental retardation:** IQ level 50–55 to approximately 70

318.0 **Moderate mental retardation:** IQ level 35–40 to 50–55

318.1 **Severe mental retardation:** IQ level 20–25 to 35–40

318.2 **Profound mental retardation:** IQ level below 20 or 25

319 **Mental retardation, severity unspecified:** when there is strong presumption of mental retardation but the person's intelligence is untestable by standard tests

view of a parent or caregiver. Age-dependent expected competency scores of adaptive skills are established for children up to age 18 years with different levels of mental retardation. Adaptive competence may be above or below the level of general intelligence.

☐ Clinical Description

Developmental slowness may appear in mental retardation across all areas of functioning but is primarily evident in cognition and intellectual functioning. Neurobiological, motor, sensory, and integrative features, parent-child attachment, self-other differentiation, and subsequent emotional development are commonly affected. Other aspects of psychological development may be impaired secondarily, but there can be a remarkable degree of preservation of psychological growth. There may be wide "scatter" among various subtests of intellectual and adaptive functions, reflecting significant strengths in particular areas.

Certain clinical findings are primary cognitive and neurobiological features of mental retardation. Cognitively, there may be concreteness, egocentricity, distractibility, and short attention span. Sensory hyperreactivity may lead to "overflow" behaviors, stimulus avoidance, and the need to process stimuli at low levels of intensity. Emotional features may include difficulty in expressing feelings and in perceiving affects in self and others. Slow development of self-other differentiation may be clinically evident in affect management. The affective expressivity may be modified by physical disabilities. There may be cognitively based difficulty in "reading" facial expressions. With delays in speech and language development, limitations in communication may inhibit expression of negative affect, leading to instances of apparent affective hyperreactivity including impulsive anger and low frustration tolerance. In extreme cases, impulse dyscontrol may lead to violence and destructiveness.

The ordinary complexities of daily human interactions may test an individual's cognitive limits (Sigman 1985). Cognitive capacities may be taxed in the parallel processing of speech production, thought communication, listening, and understanding of situational context, social cues, and emotional signals. Changes in daily situation may stretch cognitive capacities and coping abilities, sometimes leading to frustration. Resistance to novelty and environmental change may be viewed as an associated finding or a developmental consequence of mental retardation. Defensive style can include rigidity or withdrawal. Primitive reactions to frustration and tension may involve aggressive, self-injurious, self-stimulatory, or habitual behaviors.

Rehabilitation may be inhibited by the individual's difficulty in recognizing the historical and interpersonal dimensions of the behavioral and affective problems, or by limitations in memory, cognitive processing, abstract thinking, sense of time, and perspective taking. Medical problems (including associated neurological or metabolic disorders, physical disabilities, and sensory deficits) often are undertreated. Receiving adequate medical care may require organizational and social skills that exceed the easy grasp of mentally retarded persons.

☐ Epidemiology

The prevalence of mental retardation in the United States has been estimated to be 1% to 3%, depending on the definition of adaptive functioning. Approximately 90% of cases are mildly retarded (IQ 55–70). There is a male predominance at all levels of mental retardation (overall, about 1.5:1 to 6:1).

Diagnostic labeling is low before age 5 years, rises sharply in the early school years, peaks in the later school years (around age 15), and then declines during adulthood toward 1%. High prevalence rates during the school years are usually attributed to the adaptive and intellectual demands of school and the high degree of supervision in classrooms. The decline of diagnostic labeling during adulthood is usually attributed to improving social and economic skills, less supervision at work, and perhaps delayed intellectual development. Typically, there is an earlier age of diagnosis for more severe levels of mental retardation.

Socioeconomic class is a crucial variable. Severe and profound mental retardation are distributed uniformly across all socioeconomic classes, but mild mental retardation is more common in low socioeconomic classes.

☐ Etiology

The etiology is partially dependent on the level of mental retardation. Mild retardation is generally idiopathic and familial, but severe and profound retardation are typically genetic or related to brain damage.

The most common form, idiopathic mental retardation "associated with sociocultural or psychosocial disadvantage," is typically seen in the offspring of retarded parents ("familial"). Degree of retardation is generally mild (or moderate). Intellectual and adaptive deficits are presumed to be determined by a "polygenic" mechanism, though, currently, emphasis is placed on the intervening social factors. These individuals live in low socioeconomic circumstances, and their functioning is influenced by poverty, disease, deficiencies in health care, and impaired help seeking. Family size may exceed parental capacities for attention and positive stimulation of the children. Social disadvantage contributes heavily to the etiology of some forms of mild mental retardation. Nonetheless, the overrepresentation of various genetic, physical, and neurological abnormalities in persons with mild mental retardation is a reminder that social forces may not be the predominant etiological factors.

Moderate and severe forms of mental retardation are less likely to be idiopathic. Known biomedical etiologies may be identified in 25% of all cases of mental retardation, and in 60% to 80% of severe or profound mental retardation. These moderate and severe cases are usually first diagnosed in infancy or early childhood, and 90% have prenatal causes. Major mechanisms include genetic and neurodevelopmental damage. When biological causes are identifiable, the disabilities, physical limitations, and dependency are more severe. There are more than 200 recognized biological syndromes involving mental retardation (Grossman 1983), entailing disruptions in virtually any sector of brain biochemical or physiological functioning.

Chromosomal factors can be identified in 10% of institutionalized individuals with mental retardation. Apart from polygenetic inheritance, the major chromosomal mechanisms include dominantly inherited single-gene defects, recessively inherited inborn errors of metabolism, recessive chromosomal aberrations, and early developmental (i.e., embryonic) gene alterations. Trisomy 21 (Down's syndrome) is the most common and well described. Patients with trisomy 21 have neurochemical pathology including major loss of acetylcholine (nucleus basalis) and somatostatin (cerebral cortex) neurons, as well as loss in serotonin and norepinephrine pathways. Patients with Down's syndrome show progressive neuropathological changes similar to those in Alzheimer's disease, including neurofibrillary tangles and neuritic plaques, which are seen in 100% of individuals with Down's syndrome who survive beyond age 30. Chromosome 21 contains the gene for β-amyloid, the brain protein that accumulates in the neuritic plaques of patients with Down's syndrome or Alzheimer's disease. Cerebral glucose metabolism may decrease with age (Bregman and Hodapp 1991).

Fragile X syndrome is the second most common genetic cause (occurring in 1 in 1,000 males) of moderate and severe mental retardation (Bregman et al. 1987). About 80% of males with fragile X syndrome have mild to severe mental retardation, which accounts for 40% of the male predominance in cases of moderate and severe mental retardation. Affected males have large testes in 25% of cases before puberty and in 85% percent after puberty. Macroorchidism is an unusual symptom in medicine, and its high frequency in this syndrome makes it useful as a screening question. Most symptomatic males have an elongated dysmorphic face (large jaw, forehead, and ears), large head circumference, mitral valve prolapse (80%), hyperextensible joints, and a highly arched palate. Behavioral abnormalities, including hyperactivity, violence, stereotypies, resistance to environmental changes, and self-mutilatory behaviors, are present in 80% of males. Language and speech deficits include immature syntax, poor abstraction, expressive and receptive language deficits, and articulation problems. Frontal lobe symptoms may include perseverative language and behavior, attention deficits, and impaired shifting between mental sets (Mazzocco et al. 1992).

In females (who are partially protected by having two X chromosomes), a "carrier" state may be asymptomatic or associated with learning disorders or mild mental retardation. The proposed gene abnormality involves a nucleotide sequence (cytosine-guanine-guanine) that is redundantly repeated to variable degrees and becomes quite lengthy in patients with fragile X syndrome (Verkerk et al. 1991).

□ Course and Prognosis

Although biological factors of each mental retardation syndrome in each individual may determine certain aspects of development, the course and outcome of mental retardation depend largely on social, economic, health/medical, educational, and developmental circumstances. Whether the mental retardation is a mild familial form or the result of a severe inborn metabolic error, its course is influenced by interactions with environmental opportunities and barriers. Parental characteristics may entail advantages that may be compensatory, or disadvantages that may be compounding. Features of the microenvironment operate as intervening factors and may have a stronger influence on adult outcome than do causative factors, except in extreme cases. The course and prognosis of mental retardation are much less predictable than originally believed.

Neurodevelopmental evaluation during the first year can predict intellectual outcome and neurological status in later childhood in nearly 90% of premature children (Largo et al. 1990). Premature infants with intracranial hemorrhage (demonstrated on ultrasound) are especially likely to demonstrate impaired cognitive and motor abilities later, especially if there are persistent signs of periventricular abnormalities (Williams et al. 1987).

Data on the course of mental retardation reflect varying degrees of aggressivity in rehabilitative efforts. The prognosis in mental retardation may be expected to improve as therapeutic interventions become publicly available. About two-thirds of mentally retarded individuals shed their diagnoses in adulthood as adaptive skills increase (Grossman 1983). Typically, the global level of adaptive functioning changes over the course of months or years in response to changes in economic and social supports, living arrangements, work opportunities, and parental support. Generally, adaptive behavior improves over the course of a lifetime.

Complications of mental retardation are numerous. In the care structure, a lack of aggressivity in medical care and a lack of continuity of rehabilitative care hinder basic medical treatment. Common psychological complications include frequent experiencing of failure, low self-esteem, frustration in fulfillment of dependency needs and wishes for love, wavering parental support, regressive wishes for institutionalization, anticipation of failure, defensive rigidity, and excessive caution. Additional psychosocial complications are impaired communicational interactions, inappropriate social assertiveness, and vulnerability to being exploited.

A major part of the care of mentally retarded individuals includes prevention and management of the numerous medical, psychological, and family complications. Another major function is the monitoring of overall speed of progress: a lack of developmental improvement raises the possibility of concomitant psychiatric diagnoses.

☐ Evaluation

It cannot be overemphasized that all psychiatric diagnoses may co-occur with, and that all personality types may occur in, mental retardation. Approximately one-third to one-half of patients with mental retardation have ADHD. They may also have unipolar and bipolar mood disorders, anxiety disorders, psychotic reactions, autistic disorder, and learning disorders (Menolascino et al. 1986).

Medical evaluation should include physical examination (seeking physical stigmata) and laboratory tests, including chromosome analysis, amino and organic acids studies, thyroid function, lead testing, and a mucopolysaccharide screen. Roentgenograms (X rays) of long bones and wrists should be obtained. Neurological evaluation, including EEG and CT scan, should be conducted to examine for possible treatable causes of mental retardation, seizure disorders, and possibly deafness and blindness. Head and face size and symmetries, head shape (including hair patterns), eye and ear position, and asymmetries of motor and sensory function should be checked. A history of maternal miscarriage, toxic exposure or infections, and fetal size and activity should be elicited. Psychological testing, including neuropsychological evaluation, is commonly required. Social adaptive skills of the individual should be measured (using, e.g., the Vineland scales) to target areas of remediation and strength.

☐ Treatment

For treatment of the multiple handicaps and complications commonly associated with mental retardation, multimodal treatment with a developmental orientation is typical (Sigman 1985; Szymanski and Tanguay 1980). Long-term rehabilitative programs involve many specialists and agencies working collaboratively over time and across agency boundaries. The specifically psychiatric component of treatment includes the coordination of primary diagnostic evaluation of medical and psychiatric conditions and parent guidance, as well as the usual variety of psychiatric therapies when specific concomitant psychiatric disorders are diagnosed (Szymanski and Tanguay 1980).

Although treatments based on abstract thinking may not be helpful, developmentally oriented psychotherapeutic interventions may be effective for crisis management or long-term psychosocial goals. For certain adolescent or adult patients with mild mental retardation, verbal psychotherapy may be used to promote self-other differentiation, self-esteem, identity formation, interpersonal development, emotional and behavioral control, management of power, and promotion of the expression of love and sexuality. Technical modifications include the use of briefer and clearer verbalizations, focus on current events and feelings, reinforcement of reality-fantasy differentiations, management of projections, teaching about the nature of emotional life, and free use of positive reinforcement. Brief frequent sessions may be more useful than standard formats. For children, play therapy may be used.

Behavior modification is useful for treatment of aggression, defiance, overactivity, asocial behavior, self-injury, stereotypies, and pica; in some cases, toilet training, dressing and grooming, and eating skills may be taught. Educational and developmental training to enhance speech and language, motor, cognitive, and occupational skills, as well as social, recreational, sexual, and adaptive skills, is commonly provided by specialized professionals. The individual may be trained to initiate task simplifications, request communicational clarifications, and perform environmental improvements. Parent counseling and education, as well as family support, are standard.

■ PERVASIVE DEVELOPMENTAL DISORDERS

The pervasive developmental disorders are a neurobiologically diverse group of conditions characterized by deficits across many areas of functioning that lead to a pervasive disruption of developmental processes. These multiply-handicapped individuals typically show a developmental process that is not merely slow or limited, but is "atypical" or "deviant." Many of these individuals are also mentally retarded, and their treatment requires multimodal developmentally oriented long-term rehabilitation.

The DSM-IV recognizes several pervasive developmental disorders that differ in symptoms, symptom severity, and pattern of onset. *Autistic disorder* involves an early onset of impairments in social interaction, communication deficits, and restricted activities and interests. *Childhood disintegrative disorder* entails largely similar symptoms, but the symptoms follow at least 2 years of seemingly normal development; the child then loses early developmental gains and reaches a stable level of autistic-like functioning. *Rett's disorder*, an early-onset progressive neurodegenerative disorder of females, is associated with mental retardation, generalized growth retardation, and multiple neurological symptoms. This disorder appears similar to autistic disorder for a limited period during early childhood. *Asperger's disorder* is similar to "high functioning" autistic disorder, in which there is a relative preservation of language skills and intellect.

☐ Autistic Disorder

This early-onset pervasive developmental disorder entails disabilities in virtually all psychological and behavioral sectors. Most individuals with autistic disorder do not have the massively severe developmental impairments seen in classically described cases.

Clinical Description

The DSM-IV definition of autistic disorder puts particular emphasis on the impairments in social interaction and reciprocity, the difficulties with verbal and nonverbal communication (and related capacities such as symbolization), and the stereotyped pattern of behaviors and interests (Table 23–17).

Autistic disorder presents in a wide spectrum of severities. The classical form of "early infantile autism" described by Kanner (1943) was a severe infancy-onset disorder with profoundly disturbed social relations, communication disruption, motor abnormalities, affective atypicality, massive cognitive impairments, multiple behavioral oddities, distorted perception, and bizarre thoughts. However, despite the significant "disorganization" and disrupted integration of functions, autistic disorder is not associated with delusions, hallucinations, or loose associations in the manner of adult psychotic disorders. There are relatively mild forms of autistic disorder in which the social, communicative, and behavioral abnormalities may be so subtle that they merge into the range of character pathology.

Children or adults with autistic disorder show low social interactiveness, a seeming indifference to human warmth, little imitation or sharing, and rare smiling. Socially, these individuals appear passive and aloof, initially avoiding social contacts, but can come to enjoy and seek interpersonal experiences. Autistic children may have difficulty in comprehending verbal and nonverbal language. They often show persistent deficits in appreciating the feelings of other people and understanding the process and nuances of social communications. Communicative speech and gesturing are limited and may be difficult to understand

Table 23–17. DSM-IV diagnostic criteria for autistic disorder

A. A total of six (or more) items from (1), (2), and (3), with at least two from (1), and one each from (2) and (3):

1. Qualitative impairment in social interaction, as manifested by at least two of the following:

   a. Marked impairment in the use of multiple nonverbal behaviors such as eye-to-eye gaze, facial expression, body postures, and gestures to regulate social interaction

   b. Failure to develop peer relationships appropriate to developmental level

   c. A lack of spontaneous seeking to share enjoyment, interests, or achievements with other people (e.g., by a lack of showing, bringing, or pointing out objects of interest)

   d. Lack of social or emotional reciprocity

2. Qualitative impairments in communication as manifested by at least one of the following:

   a. Delay in, or total lack of, the development of spoken language (not accompanied by an attempt to compensate through alternative modes of communication such as gesture or mime)

   b. In individuals with adequate speech, marked impairment in the ability to initiate or sustain a conversation with others

   c. Stereotyped and repetitive use of language or idiosyncratic language

   d. Lack of varied spontaneous make-believe play or social imitative play appropriate to developmental level

3. Restricted repetitive and stereotyped patterns of behavior, interests, and activities, as manifested by at least one of the following:

   a. Encompassing preoccupation with one or more stereotyped and restricted patterns of interest that is abnormal either in intensity or in focus

   b. Apparently inflexible adherence to specific, nonfunctional routines or rituals

   c. Stereotyped and repetitive motor mannerisms (e.g., hand or finger flapping or twisting, or complex whole-body movements)

   d. Persistent preoccupation with parts of objects

B. Delays or abnormal functioning in at least one of the following areas, with onset prior to age 3 years:

   1) social interaction,

   2) language as used in social communication, or

   3) symbolic or imaginative play.

C. The disturbance is not better accounted for by Rett's disorder or childhood disintegrative disorder.

because of echolalia, pronoun reversals, and idiosyncratic meanings. Speech is typically late and unusual, and sometimes fails to develop. Phonological (i.e., sound production) and syntactic (i.e., grammar) functions may be relatively spared, with more significant impairments of semantics (i.e., sociocultural meanings) and pragmatics (i.e., rules of interpersonal exchange), and aspects of communication. Imaginative and symbolic functions may be deeply affected. Rituals, stereotypies, self-stimulation, self-mutilation, and unusual mannerisms are common. There is often an obsessive attachment to certain people or objects and a lack of ordinary spontaneity. Affective responses may be "shallow," overly responsive to small changes, oblivious to large changes in the environment, and unpredictably labile and odd. Cognitive deficits include impairments in abstraction, sequencing, and integration. There may be distorted perception for smell, taste, or touch, and underdevelopment of visual and auditory processing.

The majority of individuals with autistic disorder show subnormal intelligence, but a few show large "increases" in measured IQ during the course of treatment or development. There are often dramatic inconsistencies, with extraordinary "scatter" of capabilities between different subtests and over time. Unusual or special capacities ("savant" skills) may be present in particular areas such as music, drawing, arithmetic, or calendar calculation.

Epidemiology

The available prevalence estimates for autistic disorder are based on criteria that emphasize the more severe forms of this disorder. When these criteria are used, prevalence is estimated at approximately 30 to 50 per 100,000. The less severe forms are more common. There is a male predominance of approximately 3:1 to 4:1, but females may have more severe symptoms.

Etiology

Genetic and biological factors appear to predominate in autistic disorder (Folstein and Piven 1991). Neuropathological studies suggest that neurodevelopmental changes begin early in gestation, probably in the second trimester (Bauman 1991). The higher concordance in monozygotic than dizygotic twins (36% vs. 0%) suggests a genetic factor. Siblings of autistic children show a prevalence of autistic disorder of 2% (50 times over the expected prevalence). About 5% to 25% of siblings have delays in learning (usually language or speech disorder), mental retardation, or physical defects. In family studies, there are suggestions of autosomal recessive inheritance for certain cases of autistic disorder.

A specific medical cause may be identified in some individuals. There is an elevated incidence of early developmental problems, such as postnatal neurological infections, congenital rubella, and phenylketonuria. The role of perinatal asphyxia appears to be minor. About 2% to 5% of autistic individuals appear to have fragile X syndrome. Seizure disorders appear in 15% to 50% of autistic persons by age 20. Both major motor and partial complex seizures may be diagnosed.

Neuropsychological testing shows various positive findings. Low IQ is associated with a higher incidence of seizures, social impairment, self-mutilatory and bizarre behavior, and a poorer prognosis. The increase in seizure disorders during adolescence is particularly seen in those autistic individuals with low IQ. There is delayed development of cerebral dominance and an excess of non–right-handedness, primitive neurological reflexes, soft neurological signs, and physical anomalies. There is a single report indicating an 80% positivity on the dexamethasone suppression test.

Course and Prognosis

Autistic disorder is often apparent at birth or early infancy, and parents may seek a medical opinion during the child's first year (often for deafness). The DSM-IV definition requires an apparent onset of autistic disorder before age 3 years.

Predictors of good adaptive outcome for individuals with autistic disorder include higher IQ, more language skills (especially vocabulary), and greater social and communicative skills. Later onset also predicts better outcome. The general course of autistic disorder is one of gradual improvement, but there is a high degree of irregularity in the speed of improvement. Periods of rapid developmental growth alternate with periods of slow stable growth, with changes in maturational tempo occurring unpredictably. Episodes of overt regression may occur during intercurrent medical illness, during conditions of environmental stress, and especially at puberty, as well as during periods of rapid developmental progress that is unexplained by environmental factors. The availability of educational and supportive services has a marked beneficial impact. Developmental progress may be made in particular skills without improvement in other areas of functioning, or may occur pervasively across many areas of functioning.

As adults, autistic individuals continue to show a gradual clearing of symptoms but retain clinical evidence of residual organic brain damage (Rumsey et al. 1985b). Depending on the severity of the autistic disorder, perhaps 2% to 15% achieve a nonretarded level of cognitive and adaptive functioning. "Obsessive-compulsive" features remain predominant in adulthood, including stereotyped pacing, rocking, perseveration, and stuttering. Adults with autistic disorder remain socially aloof and often retain an oppositional streak.

Evaluation

In addition to standard psychiatric and behavioral evaluation, a workup of autistic disorder includes assessment of language skills, cognition, social skills, and adaptive functioning. Neurological examination would include consideration of possible inborn metabolic and degenerative diseases. Screening for phenylketonuria is probably cost-effective. MRI studies cannot be considered useful at this time for diagnosing autistic disorder, but can be helpful in some cases as a part of the neurological workup. An EEG for possible seizure disorder and a chromosome analysis (regarding fragile X syndrome) are advisable. In certain cases, audiological examination for possible deafness, and other examinations for other sensory deficits, may be considered. Psychological testing for mental retardation, juvenile psychotic disorders, and mixed receptive/expressive language disorder may be helpful. Evaluation for communication disorders may be particularly difficult if the child's nonverbal skills are also impaired. An assessment of the home environment and emotional supportiveness of the family may be valuable in certain cases. There are standardized evaluation checklists based on clinical observation and parental recall of early behavior (Parks 1983).

Treatment

Behavior therapy may be helpful for controlling unwanted symptoms, promoting social interactions, increasing self-reliance, and facilitating exploration. Special education, vocational training, teaching of adaptive skills, and support in managing major life events are basic. Environmental management, especially predictable or programmed structure, is powerfully helpful.

Psychotropic medications may be used for treatment of comorbid psychiatric disorders, management of seizures, or control of disruptive symptoms. Low doses of nonsedating neuroleptics may be helpful for promoting learning, controlling behavioral symptoms, reducing excessive activity levels, and enhancing the effect of behavior therapy. Symptoms of impulsivity or slowness in behavior or cognition may be treated with neuroleptics or psychostimulants. Psychostimulant medication may be helpful for children who are underactive or who have concurrent ADHD. Anticonvulsant medication may be useful in many of these patients, who often have clinical (15% to 50%) or subclinical seizures. Beta-blocking agents and clonidine may also be helpful for managing symptoms of impulsivity and aggression. Naltrexone, an opiate receptor blocking agent, may be helpful for improving affective availability, promoting social reciprocity, and reducing stereotyped motor and self-injurious behaviors (Campbell et al. 1990). Several preliminary reports suggest that fluoxetine can be helpful in treating obsessional and depressive symptoms in patients with autistic disorder.

Providing guidance to parents is critical when giving them support, because they sometimes make the chronically afflicted child into the emotional center of their lives. Although this attentiveness may have some beneficial effects for the child, it is often driven by unjustified guilt, unrealistic pessimism, or narcissism. Parents can contribute to the child's learning of self-care and adaptive skills, arrange for special education and management with schools and other public agencies, and make long-term plans for the child's future.

☐ Childhood Disintegrative Disorder

Childhood disintegrative disorder differs from autistic disorder in time of onset, clinical course, and prevalence. In contrast to autistic disorder, there is an early period of normal development until age 3 to 4 years. This is followed by a period of very marked deterioration of formerly gained capacities (Table 23–18). Childhood disintegrative disorder may begin with behavioral symptoms, such as anxiety, anger, or outbursts, but the general loss of functions becomes extremely pervasive and severe. Over time, the deterioration remains stable, although some capacities may be regained to a very limited degree. About 20% will regain the ability to speak in sentences, but even their communication skills will be impaired (Hill and Rosenbloom 1986). Most adults are completely dependent and require institutional care, and some have a shortened life span.

Childhood disintegrative disorder appears to be less prevalent than autistic disorder, with estimates ranging from 1 to 4 in 100,000. There appears to be a male predominance of greater than 4:1.

The evaluation and treatment of childhood disintegrative disorder are essentially comparable to the approach to autistic disorder, although much more active support, behavioral treatment, neurological care, and medical monitoring are needed.

☐ Rett's Disorder

Rett's disorder is a progressive neurological disorder of girls that resembles autistic disorder, but only for a period of several years during childhood. The disorder unfolds in stages: brief normalcy, a loss of functions, a plateau, and then serious motor decline (Hagberg and Witt-Engerstrom 1986) (Table 23–19). The estimated prevalence of Rett's disorder is 5 to 15 in 100,000 girls. The documented cases have all have been girls, but it is still possible that Rett's disorder may be found in some boys.

Table 23–18.   DSM-IV diagnostic criteria for childhood disintegrative disorder

A.   Apparently normal development for at least the first 2 years after birth as manifested by the presence of age-appropriate verbal and nonverbal communication, social relationships, play, and adaptive behavior.

B.   Clinically significant loss of previously acquired skills (before age 10 years) in at least two of the following areas:

    1.   Expressive or receptive language

    2.   Social skills or adaptive behavior

    3.   Bowel or bladder control

    4.   Play

    5.   Motor skills

C.   Abnormalities of functioning in at least two of the following areas:

    1.   Qualitative impairment in social interaction (e.g., impairment in non-verbal behaviors, failure to develop peer relationships, lack of social or emotional reciprocity)

    2.   Qualitative impairments in communication (e.g., delay or lack of spoken language, inability to initiate or sustain a conversation, stereotyped and repetitive use of language, lack of varied make-believe play)

    3.   Restricted, repetitive, and stereotyped patterns of behavior, interests, and activities, including motor stereotypies and mannerisms

D.   The disturbance is not better accounted for by another specific pervasive developmental disorder or by schizophrenia.

Table 23–19.   DSM-IV diagnostic criteria for Rett's disorder

A.   All of the following:

    1.   Apparently normal prenatal and perinatal development

    2.   Apparently normal psychomotor development through the first 5 months after birth

    3.   Normal head circumference at birth

B.   Onset of all of the following after the period of normal development:

    1.   Deceleration of head growth between ages 5 and 48 months

    2.   Loss of previously acquired purposeful hand skills between ages 5 and 30 months with the subsequent development of stereotyped hand movements (e.g., hand wringing or hand washing)

    3.   Loss of social engagement early in the course (although often social interaction develops later)

    4.   Appearance of poorly coordinated gait or trunk movements

    5.   Severely impaired expressive and receptive language development with severe psychomotor retardation

Etiological factors remain unclear. A strong genetic component is suggested by the finding of 100% concordance for Rett's disorder in eight monozygotic twins and 0% in six dizygotic twins (Hagberg 1989). Data are suggestive of a dominant X-linked inheritance, with early death of the males in spontaneous abortion.

☐ Asperger's Disorder

Asperger's disorder represents a subclass of the pervasive developmental disorders that is similar to autistic disorder except that there is a partial preservation of language skills and cognition (Table 23–20). There also tends to be a relative sparing of intelligence and a lower prevalence of

---

Table 23–20.   DSM-IV diagnostic criteria for Asperger's disorder

A. Qualitative impairment in social interaction, as manifested by at least two of the following:
   1. Marked impairment in the use of multiple nonverbal behaviors such as eye-to-eye gaze, facial expression, body postures, and gestures to regulate social interaction
   2. Failure to develop peer relationships appropriate to developmental level
   3. A lack of spontaneous seeking to share enjoyment, interests, or achievements with other people (e.g., by a lack of showing, bringing, or pointing out objects of interest to other people)
   4. Lack of social or emotional reciprocity
B. Restricted repetitive and stereotyped patterns of behavior, interests, and activities, as manifested by at least one of the following:
   1. Encompassing preoccupation with one or more stereotyped and restricted patterns of interest that is abnormal either in intensity or in focus
   2. Apparently inflexible adherence to specific, nonfunctional routines or rituals
   3. Stereotyped and repetitive motor mannerisms (e.g., hand or finger flapping or twisting, or complex whole-body movements)
   4. Persistent preoccupation with parts of objects
C. The disturbance causes clinically significant impairment in social, occupational, or other important areas of functioning.
D. There is no clinically significant general delay in language (e.g., single words used by age 2 years, communicative phrases used by age 3 years).
E. There is no clinically significant delay in cognitive development or in the development of age-appropriate self-help skills, adaptive behavior (other than in social interaction), and curiosity about the environment in childhood.
F. Criteria are not met for another specific pervasive developmental disorder or schizophrenia.

---

mental retardation in Asperger's disorder. On the other hand, persons with Asperger's disorder often misread nonverbal cues, have marked difficulties with peer interactions (especially in groups), focus repetitively on topics of interest to themselves in conversation, appear not particularly empathic, speak without normal inflection and tone variation, may be relatively unexpressive affectively, and tend to have few friends (Wing 1981). Even so, persons with Asperger's disorder are often quite sociable and talkative, and may form affectionate bonds with family members (Frith 1991).

Epidemiological data are limited, but the prevalence of Asperger's disorder is estimated at 5 to 15 in 100,000. The male predominance is 3:1 to 4:1. Onset is typically later than in autistic disorder. The course tends to be stable over time, often with some gradual gains (Szatmari et al. 1989).

The etiology of Asperger's disorder is unclear. There is an overrepresentation of this disorder in families. About 30% of patients have abnormal EEGs, and 15% show some evidence of brain atrophy (Gillberg 1989). Treatment includes social and motor skills training, remedial educational interventions when indicated, and vocational training.

■ TIC DISORDERS

Tic disorders are stereotyped abnormalities of semi-involuntary movement presumably relating to dysfunction in the basal ganglia, which are situated at a midway position among higher and lower centers within the brain. Symptoms of these disorders are subject to moment-to-moment influences from environmental and internal stimuli, and thus permit study of interacting biopsychosocial influences (Chase et al. 1992; Kurlan 1993).

Although tics are experienced as involuntary (Table 23–21), patients may consciously (though only temporarily) suppress tic movements, in contrast to choreiform (i.e., disruptions of normal synergistic movement by coordinated muscle groups) and athetoid (i.e., slow writhing) movements. Tics are distinct from dyskinesias (i.e., disruptions of voluntary and involuntary motions), dystonias (i.e., abnormal muscle tone), and other neurological movement disorders. Instead, tics are brief and repetitive, but not rhythmic, motor (muscular) or vocal (phonic) responses that are purposeless but may resemble purposeful acts. They involve recurrent movements of the same muscle groups, but their location can change gradually over time. Their form may be simple (motor: jerking movements, shrugging, eye blinking; vocal: grunting, sniffing, throat clearing) or complex (motor: grimacing, bending, banging; vocal: echolalia, odd inflections and accents).

Table 23–21.   DSM-IV diagnostic criteria for tic disorders

Transient tic disorder

A.   Single or multiple motor and/or vocal tics (i.e., sudden, rapid, recurrent, nonrhythmic, stereotyped motor movements or vocalizations).

B.   The tics occur many times a day nearly every day for at least 4 weeks, but for no longer than 12 consecutive months.

C.   The disturbance causes marked distress or significant impairment in social, occupational, or other important areas of functioning.

D.   The disturbance is not due to the direct physiological effects of a substance (e.g., stimulants) or a general medical condition (e.g., Huntington's disease or postviral encephalitis).

E.   The onset is before age 18 years.

F.   Criteria have never been met for Tourette's disorder or chronic motor or vocal tic disorder.

Specify if:

Single episode or **recurrent**

Chronic motor or vocal tic disorder

A.   Single or multiple motor or vocal tics (i.e., sudden, rapid, recurrent, nonrhythmic, stereotyped motor movements or vocalizations), but not both, have been present at some time during the illness.

B.   The tics occur many times a day nearly every day or intermittently throughout a period of more than 1 year, and during this period there was never a tic-free period of more than 3 consecutive months.

C.   The disturbance causes marked distress or significant impairment in social, occupational, or other important areas of functioning.

D.   The onset is before age 18 years.

E.   The disturbance is not due to the direct physiological effects of a substance (e.g., stimulants) or a general medical condition (e.g., Huntington's disease or postviral encephalitis).

F.   Criteria have never been met for Tourette's disorder.

Tourette's disorder

A.   Both multiple motor and one or more vocal tics have been present at some time during the illness, although not necessarily concurrently. (A *tic* is a sudden, rapid, recurrent, nonrhythmic, stereotyped motor movement or vocalization.)

B.   The tics occur many times a day (usually in bouts) nearly every day or intermittently throughout a period of more than 1 year, and during this period there was never a tic-free period of more than 3 consecutive months.

C.   The disturbance causes marked distress or significant impairment in social, occupational, or other important areas of functioning.

D.   The onset is before age 18 years.

(continued)

Table 23–21.   DSM-IV diagnostic criteria for tic disorders *(continued)*

E.   The disturbance is not due to the direct physiological effects of a substance (e.g., stimulants) or a general medical condition (e.g., Huntington's disease or postviral encephalitis).

Tic disorder not otherwise specified

This category is for disorders characterized by tics that do not meet criteria for a specific tic disorder. Examples include tics lasting less than 4 weeks or tics with an onset after age 18 years.

Tic disorders are subtyped into transient tic, chronic tic, and Tourette's disorders. These conditions appear closely related in descriptive, genetic, and developmental characteristics. They vary in intensity over time, usually increasing during psychosocial stress, intrapsychic conflict, and positive or negative emotional excitement. Psychosocial stress may be particularly symptom-inducing at the start of the school year, at times of parental separation and divorce, and during physical fatigue. Tics typically decrease in frequency and severity during focused mental activity, concentration, or sudden alerting but may not fully disappear during sleep.

☐ Tourette's Disorder

Tourette's disorder is a lifelong disease entailing vocal and multiple motor tics. If *both* motor and vocal tics are present for up to 1 year, transient tic disorder is diagnosed; beyond 1 year, the diagnosis is Tourette's disorder.

Clinical Description

Motor and vocal tics, both simple and complex, are observable. The behavioral component can be suppressed voluntarily, but then a subjective sense of tension (i.e., premonitory sensory urge) builds. This pre-tic "craving" is relieved temporarily when patients allow themselves to express their tics in action. Many patients experience their tics as a voluntary response to these premonitory urges and may feel more troubled by the continual pre-tic tension than by the tics themselves (Leckman et al. 1993).

Tourette's disorder involves a typical pattern of waxing and waning over time. Severity varies widely. Mild cases may go undiagnosed even in public speakers, and severe cases may be disabling and socially disfiguring. As in other tic disorders, anxiety and excitement lead to increased symptoms, while relaxation and focused attention reduce symptoms, and symptoms are absent during sleep. Increased symptom severity may be evident for several minutes during stressful situations, may last for months during periods of developmental anxiety and stress, or may last for years.

Clinical presentation may change during the course of development. Onset is usually between ages 2 and 13 years. Symptoms begin as a single tic in 50% of patients. At age 7 years (average age at onset), motor tics are initially evident, with a rostrocaudal progression over time (i.e., head before trunk and limbs). At age 11 years (on average), phonic and vocal tics may appear, followed by obsessive-compulsive behaviors. Vocal tics may start as a single syllable, and then progress to longer exclamations, and occasionally to complex gestures. Classical coprolalia is observed in 60% of patients with Tourette's disorder, with an initial appearance typically in early adolescence. Copropraxia (i.e., complex obscene gestures) may appear later, as copralalia resolves. Complex motor tics may appear to be purposeless, or they may be camouflaged by being blended into other purposeful movements. Obsessive-compulsive symptoms usually begin about 5 to 10 years after the first appearance of simple tics (Bruun 1988).

Neurological soft signs (50%) and choreiform movements (30%) are common. Approximately 50% of these patients show abnormal findings on the EEG, particularly immature patterns (excess slow waves and posterior sharp waves). CT scans are usually normal. Disordered sleep and enuresis may be overrepresented. Increased aggressive (Stefl 1983) or sexual (Jagger et al. 1982) behavior may each be seen in about one-third of patients with Tourette's disorder.

Epidemiology

The general prevalence of tic disorders is currently estimated at 1% to 2% but is probably higher in children and adolescents; up to 12% of children may have tic symptoms. Prevalence estimates for Tourette's disorder itself are about 1 in 1,500. There is a male predominance of 3:1 (perhaps up to as high as 10:1).

Etiology

Genetic, biological, and psychosocial factors appear operative in Tourette's disorder. Tics are noted in two-thirds of relatives of Tourette's disorder patients. Family studies of tic disorders and OCD show that both groups are associated with a similar prevalence of tics and compulsive behaviors in family members. A higher concordance of Tourette's disorder in monozygotic than dizygotic twins suggests an inheritable component. Genetic studies show a link between Tourette's disorder, chronic tics, and OCD. There may also be a link between Tourette's disorder and ADHD. The familial predisposition to tic disorders and OCD appears to be governed by a single gene with autosomal dominant transmission (Pauls and Leckman 1986).

Tourette's disorder is more common in boys, but there is a higher prevalence of chronic tic and Tourette's disorders in the relatives of Tourette's girls than Tourette's boys. When all forms of the disorder are considered, the penetrance for males is 100%, and for females, 71%. Within affected families, males are more likely to have tic disorders, and females are more likely to have OCD (Pauls and Leckman 1986).

A leading hypothesis suggests that Tourette's disorder is associated with a supersensitivity of postsynaptic dopaminergic D_2 receptors in the basal ganglia, but abnormalities of serotonin, dynorphin, gamma-aminobutyric acid (GABA), acetylcholine, and norepinephrine have also been described.

Course and Prognosis

The onset of illness is typically during childhood (ages 2 to 13 years); rarely does the disorder have a postpubertal onset. This lifelong disease shows a characteristic waxing and waning in frequency and severity, corresponding only in part to periods of increased stress or anxiety. Presentation varies during development (see clinical description). Maximal tic symptoms may be seen in the early adolescent years, although obsessive-compulsive symptoms may then become more prominent and troubling.

Complications of Tourette's disorder generally include major effects on self-esteem and social performance. Teasing, shame, self-consciousness, and social ostracism are standard features of these patients' lives. These individuals show a reluctance to involve themselves in socially demanding situations. Particularly if the symptoms are severely socially disfiguring, these patients may avoid entering intimate relationships, marriage, and other interpersonally gratifying activities. There is also a high rate of unemployment, reportedly as high as 50%, in adults with Tourette's disorder

Evaluation

A complete psychiatric evaluation of the child and parents is indicated, including assessment of possible ADHD, conduct disorder, OCD, learning disorders, pervasive developmental disorders, and mental retardation. Neurological examination is appropriate to rule out other movement disorders, including Wilson's disease. An assessment of baseline dyskinesias is needed prior to the start of neuroleptic drug treatments. An EEG is helpful in ruling out myoclonic seizures and other neurological disorders. School reports, including those addressing academic performance, general behavior, severity of tics, and social skills,

are useful. The child's self-consciousness, management of teasing and social ostracism, and assertiveness may be assessed. The possibility of concurrent mood or anxiety disorder should be evaluated. Evaluation of tic
disorders in relatives may be considered.

Treatment

Pharmacotherapy, behavior therapy, and sometimes psychotherapy and
special education may be employed. Approximately 60% to 80% of Tourette's patients improve on neuroleptic drugs. Haloperidol is typically
used in low doses for treatment of Tourette's disorder, but is probably no
more effective than other neuroleptic agents. Dosage may require gradual elevation over time, but decreases in dosage may be possible depending on life circumstances. Pimozide, a neuroleptic with side effects
similar to those of haloperidol but less cognitively blunting, might also be
useful.

　　An alternative treatment is clonidine, which appears to be helpful in
about 50% of Tourette's patients. Clonidine may be helpful particularly
for behaviorally disordered Tourette's children, whose ADHD may be
treated with clonidine. Both neuroleptics and clonidine are employed for
long-term treatments. The use of neuroleptics in low dosages reduces the
risk of tardive dyskinesia, but long-term neurological complications remain a possibility.

■ FEEDING AND EATING DISORDERS OF INFANCY OR EARLY CHILDHOOD

☐ Pica

Pica has been extensively documented in the pediatric literature, but
minimally documented in the psychiatric literature—despite its presumed biopsychosocial etiology and major behavioral, cognitive, neurological, and developmental complications. A pattern of eating nonfood
materials can be seen in young children, individuals with severe or profound mental retardation, and pregnant women. A similar phenomenon,
involving the eating of clay or soil, is an ordinary, sanctioned activity in
many cultures worldwide; such culturally determined forms of pica are
not considered a mental disorder (Table 23–22). In children, pica is rarely
diagnosed, although it might be quite common. Particularly at a younger
age, the risk of accidental poisoning is significant.

Table 23–22.   DSM-IV diagnostic criteria for pica

A.   Persistent eating of nonnutritive substances for a period of at least
     1 month.
B.   The eating of nonnutritive substances is inappropriate to the develop-
     mental level.
C.   The eating behavior is not part of a culturally sanctioned practice.
D.   If the eating behavior occurs exclusively during the course of another
     mental disorder (e.g., mental retardation, pervasive developmental
     disorder, schizophrenia), it is sufficiently severe to warrant independent
     clinical attention.

Clinical Description

Children may be found to eat paper, paint, plaster, string, rags, hair, feces, vomitus, leaves, bugs, worms, and cloth. The eating of earth, clay, sand, and pebbles (i.e., geophagia) is seen in both children and pregnant women. Pica in children is typically observed in association with behavioral and other medical problems, and is rarely brought for treatment as an isolated problem.

Epidemiology

About 10% to 20% of American children are believed to show pica as a symptom at some point in their lives. In children, boys and girls are equally involved. Epidemiological studies of children with pica show that they typically come from a low socioeconomic class, have pets at home, and display various behavioral abnormalities. Up to 50% to 70% of children in lower socioeconomic classes have pica between ages 1 and 6 years. Typically, these children are not referred for treatment unless concomitant disorders or complications are identified. Over 50% of children hospitalized for accidental ingestions have been found to have pica (Millican et al. 1968).

Prevalence estimates of pica are higher among individuals with mental retardation. Approximately 20% to 40% of institutionalized persons with severe or profound mental retardation have pica. There is an equal gender prevalence.

Etiology

Childhood pica is often described as an ordinary part of exploratory learning, or a reflection of a young child's inability to differentiate food from inedible objects. The findings of increased childhood pica in households with pets, and of the eating of pets' food by the child, suggest that imitation can also be a contributing factor. Many children with pica have parents with a history of pica, which may be passed along by a variety of mechanisms. Psychoanalytic hypotheses have emphasized impairments in aggressivity or orality. The overrepresentation of pica in lower socio-economic classes may partially be a marker for psychosocial stress or family pathology, which may be involved in the etiology. Parental depression, neglect, and inadequate supervision are related to the risk for toxic ingestions in children (Bithoney et al. 1985), and are presumed to be tangible behavioral factors that contribute to the appearance of pica. Mothers of children with pica are often described as immature, emotionally unavailable, and overwhelmed by parenting tasks.

In individuals with severe or profound mental retardation, the primary mechanisms are believed to be self-stimulatory rather than resulting from impaired judgment. These individuals tend to prefer to engage in pica with a favorite object.

A nutritional etiology has been proposed in certain adults who have an instinctive craving for vitamins and minerals (especially iron and perhaps zinc or calcium); hypothetically, the eating is an attempt to correct a nutritional deficiency.

Course and Prognosis

In children, pica usually starts at 12 to 24 months and resolves by age 6. However, pica can persist into adulthood, particularly when associated with mental retardation. In pregnant women, geophagia usually resolves at the end of the pregnancy, but may recur in subsequent pregnancies.

Ingestion of lead-containing paint, plaster, and earth can lead to toxic encephalopathy in severe cases, fatigue and weight loss (with constipation) in moderate cases, and learning impairments in mild cases. Approximately 80% of severely lead-poisoned children have pica, and at least 30% of children with pica show lead-related symptoms. Children with pica may exhibit slow motor and mental development, growth retardation, seizures, and neurological deficits, as well as behavioral abnormalities both before and after the period of pica.

Evaluation

Evaluation of children with pica involves behavioral and psychiatric evaluation of the child and parents, psychosocial evaluation of the home, nutritional status, feeding history, history of lead exposure, and cultural values. The possibility of inadequate supervision of children or parental neglect needs assessment. The diagnosis of pica is often missed, because children are typically brought for evaluation of other problems. Adults may not have directly observed pica behavior, or may volunteer their observations only reluctantly.

Treatment

Behavior therapy has been employed for children and mentally retarded individuals with pica. Rewarding appropriate eating, teaching the differentiation of edible foods, overcorrecting (i.e., enforcing immediate oral hygiene), and using negative reinforcement have been successfully employed, especially for mentally retarded persons.

Psychosocial interventions include promotion of maternal supervision and stimulation, improvement of play opportunities, and placement in day care. Concomitant medical treatments may be required. Nutritional iron and zinc treatments have been suggested to produce short-term improvements in some individuals.

☐ Rumination Disorder

Rumination disorder, a potentially fatal disorder of infants, is particularly apparent when infants are alone and appears to reflect abnormal development of early self-stimulation and physiological regulation (Table 23–23). It may be a cause or a result of disrupted parent-child attachments, and can be associated with major developmental delays and mental retardation. The symptom of rumination is also seen in adults with mental retardation.

Clinical Description

Rumination involves the continued eating of partially digested stomach contents that are regurgitated into the esophagus or mouth. It is different from vomiting, in which the stomach contents are expelled through the mouth. Certain infants show a pleasurable relaxation as they regurgitate,

---

Table 23–23.   DSM-IV diagnostic criteria for rumination disorder

A. Repeated regurgitation and rechewing of food for a period of at least 1 month following a period of normal functioning.

B. The behavior is not due to an associated gastrointestinal or other general medical condition (e.g., esophageal reflux).

C. The behavior does not occur exclusively during the course of anorexia nervosa or bulimia nervosa. If the symptoms occur exclusively during the course of mental retardation or a pervasive developmental disorder, they are sufficiently severe to warrant independent clinical attention.

---

re-chew, drool, and re-swallow their food, usually in the absence of care-givers and other sources of stimulation. These infants' continuing self-stimulation, apparent satisfaction, and langorous obliviousness highlight their full engrossment in rumination. Their obvious enjoyment and en-thusiasm occur despite malnourishment and diminished weight gain, and stand in marked contrast to their parents' disgust at this activity.

Epidemiology

There are no available prevalence figures, but rumination disorder is rare and decreasing in prevalence in the general population, perhaps due to improving child and infant care. However, rumination is not rare in mental retardation; about 10% of institutionalized mentally retarded adults show similar medically unexplained symptoms.

Etiology

There is strong evidence of both organic and environmental contribu-tions to the etiology of rumination disorder. Rumination in infants can result from gastroesophageal reflux due to esophageal sphincter disor-der (e.g., hiatal hernia). Medical conditions are thus considered exclu-sion criteria for the diagnosis for rumination disorder of infancy. In these cases, the rumination can be viewed as an attempt to clear the esopha-gus of refluxed material or as a reflexive response triggered by esopha-geal dilation. Medical or surgical intervention reduces the rumination behavior.

The majority of infants with rumination disorder are not develop-mentally delayed. A low Developmental Quotient score, associated with mental retardation or with pervasive developmental disorders, is seen in 25% of these infants. Obstetric complications are seen in one-third. This finding suggests that perinatal brain damage may contribute to the ap-pearance of rumination disorder, or, more likely, that prenatal pathology can contribute to subsequent perinatal and postnatal difficulties. In fact, the majority of infants with rumination disorder achieve milestones nor-mally and show no obvious developmental problems.

An understimulating environment can contribute to the appearance of rumination disorder. Infants with rumination disorder are often from underprivileged families, in which sensory and interpersonal stimula-tion may be low. Primary caregivers are believed to provide inappropri-ate stimulation that is due to inadequate time spent with the infant, preexisting parental anxiety or avoidance, parental psychiatric impair-ment, absence, or harsh handling. Excessive parental stimulation can also lead to rumination disorder.

Course and Prognosis

Regurgitation or vomiting (with reflux on barium fluoroscopy) is generally seen during the first 3 months of life, but rumination does not typically appear until 3 to 12 months of age. It usually resolves by the end of the second year, but may persist until the third or fourth year. More persistent cases generally have mental retardation. Persons with mental retardation can show a later onset of rumination disorder, but it typically emerges during childhood or adolescence.

Dehydration, electrolyte imbalance, slow weight gain, growth retardation, malnutrition, and tooth decay can be seen in some individuals. Spontaneous remissions are common, but there is also a high risk of developmental delay and death. The only available follow-up study of infants with rumination disorder indicates that about 50% have normal behavioral development and that 20% have major developmental or medical pathology at age 5 years (Sauvage et al. 1985).

Evaluation

Evaluation includes behavioral and psychiatric evaluation of child and parents, with an emphasis on developmental history and psychosocial assessment, as well as eating history, nutritional status, and observation of parent-child interactions during feeding. Gastrointestinal disease needs to be considered, including gastroesophageal reflux, hiatal hernia, pyloric stenosis, other congenital anomalies, and infections. Structural abnormalities (including gastrointestinal) may be particularly common in individuals with cerebral palsy, physical anomalies, or developmental disorders. Regurgitation in infants can also be due to anxiety, and these children appear openly distressed during rumination.

Treatment

There is no established treatment of rumination disorder of infancy, although various forms of behavior therapy, parent guidance, and medication (e.g., antispasmodics and tranquilizers) have been tried. Psychotherapy of the caregiver, dietary changes, and hand restraints have not been found to be particularly effective.

Behavioral techniques include cuddling and playing with the child before, during, and after mealtime to reduce social deprivation and behavioral withdrawal. Aversive conditioning produces the most rapid symptom suppression but generally elicits strong caregiver resistance and cannot usually be applied immediately or consistently. Negative attention, such as shouting or slapping the child, can actually reinforce the behavior, especially if other forms of reinforcement and attention are lacking or ineffective. A combination of a negative reinforcement with a reward for nonrumination has been used in outpatient treatment (Lavigne et al. 1981).

Temporary hospitalization is commonly used to provide a separation of the child from the primary caregiver, an alternative feeding environment for the child (to "decondition" the symptoms), and a period of relaxation for the parent.

☐ Feeding Disorder of Infancy or Early Childhood

In pediatrics, the diagnosis of *failure to thrive* (FTT) includes retardation of body growth (or milestone attainment) resulting from inadequate nutritional intake. The "organic" forms of FTT can result from chronic physical illness (e.g., congenital AIDS), neurological disease, sensory deficit, or virtually any serious pediatric disease. The "nonorganic" forms, constituting at least 80% of cases of FTT, encompass 1) homeostatic disorders of infancy (sleep and feeding dysregulation), 2) pathological food refusal, 3) protein-calorie malnutrition, and 4) social and emotional factors that interfere with adequate nutritional care (including reactive attachment disorder).

The newly created DSM-IV diagnosis of feeding disorder of infancy or early childhood does not include all forms of *nonorganic failure to thrive* (NFTT), but only those types of eating failures that occur in the context of an adequate provision of food (Table 23–24).

Clinical Description

Symptomatically, NFTT infants may gag when being fed or may refuse to open their mouths. Young children may decline to eat, or eat so slowly that their intake is drastically reduced. In infants, the retardation in weight gain is typically accompanied by motor, social, and linguistic de-

---

Table 23–24. DSM-IV diagnostic criteria for feeding disorder of infancy or early childhood

A. Feeding disturbance as manifested by persistent failure to eat adequately with significant failure to gain weight or significant loss of weight over at least 1 month.

B. The disturbance is not due to an associated gastrointestinal or other general medical condition (e.g., esophageal reflux).

C. The disturbance is not better accounted for by another mental disorder (e.g., rumination disorder) or by lack of available food.

D. The onset is before age 6 years.

---

lays as well as a problematic relationship with the feeder or caregiver (as a result, if not a cause, of the disorder). In early childhood, symptoms may include impaired interpersonal relationships and interactions, mood symptoms, behavior problems, developmental delays, unusual food preferences, excessively rigid or narrow food choices, and perhaps bizarre eating and foraging behaviors.

Epidemiology

Approximately 1% to 5% of pediatric hospital admissions are due to NFTT.

Etiology

The relative loss of weight in NFTT is due to malnutrition, but the malnutrition may be due to various causes (Woolston 1983). Both physical and psychosocial etiologies may be involved, although the definition of the disorder excludes cases that clearly result from overt medical problems or other psychiatric disorders. Various mechanisms (and potential subtypes) include difficulties with physiological homeostasis, with attachment to the caregiver, with autonomy from the caregiver, and posttraumatic responses.

Attachment problems, reflected in impaired relatedness and reciprocal interactions with the caregiver, may operate to inhibit adequate feeding. The ordinary signals involving eye contact, smiling, vocal contact, visual stimulation, and physical touching may not be provided (or responded to) by child or parent, and the reciprocal signaling that underlies effective feeding may be undermined. Apathy might replace the potential for pleasurable enjoyment of feeding experienced by child and caregiver. Additional social and emotional factors that might reduce nutritional intake and body growth include posttraumatic responses to medical procedures involving the mouth; child abuse; emotional deprivation; or family pathology.

Course and Prognosis

The untreated course of feeding disorder of infancy or early childhood may depend on the specific subtype or mechanisms involved, but the expected outcome ranges from spontaneous remission to malnutrition, infection, or death. Both nutritional or psychosocial deprivation may result in long-term behavioral changes, hyperactivity, short stature, and lowered IQ. The relationship of these feeding disorders to other psychiatric disorders, including the eating disorders of adulthood, is undetermined.

Evaluation and Treatment

A multidisciplinary team, preferably in a hospital setting, is helpful for evaluating and initiating treatment. Evaluation would include assessment of body growth as well as observations of the mother-child interactions in general and in feeding in particular.

■ ELIMINATION DISORDERS

☐ Functional Encopresis

Functional encopresis includes fecal soiling of clothes, voiding in bed, and excretion onto the floor, occurring after age 4 years when full bowel control is developmentally expected. Because "organic" causes of encopresis need to be excluded, medical evaluation for structural and other nonfunctional abnormalities must be obtained prior to labeling as functional (Table 23–25). Once medical-physical etiologies are ruled out, psychodynamic and biopsychiatric etiologies predominate. Low intelligence is not a factor in the development of most cases of encopresis.

Clinical Description

Functional encopresis during the daytime is much more common than nocturnal encopresis. In half of patients with functional encopresis, bowel control is not yet learned, so the symptom may be viewed as reflecting an early developmental fixation (i.e., primary encopresis). In the other half, the children initially learned bowel control, had been continent for at least 1 year, and then regressed (i.e., secondary encopresis). Secondary encopresis usually starts by age 8 years.

About 75% to 90% of cases involve the DSM-IV subtype designated

---

Table 23–25. DSM-IV diagnostic criteria for encopresis

A. Repeated passage of feces into inappropriate places (e.g., clothing or floor) whether involuntary or intentional.

B. At least one such event a month for at least 3 months.

C. Chronological age is at least 4 years (or equivalent developmental level).

D. The behavior is not due exclusively to the direct physiological effects of a substance (e.g., laxatives) or a general medical condition except through a mechanism involving constipation.

Code as folows:

787.6 **With constipation and overflow incontinence**

307.7 **Without constipation and overflow incontinence**

---

as "constipation and overflow incontinence." These "retentive" cases include a low frequency of bowel movements, impaction, overflow of liquid around the partially hardened stool, and leakage of liquid into the clothing. This type of encopresis may be due to chronic constipation, inadequate bowel training, pain, or phobic avoidance of toilets. These retentive episodes usually extend for several days and are followed by painful defecation.

Encopresis without constipation and overflow can involve a variety of sources, including a lack of awareness or poor sphincter control. In cases of soiling occurring after bath, physical stimulation may be causative. If soiling is deliberate, the child is typically impulsive or hostile; antisocial or major psychiatric disorders may be associated. Smearing may be accidental or purposeful. Certain encopretic children show neurodevelopmental symptoms, including inattention, hyperactivity, impulsivity, low frustration tolerance, and dyscoordination.

Epidemiology

Functional encopresis is less common than enuresis. Prevalence of encopresis is approximately 1.5% after age 5 years, diminishes with age, and is rare in adolescents. Slightly higher rates are associated with the lower socioeconomic classes. There is a 4:1 male predominance. A familial occurrence of functional encopresis has been noted, with 15% of fathers having childhood encopresis. Higher rates are observed among individuals with mental retardation, particularly in moderate and severe cases.

Etiology

Medical causes of fecal incontinence include hypothyroidism, hypercalcemia, anal fissure, rectal stenosis, lactase deficiency, overeating of fried and fatty foods, congenital aganglionic megacolon, and other neuromedical disorders. Pathophysiological mechanisms include altered colon motility and contraction patterns, stretching and thinning of colon walls (megacolon), and decreased sensation or perception (usually appearing early in illness). In infancy, encopresis may result from severe diaper rash, when fecal withholding may occur to avoid rectal pain. These medical causes of fecal soiling exclude the diagnosis of functional encopresis.

Encopresis may result from inadequate or punitive toilet training, physical discomfort associated with inadequate physical support during toilet training, or improper management of toilet-related fears. Stress-related factors appear causative in one-half of cases of secondary encopresis.

Course and Prognosis

Substantial follow-up studies are unavailable, but associated psycho-pathology or medical disorders may be the primary determinant of prognosis. Conduct disorder, the use of soiling as a direct expression of anger, and parental disinterest in dealing with the problem appear to predict a more protracted course.

Evaluation and Treatment

Initial medical evaluation is required to evaluate possible structural abnormalities (e.g., anal fissure), and may involve barium enema. Psychiatric evaluation includes assessment of associated psychiatric disorders, including mental retardation, oppositional defiant disorder, conduct disorder, mood disorders, and psychosis.

Many cases can be treated in a pediatric model by decompaction and behavioral treatment, but "resistant" cases may require psychiatric intervention. Pediatric management of "mild" cases may include bowel cleansing, daily maintenance on mineral oil, counseling, and follow-up. In pediatric practice, improvement is seen in approximately 50% to 75% of cases (Levine 1982).

☐ Functional Enuresis

Urinary incontinence may be seen in young children, and occasionally in older children after the completion of toilet training, as a normal developmental phenomenon. Enuresis is diagnosed when urinary incontinence without medical explanation is either frequent, distressing, or interfering with activities (Table 23–26). Urinary bladder control is typically attained by age 3 or 4 years, so DSM-IV diagnosis requires a minimal age of 5 years. Prior to designating these presentations as functional, a medical assessment of physical causes of enuresis is required.

Clinical Description

In enuresis, bed-wetting is more common than daytime urinary incontinence. Nocturnal enuresis typically occurs 30 minutes to 3 hours after sleep onset, with the child either sleeping through the episode or being awakened by the moisture. For some children, however, enuresis may occur at any time during the night. Children with daytime enuresis usually have nocturnal enuresis too. In 80% of enuretic children, bladder control has not yet been attained, and the enuresis is "primary." In 20%, urinary incontinence is "secondary," reappearing after competent functioning is attained.

Table 23–26.   DSM-IV diagnostic criteria for enuresis

A.   Repeated voiding of urine into bed or clothes (whether involuntary or intentional).

B.   The behavior is clinically significant as manifested by either a frequency of twice a week for at least 3 consecutive months or the presence of clinically significant distress or impairment in social, academic (occupational), or other important areas of functioning.

C.   Chronological age is at least 5 years (or equivalent developmental level).

D.   The behavior is not due exclusively to the direct physiological effect of a substance (e.g., a diuretic) or a general medical condition (e.g., diabetes, spina bifida, a seizure disorder).

Specify type:

Nocturnal only
Diurnal only
Nocturnal and diurnal

Epidemiology

Nocturnal enuresis may be seen occasionally in 25% of boys, but occurs repetitively beyond age 5 in 7% to 10% of boys and 3% of girls. The male predominance remains, but decreases with age. At age 10, 3% of boys and 2% of girls are diagnosable. In adulthood, the prevalence in the general population is 1%.

Etiology

Nonfunctional enuresis may be caused by urological, anatomic, physiological, metabolic, or neurological mechanisms. Some forms of functional enuresis may run in families, particularly in males. Approximately 70% of these children have a first-degree relative with functional enuresis. The chances of a child having enuresis are 77% if both parents have a history of enuresis, and 44% if one parent has a history (Bakwin 1973).

For many children and adults with nocturnal enuresis, hormonal factors and biological rhythms may be causative. Some children with nocturnal enuresis do not have a normal nighttime release of vasopressin and so may not have the usual nocturnal reduction in urine production (Rittig et al. 1989). A "maturational" disorder is suggested in some cases by the findings of small volume of voidings, short stature, low mean bone age for chronological age, and, in adolescence, delayed sexual maturation. In general, enuresis is associated with an overrepresentation of developmental delays (Steinhausen and Göbel 1989).

Course and Prognosis

Functional enuresis has a spontaneous remission rate of 15% per year (Forsythe and Butler 1989). Approximately 1% of boys (and fewer girls) still have this condition at age 18, generally with little associated psychopathology. The adolescent-onset form of enuresis, however, may signify more psychopathology and less favorable outcome. There is a higher prevalence of functional enuresis in cases of moderate and severe mental retardation.

Evaluation and Treatment

Initial medical assessment is required to rule out the various nonfunctional forms of enuresis. In certain cases, a sleep evaluation may be helpful, but an EEG is not routinely required. Measurement of certain maturational indices may be useful for identifying simple developmental variance. Psychiatric evaluation of the child and family includes assessment of associated psychopathology, determination of recent psychosocial stressors, and evaluation of family concern and management of the symptoms.

Most cases of functional enuresis are treated by pediatricians. Behavioral methods for treating nocturnal enuresis include restriction of prebedtime fluid intake, midsleep awakenings for voiding in the toilet, and rewards for successful nights. A device that sounds a bell connected to a moisture-sensitive blanket that arouses a child from sleep after a voiding has a high success rate (80% to 90%) but also a high relapse rate (up to 40%). If relapse occurs, reinitiation of the system is often effective (Forsythe and Butler 1989).

Antidepressants can be helpful if a case is resistant to behavioral interventions, if there is daytime as well as nighttime enuresis, or if there is an associated mood or anxiety disorder. Antidepressants have been shown to be effective in many double-blind studies, typically in low doses. Although some reports suggest that the success rate is only 15% after discontinuing antidepressants, the success rate is probably much higher if the dose is tapered gradually.

Desmopressin, an analog (1-desamino-8-D-arginine vasopressin [DDAVP]) of the antidiuretic hormone vasopressin, has been successful in several double-blind trials in treating nocturnal enuresis. Its efficacy in 70% of cases is not quite as high as that for bell alarms (Wille 1986), but the combination of desmopressin and bell alarm appears most effective (Sukhai et al. 1989). Desmopressin might be more effective in older children, especially those with a demonstrable excess of nocturnal vasopressin release. Relapse is common when treatment is discontinued.

■ OTHER DISORDERS OF INFANCY, CHILDHOOD, OR ADOLESCENCE

☐ Separation Anxiety Disorder

In addition to normal situational and developmental anxiety, children can show genuine anxiety disorders. Separation anxiety disorder is the only anxiety disorder listed in DSM-IV as a disorder usually first diagnosed in children or adolescence. Like other anxiety disorders in children, separation anxiety disorder can lead to social problems, academic underachievement, and/or interference with developing assertiveness skills and personal autonomy, possibly resulting in social awkwardness or immaturity, and perhaps a reluctance to date.

Separation anxiety, a normal developmental phenomenon at age 18 to 30 months, has been described in attachment and separation theory. In separation anxiety disorder, cognitive, affective, somatic, and behavioral symptoms appear in response to genuine or fantasied separation from attachment figures (Table 23–27). Separation anxiety disorder can present clinically in a variety of ways, including difficulty in falling asleep (prebedtime agitation) and school absenteeism (Bernstein and Borchardt 1991).

Clinical Description

Major attachment objects are usually a parent or caregiver, but can be a favorite toy or familiar place. Typically, even a young child can specify the attachment object that gives a sense of protection or safety from anxiety. Common presentations include preoccupying or morbid fear of parents' death, clinging to parents, school refusal, sleep refusal, refusal to be alone, nightmares, anticipatory worrying, cognitive disruption, or somatization. Although the anxiety is usually centered around separation from a parent, the fear can instead manifest as an anticipatory fear of being injured, kidnapped, or killed. Interference with autonomous functioning can extend to inability to sleep in one's own bed, visit friends, go on errands, or stay at camp. Homesickness may be freely described by young children, but can be hard to admit for adolescents (especially boys).

Over 92% of children with separation anxiety disorder have other DSM-IV disorders, typically anxiety or mood disorders. Many children with major depressive disorder also fulfill criteria for separation anxiety disorder. These children typically display internalizing behaviors and psychological mechanisms. Pathological compliance, perfectionism, and "nicey nice" presentation of self may be seen. The children can show somatizations in the morning on school days, a fear of teachers, or passive-

---

Table 23–27. DSM-IV diagnostic criteria for separation anxiety disorder

---

A. Developmentally inappropriate and excessive anxiety concerning separation from home or from those to whom the individual is attached, as evidenced by three (or more) of the following:

   1. Recurrent excessive distress when separation from home or major attachment figures occurs or is anticipated

   2. Persistent and excessive worry about losing, or about possible harm befalling, major attachment figures

   3. Persistent and excessive worry that an untoward event will lead to separation from a major attachment figure (e.g., getting lost or being kidnapped)

   4. Persistent reluctance or refusal to go to school or elsewhere because of fear of separation

   5. Persistently and excessively fearful or reluctant to be alone or without major attachment figures at home or without significant adults in other settings

   6. Persistent reluctance or refusal to go to sleep without being near a major attachment figure or to sleep away from home

   7. Repeated nightmares involving the theme of separation

   8. Repeated complaints of physical symptoms (such as headaches, stomachaches, nausea, or vomiting) when separation from major attachment figures occurs or is anticipated

B. The duration of the disturbance is at least 4 weeks.

C. The onset is before age 18 years.

D. The disturbance causes clinically significant distress or impairment in social, academic (occupational), or other important areas of functioning.

E. The disturbance does not occur exclusively during the course of a pervasive developmental disorder, schizophrenia, or other psychotic disorder and, in adolescents and adults, is not better accounted for by panic disorder with agoraphobia.

Specify if:

Early onset: If onset occurs before age 6 years

---

aggressive traits. In certain cases, anxiety disorders in children become the basis for disruptive behavioral symptoms. Children with separation anxiety disorder commonly experience stomachaches and palpitations, and generally have more somatic complaints than do children with any other psychiatric disorder (Livingston et al. 1988). School absenteeism is reported in about 75% of children with separation anxiety disorder, and separation anxiety disorder is reported in up to 50% to 80% of school absentees (Klein and Last 1989).

Epidemiology

Separation anxiety disorder appears to be common and tends to run in families. Epidemiological studies report a prevalence of 0.6% to 6%. Gender ratio is equal or shows some (2:1) predominance in females.

Etiology

Developmental theorists have speculated about mechanisms contributing to separation anxiety disorder. Unconscious internal conflicts regarding aggressive and sexual impulses, uncertainty regarding the location of caregivers after the toddler's initial ambulatory movements, and parent-induced anxious attachment are standard psychodynamic formulations. Learning theorists have emphasized the maintenance of symptoms by conditioned fear, based on stimulus generalization and reinforcement. Biological theorists focus on temperament factors, pharmacological features, and the possible relationship to childhood mood and adult anxiety disorders. Over half of children with separation anxiety disorder have parents with mood or anxiety disorders.

Course and Prognosis

Separation anxiety disorder may be diagnosed after the normative period of separation anxiety, but it is typically not observed before age 4 years. It is usually recognized in early or mid childhood. Separation anxiety disorder is typically a chronic disorder, but exacerbations can occur at times of actual separations, deaths, family moves, or natural disasters. Symptoms may worsen during or after medical illness, particularly chronic medical conditions. Multiple medical evaluations are commonly sought by child or parents. A follow-up study of children with separation anxiety disorder (with a communication disorder) found that after 4 years, 11% still had separation anxiety disorder, 33% had a different diagnosis (typically another anxiety disorder), and 44% no longer had an anxiety disorder (Cantwell and Baker 1989).

Evaluation and Treatment

The workup includes the assessment of the possibility of mood disorder or anxiety disorder. Clinically, it is difficult to distinguish the presenting symptoms of separation anxiety disorder from ordinary acute anxiety. Both conditions can involve distractibility, distorted cognition, depersonalization, transient impairment in reality sense, motoric overactivity, and angry outbursts. However, the presence of separation anxiety disorder implies that separation-related psychodynamics are the primary trigger of the acute anxiety.

The treatment of separation anxiety disorder involves individual psychotherapy combined with parent guidance or family therapy, and often includes an antidepressant medication. Tricyclic antidepressant treatment is indicated for the child whose school absenteeism exceeds 2 weeks and is not explained by a medical problem, truancy, overt psychosis, sociocultural conformity, or realistic fear of physical danger. The use of antidepressants for treating separation anxiety disorder is common, despite a meager literature supporting its effectiveness (Popper 1993). Antidepressants are probably effective in treating school absenteeism when the underlying etiology is separation anxiety disorder, mood disorder, phobic disorder, or panic disorder.

If a parent has an anxiety or mood disorder that causes difficulty in his or her separating from the child, then the parent should also receive direct psychiatric treatment as well as behavioral guidance. Treatment of a parent with antidepressant medication for mood or anxiety disorders is often a part of the treatment of a child with separation anxiety disorder.

Benzodiazepines have also been employed for children and parents, and are particularly helpful for the "anticipatory" anxiety that can develop secondarily around "primary" anxiety symptoms. Alternatively, buspirone or fluoxetine might be considered.

Separation anxiety disorder can also be partially alleviated by the use of a "high tech" method: the attachment figure is given an electronic "beeper," and the child is given a coin, which permits him or her to telephone the parent in the event of a surge of anxiety. Typically, the child will attempt to reach the parent once or twice, and then can use the coin as a symbol of the capacity to reach the attachment figure if needed. This technique can be useful in facilitating school attendance.

☐ Reactive Attachment Disorder of Infancy and Early Childhood

Following physical or emotional abuse by a caregiver, abnormal interpersonal behavior and emotional excitability may be observed. It is natural to infer that the abnormal social behavior results from disordered development of early interpersonal attachment (Table 23–28). Reactive attachment disorder encompasses both increased and decreased social interactiveness after trauma in infancy or early childhood. This DSM-IV diagnosis labels a variety of conditions originating in childhood, including the consequences of physical or sexual abuse, caregiving by emotionally disturbed individuals, inappropriate parental emotional involvement, neglect, enduring posttraumatic stress reactions, instability of home environments, and impaired attachment or bonding (Tibbits-Kleber and Howell 1985). The hallmark of reactive attachment disorder is the appearance of grossly disturbed interpersonal relations following

---

Table 23–28.   DSM-IV diagnostic criteria for reactive attachment disorder of infancy or early childhood

---

A.   Markedly disturbed and developmentally inappropriate social relatedness in most contexts, beginning before age 5 years, as evidenced by either (1) or (2):

1.   Persistent failure to initiate or respond in a developmentally appropriate fashion to most social interactions, as manifest by excessively inhibited, hypervigilant, or highly ambivalent and contradictory responses (e.g., the child may respond to caregivers with a mixture of approach, avoidance, and resistance to comforting, or may exhibit frozen watchfulness).

2.   Diffuse attachments as manifest by indiscriminate sociability with marked inability to exhibit appropriate selective attachments (e.g., excessive familiarity with relative strangers or lack of selectivity in choice of attachment figures).

B.   The disturbance in criterion A is not accounted for solely by developmental delay (as in mental retardation) and does not meet criteria for a pervasive developmental disorder.

C.   Pathogenic care as evidenced by at least one of the following:

1.   Persistent disregard of the child's basic emotional needs for comfort, stimulation, and affection.

2.   Persistent disregard of the child's basic physical needs.

3.   Repeated changes of primary caregiver that prevent formation of stable attachments (e.g., frequent changes in foster care).

D.   There is a presumption that the care in criterion C is responsible for the disturbed behavior in criterion A (e.g., the disturbances in criterion A began following the pathogenic care in criterion C).

Specify type:

Inhibited type: If criterion A1 predominates in the clinical presentation

Disinhibited type: If criterion A2 predominates in the clinical presentation

---

grossly inadequate early care in childhood, with the connection being inferential.

The pediatric label of NFTT includes those cases of reactive attachment disorder that involve physical growth retardation, the DSM-IV category of feeding and eating disorders of infancy or early childhood, and some cases of retarded physical growth without prominent social abnormalities.

Clinical Description

A variety of behavioral, cognitive, and affective presentations may be seen at different ages. In children, odd social responsiveness, weak interpersonal attachment, apathy or inappropriate excitability, and mood abnormalities are common. Any failure of normal development may be labeled as reactive attachment disorder if preceded by clear failures in ordinary care.

In early infancy, diagnosis is based on the failure to achieve developmental expectations: lack of eye tracking or responsive smiling by age 2 months, and failure to play simple games or reach out to be picked up by age 5 months. In normal development, an infant is expected to show overt behavioral signs of attachment and bonding to a parent by age 8 months. Infants with reactive attachment disorder appear lethargic and show little body movement or activity. Body movements are weak. Sleep is excessive and disrupted, and weight gain is slow. The infants resist being held, and there is little interactive interest in the environment.

Children or infants with reactive attachment disorder may appear withdrawn, passive, or disinterested in people, or may respond to interpersonal stimuli in odd ways. Alternately, children may display excessive interest, overly rapid familiarity, inappropriate touching, clinging, or immediate emotional involvement that may seem initially gratifying but is also experienced as weird or unusual.

Etiology

In this particular DSM-IV diagnosis, the etiology is written into the definition of the disorder: prior abuse, neglect, or impaired caregiving is definitionally required, and disruption of parent-child bonding is implied by the disease label.

Course and Prognosis

If reactive attachment disorder is untreated, the course may vary from spontaneous remission to malnutrition, infection, or death. Both nutritional or psychosocial deprivation may result in long-term behavioral changes, hyperactivity, short stature, and lowered IQ. If emotional deprivation continues but enforced feeding is provided, children may show improved weight gain. However, even when body growth is preserved, ongoing emotional deprivation can cause "depression" and developmental delays in infants (Provence and Lipton 1962). Improved body growth and emotional responsiveness do not guarantee a normal developmental outcome, but specific predictors of behavioral, cognitive, and physical sequelae have not been identified.

Evaluation and Treatment

In practice, reactive attachment disorder is diagnosed by observation of mother-child interaction, home visit, and symptomatic response to adequate care. Assessment of caregiver-child interaction involves observation of the simple capacity for physical holding, physical and interpersonal stimulation, empathy, attentiveness to the child's behavior, fear of the child, anger, or indifference. A home visit is generally indicated to evaluate the adequacy of housing, safety, nutrition, and parental involvement with the child. Multiple shifts of home environment or caregiver may be causative. Psychiatric evaluation of the parents is an essential component of the overall evaluation. Physical or sexual abuse, and neglect, may not be quickly identifiable in some cases. For infants or very young children, hospitalization may be useful for diagnosis and treatment. Medical assessment is required to rule out chronic physical illness that may result in organic failure to thrive, homeostatic sleep and feeding disorders, food refusal, malnutrition, neurological disease, and sensory deficit.

Basic medical care, provision of adequate caregiving, parental education, and parental psychiatric treatment are generally needed to treat reactive attachment disorder of infancy or early childhood. This massive intervention typically justifies medical hospitalization. Given the complexity of medical and psychiatric problems, the required sensitivity in managing the parents, and the frequent need for legal procedures, it is often helpful to have a specialized treatment team on pediatric hospital units.

A major improvement in clinical status of the child typically results from hospitalization or treatment intervention. This improvement in response to treatment is considered confirmation of the diagnosis of reactive attachment disorder. Clinical nonresponsiveness implies that a different disorder is present, or that extreme medical complications with persistent physical damage had occurred prior to treatment.

☐ Stereotypic Movement Disorder

Certain repetitive and purposeless motor behaviors may be seen in young children, sensory-deprived persons, or individuals with mental retardation, pervasive developmental disorders, and some psychotic disorders (schizophrenia, or mood disorders with psychomotor changes). Many stereotypies appear to have a self-stimulatory component, but the diagnosis of stereotypic movement disorder is made only if these repetitive behaviors cause functional interference or physical injury (Table 23–29).

Clinical Description

Examples of stereotypies or habits include head banging, body rocking, hand flapping, whirling, stereotyped laughter, thumb sucking, hair fin-

Table 23–29.   DSM-IV diagnostic criteria for stereotypic movement disorder

A.   Repetitive, seemingly driven, and nonfunctional motor behavior
     (e.g., hand shaking or waving, body rocking, head banging, mouthing of
     objects, self-biting, picking at skin or bodily orifices, hitting own body).

B.   The behavior markedly interferes with normal activities or results in self-
     inflicted bodily injury that requires medical treatment (or would result
     in an injury if preventive measures were not used).

C.   If mental retardation is present, the stereotypic or self-injurious behavior
     is of sufficient severity to become a focus of treatment.

D.   The behavior is not better accounted for by a compulsion (as in obsessive-
     compulsive disorder), a tic (as in tic disorder), a stereotypy that is part of
     a pervasive developmental disorder, or hair pulling (as in trichotillomania).

E.   The behavior is not due to the direct physiological effects of a substance
     or a general medical condition.

F.   The behavior persists for 4 weeks or longer.

Specify if:

With self-injurious behavior: If the behavior results in bodily damage that requires specific treatment (or that would result in bodily damage if protective
measures were not used)

gering, facial touching, eye poking, object biting, self-biting, self-scratch-
ing, self-hitting, grinding of teeth, and holding of breath. Although one
behavioral habit may predominate, it is typical for several stereotypies to
occur together. Different stereotypies may become prominent at different times. The rhythm of the repetitive behavior may be slow and gentle,
or fast and energetic, or even violently energized. Sometimes waves of
increasing and decreasing energy may be seen over the course of several
minutes. Frequency may increase during periods of tension, frustration,
boredom, or isolation, and just before bedtime.

Epidemiology

Approximately 15% to 20% of a normal pediatric population may have a
history of transient stereotypies or habits, but no data are available regarding the prevalence of stereotypic movement disorder with physical
injury or functional interference. Stereotypic behaviors show equal gender prevalence. There is a higher prevalence of stereotypic movement
disorder in individuals with mental retardation. Among institutionalized
persons with severe and profound mental retardation, about 60% have
stereotypic movement disorder, and 15% have self-injurious behaviors
(Schroeder et al. 1979).

Etiology

There is no clear etiology of stereotypic movement disorder, but several theories have been advanced, and multiple contributing or interacting factors are probably involved. Organic influences are supported by the increased incidence of stereotypic movement disorder in individuals with abnormal brain state or function: mental retardation, sensory deficit, brain disease (seizures, postinfection, metabolic abnormality), psychotic disorder, and drug-induced psychosis (amphetamine).

An etiological role of self-stimulation (or autoerotic stimulation) is suggested by the child's self-absorbed and apparently pleasurable appearance, and the occurrence of such activity during boredom or physical isolation. Self-stimulation through repetitive physical activity may be particularly satisfying if the usual forms of stimulation are ineffective; for patients with extreme impairments in cognition, the ordinary array of sights and sounds may not be as interpretable or pleasurable as physical activity. A tension-relieving purpose is plausible, because these behaviors increase during anxiety, tension, and frustration. An arousal factor has been proposed, since behaviors can be more evident at bedtime or upon arising in the morning. Head banging during temper tantrums may be viewed in terms of self-stimulation, tension discharge, or arousal.

Course and Prognosis

Certain stereotypies, such as head banging and body rocking, begin as early as 6 to 12 months. These behaviors typically resolve in 80% of normal children by age 4 years, although more subtle habits, such as finger tapping or teeth grinding, may then persist (DeLissovoy 1962). In persons with mental retardation and pervasive developmental disorders, such early-onset stereotypies may persist for years. Later-onset stereotypies and habits may be descriptively similar, but appear episodically during periods of anxiety or stress.

Evaluation and Treatment

When stereotypic movement disorder begins during infancy or very early childhood, evaluation for concurrent mental retardation and other developmental disabilities is appropriate. For a later-onset form of this disorder, it is necessary to evaluate for agitation associated with psychosis or mood disorders, as well as mental retardation and pervasive developmental disorders. In some cases, the use of psychostimulant medications and other dopamine agonists may aggravate or produce stereotypic behavior, so evaluation of current medication usage is appropriate.

The symptoms of stereotypic movement disorder are often treatment-resistant, but behavioral techniques (especially overcorrection) have been found most effective. Interventions involving anxiety reduction, sensory stimulation, and the offering of alternatives to self-stimulation are also helpful. Behavioral methods usually attempt to rely on reward systems whenever possible, but positive reinforcement in treating stereotypic movement disorder is usually not effective when used alone. Overcorrection has the best empirical support, but it is a coercive treatment that may invoke anger, oppositionalism, and symptom substitution. In treating coprophagy (i.e., eating of feces), a program of positive-practice overcorrection may involve oral hygiene, cleaning fingers and nails, and washing the arms for several minutes each.

Some clinicians advise simple and practical management techniques, such as directing a child to bang his or her head on a soft surface, combined with interventions for stress reduction. Blocking pleasurable feedback from self-stimulation can be useful. The particular technique used depends on the sensory mode of predominant self-stimulation. For self-stimulation based on sound, a white noise or tape-recorded music may be used. For rocking, a vibrator taped to the hand may distract from kinesthetic self-stimulation. For finger waving, beads on a string may provide proprioceptive stimulation. For visual stimulation, ambient lighting may be altered, or a bubble-blower may be provided. Such distraction from self-stimulation and the substitution of stimulation can be useful in the treatment of some individuals (Baroff 1986).

Neuroleptics or diphenhydramine may be helpful in certain cases. Psychostimulants and other dopamine agonists may aggravate or induce the appearance of stereotypic behaviors (Green 1991). Seizure disorders are commonly present in patients with self-injurious behaviors, so anticonvulsants may be considered for some of these individuals. The opiate blocker naltrexone has been effective in reducing self-injurious behaviors, particularly in mental retardation with stereotypies (Sandman 1991).

■ REFERENCES

Achenbach TM, Edelbrock C: Manual for the Child Behavioral Checklist and Revised Child Behavioral Profile. Burlington, VT, University of Vermont Psychology Department, 1983

Achenbach TM, McConaughty SH: Empirically Based Assessment of Child and Adolescent Psychopathology. Newbury Park, CA, Sage, 1987

Aichhorn A: Wayward Youth. New York, Meridian Books, 1955 [Original publication: Vienna, Internationaler Psychoanalytischer Verlag, 1925]

American Association on Mental Retardation: Mental Retardation: Definition, Classification, and Systems of Supports, 9th Edition. Washington, DC, American Association on Mental Retardation, 1992

American Psychiatric Association: Diagnostic and Statistical Manual of Mental Disorders, 4th Edition. Washington, DC, American Psychiatric Association, 1994

Anderson JC, Williams S, McGee R, et al: DSM-III disorders in preadolescent children: prevalence in a large sample from the general population. Arch Gen Psychiatry 44:69–76, 1987

Aram DM, Ekelman BL, Nation JE: Preschoolers with language disorder: 10 years later. J Speech Hear Res 27:232–244, 1984

August GJ, Stewart MA, Holmes CS: A four-year follow-up of hyperactive boys with and without conduct disorder. Br J Psychiatry 143:l92–198, 1983

Bakwin H: The genetics of enuresis, in Bladder Control and Enuresis. Edited by Kolvin RC, MacKeith RC, Meadow SR. London, W Heinemann Medical Books, 1973, pp 73–77

Barkley RA (ed): Attention Deficit Hyperactivity Disorder: A Handbook for Diagnosis and Treatment. New York, Guilford, 1990

Barkley RA, Cunningham CE: Do stimulant drugs improve the academic performance of hyperkinetic children? A review of outcome studies. Clin Pediatr (Phila) 17:85–92, 1978

Baroff GS: Mental Retardation: Nature, Cause and Management. New York, Hemisphere, 1986

Bauman ML: Microscropic neuroanatomical abnormalities in autism. Pediatrics 87(suppl):791–796, 1991

Beitchman JH, Nair R, Clegg M, et al: Prevalence of psychiatric disorders in children with speech and language disorders. Journal of the American Academy of Child Psychiatry 25:528–535, 1986

Bernstein GA, Borchardt CM: Anxiety disorders of childhood and adolescence: a critical review. J Am Acad Child Adolesc Psychiatry 30:519–532, 1991

Bithoney WG, Snyder J, Michalek J, et al: Childhood ingestions as symptoms of family distress. Am J Dis Child 139:456–459, 1985

Bregman JD, Hodapp RM: Current developments in the understanding of mental retardation, Part I: biological and phenomenological perspectives. J Am Acad Child Adolesc Psychiatry 30:707–719, 1991

Bregman JD, Dykens E, Watson M, et al: Fragile-X syndrome: variability of phenotypic expression. J Am Acad Child Psychiatry 26:463–471, 1987

Bruun RD: The natural history of Tourette's syndrome, in Tourette's Syndrome and Tic Disorders: Clinical Understanding and Treatment. Edited by Cohen D, Bruun R, Leckman J. New York, Wiley, 1988, pp 21–39

Campbell M, Anderson LT, Small AM, et al: Naltrexone in autistic children: a double-blind and placebo-controlled study. Psychopharmacol Bull 26:130–135, 1990

Cantwell DP, Baker L: Developmental Speech and Language Disorders. New York, Guilford, 1987

Cantwell DP, Baker L: Issues in the classification of child and adolescent psychopathology. J Am Acad Child Adolesc Psychiatry 27:521–533, 1988

Cantwell DP, Baker L: Stability and natural history of DSM-III childhood diagnoses. J Am Acad Child Adolesc Psychiatry 28:691–700, 1989

Chase TN, Friedhoff AJ, Cohen DJ (eds): Tourette Syndrome: Genetics, Neurobiology, and Treatment (Advances in Neurology, Vol 58). New York, Raven, 1992

Cohen D, Caparulo B, Shaywitz B: Primary childhood aphasia and childhood autism: clinical, biological and conceptual observations. Journal of the American Academy of Child Psychiatry 15:604–645, 1976

Cohen J: Learning disabilities and adolescence: developmental considerations, in Adolescent Psychiatry: Developmental and Clinical Studies, Vol 12. Edited by Feinstein SC, Sugar M, Esman AH, et al. Chicago, IL, University of Chicago Press, 1985, pp 177–196

DeLissovoy V: Head banging in early childhood. Child Dev 33:43–56, 1962

Deuel RK, Robinson D: Developmental motor signs, in Soft Neurological Signs. Edited by Tupper DE. New York, Grune & Stratton, 1987, pp 95–129

Deutsch CK, Swanson JM, Bruell JH, et al: Overrepresentation of adoptees in children with the attention deficit disorder. Behav Genet 12:231–238, 1982

Edelbrock C: Behavioral checklists and rating scales, in Basic Handbook of Child Psychiatry, Vol 5. Edited by Call JD, Cohen RL, Harrison SI, et al. (Editor-in-Chief, Noshpitz JD). New York, Basic Books, 1987, pp 153–164

Elliott DS, Huizinga D, Ageton SS: Explaining Delinquency and Drug Use. Beverly Hills, CA, Sage, 1985

Faulstich ME, Moore JR, Roberts RW, et al: A behavioral perspective on conduct disorders. Psychiatry 51:398–416, 1988

Fendrich M, Warner V, Weissman MM: Family risk factors, parental depression, and psychopathology in offspring. Dev Psychol 26:40–50, 1990

Fey M, Leonard L, Wilcox K: Speech style modification in language-impaired children. J Speech Hear Disord 46:91–96, 1981

Folstein SE, Piven J: Etiology of autism: genetic influences. Pediatrics 87(suppl): 767–773, 1991

Forsythe WI, Butler RJ: Fifty years of enuretic alarms. Arch Dis Child 64:879–885, 1989

Frith U (ed): Autism and Asperger syndrome. Cambridge, UK, University of Cambridge, 1991

Galaburda AM, Sherman GF, Rosen GD, et al: Developmental dyslexia: four consecutive patients with cortical anomalies. Ann Neurol 18:222–233, 1985

Geschwind N, Galaburda AM: Cerebral lateralization: biological mechanisms, associations, and pathology. Arch Neurol 42:428–459, 521–552, 634–654, 1985

Gillberg C: Asperger syndrome in 23 Swedish children. Dev Med Child Neurol 31:520–531, 1989

Gittelman R, Mannuzza S, Shenker R, et al: Hyperactive boys almost grown up, I: psychiatric status. Arch Gen Psychiatry 42:937–947, 1985

Green WH: Child and Adolescent Clinical Psychopharmacology. Baltimore, MD, Williams & Wilkins, 1991

Gregg N, McAlexander PA: The relation between sense of audience and specific learning disabilities: an exploration. Annals of Dyslexia 39:206–226, 1989

Grossman HJ (ed): Classification in Mental Retardation. Washington, DC, American Association on Mental Deficiency [American Association on Mental Deficiency], 1983

Hagberg BA: Rett syndrome: clinical peculiarities, diagnostic approach, and possible cause. Pediatr Neurol 5:75–83, 1989

Hagberg BA, Witt-Engerstrom I: Rett's syndrome: a suggested staging system for describing the impairment profile with increasing age toward adolescence. Am J Med Genet 24:47–59, 1986

Hare RD, McPherson LM, Forth AE: Male psychopaths and their criminal careers. J Consult Clin Psychol 56:710–714, 1988

Haslam RH, Dalby JT, Johns RD, et al: Cerebral asymmetry in developmental dyslexia. Arch Neurol 38:679–682, 1981

Hauser P, Zametkin AJ, Martinez P, et al: Attention deficit-hyperactivity disorder in people with generalized resistance to thyroid hormone. N Engl J Med 328:997–1001, 1993

Hill AE, Rosenbloom L: Disintegrative psychosis of childhood: teenage follow-up. Dev Med Child Neurol 28:34–40, 1986

Howie VM: Developmental sequelae of chronic otitis media: a review. J Dev Behav Pediatr 1:34–38, 1980

Huesmann LR, Eron LD, Lefkowitz MM, et al: The stability of aggression over time and generations. Developmental Psychology 20:1120–1134, 1984

Hunt RD, Capper L, O'Connell P: Clonidine in child and adolescent psychiatry. Journal of Child and Adolescent Psychopharmacology 1:87–102, 1990

Jagger J, Prusoff BA, Cohen DJ, et al: The epidemiology of Tourette's syndrome: a pilot study. Schizophr Bull 8:267–278, 1982

Johnson AM, Falstein EI, Szurek SA, et al: School phobia. Am J Orthopsychiatry 11:702–711, 1941

Kanner L: Autistic disturbances of affective contact. Nerv Child 2:217–250, 1943

Kazdin AE: Conduct Disorders in Childhood and Adolescence. Newbury Park, CA, Sage, 1987

Kazdin AE, Bass D, Siegel T, et al: Cognitive-behavioral therapy and relationship therapy in the treatment of children referred for antisocial behavior. J Consult Clin Psychol 57:522–535, 1989

Klein RG, Last CG: Anxiety Disorders in Children. Newbury Park, CA, Sage, 1989

Kovacs M, Paulauskas S, Gatsonis C, et al: Depressive disorders in childhood, III: a longitudinal study of comorbidity with and risk for conduct disorders. J Affect Disord 15:205–217, 1988

Kurlan R (ed): Handbook of Tourette's Syndrome and Related Tic and Behavioral Disorders. New York, Marcel Dekker, 1993

Largo RH, Graf S, Kundu S, et al: Predicting developmental outcome at school age from infant tests of normal, at-risk, and retarded infants. Dev Med Child Neurol 32:30–45, 1990

Lavigne JV, Burns WJ, Cotter PD: Rumination in infancy: recent behavioral approaches. International Journal of Eating Disorders 1:70–82, 1981

Leckman JF, Walker DE, Cohen DJ: Premonitory urges in Tourette's syndrome. Am J Psychiatry 150:98–102, 1993

Levine MD: Encopresis: its potentiation, evaluation, and alleviation. Pediatr Clin North Am 29:315–330, 1982

Levine MD, Oberklaid F, Meltzer LJ: Developmental output failure: a study of low productivity in school-aged children. Pediatrics 67:18–25, 1981

Livingston R, Taylor JL, Crawford SL: A study of somatic complaints and psychiatric diagnosis in children. J Am Acad Child Adolesc Psychiatry 27:185–187, 1988

Lou HC, Henriksen L, Bruhn P, et al: Striatal dysfunction in attention deficit and hyperkinetic disorder. Arch Neurol 46:48–52, 1989

Mannuzza S, Gittelman Klein R, Horowitz Konig P, et al: Hyperactive boys almost grown up, IV: criminality and its relationship to psychiatric status. Arch Gen Psychiatry 46:1073–1079, 1989

Marcus J, Hans SL, Mednick SA, et al: Neurological dysfunctioning in offspring of schizophrenics in Israel and Denmark: a replication analysis. Arch Gen Psychiatry 42:753–761, 1985

Martin JAM: Syndrome delineation in communication disorders, in Language and Language Disorders in Childhood. Edited by Hersov LA, Berger M. Oxford, UK, Pergamon Press, 1980

Mazzocco MMM, Hagerman RJ, Cronister-Silverman A, et al: Specific frontal lobe deficits among women with the fragile X gene. J Am Acad Child Adolesc Psychiatry 31:1141–1148, 1992

McGee R, Williams S: A longitudinal study of depression in nine-year-old children. J Am Acad Child Adolesc Psychiatry 27:342–348, 1988

Menolascino FJ, Levitas A, Greiner C: The nature and types of mental illness in the mentally retarded. Psychopharmacol Bull 22:1060–1071, 1986

Millican FK, Layman EM, Lourie RS, et al: Study of an oral fixation: pica. Journal of the American Academy of Child Psychiatry 7:79–107, 1968

Nelson KB, Ellenberg JH: Antecedents of cerebral palsy: multivariate analysis of risk. N Engl J Med 315:81–86, 1986

Nichols PL, Chen T-C: Minimal Brain Dysfunction: A Prospective Study. Hillsdale, NJ, Lawrence Erlbaum, 1981

Parks SL: The assessment of autistic children: a selective review of available instruments. J Autism Dev Disord 13:255–267, 1983

Patterson GR: Coercive Family Processes. Eugene, OR, Castalia, 1982

Paul R, Cohen DJ, Caparulo BK: A longitudinal study of patients with severe developmental disorders of language learning. Journal of the American Academy of Child Psychiatry 22:525–534, 1983

Pauls DL: Genetic factors in the expression of attention-deficit hyperactivity disorder. Journal of Child and Adolescent Psychopharmacology 1:353–360, 1991

Pauls DL, Leckman JF: The inheritance of Gilles de la Tourette's syndrome and associated behaviors. N Engl J Med 315:993–997, 1986

Popper CW: Psychopharmacologic treatment of anxiety disorders in adolescents and children. J Clin Psychiatry 54 (No 5, Suppl): 52–63, 1993

Provence S, Lipton RC: Infants and Institutions. New York, International Universities Press, 1962

Puig-Antich J: Major depression and conduct disorder in prepuberty. Journal of the American Academy of Child Psychiatry 21:118–128, 1982

Raine A, Venables PH, Williams M: Relationships between central and autonomic measures of arousal at age 15 years and criminality at age 24 years. Arch Gen Psychiatry 47:1003–1007, 1990

Raynaud C, Billard C, Tzongrig H, et al: Study of rCBF in developmental dysphasia children at rest and during verbal stimulation. Cerebral Blood Flow Metabolism 1(suppl):S323, 1989

Riddle MA, Nelson JC, Kleinman CS, et al: Sudden death in children receiving Norpramin194: a review of three reported cases and commentary. J Am Acad Child Adolesc Psychiatry 30:104–108, 1991

Rittig S, Knudsen UB, Norgaard JP, et al: Abnormal diurnal rhythm of plasma vasopressin and urinary output in patients with enuresis. Am J Physiol 256:F664–F671, 1989

Robins LN: Deviant Children Grown Up. Baltimore, MD, Williams & Wilkins, 1966

Rourke BP, Strang JD: Subtypes of reading and arithmetic disabilities: a neuropsychological analysis, in Developmental Neuropsychiatry. Edited by Rutter M. New York, Guilford, 1983, pp 473–488

Rumsey JM, Duara R, Grady C, et al: Brain metabolism in autism: resting cerebral glucose utilization rates as measured with positron emission tomography. Arch Gen Psychiatry 42:448–455, 1985a

Rumsey JM, Rapoport JL, Sceery WR: Autistic children as adults: psychiatric, social, and behavioral outcomes. Journal of the American Academy of Child Psychiatry 24:465–473, 1985b

Rutter M, Giller H: Juvenile Delinquency: Trends and Perspectives. New York, Guilford, 1984

Rutter M, Yule W: A Neuropsychiatric Study in Childhood. Suffolk, UK, Lavenhan Press, 1970

Rydelius P-A: The development of antisocial behaviour and sudden violent death. Acta Psychiatr Scand 77:398–403, 1988

Sandman CA: The opiate hypothesis in autism and self-injury. Journal of Child and Adolescent Psychopharmacology 1:237–248, 1991

Satterfield JH, Satterfield BT, Cantwell DP: Three-year multimodality treatment study of 100 hyperactive boys. J Pediatr 98:650–655, 1981

Sauvage D, Leddet I, Hameury L, et al: Infantile rumination: diagnosis and follow-up study of twenty cases. Journal of the American Academy of Child Psychiatry 24:197–203, 1985

Schroeder S, Schroeder C, Smith B, et al: Prevalence of self-injurious behaviors in a large state facility for the retarded: a three-year follow-up study. Journal of Autism and Childhood Schizophrenia 8:261–269, 1979

Shaffer D, Gould MS, Brasic J, et al: A Children's Global Assessment Scale (CGAS). Arch Gen Psychiatry 40:1228–1231, 1983

Sigman M (ed): Children With Emotional Disorders and Developmental Disabilities: Assessment and Treatment. Orlando, FL, Grune & Stratton, 1985

Smith S, Kimberling W, Pennington B, et al: Specific reading disability: identification of an inherited form through linkage analysis. Science 219:1345–1347, 1983

Sparrow SS, Balla DA, Cicchetti DV: Vineland Adaptive Behavior Scales. Circle Pines, MN, American Guidance Service, 1984

Stefl ME: The Ohio Tourette's Study. Cincinnati, OH, University of Cincinnati School of Planning, 1983

Steinhausen H-C, Göbel D: Enuresis in child psychiatric clinic patients. J Am Acad Child Adolesc Psychiatry 28:279–281, 1989

Sukhai RN, Mol J, Harris AS: Combined therapy of enuresis alarm and desmopressin in the treatment of nocturnal enuresis. Eur J Pediatr 148:465–467, 1989

Szatmari P, Bremner R, Nagy J: Asperger's syndrome: a review of clinical features. Can J Psychiatry 34:554–560, 1989

Szymanski LS, Tanguay PE (eds): Emotional Disorders of Mentally Retarded Persons: Assessment, Treatment, and Consultation. Baltimore, MD, University Park Press, 1980

Tallal P: Developmental langauge disorders, in Learning Disabilities: Proceedings of the National Conference. Edited by Kavanagh JF, Truss TJ. Parkton, MD, York, 1988, pp 181–272

Tibbits-Kleber AL, Howell RJ: Reactive attachment disorder of infancy (RAD). Journal of Clinical Child Psychology 14:304–310, 1985

Tizard J, Schofield WN, Hewison J: Collaboration between teachers and parents in assisting children's reading. Br J Educ Psychol 52:1–15, 1982

Tolan PH, Cromwell RE, Brasswell M: Family therapy with delinquents: a critical review of the literature. Fam Process 25:619–650, 1986

Tremblay RE, LeBlanc M, Schwartzman AE: The pediatric power of first-grade peer and teacher ratings of behavior: sex differences in antisocial behavior and personality at adolescence. J Abnorm Child Psychol 16:571–583, 1988

Vandenberg SG, Singer SM, Pauls DL: The Heredity of Behavior Disorders in Adults and Children. New York, Plenum, 1986

Verkerk AJMH, Piereti M, Sutcliffe JS, et al: Identification of a gene (FMR-1) containing a CGG repeat coincident with a breakpoint cluster region exhibiting length variation in fragile X syndrome. Cell 65:396–399, 1991

Voeller KKS: Right-hemisphere deficit syndrome in children. Am J Psychiatry 143:1004–1009, 1986

Weiss G, Hechtman LT: Hyperactive Children Grown Up: Empirical Findings and Theoretical Considerations. New York, Guilford, 1986

Wender PH: The Hyperactive Child, Adolescent, and Adult: Attention Deficit Disorder Through the Lifespan. New York, Oxford University Press, 1987

Wille S: Comparison of desmopressin and enuresis alarm for nocturnal enuresis. Arch Dis Child 61:30–33, 1986

Williams ML, Lewandowski LJ, Coplan J, et al: Neurodevelopmental outcome of preschool children both preterm with and without intracranial hemorrhage. Dev Med Child Neurol 29:243–249, 1987

Wing L: Asperger's syndrome: a clinical account. Psychol Med 11:115–129, 1981

Wolfgang ME, Figlio RM, Cellin T: Delinquency in a Birth Cohort. Chicago, IL, University of Chicago Press, 1972

Woolston JL: Eating disorders in infancy and early childhood. Journal of the American Academy of Child Psychiatry 22:114–121, 1983

CHAPTER 24

Sleep Disorders

Thomas C. Neylan, M.D.
Charles F. Reynolds III, M.D.
David J. Kupfer, M.D.

For the past 25 years the field of sleep medicine has striven to communicate an essential message: the symptoms of insomnia and excessive daytime sleepiness have differential diagnoses and require specific evaluation and interventions. In the DSM-IV (American Psychiatric Association 1994) classification, the sleep disorders are divided into four major headings: primary sleep disorders; sleep disorders related to another mental disorder; sleep disorder due to a general medical condition; and substance-induced sleep disorder (Table 24–1).

■ NORMAL HUMAN SLEEP

The brain has three major states of activity and function: wakefulness, rapid eye movement (REM) sleep, and non-REM sleep. Healthy sleep in humans consists of recurring 70- to 120-minute cycles of non-REM and REM sleep. Typically, sleep progresses from wakefulness through the four stages of non-REM sleep until the onset of the first REM period. In the healthy adult, the deepest stages of sleep, non-REM Stages 3 and 4 (collectively referred to as slow-wave sleep), occur in the first two

Supported in part by National Institute of Health Grants MH00295 (CFR:RSA), MH37869 (CFR), and MH30915 (DJK), and National Institute on Aging Grant AG06836 (CFR).

Table 24–1.   DSM-IV classification of sleep disorders

Primary sleep disorders

Dyssomnias

  Primary insomnia

  Primary hypersomnia

  Narcolepsy

  Breathing-related sleep disorder

  Circadian rhythm sleep disorder (sleep-wake schedule disorder)

    Delayed sleep phase type

    Jet lag type

    Shift work type

    Unspecified

  Dyssomnia not otherwise specified

Parasomnias

  Nightmare disorder (dream anxiety disorder)

  Sleep terror disorder

  Sleepwalking disorder

  Parasomnia not otherwise specified

Sleep disorders related to another mental disorder

Insomnia related to [Axis I or Axis II disorder]

Hypersomnia related to [Axis I or Axis II disorder]

Other sleep disorders

Sleep disorder due to a general medical condition

  Insomnia type

  Hypersomnia type

  Parasomnia type

  Mixed type

Substance-induced sleep disorder

  Insomnia type

  Hypersomnia type

  Parasomnia type

  Mixed type

---

non-REM periods. In contrast, the REM periods in the first half of the sleep period are brief in duration and lengthen in duration in successive cycles.

During wakefulness the EEG is characterized by low-voltage fast activity consisting of a mix of alpha (8 to 13 Hz) and beta (> 13 Hz) frequencies. *Stage 1* of non-REM sleep is a transitional stage between wakefulness and sleep during which the predominant alpha rhythm disappears, giving way to the slower theta (4 to 7 Hz) frequencies. Tonic electromyographic activity decreases, and the eyes move in a slow, rolling pattern. Stage 2 is characterized by a background theta rhythm and the episodic appearance of sleep spindles (i.e., brief bursts of 12- to 14-Hz activity) and K complexes (i.e., a high-amplitude, slow-frequency electronegative wave followed by an electropositive wave). Muscle tone remains diminished, and eye movements are rare. *Stages 3 and 4* are defined as epochs of sleep consisting of greater than 20% and 50%, respectively, of high-amplitude activity in the delta band (0.5 to 3.0 Hz). Muscle tone is nearly atonic, and eye movements are absent. REM sleep is characterized by a low-amplitude, mixed-frequency EEG, rapid eye movements, and absence of muscle tone.

Infants at birth spend up to 20 hours per day asleep. REM and non-REM stages are not fully differentiated until 3 to 6 months of age. During the first 3 years, the sleep-wake rhythm develops from an ultradian to a circadian pattern, with the principal sleep phase occurring at night. Sleep in prepubertal children is characterized by large percentages of REM and high-amplitude slow-wave sleep. During adolescence there is a precipitous drop in slow-wave sleep (Feinberg 1974). In the third through sixth decades there is a gradual and slight decline in sleep efficiency and total sleep time. With advancing age there are more transient arousals and more sleep stage shifts, as well as a gradual disappearance of slow-wave sleep (Gillin and Ancoli-Israel 1992). In addition, the diurnal sleep-wake pattern decays as sleep is redistributed into the light phase in the form of frequent naps (Buysse et al. 1992).

■ CLINICAL MANIFESTATIONS AND EVALUATION OF SLEEP DISORDERS

Disorders of sleep and wakefulness produce a wide spectrum of symptomatology that is related to disrupted or too little sleep, excessive sleepiness, or adverse events associated with the sleep period. A thorough medical and psychiatric history is essential for diagnosing conditions that impact on sleep-wake function. The entire 24-hour time period should be explored with respect to sleep-wake habits. Patients with insomnia should be questioned about their views on what constitutes healthy sleep. Very often patients who by virtue of their constitution are short sleepers are subjectively distressed by their inability to sleep for the popular standard of 8 hours. The severity of insomnia can only be understood in terms of its impact on daytime function such as mood, fatigue, muscle aches, attention, and concentration. A 2-week sleep-wake log is invaluable for obtaining a history of irregular sleep-wake patterns; napping; use of stimulants, hypnotics, or alcohol; diet; activity during the day; number of arousals; and perceived length of sleep time and its relationship to daytime mood and alertness.

Approximately 4% to 5% of the general population complain of excessive sleepiness (Bixler et al. 1979). Sleepiness relates to the propensity to sleep, such as after sleep deprivation. Clinically, it is more alarming than insomnia because of the higher degree of psychosocial impairment as well as the high rate of automobile and occupational accidents (Guilleminault and Carskadon 1977). Patients should be asked about symptoms of morning headaches, cataplexy, hypnagogic/hypnopompic hallucinations, sleep paralysis, automatic behavior, or sleep drunkenness. In addition, they should be questioned carefully about falling asleep while driving or while performing any other potentially dangerous activity. Additional history should be obtained from bedpartners for events usually not perceived by the patients, such as snoring, respiratory pauses longer than 10 seconds, unusual body movements, or somnambulism.

Patients who complain of disturbances associated with the sleep period should be questioned about nocturnal incontinence or polyuria, orthopnea, paroxysmal nocturnal dyspnea, headaches that interrupt sleep, jaw clenching or bruxism, sleep talking, somnambulism, and, in the case of males, painful nocturnal erections (Aldrich 1989).

Polysomnography remains the principal diagnostic tool in the field of sleep medicine. A thorough polysomnographic study provides data on sleep continuity, sleep architecture, REM physiology, sleep-related respiratory impairment, oxygen desaturation, cardiac arrhythmias, and periodic movements. Additional measures may include nocturnal penile tumescence, temperature, and infrared video monitoring.

The Multiple Sleep Latency Test (MSLT; Carskadon et al. 1986) is the most objective and valid measure of excessive sleepiness. In the MSLT the patient is given the opportunity to fall asleep in a darkened room for five 20-minute periods in 2-hour intervals across the patient's usual period of wakefulness. The average latency to sleep onset, measured polysomnographically, is a direct measure of the propensity to fall asleep. An average sleep latency of less than 5 minutes indicates a pathological degree of sleepiness (Carskadon et al. 1981). The detection of sleep-onset REM periods in the MSLT has become a cornerstone in the diagnosis of narcolepsy (Mitler 1982).

■ PRIMARY SLEEP DISORDERS

☐ Dyssomnias

Primary Insomnia

Primary insomnia is the term used to describe difficulty initiating or maintaining sleep, or nonrestorative sleep, lasting at least a month in duration. By definition, primary insomnia results in significant daytime impairment and is not secondary to another sleep disorder. The degree of sleep fragmentation can be externally validated by polysomnography, which shows prolonged sleep latencies, decreased sleep efficiency, and a predominance of the lighter stages of non-REM sleep (Hauri and Olmstead 1980). An overview of the evaluation of chronic insomnia is provided in Figure 24–1.

For some patients, primary insomnia represents a lifetime disorder or trait characteristic in which the patient has a constitutional predisposition for fragmented sleep (Hauri and Olmstead 1980). Other patients develop primary insomnia following a period of severe stress. In these patients the symptoms of insomnia do not remit with the resolution of the stressful event because new behaviors that disrupt sleep have been adapted. For example, some patients develop a form of performance anxiety associated with going to sleep. Their struggles to fall asleep and their anxiety about possible daytime fatigue set up a conditioned association between bedtime behavior and anxious arousal. Often environmental cues in the sleeping environment, such as clocks, become associated and paired with arousal, thus further reinforcing the sleep disturbance.

There are several effective treatment approaches to chronic insomnia that do not involve the use of hypnotics. Education about normal sleep and counseling around habits for promoting good sleep hygiene, such as

Step 1	Evaluate for a general medical condition that may adversely affect sleep.
Step 2	Evaluate if medications or substance use is disrupting sleep.
Step 3	Evaluate if another mental disorder such as depression, schizophrenia, anxiety disorder, etc., is causing sleep disruption.
Step 4	Consider a breathing-related sleep disorder particularly if the patient snores or is obese.
Step 5	Consider a sleep-wake schedule disorder if the patient has an irregular schedule or is involved in shift work.
Step 6	Consider a parasomnia diagnosis if the patient complains of behavioral or mental events that occur during sleep.
Step 7	If insomnia has persisted for over a month and is not related to the above disorders, then the diagnosis is primary insomnia.
Step 8	If insomnia is not described by the above criteria, then the diagnosis of dyssomnia not otherwise specified is used.

Figure 24–1. Evaluation of chronic insomnia. Adapted from Reynolds CF, Buysse DJ, Kupfer DJ: "Disordered Sleep: Developmental and Biopsychosocial Perspectives on the Diagnosis and Treatment of Persistent Insomnia," in *American College of Neuropsychopharmacology: Fourth Generation of Progress.* Edited by Bloom FE, Kupfer DJ. New York, Raven, 1995, pp. 1617–1629.

regular exercise and sleep times, are potentially a sufficient intervention (Hauri 1989). Various relaxation therapies such as hypnosis, meditation, deep breathing, and progressive muscle relaxation can be helpful. These techniques, in contrast to the use of hypnotics, are not immediately beneficial but require several weeks of practice to improve sleep (McClusky et al. 1991). Success is dependent on a high degree of motivation in patients, who must devote considerable time to practicing these techniques. Those who succeed in learning these techniques have a greater satisfaction with maintenance treatment than do patients chronically using hypnotics (Morin et al. 1992).

Stimulus control behavior modification focuses on eliminating environmental cues associated with arousal (Bootzin 1972). This technique is similar to implementing rules for sleep hygiene in that patients are instructed to restrict the use of their bed for sleep and intimacy, to go to bed only when sleepy, to remove clocks from sight, and to adhere to a stable sleep-wake schedule. The goal is to limit the amount of wake time spent in bed, thereby reestablishing the association between the bed and sleep.

Sleep restriction therapy is similarly aimed at reducing the amount of wake time spent in bed (Spielman et al. 1987). Patients are asked to record in a sleep diary the amount of time they estimate they are asleep. They are then instructed to restrict their time in bed to a degree commensurate to their estimate of their total sleep time. Patients often have their usual difficulties with sleep fragmentation during the first few nights and become sleep deprived. Sleep deprivation helps consolidate sleep on subsequent nights, thereby improving sleep efficiency. Increases in length of time in bed can subsequently be titrated to the presence of daytime fatigue.

Chronic use of hypnotics. Very few clinicians dispute that the use of benzodiazepines of short and intermediate half-life in appropriate doses is safe and effective in treating transient insomnia in non–substance-abusing young and middle-age adults. Elderly patients have reduced clearance of hypnotics and hence experience more sedation and cognitive side effects as compared with younger patients (Greenblatt et al. 1991). The use of hypnotics in treating chronic insomnia remains controversial, particularly in elderly patients, and is a subject of considerable debate.

Historically there have always been concerns about hypnotics, many of which were realistic concerns about the potential for overdose and addiction with barbiturates. The introduction of long–half-life benzodiazepines brought about concerns of daytime impairment and memory disturbance (Gillin 1991). Short–half-life benzodiazepines have fewer "hangover" effects (Johnson and Chernik 1982), but there are concerns about daytime anxiety, confusion, and hyperexcitability (Oswald 1989). Rebound insomnia following drug withdrawal, particularly with short–half-life benzodiazepines, is well described and represents an abstinence syndrome (Roehrs et al. 1986).

All benzodiazepines, particularly those with short half-lives, have some potential for addiction. Abrupt withdrawal of any benzodiazepine will cause some degree of rebound anxiety and insomnia (Mendelson 1990), with short–half-life compounds having the greatest effect. However, most patient groups who chronically use benzodiazepines do not escalate the dosages over time (American Psychiatric Association 1990). Further, careful tapering of benzodiazepines, including short–half-life compounds, is effective in eliminating the abstinence syndrome (Greenblatt et al. 1987).

To date there is no hypnotic available that can be used in elderly patients without risk. For example, over-the-counter hypnotics also cause amnesia and daytime sedation at a rate similar to that of prescription hypnotics (Balter and Uhlenhuth 1991). There has been a reemergence of the use of more dangerous sedative-hypnotics as evidenced by the increase in reported overdoses of meprobamate and methaqualone (Hoffman et al. 1991; Weintraub et al. 1991). Trazodone has several advantages as a hypnotic, with its sustained efficacy and its lack of anticholinergic effects (Ware and Pittard 1990); however, it can cause hypotension and increase the risk of falls and fractures. Zolpidem is a short–half-life non-benzodiazepine drug that binds selectively to the type-1 benzodiazepine receptor subtype (Langer et al. 1987). In therapeutic doses it has minimal effects on sleep architecture and does not cause rebound insomnia after discontinuation (Kryger et al. 1991; Merlotti et al. 1989).

The pros and cons of various hypnotics are overviewed in Table 24–2. The guidelines of the National Institutes of Health Consensus Development Conference Statement on the Treatment of Sleep Disorders of Older People (1991) are pertinent. Hypnotics should only be considered after making a thorough diagnostic assessment of secondary causes of insomnia, after improving sleep hygiene, and after attempting behavioral treatments. If these approaches are unsuccessful, then hypnotics can be used, starting with very low doses and limiting use for short periods.

Primary Hypersomnia

Primary hypersomnia is characterized by prolonged nocturnal sleep and severe daytime sleepiness that can be objectively documented by a short mean sleep latency on the MSLT. Primary hypersomnia is a diagnosis of exclusion, made when other disorders causing excessive sleepiness have been ruled out. A recurrent form of primary hypersomnia, Kleine-Levin syndrome, is characterized by intermittent attacks of hypersomnolence

Table 24–2.   Overview of the use of hypnotics in the treatment of elderly patients

Hypnotic	Advantages	Disadvantages
Antidepressants		
Amitriptyline	No tolerance	Anticholinergic delirium, increased risk of falls, daytime sedation
Doxepin	No tolerance	Increased risk of falls, daytime sedation
Trazodone	No tolerance, no anticholinergic effects	Increased risk of falls, daytime sedation
Antipsychotics		
Haloperidol	No tolerance, few anticholinergic effects	Extrapyramidal effects, increased risk of falls, not very sedating
Thioridazine	No tolerance	Extrapyramidal effects, increased risk of falls, anticholinergic delirium
Barbiturates	No pertinent advantages over benzodiazepines	High risk of addiction, dangerous withdrawal syndrome, overdose potential, daytime sedation
Benzodiazepines		
Estazolam	Intermediate half-life	Some daytime sedation and performance decrements
Flurazepam	Delayed rebound insomnia	Daytime sedation, high risk of falls, driving errors
Temazepam	Intermediate half-life	Some daytime sedation and performance decrements
Triazolam	No daytime sedation	Rebound insomnia
Miscellaneous		
Chloral hydrate	Less addictive than benzodiazepines	Overdose potential, tolerance to hypnotic effects over time, nausea
Diphenhydramine	No tolerance	Anticholinergic delirium, increased risk of falls, daytime sedation and memory impairment
Zolpidem	No disruption to sleep architecture, no tolerance	May cause mild daytime performance impairment

and hyperphagia, often associated with indiscrete hypersexuality, poor social judgment, mood disturbance, and hallucinations. Between episodes there can be a complete remission of symptoms. The pathophysiology of primary hypersomnia is postulated to involve an underlying disturbance of limbic and hypothalamic function. Treatment usually involves the use of stimulants for both the hypersomnolence and the increased appetite.

Narcolepsy

Narcolepsy is a common cause of daytime hypersomnolence in which REM sleep repeatedly and suddenly intrudes into wakefulness. It represents an impairment in the ability to maintain a stable neural state: REM is no longer segregated in its usual ultradian rhythm during sleep. The clinical phenomenology of narcolepsy is best understood by a consideration of normal REM physiology (e.g., activated EEG, generalized atonia, dream cognition). Both cataplexy and sleep paralysis involve muscle atonia occurring at a time when the patient is cognizant of the environment and subjectively feels awake. Hypnagogic hallucinations are not well understood but are thought to be related to the dream-like perceptual phenomenon of REM sleep. Nocturnal sleep is characterized by short REM latency and frequent arousals and shifts from non-REM to REM to wakefulness (Rechtschaffen et al. 1963).

Although the term narcolepsy (literally, "sleep seizure") suggests an ictal disorder, the pathophysiology remains unknown. There is convincing evidence of a heritable transmission of the disorder. A canine form of narcolepsy shows an autosomal recessive mode of transmission (Foutz et al. 1979). In humans, there is a close association of the disorder with the human leukocyte antigen (HLA) DR2 and DQw1 haplotypes genetically encoded on chromosome 6 (Juji et al. 1984; Langdon et al. 1986).

Therapeutic approaches include the use of stimulants such as methylphenidate, amphetamine, and pemoline to treat daytime somnolence. REM-suppressing agents such as tricyclic antidepressants and gamma-hydroxybutyrate have been found to control cataplexy. Numerous other medications have been tried and found to have modest benefit such as codeine, propranolol, L-tyrosine, and methysergide (Aldrich 1992). An important nonpharmacological approach is the use of scheduled naps throughout the wake period.

Breathing-Related Sleep Disorder

If evolution had led to the development of a stiff upper airway, the problems of snoring and obstructive apnea would never have occurred. Because it must be flexible for purposes of swallowing and production of speech, the upper airway has an inherent potential for collapse during respiration. To compensate for this vulnerability, there is a complex set of muscles that dilate the upper airway during inspiration. In addition, anatomic factors that affect lumen size (e.g., obesity) and exogenous factors that reduce phasic muscle activity of the upper airway (e.g., sedative-hypnotics [Bonora et al. 1984]) can independently lead to an increased potential for airway collapse.

Although occasionally causing insomnia, sleep apnea is typically an occult disorder that causes daytime somnolence, impaired concentration and intellectual functioning, and morning headaches. It is associated with obesity, loud snoring, systemic and pulmonary hypertension, cardiac arrhythmias, and excessive mortality. It can be caused by an impairment in central respiratory drive (central apnea), intermittent upper airway obstruction (obstructive apnea), or a combination of the two (mixed apnea). Patients with this disorder experience frequent respiratory pauses during sleep associated with oxygen desaturation. The apneic events are terminated by loud gasping, thrashing movements, and EEG arousal.

A variety of behavioral, medical, pharmacological, and surgical treatments are available for sleep apnea. Behavioral approaches include weight loss, abstinence from sedative-hypnotics, and sleep position training (which helps the patient avoid the supine position during sleep) (Cartwright et al. 1991). Mechanical approaches include tongue-retaining devices, orthodontic appliances that advance the mandible (Nakazawa et al. 1992), and nasal continuous positive airway pressure (CPAP) (Figure 24–2). Medical approaches consist of the use of tricyclic antidepressants, particularly protriptyline. Surgical techniques aim to increase the lumen size of the oropharynx and include uvulopalatopharyngoplasty (UPPP), maxillomandibular and hyoid advancement, and chronic tracheostomy (Guilleminault et al. 1989).

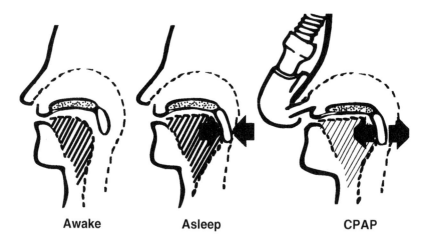

Awake   **Asleep**   **CPAP**

Figure 24–2. Continuous positive airway pressure (CPAP). CPAP prevents collapse of the oropharyngeal airway by providing a pneumatic splint during sleep. Adapted from Sullivan CE, Grunstein RR: "Continuous Positive Airway Pressure in Sleep-Disordered Breathing," in *Principles and Practice of Sleep Medicine,* 2nd Edition. Edited by Kryger MH, Roth T, Dement WC. Philadelphia, PA, WB Saunders, 1994, pp. 694–705.

Circadian Rhythm Sleep Disorder
(Sleep-Wake Schedule Disorder)

The sleep-wake cycle, under the circadian control of endogenous regulators or oscillators, can be disrupted by a misalignment between biological rhythms and external demands on waking behavior. Circadian rhythm sleep disorders present with either insomnia or hypersomnolence, depending on the juxtaposition of performance demands and the underlying circadian cycle, and are associated with significant medical comorbidity and impairment in psychosocial functioning. For example, rotating shift workers have been found to have an injury rate of two to three times that of their co-workers who work stable day, evening, or night shifts (Smith M and Colligan 1982).

Rapid shifts in the sleep-wake schedule cause an acute circadian dysrhythmia. The *jet lag type* is one of the most common of these disorders. Travelers flying across multiple time zones are met with a radical change in the cues, called *Zeitgebers,* that help entrain circadian rhythms with respect to both social schedule and the light-dark cycle. Night shift workers are usually in a state of permanent circadian misalignment because of their tendency to revert to conventional schedules on their days off. Patients with irregular sleep-wake patterns may have little to no circadian rhythmicity to their sleep cycle. For example, some institutionalized patients with dementia have a polyphasic sleep-wake cycle in which brief periods of wakefulness followed by napping persist throughout the 24-hour day.

All of these disorders give rise to sleep-wake complaints, mood disturbance, decreased work performance, and general physical malaise. The general treatment approach is to promote good sleep hygiene with the goal of properly aligning the patients' circadian system with their sleep-wake schedule.

Some circadian sleep-wake disorders are related to a diminished capacity to respond to external Zeitgebers. Congenitally blind subjects, for whom light is ineffective as a Zeitgeber, may have a sleep-wake pattern longer than 24 hours (Miles et al. 1977). Of interest is a report that shows that melatonin administration can entrain a free-running blind subject to a conventional sleep-wake schedule (Sack et al. 1990). Patients with the *delayed sleep phase type* disorder are described as night owls, with an innate preference to begin sleeping in the late hours of night and to sleep until the late morning or early afternoon. They experience sleep-onset insomnia and morning hypersomnolence when forced to comply with a conventional sleep-wake schedule. Treatment involves the realignment of the sleep-wake schedule with manipulation or augmentation of external Zeitgebers such as the use of bright light therapy.

Multiple studies have shown that exposure to light at 2,000 lux or more can shift circadian rhythms (Terman 1989). Much of the literature examining the clinical utility of bright light has focused on seasonal affective disorder (Lewy et al. 1984; Rosenthal et al. 1984). Several investigators have suggested that seasonal affective disorder is a chronobiological disturbance in which the sleep-wake rhythm, as well as other circadian factors, is phase-delayed. (Lewy et al. 1987; Terman et al. 1988). Other studies have shown light therapy to be effective independent of circadian phase or time of day (Wirz-Justice et al. 1993). Bright light has been found to be effective in treating delayed sleep phase disorder (Rosenthal et al. 1990) and jet lag (Daan and Lewy 1984). Further, it has been found to effectively improve alertness and cognitive performance in night shift workers (Czeisler et al. 1990).

Dyssomnia Not Otherwise Specified

The category of dsyssomnia not otherwise specified (NOS) includes the phenomenon of *nocturnal myoclonus,* which is characterized by the occurrence of periodic leg movements of sufficient severity to cause sleep continuity disturbance, leading to complaints of either insomnia or daytime sleepiness. Nocturnal myoclonus consists of repetitive, brief leg jerks that occur in regular 20- to 40-second intervals. These movements are frequently associated with transient arousals that lead to sleep fragmentation and a predominance of the lighter stages of non-REM sleep. Patients are usually unaware of this disorder other than having the experience of morning leg cramps and a sense of insufficient sleep. The most common treatments involve the use of benzodiazepines and L-dopa/carbidopa.

Restless legs syndrome is a syndrome that causes sleep-onset insomnia. It is characterized by the presence of deep paresthesias in the calf muscles, prompting the urge to keep the legs in motion. It is associated with uremia, anemia, pregnancy, as well as nocturnal myoclonus. The main treatment involves the use of either benzodiazepines or dopaminomimetics such as L-dopa and bromocriptine (Montplaisir et al. 1992).

☐ Parasomnias

Parasomnias are adverse events that occur during sleep. Many of these disorders have been described as disorders of partial arousal from various sleep stages (Karacan 1988). *Sleep walking* and *night terrors* are found normally in young children and are associated with psychopathology only if persisting into adulthood. Typically, they involve a partial arousal from sleep during the first third of the night, a period characterized by a predominance of slow-wave sleep. In sleep walking, subjects become partially aroused and ambulatory; they are typically difficult to awaken and have amnesia for the events. Sleep terrors involve an emergence of intense fear associated with autonomic arousal in which patients are inconsolable, difficult to fully awaken, and unable to assign specific cognitions associated with the anxiety. This condition is in contradistinction to *nightmare disorder*, in which anxiety-provoking dreams are characterized by vivid, detailed imagery, associated with good recall. Treatment is directed toward reducing stress, anxiety, and sleep deprivation, all of which are known to exacerbate these disorders. In extreme cases low-dose benzodiazepines are indicated and effective.

REM sleep behavior disorder occurs when there is incomplete or absent muscle atonia during REM sleep. The disorder is characterized by prominent motor activity during dreaming. Several dramatic cases have involved patients who suddenly assaulted their bedpartners in response to frightening dreams. Benzodiazepines, particularly clonazepam, and carbamazepine have been found to be useful in reducing these events (Bamford 1993; Mahowald and Schenk 1989). *Nocturnal paroxysmal dystonia* is characterized by stereotypical and violent movements of the trunk and limbs of short duration. These movements can resemble seizure activity and respond to treatment with carbamazepine (Lugaresi et al. 1986).

. Some parasomnias occur during sleep-wake transitions. Head banging, formerly known as *jactatio capitis nocturnus*, is a rhythmic movement disorder that is thought to be a self-soothing behavior in children during the transition from wakefulness to sleep. Sleep starts, or hypnic jerks, are sudden muscle contractions that often occur during sleep onset and are thought to be clinically insignificant.

■ SLEEP DISORDERS RELATED TO ANOTHER MENTAL DISORDER

☐ Mood Disorders

Sleep disturbance is verifiable in 90% of patients with major depression and is characterized by sleep fragmentation, decreased quantity and altered distribution of delta sleep, reduced duration of the first non-REM period (i.e., REM latency), redistribution of REM sleep into the first half of the night, and increased number of rapid eye movements per minute of REM sleep (Kupfer and Reynolds 1992; Reynolds and Kupfer 1987). Bipolar patients, in contrast, typically become hypersomnolent during depressive episodes and have comparatively increased sleep efficiency and total sleep time (Detre et al. 1972). Manic patients have polysomnographic abnormalities very similar to those of patients with unipolar depression (Hudson et al. 1992).

A review of sleep data from psychiatric patients concluded that no single variable, such as REM latency, has diagnostic specificity (Benca et al. 1992). However, REM latency has been found to be a reliable marker for particular state and trait variables as well as to have value in predicting clinical course and treatment outcome. For example, first-degree relatives of depressed patients with short REM latency have been found to be at increased risk of developing major depression (Giles et al. 1988). REM suppression by clomipramine has been found to predict response to treatment (Höchli et al. 1986). Short REM latency during an index episode of depression confers a higher risk of relapse following clinical remission (Giles et al. 1987; Reynolds et al. 1989b).

Multiple studies have shown that REM latency is related to state-dependent factors in major depression. Giles et al. (1986) found that REM latency helped distinguish endogenous versus nonendogenous depression. Short REM latency was related to appetite loss, terminal insomnia, anhedonia, and unreactive mood. Reynolds et al. showed that subjects with bereavement-related depression had more sleep continuity disturbance and shorter REM latencies than did bereaved subjects without depression (Reynolds et al. 1992). Kupfer et al. (1988) have shown, in one of the few longitudinal studies of sleep in depression, that REM latency is shorter during the earlier phases of relapse in recurrent major depression. Finally, delusional depression is distinguishable from the nondelusional subtype because the former is associated with a higher frequency of sleep-onset REM periods and decreased total REM time (Thase et al. 1986).

☐ Schizophrenia

Schizophrenic patients have been found to have prolonged sleep latencies, sleep fragmentation with multiple arousals, decreased slow-wave sleep, variability in REM latency, and decreased REM rebound after REM sleep deprivation (Ganguli et al. 1987; Keshavan et al. 1990b; Zarcone 1988). Several investigators have attempted to find correlations between clinical features of schizophrenia and specific sleep variables. For example, the variability in REM latency in schizophrenia has been found to be linked to family history of affective disorder (Keshavan et al. 1990a), presence of negative symptoms (Maggini et al. 1987; Tandon et al. 1989), tardive dyskinesia (Thaker et al. 1989), and neuroleptic withdrawal (Neylan et al. 1992; Tandon et al. 1992). Diminished slow-wave sleep is one of the most replicated findings in schizophrenia (Feinberg and Hiatt 1978). It has been found to be associated with poor performance on neuropsychological tests of attention (Orzack et al. 1977) and negative symptoms (Ganguli et al. 1987; Tandon et al. 1989). Studies have shown an inverse relationship between slow-wave sleep and cerebral atrophy as measured by the ventricular brain ratio on computed tomography scans (Benson and Zarcone 1992). Slow-wave sleep has also been found to be correlated with the serotonin metabolite 5-hydroxyindoleacetic acid (5-HIAA) (Benson et al. 1991) and delta sleep–inducing peptide–like immunoreactivity (van Kammen et al. 1992) in cerebrospinal fluid of schizophrenic volunteers.

☐ Anxiety Disorders

Sleep in patients with generalized anxiety disorder is similar to that seen in primary insomnia in that there are prolonged sleep latencies and increased sleep fragmentation. Sleep in patients with anxiety disorders differs from that seen in patients with major depression, with the former exhibiting normal REM latencies and decreased REM percentage (Reynolds et al. 1983).

A report on sleep and panic disorder by Mellman and Uhde (1989) confirmed that panic attacks can arise during non-REM sleep, particularly during transitions from Stage 2 to delta sleep. The mild hypercapnia normally found in sleep may predispose patients to sleep panic, although this hypothesis needs further testing (Mellman and Uhde 1989). Ross et al. (1989) have reviewed what is known about sleep in posttraumatic stress disorder (PTSD). These authors argue that sleep disturbance, particularly disturbing repetitive dreams, may be the essential feature of the disorder. They have suggested that dysfunctional REM sleep physiology may contribute to the pathogenesis of PTSD. Further studies are needed to delineate if intrusive memories of the traumatic event are segregated to any particular sleep stage.

☐ Dementia

Patients with dementia of the Alzheimer's type (DAT) have more sleep fragmentation, less delta and REM sleep (Reynolds 1989; Vitiello and Prinz 1988), and little to no spindle and K-complex activity (Reynolds et al. 1985a; Smirne et al. 1977) in comparison with age-matched control subjects. Vitiello et al. (1992) have suggested that the poor sleep of these patients results from the loss of neurons from areas that participate in the regulation of sleep such as the nucleus basalis of Meynert (McKinney et al. 1982; Sterman and Clemente 1974) and the brain-stem reticular formation (Hirano and Zimmerman 1962). Demented patients have more sleep-related phenomena, such as sundowning and nocturnal wanderings, that provoke attempts to consolidate nocturnal sleep with hypnotics as well as prompt families to institutionalize their elderly relatives (Sanford 1975).

Studies examining the relationship between sleep, aging, and dementia suggest an important relationship between normal sleep-wake function and cognition. Feinberg et al. (1967) suggested that EEG sleep is an indicator of the functional integrity of the cerebral cortex. An important unanswered question is whether sleep loss in aging is related to cognitive impairment, or whether the two emerge secondary to some underlying, independent biological process (Reynolds et al. 1989a). There is evidence that the prevalence of sleep apnea is higher in patients with probable Alzheimer's dementia as compared with age- and sex-matched control subjects. Further, the severity of dementia is correlated with the severity of apnea (Hoch et al. 1986; Reynolds et al. 1985b).

■ SLEEP DISORDER DUE TO A GENERAL MEDICAL CONDITION

Sleep can be adversely affected by multiple medical disorders, particularly those that compromise cardiopulmonary function or cause chronic pain. Endocrine disorders such as diabetes and hyperthyroidism can cause significant sleep continuity disturbance. Hot flashes associated with normal menopause can occur in sleep and cause arousals. Patients may complain of insomnia, hypersomnia, parasomnia, or a combination of symptoms.

□ Sleep and Seizures

Many epileptic patients have their seizures predominantly during sleep or upon arousal from sleep (Janz 1962). The clinical course depends on the type and severity of the seizure disorder. Although complaints of insomnia are unusual, sleep can be sufficiently fragmented to cause daytime hypersomnolence. Unusual nocturnal motor behavior, sleep-related incontinence, or nocturnal tongue biting warrants an evaluation for sleep seizures. Often seizure-related behavior is difficult to distinguish from parasomnias such as enuresis and somnambulism. Family history of either parasomnias or seizure disorder is useful collaborative evidence. Persons who exhibit somnambulism usually have more purposeful motor behavior and are easier to redirect. Finally, an all-night EEG may be needed to screen for epileptiform activity.

□ Sleep and Parkinson's Disease

Sleep disturbance is reported in approximately 75% of patients with Parkinson's disease. These patients' sleep is characterized by an increased number of awakenings, decreased delta and REM sleep, and a scarcity of sleep spindles. The resting tremor usually subsides with the onset of Stage 1 sleep, but, depending on the severity of the disorder, it can persist into Stage 2 or reemerge during sleep stage changes (April

1966). Nigrostriatal degeneration may have a direct or indirect impact on the neural substrate regulating sleep. Dopaminomimetic drugs such as L-dopa have dose-dependent effects on sleep, with lower doses improving sleep quality and higher doses causing decreased sleep efficiency (Bergonzi et al. 1974).

■ SUBSTANCE-INDUCED SLEEP DISORDER

Substance-induced sleep disorder is related to both direct and indirect toxic effects on sleep. Both alcohol and hypnotic-induced sleep disorders involve the development of tolerance to the sleep-inducing effects of the agent, as well as increased arousals during withdrawal periods. Many studies have shown that acute alcohol administration causes REM sleep suppression in the first half of the night followed by a rebound increase of REM sleep and arousals in the second half (Mendelson 1987). Abstinent alcoholic subjects have been shown to have decreased slow-wave sleep and increased sleep stage changes for many months following alcohol withdrawal (Adamson and Burdick 1973).

Stimulants cause sleep-onset insomnia during usage and rebound hypersomnia during withdrawal. Food allergy and toxin-induced sleep disorders presumably involve indirect toxic effects on the physiological substrate regulating sleep. In all of these disorders, careful removal of the offending agent either eliminates the problem or exposes an additional sleep disorder.

■ REFERENCES

Adamson J, Burdick JA: Sleep of dry alcoholics. Arch Gen Psychiatry 28:146–149, 1973

Aldrich MS: Cardinal manifestations of sleep disorders, in Principles and Practice of Sleep Medicine. Edited by Kryger MH, Roth T, Dement WC. Philadelphia, PA, WB Saunders, 1989, pp 313–319

Aldrich MS: Narcolepsy. Neurology 42 (suppl 6):34–43, 1992

American Psychiatric Association: Benzodiazepine Dependence, Toxicity, and Abuse: A Task Force Report of the American Psychiatric Association. Washington, DC, American Psychiatric Association, 1990

American Psychiatric Association: Diagnostic and Statistical Manual of Mental Disorders, 4th Edition. Washington, DC, American Psychiatric Association, 1994

April RS: Observations on parkinsonian tremor in all-night sleep. Neurology (New York) 16:720–724, 1966

Balter MB, Uhlenhuth EH: The beneficial and adverse effects of hypnotics. J Clin Psychiatry 52 (No 7, Suppl): 16–23, 1991

Bamford CR: Carbamazepine in REM sleep behavior disorder. Sleep 16:33–34, 1993

Benca RM, Obermeyer WH, Thisted RA, et al: Sleep and psychiatric disorders: a meta-analysis. Arch Gen Psychiatry 49:651–668, 1992

Benson KL, Zarcone VP: Slow wave sleep and brain structural imaging in schizophrenia. Sleep Research 21:250, 1992

Benson KL, Faull KF, Zarcone VP: Evidence for the role of serotonin in the regulation of slow wave sleep in schizophrenia. Sleep 14:133–139, 1991

Bergonzi P, Chiurulla C, Cianchetti C, et al: Clinical pharmacology as an approach to the study of biochemical sleep mechanisms: the action of L-dopa. Confin Neurol 36:5–22, 1974

Bixler EO, Kales A, Soldatos CR, et al: Prevalence of sleep disorders in the Los Angeles metropolitan area. Am J Psychiatry 136:1257–1262, 1979

Bonora M, Shields G, Knuths S, et al: Selective depression by ethanol of upper airway respiratory motor activity in cats. Am Rev Respir Dis 130:156–161, 1984

Bootzin RR: A stimulus control treatment for insomnia (abstract), in Proceedings of the Annual Meeting of the American Psychological Association. Washington, DC, American Psychological Association, 1972, pp 395–396

Buysse DJ, Browman KE, Monk TH, et al: Napping and 24-hour sleep/wake patterns in healthy elderly and young adults. J Am Geriatr Soc 40:779–786, 1992

Carskadon MA, Harvey K, Dement WC: Sleep loss in young adolescents. Sleep 4:299–312, 1981

Carskadon MA, Dement WC, Mitler MM, et al: Guidelines for the Multiple Sleep Latency Test (MSLT): a standard measure of sleepiness. Sleep 9:519–524, 1986

Cartwright RD, Ristanovic R, Diaz F, et al: A comparative study of treatments for positional sleep apnea. Sleep 14:546–552, 1991

Czeisler CA, Johnson MP, Duffy JF, et al: Exposure to bright light and darkness to treat physiologic maladaptation to night work. N Engl J Med 322:1253–1259, 1990

Daan S, Lewy AJ: Scheduled exposure to daylight: a potential strategy to reduce "jet lag" following transmeridian flight. Psychopharmacol Bull 20:566–568, 1984

Detre T, Himmelhoch J, Swartzburg M, et al: Hypersomnia and manic-depressive disease. Am J Psychiatry 128:1303–1305, 1972

Feinberg I: Changes in sleep cycle patterns with age. J Psychiatr Res 10:283–306, 1974

Feinberg I, Hiatt JF: Sleep patterns in schizophrenia: a selective review, in Sleep Disorders: Diagnosis and Treatment. Edited by Williams RC, Karacan I. New York, Wiley, 1978, pp 205–231

Feinberg I, Koresko RL, Heller N: EEG sleep patterns as a function of normal and pathological aging in man. J Psychiatr Res 5:107–144, 1967

Foutz AS, Mitler MM, Cavalli-Sforza LL, et al: Genetic factors in canine narcolepsy. Sleep 1:413–422, 1979

Ganguli R, Reynolds CF, Kupfer DJ: Electroencephalographic sleep in young, never-medicated schizophrenics: a comparison with delusional and nondelusional depressives and with healthy controls. Arch Gen Psychiatry 44:36–44, 1987

Giles DE, Roffwarg HP, Schlesser MA, et al: Which endogenous depressive symptoms relate to REM latency reduction? Biol Psychiatry 21:473–482, 1986

Giles DE, Jarrett RB, Roffwarg HP, et al: Reduced rapid eye movement latency: a predictor of recurrence in depression. Neuropsychopharmacology 1:33–39, 1987a

Giles DE, Biggs MM, Rush AJ, et al: Risk factors in families of unipolar depression, I: psychiatric illness and reduced REM latency. J Affect Disord 14:51–59, 1988

Gillin JC: The long and the short of sleeping pills. N Engl J Med 324:1735–1737, 1991

Gillin JC, Ancoli-Israel S: The impact of age on sleep and sleep disorders, in Clinical Geriatric Psychopharmacology, 2nd Edition. Edited by Salzman C. Baltimore, MD, Williams & Wilkins, 1992, pp 213–234

Greenblatt DJ, Harmatz JS, Zinny MA, et al: Effect of gradual withdrawal on the rebound sleep disorder after discontinuation of triazolam. N Engl J Med 317:722–728, 1987

Greenblatt DJ, Harmatz JS, Shapiro L, et al: Sensitivity to triazolam in the elderly. N Engl J Med 324:1691–1698, 1991

Guilleminault C, Carskadon M: Relationship between sleep disorders and daytime complaints, in Sleep 1976. Edited by Koeller WP, Oevin PW. Basel, S Karger, 1977, pp 95–100

Guilleminault C, Riley RW, Powell NB: Surgical treatment of obstructive sleep apnea, in Principles and Practices of Sleep Medicine. Edited by Kryger MH, Roth T, Dement WC. Philadelphia, PA, WB Saunders, 1989, pp 571–583

Hauri P: Primary insomnia, in Treatment of Psychiatric Disorders, Vol 3. Washington, DC, American Psychiatric Association, 1989, pp 2424–2433

Hauri P, Olmstead P: Childhood-onset insomnia. Sleep 3:59–65, 1980

Hirano A, Zimmerman H: Alzheimer's neurofibrillary changes: a topographic study. Arch Neurol 7:227, 1962

Hoch CC, Reynolds CF, Kupfer DJ, et al: Sleep-disordered breathing in normal and pathologic aging. J Clin Psychiatry 47:499–503, 1986

Höchli D, Riemann D, Zulley J, et al: Initial REM sleep suppression by clomipramine: a prognostic tool for treatment response in patients with a major depressive disorder. Biol Psychiatry 21:1217–1220, 1986

Hoffman RS, Wipfler MG, Maddaloni MA, et al: How the New York State triplicate benzodiazepine prescription regulation influenced sedative-hypnotic overdoses. N Y State J Med 91:436–439, 1991

Hudson JI, Lipinski JF, Keck PE Jr, et al: Polysomnographic characteristics of young manic patients: comparison with unipolar depressed patients and normal control subjects. Arch Gen Psychiatry 49:378–383, 1992

Janz D: The grand mal epilepsies and the sleeping-waking cycle. Epilepsia 3:69–109, 1962

Johnson LC, Chernik DA: Sedative-hypnotics and human performance. Psychopharmacology (Berlin) 76:101–113, 1982

Juji T, Satake M, Honda Y, et al: HLA antigens in Japanese patients with narcolepsy, Tissue Antigens 24:316–319, 1984

Karacan I: Parasomnias, in Sleep Disorder: Diagnosis and Treatment, 2nd Edition. Edited by Williams RL, Karacan I, Moore CA. New York, Wiley, 1988, pp 131–144

Keshavan MS, Reynolds CF, Ganguli R, et al: EEG sleep in familial subgroups of schizophrenia. Sleep Research 19:330, 1990a

Keshavan MS, Reynolds CF, Kupfer KJ: Electroencephalographic sleep in schizophrenia: a critical review. Compr Psychiatry 31:34–47, 1990b

Kryger MH, Steljes D, Pouliot Z, et al: Subjective versus objective evaluation of hypnotic efficacy: experience with zolpidem. Sleep 14:399–407, 1991

Kupfer DJ, Reynolds CF: Sleep and affective disorders, in Handbook of Affective Disorders, 2nd Edition. Edited by Paykel ES. New York, Guilford, 1992, pp 311–323

Kupfer DJ, Frank E, Grochocinski VJ, et al: Electroencephalographic sleep profiles in recurrent depression: a longitudinal investigation. Arch Gen Psychiatry 45:678–681, 1988

Langdon N, Lock C, Welsh K, et al: Immune factors in narcolepsy. Sleep 9:143–148, 1986

Langer SZ, Arbilla S, Scatton B, et al: Receptors involved in the mechanism of action of zolpidem, in Imidazopyridines in Sleep Disorders: A Novel Experimental and Therapeutic Approach. Edited by Sauvanet JP, Langer SZ, Morselli PL. New York, Raven, 1987, pp 55–72

Lewy AJ, Sack RA, Singer CL: Assessment and treatment of chronobiologic disorders using plasma melatonin levels and bright light exposure: the clock-gate model and the phase response curve. Psychopharmacol Bull 20:561–565, 1984

Lewy AJ, Sack RA, Miller S, et al: Antidepressant and circadian phase-shifting effects of light. Science 235:352–354, 1987

Lugaresi E, Cirignotta F, Montagna P: Nocturnal paroxysmal dystonia. J Neurol Neurosurg Psychiatry 49:375–380, 1986

Maggini C, Guazzeli M, Ciapparelli A: All-night sleep abnormalities in schizophrenia, in Schizophrenia: A Psychobiological View. Edited by Casacchia M, Rossi A. Dordrecht, The Netherlands, Kluwer Academic Publishers, 1987, pp 125–136

Mahowald MW, Schenck CH: REM sleep behavior disorder, in Principles and Practices of Sleep Medicine. Edited by Kryger MH, Roth T, Dement WC. Philadelphia, PA, WB Saunders, 1989, pp 389–409

McClusky HY, Milby JB, Switzer PK, et al: Efficacy of behavioral versus triazolam treatment in persistent sleep-onset insomnia. Am J Psychiatry 148:121–126, 1991

McKinney M, Hedreen C, Coyle JT: Cortical cholinergic innervation: implications for the pathophysiology and treatment of Alzheimer's Disease, in Alzheimer's Disease: A Report of Progress in Research. Edited by Corkin S, Davis K, Crowden J, et al. New York, Raven, 1982, pp 259–265

Mellman TA, Uhde TW: Electroencephalographic sleep in panic disorder: a focus on sleep-related panic attacks. Arch Gen Psychiatry 46:178–184, 1989

Mendelson WB: Human Sleep: Research and Clinical Care. New York, Plenum, 1987

Mendelson WB: Hypnotics in the treatment of chronic insomnia, in Handbook of Sleep Disorders. Edited by Thorpy MJ. New York, Marcel Dekker, 1990, pp 737–753

Merlotti L, Roehrs T, Koshorek G, et al: The dose effects of zolpidem on the sleep of healthy normals. J Clin Psychopharmacol 9:9–14, 1989

Miles LM, Raynal DM, Wilson MA: Blind man living in normal society has circadian rhythms of 24.9 hours. Science 198:421–423, 1977

Mitler MM: The multiple sleep latency test as an evaluation for excessive somnolence, in Disorders of Sleeping and Waking: Indications and Techniques. Edited by Guilleminault C. Menlo Park, CA, Addison-Wesley, 1982, pp 145–153

Montplaisir J, Lapierre O, Warnes H, et al: The treatment of the restless leg syndrome with or without periodic leg movements in sleep. Sleep 15:391–395, 1992

Morin CM, Gaulier B, Barry T, et al: Patients' acceptance of psychological and pharmacological therapies for insomnia. Sleep 15:302–305, 1992

Nakazawa Y, Sakamoto T, Yasutake R, et al: Treatment of sleep apnea with prosthetic mandibular advancement (PMA). Sleep 15:499–504, 1992

National Institutes of Health Consensus Development Conference Statement: the treatment of sleep disorders of older people (March 26–28, 1990). Sleep 14:169–177, 1991

Neylan TC, van Kammen DP, Kelley ME, et al: Sleep in schizophrenic patients on and off haloperidol therapy: clinically stable vs relapsed patients. Arch Gen Psychiatry 49:643–649, 1992

Orzack MH, Hartmann EL, Kornetsky C: The relationship between attention and slow-wave sleep in chronic schizophrenia. Psychopharmacol Bull 13(2):59–61, 1977

Oswald I: Triazolam syndrome 10 years on. Lancet 2:451–452, 1989

Rechtschaffen A, Wolpert EA, Dement WC, et al: Nocturnal sleep of narcoleptics. Electroencephalogr Clin Neurophysiol 15:599–609, 1963

Reynolds CF: Sleep in dementia, in Principles and Practices of Sleep Medicine. Edited by Kryger MH, Roth T, Dement WC. Philadelphia, PA, WB Saunders, 1989, pp 415–416

Reynolds CF, Kupfer DJ: Sleep research in affective illness: state of the art circa 1987. Sleep 10:199–215, 1987

Reynolds CF, Shaw DH, Newton TF, et al: EEG sleep in outpatients with generalized anxiety: a preliminary comparison with depressed outpatients. Psychiatry Res 8:81–89, 1983

Reynolds CF, Kupfer DJ, Taska LS, et al: EEG sleep in elderly depressed, demented, and healthy subjects. Biol Psychiatry 20:431–442, 1985a

Reynolds CF, Kupfer DJ, Taska LS, et al: Sleep apnea in Alzheimer's dementia: correlation with mental deterioration. J Clin Psychiatry 46:257–261, 1985b

Reynolds CF, Hoch CC, Monk TH: Sleep and chronobiologic disturbances in late life, in Geriatric Psychiatry. Edited by Busse EW, Blazer DG. Washington, DC, American Psychiatric Press, 1989a, pp 475–488

Reynolds CF, Perel JM, Frank E, et al: Open-trial maintenance nortriptyline in geriatric depression: survival analysis and preliminary data on the use of REM latency as a predictor of recurrence. Psychopharmacol Bull 25:129–132, 1989b

Reynolds CF, Hoch CC, Buysse DJ, et al: Electroencephalographic sleep in spousal bereavement and bereavement-related depression of late life. Biol Psychiatry 31:69–82, 1992

Reynolds CF, Buysse DJ, Kupfer DJ: Disordered sleep: developmental and biopsychosocial perspectives on the diagnosis and treatment of persistent insomnia, in American College of Neuropsychopharmacology: Fourth Generation of Progress. Edited by Bloom FE, Kupfer DJ. New York, Raven, 1995, pp 1617–1629

Roehrs T, Jorick NJ, Wittig RM, et al: Dose determinants of rebound insomnia. Br J Clin Pharmacol 22:143–147, 1986

Rosenthal NE, Sack DA, Gillin JC, et al: Seasonal affective disorder: a description of the syndrome and preliminary findings with light therapy. Arch Gen Psychiatry 41:72–80, 1984

Rosenthal NE, Joseph-Vanderpool JR, Levendosky AA, et al: Phase-shifting effects of bright morning light as treatment for delayed sleep phase syndrome. Sleep 13:354–361, 1990

Ross RJ, Ball WA, Sullivan KA, et al: Sleep disturbance as the hallmark of posttraumatic stress disorder. Am J Psychiatry 146:697–707, 1989

Sack RL, Stevenson J, Lewy AJ: Entrainment of a previously free-running blind human with melatonin administration. Sleep Research 19:80, 1990

Sanford JRA: Tolerance of debility in elderly dependants by supporters at home: its significance for hospital practice. BMJ 3:471–473, 1975

Smirne S, Come G, Franceschi M, et al: Sleep in presenile dementia, in Communications in EEG. International Federation of Societies for Electroencephalography and Clinical Neurophysiology, 9th Congress. 1977, E271, pp 521–522

Smith M, Colligan M: Health and safety consequences of shift work in the food processing industry. Ergonomics 25:133–144, 1982

Spielman A, Saskin P, Thorpy M: Treatment of chronic insomnia by restriction of time in bed. Sleep 10:45–56, 1987

Sterman MB, Clemente CD: Forebrain mechanisms for the onset of sleep, in Basic Sleep Mechanisms. Edited by Petre-Quadens O, Schlag JD. New York, Academic, 1974, pp 83–97

Sullivan CE, Grunstein RR: Continuous positive airway pressure in sleep-disordered breathing, in Principles and Practice of Sleep Medicine, 2nd Edition. Edited by Kryger MH, Roth T, Dement WC. Philadelphia, PA, WB Saunders, 1994, pp 694–705

Tandon R, Shipley JE, Eiser AS, et al: Association between abnormal REM sleep and negative symptoms in schizophrenia (letter). Psychiatry Res 27:359–361, 1989

Tandon R, Shipley JE, Taylor S, et al: Electroencephalographic sleep abnormalities in schizophrenia: relationship to positive/negative symptoms and prior neuroleptic treatment. Arch Gen Psychiatry 49:185–194, 1992

Terman M: Light therapy, in Principles and Practices of Sleep Medicine. Edited by Kryger MH, Roth T, Dement WC. Philadelphia, PA, WB Saunders, 1989, pp 717–722

Terman M, Terman JS, Quitkin FM, et al: Response of the melatonin cycle to phototherapy for seasonal affective disorder. J Neural Transm 72:147–165, 1988

Thaker GK, Wagman AM, Kirkpatrick B, et al: Alterations in sleep polygraphy after neuroleptic withdrawal: a putative supersensitive dopaminergic mechanism. Biol Psychiatry 25:75–86, 1989

Thase ME, Kupfer DJ, Ulrich RF: Electroencephalographic sleep in psychotic depression: a valid subtype? Arch Gen Psychiatry 43:886–893, 1986

van Kammen DP, Widerlov E, Neylan TC, et al: Delta sleep-inducing-peptide–like immunoreactivity (DSIP-LI) and delta sleep in schizophrenic volunteers. Sleep 15:519–525, 1992

Vitiello MV, Prinz PN: Aging and sleep disorders, in Sleep Disorders: Diagnosis and Treatment, 2nd Edition. Edited by Williams RL, Karacan I, Moore CA. New York, Wiley, 1988, pp 293–312

Vitiello MV, Bliwise DL, Prinz PN: Sleep in Alzheimer's disease and the sundown syndrome. Neurology 42 (suppl 6):83–94, 1992

Ware JC, Pittard JT: Increased deep sleep after trazodone use: a double-blind placebo-controlled study in healthy young adults. J Clin Psychiatry 51 (No 9, Suppl):18–22, 1990

Weintraub M, Singh S, Byrne L, et al: Consequences of the 1989 New York State triplicate benzodiazepine regulations. JAMA 266:2392–2397, 1991

Wirz-Justice A, Graw P, Kräuchi K, et al: Light therapy in seasonal affective disorder is independent of time of day or circadian phase. Arch Gen Psychiatry 50:929–937, 1993

Zarcone VP Jr: Sleep and schizophrenia, in Sleep Disorders: Diagnosis and Treatment, 2nd Edition. Edited by Williams RL, Karacan I, Moore CA. New York, Wiley, 1988, pp 165–188

Eating Disorders: Anorexia Nervosa, Bulimia Nervosa, and Obesity

Katherine A. Halmi, M.D.

The eating disorders *anorexia nervosa* and *bulimia nervosa,* and the condition of *obesity* have been known since earliest times in Western civilization. The eating disorders are entities or syndromes and not specific diseases with a common cause, course, and pathology. They are best conceptualized as syndromes and are therefore classified on the basis of the clusters of symptoms with which they present.

■ PHYSIOLOGY AND BEHAVIORAL PHARMACOLOGY OF EATING

A major conceptual revision for understanding the physiology and behavior of eating has expanded the dual-center theory of hypothalamic facilitatory and inhibitory centers for eating. The sensitive hypothalamic eating centers are part of a broad complex of neuroregulator interactions that includes a peripheral satiety system (gastrointestinal and pancreatic hormones released by food passing through the gastrointestinal tract) and a broad neural network affecting feeding within the brain. Eating behavior is now known to reflect an interaction between an organism's physiological state and environmental conditions. Salient physiological variables include the balance of various neuropeptides and neurotransmitters, metabolic state, metabolic rate, condition of the gastrointestinal tract, amount of storage tissue, and sensory receptors for taste and smell. Environmental conditions include features of the food such as taste, texture, novelty, accessibility, and nutritional composition, and other external conditions such as ambient temperature, presence of other people, and stress (Blundell and Hill 1986). It is important to remember that when an exogenous agent such as a drug or peptide is given to an animal or human, it does not simply activate a specific set of receptors that induce specific responses, but intervenes into a complex transactional fabric (Blundell and Hill 1986).

☐ Neurotransmitters—Biogenic Amines

The study of catecholaminergic pathways in the hypothalamus by Leibowitz and associates led to the discovery of the role of alpha$_2$-adrenergic receptors (α_2) in the paraventricular nucleus (PVN) and the beta$_2$-adrenergic receptors (β_2) in the perifornical hypothalamus (PFH) in feeding (Leibowitz 1980). Microinjection of α_2 agonists to the PVN produces hyperphagia and causes a preferential ingestion of carbohydrate. This adrenergic β_2-responsive circuit in the PFH inhibits feeding.

Serotonin, an indoleamine, has been demonstrated to facilitate satiety (Hoebel 1977) and may at least in part control the intake of carbohydrate (Wurtman and Wurtman 1979). Serotonin injected peripherally and centrally into the PVN suppresses deprivation-induced and norepinephrine-induced eating (Leibowitz 1980). Low doses of dopamine and dopamine agonist stimulate feeding, whereas higher doses inhibit feeding (Leibowitz 1980). There is evidence of increased hypothalamic dopamine turnover during feeding, suggesting that central dopaminergic mechanisms mediate the rewarding effects of food as they mediate the rewarding effects of intracranial self-stimulation and the self-stimulation of psychoactive drugs.

☐ Peptides and Opioids

Corticotropin-releasing factor (CRF) acts within the PVN to inhibit feeding. Norepinephrine seems to inhibit the CRF inhibitory feeding effect. The pancreatic polypeptide neuropeptide Y increases both food and water intake when injected into the PVN. Another pancreatic polypeptide, peptide YY, is a more potent stimulator of feeding than neuropeptide Y (Morley and Levine 1985).

Opioid antagonism decreases feeding in many species but has no effect in reducing food intake in other species. Under some physiological conditions, such as starving or insulin-induced hypoglycemia, naloxone fails to inhibit feeding. Stress-induced eating is probably driven by activation of the opioid system. Dynorphin, an endogenous kappa opioid receptor ligand, enhances feeding. Again the major site of action for dynorphin appears to be the PVN (Morley and Levine 1985).

☐ Peripheral Satiety Network

Several peptides are released by ingested food from the gastrointestinal tract. Some of these inhibit feeding by activating ascending vagal fibers. Cholecystokinin (CCK) is the most extensively studied of these peptides. Its effects, mediated by vagal fibers, have been traced to the PVN of the hypothalamus, where lesions will abolish CCK's effect on feeding. Low doses of CCK infused into the PVN attenuate feeding, and central infusions of CCK antibodies enhance feeding. There is variability of the potency of the satiety effect of CCK across various animal species. Other peptides that appear to inhibit feeding via vagal fibers are glucagon, somatostatin, and thyrotropin-releasing hormone.

■ ANOREXIA NERVOSA

Anorexia nervosa is a disorder characterized by preoccupation with body weight and food, behavior directed toward losing weight, peculiar patterns of handling food, weight loss, intense fear of gaining weight, disturbance of body image, and amenorrhea. Criteria from DSM-IV (American Psychiatric Association 1994) for anorexia nervosa are contained in Table 25–1.

☐ Clinical Features

Anorexic individuals typically express an intense fear of gaining weight, tend to be preoccupied with thoughts of food, and irrationally worry about fatness. Denial of their own clearly observable symptoms is characteristic of anorexic patients. They frequently look in mirrors to make sure they are thin and incessantly express concern about looking fat and feeling flabby.

Anorexic patients fear that they are gaining weight exists even in the face of increasing cachexia, and these individuals characteristically display disinterest in and even resistance to treatment. Anorexic patients lose weight by drastically reducing their total food intake and disproportionately decreasing the intake of high carbohydrate and fatty foods. Some anorexic persons will develop rigorous exercising programs, and others will simply be as active as possible at all times. Self-induced vomiting, laxatives, and diuretic abuse are other purging behaviors by which anorexic individuals attempt to lose weight. Persons with anorexia have a disturbance in the way in which they experience their body weight and

---

Table 25–1. DSM-IV diagnostic criteria for anorexia nervosa

A. Refusal to maintain body weight at or above a minimally normal weight for age and height (e.g., weight loss leading to maintenance of body weight less than 85% of that expected; or failure to make expected weight gain during period of growth, leading to body weight less than 85% of that expected).

B. Intense fear of gaining weight or becoming fat, even though underweight.

C. Disturbance in the way in which one's body weight or shape is experienced; undue influence of body weight or shape on self-evaluation, or denial of the seriousness of current low body weight.

D. In postmenarchal females, amenorrhea, i.e., the absence of at least three consecutive menstrual cycles. (A woman is considered to have amenorrhea if her periods occur only following hormone, e.g., estrogen, administration.)

Specify type:

Restricting type: During the episode of anorexia nervosa, the person has not regularly engaged in binge-eating or purging behavior (i.e., self-induced vomiting or the misuse of laxatives, diuretics, or enemas).

Binge eating/purging type: During the current episode of anorexia nervosa, the person has regularly engaged in binge-eating or purging behavior (i.e., self-induced vomiting or the misuse of laxatives, diuretics, or enemas).

---

shape. They often fail to recognize that their degree of emaciation is dangerous. Their cognition is so distorted that they judge their self-worth predominantly by body shape and weight.

Obsessive-compulsive behavior often develops after the onset of anorexia nervosa. An obsession with cleanliness, an increase in house cleaning activities, and a more compulsive approach to studying are not uncommonly observed in these patients. Amenorrhea can appear before noticeable weight loss has occurred. Poor sexual adjustment is frequently present in anorexic patients. Many adolescent anorexic patients have delayed psychosocial sexual development, and adults often have a markedly decreased interest in sex with the onset of anorexia nervosa.

Anorexia nervosa patients can be subdivided into those who binge and purge and those who merely restrict food intake in order to lose weight. There is a relatively frequent association with impulsive behavior such as suicide attempts, self-mutilation, stealing, and substance abuse (including alcohol abuse) in the bulimic anorexic patients, who are also less likely to be regressed in their sexual activity, and in fact may be promiscuous. Bulimic anorexic patients are more likely to have discrete personality disorder diagnoses (Halmi 1987).

Most of the physiological and metabolic changes in anorexia nervosa are secondary to the starvation state or purging behavior, and include abnormalities in hematopoiesis, such as leukopenia and relative lymphocytosis, in acutely emaciated anorexic patients. Anorexia nervosa patients who engage in self-induced vomiting or who abuse laxatives and diuretics are liable to develop hypokalemic alkalosis. These patients often have elevated serum bicarbonate, hypochloremia, and hypokalemia. Patients with electrolyte disturbances have physical symptoms of weakness, lethargy, and, at times, cardiac arrhythmias. The latter condition may threaten sudden cardiac arrest, a not infrequent cause of death in patients who purge. Elevation of serum enzymes reflects fatty degeneration of the liver and is observed both in the emaciated anorexic phase and during refeeding. Elevated serum cholesterol levels tend to occur more frequently in younger patients.

☐ Epidemiology, Course, and Prognosis

The incidence of anorexia nervosa has increased in the past 30 years both in the United States and in Western Europe. In Monroe County, New York, an average annual incidence rate of 0.35 per 100,000 population in the 1960s increased to 0.64 per 100,000 in the 1970s (Jones et al. 1980). In London, the prevalence of anorexia nervosa was one severe case in about 200 girls ages 12 to 18 in the 1970s (Crisp et al. 1976). The most recent incidence study in northeastern Scotland found four cases of anorexia nervosa per 100,000 population per annum (Szmukler 1985). Only 4% to 6% of the anorexia nervosa population are males (Halmi 1974).

The course of anorexia nervosa varies from a single episode with weight and psychological recovery, to nutritional rehabilitation with relapses, to an unremitting course resulting in death. Two of the most methodologically satisfying long-term follow-up studies have shown a death rate of 6.6% at 10 years after a well-defined treatment program and a death rate of 18% at 30 years follow-up (Halmi et al. 1991; Theander 1970).

☐ Etiology and Pathogenesis

A specific etiology and pathogenesis leading to the development of anorexia nervosa are unknown. Anorexia nervosa begins after a period of severe food deprivation, which may be due to

1. Willful dieting for the purpose of being more attractive
2. Willful dieting for the purpose of being more professionally competent (e.g., ballet dancers, gymnasts, jockeys)
3. Food restriction secondary to severe stress
4. Food restriction secondary to severe illness and/or surgery
5. Involuntary starvation

The psychological theories concerning the causes of anorexia have centered mostly on phobic mechanisms and psychodynamic formulations. Crisp (1967) postulated that anorexia nervosa constitutes a phobic avoidance response to food resulting from the sexual and social tension generated by the physical changes associated with puberty. Psychodynamic theories have focused on fantasies of oral impregnation and dependent seductive relationships with warm, passive fathers and guilt over aggression toward ambivalently regarded mothers.

A cognitive and perceptual developmental defect was postulated by Bruch (1962) as the cause of anorexia nervosa. She described the disturbances of body image (i.e., denial of emaciation), disturbances in perception, (i.e., lack of recognition or denial of fatigue, weakness, hunger), and a sense of ineffectiveness as being caused by untoward learning experiences.

Russell (1969) suggested that the amenorrhea may be caused by a primary disturbance of hypothalamic function, and that the full expression of this disturbance is induced by psychological stress. Further support for the theory of disturbed hypothalamic function in anorexia nervosa comes from recent neurotransmitter studies. The increased cortisol production present in anorexia nervosa has recently been traced to the hypothalamus. Two groups of investigators (Gold et al. 1986; Hotta et al. 1986) have shown that anorexic patients have increased CRF in their cerebrospinal fluid (CSF), which probably means that increased CRF production from the hypothalamus is causing the cortisol changes observed in anorexia.

Although there are serious methodological problems in assessing neurotransmitter function in the brain in humans, preliminary indirect studies indicate that there is probably a dysregulation of all three of these neurotransmitters. Kaye et al. (1984a) have shown a decreased serotonin turnover in bulimic anorexic patients compared with restricting anorexic patients. In addition, Kaye et al. (1984b) have found low CSF norepinephrine levels in long-term anorexic patients who have obtained a weight within at least 15% of their normal weight range. Neuropeptide Y, a powerful endogenous stimulant of eating behavior in the central nervous system, was found to be significantly elevated in the CSF of emaciated anorexic patients (Kaye et al. 1990).

Family studies of anorexia nervosa have shown a tendency to familial occurrence of this disorder and a high association with affective disorder. Theander (1970) calculated the morbidity risk for a sister of an anorexic patient to be 6.6%, which greatly exceeds normal expectation. In 30 female twin pair studies in London, 9 out of 16 of the monozygotic and 1 out of 14 of the dizygotic pairs were concordant for anorexia nervosa (Holland et al. 1984). In a later expansion of this study, Holland et al. (1988) concluded that their data indicated a genetic predisposition that could become manifest under adverse conditions, such as inappropriate dieting or emotional stress. Other family studies have shown an increased frequency of affective disorder in the first-degree relatives of the anorexic probands compared with the first-degree relatives of normal control subjects. In two controlled studies there was no higher prevalence of eating disorder in the first-degree relatives of probands with affective disorder. This suggests that an independent predisposition to anorexia must be superimposed on a predisposition to affective disorder for anorexia nervosa to be manifest. Strober et al. (1985) found increased rates of anorexia nervosa, bulimia nervosa, and subclinical anorexia nervosa in first- and second-degree relatives of anorexic probands compared with the relatives of nonanorexic psychiatrically ill control probands. He proposed that the pattern of familial clustering of these disorders represents variable expressions of a common underlying psychopathology.

☐ Treatment

A multifaceted treatment endeavor with medical management and behavioral, individual, cognitive, and family therapy is necessary to treat anorexia nervosa. The immediate treatment aim should be to restore the patient's nutritional state to normal. Mere emaciation or the state of being mildly underweight (15% to 25%) can cause irritability, depression, preoccupation with food, and sleep disturbance. Outpatient therapy as an initial approach has the best chance for success in anorexic patients who 1) have had the illness for less than 6 months, 2) are not bingeing and vomiting, and 3) have parents who are likely to cooperate and effectively participate in family therapy.

The more severely ill anorexic patient may present an extremely difficult medical-management challenge and should be hospitalized, with daily monitoring of weight, food, and calorie intake and of urine output. In the patient who is vomiting, frequent assessment of serum electrolytes is necessary.

Behavior therapy can be used in both outpatient and inpatient settings. The operant conditioning paradigm has been the most effective form of behavior therapy for the treatment of anorexia nervosa. This approach can be used both in the context of a structured ward milieu setting and in an individualized treatment program set up after a behavioral analysis of the patient is completed. Positive reinforcements are used, consisting of increased physical activity, visiting privileges, and social activities contingent on weight gain. An individual behavioral analysis may show other positive reinforcements to be more clinically relevant in a particular case. In addition to effectively inducing weight gain, behavior therapy can be used to stop vomiting. A response-prevention technique is used when bingeing and purging patients are required to stay in an observed dayroom area for 2 to 3 hours after every meal. Very few patients vomit in front of other people, and thus the emesis response is prevented and, after a period of time, extinguished.

Cognitive therapy techniques for treating anorexia nervosa were developed by Garner and Bemis (1982). The assessment of cognition is a first step in cognitive therapy. Patients are asked to write down their thoughts on an assessment form so that cognitions can be examined for systematic distortions in the processing and interpretation of events.

A family analysis should be done on all anorexic patients who are living with their families. On the basis of this analysis a clinical judgment should be made as to what type of family therapy or counseling is clinically advisable. A controlled family therapy study by Russell et al. (1987) showed that anorexic patients under the age of 18 benefited from family therapy, whereas patients over the age of 18 did worse in family therapy compared with the control therapy.

Drugs can be useful adjuncts in the treatment of anorexia nervosa. The first drug used in treating anorexic patients was chlorpromazine, which is especially effective in the severely obsessive-compulsive anorexic patients. Another category of drugs frequently used in the treatment of anorexia nervosa is the antidepressants. A study in which 72 anorexic patients were randomly assigned to amitriptyline, cyproheptadine (an antihistaminic drug), and placebo showed that both cyproheptadine and amitriptyline had a marginal effect in decreasing the number of days necessary to achieve a normal weight (Halmi et al. 1986). With the bulimic subgroups of anorexic patients, cyproheptadine had a negative effect compared with both placebo and amitriptyline. This differential effect within the bulimic anorexic subgroups indicates an actual medical distinction and appears to justify this subgrouping. Cyproheptadine has the advantage of not having the tricyclic antidepressant side effects of reducing blood pressure and increasing heart rate. This characteristic makes this drug especially attractive for use in emaciated anorexic patients.

■ BULIMIA

Bulimia is merely a term that means binge eating. This is a behavior that has become a common practice among female students in universities and, more recently, in high schools. Not all persons who engage in binge eating require a psychiatric diagnosis. Bulimia can occur in anorexia nervosa, and when that happens the patient, under the DSM-IV system, should have a diagnosis of *anorexia nervosa—binge eating/purging type*. Bulimia can also occur in a normal weight condition associated with psychological symptomatology. In that case, a diagnosis of bulimia nervosa will apply (Table 25–2). Normal-weight bingeing and purging patients can fall into two categories: 1) normal-weight bulimic patients who have never had a previous history of anorexia nervosa, and 2) those who have had a previous history of anorexia nervosa.

Bulimia nervosa is a disorder in which the behavior of bulimia or binge eating is the predominant behavior. Abdominal pain or discomfort, self-induced vomiting, sleep, or social interruption terminates the bulimic episode, which is followed by feelings of guilt, depression, or self-disgust. Bulimic patients often use cathartics for weight control and have an eating pattern of alternate binges and fasts. Bulimic patients have a fear of not being able to stop eating voluntarily. Frequent weight fluctuations occur, but without the severity of weight loss present in anorexia nervosa.

Bulimia is also encountered in the newly defined *binge-eating disorder* (BED), which did not exist in DSM-III-R (American Psychiatric Association 1987). This disorder is listed as an example under the category of "Eating Disorders—Not Otherwise Specified" (Tables 25–3 and 25–4).

Table 25–2.   DSM-IV diagnostic criteria for bulimia nervosa

A. Recurrent episodes of binge eating. An episode of binge eating is characterized by both of the following:

1. Eating, in a discrete period of time (e.g., within any 2-hour period), an amount of food that is definitely larger than most people would eat during a similar period of time and under similar circumstances

2. A sense of lack of control over eating during the episode (e.g., a feeling that one cannot stop eating or control what or how much one is eating)

B. Recurrent inappropriate compensatory behavior in order to prevent weight gain, such as self-induced vomiting; misuse of laxatives, diuretics, enemas, or other medications; fasting; or excessive exercise.

C. The binge eating and inappropriate compensatory behaviors both occur, on average, at least twice a week for 3 months.

D. Self-evaluation is unduly influenced by body shape and weight.

E. The disturbance does not occur exclusively during episodes of anorexia nervosa.

Specify type:

Purging type: During the current episode of bulimia nervosa, the person has regularly engaged in self-induced vomiting or the misuse of laxatives, diuretics, or enemas.

Nonpurging type: During the current episode of bulimia nervosa, the person has used other inappropriate compensatory behaviors, such as fasting or excessive exercise, but has not regularly engaged in self-induced vomiting or the misuse of laxatives, diuretics, or enemas.

Table 25–3.   DSM-IV diagnostic criteria for eating disorder not otherwise specified

---

This category is for disorders of eating that do not meet the criteria for any specific eating disorder. Examples include

1.   For females, all of the criteria for anorexia nervosa are met except that the individual has regular menses.

2.   All of the criteria for anorexia nervosa are met except that, despite significant weight loss, the individual's current weight is in the normal range.

3.   All of the criteria for bulimia nervosa are met except that the binge eating and inappropriate compensatory mechanisms occur at a frequency of less than twice a week or for a duration of less than 3 months.

4.   The regular use of inappropriate compensatory behavior by an individual of normal body weight after eating small amounts of food (e.g., self-induced vomiting after the consumption of two cookies).

5.   Repeatedly chewing and spitting out, but not swallowing, large amounts of food.

6.   Binge-eating disorder: recurrent episodes of binge eating in the absence of the regular use of inappropriate compensatory behaviors characteristic of bulimia nervosa [see Table 25–4].

There are not enough data available at the present time to make BED a distinct Axis I diagnosis. Preliminary field studies show that the majority of persons who meet criteria for BED are obese.

☐ Clinical Features

Bulimia nervosa usually begins after a period of dieting of a few weeks to a year or longer. The dieting may or may not have been successful in achieving weight loss. Most binge-eating episodes are followed by self-induced vomiting and, less frequently, by the use of laxatives. A minority of bulimic individuals use diuretics for weight control. Most bulimic patients do not eat regular meals and have difficulty feeling satiety at the end of a normal meal. Bulimic patients usually prefer to eat alone and at their homes. About one-third to one-fifth of bulimic patients will choose a weight within a normal weight range as their ideal body weight. About one-fourth to one-third of bulimia nervosa patients have had a previous history of anorexia nervosa.

The majority of bulimic patients have depressive signs and symptoms. They have problems with interpersonal relationships, self-concept, and impulsive behaviors, and show high levels of anxiety and compulsivity. Chemical dependency is not unusual in this disorder, alcohol abuse being the most common. Bulimic patients will abuse amphetamines to reduce their appetite and to lose weight. Impulsive stealing

Table 25–4.   DSM-IV (appendix) research criteria for binge-eating disorder

A. Recurrent episodes of binge eating. An episode of binge eating is characterized by both of the following:

1. Eating, in a discrete period of time (e.g., within any 2-hour period),
an amount of food that is definitely larger than most people would
eat in a similar period of time under similar circumstances.

2. A sense of lack of control over eating during the episode (e.g., a feeling
that one cannot stop eating or control what or how much one is eating).

B. The binge-eating episodes are associated with three (or more) of the
following:

1. Eating much more rapidly than normal

2. Eating until feeling uncomfortably full

3. Eating large amounts when not feeling physically hungry

4. Eating alone because of being embarrassed by how much one is eating

5. Feeling disgusted with oneself, depressed, or very guilty after overeating

C. Marked distress regarding binge eating is present.

D. The binge eating occurs, on average, at least 2 days a week for 6 months.

Note: The method of determining frequency differs from that used for
bulimia nervosa; future research should address whether the preferred
method of setting a frequency threshold is counting the number of days
on which binges occur or counting the number of episodes of binge eating.

E. The binge eating is not associated with the regular use of inappropriate
compensatory behaviors (e.g., purging, fasting, excessive exercise) and
does not occur exclusively during the course of anorexia nervosa or bulimia
nervosa.

usually occurs after the onset of binge eating; however, about one-fourth
of patients actually begin stealing before the onset of bulimia.

Bulimia nervosa patients who engage in self-induced vomiting and
abuse purgatives or diuretics are susceptible to hypokalemic alkalosis.
These patients have electrolyte abnormalities, including elevated serum
bicarbonate, hypochloremia, hypokalemia, and, in a few cases, a low serum bicarbonate, indicating metabolic acidosis. The latter is particularly
true in those individuals who abuse laxatives. It is important to remember that fasting can promote dehydration, which results in volume depletion. Patients with electrolyte disturbances have physical symptoms
of weakness, lethargy, and at times cardiac arrhythmias. The latter, of
course, can lead to a sudden cardiac arrest. Bulimia nervosa patients can
have severe attrition and erosion of the teeth, causing an irritating sensitivity, pathological pulp exposures, loss of integrity of the dental arches,
diminished masticatory ability, and an unaesthetic appearance.

Parotid gland enlargement associated with elevated serum amylase
levels is commonly observed in patients who binge and vomit. In fact,

the serum amylase level is an excellent way to follow reduction of vomiting in eating disorder patients who deny purging episodes. Acute dilatation of the stomach is a rare emergency condition for patients who binge. Esophageal tears can also occur in the process of self-induced vomiting. A complication of shock can result subsequent to the esophageal tear and should be treated by experienced medical and surgical personnel. Severe abdominal pain in the bulimia nervosa patient should alert the physician to a diagnosis of gastric dilatation and the need for nasogastric suction, X rays, and surgical consultation.

Cardiac failure caused by cardiomyopathy from ipecac intoxication is a medical emergency that is being reported more frequently, and usually results in death. Symptoms of precordial pain, dyspnea, and generalized muscle weakness associated with hypotension, tachycardia, and abnormalities on the electrocardiogram should alert one to possible ipecac intoxication.

☐ Epidemiology, Course, and Prognosis

No satisfactory incidence studies on bulimia nervosa have been reported. The bulimia nervosa diagnostic criteria have been revised every few years, and this may account for the disparity in reported prevalence rates for this disorder. Studies that used strict criteria found prevalence rates between 1 and 3.8 per 100 females (Schotte and Stunkard 1987; Timmerman et al. 1990; Whitaker et al. 1989). The prevalence of males in the bulimia nervosa population varies between 10% and 15%. The average age at onset of bulimia nervosa in most studies is 18, with a range between 12 and 35.

☐ Etiology and Pathogenesis

Fairburn and Cooper (1984) found that a rigid diet was the most commonly reported precipitant of binge-eating behavior, and a gross bingeing bout was the most common precipitant for vomiting behavior. In another study of clinical features, Hatsukami et al. (1984) found in a sample of 108 women with bulimia nervosa that 43.5% had affective disorder at some time in their lives and 18.5% had a history of alcohol or drug abuse. Although there is a high association of affective disorder with bulimia nervosa, at the present time not enough evidence is available to regard bulimia nervosa as a mere forme fruste of affective disorder. Bulimia nervosa theoretically fits well into an addictive model (Szmukler and Tantam 1984).

There is substantial evidence that personality disorders are commonly associated with bulimia nervosa. A study that compared bulimia nervosa women with alcohol- and drug-abusing women found that the two groups had similar profiles on the Minnesota Multiphasic Personality Inventory. They had elevations on the scales denoting depression, impulsivity, anger, rebelliousness, anxiety, rumination, social withdrawal, and idiosyncratic thinking (Hatsukami et al. 1982). Two studies using the Social Adjustment Scale found that bulimia nervosa women were significantly worse in all areas of adjustment (work, social, and leisure activities; relationship with extended family; role as spouse; role as parent; and membership in a family unit) than were women in a normal control sample (Johnson and Berndt 1983; Norman and Herzog 1984).

☐ Treatment

Treatment studies of bulimia nervosa have proliferated in recent years, in contrast to the relatively few treatment studies of anorexia nervosa. Specific therapy techniques such as behavior therapy, cognitive therapy, psychodynamic therapy, and "psychoeducation therapy" have been conducted both in individual and group therapies. Often a variety of therapy techniques such as cognitive, behavioral, and drug treatment may be used together in either individual or group therapy.

Psychodynamic Therapy

Lacey (1983) described the use of psychodynamic therapy with cognitive and behavioral techniques in both the individual and group therapy formats. Common themes that need to be dealt with are poor self-esteem, dependency problems, and a sense of ineffectiveness.

Cognitive-Behavior Therapy

Various controlled studies have examined the efficacy of cognitive-behavior therapy (CBT) in bulimia nervosa (Fairburn 1981). Nearly all of the studies used a psychoeducational component that included information on the social-cultural emphasis on thinness; set point theory; the physical effects and medical complications of bingeing, purging, laxative, and diuretic abuse; and information on how dieting and fasting precipitate binge-purge cycles. Self-monitoring is an important part of all these studies and usually consists of a daily record of the times and durations of meals and a record of binge eating and purging episodes along with descriptions of the moods and circumstances surrounding the binge-purge episodes. The studies all stress the importance of eating regular meals.

Cognitive restructuring is the basis of all the CBT programs. The first step in cognitive therapy is the assessment of cognition. Patients are asked to write their thoughts on an assessment form so that cognitions can be examined for systematic distortions in the processing and interpretation of events. Two recent reviews of controlled studies of CBT for bulimia nervosa concluded that CBT benefits the majority of patients (Fairburn et al. 1992; Gotestam and Agras 1989). CBT was found to be more effective when compared with treatment with antidepressants alone, self-monitoring plus supportive psychotherapy, and behavioral treatment without the cognitive treatment component. One-year follow-up studies with CBT have shown a good maintenance of change, superior to that following treatment with antidepressants.

Behavior therapy is used to specifically stop the binge eating and purging behaviors. Behavioral approaches include restricting exposure to cues that trigger a binge-purge episode, developing a strategy of alternate behaviors, and delaying the vomiting response to eating. Response prevention is a technique used specifically to prevent vomiting. After eating, a patient is placed in a situation where it is very difficult for him or her to comfortably vomit.

Two studies have examined the combined effects of CBT and antidepressant medication for treatment of bulimia nervosa. Mitchell et al. (1990) found that group CBT was superior to imipramine for decreasing binge eating and purging, and the combined treatment demonstrated no additive effects to those of the group CBT alone. Agras et al. (1992) had similar results comparing individual CBT, desipramine, or the combination at 16 weeks. However, at 32 weeks, only the combined treatment given for 24 weeks was superior to medication given for 16 weeks. A study with interpersonal psychotherapy (IPT), which targets interpersonal functioning, showed that IPT was equivalent to CBT in reducing bulimic symptoms and psychopathology; at follow-up it was actually *superior* to CBT (Fairburn et al. 1992).

Drug Therapy

Studies of antidepressant medications have consistently shown some efficacy in the treatment of bulimia nervosa. These studies were prompted by observations that patients with bulimia nervosa also had significant mood disturbances. In the past decade over a dozen double-blind, placebo-controlled trials of various antidepressants were conducted in normal-weight outpatients with bulimia nervosa. All of these trials demonstrated a significantly greater reduction in binge eating under antidepressant medication compared with placebo. Antidepressants improved mood and reduced psychopathological symptoms such as preoccupation with shape and weight. These studies provide evidence for the short-term efficacy of antidepressant medication, but its long-term efficacy remains unknown. The average abstinence rate from bingeing and purging in these studies was 22%, indicating that the majority of patients remain symptomatic at the end of antidepressant drug treatment. Both of the systematic studies conducted to evaluate maintenance of change in bulimic symptomatology yielded disappointing results: most subjects did not maintain improvement (Pyle et al. 1990; Walsh et al. 1991). The current data suggest that the treatment of choice for bulimia nervosa should be CBT and that a single antidepressant in the absence of psychotherapy cannot be considered an adequate treatment.

■ OBESITY

In contrast with anorexia nervosa and bulimia nervosa, obesity is classified not as a psychiatric disorder but as a medical disorder. Obesity is an excessive accumulation of body fat and operationally is defined as the patient's being overweight. The body mass index (BMI), which is weight (kg)/height (m^2), has the highest correlation, 0.8, with body fat measured by other more precise laboratory methods. Mildly overweight is defined as a BMI of 25 to 30, or body weight between the upper limit of normal and 20% above that limit on standard height-weight charts. Obesity is defined as a BMI above 30, or body weight greater than 20% above the upper limit for height (Bray 1978).

☐ Clinical Features

The most obvious clinical features of obesity are physical and are discussed below in the subsection on medical complications. The psychological and behavioral aspects of obesity are best considered in two categories: *eating behavior* and *emotional disturbance.* There is considerable heterogeneity in eating patterns. Most commonly, obese persons complain that they cannot restrain their eating and that they have difficulty achieving satiety. Some obese persons cannot distinguish hunger from other dysphoric states and will eat when they are emotionally upset. The most methodologically satisfying studies have shown no distinct or excess psychopathology in obesity. Because health risks and mortality vary with degree of adiposity, Bray (1986) proposed a classification into low risk (BMI of 25 to 30), moderate risk (BMI of 31 to 40), and high risk (BMI greater than 40) individuals.

Obesity affects a great variety of physiological functions. Blood circulation may be overtaxed as body weight increases, and congestive heart failure may occur in grossly obese individuals. There is a high association of hypertension with obesity, and the prevalence of carbohydrate intolerance in grossly obese subjects is about 50%. Increased body fat in the upper region of the body as opposed to the lower region is more likely to be associated with the onset of diabetes mellitus. The impairment of pulmonary function becomes extreme in severe obesity with hypoventilation, hypercapnia, hypoxia, and somnolence. Obesity may accelerate the development of osteoarthritis and of dermatological problems from stretching of the skin, intertrigo, and acanthosis nigricans. Obese women are at obstetrical risk, with special susceptibility to toxemia and hypertension.

Obesity has been associated with several types of cancer. Obese males have a higher rate of prostate and colorectal cancer, and obese females have increased rates of gall bladder, breast, cervical, endometrial, uterine, and ovarian cancer. Most studies on the topic suggest that obesity influences the development and progression of both endometrial and breast cancer through influences on estrogen production. Low-density lipoproteins are increased in obesity, and high-density lipoproteins (HDL cholesterol) are reduced. The low levels of HDL may be one mechanism by which obesity is associated with an increased risk for cardiovascular disease.

☐ Epidemiology, Course, and Prognosis

If obesity is defined as being 20% above ideal weight, close to a quarter of the United States population would be considered obese (VanItallie 1985). Socioeconomic status is highly correlated with obesity: it is much more common among women (less so among men) of low status. This relationship is also present in obese children. Increasing age and obesity are associated until age 50. There is a higher prevalence of obesity in women compared with men; over the age of 50 this may be due to the increased mortality rate among obese men with advancing age.

☐ Etiology and Pathogenesis

It is unlikely that there is a single etiology for obesity. Lipid, amino acid, and glucose metabolism all seem to have some feedback to central neural regulatory mechanisms that influence eating behavior. Obesity is regarded today by most investigators as a disorder of energy balance, a disorder with a strong genetic component that is modulated by cultural and environmental influences.

Obesity has a definite familial component. Eighty percent of the offspring of two obese parents are obese, compared with 40% of the offspring of one obese parent and only 10% of the offspring of lean parents. Twin studies and adoption studies suggest that genetic factors play a strong role in the development of obesity.

☐ Treatment

For mild obesity (20% to 40% overweight), the most efficient treatment to date consists of behavior modification in groups, a balanced diet, and exercise. For moderate obesity (41% to 100% overweight), a medically supervised protein-sparing modified fast with 400 to 700 calories a day is often necessary. This diet may or may not be combined with behavior modification techniques.

The use of medication such as phenylpropanolamine hydrochloride and fenfluramine may be helpful. The problem with these drugs is that upon withdrawal there is a rebound ballooning up of weight, and in some patients a concomitant lethargy and depression.

Severe obesity (greater than 100% over a normal weight) is the least common form of obesity and is most effectively treated by surgical procedures that reduce the size of the stomach. These procedures produce a large weight loss and show a good record of weight loss maintenance.

Behavior modification is the treatment of choice for overweight children and should include involvement of the parents and the schools. Psychotherapy is not recommended as a treatment per se for obesity, although it is possible that some patients may have particular problems that may be effectively treated or helped with psychotherapy.

■ REFERENCES

Agras WS, Rossiter EM, Arnow B, et al: Pharmacologic and cognitive-behavioral treatment for bulimia nervosa: a controlled comparison. Am J Psychiatry 149:82–87, 1992

American Psychiatric Association: Diagnostic and Statistical Manual of Mental Disorders, 3rd Edition, Revised. Washington, DC, American Psychiatric Association, 1987

American Psychiatric Association: Diagnostic and Statistical Manual of Mental Disorders, 4th Edition. Washington, DC, American Psychiatric Association, 1994

Blundell JE, Hill A: Behavioral pharmacology of feeding: relevance of animal experiments for studies in man, in Pharmacology of Eating Disorders. Edited by Blundell J, Hill A. New York, Raven, 1986

Bray GA: Definitions, measurements and classification of the syndromes of obesity. Int J Obes 2:99–112, 1978

Bray GA: Effects of obesity on health and happiness, in Handbook of Eating Disorders: Physiology, Psychology, and Treatment. Edited by Brownell KD, Foreyt JP. New York, Basic Books, 1986, pp 3–44

Bruch H: Perceptual and conceptual disturbance in anorexia nervosa. Psychosom Med 24:187–195, 1962

Crisp AH: The possible significance of some behavioral correlates of weight and carbohydrate intake. J Psychosom Res 11:117–123, 1967

Crisp AH, Palmer RL, Kalucy RS: How common is anorexia nervosa? A prevalence study. Br J Psychiatry 128:549–554, 1976

Fairburn CG: A cognitive behavioral approach to the management of bulimia. Psychol Med 11:707–711, 1981

Fairburn CG, Cooper PJ: The clinical features of bulimia nervosa. Br J Psychiatry 144:238–246, 1984

Fairburn CG, Jones R, Peveler RC, et al: Three psychological treatments for bulimia nervosa: a comparative trial. Arch Gen Psychiatry 48:463–469, 1992

Garner DM, Bemis KM: A cognitive-behavioral approach to anorexia nervosa. Cognitive Therapy and Research 6:1223–1250, 1982

Gold PW, Gwirtsman H, Kaye W, et al: Pathophysiologic mechanisms in underweight and weight corrected patients. N Engl J Med 314:335–342, 1986

Gotestam KG, Agras WS: Bulimia nervosa: pharmacologic and psychologic approaches to treatment. Nordisk Psykiatrisk Tidsskrift 43:543–551, 1989

Halmi KA: Anorexia nervosa: demographic and clinical features in 94 cases. Psychosom Med 36:18–26, 1974

Halmi KA: Anorexia nervosa and bulimia, in Handbook of Adolescent Psychology. Edited by Hersen M, Van Hasselt T. New York, Pergamon, 1987, pp 265–287

Halmi KA, Sunday SR: Temporal patterns of hunger and satiety ratings and related cognitions in anorexia and bulimia. Appetite 16:219–237, 1991

Halmi KA, Eckert E, LaDu TJ, et al: Anorexia nervosa: treatment efficacy of cyproheptadine and amitriptyline. Arch Gen Psychiatry 43:177–181, 1986

Halmi KA, Eckert E, Marchi P, et al: Comorbidity of psychiatric diagnoses in anorexia nervosa. Arch Gen Psychiatry 48:712–718, 1991

Hatsukami J, Mitchell J, Eckert E: Similarities and differences on the MMPI between women with bulimia and women with alcohol and drug abuse problems. Addict Behav 7:435–439, 1982

Hatsukami J, Mitchell J, Eckert E, et al: Affective disorder and substance abuse in women with bulimia. Psychol Med 14:704–710, 1984

Hoebel BG: Pharmacological control of feeding. Annu Rev Pharmacol Toxicol 17:605–621, 1977

Holland AJ, Hall A, Murray R, et al: Anorexia nervosa: a study of 34 twin pairs and one set of triplets. Br J Psychiatry 145:414–419, 1984

Holland AJ, Sicotte N, Tresure J: Anorexia nervosa: evidence for a genetic basis. J Psychosom Res 32:561–571, 1988

Hotta M, Chibasaki T, Masuda A, et al: The responses of plasma adrenal corticotropin and cortisol to corticotropin-releasing hormone and cerebral spinal fluid immunoreactive CRH in anorexia nervosa patients. J Clin Endocrinol Metab 62:319–321, 1986

Johnson C, Berndt DJ: Preliminary investigation of bulimia and life adjustment. Am J Psychiatry 140:774–777, 1983

Jones D, Fox MM, Babigian HM, et al: Epidemiology of anorexia nervosa in Monroe County, N.Y., 1960–1976. Psychosom Med 42:551–558, 1980

Kaye WH, Ebert MH, Gwirtsman HE, et al: Differences in brain serotonergic metabolism between nonbulimic and bulimic patients with anorexia nervosa. Am J Psychiatry 141:1598–1601, 1984a

Kaye WH, Ebert MH, Raleigh M, et al: Abnormalities in CNS monoamine metabolism in anorexia nervosa. Arch Gen Psychiatry 41:350–355, 1984b

Kaye WH, Berrettini W, Gwirtsman HE, et al: Altered cerebrospinal fluid neuropeptide Y and peptide YY immunoreactivity in anorexia and bulimia nervosa. Arch Gen Psychiatry 47:548–556, 1990

Lacey JH: An outpatient treatment program for bulimia nervosa. International Journal of Eating Disorders 2:209–241, 1983

Leibowitz SF: Neurochemical systems of the hypothalamus: control of feeding and drinking behavior and water electrolyte excretion, in Handbook of the Hypothalamus, Vol 3. Edited by Morgane PJ, Panksepp J. New York, Raven, 1980, pp 299–437

Mitchell JE, Pyle RL, Eckert ED, et al: A comparison study of antidepressants and structured intensive group therapy in the treatment of bulimia nervosa. Arch Gen Psychiatry 47:149–157, 1990

Morley J, Levine AS: Pharmacology of eating behavior. Annu Rev Pharmacol Toxicol 25:127–146, 1985

Norman DK, Herzog DB: Persistent social maladjustment in bulimia: a 1-year follow-up. Am J Psychiatry 141:444–446, 1984

Pyle RL, Mitchell JE, Eckert ED, et al: Maintenance treatment and 6-month outcome for bulimia patients who respond to initial treatment. Am J Psychiatry 147:871–875, 1990

Russell GFM: Metabolic, endocrine and psychiatric aspects of anorexia nervosa. Scientific Basis of Medicine Annual Review 14:236–255, 1969

Russell GFM, Szmukler GI, Dare C, et al: An evaluation of family therapy in anorexia nervosa and bulimia nervosa. Arch Gen Psychiatry 44:1047–1056, 1987

Schotte D, Stunkard A: Bulimia vs bulimic behaviors on a college campus. JAMA 9:1213–1215, 1987

Strober M, Morell W, Burroughs J, et al: A controlled family study of anorexia nervosa. J Psychiatr Res 19:329–346, 1985

Szmukler GI: The epidemiology of anorexia nervosa and bulimia. J Psychiatr Res 19:1243–1253, 1985

Szmukler GI, Tantam D: Anorexia nervosa: starvation dependence. Br J Med Psychol 57:303–310, 1984

Theander S: Anorexia nervosa. Acta Psychiatr Scand 214:1–300, 1970

Timmerman MG, Wells LA, Chen S: Bulimia nervosa and associated alcohol abuse among secondary school students. J Am Acad Child Adolesc Psychiatry 29:118–122, 1990

VanItallie TB: Health implications of overweight and obesity in the United States. Ann Intern Med 103:983–988, 1985

Walsh BT, Hadigan CM, Devlin MJ, et al: Long-term outcome of antidepressant treatment for bulimia nervosa. Am J Psychiatry 148:1206–1212, 1991

Whitaker A, et al: The struggle to be thin: a survey of anorectic and bulimic symptoms in a non-referred adolescent population. Psychol Med 19:143–146, 1989

Wurtman JJ, Wurtman RJ: Drugs that enhance central serotonergic transmission diminished elective carbohydrate consumption by rats. Life Sci 24:895–904, 1979

CHAPTER 26

Pain Disorders

Steven A. King, M.D.
James J. Strain, M.D.

Of all the problems faced by physicians, pain is among the most pervasive and difficult to diagnose and treat. It is not only one of the most frequently encountered complaints in medicine in general but also a common symptom of mental disorders. The scope of the problem is reflected by the fact that in any given year, 10% to 15% of adults in the United States have some form of work disability due to back pain alone (Osterweis et al. 1987). Unfortunately, psychiatry's involvement in the field of of pain has been markedly limited by misconceptions and misunderstandings about the nature of pain and its assessment and management.

Although pain has not traditionally been considered a mental disorder, the current definitions of pain accept the primacy of psychological factors in the pain experience. The most commonly accepted definition is that presented by the Task Force on Taxonomy of the International Association for the Study of Pain: "An unpleasant sensory and emotional experience associated with actual or potential tissue damage, or described in terms of such damage . . . activity induced in the nociceptor and nociceptive pathways by a noxious stimulus is not pain, *which is always a psychological state*, even though we may well appreciate that pain most often has a proximate physical cause" (Merskey and Bogduk 1994, p. 210; emphasis added). This definition indicates the necessity of terminating the dualistic concept that pain should be divided into that which is associated with identifiable organic pathology and that which is considered to be secondary to psychological factors.

■ DIAGNOSTIC CLASSIFICATION OF PAIN

The literature reveals that pain disorder categories in earlier versions of the DSM were rarely used for patients with pain (King and Strain 1994). The apparent deficiencies in the diagnoses of psychogenic and somatoform pain disorders prompted a new, more broadly defined diagnostic grouping for pain in DSM-IV (American Psychiatric Association 1994): *pain disorder*. The diagnostic criteria for this disorder are presented in Table 26–1.

The DSM-IV diagnostic category of pain disorder is compatible with current theories of pain and establishes the concept that the psychological state of patients is important. Furthermore, it 1) allows a much greater opportunity for specification of the clinician's judgment of presumed etiological factors responsible for pain, and thus provides for the development of treatment programs tailored to addressing them; 2) offers a clinically useful schema for differential diagnosis; 3) eliminates the requirement that there be a correlation between physical findings and pain; and 4) includes both acute and chronic pain. This classification is more relevant than simply one category—somatoform pain disorder—to the clinical practice of medicine; it provides greater assistance in the evaluation and treatment of patients with pain for the psychiatrist as well as those in other disciplines of medicine.

Although it is not contained in any formal diagnostic classification systems for pain, the term *chronic pain syndrome* is frequently applied to patients suffering from extended pain. Although there are different views as to what should be subsumed under this syndrome, most clinicians employ Black's (1975) criteria: "intractable, often multiple pain complaints, which are usually inappropriate to existing somatogenic problems; multiple physician contacts and many nonproductive diagnostic procedures; excessive preoccupation with the pain problem; [and] an altered behavior pattern with some of the features of depression, anxiety, and neuroticism" (p. 1000).

Because of the extremely subjective nature of many of the criteria, the validity of this diagnosis is questionable. Furthermore, some of the factors described, such as the overuse of diagnostic procedures, may be related as much to limitations in training and knowledge about pain among medical professionals as to patient behavior. Because of these limitations and the pejorative connotations that have surrounded its use, the diagnostic category chronic pain syndrome is best avoided.

■ GATE CONTROL THEORY OF PAIN

A variety of theories have been promulgated to explain pain. While there is no universal acceptance of any one concept, the *gate control theory* de-

---

Table 26–1.   DSM-IV diagnostic criteria for pain disorder

A.   Pain in one or more anatomical sites is the predominant focus of the clinical presentation and is of sufficient severity to warrant clinical attention.

B.   The pain causes clinically significant distress or impairment in social, occupational, or other important areas of functioning.

C.   Psychological factors are judged to have an important role in the onset, severity, exacerbation, or maintenance of the pain.

D.   The symptom or deficit is not intentionally produced or feigned (as in factitious disorder or malingering).

E.   The pain is not better accounted for by a mood, anxiety, or psychotic disorder and does not meet criteria for dyspareunia.

Code as follows:

307.80   Pain disorder associated with psychological factors: Psychological factors are judged to have the major role in the onset, severity, exacerbation, or maintenance of the pain. (If a general medical condition is present, it does not have a major role in the onset, severity, exacerbation, or maintenance of the pain.) This type of pain disorder is not diagnosed if criteria are also met for somatization disorder.

 Specify if:

 Acute: duration of less than 6 months

 Chronic: duration of 6 months or longer

307.89   Pain disorder associated with both psychological factors and a general medical condition: Both psychological factors and a general medical condition are judged to have important roles in the onset, severity, exacerbation, or maintenance of the pain. The associated general medical condition or anatomical site of the pain (see below) is coded on Axis III.

 Specify if:

 Acute: duration of less than 6 months

 Chronic: duration of 6 months or longer

Note: The following is not considered to be a mental disorder and is included here to facilitate differential diagnosis and should be coded on Axis III.

Pain disorder associated with a general medical condition: A general medical condition has a major role in the onset, severity, exacerbation, or maintenance of the pain. (If psychological factors are present, they are not judged to have a major role in the onset, severity, exacerbation, or maintenance of the pain.)

---

veloped by Melzack and Wall (1965) has received much attention. They believe that the transmission of nerve impulses from the periphery to the spinal cord is modified by a gate-like mechanism in the dorsal horn. The position of the gate and the amount of information that subsequently is conveyed to the brain are determined by several factors. Large A-beta fibers as well as small A-delta and C fibers carry impulses from the periphery to the substantia gelatinosa and spinal cord transmission (T) cells. When the large fibers are activated, transmission to the T cells is inhibited, thus closing the gate, whereas activation of the small fibers increases transmissions, or opens the gate. The impact of the large and small fibers on the T cells is mediated by the substantia gelatinosa.

In addition to the impulses from the periphery, the gating mechanism is also influenced by descending messages from the brain and by a "central control" mechanism that is activated by the large-diameter fibers and involves certain cognitive processes. Thus, according to this theory, pain is determined not only by peripheral stimulation but also by information traveling from the brain to the spinal cord, reaffirming the role of the mind-body interaction. Although research indicates that the gating system is more complicated than first conceived and that there may be more than one such mechanism involved, the basic concept remains intact (Melzack and Wall 1983).

■ PAIN DISORDERS AND OTHER MENTAL DISORDERS

Although there is unquestionably a relationship between pain and other mental disorders, the exact nature of this relationship is unclear. Most research on this issue has focused on the frequency of psychiatric disorders among patients whose primary complaint is pain, but the few studies that addressed pain among psychiatric patients reported it to be a common problem. Delaplaine et al. (1978) found that 38% of 227 patients admitted to a psychiatric hospital complained of pain. Chaturvedi (1987) identified pain in 18% of patients attending a psychiatric clinic.

Chronic pain appears to be most frequently associated with various forms of depressive disorders, including major depression, dysthymia, and adjustment disorder with depressed mood. The current literature describes a range in the prevalence of depression in chronic pain patients of 10% to 100% (King and Strain 1989; Romano and Turner 1985). While the variability of these results may reflect difficulties in applying these diagnoses to patients with pain, it may also be due to differences in the patient populations studied.

Although it is often conceived that patients develop depression as a response to pain, other opinions regarding this have been voiced. Engel (1959) proposed that there are individuals who, because of the presence of certain psychological factors, could be considered "pain-prone." Blumer and Heilbronn (1982) similarly suggested that the associated mental disorder may precede the pain and possibly predispose one to it, and described the pain-prone individual whose pain is a form of masked depression. Depressive disorders and alcohol dependence may be more common in the first-degree relatives of persons with chronic pain, suggesting a possible environmental or genetic predisposition for developing pain (Hudson et al. 1985; Katon et al. 1985; Magni 1987). Other studies suggest that depression is secondary to the pain (Atkinson et al. 1991), or that these two problems may coexist either independently or as the result of a common psychological or neurochemical pathway (Gamsa 1990; Magni 1987). Certain forms of acute pain also appear to be frequently associated with other mental disorders. Beitman et al. (1989) observed that greater than 30% of patients with chest pain and normal coronary arteries by cardiac catheterization fit the criteria for panic disorder.

■ ASSESSMENT OF PAIN

Because pain is a complex, subjective experience, many different methods for assessing and measuring it have been promulgated (Chapman et al. 1985). Although no single method has been found to be universally valid or reliable, the following are among the most commonly employed. The simplest pain measurement is the *numerical rating scale,* in which the patient is asked to assign a numerical score to the pain. A typical scale ranges from 0 to 10, where "0" represents no pain and "10" corresponds to the worst pain imaginable. The *visual analog scale* requires the patient to mark a place on a 10-centimeter line, the ends of which are labeled similar to those of the numerical rating scale (Scott and Huskisson 1976).

The McGill Pain Questionnaire offers a more in-depth analysis of the pain the patient is experiencing (Melzack 1975). The test lists 20 sets of words that describe pain. These words are assigned to sensory, affective, and evaluative scales. The test can be scored based on the total number of words chosen or by the rank order of the words. Research indicates that patterns of response vary according to the type of pain experienced (Reading et al. 1982). The McGill Pain Questionnaire has been criticized for its reliance on language skills. Consequently, results may reflect the patient's intelligence level, education, or cultural background.

A commonly employed alternative is the West Haven–Yale Multidimensional Pain Inventory, a 52-question instrument that measures the patient's perception of how others respond to his or her pain; participation in daily activities; and the effect of pain on the patient's overall lifestyle (Kerns et al. 1985). Other, more traditional psychological testing instruments have also been employed with pain patients, most notably the Minnesota Multiphasic Personality Inventory (MMPI). However, the validity of this and similar psychological instruments is controversial when applied to patients with pain (Hegel and Ahles 1994).

□ The Problem of Pain in Special Populations

Because pain is a subjective problem, physicians must rely on patient self-report. However, in certain groups of patients whose verbal skills may be diminished, most notably very young and elderly populations, this does not suffice. Unfortunately, failure to recognize limitations of patients' self-reporting has resulted in the undertreatment of pain for both these groups. Furthermore, because these patients are often unable to complain of pain, myths have developed that they suffer less pain than do nongeriatric adults (Acute Pain Management Guideline Panel 1992). Physicians who are caring for these patients must be especially vigilant in observing for signs that they are in pain, and to use their experience to identify conditions and procedures that are likely to cause pain and treat it appropriately (Sengstaken and King 1993). Assessment of pain may at times require the use of different tools—for example, the substitution of nonverbal scales of pain measurement, such as one employing faces ranging from happy to sad, developed for small children in place of the numerical rating and visual analog scales. The recommendations for pain management in these two groups are similar to those for nongeriatric adults, although extra caution must be employed when providing medications to children and geriatric patients.

☐ Effect of Litigation

Because many patients who suffer chronic pain have developed the problem as the result of an injury, psychiatrists who evaluate and treat such patients must be aware of the potential effects that involvement in the judicial system may have on the patient and his or her pain. When there is financial gain from having pain, the possibility of malingering is often paramount; however, concerns about this are overstated. Patients may exaggerate symptoms and the extent of disability in order to attain secondary gains, but these usually arise after the presence of the illness that initiated the pain is established. Actual falsification of pain and injury appears to be infrequent. The Commission on the Evaluation of Pain (Social Security Administration 1987) found that malingering was not a significant problem in the Social Security Administration's disability system. Leavitt and Sweet (1986) similarly found malingering to be rare in individuals complaining of low back pain.

■ MANAGEMENT OF PAIN

Though acute and chronic pain are often managed with similar therapeutic modalities, there are significant differences in how these two types are approached and in the goals that the treating clinician should endeavor to attain. No method of differentiating acute from chronic pain has yet received universal acceptance. In the literature, the definition most frequently employed is pain of 6 months' or longer duration.

□ Approaches to Management

Acute Pain

The goal of treatment for acute pain is primarily to relieve the pain. Although the methods for effectively treating most cases of this form of pain appear to be available, it is often undertreated. Marks and Sachar (1973) found that of 37 medical inpatients being treated for pain with narcotic analgesics, 32% were continuing to experience severe distress and another 41% moderate distress despite the medication regimen. The authors observed that misconceptions among physicians regarding the pharmacokinetics of these medications and concern about the potential for addiction were major factors in the physicians' failing to adequately address their patients' pains. Contrary to the concern about starting the patient on the road to addiction by treating acute pain with opioid analgesics, the potential for developing opioid dependence after receiving one of these medications iatrogenically for acute pain is uncommon. Porter and Jick (1980) reported that among almost 12,000 patients, only four who had no previous history of dependence developed this problem.

Although the management of postoperative and other forms of acute pain will usually be provided by surgeons, anesthesiologists, and other physicians directly involved in the care of the patient, psychiatrists should be aware that there is much they can contribute to the care of pain patients. The Acute Pain Management Guideline Panel (1992) of the Agency for Health Care Policy and Research highlighted the importance of employing cognitive and behaviorally based interventions such as relaxation, guided imagery, biofeedback, and education and instruction in the management of postoperative and other acute pain. However, many nonpsychiatric physicians involved in caring for patients with these forms of pain may lack the training and experience possessed by psychiatrists that are required to provide these therapeutic modalities. Guidelines for the psychiatric approach to acute pain are presented in Table 26–2.

Chronic Pain

In treating chronic pain, the goal should be to "manage" the pain as opposed to "curing" it. In many cases, this requires refocusing the patient away from the pain. In essence, patients with chronic pain must wrest control of their lives back from the pain. Much of the benefit attained from the use of psychologically based treatment modalities may relate more to their effect on the patient as a whole than to directly reducing the pain itself (Malone and Strube 1988).

Only a small percentage of patients with acute pain develop chronic pain, and it is still unclear who these individuals are and whether there

---

Table 26–2.   Guidelines for the psychiatric approach to acute pain

1. In acute pain, the primary goal is to alleviate the pain as much as possible.
2. While the appropriate use of analgesic medications is the mainstay of the effective management of acute pain, psychologically based interventions are also efficacious and should be employed.
3. The pain and the effectiveness of the therapeutic modalities being used to treat it should be frequently assessed.
4. Problems for which psychiatric consultations are often obtained on patients with acute pain, such as anxiety, depression, and problems coping with the illness, may reflect poor pain management.
5. When acute pain is accompanied by other mental disorders, relief of the pain may improve the mental state of the patient.
6. The physician should be aware of the special issues that may be encountered in the management of acute pain. For example, patients with cancer pain may develop suicidal ideation.
7. Opioid analgesics may be safely used for the management of acute pain with minimal risk of abuse or dependence.

---

is any way to predict long-term disability. The current literature supports the importance of psychosocial factors rather than organic variables in determining whether a person will recover from his or her pain (Osterweis et al. 1987).

In approaching the patient with chronic pain, the psychiatrist faces a number of obstacles. Unfortunately, many patients with this problem tend to view referrals to psychiatrists and other mental health practitioners negatively. They fear that such a referral may indicate that their treating physicians do not believe that the pain is "real." Furthermore, many believe that by making such referrals, the physicians are "giving up" and that acceptance of the referrals forces patients to acquiesce in this condition. Physicians, too, may mistakenly assume that psychiatrists have a role to play only when there is no organic pathology and may ask them to assist in determining whether the pain is "real."

One of the obstacles that frequently must be overcome in cases of chronic pain consists of the common fears that the pain indicates the presence of a severe underlying condition that must be detected and that an increase in activity will exacerbate rather than improve the pain. Patients who manage to avoid or conquer these concerns tend to do better than those who retain them (Jensen et al. 1991). Guidelines for the psychiatric approach to chronic pain are presented in Table 26–3.

☐ Psychologically Based Modalities

Psychologically based treatment approaches are considered to be a vital part of pain management programs (Fordyce et al. 1985). A wide variety

---

Table 26–3. Guidelines for the psychiatric approach to chronic pain

---

1. The focus of the management of chronic pain should be on improving function rather than alleviation of the pain.

2. Unless there is clear evidence that the patient is malingering, accept that the reported pain is present.

3. When evaluating patients with chronic pain, explain that psychiatrists' involvement in their care in no way suggests that they do not have "real" pain or that "it is all in their head."

4. In order to determine an appropriate treatment plan, attempt to discern the roles that psychological factors and a general medical condition are playing in the onset and maintenance of the pain. Be aware that even when a general medical condition has a major role in the pain, psychologically based therapeutic approaches are often efficacious.

5. Because psychosocial factors often determine the responses of patients with chronic pain to many therapeutic modalities, psychiatrists should endeavor to assist their nonpsychiatric physician colleagues in evaluating these patients before treatment plans are created.

6. Recognize that pain is often comorbid with other mental disorders. The pain may be a symptom of these mental disorders, lead to them, or coexist with them.

7. Be aware that the effective management of chronic pain often depends on the willingness and ability of patients with this problem to learn and practice strategies that will assist them in coping with their pain.

8. Be supportive. Patients with chronic pain often feel angry and frustrated about many issues including interactions with the health care and legal systems.

9. Avoid therapeutic modalities such as the extended use of benzodiazepines or opioid analgesics that may worsen the patient's problems.

---

of psychotherapies have been reported to be beneficial for pain, including many forms of individual, group, and family therapies. The most commonly used approaches fall into two major categories: operant conditioning and cognitive-behavior therapies that include biofeedback, relaxation training, and hypnosis.

Operant conditioning is based on the concept that there are certain operant or learned behaviors that develop in response to environmental cues. Common examples among pain patients include complaints of pain and reluctance to indulge in certain activities. The anticipated response to pain is often receipt of medication and being excused from work or normal daily tasks. The goal of operant conditioning is to reinforce the positive, or "healthy," behaviors and to diminish the destructive behaviors that maintain the patient's pain.

Cognitive-behavior therapy involves identifying and correcting the patient's distorted attitudes, beliefs, and expectations. The goal of this therapy is to make the patient more aware of factors that exacerbate and diminish the pain and to modify behavior accordingly. A variety of therapeutic modalities may be used to achieve this. In biofeedback, electronic equipment is employed to measure certain physiological functions of which the patient is usually unaware, and to convey this information back to the patient. A wide variety of relaxation techniques can be taught to patients. Among the most common methods is progressive muscle relaxation, in which the patient learns to relax different muscle groups by contracting and then relaxing each one (Jacobson 1970).

Although hypnosis involves relaxation, its efficacy in the treatment of pain extends beyond this. Patients can be taught to reduce the pain through hypnotic suggestions such as forming a visual image of the pain and changing it or dissociating the painful part from the rest of the body. The benefits of hypnosis for acute pain are well documented, but, unfortunately, support for its efficacy in chronic pain is primarily based on anecdotal evidence (Hilgard and Hilgard 1983).

Research suggests certain general guidelines regarding how each of these techniques is best utilized. Based on their reviews of the literature, Turner and Chapman (1982a, 1982b) and Linton (1986) found operant therapy to be especially useful in decreasing patients' medication use and increasing their activity levels. In contrast, cognitive-behavior therapy was observed to be helpful in reducing pain complaints. Each of these therapies may be employed when pain is the primary problem. However, when pain is the symptom of a mental disorder, that disorder should be addressed: appropriate treatment with psychotherapy and/or psychotropic medications must be initiated.

☐ Pharmacological Management of Pain

Opioid Analgesics

Although opioid analgesics play a primary role in the management of acute pain and the pain associated with cancer, the prescribing of opioid analgesics for patients with noncancer chronic pain is the subject of controversy. Studies have shown that these medications can be safely prescribed and are effective for this form of pain (Portenoy and Foley 1986; Zenz et al. 1992). Furthermore, there is evidence that many painful conditions are undertreated and mismanaged because of physicians' concerns about the use of these drugs. However, physicians must also be aware that these medications are subject to abuse and can have potentially life-shattering side effects, the most notable being the development of dependence.

Other potential problems must also be considered. Because patients can obtain medications from multiple sources, it may be difficult to determine if they are being honest about their drug use. Furthermore, the issue of deciding what constitutes abuse and dependence for drugs that are prescribed is complex. At the present time, the best recommendation is to consider the prescription of opioid analgesics for chronic noncancer pain on a case-by-case basis, with close monitoring of patients and continuous scrutiny for signs of abuse. Whether opioid analgesics are being instituted for cancer pain or for other chronic pain, the following guidelines should be employed:

Guideline 1. Nonopioid analgesics, such as the nonsteroidal antiinflammatory drugs and tricyclic antidepressants, and other forms of pain management should be tried first. The World Health Organization Expert Committee on Cancer Pain Relief and Active Supportive Care (1990) recommended a stepwise approach starting with nonopioid analgesics, with the addition of opioid analgesics if pain is not controlled. Even if the non-narcotic analgesics are insufficient for pain relief, they should be continued after the introduction of an opioid. They may enable analgesia to be attained at a lower dosage of the opioid than would be required if it were used alone.

Guideline 2. When initiating treatment with narcotic analgesics, the milder ones should be used first. These include codeine, oxycodone, and hydrocodone. If these are insufficient, the stronger narcotics, including morphine, methadone, and hydromorphone, should be considered. These medications are all μ opioid agonists. The other basic class of opioid analgesics consists of the mixed agonist-antagonists. Patients who take a mixed agonist-antagonist after receiving μ agonists may go into withdrawal. Furthermore, pentazocine—a commonly used mixed agonist-antagonist—can cause psychotomimetic effects including hallucinations. The use of the mixed agonist-antagonist is therefore not generally recommended.

Mu opioid analgesics also have individual properties that affect their efficacy. Propoxyphene is a mild opioid that appears to possess a lesser analgesic effect than do similar opioids such as codeine. When methadone is employed, it must be remembered that, because its duration of analgesia is shorter than its half-life, it must be given on a tid or qid schedule to be effective. Also because of its long half-life, methadone may take 2 to 3 days before it provides effective analgesia. Therefore, another shorter-acting opioid analgesic should be provided for "breakthrough pain" during this period. These recommendations also apply to levorphanol.

Meperidine is a strong opioid analgesic that is used in a variety of pain settings. Although it is an effective treatment for acute pain, the Acute Pain Management Guideline Panel (1992) indicates that it is overused even for this and that other opioid analgesics are more effective. The extended use of meperidine is contraindicated, because repeated dosing may result in the accumulation of a toxic metabolite, normeperidine, a cerebral irritant that can cause problems ranging from marked anxiety to convulsions. The oral bioavailability of meperidine is also quite poor, necessitating the switch to an alternative analgesic when parenteral administration is no longer required. Psychiatrists should be aware that, apparently alone among the opioid analgesics, meperidine can have a lethal interaction with monoamine oxidase inhibitors (MAOIs) (Browne and Linter 1987).

Guideline 3.　　The medications should be given on a fixed schedule rather than on an as-needed (i.e., prn) basis. Among the advantages of a fixed schedule are 1) better analgesia is often provided and 2) the patient is freed from a multitude of decisions that prn dosing engenders. The patient does not have to decide if the pain is sufficient to take the medication, whether to take it as the pain is beginning or to wait until it becomes unbearable, or whether to delay taking it so that it will remain available. Unfortunately, these decisions tend to focus the patient's mind on the pain rather than away from it, the opposite of what is desired in the management of most cases of pain.

Guideline 4.　　Physicians who prescribe opioid analgesics should be aware of the various ways they can be administered and of the potential side effects associated with them. These medications can be provided by multiple routes of administration including orally; intramuscularly; intravenously either by bolus, continuous infusion, or pumps such as patient-controlled analgesic (PCA) devices; rectally; by epidural and intrathecal infusion; and transdermally. Fentanyl administered by a transdermal patch may provide a useful alternative to other forms of parenteral administration in patients who are unable to ingest oral medications. However, in general, because it is the simplest and usually the least expensive, oral administration is usually preferred unless the patient is unable to tolerate it or this method of administration has ceased to be effective. A major advantage of parenteral medication is more rapid onset of peak analgesia.

The side effects most commonly associated with the opioid analgesics are constipation, nausea and vomiting, and sedation. Treatment with stool softeners and laxatives should be initiated prophylactically to prevent constipation. Nausea and vomiting can be treated with hydroxyzine or a phenothiazine antiemetic. Respiratory depression may develop with the administration of opioids. This is the most frequent cause of mortality associated with this class of drugs. It may occur acutely as the result of an overdose, but in clinical situations it more commonly results from the gradual accumulation of the opioid. Because their half-lives are much longer than the duration of analgesia, methadone and levorphanol are most likely to cause this problem. Although these medications can be safely administered to most patients, the physician needs to be especially observant when prescribing them for patients with preexisting respiratory disease, geriatric patients, and other patients whose physical condition is markedly impaired.

When treating patients who are receiving opioid analgesics, the recognition of withdrawal syndromes is vital. Multiple protocols for detoxifying patients from opioid analgesics are available. The simplest method is a gradual tapering schedule of the opioid being used. This is usually accomplished by placing the patient on a fixed schedule followed by a reduction in dose. Generally, the dose of the opioids can be safely reduced by 10% to 20% each day with minimal risk of withdrawal. Although detoxification can be performed quickly and safely, most patients with chronic pain require the institution of other forms of pain management in order to prevent relapse. Simply detoxifying such patients without addressing the reasons why they required an opioid analgesic in the first place may make physicians feel they have accomplished something but offers little long-term benefit for the patients.

Nonsteroidal Anti-inflammatory Drugs

Nonsteroidal anti-inflammatory drugs (NSAIDs) are effective analgesics for a wide range of pain conditions. They are especially effective for the pain associated with bone metastases, one of the most common cancer-related pains. The NSAIDs, other than acetaminophen, appear to exert their analgesic actions primarily through the inhibition of cyclooxygenase and, in turn, the synthesis of prostaglandins. As others have noted, the selection of an NSAID appears to be more an art than a science (Gottlieb 1985). Aspirin is one of the most widely used, but it appears to be tolerated less well than other NSAIDs (Brooks and Day 1991). Because of its availability in over-the-counter preparations, making it relatively inexpensive, ibuprofen is often considered to be the first-line NSAID. If one NSAID is not beneficial after a 1- to 2-week period at a sufficient dose, an alternative should be considered.

Although NSAIDs are very effective analgesics, a significant number of patients are unable to tolerate the associated side effects, primarily gastrointestinal distress that is related to the inhibition of prostaglandin synthesis. At this time there does not appear to be any substantial difference between the various NSAIDs regarding their potential for causing gastrointestinal problems. As a result of their inhibition of prostaglandin synthesis, NSAIDs must be prescribed quite carefully to patients with impaired renal function.

Antidepressants

A growing body of evidence supports the analgesic properties of antidepressant medications, most notably the tricyclics, for both cancer pain and chronic nonmalignant pain. Although this effect was initially thought to be related to the antidepressant properties of these medications, substantial research indicates that they have separate analgesic effects that are unrelated to the emotional state of the patient.

While the antidepressants appear to be efficacious for a wide range of painful conditions, Magni (1991), in a review of 40 placebo-controlled studies, found that they appear to be especially effective for neuropathic pain, headache including migraines, facial pain, fibrositis, osteoarthritis, and rheumatoid arthritis. The tricyclic antidepressants are now considered to be first-line drugs for the treatment of pain related to neuropathies, including postherpetic neuralgia and diabetic neuropathy. Even when the antidepressants themselves are not sufficient to control pain, as in many cases of cancer pain, they may enable reduction in the dose of opioids required, with a concomitant decrease in the side effects caused by the latter.

The mechanism of the analgesic effect of the antidepressants is unclear. Although it has been suggested that it is an increase in the bioavailability of serotonin that results in analgesia, it has been shown that antidepressants that primarily act on the noradrenergic system also reduce pain. There have been reports of the analgesic effects of the MAOIs and other antidepressants, including the selective serotonin reuptake inhibitors; however, the tricyclics are considered to be the most efficacious of the antidepressants for pain.

Determining which tricyclic has the most analgesic effects is a matter of controversy. Amitriptyline appears to be the one most widely used for pain. However, it is unclear if this reflects its having a true advantage or simply that it has been the one most studied in the literature. A major advantage of amitriptyline is its sedative effect. Because problems with sleep often accompany chronic pain and such problems may be treated with benzodiazepines that may exacerbate the pain, amitriptyline may be especially beneficial.

While the tricyclic antidepressants appear to exert their analgesic effects at lower dosage levels than are required for their antidepressant actions, analgesia appears to be dose related. The best way to initiate treatment for analgesia with a tricyclic antidepressant is to start at a dose smaller than the usual initial dose for depression and then to gradually increase the dose until side effects, most commonly daytime sedation, develop. Because the duration of analgesia appears to be similar to that of the antidepressant effect, once-a-day dosing is usually sufficient. However, some patients may obtain a better analgesic effect with divided doses. Although patients may show improvement within several days, as with depression, the analgesic effects of the tricyclics may take several weeks to develop. As in the treatment of depression, the recommended length of maintenance therapy of antidepressants for chronic pain varies from patient to patient. Every few months, physicians should reassess the continuing need for an antidepressant and should consider tapering and discontinuing it after the patient's condition has stabilized.

Benzodiazepines

As with the narcotics, the use of benzodiazepines for patients with chronic noncancer pain is controversial. These medications appear to provide little benefit in most cases of cancer pain. There is evidence to support the efficacy of clonazepam and alprazolam for neuropathic pain, but there is little to indicate that they are more effective than the tricyclic antidepressants for treatment of these conditions. Apart from these two medications, it is generally recommended that benzodiazepines be avoided when chronic pain is a problem. It has been noted that because of their GABAergic effects, benzodiazepines may actually exacerbate pain rather than reduce it. Despite this, King and Strain (1990) found that these medications are frequently employed in the management of chronic pain. They also observed that the most frequent reason that patients were taking these medications was to improve sleep. Because of the additional analgesic effects provided by the tricyclic antidepressants, it is recommended that they be used to treat the insomnia that may accompany pain.

Neuroleptics, Anticonvulsants, and Lithium

In addition to the antidepressants, other psychotropic medications also appear to have analgesic effects. Several of the neuroleptics, including haloperidol and chlorpromazine, have been reported to provide analgesia, most notably for neuropathic pain. However, methotrimeprazine, a phenothiazine, is the only neuroleptic that has been found in controlled studies to have analgesic effects.

Anticonvulsants, including phenytoin, carbamazepine, and sodium valproate, have also been found to be beneficial in pain that is due to peripheral nerve syndromes, including postherpetic neuralgia and diabetic neuropathy. However, because the tricyclic antidepressants also are efficacious for these syndromes and are less likely to result in significant side effects, it is recommended that they be tried first before proceeding to the anticonvulsants.

Lithium has been shown to be beneficial in cases of acute and cluster headaches. Therapeutic dosage is usually similar to that required when this medication is used to treat bipolar disorder.

☐ Other Treatment Modalities

Among the other therapies that have been found to be beneficial are various surgical interventions, nerve blocks, trigger point injections, acupuncture, physical therapy, and transcutaneous electrical nerve stimulation (TENS). The provision of each of these therapies requires clinicians with specific training and experience. As with the psychologically based modalities, support in the literature for the efficacy of each of these therapies is variable. The best recommendation is that, in the absence of a medical emergency, conservative therapies be tried before proceeding to more invasive ones such as nerve blocks and surgery. Therapeutic interventions such as physical therapy, acupuncture, and TENS carry little risk of side effects or of worsening the patient's pain. It has often been noted that there is a dearth of well-performed research supporting the efficacy of these treatments. However, it should be remembered that this statement can be applied to most of the therapies employed for chronic pain, including surgery. When any of the organic therapies are employed, they should be used in addition to, not in place of, the interventions that address the psychosocial aspects of the pain.

As the interest in pain has grown, various forms of pain services, clinics, and treatment centers have been created. These vary from true multidisciplinary establishments to those offering single forms of treatment provided by one or more clinicians. Because of the importance in improving the functioning of patients with chronic pain, the best multidisciplinary pain programs offer services that focus on this. Central to such programs are physical therapy, occupational therapy, and behaviorally oriented therapies. Although patients may prefer programs in which treatment is done *on* them, lasting improvement appears to depend on health care professionals teaching patients how to cope with and manage their pain and patients' willingness to do this.

■ REFERENCES

Acute Pain Management Guideline Panel: Acute Pain Management: Operative or Medical Procedures and Trauma. Clinical Practice Guideline, AHCPR Publ No 92-0032. Rockville, MD, Agency for Health Care Policy and Research, Public Health Service, U.S. Department of Health and Human Services, February 1992

American Psychiatric Association: Diagnostic and Statistical Manual of Mental Disorders, 4th Edition. Washington, DC, American Psychiatric Association, 1994

Atkinson JH, Slater MA, Patterson TL, et al: Prevalence, onset and risk of psychiatric disorders in men with chronic low back pain: a controlled study. Pain 45:111–122, 1991

Beitman BD, Mukerji V, Lamberti JW, et al: Panic disorder in patients with chest pain and angiographically normal coronary arteries. Am J Cardiol 63:1399–1403, 1989

Black RG: The chronic pain syndrome. Surg Clin North Am 55:999–1011, 1975

Blumer D, Heilbronn M: Chronic pain as a variant of depressive disease: the pain-prone disorder. J Nerv Ment Dis 170:381–406, 1982

Brooks PM, Day RO: Nonsteroidal antiinflammatory drugs–differences and similarities. N Engl J Med 324:1716–1725, 1991

Browne B, Linter S: Monoamine oxidase inhibitors and narcotic analgesics: a critical review of the implications for treatment. Br J Psychiatry 151:210–212, 1987

Chapman CR, Casey KL, Dubner R, et al: Pain measurement: an overview. Pain 22:1–31, 1985

Chaturvedi SK: Prevalence of chronic pain in psychiatric patients. Pain 19:231–237, 1987

Delaplaine R, Ifabumuyi OI, Merskey H, et al: Significance of pain in psychiatric hospital patients. Pain 4:361–366, 1978

Engel GL: "Psychogenic" pain and the pain-prone patient. Am J Med 26:899–918, 1959

Fordyce WE, Roberts AH, Sternbach RA: The behavioral management of chronic pain: a response to critics. Pain 22:113–125, 1985

Gamsa A: Is emotional disturbance a precipitator or a consequence of chronic pain? Pain 42:183–195, 1990

Gottlieb NL: The art and science of non-steroidal anti-inflammatory drug selection. Semin Arthritis Rheum 15 (Suppl 2):1–3, 1985

Hegel MT, Ahles TA: Appropriateness of the MMPI-2 in the psychological assessment of chronic pain (letter). J Pain Symp Manag 9:1–2, 1994

Hilgard ER, Hilgard JR: Hypnosis in the Relief of Pain, Revised Edition. Los Altos, CA, William Kaufman, 1983

Hudson JI, Hudson MS, Pliner LF, et al: Fibromyalgia and major affective disorder: a controlled phenomenology and family history study. Am J Psychiatry 142:441–446, 1985

Jacobson E: Modern Treatment of Tense Patients. Springfield, IL, Charles C Thomas, 1970

Jensen MP, Turner JA, Romano JM, et al: Coping with chronic pain: a critical review. Pain 47:249–283, 1991

Katon W, Egan K, Miller D: Chronic pain: lifetime psychiatric diagnoses and family history. Am J Psychiatry 142:1156–1160, 1985

Kerns RD, Turk DC, Rudy TE: The West Haven–Yale Multidimensional Pain Inventory (WHYMPI). Pain 23:345–356, 1985

King SA, Strain JJ: The problem of psychiatric diagnosis for the pain patient in the general hospital. Clinical Journal of Pain 5:329–335, 1989

King SA, Strain JJ: Benzodiazepine use by chronic pain patients. Clinical Journal of Pain 6:143–147, 1990

King SA, Strain JJ: Somatoform pain disorder, in The DSM-IV Sourcebook. Edited by American Psychiatric Association. Washington, DC, American Psychiatric Press, 1994

Leavitt F, Sweet JJ: Characteristics and frequency of malingering among patients with low back pain. Pain 25:357–374, 1986

Linton SJ: Behavioral remediation of chronic pain: a status report. Pain 24:125–141, 1986

Magni G: On the relationship between chronic pain and depression when there is no organic lesion. Pain 31:1–21, 1987

Magni G: The use of antidepressants in the treatment of chronic pain: a review of the current evidence. Drugs 42:730–748, 1991

Malone MD, Strube MJ: Meta-analysis of non-medical treatments for chronic pain. Pain 34:231–244, 1988

Marks RM, Sachar EJ: Undertreatment of medical inpatients with narcotic analgesics. Ann Intern Med 78:173–181, 1973

Melzack R: The McGill Pain Questionnaire: major properties and scoring methods. Pain 1:277–299, 1975

Melzack R, Wall PD: Pain mechanisms: a new theory. Science 150:971–979, 1965

Melzack R, Wall PD: The Challenge of Pain. New York, Basic Books, 1983

Merskey H, Bogduk N: Classification of Chronic Pain, 2nd Edition. Seattle, WA, IASP Press, 1994

Osterweis M, Kleinman A, Mechanic D (eds): Pain and Disability. Washington, DC, National Academy Press, 1987

Portenoy RK, Foley KM: Chronic use of opioid analgesics in non-malignant pain: report of 38 cases. Pain 25:171–186, 1986

Porter J, Jick H: Addiction rare in patients treated with narcotics (letter). N Engl J Med 302:123, 1980

Reading AE, Everitt BS, Sledmere CM: The McGill Pain Questionnaire: a replication of its construction. Br J Clin Psychol 21:339–349, 1982

Romano JM, Turner JA: Chronic pain and depression: does the literature support a relationship? Psychol Bull 97:18–34, 1985

Scott J, Huskisson EC: Graphic representation of pain. Pain 2:175–184, 1976

Sengstaken EA, King SA: The problems of pain and its detection among geriatric nursing home residents. J Am Geriatr Soc 41:541–544, 1993

Social Security Administration: Report of the Commission on the Evaluation of Pain (DHHS Publ No 64-031). Social Security Administration, Office of Disability, U.S. Department of Health and Human Services, 1987

Turner JA, Chapman CR: Psychological interventions for chronic pain: a critical review, I: relaxation training and biofeedback. Pain 12:1–21, 1982a

Turner JA, Chapman CR: Psychological interventions for chronic pain: a critical review, II: operant conditioning, hypnosis, and cognitive-behavioral therapy. Pain 12:23–46, 1982b

World Health Organization, Expert Committee on Cancer Pain Relief and Active Supportive Care: Cancer pain relief and palliative care: report of a WHO expert committee (WHO Technical Series 804). Geneva, World Health Organization, 1990

Zenz M, Strumpf M, Tryba M: Long-term oral opioid therapy in patients with chronic nonmalignant pain. Journal of Pain and Symptom Management 7:69–77, 1992

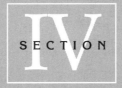

SECTION

IV

Psychiatric Treatments

CHAPTER 27

Psychopharmacology and Electroconvulsive Therapy

Jonathan M. Silver, M.D.
Stuart C. Yudofsky, M.D.
Gerald I. Hurowitz, M.D.

■ SOMATIC TREATMENTS: AN INTRODUCTION

Somatic treatments of psychiatric illnesses include the use of medication, electroconvulsive therapy (ECT), light therapy, sleep modification techniques, and psychosurgery. Although there is convincing evidence that the proper application of each of these categories of somatic treatment is beneficial in selected clinical situations, this chapter focuses predominantly on psychopharmacology and ECT, which constitute the most commonly utilized somatic interventions. The use of a somatic treatment for a psychiatric illness is a decision that should be made only after careful consideration of many factors for that individual patient. A medication, per se, is never the treatment of a patient; rather, medications may be important components of a larger treatment plan ranging from com-

---

In this chapter we provide specific guidelines for the safe and effective use of psychopharmacological agents and electroconvulsive therapy (ECT). Some of these recommendations have been supported by an official American Psychiatric Association (APA) task force. Others have been developed by the authors after careful review of the literature and in consultation with recognized experts in psychopharmacology. Future research may necessitate the revision of some of these guidelines. Additionally, the reader must consider the unique state of each patient and modify the recommendations according to that individual's needs.

prehensive medical evaluation to continuous assessment of the treatment plan and outcome. The clinician must be guided by sound therapeutic principles to ensure adequate diagnosis, correct choice of a drug or other somatic treatment, proper communication with the patient and the family related to risks and benefits of the approach, and clear instructions related to administration, side effects, evaluation of response, and discontinuation of treatment.

☐ Decision to Use a Somatic Treatment

All psychiatric patients require a skilled and thorough psychiatric, neurological, and physical evaluation (MacKinnon and Yudofsky 1991). Organic etiologies of psychological symptoms must be considered for all patients. Frequent organic causes of psychiatric symptoms include the effects of 1) concomitant medications, 2) abused substances, 3) central nervous system (CNS) dysfunction, and 4) endocrine disorders.

☐ Target Symptoms

A key component of a well-considered decision to utilize a somatic treatment is the delineation of target symptoms. The psychiatrist should determine and list those specific symptoms that are designated for treatment, and monitor response of these symptoms to treatment. A frequent and dangerous clinical error is the treatment of specific symptoms of a disorder with multiple drugs, rather than treating, more specifically, the underlying disorder. Often, the somatic complaints, insomnia, and anxiety are components of the underlying depression that is aggravated by the polypharmaceutical approach inherent to symptomatic treatment. In such circumstances, full explanation to the patient of the syndrome of depression with emphasis on the necessity of adequate doses and duration of treatment with an antidepressant should precede discontinuation of the benzodiazepine and analgesic medications and the proper administration of an antidepressant agent. On the other hand, there are many patients whose psychiatric conditions require the concomitant use of several psychotropic agents. We call this carefully considered rational utilization of several psychiatric medications "combined treatment" to distinguish it from ill-considered polypharmacy.

☐ Choice of Drug

After the decision has been made to initiate psychopharmacological treatment, the clinician must select the specific drug. Usually, this choice is made on the basis of the patient's prior history of response to medication (if possible), the side-effect profile of the drug chosen, and the patient's current physical status and life circumstances that will likely be affected by the specific side effects of the chosen agent. Choice of a medication also involves an understanding of the pharmacokinetics of a particular drug, as well as a familiarity with the relative benefits of the available routes of administration of that medication. Most antidepressant and antipsychotic drugs have sufficiently long half-lives to permit a once-a-day dosing regimen, which may increase compliance. The choice of a particular medication may depend on whether that drug is available in injection and liquid forms in addition to tablet, pill, or capsule forms.

☐ Patient Information and Patient-Physician Communication

Once the physician has established a diagnosis and determined the target symptoms most likely to respond to medication, time and attention must be devoted to imparting information and discussing with the patient and family the indications for and risks and benefits of the medications. A general principle is that the more the patient and his or her family understands about the illness and the reason that medications have been chosen to treat the illness, the more compliant the patient and the more supportive the family will be. Failure to devote adequate time to patient information discussion and instruction prior to the recommendation of a medication may result in poor therapeutic response, poor compliance by the patient, areas of mistrust and miscommunication, and the requirement, at a later time, of extensive professional time and effort. We believe that excellent communication among the physician, the patient, and the family *prior* to the selection of a medication will increase the likelihood that the most therapeutically effective agent with the safest side-effect profile will be chosen.

The clinician must also consider the physical, intellectual, and psychological capacities of the patient and of his or her caregivers when selecting a new medication. For example, impulsive patients with histories of suicide attempts and alcohol abuse may not safely or reliably be treated with a monoamine oxidase inhibitor, wherein it is important to follow a strict dietary regimen. In general, the more complicated the instructions or the more medications that are prescribed, the more difficulty the patient will have in complying with the therapeutic regimen.

☐ Evaluation of Response

Once target symptoms have been determined and measured, a treatment plan should be established that is subject to continuous reassessment and revision. A component of the treatment plan should comprise the evaluation of response and criteria for discontinuation of the medication. Included among these criteria should be the dose and duration that have been predetermined for an adequate trial of the medication. Far too frequently, medications are discontinued with the assumption of "failure of response" without the benefit of an adequate drug trial (e.g., inadequate dosage or duration of treatment). A patient's treatment plan should be revised if the patient has an unusual sensitivity to the medication, if dangerous or disabling side effects emerge, or if the patient does not respond to an adequate drug trial. In such cases, a diagnostic reevaluation of the patient may be indicated, with further tests to detect any underlying physical illness that did not appear during the initial assessment but that may be related to the persistence of the symptoms. Different treatment approaches range from a second trial with a related class of medication to the utilization of complementary or different treatment modalities. Finally, for those patients whose specific target symptoms do respond to somatic intervention, an end point for treatment must be determined. Far too frequently, patients are continued on medications beyond the point that therapeutic benefit is derived.

■ ANTIPSYCHOTIC DRUGS

Since the introduction of chlorpromazine in the 1950s, the efficacy of the antipsychotic drugs has been clear and dramatic (National Institute of Mental Health Psychopharmacology Service Center Collaborative Study Group 1964). Although antipsychotic medications have been termed "major tranquilizers," their principal treatment effect is to organize psychotic thinking. Antipsychotic agents may treat delusions, hallucinations, and other thought disorders that stem from a wide range of functional and organic etiologies. It is important to note that the sedation that frequently occurs with the use of these drugs is a side effect that may have specific therapeutic advantages or disadvantages distinct from the antipsychotic actions.

Available antipsychotic drugs may be categorized into several classes: the phenothiazines (including their derivatives), the thioxanthenes, the butyrophenones, and the dibenzoxazepine and indole derivatives (Table 27–1). Although there are many therapeutic agents available in parenteral, oral, and depot preparations, the choice of a drug in treating psychosis is determined largely by the side-effect profile of the specific drug and the ability of the individual patient to tolerate or benefit from those side effects.

☐ Indications and Efficacy

The most common indication for the use of antipsychotic drugs is in the treatment of acute psychotic exacerbations and to maintain a remission

Table 27–1.   Selected antipsychotic drugs: dosages

Class/ Generic name	Trade name	Dose equivalent (mg)	Usual daily oral dose (mg)	Parenteral single dose (mg)
Phenothiazines				
Chlorpromazine hydrochloride	Thorazine	100	200–600	25–100
Triflupromazine hydrochloride	Vesprin	26–30	50–150	60–150
Piperidines				
Thioridazine hydrochloride	Mellaril	90–104	200–600	NA
Mesoridazine besylate	Serentil	50–62	150	25–175
Piperacetazine	Quide	11	20–40	NA
Pimozide	Orap	NA	2–10	NA
Piperazines				
Trifluoperazine	Stelazine	2.4–3.2	2–4	1–2
Fluphenazine hydrochloride	Prolixin Permitil	1.1–1.3	2.5–10	2–5
decanoate enanthate	Prolixin	0.61	10 mg/day oral fluphenazine equals 12.5– 25 mg/2 weeks fluphenazine decanoate	
Perphenazine	Trilafon	8.4–9.6	16–64	5–10
Acetophenazine maleate	Tindal	22–24	60	NA
Thioxanthenes				
Chlorprothixene	Taractan	36–52	75–200	75–200
Thiothixene	Navane	3.4–5.4	6–30	4
Butyrophenones				
Haloperidol decanoate	Haldol	1.1–2.1	2–12 10 mg/day oral haloperidol equals 100– 200 mg/4 weeks haloperidol decanoate	2–5
Dibenzoxazepine				
Loxapine	Loxitane	10	20	12.5–50
Dibenzodiazepine				
Clozapine	Clozaril	NA	200–900	NA
Indole derivatives				
Molindone hydrochloride	Moban Lidone	5.1–6.9	15–60	NA
Benzisoxazole				
Risperidone	Risperidal		2–6	

Note.   NA = not available.
Source.   Dose equivalents from Davis 1976.

of these psychotic symptoms in patients with schizophrenia. Psychotic symptoms include abnormal thought content such as delusions, perceptual abnormalities such as hallucinations, and abnormal thought form as reflected in disorganized speech.

The different effects of antipsychotics on the positive and negative symptoms of schizophrenia have been studied. Among the older antipsychotics, pimozide has shown special promise in the treatment of both positive and negative symptoms (Feinberg et al. 1988). And finally, clozapine, in addition to its effectiveness in treating refractory schizophrenia (Kane et al. 1988), has been demonstrated to improve negative symptoms as well (Meltzer 1990).

The impressive data on the effectiveness of antipsychotic drugs as maintenance treatment for schizophrenia have been reviewed thoroughly by Davis and Andriukaitis (1986). Without continued treatment with antipsychotic medication after remission of acute psychotic symptoms, there is relapse rate of approximately 8% to 15% per month for patients with schizophrenia (Davis and Andriukaitis 1986). Patients maintained on drug have a relapse rate ranging from 1.5% to 3% per month (Davis 1985). A review of 35 placebo-controlled studies on the long-term prognosis of schizophrenia revealed that there was a relapse rate of 57.6% in placebo-treated patients compared with a rate of 16.2% in patients treated with antipsychotic drugs (Davis and Andriukaitis 1986).

Antipsychotic drugs are effective in ameliorating psychotic symptoms that result from many diverse etiologies: mood disorders with psychotic features, drug toxicities such as steroid psychoses, and brain disorders such as Huntington's disease or traumatic brain injury. The delusional disorders, including paranoia, delusional jealousy, erotomania, and monosymptomatic hypochondriacal psychosis, have been shown to respond best to pimozide (Opler and Feinberg 1991). Acute manic symptoms are effectively treated with antipsychotic drugs, with a more rapid response than with lithium carbonate (Prien et al. 1972). Patients with borderline or schizotypal personality disorder have been treated with antipsychotic drugs. Brief treatment with antipsychotic drugs may be effective in alleviating the symptoms of somatization, anxiety, and psychotic ideation in these patients (Gunderson 1986). In the treatment of severe obsessive-compulsive disorder (OCD), neuroleptics have been used effectively to augment antiobsessional agents (McDougle et al. 1990). Patients with psychotic or delusional depression may be successfully treated with a combination of antipsychotic and antidepressant drugs, but not with antipsychotic drugs alone (Spiker et al. 1985).

Phenothiazines (e.g., prochlorperazine) and other drugs with dopamine receptor–blocking action (e.g., metoclopramide) are also used for their antimimetic effect. The neurological disorder Gilles de la Tourette's syndrome may be controlled with antipsychotic agents, with haloperidol being the most frequently used drug for this disorder. However, pimozide may be more effective than haloperidol in treatment of Tourette's syndrome and may produce fewer side effects (Shapiro et al. 1983).

The sedative side effect of antipsychotic medications may lead to their misuse in several clinical situations. Antipsychotics frequently are improperly prescribed as hypnotic or anxiolytic agents. In addition, antipsychotic drugs are administered to patients who are chronically agitated and violent. Because of the potential long-term risks of these drugs, antipsychotics are not recommended for the treatment of anxiety or insomnia. We emphasize that although valuable for acute episodes of agitation and aggression, these drugs should not be used for the treatment of chronic aggression and agitation.

☐ Use of Antipsychotic Drugs

The choice of medication in the treatment of psychosis is determined, in large part, by the side effects that either are desired or must be avoided in the treatment of the patient. *Drug potency* refers to the milligram equivalence of drugs, not to the relative efficacy. For example, although haloperidol is more potent than chlorpromazine (haloperidol, 2 mg = chlorpromazine, 100 mg), therapeutically equivalent doses are equally effective (haloperidol, 12 mg = chlorpromazine, 600 mg). By convention, the potency of antipsychotic drugs is compared to a standard 100-mg dose of chlorpromazine. As a rule, the high-potency antipsychotic drugs with an equivalent dose of less than 5 mg have a high degree of extrapyramidal side effects (EPS) and a low level of sedation and autonomic side effects. Low-potency antipsychotic drugs have an equivalent dose of greater than 40 mg. These have a high level of sedation and autonomic side effects and a low degree of EPS. Those antipsychotic drugs with intermediate potency (i.e., equivalent dose between 5 and 40 mg) have a side-effect profile that lies between the profiles of these two groups.

Carefully controlled studies confirm that lower dosages of antipsychotic drugs have equal efficacy in treating psychosis as compared with high-dose treatment. For example, treatment of the acutely psychotic patient with parenteral haloperidol was as effective at a dosage of 2 mg per hour as at a dosage of 10 mg per hour (Neborsky et al. 1981). Fluphenazine decanoate is effective at dosages of 5 mg every 2 weeks (Marder et al. 1984). McEvoy et al. (1986) reported that haloperidol doses at a threshold dose (i.e., the point at which slight hypokinesia-rigidity first appeared) resulted in significant therapeutic improvement in two-thirds of the patients in the study.

Each psychiatric clinician should be familiar with the use of at least three oral antipsychotic drugs, two parenteral preparations, and one long-acting depot preparation. Special circumstances may call for a drug that has a low incidence of a particular side effect, such as weight gain (e.g., molindone), or one that has little effect on the seizure threshold (e.g., molindone or fluphenazine). If a patient requires intramuscular medication for acute exacerbations of psychosis, but in general is treated effectively with oral medications, an antipsychotic with both oral and parenteral availability is desirable (i.e., chlorpromazine, haloperidol). For the patient with chronic psychotic symptoms who does not comply with a daily medication regimen, a long-acting depot neuroleptic should be considered (e.g., fluphenazine decanoate or haloperidol decanoate).

In the initial stages of treatment with antipsychotic medication, sedation caused by the drug may predominate over the specific antipsychotic effects. Although it is widely recognized that antidepressant drugs may take 3 to 4 weeks before the patient shows clinical improvement, many psychiatrists incorrectly believe that if psychosis does not rapidly respond with the use of antipsychotics, higher doses are necessary. In fact, as with antidepressant therapy, reversal of psychosis often may be gradual and may occur over several weeks to several months. Unless this fact is recognized by the clinician, a patient may be exposed to higher-than-required doses of antipsychotic medication. Treatment with antipsychotic medication must be tailored to the individual patient. Flexible guidelines that are supported by scientific principles and research data should be followed. These guidelines are outlined in Table 27–2.

Several points require special emphasis. There is evidence that long-term outcome of a patient with schizophrenia is better when treatment of the acute episode is initiated rapidly. Davis and Andriukaitis (1986) observed that discharged patients treated with placebo and psychotherapy subsequently were hospitalized for longer periods of time than those patients who received pharmacotherapy alone after the initial release from the hospital. It has been shown, however, that psychosocial therapy may also be beneficial in the maintenance treatment of the patient with schizophrenia (Schooler 1986). This therapy involves education of the patient about his or her disorder; family treatments; and social skills training for the patient (Hogarty et al. 1986). For the patient with schizophrenia, after a first psychotic episode the antipsychotic medication should be continued for approximately 1 year after a full remission of psychotic symptoms (Johnson 1985). At that time, the medication should be gradually tapered and discontinued. The patient and his or her family should be educated as to early signs and symptoms of relapse, such as suspiciousness, difficulty sleeping, and argumentativeness.

For the patient with a chronic, relapsing form of schizophrenia, antipsychotic medication should be continued for up to 5 years before discontinuation (Johnson 1985). Kane et al. (1983) have done careful studies of patients maintained on high-dose (12.5 to 50.0 mg every 2 weeks) and

Table 27–2.   Guidelines for antipsychotic drug therapy

1. Conduct a thorough medical evaluation, including evaluation for tardive dyskinesia.
2. Select drug on the basis of side-effect profile, risk-benefit ratio, and history of prior use and response by patient.
3. Inform the patient and family of risk of tardive dyskinesia.
4. Initiate drug therapy at low dose (chlorpromazine equivalent 50 mg orally three times a day).
5. Use prophylactic anticholinergic medication with high-potency antipsychotic drugs or in patients younger than 40 years of age.
6. Gradually increase dose (50–100 mg chlorpromazine equivalent every other day) until improvement or usual maximum dose of 600 mg chlorpromazine equivalent is reached.
7. Maintain maximum dose for 2 to 4 weeks.
8. Use sedative drugs or beta-blockers for agitation.
9. If response is inadequate, obtain plasma level of drugs.
10. If level is low, increase dose to 1,000 mg chlorpromazine equivalent.
11. Maintain dose for 2 to 4 weeks. If improvement is inadequate, gradually decrease drug, and substitute an antipsychotic from a different class.
12. Monitor patient closely for both therapeutic effects and side effects of treatment.
13. Decrease dosage of antipsychotic medications as soon as possible after initial control of psychotic symptoms.

low-dose (1.25 to 5.0 mg every 2 weeks) fluphenazine decanoate treatment. Although the high-dose medication prevented relapse better than the low-dose treatment, those patients treated with low-dose medication had fewer extrapyramidal side effects. Additionally, the mild exacerbations of their psychoses were successfully treated with periodic increases in medication, without the necessity of hospitalization. Marder et al. (1984) compared the clinical course in patients with schizophrenia treated with 5 or 25 mg of fluphenazine decanoate administered every 2 weeks. They found no difference in relapse rates between the two groups, although the higher-dose group had evidence of more side effects. In light of these important studies, we recommend that patients be maintained on the lowest dose of antipsychotic drugs possible. In addition, patients should be monitored closely for symptoms of relapse. If the patient is compliant with treatment, oral medications are usually sufficient. However, if there is concern that the patient may not reliably take daily oral medication (based upon previous treatment history), a long-acting depot preparation may be indicated.

Risks, Side Effects, and Their Management

Extrapyramidal reactions.   Many serious side effects of antipsychotics result from the blockade of the postsynaptic dopamine receptor. A variety of extrapyramidal symptoms may emerge, including acute dystonic reactions, parkinsonian syndrome, akathisia, akinesia, tardive dyskinesia, and neuroleptic malignant syndrome.

Acute dystonic reactions.   Among the most disturbing and acutely disabling adverse drug reactions that can occur with the administration of antipsychotic drugs is an acute dystonic reaction. This reaction most frequently occurs within hours or days of the initiation of antipsychotic therapy. The most common feature of this syndrome includes uncontrollable tightening of the face and neck, and spasm and distortions of the patient's head and/or back (i.e., opisthotonus). If the extraocular muscles are involved, an oculogyric crisis may occur, wherein the eyes are elevated and "locked" in this position. Laryngeal involvement may lead to respiratory and ventilatory difficulties. These reactions are often terrifying to the patient who has no prior experience with these problems or knowledge of this side effect. When a patient with psychosis experiences a dystonic reaction, the fragile trust developed between psychiatrist and patient may be irrevocably damaged.

Intravenous or intramuscular administration of anticholinergic medication is a rapid and effective treatment of acute dystonia, so rapid, in fact, that the dystonia may even disappear before the injection is completed. The drugs and dosages that must be used to treat dystonic reactions are listed in Table 27–3. Note that the anticholinergic drug given to reverse the dystonia will wear off after several hours. Because many antipsychotic drugs may have long half-lives and durations of action, additional oral anticholinergic drugs should be prescribed for several days after the dystonic reaction has occurred.

Parkinsonian syndrome (or pseudoparkinsonism).   The parkinsonian syndrome has many of the features of classic idiopathic Parkinson's disease: diminished range of facial expression (masked facies), cogwheel rigidity, slowed movements (bradykinesia), drooling, small handwriting (micrographia), and "pill-rolling" tremor. The onset of this side effect is gradual and may not appear for weeks after neuroleptics have been administered. Treatment relies upon anticholinergic drugs, which include trihexyphenidyl, benztropine mesylate, and diphenhydramine. Amantadine, which is a dopamine agonist, is also effective. Drugs used in the treatment of the parkinsonian side effects of antipsychotic agents are listed in Table 27–3.

Table 27–3. Drugs for treatment of extrapyramidal disorders

Generic name (trade name)	Starting dose	Used to treat
Anticholinergic drugs		
Benztropine (Cogentin)	po 0.5 mg tid	Dystonic reaction, akinesia, parkinsonian syndrome, rabbit syndrome, prophylactic treatment
	im/iv 1 mg	Dystonic reaction
Biperiden (Akineton)	po 2 mg tid	Dystonic reaction, akinesia, parkinsonian syndrome, rabbit syndrome, prophylactic treatment
	im/iv 2 mg	Dystonic reaction
Diphenhydramine (Benedryl)	po 25 mg qid	Dystonic reaction, akinesia, parkinsonian syndrome, rabbit syndrome, prophylactic treatment
	im/iv 25 mg	Dystonic reaction
Ethopropazide (Parsidol)	po 50 mg bid	Dystonic reaction, akinesia, parkinsonian syndrome, rabbit syndrome, prophylactic treatment
Orphenadrine (Norflex, Disipal)	po 100 mg bid	Dystonic reaction, akinesia, parkinsonian syndrome, rabbit syndrome, prophylactic treatment
	iv 60 mg	Dystonic reaction
Procyclidine (Kemadrin)	po 2.5 mg tid	Dystonic reaction, akinesia, parkinsonian syndrome, rabbit syndrome, prophylactic treatment
Trihexyphenidyl (Artane)	po 1 mg tid	Dystonic reaction, akinesia, parkinsonian syndrome, rabbit syndrome, prophylactic treatment
Dopamine agonists		
Amantadine (Symmetrel)	po 100 mg bid	Akinesia, parkinsonian syndrome, rabbit syndrome, prophylactic treatment
Bromocriptine (Parlodel)	po 1.25 mg bid	Neuroleptic malignant syndrome
Beta-blockers		
Propranolol (Inderal)	po 20 mg tid	Akathisia
Muscle relaxant		
Dantrolene (Dantrium)	po 4 mg/kg/day in four divided doses iv 1 mg/kg, maximum 10 mg/kg	Neuroleptic malignant syndrome; should not be used in patients with hepatic dysfunction
Antidopaminergic drugs		
Reserpine (Serpasil)	po 1 mg	Tardive dyskinesia

Note. All doses are initial doses. These should be titrated to response or side effects, unless otherwise noted. po = orally; im = intramuscularly; iv = intravenously; tid = three times a day; qid = four times a day; bid = twice a day.

Akathisia.   Akathisia is an extrapyramidal disorder consisting of an unpleasant feeling of restlessness and the inability to sit still. It is a common reaction and most often occurs shortly after the initiation of antipsychotic drugs. Unfortunately, akathisia is frequently mistaken for an exacerbation of psychotic symptoms, anxiety, and/or depression. The patient may pace or become agitated or angry when he or she is unable to control the feeling of restlessness. Consequently, akathisia is a major cause of neuroleptic noncompliance. If the dosage of antipsychotic medication is increased, the restlessness continues and eventually worsens. Lowering the dosage may improve the symptoms.

Unfortunately, akathisia is among the most treatment resistant of the acute extrapyramidal side effects. The treatment of choice is beta-adrenergic blocking drugs, particularly propranolol. Several well-controlled studies have documented that propranolol, in doses up to 120 mg/day, is an effective treatment for akathisia (Adler et al. 1985, 1989). In general, the lipophilic beta-blockers are more effective in treating akathisia than the hydrophilic ones (Reiter et al. 1987). Nonselective beta-blockers, such as propranolol, and beta$_2$-selective agents are equally effective (Adler et al. 1989).

Akinesia.   Akinesia is defined as "a behavioral state of diminished spontaneity characterized by few gestures, unspontaneous speech, and, particularly, apathy and difficulty with initiating usual activities" (Rifkin et al. 1975, p. 672). As with the parkinsonian syndrome, akinesia may appear only after several weeks of therapy. Among patients treated with antipsychotic agents this syndrome may be mistaken for depression. The anticholinergic drugs in dose ranges suggested in Table 27–3 are effective. However, akinesia may also be a manifestation of negative symptomatology in a patient with schizophrenia. In this circumstance, treatment strategies aimed at improving the negative symptoms will be necessary.

Prophylactic treatment of acute dystonic reactions, parkinsonian syndrome, akathisia, akinesia, and rabbit syndrome.   These extrapyramidal syndromes may be treated prophylactically with variable efficacy with anticholinergic medications. Trihexyphenidyl, 2 mg bid, may be initiated at the same time as the antipsychotic agent haloperidol is prescribed in the treatment of a patient with schizophrenia. Although prophylactic treatment will expose patients to the side effects of anticholinergic drugs, the development of extrapyramidal reactions may reduce patient compliance. Some patients, such as the young male patient treated with high-potency antipsychotic drugs, are at particularly high risk for the development of extrapyramidal side effects. We suggest that prophylactic treatment is indicated for patients for whom the risk of developing extrapyramidal reactions is high (e.g., prolonged use of high-potency antipsychotic drugs in patients younger than 40 years old), or for patients for whom the development of these reactions is likely to diminish compliance (e.g., the angry, paranoid patient). Patients for whom anticholinergic drugs are contraindicated require careful assessment of risk-benefit ratios before initiation of medications. For such patients, amantadine should be considered if extrapyramidal side effects occur.

Tardive dyskinesia.   Tardive dyskinesia (TD) is a disorder characterized by involuntary movements of the face, trunk, or extremities (Table 27–4). The syndrome is usually associated with prolonged exposure to dopamine receptor blocking agents, most frequently, antipsychotic drugs. However, the use of drugs such as the antidepressant amoxapine, the antiemetic agents metoclopramide and prochlorperazine, and other drugs with dopamine receptor blocking properties can result in TD. The newer, atypical antipsychotic drugs, such as sulpiride, risperidone, and, especially, clozapine, seem to carry little or no risk of inducing TD.

Reports regarding the prevalence and incidence of TD have varied widely depending upon the population studied. However, the APA Task

---

Table 27–4. Clinical features of tardive dyskinesia

The following abnormal movements may be seen in tardive dyskinesia:

Facial and oral movements

a. *Muscles of facial expression:* involuntary movement of forehead, eyebrows, periorbital area, cheeks; involuntary frowning, blinking, smiling, grimacing.

b. *Lips and perioral area:* involuntary puckering, pouting, smacking.

c. *Jaw:* involuntary biting, clenching, chewing, mouth opening, lateral movements.

d. *Tongue:* involuntary protrusion, tremor, choreoathetoid movements (i.e., rolling, wormlike movement without displacement from the mouth).

Extremity movements

a. *Involuntary movement of upper arms, wrists, hands, fingers:* choreic movements (i.e., rapid, objectively purposeless, irregular, spontaneous), athetoid movements (i.e., slow, irregular, complex, serpentine), tremor (i.e., repetitive, regular, rhythmic).

b. *Involuntary movement of lower legs, knees, ankles, toes:* lateral knee movement, foot tapping, foot squirming, inversion and eversion of foot.

Trunk movements

Involuntary movement of neck, shoulders, hips: rocking, twisting, squirming, pelvic gyrations.

Source.   Adapted from the Abnormal Involuntary Movement Scales (AIMS) from the National Institute of Mental Health.

Force on Tardive Dyskinesia (American Psychiatric Association 1992) estimated that among patients receiving chronic neuroleptic treatment, 15% to 20% will have some evidence of this condition. Incidence rates seem to correlate with time of exposure to the causative agent. Kane and Smith (1982) found a 12% incidence after 4 years of treatment, and the APA Task Force on TD estimates an incidence of 5% per year of exposure among young adults, and 30% after 1 year of treatment among elderly patients.

The most significant and consistently documented risk factor for the development of TD is increasing age of the patient (Kane and Smith 1982). Women have been found to be at a greater risk for severe TD, although the evidence to date suggests that this finding is limited to geriatric populations (Kennedy et al. 1971).

Treatment of any patient with antipsychotic medication requires an evaluation for abnormal movements before treatment has begun, and every 6 months thereafter. In the most mild stages, the patient may not be aware of the involuntary movements. As the movements become more severe, the patient may become dysfunctional to the point of experiencing difficulty eating or resting. Although the most common form of tardive disorder is the dyskinetic variety, other types have been observed. These include tardive akathisia, tardive dystonia, and tardive tics (Fahn 1985).

Prevention is the most important aspect of TD management. Periodic assessments must be made to determine the patient's requirement for continuing antipsychotic drug therapy. In addition, every several months, attempts must be made to decrease the dose of neuroleptic. Even if the patient is psychotic, reevaluation is required to ascertain the lowest possible dose of antipsychotic drug that is effective for the treatment of his or her psychotic symptoms.

Because neuroleptics remain the most effective treatment for most patients with schizophrenia, the case often arises in which a patient develops TD but still requires the neuroleptic treatment to function. If discontinuation of the antipsychotic drug is clinically possible, improvement in the TD may be gradual. Worsening of the involuntary movements often initially occurs with tapering of neuroleptics. These movements also may be masked temporarily by increasing the dosage of neuroleptic medications; but eventually the symptoms will reemerge, often in a more severe form. In other clinical situations TD may not occur until months after the discontinuation of a long-acting depot neuroleptic. However, a 50% reduction in dyskinetic movement is documented in most patients by 18 months after discontinuation of antipsychotic agents (Glazer et al. 1984).

For patients who develop TD and yet cannot be taken off neuroleptics, the most promising treatment is clozapine. In an open trial,

Lieberman et al. (1991) found at least 50% improvement in TD among 43 percent of patients switched from another neuroleptic to clozapine. Severe TD, and especially tardive dystonia, seem to respond best. In view of the risks of agranulocytosis with clozapine treatment, this strategy must be investigated further.

Alpha-tocopherol (vitamin E) has been shown to also be of some benefit (Elkashef et al. 1990) in the treatment of TD, especially in cases of buccolingual dyskinesia. Vitamin E is a relatively nontoxic antioxidant that may protect neurons from the damaging effects of free radicals, which have been implicated in the etiology of TD. The typical dose of vitamin E is 400 mg tid. In addition to the treatment of existing TD, prophylaxis with vitamin E has been recommended for patients taking a neuroleptic for the first time.

The issue of informed consent with respect to antipsychotic medications and the risk of TD has been extensively reviewed (Munetz and Roth 1985). It is usually difficult, if not impossible, to obtain informed consent from a patient with acute psychosis. A general guideline is to inform and educate the family of the patient about the risks of TD before starting the antipsychotic and to educate the patient gradually about this disorder as soon as possible after agitation and psychosis remit. In many circumstances, true informed consent may not be obtainable from a patient with acute psychosis for several weeks. The psychiatrist also needs to be aware that some states (e.g., California and New Jersey) legally mandate that "informed consent" be obtained from patients prior to the initiation of antipsychotic treatment. All such discussions with patients and their families should be documented in the patients' records. Informed consent that is exclusively in the written form has been shown to be less effective in communicating information to the patient than verbal communication combined with written information (Munetz and Roth 1985). The psychiatrist must allocate adequate time to the provision of informed consent consistent with the confusional state and cognitive capabilities of the patient.

Neuroleptic malignant syndrome. In rare instances, patients on antipsychotic medications may develop a potentially life-threatening disorder known as *neuroleptic malignant syndrome* (NMS). Although occurring most frequently with the use of high-potency neuroleptics, this condition may accompany the use of any antipsychotic agent. The patient with NMS becomes severely rigid and frequently manifests mental status changes, including delirium, severe anxiety, hypophonia or mutism, and, at times, catatonia. The patient with NMS also has fever, elevated white blood cell count, tachycardia, abnormal blood pressure fluctuations, tachypnea, and diaphoresis (Levenson 1985). Creatinine phosphokinase (CPK) levels are elevated due to muscle breakdown (we have evaluated one patient with a CPK of 75,000), and this can lead to myoglobinuria (detected on urinalysis as positive for blood by dipstick, but no red cells are seen) and to acute renal failure. Pope et al. (1986) have proposed specific operational criteria for NMS, the key features of which are listed in Table 27–5.

The key treatment steps after recognition of the syndrome are discontinuation of all medications, thorough medical evaluation, intravenous fluids, antipyretic agents, and cooling blankets. Several treatments have been suggested to control NMS, including amantadine, ECT, benzodiazepines, and anticholinergic drugs (Levenson 1985). Dantrolene and bromocriptine have received the most attention and are, apparently, the most successful agents. However, their efficacy over supportive care has not been proven (Levenson 1985). Because these two agents may treat different symptoms of NMS and act through distinct mechanisms, they may also be useful in combination. Unfortunately, no controlled prospective clinical trials have yet been conducted related to the somatic treatment of NMS. Rosebush et al. (1991) found, in a retrospective controlled study comparing supportive treatment alone with supportive treatment plus dantrolene and/or bromocriptine, that these two agents may, in fact, prolong recovery. The most rational approach at present is to begin with supportive treatment and to initiate a trial of either dantrolene or bromocriptine only if supportive treatment proves inadequate.

Anticholinergic side effects.   In the treatment of a patient with antipsychotic drugs, anticholinergic side effects may be caused by the neu-

---

Table 27–5.   Clinical features of neuroleptic malignant syndrome

1. *Hyperthermia:* oral temperature of at least 37.5°C in the absence of another known etiology.

2. *Severe extrapyramidal effects characterized by the following:* lead-pipe muscle rigidity, pronounced cogwheeling, sialorrhea, oculogyric crisis, retrocollis, opisthotonos, trismus, dysphagia, choreiform movements, dyskinetic movements, festinating gait, and flexor-extensor posturing.

3. *Autonomic dysfunction characterized by the following:* hypertension (at least 20 mm rise in diastolic pressure above baseline), tachycardia (at least 30 beats per minute above baseline), tachypnea (at least 25 respirations per minute), prominent diaphoresis, and incontinence.

4. *Characteristic signs:* clouded consciousness as evidenced by delirium, mutism, stupor, or coma; leukocytosis (more than 15,000 WBC/mm^3); and serum creatinine kinase level greater than 300 U/ml.

Source.   Adapted from Pope et al. 1986.

roleptic, by the anticholinergic drug that has been prescribed to alleviate extrapyramidal side effects, or by the additive effects of both. In general, the anticholinergic potency of the antipsychotic drugs is less than that of the anticholinergic drugs. However, when certain antipsychotic drugs (especially chlorpromazine and thioridazine) are given in high dosages, anticholinergic side effects often become pronounced.

Anticholinergic effects are categorized as peripheral or central. The most common peripheral side effects are dry mouth, decreased sweating, decreased bronchial secretions, blurred vision (due to inhibition of accommodation), difficulty in urination, and constipation. Central side effects of anticholinergic drugs include impairment in concentration, attention, and memory. Certain patients may be subject to these symptoms at relatively low doses of medication, and the psychiatrist must endeavor to differentiate these side effects from symptoms caused by the patient's psychosis. In cases of toxicity, anticholinergic delirium, which includes hot dry skin, dry mucous membranes, dilated pupils, absent bowel sounds, and tachycardia, may appear. Anticholinergic delirium constitutes a medical emergency and requires full supportive medical care. Physostigmine, a centrally and peripherally acting reversible anticholinesterase, may be used as a diagnostic agent in cases of suspected anticholinergic toxicity.

Adrenergic side effects.   Neuroleptics also can block alpha-adrenergic receptors, and this can result in orthostatic hypotension and dizziness. Mesoridazine, chlorpromazine, and thioridazine are the most potent alpha$_1$ blockers of the antipsychotic drugs (Richelson 1984). The administration of epinephrine, which stimulates both alpha- and beta-adrenergic receptors, will result in a paradoxical drop in blood pressure. This lowering of blood pressure is explained by the stimulation of beta receptors in the presence of alpha receptor blockade. In the asthmatic patient who requires treatment with antipsychotics, as well as episodic treatment with alpha-adrenergic drugs, specific warnings are necessary regarding the dangers inherent in the use of epinephrine in the treatment of an acute asthmatic attack. In such cases, open channels of communication among the patient, family, internist, and psychiatrist are essential.

Endocrine and sexual side effects.   Changes in hormonal function occur with neuroleptic treatment. Correa et al. (1987) proposed that, in addition to gynecomastia and galactorrhea, other neuroendocrine side effects of neuroleptics mediated by hyperprolactinemia include amenorrhea, weight gain, breast tenderness, and decreased libido. Amantadine may be an effective treatment for these side effects. Many patients experience weight gain while on neuroleptic treatment. Molindone may be different from other antipsychotic drugs in that weight gain is reported to be rare (Gardos and Cole 1977). Molindone should be considered in patients who cannot tolerate additional weight and in whom weight gain would compromise compliance.

Sexual dysfunction also may be caused by neuroleptic therapy. A combination of anticholinergic effects, alpha-adrenergic receptor blockade, and hormonal effects may lead to several types of sexual difficulty. In men, inability to achieve or maintain erections, decreased ability to achieve orgasm, and changes in the pleasurable quality of orgasm are reported (Ghadirian et al. 1982). Thioridazine may cause painful retrograde ejaculation, in which semen is ejected into the bladder (Shader 1964). Many patients and even some psychiatrists are reluctant to discuss sexual side effects. Within the context of severe psychotic symptomatology some psychiatrists may even trivialize sexual side effects. Yet, sexual side effects are usually highly troubling to the patient and often interfere with treatment compliance. Therefore, regular assessment by the clinician of sexual side effects is mandatory. Reducing the dose or changing the type of the antipsychotic agent usually reverses these symptoms.

Eye and skin effects.   Antipsychotics may cause pigmentary changes in the skin and in the lens and retina, especially with long-term treatment. Pigment deposition in the lens of the eye does not affect vision. However, pigmentary retinopathy, which can lead to irreversible blindness, has been associated specifically with the use of thioridazine. Because of these effects, regular ophthalmological examinations are required in patients maintained on neuroleptics. Almost all patients on neuroleptics, especially the aliphatic phenothiazines (e.g., chlorpromazine), become more sensitive to the effects of sunlight, which can lead to severe sunburn. Especially in the summer months, patients should avoid excess sun exposure and use ultraviolet-blocking agents such as sunscreens that contain fully protective levels of p-aminobenzoic acid (PABA). In our experience, clinicians commonly fail to advise patients of this painful and potentially dangerous side effect. As with many other medications, allergic maculopapular skin eruptions may occur. These are best treated by discontinuation of the agent, accompanied by symptomatic treatment with antihistamines, such as diphenhydramine. For subsequent treatment of psychosis, the patient should be given a drug from another family of antipsychotics.

Effects on hepatic function.   Increases in liver function tests have been associated with antipsychotic treatment. Many cases of this reaction were linked to impurities in the original formulation of chlorpromazine, and the incidence has decreased over the years. When the abnormalities occur, this usually suggests obstructive liver disease, with increases in bilirubin and alkaline phosphatase. In such circumstances the drug must be immediately discontinued and a different antipsychotic drug initiated.

Hematologic effects.   Transient leukopenia and, in rare cases, agranulocytosis have been associated with neuroleptic treatment (Balon and Berchou 1986). Although agranulocytosis is strictly defined as a complete absence of all granulocytes in the blood, it may also refer to severe neutropenia, with a neutrophil count of less than 500 per ml. This is an idiosyncratic reaction that usually occurs within the first 3 to 4 weeks after the initiation of treatment with an antipsychotic drug. However, the period of risk for agranulocytosis and leukopenia continues for 2 to 3 months of treatment. A higher risk for agranulocytosis is associated with the following: middle age, Caucasian race, female, and treatment with low-potency antipsychotic drugs, including chlorpromazine and clozapine (Balon and Berchou 1986). The risk of agranulocytosis is particularly high with clozapine treatment. Signs and symptoms of this reaction include high fever, stomatitis, severe pharyngitis, lymphadenopathy, and malaise. This reaction requires immediate discontinuation of all medications and immediate medical evaluation and treatment. Agranulocytosis usually resolves after discontinuation of the causative agent. There must be vigorous treatment of any infections that develop. Further treatment of psychosis must be with an agent of a completely different chemical class of antipsychotic drugs (e.g., haloperidol instead of chlorpromazine).

Effects on seizure threshold.   The antipsychotic drugs have been shown to lower seizure threshold, a phenomenon that has been confirmed in animal models. Of all the antipsychotics, molindone and fluphenazine have been most consistently shown to have the lowest potential for lowering the seizure threshold (Oliver et al. 1982). Special precautions must be taken with the use of antipsychotic agents for those patients with a history of seizure disorder and for those patients with brain lesions associated with abnormal EEG findings.

Effects on temperature regulation.   Antipsychotic drugs directly affect the hypothalamus and suppress temperature regulation. In combination with the alpha-adrenergic receptor and cholinergic receptor blocking effects of antipsychotics, this effect becomes particularly serious in hot, humid weather. Severe hyperthermia, rhabdomyolysis, and renal failure may result, a potentially life-threatening condition that requires immediate medical intervention and supportive treatment (Mann and Roger 1978). It is mandatory that cool environments and adequate amounts of fluids be provided for patients taking antipsychotic agents. Also, care must be taken that patients not overexert themselves in warm weather or hot environments. Special monitoring is also required for the acutely agitated or manic patient and for patients in restraints, as they are prone to this dangerous condition.

Use in Pregnancy

As with most other drugs, antipsychotic agents, if possible, should be avoided during pregnancy and during lactation periods for mothers who breast feed their infants. There is a possible increase in birth defects among infants born to mothers who were first exposed to antipsychotic drugs during the 6th to 10th week of gestation (Edlund and Craig 1984). Edlund and Craig (1984) pointed out that because there is an increased risk of fetal death in psychotic mothers, the small risk of neuroleptic-induced teratogenesis must be assessed carefully and balanced against the risks involved in withholding treatment. In addition to the risks of first trimester use, antipsychotic agents should be prescribed with great caution in the peripartum period. As a general guideline, antipsychotic drugs should be used in pregnant patients only if absolutely necessary, at the minimal dose required, and for the briefest possible time. Documentation of informed consent from the mother and the father is necessary. Use of ECT to treat acute psychosis in pregnant mothers must also be considered.

Drug Interactions

When other drugs are used concomitantly with antipsychotic agents, the clinician should be ever alert for the possibility of drug-drug interactions. When an antipsychotic drug is used with an antidepressant or anticonvulsant, the plasma level of the concomitantly administered drug can change when the antipsychotic drug is added, increased, or decreased. Drugs with potentially serious adverse effects (such as retinopathy with thioridazine) should be monitored through plasma level determinations when other medications are used concurrently. Antipsychotic drugs have profound effects on multiple CNS receptors, and these effects are compounded when other medications are added.

☐ Clozapine and the Treatment of Refractory Psychosis

The treatment of refractory psychosis had been constrained for many years by the fact that all of the available antipsychotic medications, when used correctly, were equally effective. A patient who failed to respond to one antipsychotic medication was, therefore, unlikely to respond to another. The introduction of the atypical neuroleptic clozapine for use in treatment-resistant schizophrenia has changed this situation. Clozapine is atypical because it causes significantly less extrapyramidal side effects, does not elevate serum prolactin, and, to date, has not been proved to induce TD. Unfortunately, clozapine has a 1% to 2% risk of producing a potentially fatal agranulocytosis (apparently the risk is higher among Ashkenazic Jews), which delayed its use in the United States for many years (Lieberman et al. 1988).

A large, multicenter, double-blind prospective study of neuroleptic refractory patients with schizophrenia confirmed that clozapine is superior to chlorpromazine in this group: a significant improvement was demonstrated in 30% of the patients enrolled (Kane et al. 1988). Improvement was found to be significant for the treatment of both positive and negative symptoms. Furthermore, the institution of weekly white blood cell monitoring provided sufficient time for withdrawal of the drug prior to the development of a life-endangering neutropenia.

Clozapine is now available for use in the U.S., and a weekly CBC is required. Based on the patient's absolute neutrophil count, strict guidelines have been set requiring discontinuation of the clozapine if the count is reduced below certain levels. Despite these precautions, however, some fatalities with clozapine have been reported, each occurring within 5 to 10 weeks after the initiation of clozapine treatment. These reports indicate that a small mortality risk remains in clozapine-treated patients, despite weekly blood count monitoring. However, the risk of agranulocytosis diminishes significantly after 6 months of continuous treatment (Alvir et al. 1993), and so the requirement for a weekly CBC beyond 6 months may eventually be revised. Patients being considered for clozapine treatment must be screened for illnesses associated with immunocompromise, including tuberculosis and HIV infection. At the present time, despite the risks, the proven efficacy of clozapine in refractory schizophrenia makes this drug the treatment of choice in cases of severely disabling psychotic illness that has not responded to "standard" antipsychotic medications.

In addition to its value for the patient with chronic refractory schizophrenia, clozapine has been shown to be useful in refractory cases of schizoaffective disorder and psychotic mood disorders (McElroy et al. 1991). Moreover, because clozapine appears to be devoid of parkinsonian side effects, its usefulness in low doses for Parkinson's patients with drug (i.e., dopamine agonist)–induced psychoses is becoming recognized (Ostergaard and Dupont 1988). Despite the absence of EPS in clozapine-treated patients, there have been reports of NMS in patients medicated with clozapine alone (Miller et al. 1991).

Clozapine treatment is also associated with significant risk of seizures. The overall cumulative risk to patients has been estimated to be 10% after 3.8 years of treatment. However, the risk appears to be dose related (Devinsky et al. 1991). On the basis of four cases, Haller and

Binder (1990) recommended avoiding doses greater than 600 mg/day unless the patient has failed to respond at lower doses. Once a seizure has occurred, the question of whether or not to continue the clozapine requires clinical judgment, including an assessment of the risk-benefit ratio. If the choice is made to continue the clozapine, this should commence only after additional informed consent from the patient and family is secured. Cotreatment with anticonvulsants may be warranted, *but carbamazepine must be avoided because of the risk of bone marrow suppression.* There are reports of successful treatment combining clozapine and phenytoin, but Miller (1991) warned that this anticonvulsant can lower serum clozapine levels. Even worse, phenytoin carries its own risk of bone marrow suppression. For this reason, at the present time, phenobarbital and valproate would appear to be the safest anticonvulsants for patients taking clozapine.

☐ Other Antipsychotic Drugs

Risperidone, a novel benzisoxazole derivative, is another atypical neuroleptic now approved for use in the United States. In addition to its D_2 receptor antagonism, risperidone is a potent serotonin $5\text{-}HT_2$ receptor antagonist, an effect that some investigators believe accounts for clozapine's superior therapeutic action, especially in treating the negative symptomatology of schizophrenia (Chouinard et al. 1993). A double-blind, placebo-controlled study of 135 patients with chronic schizophrenia found that risperidone, 6 mg/day, was globally superior to haloperidol, 20 mg/day (Chouinard et al. 1993). Negative symptoms of schizophrenia also responded to risperidone, whereas haloperidol was ineffective in treating these symptoms.

■ ANTIDEPRESSANT DRUGS

The modern era of the treatment of depression with medication began in the 1950s when iproniazid, a monoamine oxidase inhibitor (MAOI) used for the treatment of tuberculosis, was noted to elevate mood (Selikoff et al. 1952). Efficacy in the treatment of depressed patients was subsequently shown in studies by Crane (1957) and Kline (1958). Imipramine, the first of the tricyclic antidepressants (TCAs), was developed as a derivative of chlorpromazine with the hope that imipramine would be more effective as an antipsychotic agent. Although imipramine did not exhibit antipsychotic efficacy, it was shown to be effective in the treatment of depression (Kuhn 1958). Subsequently, many other antidepressants have been approved for use in the United States. Among this group are the secondary amine TCAs, drugs of the MAOI family, selective serotonin reuptake inhibitors (SSRIs), and the so-called atypical antidepressants, trazodone (a triazolopyridine) and bupropion (an aminoketone). Currently available antidepressants and those that may soon be approved in the United States are listed in Table 27–6.

☐ Indications and Efficacy

Although the antidepressants have many potential therapeutic uses, the primary approved indication for these drugs is the treatment of depression in patients who suffer from major depressive disorder, as defined by DSM-III-R (American Psychiatric Association 1987). Additionally, antidepressants are indicated for patients with dysthymia and bipolar patients suffering a major depressive episode. Overall, approximately 70% of patients with depression respond to an adequate trial of an antidepressant. Patients with psychotic depression, however, respond poorly to treatment with antidepressants alone (Spiker et al. 1985). Several other disorders also respond to antidepressants, although, in most cases, the Food and Drug Administration (FDA) has not approved antidepressants to treat these conditions. Among these other disorders are panic disorder, social phobia (MAOIs and SSRIs), posttraumatic stress disorder, obsessive-compulsive disorder (SSRIs), peptic ulcer disease (TCAs), irritable bowel syndrome, enuresis (TCAs), chronic pain (TCAs), migraine headache (TCAs and MAOIs), bulimia (SSRIs), and attention-deficit/hyperactivity disorder (Goodman and Charney 1985).

Patients with a depressive syndrome that is characterized by mood reactivity (i.e., mood that is responsive acutely to favorable and unfavorable life experiences), oversleeping, overeating, extreme lethargy, and extreme sensitivity to rejection, the so-called atypical subtype, may show a preferential response to MAOI therapy (Quitkin et al. 1979; Zisook 1985). These atypical symptoms may, in fact, provide a marker for the patient who is likely to respond to MAOIs. McGrath et al. (1992) reported that patients with mood reactivity and only one of the other four atypical symptoms were less likely to respond to TCAs than to MAOIs. Thase et al. (1991) disputed the importance of mood reactivity and rejection sensitivity in identifying the MAOI-responsive patient, but agreed that the "reverse" neurovegetative symptoms cluster (i.e., hyperphagia, hypersomnia, anergy, and psychomotor retardation) is a marker for selective response to the MAOIs. As a result, MAOIs have been suggested as the treatment of choice for atypical depression, but this recommendation must be considered relative to the increased risks inherent to MAOI therapy (Liebowitz et al. 1988).

For patients with recurrent unipolar depressions, tricyclic antidepressants are effective in preventing future episodes of depression (Consensus Development 1985). Kupfer and Frank (1987) suggested that

Table 27–6. Selected antidepressant drugs: dosages

Class/Generic name	Trade name	Usual daily maximum oral dose (mg)
Tricyclics		
Tertiary amine tricyclics		
Imipramine	Tofranil	300
	Tofranil PM	
	SK-Pramine	
	Janimine	
Amitriptyline	Elavil	300
	Endep	
Doxepin	Adapin	300
	Sinequan	
Trimipramine	Surmontil	300
Clomipramine	Anafranil	250
Secondary amine tricyclics		
Desipramine	Norpramin	300
	Pertofrane	
Nortriptyline	Aventyl	150
	Pamelor	
Protriptyline	Vivactil	60
Tetracyclic		
Maprotiline	Ludiomil	225
Bicyclic		
Venlafaxine	Effexor	375
Dibenzoxazepine		
Amoxapine	Asendin	600
Aminoketone		
Bupropion	Wellbutrin	450
Triazolopyridine		
Trazodone	Desyrel	400
Phenylpiperazine		
Nefazodone	Serzone	500
Selective serotonin reuptake inhibitors		
Fluoxetine	Prozac	80
Sertraline	Zoloft	150
Paroxetine	Paxil	60
Monoamine oxidase inhibitors		
Hydrazines		
Isocarboxazid	Marplan	50
Phenelzine	Nardil	90
Nonhydrazines		
Tranylcypromine	Parnate	50
Pargyline	Eutonyl	150

combined pharmacological and psychotherapeutic treatments result in lower relapse rates. It should be noted that antidepressants may increase the cycling of recurrent mood disorders (especially bipolar disorder) and result in more frequent episodes (Wehr and Goodwin 1979).

☐ Clinical Use of Antidepressants

Selection of Patients

The psychiatric history, current symptoms, physical examination, and mental status of patients with depressed mood are key factors in the choice of the appropriate therapeutic modality. The clinician must evaluate the patient in the context of his social, psychological, and biological state in order to choose the optimum treatment (MacKinnon and Yudofsky 1991). For some patients, treatment could consist of psychotherapy alone, whereas for others it may involve individual and family therapy, occupational counseling, and treatment with more than one medication or ECT. Diagnostic factors that may influence the choice of antidepressant drug include a history of manic or hypomanic episodes, the presence of psychosis, the prior course of episodes of depression, prior response to antidepressant treatment, and the presence of "atypical" symptoms. A history of previous episodes of mania or hypomania should alert the clinician to the possible precipitation of these episodes with antidepressants. Among the antidepressants, bupropion may be less likely to induce hypomania or mania in susceptible bipolar patients (Haykal and Akiskal 1990). If hypomania occurs while a patient is on antidepressant therapy, a reduction in dosage should be attempted as a first effort to control these symptoms.

Pretreatment with a mood stabilizer (e.g., lithium, carbamazepine, valproate) before the administration of antidepressant drugs should be considered for depressed patients who have experienced previous manic episodes. Antidepressants have been shown to decrease the interval between affective episodes and to increase "cycling" in bipolar patients (Wehr and Goodwin 1979). In addition, certain patients with no prior history of mood cycles may begin to manifest a rapid-cycling course after receiving antidepressants. A subclass of patients with antidepressant-induced rapid cycling do not respond well to the addition of a mood stabilizer, and this necessitates that the antidepressant be discontinued (Wehr et al. 1988).

Patients with delusional depression respond poorly to treatment when antidepressant medications are used as the sole agents (Glassman and Roose 1981). Patients with delusional depression are also at an increased risk of suicide (Roose et al. 1983) and, therefore, often require hospitalization. Patients with delusional depression have been reported to respond to combined treatment of antidepressants and antipsychotics (Nelson and Bowers 1978) and also show dramatic response to ECT, which is often the treatment of choice in this disorder (Yudofsky 1981). The addition of lithium carbonate to the pharmacotherapy of psychotic depression that is refractory to combined treatment with an antipsychotic and an antidepressant may be effective for bipolar but not unipolar patients (Nelson and Mazure 1986).

Psychotherapy is vitally important in the treatment of patients with depression. Studies have demonstrated that the response to the combination of psychotherapy and medication is superior to either treatment used alone (Conte et al. 1986). Psychotherapy and medication may affect different symptoms of depression. DiMascio et al. (1979) demonstrated that pharmacological treatment has its principal effects on somatic symptoms such as sleep and appetite, and that psychotherapy (short-term interpersonal) was shown to affect mood, suicidal ideation, and social functioning, usually after 1 to 2 months of treatment.

Plasma Levels and Therapeutic Monitoring

Most patients respond to usual doses of antidepressants and do not require monitoring of plasma levels. Nonetheless, there are times when a plasma level determination can be useful. Specific guidelines for the appropriate use of antidepressant plasma levels are outlined in Table 27–7. Many studies have been conducted to assess the value of plasma level monitoring for the therapeutic use of the antidepressant drugs (MacKinnon and Yudofsky 1991; Preskorn and Fast 1991). The most useful findings to date derive from studies of three TCAs: imipramine, desipramine, and nortriptyline. The APA Task Force on the Use of Laboratory Tests in Psychiatry (1985) has developed guidelines for the use of plasma level monitoring. For an adequate therapeutic trial, the combined sum of the plasma levels of imipramine and the desmethyl metabolite (desipramine) should be greater than 200 to 250 ng/ml, and desipramine levels should be greater than 125 ng/ml. A therapeutic window has been observed for nortriptyline, with optimal response between 50 to 150 ng/ml. The task force emphasized several aspects of plasma level monitoring that require special attention. Levels should be monitored after the drug has reached steady state (5 to 7 days for most TCAs) and approximately 10 to 14 hours after the last dose has been ingested.

Initiation of Antidepressant Treatment

The TCAs and SSRIs constitute the "first line" of antidepressant treatment. As with antipsychotic drugs, the choice of which TCA or SSRI is

Table 27–7.   Indications for use of antidepressant plasma levels

1. Patient has not responded to an adequate trial of nortriptyline, desipramine, or imipramine.
2. Patient is at high risk because of age or medical illness, and requires treatment with the lowest possible effective dose.
3. Patient requires rapid increases in dose because of extraordinary suicide risk.
4. Concern about patient compliance with medication regimen.
5. Documentation of plasma level to which the patient responded for use in future treatment.
6. Potential of drug interactions that may lead to an increase or decrease in plasma levels.

Source.   Adapted from American Psychiatric Association 1985.

usually determined by the side-effect profile of the drug. Other factors involved in this decision include the patient's history of previous treatment response, the anticipation of the need for useful plasma levels, the medical status of the patient, and the risk of suicide by overdose. Finally, consideration of the overall treatment strategy, including the possibility of a future trial of an MAOI, and other drug interactions play a role in the initiation of treatment.

The side effects that impact on the choice of antidepressant most often are the anticholinergic effects, cardiovascular effects, sedation, and stimulation. General guidelines for the use of TCAs are listed in Table 27–8. The SSRIs are more stimulating than the TCAs, but they are devoid of antihistaminic and anticholinergic effects. Therefore, as with the more stimulating TCAs, the use of SSRIs often must be avoided for patients with marked anxiety or agitation, but may be of particular use in the anergic patient.

Although monitoring of plasma levels may not be necessary for the treatment of most patients, the clinician may prefer that an antidepressant with therapeutically meaningful levels be used. This may prove to be invaluable if a patient does not respond to a trial with standard doses of an antidepressant. The TCAs have the advantage in this regard inasmuch as a relationship between plasma levels and therapeutic response has been established for several of these agents. To date, the efficacy of the SSRIs has been established only for the treatment of depressed outpatients, in whom they have proven to be equivalent to the TCAs. This leaves open the question of whether the SSRIs are an appropriate first-line treatment for the severely depressed, melancholic patient, who statistically is likely to respond well to a TCA.

Antidepressant drugs are initiated at a low dose and gradually in-

Table 27–8.   Guidelines for use of tricyclic antidepressant drugs

1. Complete a thorough medical evaluation, especially with regard to cardiovascular and thyroid status.
2. Select drug on the basis of side-effect profile (i.e., stimulating effect, sedating effect, anticholinergic effect, and cardiovascular effect), availability of relevant therapeutic levels, and history of previous response.
3. Inform the patient and family of risks and benefits. Emphasize the expected "delay" in therapeutic response, anticipated side effects, etc.
4. Initiate and increase dose of tricyclic antidepressant slowly. (For example, for imipramine, start at 25 mg tid and increase by 25 mg every day.)
5. Increase dosage until dose equivalent of 200 mg imipramine is reached. Stabilize at that dose for 1 week.
6. If there is no significant therapeutic effect after 1 week, increase dosage to maximum recommended dose (e.g., imipramine 300 mg).
7. If there is no significant improvement after 1 week, obtain plasma level (if appropriate) and electrocardiogram (ECG), and adjust dose (e.g., increase by 50 mg per week). Obtain level and ECG before each dose increase.
8. Remember that a therapeutic trial is defined as a 6-week treatment with antidepressant, with at least 4 weeks on the highest tolerated, safe dose.

creased to a standard treatment dose over a 2- to 3-week period, depending upon side effects and clinical response. The clinician should be contact the patient within the first 2 days of initiation of antidepressant therapy in order to check for idiosyncratic reactions and side effects. For example, imipramine would be initiated for a healthy adult at a dosage of 25 mg tid, and increased by 25 mg/day until a total dose of 200 mg/day is reached, at which point once-a-day dosing is recommended. The patient should remain at this dose for approximately 1 week before the dose is increased further. If only minor or no therapeutic effect has occurred, the clinician should increase the dose to 250 to 300 mg/day over the next week. If there is no further improvement over the next week (i.e., week 4 of treatment), the clinician should obtain a plasma level of the antidepressant and an ECG. If the plasma level is below that indicated for efficacy, the dose should be increased by 50-mg increments approximately every 1 to 2 weeks, with electrocardiographic and plasma level monitoring between increments. There are patients who, for a variety of reasons, cannot tolerate dosage increments at this suggested rate. For these patients, the dose may be initiated at a lower dose and increased at a slower rate.

It is recommended that fluoxetine be started at 10 to 20 mg a day and maintained at that dose for 6 to 8 weeks before considering an increase in dose. Yet, because of its stimulating effects, many patients cannot tolerate this level of the drug at the initiation of treatment. For this reason, we often begin treatment in doses as low as 2.5 mg/day and slowly increase the dose over several weeks. An antidepressant effect is sometimes observed at doses of 5 mg to 10 mg/day. On the other hand, increasing the drug to 40 mg/day and higher may be required when the lower dosages are not effective. There is some evidence that doses above 40 mg/day are rarely effective for the treatment of depression that has been refractory to lower doses. Sertraline is begun at 50 mg/day (although, as in the case of fluoxetine, lower doses are occasionally required) and held at that dose for 4 to 6 weeks. Doses of 100 mg or 150 mg may be prescribed sequentially for patients who fail to respond to the lower dosage.

Paroxetine treatment is initiated at a dose of 10 or 20 mg/day, maintained at 20 to 30 mg until response or, after 4 to 6 weeks, increased sequentially to 60 mg/day.

For treatment with the MAOIs, an initial dose of 15 mg bid of phenelzine is standard, and this is increased by 15 mg every other day until a total daily dose of 60 mg is reached. If no response occurs within in 2 weeks, the dose may be increased to 75 mg/day, and then to 90 mg/day. After the patient has reached a steady state of antidepressant treatment (a treatment dose for approximately 1 week), the patient may take all the medications as a single daily dose. In fact, once-a-day dosing of the MAOIs may be therapeutically superior to a multiple dosage regimen (Weise et al. 1980).

Nefazodone is begun at 100 mg bid, and after 1 week the dose is increased to 150 mg bid. The usual therapeutic dosage is between 300 and 500 mg/day. The therapeutic range for elderly patients is slightly less (i.e., between 200 and 400 mg/day in two equally divided doses).

Bupropion is initiated at a dose of 75 mg tid and increased by 25-mg increments every other day until a dose of 100 mg tid is reached. A maximum daily dosage of 450 mg has been recommended because of the finding of an increased risk of seizures in patients taking greater amounts. This risk of seizure also limits the amount of drug that may be taken per dose to 150 mg. Therefore, a maximum regimen of 150 mg tid is recommended. The most commonly experienced side effect of bupropion is excessive stimulation. Trazodone is prescribed in much the same manner as the TCAs, although there is less danger of toxicity at higher doses. The recommended therapeutic dose range is 200 mg to 400 mg/day. Excessive sedation is the most commonly encountered side effect with trazodone.

The initial therapeutic response of the depressed patient to medications may be detected as early as the first week, with the patient showing improvement in sleep and energy. For patients with severe anxiety or insomnia, the concurrent use of a benzodiazepine may be considered. However, we restrict this practice solely to the treatment of depressed patients with marked anxiety, and discontinue by tapering the benzodiazepine as the antidepressant begins to exert its therapeutic effect, usually between the third and fifth week of treatment. The patient's mood may not improve at the same time as the neurovegetative symptoms do, an improvement in mood often taking 2 to 4 weeks to become apparent once an effective dose has been reached. The clinician must inform the patient of the potential for this latency in therapeutic response, as many patients expect antidepressants to be effective with the first dose. A patient may experience a return of energy and motivation while still experiencing the subjective symptoms of hopelessness and excessive guilt. For such patients at this key juncture of treatment, there may be an increased risk of suicide, as a return of energy in a still very dysphoric individual may provide the impetus and wherewithal for an act of self-destruction.

A complete trial of antidepressant medication consists of treatment with therapeutic doses of a drug for a total of 6 to 8 weeks. At the completion of such a trial the patient can be conceptualized as falling into one of three groups, depending upon whether there has been 1) a full response, 2) a partial response, or 3) no response at all. For those fortunate patients who achieve full remission, treatment should continue for a minimum of 6 months, or longer when there is a history of a recurrent course. Nonresponders should be switched to a drug in the other first-line class of antidepressants—that is, from a TCA to an SSRI, or vice versa.

Augmentation strategies are often the best approach when a severely depressed patient has already achieved a moderate response. In other cases a switch to the other first-line class of antidepressants may be preferable. For patients who fail to respond to sequential trials of a TCA and an SSRI, and when augmentation strategies have also been ineffective, a second-line antidepressant is warranted. Bupropion has been recommended as the most promising second-line antidepressant based on its unique mechanism of action and on empirical evidence that it may be especially effective for the TCA nonresponder (Preskorn and Burke 1992). The MAOIs have also been recommended as a second-line treatment. Thase et al. (1992) administered phenelzine or tranylcypromine to patients with TCA-resistant major depression and documented a response rate of 58%. Nonetheless, the patient's clinical presentation is the best predictor of response to MAOI therapy. The atypical depressive features—mood reactivity, hypersomnia, hyperphagia, severe anergy, and increased sensitivity to rejection—are indicative of preferential response to the MAOIs (Liebowitz et al. 1988; McGrath et al. 1992). The converse, however, is not true: patients with classic melancholia have been shown to respond to MAOIs at an overall rate equal to that of the TCAs (McGrath et al. 1984). Trazodone has been shown to be clearly superior to placebo and roughly equivalent to the TCAs in systematic studies; nonetheless, many clinicians believe that trazodone has less potent antidepressant effects than the TCAs and SSRIs (Preskorn and Burke 1992).

Maintenance Therapy

Once the patient's depressive symptoms have resolved, the dose of the antidepressant and the appropriate length of treatment on medication must be determined. If the dose required for treatment of the initial acute episode is associated with side effects, the dose for maintenance may be decreased gradually to a better tolerated level, with close monitoring for recurrence of depressive symptoms. However, without the presence of disabling side effects, the routine use of lower "maintenance levels" of antidepressants is no longer justifiable, because there is evidence that relapse is more likely when the antidepressant dose is lowered from acute treatment levels (Frank et al. 1990).

Results from the National Institute of Mental Health (NIMH) collaborative study indicated that antidepressant therapy should not be discontinued before there have been four to five symptom-free months (Prien and Kupfer 1986). Most clinicians treat single episodes of depression for a minimum of 6 months in the maintenance phase. However, many patients have histories of chronic recurrent depressions. For such patients, longer periods of antidepressant treatment are warranted in order to protect against recurrence (Frank et al. 1990).

When the decision has been made that it is safe to discontinue the antidepressant, it should be gradually tapered. We recommend that doses of antidepressants should be decreased slowly (e.g., reduce imipramine by 25 mg per week) over several months, with careful monitoring of the patient's sleep, energy, and mood. If an increase in depressive symptoms is detected, the medication should be increased until therapeutic response returns.

Rapid discontinuation of antidepressant medication (i.e., over several days) should be avoided, because withdrawal symptoms may occur. (This is less of a problem with fluoxetine, which, because of its very long half-life, in effect tapers itself.) In the case of the TCAs and MAOIs, withdrawal symptoms may be due to rebound "cholinergic overdrive" (Dilsaver et al. 1983). Withdrawal symptoms may occur in as many as 50% of patients who are being tapered from antidepressants, and these include a range of somatic, gastrointestinal, and behavioral difficulties. The most common withdrawal symptoms are insomnia, increased anxiety, a flu-like malaise, diarrhea, and recurrence of depressed mood. Management of severe withdrawal symptoms consists of reinstituting an adequate dose of antidepressants and, when symptoms resolve, reducing medication dose according to a much more gradual regimen (e.g., 10 mg per week of imipramine).

Refractory Depression

Careful review of the clinical history and response to previous treatment often reveals that the depressed patient who has been refractory to standard antidepressant treatment has had an inadequate therapeutic trial with the antidepressant (Lydiard 1985). The clinician should obtain details regarding the medications prescribed, the dosages taken, the duration of the therapeutic trial, and any plasma level data obtained. Other common sources of treatment "resistance" include patient compliance and physician factors such as failure to adequately educate the patient and family about doses and side effects. Failure to complete an adequate therapeutic trial with an antidepressant drug does not constitute a depression that is resistant to pharmacotherapy. Many patients will require treatment trials with more than one antidepressant drug before a drug is found that is well tolerated and can be increased to a therapeutic dose, and that is effective for a particular patient. Another "pseudorefractory" presentation is the patient who reports a history of robust but short-lived responses to several antidepressants. Mixed mood states may ultimately develop if the patient remains on antidepressants, and the diagnosis of a refractory, agitated depression may be made erroneously. The treatment may require that antidepressants be discontinued, usually after a trial of combined treatment with a mood stabilizer (Hurowitz and Liebowitz 1993; Wehr et al. 1988). For the patient whose depression does not respond to this approach, a trial of bupropion or low-dose MAOI therapy may be effective without engendering a rapid-cycling course.

For patients who do not respond to adequate trials of first- and second-line antidepressant treatment, or who achieve only partial response, several augmentation strategies are advised. Augmentation involves the concurrent use of two antidepressants or the use of a single antidepressant in combination with lithium, thyroid hormone, or a psychostimulant. Of these strategies, lithium augmentation has received the most attention; many patients who fail to respond to TCA or SSRI treatment alone are reported to improve when the antidepressant was combined with lithium (Thase et al. 1989). Some of these patients manifested a rapid and dramatic response when lithium was added with their antidepressant, but improvement may require 6 weeks. Patients will often respond to doses of lithium that would be insufficient for the treatment of bipolar disorder. Thyroid supplementation has received a more mixed endorsement in the scientific literature (Goodwin et al. 1982). Before adjunctive thyroid hormone is prescribed, baseline thyroid function tests, including thyroid-stimulating hormone (TSH), should be obtained in order to document possible underlying hypothyroidism.

The use of more than one antidepressant for cases of refractory depression is potentially beneficial in the treatment of refractory depression. Fluoxetine plus TCA combinations have been reported to be effective for patients who fail to respond to monotherapy, and, perhaps, to bring a more rapid antidepressant effect (Nelson et al. 1991). Fluoxetine causes tricyclic levels in the blood to rise (Downs et al. 1989), but this effect likely does not account for the synergism between the two antidepressants. However, because of fluoxetine's elevation of tricyclic levels, augmentation of TCAs with fluoxetine raises the risk of TCA toxicity. If this approach is clinically indicated, we recommend beginning with low TCA doses (e.g., imipramine, 25 mg) and proceeding only after plasma levels have been measured.

Despite concerns over severe reactions that may occur with concomitant treatment with tricyclic antidepressants and MAOIs, the combination may be safely prescribed, provided specific precautions are taken. It has been firmly established that it is hazardous to add a TCA to ongoing MAOI therapy. However, there are now many reports of the safe addition of MAOIs to ongoing treatment with a TCA (Pande et al. 1991). There is some evidence that such a combination may prove effective in depressed patients who have failed monotherapy with TCAs and SSRIs (Schmauss et al. 1988). There are two general strategies for combined therapy with MAOIs: a) the MAOI is added to the TCA, or b) the two drugs are begun concurrently. If the MAOI is to be added, the TCA should be raised, as usual, to a therapeutic level. The MAOI should be added in small increments over protracted periods of time until a therapeutic response occurs or until side effects intervene. When the MAOIs and TCAs are initiated concurrently, we also recommended that gradual and small incremental adjustments be made until an effect is obtained. If the patient's depression responds, the clinician eventually may wish to determine whether it is the combined therapy or the MAOI alone that is responsible for the improvement. This can be accomplished by gradually reducing the TCA dose. If the depressive symptoms reappear, this would indicate that the combined treatment is, indeed, necessary. Feighner et al. (1985) have suggested that psychostimulants may also be added safely to MAOI-TCA combinations. However, because of the risk of the serotonin syndrome, TCAs with strong serotonin reuptake inhibition, especially clomipramine, should be avoided in combination with MAOIs (Marley and Wozniak 1984). This caveat must be extended to the entire class of SSRIs, *which must never be administered together with an MAOI.*

Stimulants such as amphetamine and methylphenidate have been used to treat depression for many years. Although such drugs have activating properties, their use has generally fallen into disfavor among many clinicians who have valid concerns about the development of tolerance to the antidepressant effects; dependence; psychiatric side effects, including psychosis; and the high rate of relapse after discontinuation of the drug (Satel and Nelson 1989). Stimulants have been shown to be useful in the treatment of patients with mild to moderate depression with prominent fatigue or apathy, depressed geriatric patients with prominent apathy, and for medically ill patients with depression. Several studies document the benefit of stimulants for the treatment of post-stroke depression (Lingam et al. 1988). Psychostimulants are useful for augmentation of antidepressants in the treatment of refractory depression.

Another "stimulant-like" drug that has shown promise in the treatment of depression is fenfluramine, a serotonin reuptake inhibitor and presynaptic serotonin releaser. The latter mechanism is likely responsible for ferfluramine's "stimulant-like" effects. O'Rourke et al. (1989) reported success in treating seasonal depression with fenfluramine alone, but fenfluramine may also be useful as an adjunct to TCAs and SSRIs in the treatment of both depression and obsessive-compulsive disorder. Price and Grunhaus (1990) added fenfluramine to desipramine in a group of depressed patients with no response to this TCA alone, and found that there was no benefit. However, among a group of obsessive-compulsive patients with partial response to SSRI therapy, Hollander et al. (1990) found that adjunctive fenfluramine, 20 to 60 mg/day, brought additional antiobsessional effects. Thus, it remains to be proved whether fenfluramine would benefit patients as an adjunct to SSRI or TCA therapy for depression.

Risks, Side Effects, and Their Management

Antidepressant side effects play a major role in determining the selection of the most appropriate drug for an individual patient. Patients have varied reactions to side effects when they do occur. Many of the TCAs have cardiovascular effects, including orthostatic hypotension and cardiac conduction delays, that may be highly dangerous in patients with pre-existing cardiovascular problems but far less dangerous for younger, healthier populations. Similarly, sedation and overstimulation from antidepressant side effects may be tolerable, or even therapeutic, to varying degrees depending on the individual and the particular manifestations of the depressive episode being treated.

Anticholinergic effects. Antidepressant drugs vary widely in their relative potential to produce anticholinergic side effects. Drugs such as amitriptyline and protriptyline have high affinity for the muscarinic receptors, whereas desipramine has approximately one-tenth and trazodone has 1/20,000 the muscarinic affinity of amitriptyline (Richelson 1983). In practical terms, trazodone, nefazodone, and the SSRIs have virtually no anticholinergic effects, yet dry mouth and blurred vision occur more frequently with trazodone treatment than with placebo. Bupropion has no effect on the cholinergic system.

Cholinergic medications have been reported to relieve some of the anticholinergic side effects (Yager 1986). Bethanechol chloride may alleviate dry mouth, constipation, urinary hesitancy and retention, and erectile and ejaculatory dysfunction. The addition of a medication to treat side effects should be used only after dosage reduction and alternative antidepressants with fewer anticholinergic side effects have been attempted. The use of antidepressants, because of their anticholinergic side effects, must proceed with great caution when treating patients with prostatic hypertrophy and narrow angle glaucoma.

Sedation.   With the exception of trazodone, the relative sedating properties of the antidepressant drugs appear to parallel their respective histamine receptor binding affinities. Trazodone, trimipramine, amitriptyline, and doxepin are the most sedating antidepressants. Less-sedating antidepressants include desipramine, protriptyline, and bupropion and the SSRIs. However, even antidepressants known for their activating properties (such as SSRIs) may induce extreme sedation in some patients. Several reports have indicated that fluoxetine and the MAOIs have had just such an effect (Joffe 1990; Teicher et al. 1988).

Stimulation/insomnia.   The SSRIs, bupropion, MAOIs, and some TCAs are associated with side effects involving excess stimulation. (Nefazodone does not produce significant stimulation or insomnia.) Patients complain of "jitteriness," restlessness, tense feelings, and disturbed sleep. These side effects can occur early in the treatment, prior to the antidepressant effect. Therefore, all patients should be informed of the symptoms of overstimulation prior to the initiation of treatment. In particular, SSRIs with a long half-life should be started at low doses and increased slowly. In this way, if overstimulation occurs, it will not be so severe and persistent that it will discourage the patient from accepting an antidepressant from another category. The short-term use of a benzodiazepine may also help the patient cope with overstimulation in the early stages of treatment, until tolerance to this side effect occurs. For some patients, however, this side effect is so severe and persistent that an antidepressant from another category must be used. Another strategy for antidepressant-induced or depression-related insomnia is to prescribe low-dose trazodone (e.g., 50 to 150 mg) at bedtime (Jacobsen 1990). Some caution should be observed, however, when trazodone is prescribed in combination with MAOIs and SSRIs. There have been several reported instances of the serotonin syndrome, which is characterized by nausea, dizziness, ataxia, myoclonic jerks, and confusion (Metz and Shader 1990).

Cardiovascular effects.   For many patients, especially those with pre-existing heart disease, tricyclic antidepressants have clinically relevant effects on blood pressure, heart rate, cardiac conduction, and cardiac rhythm (Goldman et al. 1986). MAOIs, SSRIs, and bupropion do not affect cardiac conduction, yet each has the potential to affect heart rate and blood pressure (Feder 1991).

Orthostatic hypotension is the cardiovascular side effect that most commonly results in serious morbidity, especially in elderly patients and in patients with congestive heart failure (Glassman et al. 1983). Melancholia, itself, may be a significant risk factor for the development of orthostatic hypotension (Giardina et al. 1985). The symptoms of orthostatic hypotension usually consist of dizziness or lightheadedness when the patient changes from lying to sitting or from sitting to standing positions. Glassman et al. (1979) reported an injury rate of 4% for patients with an average age of 60 years who were treated with imipramine. Although orthostatic hypotension may occur with any TCA, nortriptyline is the least likely TCA to cause this side effect (Roose et al. 1981). Trazodone can cause orthostatic hypotension and dizziness as well (Spivak et al. 1987). Rabkin et al. (1985) found a greater than 10% incidence of severe orthostatic hypotension among patients treated with MAOIs. Although the incidence is much lower than that associated with TCAs and MAOIs, fluoxetine has been reported to cause postural hypotension, bradycardia, and syncope in patients with no history of cardiovascular disease (Feder 1991). Of the newer antidepressants, bupropion does not cause orthostatic hypotension (Roose et al. 1991).

Increases in heart rate that occur with TCAs rarely result in morbidity or mortality (Glassman and Bigger 1981); however, patients often find tachycardia frightening or distracting. Antidepressants with greater anticholinergic properties, such as amitriptyline, are associated with a higher incidence of this side effect (Goldman et al. 1986). Because TCAs at toxic levels can cause life-threatening arrhythmias, many clinicians believe that TCAs can cause dangerous arrhythmias at treatment doses. In actuality, TCAs are potent antiarrhythmic agents, possessing quinidine-like properties (Glassman and Bigger 1981). The particular effects of the tricyclic antidepressants on the cardiac conduction system are of great clinical relevance. Prolongation of the PR and QRS intervals can occur with TCA use, and thus these drugs should not be used in patients with preexisting heart block (especially right bundle branch block and left bundle branch block). In such patients TCAs can and often do lead to second- or third-degree heart block, both life-threatening conditions (Roose et al. 1987). Because trazodone does not cause significant change in cardiac conduction, for some time it was felt to be the antidepressant of choice among patients with cardiac conduction defects. However, there are now several reports of increased ventricular irritability among patients with conduction defects and preexisting ventricular arrhythmias (Jankowsky et al. 1983; Vitullo et al. 1990). The information available to date suggests that bupropion and the SSRIs are free of the risk of conduction abnormalities.

Medical evaluation and management of cardiovascular side effects.   Before initiation of treatment with TCAs, the clinician must obtain a comprehensive cardiovascular history and review of symptoms. Blood pressure and pulse must be checked, both with the patient sitting and standing. The clinician must evaluate other potential sources of hypotension, including diet, dehydration, and concomitant medications. Patients should be instructed to change from the sitting or lying to the standing position in a slow, continuous fashion. The patient is instructed to stand in place for 30 seconds before ambulating, and warned against "popping upright" from prone or sitting positions to answer the phone, respond to the doorbell, and the like. Patients are advised to walk up and down stairs slowly with ample support from a secure handrail.

Orthostatic hypotension from TCAs may not be dose dependent; therefore, lowering the dose of antidepressant may not lessen the dizziness or the changes in blood pressure. If the orthostatic hypotension is caused by MAOIs, the dosing regimen may be altered by reducing the administration of the drug to once or twice daily. Additionally, the dose may be lowered and then gradually increased. Expansion of the intravascular volume by using salt tablets or fluocortisone may also be an effective treatment. The addition in low dosage of a psychostimulant medication has been shown to alleviate this side effect, as well.

For patients with preexisting heart disease and for all patients over age 35, an ECG should be taken before the initiation of antidepressant treatment. If the initial ECG reveals clinically significant abnormalities, another ECG must be taken after the patient's medication has reached a steady state level. For patients with bundle branch block, TCAs should be used only when SSRIs, bupropion, and ECT prove ineffective. In such cases, TCA treatment should then commence only with the patient being monitored in the hospital with frequent ECGs, including a prolonged ambulatory study.

Sexual side effects.   Sexual side effects may occur with any antidepressant. The psychiatrist should elicit a careful history in order to distinguish the sexual problems that may originate from depression from those problems caused by medication. Sexual dysfunction, which includes impotence, ejaculatory dysfunction, anorgasmia, and reduced libido, has been reported in every antidepressant class (Seagraves 1992). Trazodone (Scher et al. 1983) is the only antidepressant that has been associated with priapism, which may be irreversible and require surgical intervention (Mitchell and Popkin 1983). Nefazodone, on the other hand, has not been reported to produce priapism.

Whenever possible, the management of sexual side effects should be postponed until the patient has completed an adequate trial of the antidepressant. When significant sexual dysfunction persists for more than 1 month despite a positive response to treatment, a reduction in the dosage should be considered. In many cases, this results in a diminution of the symptoms, without loss of therapeutic benefit. When there is no therapeutic dose that does not cause the sexual side effect, two strategies are available: the original antidepressant can be replaced with an alternative, or other drugs can be prescribed to counteract the side effect.

Although there are reports of success after patients have been switched from one TCA to another, or from one antidepressant class to another, every antidepressant has been associated with sexual side effects. Only bupropion, which has an atypical mode of action, appears to carry a lower risk overall (Gardner and Johnston 1985). Several medications have been suggested as antidotes for the sexual side effects associated with antidepressants. Bethanechol, a cholinergic drug, has been used for anorgasmia in doses of 10 to 30 mg, taken 1 to 2 hours before coitus (Seagraves 1987). Similarly, yohimbine, an inhibitor of the alpha$_2$-noradrenaline autoreceptor, has been successful in treating impotence, in a 10-mg dose 1 hour prior to sex (Price and Grunhaus 1990). Cyproheptadine, an antihistamine with antiserotonergic properties, has been successful in reversing anorgasmia, in doses of 4 to 12 mg, also taken 1 to 2 hours before sex (Zajecka et al. 1991).

Weight gain/loss.   Patients treated with TCAs may experience undesirable weight gain. This side effect appears to be unrelated to improvement in the patient's mood (Fernstrom et al. 1986). The MAOIs are particularly associated with a risk of significant weight gain during treatment, although it appears that this reaction occurs less frequently with tranylcypromine than it does with phenelzine (Rabkin et al. 1985). In addition, some patients manifest a peripheral edema, which may respond to a reduction of salt intake. Treatment with fluoxetine has been associated with weight loss (Ferguson 1986), although it also has potential to cause weight gain in some individuals. It appears that bupropion and nefazodone do not cause weight gain as a side effect.

Allergic reactions.   As with most drugs, allergic and hypersensitivity reactions may occur with antidepressants. If a mild rash develops, the drug may be continued and symptomatic treatment instituted. For more serious skin eruptions, the drug should be discontinued, preferably over several days to reduce the possibility of antidepressant withdrawal symptoms. If further antidepressant treatment is necessary, it is preferable to avoid drugs that are metabolites of the offending drug. Elevated temperature or signs of infection associated with the rash necessitate a complete medical evaluation, including complete blood count and liver function tests.

Neurological effects. Tremor is a common side effect of tricyclic antidepressants, such as imipramine and desipramine, that affect predominantly the noradrenergic system. In these circumstances, a dose reduction or a change to a different type of antidepressant may ultimately be required to alleviate the tremor. However, treatment with a beta-adrenergic blocking drug (e.g., propranolol) will often provide symptomatic relief (Kronfol et al. 1983). Although devoid of direct noradrenergic activity, SSRIs may also cause a tremor that will respond to a beta-blocker. If propranolol is added to the therapeutic regimen, we suggest that the antidepressant level be monitored more closely, because propranolol has been reported to increase levels of other psychotropic medications (Silver et al. 1986).

The prevailing impression among clinicians is that antidepressants lower the seizure threshold, but this belief is far from being proved scientifically. Indeed, there is evidence that at certain plasma levels some of the TCAs have an anticonvulsant effect (Jobe et al. 1984). There is also a report that fluoxetine improved seizure control in epileptic patients when it was added to their existing anticonvulsant regimen (Leander 1992). Reports of an increased risk of seizures in patients treated with bupropion have been confirmed (Sheehan et al. 1986); this antidepressant was approved by the FDA with the caveat that individual doses should not exceed 150 mg and that the total daily dose should not be greater than 450 mg. Similarly, a dose-related risk of seizures has been found with clomipramine, and this has led to the recommendation that its daily dosage should not exceed 250 mg (Clomipramine Collaborative Study Group 1991). Among the remaining TCAs, amoxapine and desipramine may have a higher risk of seizures after overdosage (Wedin et al. 1986).

Risk of suicide. Teicher et al. (1990) reported that six depressed patients prescribed fluoxetine became intensely preoccupied with suicidal ideation. The resulting debate in the literature has led to several hypotheses that seek to account for the report and several others that contradict it. Fluoxetine-induced akathisia has been implicated in several cases, based on both the phenomenology of the symptom and a positive response to antiakathisia treatments (Hamilton and Opler 1992). Other cases of increased suicidality with SSRIs have been attributed to a well-known condition among severely depressed patients initiating treatment with antidepressants: relief from dysphoria may lag behind while energy levels begin to increase, with the result that the patient's motivation to complete suicide is greater than prior to treatment. Whatever the final explanation for the reports, studies of suicide rates among fluoxetine users have not indicated an increased risk of suicide attempts or of completions relative to other antidepressants (Fava and Rosenbaum 1992). More importantly, suicide rates among depressed patients treated with fluoxetine (and all other antidepressants) are markedly reduced from that of depressed patients who do not receive antidepressants.

The serotonin syndrome.   There have been several reports of a medication-induced syndrome that has been attributed to excessive stimulation of the serotonergic system. This condition arises more commonly among patients treated concurrently with two or more serotonergic drugs (e.g., fluoxetine or an MAOI with trazodone). However, it also occurs in patients who take a single SSRI. Affected individuals suffer from the constellation of lethargy, restlessness, confusion, flushing, diaphoresis, tremor, and myoclonic jerks. As the condition progresses, hyperthermia, hypertonicity, myoclonus, and rigor may develop. The latter may lead, ultimately, to rhabdomyolysis, acidosis, respiratory compromise, disseminated intravascular coagulation, and renal failure secondary to myoglobinuria (Metz and Shader 1990). The syndrome must be identified as rapidly as possible, as discontinuation of the serotonergic medications is the first step in treatment, followed by emergency medical treatment, as required.

Overdose.   Because the incidence of suicide and suicide attempts is high in depressed patients, deliberate overdosage with antidepressant drugs is a common occurrence. The major complications from overdose with tricyclic antidepressant drugs include those that arise from neuropsychiatric impairment, hypotension, cardiac arrhythmias, and seizures. The psychiatrist must be familiar with the signs and symptoms of tricyclic toxicity, as well as with the basic management principles of tricyclic overdose. Because most antidepressants have significant anticholinergic activity, anticholinergic delirium often occurs when the TCAs are taken in high doses. This is particularly true for elderly patients and for patients with neuropsychiatric conditions. Other complications of anticholinergic overdose include agitation, supraventricular arrhythmias, hallucinations, severe hypertension, and seizures (Goldfrank et al. 1986). Ventricular arrhythmias that occur secondary to overdose are typical of the arrhythmias that occur with high doses of quinidine-like agents, and these begin within the first 24 hours after hospital admission (Goldberg et al. 1985).

The SSRIs and nefazodone are much safer in overdose than the TCAs, because they do not have life-threatening effects at high plasma concentrations. Trazodone is similar in this regard, although there is the risk of myocardial irritation in patients with preexisting ventricular conduction abnormalities. The danger of bupropion overdose is, for the most part, limited to the risk of seizures. However, seizures are seldom a life-threatening event, unless they result in motor vehicle accidents, falls, or other trauma-related events. On the other hand, bupropion's lack of significant cardiovascular or respiratory toxicity means that it is rarely lethal in overdose.

The MAOIs fall between the TCAs and the SSRIs in terms of lethality in overdose. Most complications related to MAOI overdose arise from its stimulation of the sympathetic nervous system. MAOIs are most dangerous when patients suffer from hypertensive crises as the result of ingesting foods with high tyramine content. Treatment of hypertensive crises with intravenous nitroprusside or phentolamine is recommended (Goldfrank et al. 1986).

Drug interactions. Because the TCAs are metabolized by the liver, drugs that induce hepatic microsomal enzymes will result in a lowering of plasma tricyclic levels. These agents include alcohol, anticonvulsants, barbiturates, chloral hydrate, glutethimide, oral contraceptives, and cigarette smoking (Lydiard 1985). Antipsychotic drugs, methylphenidate, and increasing age are associated with increased plasma levels of TCAs (Lydiard 1985). Plasma levels of TCAs may change unexpectedly in patients who change their smoking patterns during treatment. As a general rule, plasma levels should be monitored when there are any changes in concomitant medications, smoking habits, or drinking patterns.

Although tricyclic levels are affected by several agents, usually this is not a reciprocal effect: the TCAs rarely affect the metabolism of other drugs. A notable exception to this general rule is the drug sodium valproate, levels of which may drop when a TCA is administered concurrently (Preskorn and Burke 1992). Both guanethidine and clonidine lose effectiveness if administered concomitantly with drugs, such as TCAs, that block reuptake of catecholamines into adrenergic neurons.

Fluoxetine has the effect of increasing plasma tricyclic levels by inhibiting their hepatic metabolism (Brosen et al. 1986). In some individuals this interaction may cause dangerously high levels of the TCA (Vaughan 1988), and, because of its very long half-life, fluoxetine may cause this effect even after it has been discontinued for several weeks. When the TCA involved is clomipramine, excessive plasma levels are particularly troubling, because an increased seizure risk occurs at only slightly elevated levels of this drug. Plasma TCA levels must be followed closely when a TCA and fluoxetine are prescribed together, or when a TCA is initiated shortly after the withdrawal of fluoxetine. Sertraline may also increase tricyclic levels, but the effect is far less pronounced. Paroxetine has an effect on TCA level that falls somewhere between sertraline's and fluoxetine's (Brosen et al. 1992). Plasma concentrations of carbamazepine (which is chemically similar to the TCAs) may also increase when fluoxetine is added (Grimsley et al. 1991).

Bupropion, which in itself has little effect on the metabolism of other drugs, may be increased in the plasma when coadministered with fluoxetine (Preskorn 1991). This is a clinically significant effect because of the increased risk of seizures. When fluoxetine is coadministered, seizures are induced with bupropion at doses 50% lower than doses that cause seizures when bupropion is used alone.

Particular care must be exercised in switching patients from an MAOI to other antidepressant classes. For the patient who has completed an MAOI trial without therapeutic response, TCAs, SSRIs, bupropion, nefazodone, and other MAOIs should not be started until 10 to 14 days after the original MAOI has been discontinued. Although not currently designated an antidepressant, the serotonin agonist anxiolytic buspirone should also be included on this list. If possible, a similar waiting period should follow the discontinuation of a TCA or bupropion when an MAOI is to be administered. Switching from an SSRI to an MAOI is of special concern because of the risk of the serotonin syndrome. We recommend a 5-week washout period when switching from fluoxetine to an MAOI. Because of their briefer half-life, the waiting period after sertraline and paroxetine discontinuation is only 14 days prior to the initiation of an MAOI.

Monoamine oxidase inhibitors, the tyramine reaction, and the serotonin syndrome. The tyramine reaction with an MAOI stems from ingested tyramine that is not metabolized because of the MAOI's inactivation of intestinal monoamine oxidase. This reaction has also been called the "cheese reaction," because tyramine is present in relatively high concentrations in aged cheese. Tyramine can act as a false transmitter and displace norepinephrine from presynaptic storage granules. Although life-threatening hypertensive reactions are infrequent, in a chart review study of patients receiving MAOIs in a research center, Rabkin and colleagues (1985) reported that less severe hypertensive reactions are as high as 8%.

The key foods patients receiving MAOI treatment should be instructed to avoid include cheeses (except cottage cheese, ricotta, and cream cheese), beers and ales (including nonalcoholic varieties), yeasts and protein extracts (which are ingredients in many soups, gravies, and sauces), broad beans, fermented sausage, sauerkraut, shrimp paste, soy sauce, and overripe or stewed figs, raisins, dates, and bananas. Several foods that were formerly considered a danger are no longer included on the list of prohibited substances. For example, in moderation, most wines and liquors are safe (although alcohol often aggravates depression and may interfere with antidepressant levels and actions). Liver, if fresh, is also probably safe, and caffeine and chocolate are of concern only when consumed in large amounts.

Certain drugs with sympathomimetic or serotonergic activity, including certain decongestants and cough syrups, should be avoided while a patient is being treated with an MAOI. However, pure antihistamine drugs, such as diphenhydramine, and pure expectorants without dextromethorphan (e.g., guaifenesin) are permissible. Synthetic opioids should be used with caution, because they may induce the serotonin syndrome. Meperidine must be avoided entirely for this reason. Aspirin, nonsteroid anti-inflammatory drugs, and acetaminophen should be used for mild to moderate pain. Among narcotic agents, morphine is known to be safe in combination with MAOIs, although lower-than-usual doses may be necessary, because there is some evidence that the MAOIs increase morphine levels slightly.

Despite warnings and education regarding the risks of this reaction, strict compliance to dietary guidelines is followed by fewer than one-third of patients taking MAOIs (Neil et al. 1979). We often recommend that our patients taking MAOIs read the chapter on antidepressants in books written specifically for patients and their families (Yudofsky et al. 1991). Unfortunately, even perfect compliance with the dietary and other restrictions does not guarantee complete protection from MAOI-induced hypertensive crises. Rare reports of spontaneous hypertension associated with MAOI use have come from several independent sources. Most of these reports involved the use of tranylcypromine, but phenelzine has also been implicated (daMotta and Cordas 1990).

The tyramine reaction can range from mild to severe. In the most mild form, the patient may complain of sweating, palpitations, and a mild headache. The most severe form manifests as a hypertensive crisis, with severe headache, increases in blood pressure, and possible intracerebral hemorrhage. The severity of this reaction cannot be predicted by MAOI dose, by food type or amount ingested, or even by prior history of a crisis. Patients should be warned against gaining a false sense of confidence if dietary guidelines are broken without consequences.

The calcium channel blocker nifedipine is gaining increasing acceptance as a treatment for mild to moderate cases of MAOI-induced hypertension. An oral dose of 10 mg of nifedipine will often normalize blood pressure in 1 to 5 minutes with little risk of overshoot hypotension (Schenk and Remick 1989). It is now recommended that the patient bite the gelatin capsule containing the nifedipine and then swallow the capsule (Ward and Davidson 1991).

If the patient on an MAOI experiences a severely painful or unremitting occipital headache, he or she should immediately seek medical assessment that will include having his or her blood pressure monitored. If the blood pressure is severely elevated, a drug with alpha-adrenergic blocking properties, such as intravenous phentolamine (Regitine) 5 mg, or intramuscular chlorpromazine, 25 to 50 mg, may be administered.

Because treatment with phentolamine may be associated with cardiac arrhythmias or severe hypotension, this approach should only be carried out in an emergency room setting by qualified medical personnel with proper monitoring equipment (Tollefson 1983). It is advisable to have patients on MAOIs carry an identification card or Medic Alert bracelet as notification to emergency medical personnel that the patient is currently taking MAOIs.

☐ Other Antidepressant Treatments

There are several new drugs with antidepressant effects. For example, fluvoxamine is an SSRI with antidepressant and antiobsessional effects. Venlafaxine is a structurally novel phenethylamine antidepressant that is a potent inhibitor of norepinephrine and serotonin reuptake, as well as a less potent dopamine reuptake inhibitor. In several placebo-controlled, double-blind studies, it has demonstrated an antidepressant effect comparable to that of currently available agents when given in the dose range of 75 to 375 mg/day (Khan et al. 1991; Schweizer et al. 1991). Moreover, in animal studies, venlafaxine has been shown to produce a rapid-onset downregulation of beta-adrenergic receptors (Muth et al. 1986), an effect that is more delayed with other antidepressants and that seems to correspond to the observed delay in therapeutic effect. Clinical trials have provided some evidence to suggest that venlafaxine may have a more rapid onset of action (Khan et al. 1991). It is generally well tolerated in adult and geriatric patients, with the most commonly encountered side effects being nausea, sweating, and nervousness (Schweizer et al. 1991).

The 5-HT$_2$ antagonist nefazodone was found to be equivalent to imipramine under double-blind, placebo-controlled conditions (Feighner et al. 1989). Unlike trazodone, nefazodone has few sedating and no hypotensive effects. In comparison with the SSRIs, nefazodone has fewer activating side effects, does not produce weight gain, and is not associated with insomnia.

Several nondrug modalities have been investigated for the treatment of depression. There is now strong evidence that patients with seasonal affective disorder (SAD) respond to phototherapy. Morning exposure to bright light appears to be the most efficacious (Terman et al. 1989), with current recommendations for a minimum of 2,500 lux for 2 hours each day for 1 week. Doses as high as 10,000 lux, for briefer daily periods of exposure, may be even more effective. Patients with milder depressions respond best to this form of treatment (Terman et al. 1989).

■ ANXIOLYTICS, SEDATIVES, AND HYPNOTICS

Before 1950, barbiturates were frequently utilized to treat the anxiety disorders and insomnia. Yet, because of the narrow range between therapeutic and fatal doses, and because of the significant potential for patients to become dependent, there ensued an active search for alternative compounds with anxiolytic and hypnotic properties with increased safety. This search resulted in the discoveries of meprobamate and the benozodiazepines chlordiazepoxide and diazepam. The increased safety of the benzodiazepines when ingested in overdose and the decrease in the potential for dependence has resulted in this class of compounds generally replacing other available anxiolytic and sedative drugs. Buspirone, a newer-generation anxiolytic in the azapirone class, is chemically distinct from other anxiolytic medications. It is devoid of sedating properties, has no dangerous interactions with alcohol, has no abuse potential, and does not impair psychomotor performance. However, buspirone also has a relatively slow onset of action, which can result in its being impractical in cases of transient anxiety or in clinical situations that require rapid treatment of anxiety.

In the search for agents that avoid some of the problems associated with the benzodiazepines (e.g., ataxia and rebound effects), several newer nonbenzodiazapine drugs are currently being investigated. The first of these to be marketed in the United States is zolpidem, a nonbenzodiazepine that acts at the type 1 benzodiazepine receptor site. However, to date there has been little evidence that clinically significant side effects are less with these agents when compared directly to the benzodiazepines (Jonas et al. 1992). The commonly used anxiolytics and hypnotics are listed in Table 27–9.

□ Indications and Efficacy

Benzodiazepines

Generalized anxiety disorder.   The efficacy of the benzodiazepines in the treatment of anxiety, including symptoms of worry, psychic anxiety, and somatic symptoms (gastrointestinal and cardiovascular), has been clearly and repeatedly demonstrated in many well-controlled studies (Elie and Lamontagne 1985; Rickels et al. 1983).

Panic disorder.   Benzodiazepines have demonstrated effectiveness in the treatment of panic attacks. Although the high-potency benzodiazepines alprazolam and clonazepam have received more attention as antipanic agents (Tesar 1990; Tesar et al. 1991), double-blind studies have

Table 27–9.   Anxiolytic and hypnotic drugs

Class/ Generic name	Trade name	Usual daily dose (mg)	Absorption	Approximate elimination $T_{1/2}$ including metabolites
Benzodiazepine **anxiolytics**				

Alprazolam	Xanax	0.75–1.5,
		  GAD;
		2–6,
		  Panic
		  disorder
			Rapid	12 hours

Chlordiazepoxide hydrochloride	Librium Libritabs	15–100	Rapid	1–4 days
Clorazepate dipotassium	Tranxene	15–60	Very rapid	2–4 days
Clonazepam	Klonopin	1–4	Very rapid	1–2 days
Diazepam	Valium Valrelease	4–40 15–45	Very rapid Slow	2–4 days
Halazepam	Paxepam	40–160	Rapid	2–4 days
Lorazepam	Ativan	2–6	Intermediate	12 hours
Benzodiazepine **hypnotics**				
Oxazepam	Serax	30–120	Slow	12 hours
Prazepam	Centrax	20–60	Very slow	2–4 days
Flurazepam hydrochloride	Dalmane	30	Rapid	3 days
Estazolam	ProSom	1–2	Intermediate	10–24 hours
Quazepam	Doral	7.5–15	Intermediate	3 days
Temazepam	Restoril	30	Intermediate	12 hours
Triazolam	Halcion	0.125–0.5	Rapid	6 hours
Barbiturates				
Phenobarbital		30–120	Very slow	2–4 days
Amobarbital	Amytal	50–300	Rapid	1–2 days
Secobarbital	Seconal	100–200	Rapid	1–2 days
Nonbenzodiazepine/ **nonbarbiturates**				

Hydroxyzine
  hydrochloride
  pamoate
	Atarax
	Vistaril
		75–400
		200–400
			Rapid	Less than
				  4 hours

Chloral hydrate		750
		  (sedation);
		500–1,000
		  (hypnotic)
			Rapid	Less than
				  12 hours

Buspirone	BuSpar	15–30	See text for
			  onset of
			  action	

Imidazopyridine				
Zolpidem	Ambien	5–10	Rapid	2.5 hours

Note.   GAD = generalized anxiety disorder.
Source.   Adapted from American Medical Association 1986; Greenblatt 1983; Greenblatt and Shader 1985.

also confirmed the efficacy of diazepam (Dunner et al. 1986) and of lorazepam (Charney and Woods 1989) in the treatment of panic disorder.

Insomnia.   Although only a few benzodiazepines have specific FDA-approved indications for the treatment of insomnia, almost all benzodiazepines may be used for this purpose. In the late 1980s, the benzodiazepines most commonly used as hypnotics were temazepam and triazolam. However, triazolam has received much negative attention in the lay press, based on reports of severe rebound insomnia, withdrawal, and amnestic effects, and assertions that episodes of aggression were precipitated by this agent. Although psychiatrists have, in many cases, found these reports of dangerousness exaggerated, public pressure has influenced prescribing practices significantly. Between 1988 and 1989, triazolam use dropped 20% (Wysowski and Baum 1991), and the medication has been removed from the market in Great Britain. There remains no doubt, however, that the benzodiazepines are effective in the treatment of insomnia (Greenblatt 1992).

Benzodiazepines are most clearly valuable as hypnotics in the general hospital setting, where high levels of sensory stimulation, pain, and acute stress may interfere with sleep. We advocate the use of the lowest effective dose of the benzodiazepine for the briefest possible period of time (usually several days). The safe and effective use of benzodiazepine hypnotics may, in fact, *prevent* chronic sleep difficulties from taking hold (NIMH Consensus Development Conference 1984).

Buspirone

Double-blind, controlled studies have shown that buspirone is effective in the treatment of anxiety and that, although it has a longer onset of action, its efficacy is not statistically different from that of the benzodiazepines (Cohn and Wilcox 1986; Goldberg and Finnerty 1979). However, despite its successes in the treatment of generalized anxiety disorder, buspirone does not appear to be ineffective in the treatment of panic attacks (Sheehan et al. 1990), except perhaps in an auxiliary role for the treatment of anticipatory anxiety (Gastfried and Rosenbaum 1989). On the other hand, there is some evidence that buspirone is an effective treatment for social phobia (Schneier et al. 1992).

Antidepressants

Klein and Fink (1962) described the response of panic attacks to treatment with imipramine. Since then, many antidepressants have been demonstrated to be effective in the treatment of panic disorder, including others in the TCA class (Zitrin et al. 1983), the MAOIs (Sheehan et al.

1980), and the SSRIs (Schneier et al. 1990). Patients with generalized anxiety disorder also respond to antidepressant treatment (Hoehn-Saric et al. 1988). Furthermore, patients with social phobia respond extremely well to certain antidepressant agents. The most compelling evidence is derived from a double-blind, placebo-controlled study that indicates that the MAOI phenelzine is an effective treatment for social phobia (Liebowitz et al. 1988). The SSRI fluoxetine may also be effective in treating social phobia (Van Ameringen et al. 1993).

Double-blind, placebo-controlled studies have demonstrated the effectiveness of clomipramine (Clomipramine Collaborative Study Group 1991) and fluvoxamine (Goodman et al. 1990) in the treatment of obsessive-compulsive disorder (OCD). In addition, several investigators have reported evidence in support of the efficacy of fluoxetine in the treatment of OCD (Liebowitz et al. 1989; Pigott et al. 1990). Sertraline has shown less promise as an antiobsessional agent (Chouinard et al. 1990).

Beta-Adrenergic Blocking Drugs

While beta-blockers are often effective in treating the peripheral manifestations of anxiety, such as palpitations, tachycardia, tremor, and sweating, they are less beneficial than benzodiazepines in alleviating the psychic experience—the worrying and apprehension that is the cognitive manifestation of anxiety (Tyrer and Lader 1984). Yet, in particular social situations, the ability of beta-blockers to suppress peripheral manifestations of anxiety appears to prevent the escalation of anxiety. There are persuasive anecdotal reports of success in treating social phobia with beta-blockers, but these findings have not stood up well in controlled studies (Liebowitz et al. 1991). However, in certain specialized performance situations (e.g., musical performance), there is good evidence that propranolol is an effective acute treatment of social anxiety (Liebowitz et al. 1985).

☐ Clinical Use of Anxiolytic and Sedative Drugs

Pharmacotherapy of Generalized Anxiety Disorder

Medications should be considered as only one component in a comprehensive treatment plan of anxiety. Psychotherapy, whether psychodynamic, behavioral, or supportive, is usually required to help the patient understand and control the sources and circumstances that surround the anxiety. For most patients anxiolytic medications are indicated for only relatively short-term use (i.e, 1 to 2 months); however, a small percentage of patients may require, and will continue to benefit from, more prolonged treatment (Rickels et al. 1983).

Benzodiazepines.   Benzodiazepines frequently cause sedation, may lead to physical dependence, and may impair memory and the performance of tasks requiring a high degree of mental alertness. Therefore, this class of drugs should be used for as brief a time as possible at the lowest effective dose (Table 27–10). Despite the liabilities of their use in treatment, benzodiazpines have been shown in general to be safe and effective for long-term use for the minority of patients who require such medication. Whereas tolerance to sedation often develops, the same is not true of the anxiolytic effects of these agents. When benzodiazepines are properly prescribed and closely monitored, the potential for abuse is minimized (Sellers et al. 1992). A dose equivalent to diazepam 5 mg tid is average for anxiolysis. All patients being considered for benzodiazepine treatment must be cautioned about the dangers of concomitant sedative drugs and alcohol use.

All benzodiazepines indicated for the treatment of anxiety are equally efficacious. Choice of a specific agent usually depends on the pharmacokinetics and pharmacodynamics of the drug. Diazepam, chlordiazepoxide, and clorazepate, for example, have half-lives that are several days in length. This should allow less frequent dosing than when is necessary when benzodiazepines with half-lives of 6 to 12 hours are used, such as lorazepam and alprazolam. However, single-dose administration of prazepam, a drug with a prolonged elimination half-life, was found to be less effective than with multiple-dose administration (Ansseau et al. 1984). Thus, in circumstances of severely disabling anxiety, the clinician may wish to prescribe a rapidly acting benzodiazepine; but it should be borne in mind that this rapid action may also result in rapid sedation or dizziness that may be unpleasant for some patients.

One frequently misunderstood issue is the relationship between

---

Table 27–10.   Guidelines for anxiolytic treatment with benzodiazepines

1. Complete a thorough medical evaluation, especially with regard to thyroid status, caffeine intake, and current medications.
2. Evaluate patient for psychodynamic and social factors that may contribute to or precipitate anxiety.
3. Initiate benzodiazepines at a low dose (e.g., diazepam 2 mg three times a day) and increase every few days until sedation or therapeutic effect is obtained (up to 15 mg three times a day).
4. Caution patient on sedative properties, performance impairment, dependence properties, and drug and alcohol interactions.
5. Reevaluate need for medication every month.
6. Taper medication as soon as possible, by approximately 10% per week for patients on long-term treatment (i.e., greater than 3 months).

pharmacokinetic half-life and pharmacodynamic effect. The pharma-codynamics (i.e., the effects of the drug on the CNS) depend on several factors, including pharmacokinetic half-life, affinity of the drug for the benzodiazepine receptor, and lipid solubility of the drug. For example, lorazepam has a higher binding affinity for the benzodiazepine receptor than does diazepam (Jack et al. 1982), and therefore lorazepam binds to the receptor for a longer time. Lipid solubility is another important factor in determining pharmacodynamic effects of benzodiazpines. A drug that is highly lipid soluble will rapidly distribute to fat tissues, including those within the brain; whereas a drug with a lower lipid solubility will reach the brain more slowly but maintain brain levels longer. Thus, although diazepam (high lipid solubility) has a more rapid onset of action than lorazepam (moderate lipid solubility), the acute therapeutic effects will not last as long as those of lorazepam. When compared with diazepam, a single dose of lorazepam will take longer to produce sedation, but this sedation will persist longer (Ellinwood et al. 1985). This occurs despite the fact that lorazepam has a markedly briefer pharmacokinetic half-life than do diazepam and its metabolites (8 hours vs. 48 hours, respectively).

The metabolism of benzodiazepines also is important in the choice of the specific therapeutic agent. For example, diazepam is metabolized in the liver to desmethyldiazepam, a metabolite with a long half-life. Lorazepam and oxazepam are not converted to active metabolites by the liver. Therefore, for patients with hepatic dysfunction, lorazepam and oxazepam are clinically indicated for relief of anxiety because their elimi-nation from the body will not be significantly affected (Abernethy et al. 1984). Sedative effects of diazepam have been demonstrated to persist for up to 2 weeks following discontinuation, after only 14 days of admin-istration of diazepam 3 mg tid (Salzman et al. 1983). For patients with brain disorders and for elderly patients, benzodiazepines that are brief-acting and devoid of active metabolites are usually indicated. As with the other psychotropic medications, the most critical issue is that the lowest effective doses should be used in elderly patients with careful and con-tinuous monitoring of side effects.

Buspirone.   Several clinically important facets of the anxiolytic re-sponse to buspirone differentiate it from the benzodiazepines. Studies suggest that response to buspirone occurs in approximately 2 weeks, compared with the more rapid onset associated with benzodiazepines. Because buspirone is not sedating (Seidel et al. 1985) and has no psycho-motor effects, it has a distinct advantage over the benzodiazepines when optimal alertness and motor performance are necessary. There is also evidence that the azapirones have antidepressant effects, perhaps at high doses (Lucki 1991). Such an effect is of value in the treatment of chronically anxious patients, who often suffer from concomitant depression. The maximum suggested dose of buspirone is 20 mg tid. Buspirone does not exhibit cross tolerance with benzodiazepines and other sedative/hypnotic drugs such as alcohol, barbiturates, and chloral hydrate. Thus, buspirone will not suppress benzodiazepine withdrawal symptoms (Lader and Olajide 1987). For the anxious patient treated with a benzodiazepine who requires a switch to buspirone, the clinician must remember that benzodiazepines must be tapered gradually in order to avoid withdrawal symptoms, despite the fact that the patient is receiving buspirone.

Antidepressants.   The clinical utility of antidepressants in the treatment of generalized anxiety disorder is still largely an uncharted territory. Kahn et al. (1986) reported success, comparable to that with chlordiazepoxide, in treating patients with generalized anxiety disorder patients with 75 to 150 mg/day of imipramine. As with buspirone, this anxiolytic effect was noted to have a delayed onset of approximately 2 weeks.

Pharmacotherapy of Panic Disorder

Breier et al. (1986) reported that over 80% of patients with panic disorder, with and without agoraphobia, have generalized/anticipatory anxiety responsive to treatment with benzodiazepines. Gastfried and Rosenbaum (1989) reported the successful treatment of anticipatory anxiety in panic disorder patients with adjunctive buspirone.

Benzodiazepines.   Benzodiazepines, as a class, are effective antipanic agents, with the higher-potency agents alprazolam and clonazepam receiving the most attention in the scientific literature (Spier et al. 1986; Tesar 1990). Both of these agents have a relatively rapid onset of action and are well tolerated in the higher dose ranges required to treat panic disorder. Clonazepam has the advantage of a longer elimination half-life, which provides more stable plasma drug levels and twice-a-day dosing. For many clinicians this feature of clonazepam makes it the benzodiazepine of choice in the treatment of panic disorder. For patients who are intolerant to the side effects of the antidepressants, alprazolam may have a special role to play when there is comorbid panic and depression.

For the treatment of panic disorder, begin clonazepam at 0.25 or 0.5 mg once a day, and increase to a total of 1 to 2 mg/day in two divided doses. Higher dosage levels may be necessary for complete relief of symptoms. The starting dosage of alprazolam is usually 0.25 or 0.5 mg tid; but typically, 3 to 4 mg/day in three or four divided doses is required for full response (Tesar 1990). Following successful treatment of panic disorder with alprazolam, the withdrawal and discontinuation of the medication may be complicated by the appearance of rebound anxiety and other withdrawal symptoms, including malaise, weakness, insomnia, tachycardia, lightheadedness, and dizziness (Fyer et al. 1987). For this reason, alprazolam should be tapered slowly, roughly 10% of the total dose per week, prior to discontinuation. Because clonazepam has a longer half-life and a demonstrated utility as a detoxifying agent in cases of benzodiazepine withdrawal (Patterson 1988), the termination of treatment with clonazepam is often less problematic (Herman et al. 1987).

Antidepressants.   Patients with panic disorder may require months of treatment before achieving remission, during which time their exposure to high-dose benzodiazepines may place them at risk of physical and/or psychological dependence. We therefore recommend the use of antidepressants as the initial treatment for panic disorder. For most patients, imipramine, desipramine, or nortriptyline should be considered first-line agents. Evidence to date seems to indicate that the SSRIs also possess significant antipanic effects, so these agents may be considered for the patient who cannot tolerate TCA-associated side effects. We anticipate that SSRIs will likely become a first-line treatment for panic disorder as more experience is gained with their use for this purpose. A decision as to which of these drugs to choose should be based on the same factors discussed in the section on antidepressant drugs. MAOIs are usually reserved for patients who have not responded to TCAs and SSRIs. A major caveat is that patients with panic disorder initially may be highly sensitive to the stimulant effects of small doses of antidepressants, especially desipramine and fluoxetine.

With highly anxious patients with panic disorder we often initiate treatment with clonazepam or alprazolam, and add low-dose antidepressant, which is then increased slowly. The rapid onset of action of benzodiazpines is helpful to the patient until such time that the antidepressant becomes effective. In addition, the benzodiazepine will treat any stimulating effects of the antidepressant until tolerance to this side effect develops (which may require several weeks). When panic symptoms have not been present for several weeks, the benzodiazepine is slowly tapered. In patients with marked residual anticipatory anxiety, longer-term use of a benzodiazepine or buspirone should be considered as an adjunct to the antidepressant. Buspirone is recommended for patients with a high potential for substance abuse, in which case benzodiazepines should generally be avoided.

Although patients with panic disorder respond to low-dose antidepressant therapy, in general, the doses, durations, and side effects of the antidepressants used for the treatment of depression are effective in the treatment of panic. For many patients, pharmacotherapy and brief psychotherapy may be sufficient for treatment of panic symptoms and for significant improvement in functioning. However, for certain patients with phobic or avoidant behaviors, such as agoraphobia, concurrent psychological and behavioral treatments are often required as well.

Pharmacotherapy of Insomnia

We advise dietary change, exercise, stress reduction, and, when indicated, psychotherapy before considering a hypnotic to treat persistent insomnia. While all of the currently available benzodiazepine hypnotics are absorbed relatively rapidly from the gastrointestinal tract and achieve peak plasma levels in approximately 1.5 hours (Greenblatt 1992), affinity for the benzodiazepine receptor and elimination half-life both affect the clinical utility of these agents. For example, flurazepam and the newly available quazepam are both ultimately metabolized into a clinically active compound, desalkylflurazepam, which has an elimination half-life of 40 to 50 hours (Greenblatt 1992). With successive days of treatment, the accumulation of this compound in the body may adversely affect motor performance and cause daytime drowsiness, a so-called "hangover" effect. Although tolerance to the daytime sedation may develop with time (Greenblatt et al. 1977b), we believe that for elderly patients and many others the risks of CNS side effects are too great with flurazepam and quazepam. On the other hand, a long elimination half-life reduces the risk of early morning awakening and rebound insomnia after drug discontinuation and may be appropriate for brief-term treatment. With a half-life of just 1.5 to 5 hours, triazolam is at the opposite end of the spectrum among the benzodiazepines (Greenblatt et al. 1984). The risks of accumulation of triazolam in the body are avoided in the healthy patient, but the risk of rebound insomnia makes triazolam less useful for patients with early morning awakening. Temazepam and estazolam have intermediate half-life values (Greenblatt 1992), and, as a result, these agents have fewer day-after and rebound insomnia side effects.

Quazepam is unique among the benzodiazepines in that it is selective for the type 1 benzodiazepine receptor (Wamsley and Hunt 1991). The new, nonbenzodiazapine hypnotic agent zolpidem also acts selectively at the type 1 benzodiazepine receptor, although, unlike quazepam, it has no nonselective metabolites. It is known that zolpidem has only minor anticonvulsant and muscle relaxant effects. However, when compared with the benzodiazepines, zolpidem (20 mg/day dose) has been shown to cause somewhat more CNS side effects, such as daytime drowsiness, dizziness, fatigue, depression, amnesia, and falls. Lower doses (5 to 10 mg/day) have associated adverse effects at a rate very similar to that of short-acting benzodiazepines (Palminteri and Narbonne 1988). Despite claims of fewer withdrawal effects (Sauvanet et al. 1988), there is evidence that 24-hour rebound effects do occur in much the same way as with the benzodiazepines (Jonas et al. 1992).

Hypnotic agents should be administered in the lowest effective dose. Day-after effects, in particular, may be mitigated by lowering the dose. Although the benzodiazepines are the mainstay of pharmacotherapy for insomnia, other sedating drugs, such as antihistamines, chloral hydrate, or barbiturates, may also be used. However, although these agents may be effective for special clinical situations for a number of days, long-term efficacy and/or safety issues generally result in their being inferior to the benzodiazepines. Many clinicians rely on the more sedating antidepressants as alternative hypnotics, in part as a reaction to public concern over the safety of the benzodiazepines, especially triazolam (Walsh and Engelhardt 1992). In the appropriate clinical circumstances, trazodone 50 to 100 mg at sleep is an excellent hypnotic. The clinician must be aware, however, that the use of antidepressants for sedation is not devoid of significant risks and side effects.

Pharmacotherapy of Simple Phobia, Social Phobia, and Performance Anxiety

Valid research into the causes and pharmacological treatment of social phobia continues to lag behind that for panic disorder (Uhde et al. 1991). As with panic disorder, social phobia appears to respond selectively to particular benzodiazepines: to date, the high-potency agents alprazolam (Gelernter et al. 1991) and clonazepam (Davidson et al. 1991) appear to be most effective. The MAOI phenelzine is an effective treatment for this condition (Liebowitz et al. 1988), and there are now reports of success in treating both panic disorder and social phobia with the SSRI fluoxetine (Schneier et al. 1990; Sternbach 1990). Imipramine, although highly effective in the treatment of panic disorder, appears to be ineffective for most patients with social phobia. The beta-blocker atenolol is ineffective in treating panic disorder, but it is used by many clinicians and is likely effective in treating discrete forms of social phobia, such as in performance anxiety.

Because the anxiety associated with social phobia is associated with a cluster of signs and symptoms (e.g., dry mouth, palpitations, flushing, etc.) suggestive of increased adrenergic activity, beta-blockers have long been considered as a potential form of treatment of this condition. Despite success in an early open trial of atenolol in 10 patients with generalized social phobia (Gorman et al. 1985), a poor response to atenolol was later shown when this drug was compared, under double-blind conditions, with phenelzine (Liebowitz et al. 1988). Taken within 2 hours of the stressor, propranolol, in doses ranging from 20 to 80 mg, may improve performance on examinations (Drew et al. 1985), in public speaking

(Hertley et al. 1983), and in musical performances (Brantigan et al. 1982). Before a patient is prescribed a beta-blocker, a thorough medical and physical examination should be conducted to detect any cardiovascular, pulmonary, or endocrine (diabetes or hyperthyroidism) disorder that would contradict the safe use of beta-blockers. A trial dose of 40 mg of propranolol should be administered before the specific performance situation where the patient would anticipate anxiety. Subsequently, doses of propranolol should be administered approximately 2 hours before the situation where disabling performance anxiety is expected. The dose may be increased gradually by 20-mg increments during successive performances until such time as adequate relief of performance distress is achieved (Yudofsky and Silver 1987).

Pharmacotherapy of Obsessive-Compulsive Disorder

In the 1980s, curiosity over clomipramine, a tricyclic with potent serotonin reuptake inhibition, was rekindled with new reports of success in the treatment of OCD (Flament et al. 1985; Stroebel et al. 1984). Since that time, a large multicenter study of clomipramine has established the efficacy of this drug for the treatment of OCD (Clomipramine Collaborative Study Group 1991). Before initiating clomipramine treatment, the clinician must heed all of the precautions associated with the use of any TCA. Initial dosing and titration of clomipramine must also follow the guidelines for TCAs, with the additional caveat that 250 mg is the maximum recommended dose because of an increased risk of seizures above this level. Most patients with OCD will respond to doses of clomipramine between 150 and 200 mg/day. Side effects associated with the anticholinergic, antihistaminic, and alpha$_2$-adrenergic actions of clomipramine may occur, so patients must be monitored for and made aware of the potential for constipation, dry mouth, urinary hesitancy, sedation, orthostatic hypotension, and so forth.

Fluoxetine has been compared with clomipramine under double-blind conditions and found to have an approximately equivalent antiobsessional effect (Pigott et al. 1990). It has been suggested that an effective antiobsessional dose of fluoxetine may be higher than its usual antidepressant dose. Many clinicians will seek to establish a daily dose of 60 to 80 mg in treating patients with OCD. No systematic study of this issue has confirmed this common impression and widely used practice. In fact, a preliminary report by Wheadon (1991) found no greater antiobsessional effect when fluoxetine 40 or 60 mg/day was compared with 20 mg/day. Still, on the basis of the current knowledge, in the treatment of OCD, a trial of fluoxetine should not be considered complete until the patient has failed to respond to 80 mg/day after 8 weeks (Jenike 1990).

Fluvoxamine has been the most studied SSRI for the treatment of

OCD, and its efficacy has been firmly established (Goodman et al. 1990). Effective doses of fluvoxamine range from 100 to 300 mg a day. Sertraline and paroxetine are now being investigated in large-scale studies aimed at establishing their efficacy in the treatment of OCD (Goodman et al. 1992). In open trial studies, paroxetine has shown some promise, but similar studies have thus far suggested that sertraline is less effective than the other SSRIs in treating OCD (Jenike et al. 1990).

Reviews of treatment-refractory OCD (Goodman et al. 1992; Jenike 1990) have been careful to note that because a response to medication may not appear until at least 8 to 12 weeks, a medication trial should not be considered a failure until this much time has elapsed with no observed benefit. Moreover, whereas some patients respond to pharmacotherapy with a nearly total resolution of symptoms, most achieve only a 35% to 60% reduction in their obsessions and compulsions (Jenike 1990). Therefore, without concurrent behavior therapy, pharmacotherapy should not be considered optimal. Patients receiving behavior therapy who are truly refractory to treatment trials with more than one SSRI may be treated with several augmentation strategies. A number of combination therapies have been suggested, including the addition to an SSRI of fenfluramine (Hollander et al. 1990), lithium (Ruegg et al. 1990), a neuroleptic (McDougle et al. 1990), clonazepam (Hewlett et al. 1990), or buspirone (Jenike et al. 1991).

☐ Risks and Side Effects of Anxiolytic and Hypnotic Drugs

Sedation and Impairment of Performance

Benzodiazepine-induced sedation may be considered either a therapeutic action or a side effect. Hypnotics are expected and required to produce sedation in order to be efficacious. However, when the patient complains of sleepiness the following day, this therapeutic action becomes a disabling side effect. Residual daytime somnolence is a function of two variables: drug half-life and dosage (Roth and Roehrs 1992). With longer-acting agents, such as flurazepam and quazepam, a morning-after "hangover" is common, although some tolerance to this effect may develop with time. On the other hand, any benzodiazepine, short or long acting, can cause daytime drowsiness if the nighttime dosage is too great.

Impairment of performance in sensitive psychomotor tests has been well documented after the administration of benzodiazepines. Patients must be warned that driving, engaging in dangerous physical activities, and using hazardous machinery should be avoided during the acute stages, and possibly during the later stages, of treatment with benzodiazepines. Buspirone is not sedating and does not impair mechanical performance, such as driving (Moskowitz and Smiley 1982). However, because side effects in any individual patient cannot be predicted, these activities should be avoided during the initial stages of buspirone therapy as well.

Dependence, Withdrawal, and Rebound Effects

Concerns about physical and psychological dependence on benzodiazepines are frequently raised by patients and often affect a clinician's choice of treatment. However, based on the criterion of self-reinforcement, most of the benzodiazepines, with the possible exception of diazepam, have low abuse potential when properly prescribed and supervised (American Psychiatric Association 1990; Sellers et al. 1992). Physical dependence may occur when benzodiazepines are taken in higher than usual dosages or for prolonged periods of time (Busto et al. 1986; Tyrer et al. 1983). If benzodiazepines are discontinued precipitously, withdrawal effects that include hyperpyrexia, seizures, psychosis, and even death may occur. Numerous studies have established that physical dependence may occur even when benzodiazepines are taken in usual clinical doses prolonged for periods beyond several weeks, and that the symptoms of withdrawal may arise even when drug discontinuation is not abrupt (Noyes et al. 1988). Signs and symptoms of withdrawal may include tachycardia, increased blood pressure, muscle cramps, anxiety, insomnia, panic attacks, impairment of memory and concentration, and perceptual disturbances. There is evidence that withdrawal reactions peak more rapidly and more intensely with the briefer-half-life benzodiazepines (Busto et al. 1986). These withdrawal effects are rapidly reversed with the readministration of benzodiazepines. Although it is generally believed that there is cross-tolerance for all benzodiazepines, there has been a report of withdrawal symptoms from alprazolam that were not reversed with diazepam (Zipursky et al. 1985).

For patients treated with benzodiazepines for longer than 2 to 3 months, we suggest that the dose be decreased by approximately 10% per week. Thus, for a patient receiving 4 mg/day of alprazolam, the dose should be tapered by 0.5 mg per week for 8 weeks. The last few dosage levels may be the most difficult to discontinue, and the patient will require increased attention and support from the physician during this time. Buspirone, when administered to subjects who had histories of recreational sedative abuse, showed no abuse potential (Cole et al. 1982), a finding confirmed by subsequent studies (Sellers et al. 1992). Furthermore, no withdrawal syndrome was found when patients who had been prescribed buspirone for 6 months were abruptly switched to a placebo for 4 weeks (Rickels et al. 1988).

Rebound anxiety is defined as the return, upon discontinuation of a benzodiazepine, of the anxiety signs and symptoms with greater intensity than existed before treatment. For this diagnosis, accurate documentation of specific symptoms and operationalized measures of the severity of preexisting anxiety are required.

Memory Impairment

Intravenous use of the benzodiazepines is associated with significant anterograde amnesia (Dixon et al. 1984; Reitan et al. 1986). For midazolam, diazepam, and lorazepam, this phenonemon may have certain clinical benefits, because amnesia for surgical or other invasive therapeutic procedures is often desired. When benzodiazepines are utilized to treat insomnia or anxiety, amnesia may be a serious liability. Several studies have documented the deleterious effects on memory of oral benzodiazepines (Angus and Romney 1984; Mac et al. 1985). Tolerance to these amnestic effects may not develop. The degree of anterograde amnesia appears to be related to dosage, and the amnesia may occur in the first several hours after each dose of benzodiazepine, even after repeated use (Lucki et al. 1986).

Disinhibition and Dyscontrol

Another area of recent controversy involving benzodiazepines is the allegation that triazolam, and benzodiazepines as a class, may cause behavior disinhibition leading to acts of aggression (Medawarn and Rassaby 1991; Regestein and Reich 1985). Greenblatt et al. (1984), in their review of double-blind, controlled studies of triazolam and flurazepam, found no reports of bizarre, disinhibitory reactions. However, a long history of anecdotal reports suggests that many of the benzodiazepines can cause paradoxical anger and behavioral disinhibition that is dose related (Rothschild 1992). A history of hostility, impulsivity, or borderline or antisocial personality disorder has been implicated as a potential predictor of this reaction. In light of the heightened attention focused on triazolam and the resulting potential for a significant reporting bias, the increase in anecdotal reports citing this particular agent is difficult to interpret. At the present time, some caution should be exercised when benzodiazepines are prescribed to patients with a history of poor impulse control and aggression, and communications about this possibility should be made to patients and documented in the medical record.

Side Effects of Buspirone

The side effects that are more common with buspirone than with the benzodiazepines are nausea, headache, nervousness, insomnia, dizziness, and lightheadedness (Rakel 1990). Restlessness has also been reported, which theoretically may be related to buspirone's activity at the dopamine receptor.

Overdosage

Benzodiazepines are remarkably safe when taken in overdosage. Dangerous effects occur when the overdose includes several sedative drugs, especially alcohol (Greenblatt et al. 1977a). When an overdose occurs in combination with other drugs, however, the complications depend upon the type and quantity of the nonbenzodiazepines (Finkle et al. 1979). The diagnosis of benzodiazepine overdose is usually made by the clinician's asking the patient or family or friends what drugs were ingested. This is confirmed by physical examination revealing signs and symptoms of toxicity with a CNS depressant and by either urine or blood drug screens. Because the standard urine drug screen assay may not detect the presence of many commonly prescribed benzodiazepines, including lorazepam, alprazolam, clonazepam, temazepam, and triazolam, the clinician should actively research the presence and accuracy of these tests in the laboratory that he or she uses. The benzodiazepine antagonist flumazenil can be used via intravenous injection in an emergency setting to reverse the effects of any potential overdose with a benzodiazepine (Votey et al. 1991). However, medical management of an overdose will often still require physical supportive measures, such as ensuring proper respiratory function.

Drug Interactions

Most sedative drugs, including narcotics and alcohol, potentiate the sedation of benzodiazepines. Cimetidine, oral contraceptives, acute alcohol intake, propranolol, and disulfiram inhibit the hepatic metabolism and increase the elimination half-life of those benzodiazepines that are metabolized by oxidation, which includes diazepam and chlordiazepoxide (Abernethy et al. 1984). However, benzodiazepines such as lorazepam and oxazepam are less affected by the inhibition of hepatic metabolism associated with the drugs just cited. Buspirone does not appear to interact with alcohol or other CNS depressants to increase sedation and motor impairment (Moskowitz and Smiley 1982).

Use in Pregnancy

As with most medications, usage of anxiolytics during pregnancy or breast-feeding should be avoided when possible. Although there have been concerns that benzodiazepines, when ingested during the first trimester of pregnancy, may increase the risk of the development of cleft palate, this has not been substantiated in controlled studies (Rosenberg et al. 1983).

■ ANTIMANIC DRUGS

Clinical investigations by Baastrup and Schou (1967) conclusively demonstrated that lithium was effective in the prophylaxis of recurrent affective disorders. For the patient with acute manic psychosis, treatment with antipsychotic drugs or ECT is efficacious. In fact, these treatments elicit responses more rapidly than does lithium carbonate, and they are often administered while awaiting the therapeutic response to lithium. Other classes of drugs with different chemical structures and with apparently different mechanisms of actions have been reported to be effective in the prophylaxis and treatment of mania. Among these are the anticonvulsant drugs carbamazepine and valproic acid; the calcium channel blocking drug verapamil; the alpha-adrenergic agonist clonidine; the benzodiazepine anticonvulsant clonazepam; and the beta-adrenergic receptor blocking drug propranolol. The antimanic drugs that have been most frequently investigated are listed in Table 27–11.

☐ Lithium

Indications and Efficacy

Lithium, usually administered as the carbonate salt, has been shown to be efficacious in the treatment of many mood disorders. Acute manic episodes respond to treatment with lithium within 7 to 14 days. Because manic episodes have so great a potential for psychosocial disruption, behavioral control is usually desired sooner than when lithium becomes effective. For this purpose, supplemental medication, most often an antipsychotic drug, is coadministered with lithium on an acute basis. Lithium has been proved effective and is the drug of choice for preventing both manic and depressive episodes in patients with bipolar illness (Consensus Development Panel 1985). Patients with less severe bipolar illness, such as cyclothymia (Akiskal et al. 1979) or bipolar II disorder (i.e., major depressions alternating with hypomanic episodes) (Kane et al. 1982) also exhibit significant improvement with lithium therapy. However, patients with rapid-cycling bipolar disorder (i.e., four or more mood disorder episodes per year) have been reported to respond less well to lithium treatment (Wehr et al. 1988).

Lithium is also effective in the prevention of future depressive episodes in those patients with recurrent unipolar depressive disorder (Consensus Development Panel 1985) and as an adjunct to antidepressants in depressed patients partially refractory to treatment with antide-

Table 27–11. Antimanic drugs

Generic name	Trade name	Usual dose range (mg/day)	Plasma level
Lithium			
Lithium carbonate	Eskalith Lithane Lithonate Lithotabs	600–1,800	0.7–1.5 mEq/L (acute); 0.4–1.0 mEq/L (maintenance)
Time-release	Lithobid Eskalith CR		
Lithium citrate (syrup)	Cibalith-S		
Anticonvulsants			
Carbamazepine	Tegretol	800–1,200	4–12 µg/ml
Clonazepam	Klonopin	1.5–20	
Valproic acid	Depakene	30–60 mg/kg/day	50–100 µg/ml
Calcium channel blockers			
Verapamil	Isoptin Calan	240–360	
Alpha-adrenergic agonist			
Clonidine	Catapres	0.2–0.8	
Beta-adrenergic receptor blocker			
Propranolol	Inderal	400–2,000	

pressants alone. Furthermore, it may be useful in the maintenance of remission of depressive disorder after ECT (Coopen et al. 1981) and in the maintenance of the antidepressant effect of sleep deprivation (Baxter et al. 1986). Lithium has also been used effectively in some cases of aggression and behavioral dyscontrol.

Clinical Use

Before initiating treatment with lithium, patients should be told to expect side effects that occur commonly, including nausea, diarrhea, polyuria, increased thirst, fine hand tremor, and fatigue. These may be transient, or, in some patients, may persist with therapeutic lithium levels. Because of a narrow range between the therapeutic and toxic doses of lithium, and the wide variability of lithium pharmacokinetics among different individuals, the optimum dose for an individual patient cannot be based on the dosage administered. Rather, lithium dosing should be based on

the concentration of lithium in the plasma. Lithium carbonate is completely absorbed by the gastrointestinal tract and reaches peak plasma
levels in 1 to 2 hours. The elimination half-life is approximately 24 hours.
Steady-state lithium levels are obtained in approximately 5 days. These
levels are measured accurately and inexpensively by atomic absorption
spectrophotometry.

Therapeutic plasma levels for patients on lithium therapy range from
0.5 to 1.5 mEq/L. Although lower plasma levels are associated with less
troubling side effects, there is strong evidence that levels in the range of
0.8 to 1.0 mEq/L provide better prophylaxis against relapse (Gelenberg et
al. 1989). Therefore, most clinicians now seek to establish levels of at least
0.8 mEq/L in treating acute manic episodes. When intolerable side effects
have not intervened, treatment with lithium should not be considered a
failure in acute mania until plasma levels of 1.2 to 1.5 mEq/L have been
reached and maintained for 2 weeks. However, when levels this high are
necessary for acute treatment, the dosage often may be reduced to the
0.8–1.0 mEq/L range for maintenance therapy.

Lithium has a serum half-life of approximately 24 hours, and, therefore, it may be administered as a single daily dose. The results of several
investigations favor such a dosing schedule. Divided daily doses with
the usual carbonate salt will result in several peak levels throughout the
day, with a relatively rapid decrease between doses. The multiple dose
regimen will therefore expose the kidney to multiple peak levels of intermediate concentration, whereas single daily dosing exposes the kidney
to a single peak of higher absolute concentration. It has been suggested
that nephrotoxicity is related to the duration of exposure to peak lithium
levels, and not to the absolute level of any particular peak (Bowen et al.
1991; Hetmar et al. 1987). It is for this reason that single daily dosing is
recommended. Although slow-release preparations of lithium are available, these are not necessary for adequate 24-hour levels. The main advantage of sustained release is that less lithium ion is released in the
stomach, where it can act as an irritant, while more is released in the
small intestines (Schatzberg and Cole 1991). For patients who experience
nausea and gastric irritation, the slow-release formulations may protect
them from this unpleasant side effect. General guidelines for lithium
treatment are listed in Table 27–12.

Contraindications

Although the clinical significance of renal side effects toxicity with
chronic lithium use has stirred scientific debate for over three decades,
there is sufficient evidence to indicate that, in general, lithium should be
avoided in patients with preexisting renal impairment. For patients with
mania and renal dysfunction who are unresponsive to alternate treat-

Table 27–12. Guidelines for lithium treatment

1. Complete a thorough medical evaluation.

2. Follow appropriate medical laboratory evaluations, as outlined in Tables 27–3, 27–4, and 27–7 and in Silver et al. 1994, Tables 27–3, 27–6, and 27–8.

3. Inform patient and family of proper use of lithium. Include common side effects, importance of monitoring of lithium levels, exact procedures for accurate lithium monitoring, early signs and symptoms of toxicity, potential long-term side effects, and (if patient is female) warnings regarding pregnancy during treatment.

4. Initiate therapy at 300 mg twice a day, and increase by 300 mg every 3 to 4 days.

5. Obtain lithium levels (12 hours after last dose) twice a week, until lithium level is approximately 1.0 mEq/L.

6. Keep in mind that treatment of acute manic symptoms may require concomitant therapy with antipsychotic medications.

7. Repeat lithium levels every month for the first 6 months, then every 2 to 3 months.

ments, the use of lithium must be approved by a nephrologist. Lithium also has acute and chronic effects on the thyroid. However, patients with hypothyroidism may receive lithium if the thyroid disease is adequately treated and monitored. Because lithium may affect functioning of the cardiac sinus node, patients with sinus node dysfunction (i.e., sick sinus syndrome) should not receive lithium. Lithium may result in severe developmental abnormalities, especially on the cardiovascular system of the developing fetus. Therefore, the drug is strictly contraindicated during the first trimester of pregnancy, and is prescribed only under the most "desperate" clinical circumstances during the second and third trimesters. For women of childbearing potential, lithium should be prescribed only with full informed consent and careful and regular clinical follow-up and pregnancy monitoring.

Risks, Side Effects, and Their Management

Renal effects. Most of the effects of lithium on the kidney are reversible after discontinuaton of the drug. Although permanent morphological changes in renal structure have been reported, the clinical implications of these changes have yet to be established (Hetmar et al. 1987). An evaluation of renal function is required before lithium therapy is initiated and at regular intervals throughout the course of treatment.

The most noticeable effect of lithium upon renal function is the vasopressin-resistant impairment in the kidney's ability to concentrate urine.

Termed *nephrogenic diabetes insipidus* (NDI), this condition often results in polyuria. Up to 60% of patients on lithium therapy complain of increased frequency of urination (Lokkegaard et al. 1985). NDI may result in serious complications, including dehydration, lithium toxicity, and electrolyte imbalance. Although clinically significant polyuria usually reverses itself after discontinuation of lithium therapy, it may persist for many months (Ramsey and Cox 1982).

Preventive and management strategies for NDI include increasing the patient's fluid intake and decreasing the lithium to the lowest effective dose. In the maintenance phase of treatment, a plasma level of 0.8 mEq/L is now the acceptable lower limit for the healthy, nongeriatric patient with bipolar disorder. Once-a-day dosing will also result in lower urinary output than the multiple dosing schedule (Hetmar et al. 1991). If these simpler management strategies fail to correct the polyuria, potassium supplementation, 10 to 20 mEq/day, may be effective (Martin 1993). The nonthiazide diuretic amiloride is now the preferred treatment for lithium-induced NDI, because it does not appear to increase plasma lithium levels (Battle et al. 1985). Amiloride apparently acts by blocking the absorption of lithium in the renal tubules, where the lithium would otherwise interfere with the action of vasopressin (Billings 1985). For lithium-induced NDI, amiloride is prescribed in doses of 5 mg bid, and increased to 10 mg bid if necessary. It is prudent to continue to monitor serum lithium levels with greater frequency (every 2 months at minimum) when amiloride is combined with lithium.

Characterized by tubular interstitial nephritis, *lithium nephropathy* has been reported to be a consequence of long-term lithium therapy. Hetmar et al. (1987) performed renal biopsies on 46 bipolar patients with a mean of 8 years of lithium therapy and found that the proportion of sclerotic glomeruli, atrophic tubules, and interstitial fibrosis was significantly greater in patients who had received a multiple daily dosing schedule, compared with patients with a history of once-daily dosing and with a control group with no history of lithium exposure. Lokkegaard et al. (1985) reported that decreases in the glomerular filtration rate (GFR) are only detectable after many years of lithium therapy; however, most investigators have found no clinically significant effect on the GFR (Hetmar et al. 1991; Schou 1989).

For all patients treated with lithium, laboratory tests assessing renal function should be monitored regularly. The clinician should also obtain a medical and family history of hereditary renal disorders such as polycystic kidney disease. A genitourinary review of systems should be obtained, including any systemic disorders that are associated with renal difficulties, such as diabetes mellitus, hypertension, and ingestion of renal toxins (e.g. phenacetin, nonsteroidal anti-inflammatory drugs). A 24-hour creatinine clearance test is no longer believed to be necessary

(Schou 1989). Aside from the difficulties involved in obtaining a reliable 24-hour collection of urine, there are simpler tests of renal function that can serve as adequate alternatives. Moreover, because a small change in GFR is not indicative of imminent renal failure, a high level of accuracy in assessing the GFR is no longer a priority. Serum creatinine and the plasma lithium level are sufficient measures of kidney function.

The ability of the kidney to concentrate urine, a function of the renal tubules, is now regarded to be of greater clinical significance than the GFR for patients receiving lithium. Impairment in concentrating urine may be assessed through two tests of renal function. A measurement of 24-hour urinary volume will give an indication of the severity of diabetes insipidus. As with the creatinine clearance test, this option requires that the patient be able to comply with a 24-hour urine collection. Another, perhaps simpler test is the 12-hour fluid deprivation test, wherein the patient first refrains from drinking any fluid for 12 hours. After this time, a urine specimen is collected and the urine osmolality is measured. Gelenberg et al. (1981) have suggested that a urine concentration of less than 500 mOsm/kg implies disordered kidney function and indicates that further specific renal function studies are required.

For all patients on lithium, measure of serum BUN and creatinine should be obtained at baseline and every 3 to 6 months after lithium therapy has commenced, with more frequent testing if there are specific complaints or signs of renal dysfunction. We recommend a 12-hour fluid deprivation test at baseline as well, to be repeated at a later date only when indicated for suspected polyuria. Any progressive changes in creatinine clearance or gradual increases in lithium levels (despite constant administered dosage) may indicate a decrease in renal function and require referral of the patient to a nephrologist for further renal function testing and assessment. The urine concentration test should not be repeated in clear cases of polyuria; the 12-hour fluid deprivation may cause dehydration and lithium toxicity in patients with severe diabetes insipidus.

Thyroid dysfunction.   Hypothyroidism may occur in as many as 20% of patients treated with lithium (Myers et al. 1985). Although this occurrence is hypothesized to be related to the effect of lithium on TSH adenylate cyclase, lithium may have other important effects on other key areas of thyroid function (Waller 1985). Lithium-induced hypothyroidism occurs more frequently in women, in patients with thyroid antibodies, and in patients with exaggerated TSH response to thyrotropin-releasing hormone (TRH) (Calabrese et al. 1985; Myers et al. 1985). Because the development of hypothyroidism in bipolar patients is associated with intractable depression (Yassa et al. 1988) and with the development of a rapid-cycling course (Bauer and Whybrow 1989), thyroid function must be monitored regularly during lithium treatment.

Before the initiation of treatment, a complete review of symptoms of thyroid dysfunction should be obtained. Other endocrinological disorders, especially diabetes mellitus, may also be associated with the presence of thyroid antibodies. Initial laboratory tests include T_3RU (resin uptake), T_4 RIA (radio immunoassay), FTI (free thyroxine index), and TSH. Thyroid-stimulating hormone is the most sensitive of these tests for detecting hypothyroidism. Because of the association between the presence of antithyroid antibodies and the subsequent development of hypothyroidism, antithyroid antibodies should also be measured before lithium treatment. TSH should be reassessed after every 6 months of lithium therapy. If laboratory tests indicate the development of hypothyroidism, the patient should be evaluated clinically for signs and symptoms of hypothyroidism and be referred to an endocrinologist for any further tests, such as the TRH stimulation test. In collaboration with the endocrinologist, the psychiatrist should decide on the appropriate treatment, such as thyroid hormone replacement with thyroxine, 0.05 to 0.2 mg/day, or discontinuation of lithium therapy.

Neurotoxicity. Lithium therapy may be associated with several types of neurological dysfunction. Fine resting tremor is a neurological side effect that may be detected in as many as one-half of patients taking lithium (Vestergaard et al. 1980). Beta-adrenergic blocking drugs, such as propranolol in divided daily dosages below 80 mg/day, are effective in treating this tremor (Zubenko et al. 1984). Toxic lithium levels can produce severe neurotoxic reactions, with symptoms such as dysarthria, ataxia, and intention tremor. These symptoms may also occur in some patients with lithium levels in the standard therapeutic range (Lewis 1983). Cases of delirium and hyperreflexia (Kemperman et al. 1989) and seizures—tonic-clonic and myoclonic (Julius and Brenner 1987)—have been reported in several patients with suspected or subsequently established CNS pathology. ECT-induced confusion is likely to be worsened by concurrent lithium administration, and this has led some investigators to consider lithium to be relatively contraindicated for patients who are receiving a course of ECT (Consensus Conference 1985).

Cardiac effects. Mitchell and Mackenzie (1982) reported changes in T-wave morphology on the ECG (flattening or inversion) in 20% to 30% of patients on lithium. Although these changes are most likely benign, a medical evaluation should be completed to assess other possible etiologies. Lithium also may suppress the function of the sinus node and result in sinoatrial block. Patients with sinus disease or conduction defects, therefore, should not be treated with lithium. Cases have also been reported of aggravation of preexisting ventricular arrhythmias with lithium therapy.

Prior to the initiation of treatment with lithium, all patients should have a complete cardiac evaluation, including history and physical examination pertinent to the cardiovascular system, and an ECG. The ECG should be repeated 1 month after obtaining a therapeutic level of lithium, and at yearly intervals thereafter. If, at any time, there are any changes in cardiovascular status or any complaints of cardiac symptoms, the patient should be evaluated by a qualified cardiologist.

Weight gain.   Weight gain is a frequent side effect of lithium treatment. Vendsborg et al. (1976) found a correlation between liquid intake and weight gain. Patients with polydipsia may drink fluids with a high caloric content, such as carbonated soft drinks, and thereby gain weight. These patients should be instructed to drink low-calorie liquids. Weight gain may also be a direct effect of lithium therapy. Possible mechanisms include influences on carbohydrate metabolism, changes in glucose tolerance, or changes in lipid metabolism (Peselow et al. 1980). Prior to the initiation of lithium therapy, fasting blood glucose levels and tests for the presence of ketones in the urine should be obtained.

Dermatologic reactions.   Dermatologic reactions to lithium include acneform and follicular eruptions and psoriasis (Deandrea et al. 1982). The most frequent of these reactions is skin rash, which is reported in up to 7% of lithium-treated patients (Bone et al. 1980). Changes in hair, including hair loss, hair thinning, and loss of wave, have also been reported (Yassa 1986). Except for cases of exacerbation of psoriasis, these reactions are usually benign and may not warrant discontinuation of lithium treatment.

Gastrointestinal side effects.   Gastrointestinal difficulties occur frequently with lithium treatment, especially nausea and diarrhea. While these side effects may be manifestations of toxicity, they also occur at lithium levels within the therapeutic range. Gastrointestinal symptoms may improve by reducing dosage, changing to a slow-release formulation, or patient's ingesting lithium with meals. Complaints about lithium therapy may also be related to the patient's mood state or to problems associated with gastrointestinal effects of other psychotropic medications (Bone et al. 1980).

Hematologic side effects.   The most frequent hematologic change detected in patients on lithium is leukocytosis. As reviewed by Brewerton (1986), this change is generally benign and may, in fact, be used to treat several conditions associated with granulocytopenia. Lithium-induced leukocytosis is readily reversible with discontinuation of lithium therapy. Before initiation of therapy with lithium, a white blood cell count with differential should be obtained, and it should be repeated at yearly intervals thereafter.

Overdosage and Toxicity

Because of the narrow range between therapeutic and toxic plasma lithium levels, the psychiatrist must devote sufficient time to inform the patient and the family about the signs, symptoms, and treatment of lithium toxicity (Table 27–13). The patient must be made aware of circumstances

---

Table 27–13.   Signs and symptoms of lithium toxicity

Mild to moderate intoxication (lithium level = 1.5–2.0 mEq/L)

Gastrointestinal:	Vomiting
	Abdominal pain
	Dryness of mouth
Neurological:	Ataxia
	Dizziness
	Slurred speech
	Nystagmus
	Lethargy or excitement
	Muscle weakness

Moderate to severe intoxication (lithium level = 2.0–2.5 mEq/L)

Gastrointestinal:	Anorexia
	Persistent nausea and vomiting
Neurological:	Blurred vision
	Muscle fasciculations
	Clonic limb movements
	Hyperactive deep tendon reflexes
	Choreoathetoid movements
	Convulsions
	Delirium
	Syncope
	Electroencephalographic changes
	Stupor
	Coma
	Circulatory failure (lowered blood pressure, cardiac arrhythmias, and conduction abnormalities)

Severe lithium intoxication (lithium level > 2.5 mEq/L)

Generalized convulsions
Oliguria and renal failure
Death

that may increase the chances of toxicity, such as drinking insufficient amounts of fluids, becoming overheated with increased perspiration, or ingesting too much medication. The psychiatrist must emphasize the prevention of lithium toxicity through the maintenance of adequate salt and water intake, especially during hot weather and exercise. The recommended management of lithium toxicity is reviewed in Table 27–14.

Drug Interactions

Diuretics increase lithium levels and should be used with caution when treating lithium-induced diabetes insipidus. Specific nonsteroidal anti-inflammatory drugs (NSAIDs), such as indomethacin, also can increase the plasma lithium level. However, sulindac has not been shown to affect serum lithium levels (Ragheb and Powell 1986). Theophylline will increase renal clearance and result in a lower lithium level (Cook et al. 1985). Lithium has been reported to increase the intracellular levels of some antipsychotic drugs and may thereby aggravate the inherent neurotoxicity of these agents. Concerns about increased risk of delirium and symptoms of neuroleptic malignant syndrome have been raised for the combination of lithium and neuroleptic drugs. Cohen and Cohen (1974) re-

---

Table 27–14.   Management of lithium toxicity

1. The patient should immediately contact his or her personal physician or go to a hospital emergency room.
2. Lithium should be discontinued, and the patient instructed to ingest fluids, if possible.
3. Physical examination, including vital signs, and a neurological examination with complete formal mental status examination should be completed.
4. Lithium level, serum electrolytes, renal function tests, and electrocardiogram should be obtained as soon as possible.
5. For significant acute ingestions, residual gastric contents should be removed by induction of emesis, gastric lavage, and absorption with activated charcoal.[a]
6. Vigorous hydration and maintenance of electrolyte balance are essential.
7. For any patient with a serum lithium level greater than 4.0 mEq/L within 6 hours of ingestion, or for any patient with serious manifestations of lithium toxicity, hemodialysis should be initiated.[a]
8. Repeat dialysis may be required every 6 to 10 hours, until the lithium level is within nontoxic range, and the patient has no signs or symptoms of lithium toxicity.

---

[a]Goldfrank et al. 1986.

ported several cases of irreversible brain damage with the combination of lithium carbonate and haloperidol. Goldney and Spence (1986), however, found no difference in side effects and complications in a group of patients with mania treated with antipsychotic medications alone compared with a group of patients with mania treated with antipsychotic drugs and lithium. Lassen et al. (1986) reported that neuroleptics and antidepressants had no effect on lithium clearance. We suggest that whenever lithium is added to the medication regimen the clinician should be alert to any new side effects that may result from drug interactions.

☐ Anticonvulsant Mood Stabilizers

Takezaki and Hanaoka (1971) reported that carbamazepine was effective in controlling manic behavior, and the first report from the United States of its efficacy for mania was by Ballenger and Post (1980). Subsequently, evidence from controlled studies has indicated that carbamazepine is effective in both the acute treatment and the prophylactic treatment of mania, with overall response rates comparable to those of lithium treatment (Gerner and Stanton 1992). These findings have been confirmed for patients with bipolar illness who fail to respond to lithium, and, indeed, some bipolar subtypes (dysphoric mania, rapid cycling, and schizoaffective) are now believed to respond preferentially to the anticonvulsant mood stabilizers carbamazepine and valproate (Placidi et al. 1986; Post et al. 1987). There is less evidence, however, to support the efficacy of carbamazepine in the acute treatment of depression and in the prophylactic treatment of unipolar depression. Two controlled studies found carbamazepine treatment effective in a subgroup of patients with refractory depression, with response rates greater among the bipolar depressive patients than among the unipolar depressive patients (Post et al. 1986; Small 1990). A systematic, controlled study of the antidepressant effects of carbamazepine in a more typical group of patients with depression remains to be conducted.

Since the early 1980s, several controlled studies have established that valproate is effective in acute mania (Gerner and Stanton 1992; Keck et al. 1992). As with carbamazepine, valproate is often effective for patients who fail to respond to lithium (Pope et al. 1991), and for the "non-classic" bipolar disorder subtypes, including rapid cycling and dysphoric mania (Calabrese et al. 1992; McElroy et al. 1992). Valproate has been reported to be especially effective for mania occurring in patients with a history of closed-head trauma (McElroy et al. 1989), and in patients with EEG abnormalities (Pope et al. 1988). Although several open-trial studies suggest that valproate is also effective for prophylaxis in bipolar disorder, no controlled studies have confirmed this finding to date (Keck et al. 1992).

Carbamazepine

Carbamazepine should be initiated at a dosage of 200 mg twice a day. Dose increments of 200 mg/day every 3 to 5 days should be made until a plasma level of 8 to 12 µg/ml is obtained. During this titration phase, patients may be particularly prone to side effects such as sedation, dizziness, and ataxia, which indicates that a more gradual titration should be instituted. Although the maximum recommended dose of carbamazepine is 1,200 mg/day, higher dosages are frequently required based on plasma level determinations and clinical response (Placidi et al. 1986). Carbamazepine will induce its own metabolism, and, therefore, dose adjustments may be required for weeks or months after the initiation of treatment in order to maintain therapeutic plasma levels (Eichelbaum et al. 1985). Treatment principles for the use of carbamazepine are listed in Table 27–15.

Contraindications. Because of the potential for hematologic and hepatic toxicity, carbamazepine should not be administered to patients with leukopenia, thrombocytopenia, or liver disease. Also for this reason, carbamazepine is strictly contraindicated for patients receiving clozapine. Because of reports of teratogenicity, including increased risks of spina bifida (Rosa 1991), microcephaly (Bertollini et al. 1987), and cranio-

---

Table 27–15. Evaluation and monitoring of anticonvulsant treatment of bipolar disorder

1. Complete medical evaluation (see numbers 7 and 8).
2. Inform patient and his or her family of potential side effects of treatment and of the importance of monitoring serum levels.
3. Initiate carbamazepine (CBZ) at 200 mg twice a day. Initiate valproic acid (VPA) at 250 mg twice a day.
4. Increase CBZ dose by 200 mg or VPA dose by 250 mg every 3 to 5 days.
5. Obtain serum levels every week until therapeutic levels are obtained (CBZ: 8–12 µg/ml; VPA: 50–100 ng/ml).
6. Monitor levels every month for the first 3 months and every 3 months thereafter.
7. Hematologic monitoring (for CBZ): Obtain complete blood count and platelet count every 2 weeks for the first 2 months of treatment and every 3 months thereafter.
8. Liver function monitoring (for CBZ and VPA): Obtain SGOT, SGPT, LDH, and alkaline phosphatase every month for the first 2 months of treatment and every 3 months thereafter.

Note. SGOT = serum glutamate oxaloacetate transaminase; SGPT = serum glutamate pyruvate transaminase; LDH = lactic dehydrogenase.

facial defects (Jones et al. 1989), carbamazepine is relatively contraindicated for use in pregnant women. Women of childbearing age who take carbamazepine should be monitored regularly for pregnancy.

Risks, side effects, and their management.   A thorough evaluation of the patient's hematologic and hepatic functioning should be completed before treatment with carbamazepine is initiated (Table 27–15). The most serious toxic hematologic side effects of carbamazepine are agranulocytosis and aplastic anemia, which may be fatal. While carbamazepine-induced agranulocytosis or aplastic anemia is extremely rare, leukopenia is more common, with a prevalence of approximately 10%. Persistent leukopenia as well as thrombocytopenia occurs in approximately 2% of patients, and mild anemia occurs in fewer than 5% of patients.

Hart and Easton (1982) recommended obtaining blood and platelet counts before carbamazepine therapy, and complete blood counts every 2 weeks for the first 2 months, and quarterly thereafter (Table 27–15). Patients with abnormal results on baseline tests should be considered at high risk and require a risk-benefit assessment before treatment is initiated. During ongoing carbamazepine therapy, the development of leukopenia necessitates follow-up laboratory evaluations every 2 weeks. If the counts do not return to normal in 2 weeks, the drug dose should be reduced. Interestingly, the use of lithium to counteract leukopenia induced by carbamazepine has been suggested (Brewerton 1986). However, lithium does not reverse the underlying pathophysiological effects of carbamazepine, and so the clinician should monitor patients on carbamazepine as they are being withdrawn from lithium, because a clinically significant leukopenia may be unmasked. If a patient on carbamazepine develops fever, infection, petechiae, weakness or pallor, a white blood cell count of fewer than 3,000 per mm^3, or an absolute neutrophil count of fewer than 2,000, all drugs should be discontinued immediately. Consultation with a hematologist is also required at this point. Serious complications should be reported to the drug manufacturer to ensure an accurate database for evaluation of the risks of this therapy.

Carbamazepine occasionally may result in hepatic toxicity (Gram and Bentsen 1983). This is usually a hypersensitivity hepatitis that appears after a latency period of several weeks and is associated with elevations in SGOT (serum glutamate oxaloacetate transaminase), SGPT (serum glutamate pyruvate transaminase), and LDH (lactic dehydrogenase). Cholestasis is also possible, with increases in bilirubin and alkaline phosphatase. Mild, transient elevations in LDH and the transaminases can generally be monitored without discontinuation of the carbamazepine. We recommend regular monitoring of liver enzymes for patients receiving carbamazepine (Table 27–15).

An exanthematous rash is one of the more common side effects associated with carbamazepine, occurring in 3% to 17% of patients (Warnock and Knesevich 1988). This reaction typically begins within 2 to 20 weeks after the start of treatment. Carbamazepine also may induce an exfoliative dermatitis characterized by an extensive erythematous rash with scaling. This side effect is often associated with systemic symptoms such as fever and arthritis. This condition can often be diagnosed with a patch test (Camarasa 1985), and, when found, it should lead to a cessation of treatment. Stevens-Johnson syndrome, a severe, bullous form of erythema multiforme, has also been reported in association with carbamazepine use (Patterson 1985).

Carbamazepine may cause a reduction in the circulating levels of T_3 and T_4, possibly by inducing their hepatic metabolism (Bentsen et al. 1983), although rarely does this effect have clinical significance. However, when carbamazepine is used in combination with other agents that antagonize thyroid function, such as lithium, a clinically significant synergistic effect may emerge (Kramingler and Post 1990). Carbamazepine may simultaneously reduce TSH levels, as it appears to diminish the pituitary response to TRH (Joffe et al. 1984). Patients with borderline thyroid function, and those who already receive thyroid supplement, may be at risk for the development of frank hypothyroidism when taking carbamazepine, and should therefore undergo periodic thyroid function tests to rule out such an occurrence.

The syndrome of inappropriate antidiuretic hormone (SIADH) may be induced by carbamazepine treatment. When hyponatremia develops it is often transient; but even more severe cases of this condition can often be managed by fluid restriction or the addition of lithium. Because of the risk of SIADH, baseline and follow-up sodium levels and urine specific gravity are indicated for patients receiving carbamazepine.

Drug interactions.   Carbamazepine may reduce circulation levels of several medications through the induction of hepatic metabolism. Most important among such interactions are the effects of carbamazepine on benzodiazepine and antidepressant levels. For example, alprazolam levels have been reported to drop by 50% after the addition of carbamazepine (Arana et al. 1988). Likewise, clinically significant reductions in tricyclic antidepressant levels can occur with carbamazepine co-treatment (Leinonen et al. 1991). Therefore, plasma antidepressant levels should be monitored in cases when carbamazepine has been added. Through the same mechanism of hepatic enzyme induction, carbamazepine has been implicated in oral contraceptive failure (Coulam and Annegers 1979). On the other hand, the calcium channel blockers diltiazem and verapamil, but not nifedipine, have been reported to cause potentially dangerous elevations in plasma carbamazepine levels (Brodie and MacPhee 1986).

Valproate

Valproate treatment is initiated at a dosage of 250 mg twice or three times a day, and subsequently increased by 250 mg every 3 days, with the goal of reaching a plasma level of between 50 and 100 mg/ml. Most patients will require a daily dose of 1,250 to 1,500 mg to achieve such a level. There are patients, however, who require relatively high doses of valproate, sometimes greater than 3,000 mg a day, in order to achieve sufficient plasma levels; however, daily dosage should not in any case exceed 60 mg/kg (Dean and Penry 1992). On the other hand, plasma valproate levels greater than 100 mg/ml are not often associated with side effects or toxicity, and as a result, this threshold may be crossed when clinically indicated. As with carbamazepine, the relationship between plasma levels and therapeutic effect has not been established for acute or prophylactic therapy with valproate.

Contraindications.   Valproate should be used with extreme caution in patients with disturbances of liver or renal function. The free fraction of valproate increases two to three times among patients suffering from alcoholic cirrhosis, acute hepatitis, or renal disease (Dean and Penry 1992). Valproate has been linked to spina bifida and other neural tube defects in the offspring of patients exposed to this medication in the first trimester (Lammer et al. 1987). The relative risk of teratogenensis with valproate is greater than with other anticonvulsants, including carbamazepine (Dean and Penry 1992), and, therefore, this agent should be avoided during pregnancy. Careful monitoring of female patients of childbearing age, through repeated checking for the signs and symptoms of pregnancy and episodic pregnancy tests, is required.

Risks, side effects, and their management.   Unlike with carbamazepine, reports of valproate-induced hematologic disorders are rare. However, valproate is associated with significant hepatic toxicity. While there have been reports of rare, non-dose-related hepatic failure with fatalities, estimated to occur in 1 out of 10,000 patients, none has occurred in patients over 10 years of age who were receiving valproate monotherapy (Dreifuss et al. 1987). Nonetheless, in otherwise healthy adult patients, baseline and follow-up liver function tests are indicated. Transient, mild elevations in the liver enzymes, up to twice the upper limit of normal, do not require the discontinuation of valproate. Although GGT (gamma-glutamyl transferase) levels are often checked by clinicians, this test is too sensitive a measure of hepatotoxicity in patients receiving valproate and carbamazepine, as it is often elevated without clinical significance (Dean and Penry 1992). Likewise, plasma ammonia levels are often elevated transiently with valproate treatment, but this finding does not require that the treatment be interrupted (Jaeken et al. 1980). For patients with a prior history of hepatitis, valproate is relatively contraindicated; it may be pursued as treatment only as a last resort and with the approval and continuous involvement of a gastroenterologist.

Valproate has been associated with changes in platelet count, but clinically significant thrombocytopenia has rarely been documented (Dean and Penry 1992). Coagulation defects have also been reported. Overall, the risk of inducing a coagulation disturbance in an otherwise healthy adult is very low when the daily dose of valproate used is below 3,000 mg/day. However, in patients for whom anticoagulation is strictly contraindicated, or for patients who already receive anticoagulation therapy, continuous monitoring of the coagulation profile and whole bleeding time is required.

Indigestion, heartburn, and nausea are common side effects with valproate therapy. We recommend the enteric coated Depakote preparation to help mitigate these effects. Patients may also be encouraged to take their dose with food. In most cases, however, dyspepsia is transient and not severe. Appetite may be adversely affected during the early stages of treatment, but ongoing therapy is more often associated with an increase in appetite. Weight gain, unassociated with increased intake of food, occurs in 18% of patients overall and is more common among women than men (Clark et al. 1980). Pancreatitis has been reported as a rare occurrence among some patients receiving relatively high doses of valproate (Murphy et al. 1981). Therefore, if vomiting and abdominal pain persist after 5 to 6 weeks of therapy, a serum amylase level, together with prothrombin time and partial thromboplastin time, should be obtained (Dean and Penry 1992).

One of the most common side effects associated with valproate use is benign essential tremor. This tremor is apparently not dose related and may first occur as long as 1 year after the initiation of therapy (Hyman et al. 1979). Drowsiness is another common side effect of valproate treatment, but tolerance often develops once a steady-state level of the drug is reached. A more gradual initial titration of valproate may be indicated for patients who complain of marked daytime sleepiness.

Both transient and persistent hair loss have been associated with valproate use. When hair loss occurs, it often begins 3 months or longer after the initiation of treatment and is probably not dose related. Regrowth may result in hair that is more wavy or curly than before (Jeavons et al. 1977). It is our observation that patients with thyroid abnormalities who receive valproate are more likely to suffer hair loss, even when ongoing thyroid replacement treatment has normalized their thyroid function tests.

Overdosage. Valproate overdose results in increasing sedation, confusion, and, ultimately, coma. The patient may also manifest hyperreflexia or hyporeflexia, seizures, respiratory suppression, and superventricular tachycardia (Labar 1992). Treatment should include gastric lavage, ECG monitoring, treatment of emergent seizures, and respiratory support as indicated.

Drug interactions. When coadministered, other anticonvulsants will result in increased clearance of valproate, and, hence, a reduction of plasma valproate levels occurs. Conversely, when such agents are withdrawn from a regimen that includes valproate, the clinician must be prepared for plasma valproate levels to rise, and for potential toxicity. Valproate does not have this effect on other anticonvulsants, since it does not induce hepatic enzymes. Unlike carbamazepine, therefore, valproate has not been associated with oral contraceptive failure. Valproate may actually inhibit hepatic enzymes, and so there is the potential for increases in the levels of some of the other anticonvulsants (Dean and Penry 1992).

☐ Other Pharmacological Treatments of Mania

For the patient with mania who responds poorly to sequential trials of lithium, carbamazepine, and valproate, there are several available strategies. Combined treatment with two of these three agents may succeed in patients fo whom monotherapy has failed. The combination of lithium and carbamazepine, for example, has been shown to be superior to lithium-neuroleptic treatment in the prophylaxis of bipolar patients (Shukla et al. 1985). Lithium in combination with carbamazepine (Moss and James 1983) and with valproate (McElroy et al. 1989) brought remission for some patients with acute mania who were unresponsive to lithium alone. Although combined carbamazepine-valproate therapy has received less attention, there are reports of response in otherwise refractory cases (McElroy et al. 1989).

Patients with bipolar illness who suffer from rapid cycling (i.e., more than four mood disorder episodes per year) are often refractory to lithium therapy. Among this group of patients with atypical bipolar illness, several investigators have reported higher rates of thyroid dysfunction, often subclinical, in comparison with non-rapid-cycling bipolar patients (Bauer et al. 1989; Cowdry et al. 1983; Wehr et al. 1988). For example, rapid-cycling patients, who may be clinically euthyroid at baseline, are more prone to lithium-induced hypothyroidism (Cho et al. 1979). There is evidence that high-dose levothyroxine (T_4), as high as 400 μg/day, added to lithium or other mood stabilizers may convert partial or nonresponders to responders (Bauer and Whybrow 1989). Bauer and Whybrow (1989) recommend as a guideline that the T_4 dose be increased until the patient's free thyroid index reaches 150% of the normal value. Patients receiving high-dose T_4 must be monitored for signs of thyroid toxicity, with special attention made to cardiac function.

Verapamil, a calcium channel blocking drug used for the treatment of arrhythmias and hypertension, has been reported to be effective in the treatment of mania (Brotman et al. 1986). Verapamil proved to be highly effective, comparable to lithium and neuroleptics, in patients with acute mania (Hoschl and Kozeny 1989). However, although these results are quite promising, it remains to be determined whether lithium-refractory patients, in particular, will respond to verapamil. The doses of verapamil used are in the range of 360 to 480 mg/day, taken in a divided tid regimen. Once patients are stabilized, they may be switched to the slow-release verapamil preparation, which allows for once-daily dosing.

Finally and importantly, ECT has well-documented effects on manic symptomatology. Bilateral stimulation may be required to obtain the antimanic effects (Small et al. 1985). This modality is indicated when a patient's physical condition, inability to tolerate medication side effects, and failure to respond to other modalities so dictate.

■ ANTIAGGRESSIVE DRUGS

The initial steps in the treatment of aggressive behavior include diagnosis and treatment of underlying causes of aggression (e.g., brain tumor), and evaluation and documentation of aggressive behaviors with objective measures such as the Overt Aggression Scale (Silver and Yudofsky 1991). Although no medication has been approved by the FDA specifically for the treatment of aggression, medications are widely used (and commonly misused) in the management of patients with acute or chronic aggression. The use of pharmacological interventions for aggression can be considered in two categories: 1) the use of the sedating effects of medications, as required in acute situations, so that the patient does not harm himself or herself, or others; and 2) the use of nonsedating antiaggressive medications for the treatment of chronic aggression (Silver and Yudofsky 1994).

Our recommendations for the utilization of various classes of medication in the treatment of aggressive disorders are summarized in Table 27–16. If aggression is related to active psychosis, antipsychotic agents should be used. In patients with aggression related to mania, lithium carbonate is the drug of choice in most cases. When aggression is related to seizure disorder, carbamazepine or valproic acid is indicated. Patients with mood lability or depression with concomitant irritability or rage attacks should be treated with a serotonergic antidepressant. Finally, for those patients whose aggression is secondary to organic brain syndromes, we recommend the use of beta-blockers. Beta-blockers should

Table 27–16. Psychopharmacological treatment of chronic aggression

Clinical agent(s)	Indications	Special considerations
Antipsychotics	Psychosis	Oversedation and multiple side effects
Benzodiazepines	Anxiety	Possible induction of paradoxical rage; over-sedation; cognitive impairment
Anticonvulsants		
Carbamazepine (CBZ)	Seizure disorder	Bone marrow suppression
Valproic acid (VPA)	or EEG changes	(CBZ) and hepatoxicity (CBZ and VPA)
Lithium	Manic excitement or bipolar disorder	Neurotoxicity and confusion
Buspirone	Persistent anxiety and/or depression	Latency of action of 3 to 5 weeks
Propranolol (and other beta-blockers)	Chronic or recurrent aggression	Latency of action of 4 to 6 weeks
Serotonergic anti-depressants	Depression or mood lability with irritability	May require higher than usual doses for treatment of depression

Source. Adapted from Yudofsky SC, Silver JM, Schneider SE: "Pharmacologic Treatment of Aggression." *Psychiatric Annals* 17:397–407, 1987. Copyright 1987, Slack, Inc. Used with permission.

also be considered for agitation and aggression of patients with schizophrenia whose aggression is not directly related to psychotic ideation.

☐ Acute Aggression and Agitation

In the treatment of agitation and for treating acute episodes of aggressive behavior, medications that are sedating may be indicated. However, as these drugs are not specific in their ability to inhibit aggressive behaviors, there may be detrimental effects on arousal and cognitive function. Therefore, the use of sedation-producing medications must be time-limited to avoid the emergence of seriously disabling side effects ranging from oversedation to tardive dyskinesia.

Antipsychotic Drugs

Antipsychotics are the most commonly used medications in the treatment of aggression. Although these agents are appropriate and effective when aggression is derivative of active psychosis, the use of neuroleptic agents to treat chronic aggression, especially secondary to organic brain injury, is often ineffective and entails significant risks that the patient will develop serious complications. Usually, it is the sedative side effects rather than the antipsychotic properties of antipsychotics that are used (i.e., misused) to "treat" (i.e., mask) the aggression. Often, patients develop tolerance to the sedative effects of the neuroleptics and, therefore, require increasing doses. As a result, extrapyramidal and anticholinergic-related side effects occur. Paradoxically (and frequently), because of the development of akathisia, the patient may become more agitated and restless as the dose of neuroleptic is increased, especially when a high-potency antipsychotic such as haloperidol is administered. The akathisia is often mistaken for increased irritability and agitation, and a "viscious cycle" of increasing neuroleptics and worsening akathisias occurs. Herrera et al. (1988) demonstrated that there was a marked increase in violent behavior when patients with schizophrenia were treated with haloperidol (doses up to 60 mg/day) compared with the behaviors that occurred during treatment with chlorpromazine (1,800 mg/day) or clozapine (900 mg/day), two drugs that are associated with less akathisia than is haloperidol.

There is some evidence from studies of injury to motor neurons in animals that haloperidol decreases recovery. This effect was only seen when animals actively participated in a behavioral task, and not when the animals were restrained after drug administration (Feeney et al. 1982). It is possible that haloperidol's effect of decreasing dopamine and inhibiting neuronal function, which may be the mechanism of action to treat aggression, may have other detrimental effects on recovery. This raises important potential risk-benefit issues that must be considered before antipsychotic drugs are used to treat aggressive behavior in patients with neuronal damage.

In patients with brain injury and acute aggression, we recommend starting a neuroleptic such as haloperidol at low dosages of 1 mg orally or 0.5 mg intramuscularly, with repeated administration every hour until control of aggression is achieved (Yudofsky et al. 1990). If after several administrations of haloperidol, the patient's aggressive behavior does not improve, the hourly dose may be increased until the patient is sufficiently sedated that he or she no longer exhibits agitation or violence. Once the patient is not aggressive for 48 hours, the daily dosage should be decreased gradually (i.e., by 25% per day) to ascertain whether aggressive behavior reemerges. If it does, consideration should then be made about whether it is best to increase the dose of haloperidol and then to initiate treatment with a more specific antiaggressive drug.

Sedatives and Hypnotics

There is an inconsistent literature on the effects of the benzodiazepines in the treatment of aggression. The sedative properties of benzodiazepines are especially helpful in the management of acute agitation and aggression (Yudofsky et al. 1987). Most likely, this is due to the effect of benzodiazepines on increasing the inhibitory neurotransmitter GABA. Paradoxically, several studies reported increased hostility and aggression, and the induction of rage in patients treated with benzodiazepines (Yudofsky et al. 1987). However, these reports are balanced by the observation that this phenomenon is rare (Dietch and Jennings 1988). Benzodiazepines can produce amnesia (Angus and Romney 1984) and can exacerbate preexisting memory dysfunction. Patients with brain injury may also experience increased problems with coordination and balance with benzodiazepine use.

For treatment of acute aggression, lorazepam, 1 to 2 mg, may be administered every hour by either oral or intramuscular route until sedation is achieved (Yudofsky et al. 1990). Intramuscular lorazepam has been suggested as an effective medication in the emergency treatment of the violent patient (Bick and Hannah 1986). Intravenous lorazepam is also effective, although the onset of action is similar when adminstered intramuscularly. Caution must be taken with intravenous administration of lorazepam, and it should be injected in doses of less than 1 cc (1 mg) per minute to avoid laryngospasm. As with neuroleptics, gradual tapering of lorazepam may be attempted when the patient has been in control for 48 hours. If aggressive behavior reoccurs, medications for the treatment of chronic aggression may be initiated. Lorazepam in 1- or 2-mg doses, administered either orally or by injection, may be administered, if necessary, in combination with a neuroleptic medication (haloperidol, 2 to 5 mg). Other sedating medications such as paraldehyde, chloral hydrate, or diphenhydramine may be preferable to sedative antipsychotic agents.

☐ Chronic Aggression

If a patient continues to exhibit periods of agitation or aggression beyond several weeks, the use of specific antiaggressive medications should be initiated to prevent these episodes from occurring. The choice of medication may be guided by the underlying hypothesized mechanism of action (i.e., effects on serotonergic system, adrenergic system, kindling, etc.), or in consideration of the underlying disease process (i.e., traumatic brain injury, seizure disorder, bipolar disorder). Because no medication has been approved by the FDA for treatment of aggression, the clinician must use medications that may be antiaggressive but that have been approved for other uses (i.e., seizure disorders, depression, hypertension, etc.).

Antipsychotic Medications

If, after thorough clinical evaluation, it is determined that the aggressive episodes result from psychosis, such as paranoid delusions or command hallucinations, then antipsychotic medications will be the treatment of choice. Clozapine may have greater antiaggressive effects than other antipsychotic medications (Ratey et al. 1993). The clinician should choose neuroleptics and utilize doses in the same fashion that were recommended for the treatment of psychosis.

Antianxiety Medications

In preliminary reports, buspirone has been reported to be effective in the management of aggression and agitation for patients with head injury (Ratey et al. 1992a), dementia (Tiller et al. 1988), and developmental disabilities and autism (Ratey et al. 1989). We have also noted that some patients become more aggressive when treated with buspirone. Therefore, buspirone should be initiated at low dosages (i.e., 5 mg bid) and increased by 5 mg every 3 to 5 days. Dosages of 45 to 60 mg/day may be required before there is improvement in aggressive behavior. Freinhar and Alvarez (1986) found that clonazepam decreased agitation in three elderly patients with organic brain syndromes. Keats and Mukherjee (1988) reported antiaggressive effects of clonazepam in a patient with schizophrenia and seizures. We use clonazepam when pronounced aggression and anxiety occur together, or when aggression occurs in association with neurologically induced tics and similarly disinhibited motor behaviors. Doses should be initiated at 0.5 mg bid and may be increased to as high as 2 to 4 mg bid, as tolerated. Sedation and ataxia are frequent side effects.

Anticonvulsive Medications

The anticonvulsant carbamazepine has been proved to be effective for the treatment of bipolar disorders and has also been advocated for the control of aggression in both epileptic and nonepileptic populations (Yudofsky et al. 1987). The mechanism of action of the anticonvulsants in the treatment of organic aggression may be through their effect on inhibiting kindling. Open studies have indicated that carbamazepine may be effective in decreasing aggressive behavior associated with dementia (Gleason and Schneider 1990), developmental disabilities (Yatham and McHale 1988), and schizophrenia (Luchins 1983), as well as with a variety of other organic brain disorders (Mattes 1988). Carbamazepine can be a highly effective medication to treat aggression in patients with brain injury, and we believe it is the drug of choice for those patients who have aggressive episodes with concomitant seizures or epileptic foci. Reports also indicate that the antiaggressive response of carbamazepine can be found in patients with (Yatham and McHale 1988) and without EEG abnormalities (Mattes 1988).

The anticonvulsant valproic acid may also be helpful to some patients with organically induced aggression (Mattes 1992). For those patients with aggression and epilepsy whose seizures are being treated with anticonvulsant drugs such as phenytoin and phenobarbital, switching to carbamazepine or to valproic acid may treat both conditions.

Antimanic Medications

While lithium is known to be effective in controlling aggression related to manic excitement, many studies suggest that it may also have a role in the treatment of aggression in selected, nonbipolar patient populations (Yudofsky et al. 1987). Included are patients with traumatic brain injury (Haas and Cope 1985); patients with mental retardation who exhibit self-injurious (Luchins and Dojka 1989) or aggressive behavior (Craft et al. 1987); children and adolescents with behavioral disorders (Vetro et al. 1985); prison inmates (Sheard et al. 1976); and patients with other organic brain syndromes (Williams and Goldstein 1979). Primary antiaggressive effects may be due to lithium's effect on the serotonergic system, although lithium also affects other important neuronal systems, such as inositol phosphate metabolism and kindling (Berridge et al. 1989).

Patients with brain injury have increased sensitivity to the neurotoxic effects of lithium (Moskowitz and Altshuler 1991). Because of lithium's potential for neurotoxicity and its relative lack of efficacy in many patients with aggression secondary to brain injury, we limit the use of lithium in those patients whose aggression is related to manic effects or recurrent irritability related to cyclic mood disorders.

Antidepressant Medications

Antidepressants may have effects on the serotonergic, noradrenergic, and other neurotransmitter systems. The antidepressants that have been reported to control aggressive behavior are those that act preferentially (amitriptyline) or specifically (trazodone and fluoxetine) on serotonin. Mysiw and co-workers (1988) reported that amitriptyline (maximum dose 150 mg/day) was effective in the treatment of patients with recent severe brain injury whose agitation had not responded to behavioral techniques. Trazodone has also been reported effective in treating aggression that occurs with organic mental disorders (Pinner and Rich 1988). Fluoxetine, a potent serotonergic antidepressant, has been reported to be effective in the treatment of aggressive behavior in a patient who suffered brain injury (Sorbin et al. 1989), as well as in patients with personality disorders (Coccaro et al. 1990) and depression (Fava et al. 1993). There have also been reports on the therapeutic effect of fluoxetine for adolescents with mental retardation and self-injurious behavior (King 1991). We have used fluoxetine with considerable success in aggressive patients with brain lesions. The dosage may be started with 10 mg/day, and increased to 20 mg after 1 week. For some patients with aggression related to brain disorders, response to treatment with fluoxetine occurs in the 60–80 mg/day range.

We have evaluated and treated many patients with emotional lability that is characterized by frequent episodes of tearfulness and irritability, and the full symptomatic picture of organic aggressive syndrome (Silver and Yudofsky 1994). These patients, who would be diagnosed under DSM-IV as having personality change due to a general medical condition, labile type, have responded well to antidepressants. These therapeutic results are consistent with the reports of Schiffer et al. (1985), who used amitriptyline for patients with multiple sclerosis (MS), and Seliger et al. (1992), who used fluoxetine to treat patients after brain injury, stroke, or MS. In addition, it appears that sertraline, a newer SSRI, is effective as well to treat aggression related to these disorders. It is usually necessary to administer these medications at standard antidepressant dosages to achieve full therapeutic effects.

Antihypertensive Medications (Beta-Blockers)

Since the first report of the use of beta-adrenergic receptor blockers in the treatment of acute aggression in 1977, many papers have appeared in the neurological and psychiatric literature reporting experience in using beta-blockers with patients with aggression (Yudofsky et al. 1987). Most of these patients had been unsuccessfully treated with antipsychotics, minor tranquilizers, lithium, and/or anticonvulsants before treatment with beta-blockers. The beta-blockers that have been investigated in controlled prospective studies include propranolol (Mattes 1988); nadolol (Ratey et al. 1992b); and pindolol (Greendyke et al. 1989). A growing body of preliminary evidence suggests that beta-adrenergic receptor blockers are effective agents for the treatment of aggressive and violent behaviors, particularly those related to organic brain syndrome. Guidelines for the use of propranolol are listed in Table 27–17. When a patient requires the use of a once-a-day medication because of compliance difficulties, long-acting propranolol or nadolol can be utilized in once-per-day regimens. When patients develop bradycardia that prevents prescribing of therapeutic dosages of propranolol, pindolol can be substituted, using one-tenth the dosage of propranolol. Pindolol's intrinsic sympathomimetic activity stimulates the beta receptor and restricts the development of bradycardia.

Table 27–17.   Clinical use of propranolol

1. Conduct a thorough medical evaluation.

2. Exclude patients with the following disorders: bronchial asthma, chronic obstructive pulmonary disease, insulin-dependent diabetes mellitus, congestive heart failure, persistent angina, significant peripheral vascular disease, hyperthyroidism.

3. Avoid sudden discontinuation of propranolol (particularly in patients with hypertension).

4. Begin with a single test-dose of 20 mg per day in patients for whom there are clinical concerns with hypotension or bradycardia. Increase dose of propranolol by 20 mg per day every 3 days.

5. Initiate propranolol on a 20 mg tid schedule for patients without cardiovascular or cardiopulmonary disorder.

6. Increase the dosage of propranolol by 60 mg per day every 3 days.

7. Increase medication unless the pulse rate is reduced below 50 beats per minute, or systolic blood pressure is less than 90 mmHg.

8. Do not administer medication if severe dizziness, ataxia, or wheezing occurs. Reduce or discontinue propranolol if such symptoms persist.

9. Increase dose to 12 mg/kg or until aggressive behavior is under control.

10. Doses of greater than 800 mg are not usually required to control aggressive behavior.

11. Maintain the patient on the highest dose of propranolol for at least 8 weeks prior to concluding that the patient is not responding to the medication. Some patients, however, may respond rapidly to propranolol.

12. Utilize concurrent medications with caution. Monitor plasma levels of all antipsychotic and anticonvulsive medications.

Source.   Reprinted from Yudofsky SC, Silver JM, Schneider SE: "Pharmacologic Treatment of Aggression." *Psychiatric Annals* 17:397–407, 1987. Copyright 1987, Slack, Inc. Used with permission.

The major side effects of beta-blockers when these agents are used to treat aggression are a lowering of blood pressure and pulse rate. Because peripheral beta receptors are fully blocked in doses of 300 to 400 mg/day, further decreases in these vital signs usually do not occur even when doses are increased to much higher levels. Despite reports of depression associated with the use of beta-blockers, controlled trials and our experience indicate that this rarely occurs (Yudofsky 1992). Because the use of propranolol is associated with significant increases in plasma levels of thioridazine, which has an absolute dosage ceiling of 800 mg/day, the combination of these two medications should be avoided whenever possible (Silver et al. 1986).

■ ELECTROCONVULSIVE THERAPY

Electroconvulsive therapy (ECT) is the utilization of electrically induced repetitive firings of the neurons in the CNS (i.e., grand mal seizures) to treat psychiatric illnesses such as depression and mania, or psychiatric symptoms such as psychosis or catatonia. Although ECT was first used in the late 1930s, the treatment today remains clinically relevant because of its high degree of efficacy, safety, and utility. There have been six published controlled trials since 1968 in which ECT has been shown to be superior to simulated treatment. Surveys conducted by the American Psychiatric Association in the 1970s showed that while only 3% to 5% of psychiatric inpatients in the United States receive ECT, 72% of a large group of psychiatrists believe that there are many patients for whom ECT is the safest, least expensive, and most effective form of treatment (American Psychiatric Association 1978). Only 7% of those psychiatrists surveyed believed that the use of ECT is now obsolete. In the United States, ECT is primarily used in the private sector for patients who do not receive prolonged inpatient care (Asnis et al. 1978).

☐ Indications

The principal indications for ECT are major depression, mania, and schizophrenia (American Psychiatric Association 1990). The APA Task Force on Electroconvulsive Therapy has recommended the following primary clinical situations for the use of ECT: 1) when there is a need for a rapid, definitive response for either medical or psychiatric grounds, 2) when the risks of other treatments outweigh the risks of ECT, 3) when there is a history of poor drug response and/or good ECT response, and 4) when it is the patient's preference. Yudofsky (1981) outlined special clinical situations in which ECT may be advantageous over other treatment approaches. Among these situations, which are by no means all-inclusive, are the following:

1. Patients whose severe affective disorders have not responded to adequate (i.e., appropriate dose and duration of treatment) psychopharacological treatment.
2. Patients with delusional depression (Glassman and Roose 1981).
3. Patients—particularly elderly patients—who cannot tolerate the cardiovascular, genitourinary, or CNS side effects of antidepressant or antipsychotic agents.
4. Patients whose acute symptoms are so severe (i.e., manic excitement, active suicidal behavior, psychomotor retardation, or catatonia) that a rapid and dramatic response is required.

5. Patients with histories of depressive episodes that have responded successfully to previous electroconvulsive treatments.

Depressed patients adequately treated with either drugs or ECT have significantly lower mortality rates—not just related to suicide, but also from natural causes—than those patients with depression who are not treated with such modalities (Avery and Winokur 1976). In a report that analyzed rigorously controlled studies that compared the efficacy of ECT with that of simulated ECT, placebo, and antidepressants, ECT had a clear superiority over all these forms of treatment for severe depression (Janicak et al. 1985). Although ECT and antidepressant agents are effective in similar patient populations with depression (except for patients with delusional depression, in whom ECT is superior), a number of comparative studies have shown that ECT is significantly more effective, with marked improvement generally occurring in 80% to 90% of patients (Weiner 1979). ECT may also be of benefit in the treatment of manic excitement that is not responsive to antipsychotic drugs or lithium treatment, as well as in the treatment of acute psychotic and affective symptoms of schizophrenia. The production of serious drug-related side effects in the population of patients with schizophrenia, particularly tardive dyskinesia, has made the question of the role of ECT in the treatment of schizophrenia more relevant. Salzman (1980) found that the few acceptable published studies showed that clinical response to ECT was inversely proportional to the duration of the schizophrenic symptoms. In general, patients with schizophrenia with affective and catatonic symptoms respond the best to ECT, whereas those patients who have chronic symptoms of amotivation and bizarre behavior often fail to respond to ECT.

☐ Contraindications

The contraindications to ECT are relatively few (American Psychiatric Association 1990). First, patients with clinically significant space occupying cerebral lesions or conditions with increased intracranial pressure must not receive this treatment because of the risk of brain-stem herniation (Maltbie et al. 1980). Second, patients with significant cardiovascular problems that may include recent myocardial infarction, severe cardiac ischemia, and significant hypertension (including pheochromocytoma) are more prone to the transient fluctuations in the cardiovascular system that occur during and shortly following ECT. Such patients may or may not be safely given ECT, and they must be evaluated before treatment by a cardiologist familiar with the potential side effects of ECT. Patients with recent intracerebral hemorrhage are at increased risk, as are those with bleeding or unstable vascular aneurisms or abnormalities, or retinal detachment. Adequate anesthetic and muscle relaxant techniques render ECT generally safe in patients with these disorders. While it is suggested that patients be discontinued from their MAOIs for at least 2 weeks prior to the initiation of ECT to prevent dangerous increases in blood pressure during treatment, ECT has been administered to patients currently treated with MAOIs without adverse effects (Wells and Bjorkstein 1989).

☐ Medical Evaluation Before Treatment

Prior to receiving ECT, a patient should have a complete medical and neurological examination, complete blood count, serum electrolyte analysis, and an ECG. An X ray of the lumbosacral region should be obtained if spinal orthopedic problems are suspected. A chest X ray must be obtained because of the use of positive pressure respiration during general anesthesia. Evaluation by an anesthesiologist to determine risk of anaesthesia (ASA class) is recommended. In specific clinical situations, such as when there is clinical evidence of a brain tumor or intracerebral bleed, or if there is the presence of CNS symptoms of uncertain etiology, an electroencephalogram and a brain computed tomographic scan or magnetic resonance imaging are also required. Informed consent of a competent patient is essential. Because of the high degree of fear and misinformation related to ECT, we encourage that ample time be devoted to the discussion of the risks, benefits, and techniques of ECT and of all treatment alternatives with both the patient and his or her family (Yudofsky et al. 1991).

☐ Technique

Anesthesia and Muscle Relaxation

Electroconvulsive therapy is a procedure used primarily for psychiatric inpatients, and there is an increasing practice in psychiatry for an anesthetist or anesthesiologist to assist the psychiatrist in administering the treatment. The APA Task Force on Electroconvulsive Therapy (American Psychiatric Association 1990) recommended pretreatment with an anticholinergic drug such as atropine (0.4 to 1.0 mg iv) or glycopyrrolate (0.2 to 0.4 mg iv) to decrease the morbidity of cardiac bradyarrhythmias and aspiration. General anesthesia is induced only to such a degree as to provide light coma with fast-acting anesthetics such as methohexital, which has fewer cardiac side effects than slower-acting barbiturates such as thiopental. A starting dose of approximately 0.75 to 1.0 mg/kg of intravenous methohexital is recommended, but the amount required to induce safe and brief anesthesia may vary from considerably lower amounts to considerably higher dosages depending on a patient's meta-bolism of the drug. Once the patient is anesthetized, intravenous succinylcholine is utilized for muscular relaxation. In general, approximately 0.5 to 1 mg per kilogram of intravenous succinylcholine is administered rapidly, immediately after the onset of general anesthesia. Presence of preexisting skeletal problems or other orthopedic problems may require the use of a higher dose of succinylcholine, whereas a history or evidence of pseudocholinesterase deficiency would call for a lower dose. Once the succinylcholine is administered, the patient is ventilated with 100% oxygen until muscle fasciculations and motoric relaxation of the patient are accomplished. Modern ECT devices allow for simultaneous monitoring of the EEG and ECG before, during, and after the ECT procedure. In addition, there should be frequent monitoring of blood pressure, pulse rate, and blood oxygen saturation (with pulse oximetry).

Devices

The electrical stimulation of ECT devices is classified on the basis of wave form. Mechanisms using sine wave stimulus were historically the most commonly used to initiate grand mal seizures. Newer devices using brief pulse stimulation are being increasingly used. With the latter technique, grand mal seizures usually can be initiated with an amount of electrical energy significantly lower than that required with devices utilizing sine wave stimuli (Malitz and Sackheim 1986).

Parameters

Two major issues in the administration of the electrical stimulus include the stimulus dose and the electrode placement (i.e., nondominant unilateral or bilateral). It has been documented that seizure threshold, which is defined as the minimal electrical intensity needed to produce a generalized seizure, increases with age and is greater in men than in women. However, the threshold can vary by 40-fold among patients (Sackheim et al. 1991). Electrodes may be placed unilaterally on the nondominant hemisphere (i.e., the electrodes over the right hemisphere for a right-handed individual) or bilaterally. While there have been observations that unilateral electrode placement has fewer cognitive side effects compared with bilateral stimulus, studies also suggest that unilateral placement is less efficacious (American Psychiatric Association 1990).

Sackheim et al. (1993) compared low-dose (i.e., just above threshold) unilateral ECT, high-dose (i.e., 2.5 times the threshold) unilateral ECT, low-dose bilateral ECT, and high-dose bilateral ECT for efficacy and cognitive effects. While high-dose unilateral treatment is more efficacious than low-dose unilateral stimulation, bilateral treatment is superior. In measures of time to recover orientation, unilateral stimulation had fewer deleterious effects than did bilateral stimulus, regardless of dosage.

The decision to initiate treatment with unilateral or bilateral electrode placement may be influenced by a variety of factors, including preexisting cognitive impairment and the clinical requirement for rapid improvement. However, in our practice, we determine seizure threshold during the first treatment session, and subsequent treatment dosages are increased to ensure that ECT is above threshold (American Psychiatric Association 1990).

Course of Treatment

ECT treatments are generally given on an every-other-day basis for 2 to 3 weeks. Seizure lengths of durations of greater than 20 seconds per each treatment (as assessed by motor activity, not EEG seizure activity) are considered adequate for therapeutic purposes. The number of treatments administered is generally determined by a patient's clinical response—that is, when successive treatments do not elicit further beneficial effects (Weiner 1979). With depressed patients, a typical course of ECT consists of 6 to 10 treatments. After a course of treatment and, hopefully, after a successful response to ECT, ample time and "permission" must be given for the patient to discuss with the professional his or her feelings about having been depressed and having received ECT. Occasionally, a patient will erroneously attribute his or her inability to recall a name to "permanent" side effects of the procedure. In this situation, the normal forgetting process to which most people are subject would become a frightening and unwarranted symbol of depression and ECT. In addition, there must be the recognition that ECT is a specific therapeutic tool that should be used as a component of a larger therapeutic strategy (Yudofsky et al. 1991). Because the beneficial response to ECT is often so rapid and dramatic, occasionally insufficient emphasis is placed on the sociological and intrapsychic stresses that may have contributed to the initial depression. It is only after the patient's affective illness has been improved by ECT that the patient is able to utilize psychotherapy, family therapy, and behavior therapy effectively to address those conditions that contributed to the depression.

Post ECT Treatment

Despite the efficacy of ECT, appropriate treatment after ECT is required to prevent relapse. Unfortunately, many patients who receive ECT have been previously refractory to standard medications. The efficacy of these treatments is not clear after ECT (Sackheim et al. 1990). Following a course of treatment, patients should be maintained on either a hetero-cyclic antidepressant or lithium carbonate. Continuation drug therapy was demonstrated to prevent relapses in unipolar depressive patients in the 6 months to 1 year following ECT (Coppen et al. 1981). Some patients with delusional depression require combined antipsychotic and anti-depressant continuation drug therapy after ECT. It is our practice to maintain patients on therapeutic levels of antidepressants for at least 6 months following a course of ECT, whereafter we gradually taper the antidepressants over a period of 4 to 8 weeks. We believe that mainte-nance ECT is highly valuable for certain patients with chronic affective disorder that does not respond to medications and other treatments.

☐ Risks

In general, ECT is an unusually safe procedure, with morbidity and mor-tality not significantly more than that associated with general anesthesia itself. The mortality rate of patients with ECT is 2 per 100,000 treatments (Fink 1978). The most frequent complaints of patients are memory im-pairment, headaches, and muscle aches (Gomez 1975), while the most significant risks associated with ECT are cardiovascular and intracerebral (Abrams 1992).

Ictal and postictal fluctuations in autonomic tone can elicit cardiac arrhythmias of many varieties, including premature ventricular contrac-tions during the immediate postictal period. Increase in vagal tone may result in sinus bradycardia or sinus arrest, while increases in sympathetic tone can elicit ventricular ectopy and increases in blood pressure and heart rate (Abrams 1992). In order to evaluate the safety of ECT in the cardiovascular realm, Dec et al. (1985) assessed serial ECGs and serum cardiac enzyme values of 29 patients who received ECT. The investiga-tors could not find persistent electrocardiographic changes, elevations in creatinine phosphokinase, or elevations in SGOT levels following 85 treatments in these patients. It is important that 24% of those patients sampled had stable, preexisting cardiovascular disease, which included conduction system disease, recent myocardial infarction, and depressed ventricular function. The authors concluded that with careful cardiac monitoring before and after the procedure, with frequent checks of elec-trolyte values, and with careful tailoring of the anesthetic regimen to the individual patient, cardiovascular morbidity and mortality can be mini-mized, even for patients with known cardiovascular disease. Patients with prexisting disorders that increase intracranial pressure, such as space-occupying brain lesions, or with other CNS dysfunctions, or pa-tients with hypertension, degenerative bone disease, or severe cardiac disease, are at increased risk for serious side effects related to ECT.

☐ Side Effects

For each treatment, there is an initial confusional period that lasts for approximately 30 minutes. Memory impairment that occurs with ECT is highly variable. Whereas certain patients report no problems with their memory, others report that their memory "is not as good as it used to be" before receiving ECT (Squire and Slater 1983). When memory of patients receiving ECT is carefully studied, it has been found that patients who experience retrograde amnesia (i.e., diminished ability to recall information that was recently learned before ECT was administered) following bilateral ECT seem to have recovered complete memory functions by 6 months after treatment, with little evidence that new learning ability is still deficient at that time (Squire et al. 1975). In those patients who do have memory impairment following bilateral ECT, information acquired during the days and weeks prior to, during, and for several weeks following ECT may be permanently lost. The use of brief pulse stimulation, instead of sine wave stimulation, can reduce the memory impairment still further (Squire et al. 1975). Unilateral stimulation results in fewer cognitive problems, although its efficacy also may be less (Sackheim et al. 1993). Other cognitive deficits include memory deficits for nonverbal information and transient disorientation.

■ REFERENCES

Antipsychotic Drugs

Adler LA, Angrist B, Peselow E, et al: Efficacy of propranolol in neuroleptic-induced akathisia. J Clin Psychopharmacol 5:164–166, 1985

Adler LA, Angrist B, Reiter S, et al: Neuroleptic-induced akathisia: a review. Psychopharmacology (Berl) 97:1–11, 1989

Alvir JMJ, Lieberman JA, Safferman AZ: Clozapine-induced agranulocytosis: incidence and risk factors in the United States. N Engl J Med 329:162–167, 1993

American Psychiatric Association: Tardive Dyskinesia: A Task Force Report of the American Psychiatric Association. Washington, DC, American Psychiatric Association, 1992

Balon R, Berchou R: Hematologic side effects of psychotropic drugs. Psychosomatics 27:119–127, 1986

Chouinard G, Jones BD, Remington G, et al: A Canadian multicenter, placebo-controlled study of fixed doses of resiperidone and haloperidol in the treatment of chronic schizophrenic patients. J Clin Psychopharmacol 13:25–40, 1993

Correa N, Opler LA, Kay SR, et al: Amantadine in the treatment of neuroendocrine side effects of neuroleptics. J Clin Psychopharmacol 7:91–95, 1987

Davis JM: Comparative doses and costs of antipsychotic medication. Arch Gen Psychiatry 33:858–861, 1976

Davis JM: Maintenance therapy and the natural course of schizophrenia. J Clin Psychiatry 46 (No 11, Sec 2):18–21, 1985

Davis JM, Andriukaitis S: The natural course of schizophrenia and effective maintenance drug treatment. J Clin Psychopharmacol 6:2S–10S, 1986

Devinsky O, Honigfeld G, Patin J: Clozapine-related seizures. Neurology 41:369–371, 1991

Edlund MJ, Craig TJ: Antipsychotic drug use and birth defects: an epidemiologic reassessment. Compr Psychiatry 25:32–37, 1984

Elkashef AM, Ruskin PE, Bacher N, et al: Vitamin E in the treatment of tardive dyskinesia. Am J Psychiatry 147:505–506, 1990

Fahn S: A therapeutic approach to tardive dyskinesia. J Clin Psychiatry 46 (No 4, Sec 2):19–24, 1985

Feinberg SS, Kay SR, Elijovich LR, et al: Pimozide treatment of the negative schizophrenic syndrome: a open trial. J Clin Psychiatry 49:235–238, 1988

Gardos G, Cole JO: Weight reduction in schizophrenia by molindone. Am J Psychiatry 134:302–304, 1977

Ghadirian AM, Chouinard G, Annable L: Sexual dysfunction and plasma prolactin levels in neuroleptic-treated schizophrenic outpatients. J Nerv Ment Dis 170:463–467, 1982

Glazer WM, Moore DC, Schooler NR, et al: Tardive dyskinesia: a discontinuation study. Arch Gen Psychiatry 41:623–627, 1984

Gunderson JG: Pharmacotherapy for patients with borderline personality disorder. Arch Gen Psychiatry 43:698–700, 1986

Haller E, Binder RL: Clozapine and seizures. Am J Psychiatry 147:1069–1071, 1990

Hogarty GE, Anderson DM, Reiss DJ, et al: Family psychoeducation, social skills training, and maintenance chemotherapy in the aftercare treatment of schizophrenia: one-year effects of a controlled study on relapse and expressed emotion. Arch Gen Psychiatry 43:633–642, 1986

Johnson DAW: Antipsychotic medication: clinical guidelines for maintenance therapy. J Clin Psychiatry 46 (No 5, Sec 2):6–15, 1985

Kane JM, Smith JM: Tardive dyskinesia: prevalence and risk factors, 1959 to 1979. Arch Gen Psychiatry 39:473–481, 1982

Kane JM, Rifkin A, Woerner M, et al: Low-dose neuroleptic treatment of outpatient schizophrenics, I: preliminary results for relapse rates. Arch Gen Psychiatry 40:893–896, 1983

Kane J, Honigfeld G, Singer J, et al: Clozapine for the treatment-resistant schizophrenic: a double-blind comparison vs chlorpromazine/benztropine. Arch Gen Psychiatry 45:789–796, 1988

Kennedy PF, Hershon HI, McGuire RJ: Extrapyramidal disorders after prolonged phenothiazine therapy. Br J Psychiatry 118:509–518, 1971

Levenson JL: Neuroleptic malignant syndrome. Am J Psychiatry 142:1137–1145, 1985

Lieberman JA, Johns CA, Kane JM, et al: Clozapine-induced agranulocytosis: non-cross-reactivity with other psychotropic drugs. J Clin Psychiatry 49:271–277, 1988

Lieberman JA, Saltz BL, Johns CA, et al: The effects of clozapine on tardive dyskinesia. Br J Psychiatry 158:503–510, 1991

MacKinnon R, Yudofsky SC: Principles of Psychiatric Evaluation. Philadelphia, PA, JB Lippincott, 1991

Mann SC, Roger WP: Psychotropic drugs, summer heat and humidity, and hyperpyrexia: a danger restated. Am J Psychiatry 135:1097–1100, 1978

Marder SR, Van Putten T, Mintz J, et al: Costs and benefits of two doses of fluphenazine. Arch Gen Psychiatry 41:1025–1029, 1984

McDougle CJ, Goodman WK, Price LH, et al: Neuroleptic addition in fluvoxamine-refractory obsessive-compulsive disorder. Am J Psychiatry 147:652–654, 1990

McElroy SL, Dessain EC, Pope HG Jr, et al: Clozapine in the treatment of psychotic mood disorders, schizoaffective disorder, and schizophrenia. J Clin Psychiatry 52:411–414, 1991

McEvoy JP, Stiller RL, Farr R: Plasma haloperidol levels drawn at neuroleptic threshold doses: a pilot study. J Clin Psychopharmacol 6:133–138, 1986

Meltzer HY: The role of serotonin in the action of atypical antipsychotic drugs. Psychiatric Annals 20:571–579, 1990

Miller DD: Effect of phenytoin on plasma clozapine concentrations in two patients. J Clin Psychiatry 52:23–25, 1991

Miller DD, Sharafuddin MJA, Kathol RG: A case of clozapine-induced neuroleptic malignant syndrome. J Clin Psychiatry 52:99–101, 1991

Munetz MR, Roth LH: Informing patients about tardive dyskinesia. Arch Gen Psychiatry 42:866–871, 1985

National Institute of Mental Health, Psychopharmacology Service Center Collaborative Study Group: Phenothiazine treatment in acute schizophrenia. Arch Gen Psychiatry 10:246–261, 1964

Neborsky R, Janowsky D, Munson E, et al: Rapid treatment of acute psychotic symptoms with high- and low-dose haloperidol. Arch Gen Psychiatry 38:195–199, 1981

Oliver AP, Luchins DJ, Wyatt RJ: Neuroleptic-induced seizures: an in vitro technique for assessing relative risk. Arch Gen Psychiatry 39:206–209, 1982

Opler LA, Feinberg SS: The role of pimozide in clinical psychiatry: a review. J Clin Psychiatry 52:221–233, 1991

Ostergaard K, Dupont E: Clozapine treatment of drug-induced psychotic symptoms in late stages of Parkinson's disease (letter). Acta Neurol Scand 78:349–350, 1988

Pope HG Jr, Keck PE Jr, McElroy SL: Frequency and presentation of neuroleptic malignant syndrome in a large psychiatric hospital. Am J Psychiatry 143:1227–1233, 1986

Prien RF, Caffey EM Jr, Klett CJ: Comparison of lithium carbonate and chlorpromazine in the treatment of mania: report of the Veterans Administration and National Institute of Mental Health Collaborative Study Group. Arch Gen Psychiatry 26:146–153, 1972

Reiter S, Adler L, Angrist B, et al: Atenolol and propranolol in neuroleptic-induced akathisia (letter). J Clin Psychopharmacol 7:279–280, 1987

Richelson E: Neuroleptic affinities for human brain receptors and their use in predicting adverse effects. J Clin Psychiatry 45:331–336, 1984

Rifkin A, Quitkin F, Klein DF: Akinesia: a poorly recognized drug-induced extrapyramidal behavioral disorder. Arch Gen Psychiatry 32:672–674, 1975

Rosebush PI, Stewart T, Mazurek MF: The treatment of neuroleptic malignant syndrome: are dantrolene and bromocriptine useful adjuncts to supportive care? Br J Psychiatry 159:709–712, 1991

Schooler NR: The efficacy of antipsychotic drugs and family therapies in the maintenance treatment of schizophrenia. J Clin Psychopharmacol 6:11S–19S, 1986

Shader RI: Sexual dysfunction associated with thioridazine hydrochloride. JAMA 188:1007–1009, 1964

Shapiro AK, Shapiro E, Eisenkraft GJ: Treatment of Gilles de la Tourette syndrome with pimozide. Am J Psychiatry 140:1183–1186, 1983

Antidepressant Drugs

American Psychiatric Association, Task Force on the Use of Laboratory Tests in Psychiatry: Tricyclic antidepressants—blood level measurements and clinical outcome: an APA Task Force report. Am J Psychiatry 142:155–162, 1985

American Psychiatric Association: Diagnostic and Statistical Manual of Mental Disorders, 3rd Edition, Revised. Washington, DC, American Psychiatric Association, 1987

Brosen K, Otton S, Gram L: Imipramine demethylation and hydroxylation: impact on the sporteine oxidation phenotype. Clin Pharmacol Ther 40:543–549, 1986

Brosen K, Gram L, Sihdruy S, et al: Pharmacogenetics of tricyclic antidepressants and novel antidepressants: recent developments. Clin Neuropharmacol 15 (suppl 1):80A–81A, 1992

Clomipramine Collaborative Study Group: Clomipramine in the treatment of patients with obsessive-compulsive disorder. Arch Gen Psychiatry 48:730–738, 1991

Consensus Development: Mood disorders: pharmacologic prevention of recurrence. Am J Psychiatry 142:469–476, 1985

Conte HR, Plutchik R, Wild KV, et al: Combined psychotherapy and pharmacotherapy for depression: a systematic analysis of the evidence. Arch Gen Psychiatry 43:471–479, 1986

Crane GE: Iproniazid (Marsilid) phosphate, a therapeutic agent for mental disorders and debilitating disease. J Psychiatr Res 8:142–152, 1957

daMotta T, Cordas TA: Autoinduction of hypertensive reactions by tranylcypromine. J Clin Psychopharmacol 10:232, 1990

Dilsaver SC, Kronfol Z, Sackellares JC, et al: Antidepressant withdrawal syndromes: evidence supporting the cholinergic overdrive hypothesis. J Clin Psychopharmacol 3:157–164, 1983

DiMascio A, Weissman MM, Prusoff BA, et al: Differential symptom reduction by drugs and psychotherapy in acute depression. Arch Gen Psychiatry 36:1450–1456, 1979

Downs JM, Downs AD, Rosenthal TL, et al: Increased plasma tricyclic antidepressant concentrations in two patients currently treated with fluoxetine. J Clin Psychiatry 50:226–227, 1989

Fava M, Rosenbaum JF: Suicidality and fluoxetine: is there a relationship? J Clin Psychiatry 52:108–111, 1992

Feder R: Bradycardia and syncope induced by fluoxetine. J Clin Psychiatry 52:139, 1991

Feighner JP, Herbstein J, Damlour N: Combined MAOI, TCA, and direct stimulant therapy of treatment-resistant depression. J Clin Psychiatry 46:206–209, 1985

Feighner JP, Pambakian R, Fowler RC, et al: A comparison of nefazodone, imipramine, and placebo in patients with moderate to severe depression. Psychopharmacol Bull 25:219–221, 1989

Ferguson JM: Fluoxetine-induced weight loss in overweight, nondepressed subjects (letter). Am J Psychiatry 143:1496, 1986

Fernstrom MH, Krowinski RL, Kupfer DJ: Chronic imipramine treatment and weight gain. Psychiatry Res 17:269–273, 1986

Frank E, Kupfer DJ, Perel JM, et al: Three-year outcomes for maintenance therapies in recurrent depression. Arch Gen Psychiatry 47:1093–1099, 1990

Gardner EA, Johnston JA: Bupropion: an antidepressant without sexual pathophysiological action. J Clin Psychopharmacol 5:24–29, 1985

Giardina EGV, Johnson LL, Vita J, et al: Effect of imipramine and nortriptyline on left ventricular function and blood pressure in patients treated with arrhythmias. Am Heart J 109:992–998, 1985

Glassman AH, Bigger JT: Cardiovascular effects of therapeutic doses of tricyclic antidepressants: a review. Arch Gen Psychiatry 39:815–820, 1981

Glassman AH, Roose SP: Delusional depression: a distinct clinical entity? Arch Gen Psychiatry 38:424–427, 1981

Glassman AH, Bigger JT, Giardina EGV, et al: Clinical characteristics of imipramine-induced orthostatic hypotension. Lancet 1:468–472, 1979

Glassman AH, Johnson LL, Giardina EGV, et al: Psychotropic drug use in depressed patients with congestive heart failure. JAMA 250:1997–2001, 1983

Goldberg RJ, Capone RJ, Hunt JD: Cardiac complications following tricyclic antidepressant overdose: issues for monitoring policy. JAMA 254:1772–1775, 1985

Goldfrank LR, Lewin NA, Flomenbaum NE, et al: Antidepressants: tricyclics, tetracyclics, monoamine oxidase inhibitors, and others, in Goldfrank's Toxicologic Emergencies, 3rd Edition. Edited by Goldfrank LR, Flomenbaum ME, Lewis NA, et al. Norwalk, CT, Appleton-Century-Crofts, 1986, pp 351–363

Goldman LS, Alexander RD, Luchins DJ: Monoamine oxidase inhibitors and tricyclic antidepressants: comparison of their cardiovascular effects. J Clin Psychiatry 47:225–229, 1986

Goodman WK, Charney DS: Therapeutic applications and mechanisms of action of monoamine oxidase inhibitor and heterocyclic antidepressant drugs. J Clin Psychiatry 46(No 10, Suppl 2):6–22, 1985

Goodwin FK, Prange AJ, Post RM, et al: Potentiation of antidepressant effects by L-triiodothyronine in tricyclic nonresponders. Am J Psychiatry 139:34–38, 1982

Grimsley SR, Jann MW, Carter JG, et al: Increased carbamazepine plasma concentrations after fluoxetine coadministration. Clin Pharmacol Ther 50:10–15, 1991

Hamilton MS, Opler LA: Akathisia, suicidality, and fluoxetine. J Clin Psychiatry 53:401–406, 1992

Haykal RF, Akiskal HS: Bupropion as a promising approach to rapid-cycling bipolar II patients. J Clin Psychiatry 51:450–455, 1990

Hollander E, DeCaria CM, Franklin FR, et al: Fenfluramine augmentation of serotonin reuptake blockade antiobsessional treatment. J Clin Psychiatry 51:119–123, 1990

Hurowitz GI, Liebowitz MR: Antidepressant-induced rapid cycling: six case reports. J Clin Psychopharmacol 13:52–56, 1993

Jacobsen FM: Low-dose trazodone as a hypnotic in patients treated with MAOIs and other psychotropics: a pilot study. J Clin Psychiatry 51:298–302, 1990

Jankowsky D, Curtis G, Zisook S, et al: Trazodone-aggravated ventricular arrhythmias. J Clin Psychopharmacol 3:372–376, 1983

Jobe PC, Woods TW, Dailey JW: Proconvulsant and anticonvulsant effects of tricyclic antidepressants in genetically epilepsy-prone rats, in Advances in Epileptology: The XVth Epilepsy International Symposium. Edited by Porter RJ, Mattson RH, Ward AA Jr, et al. New York, Raven, 1984, pp 187–191

Joffe RT: Afternoon fatigue and somnolence associated with tranylcypromine treatment. J Clin Psychiatry 51:192–193, 1990

Khan A, Fabre LF, Rudolph R: Venlafaxine in depressed outpatients. Psychopharmacol Bull 27:141–144, 1991

Kline NS: Clinical experience with iproniazid (Marsilid). J Clin Exp Psychopathol 19 (suppl 1):72–78, 1958

Kronfol Z, Greden JF, Zis AP: Imipramine-induced tremor: effects of a beta-adrenergic blocking agent. J Clin Psychiatry 44:225–226, 1983

Kuhn R: The treatment of depressive states with G 22355 (imipramine hydrochloride). Am J Psychiatry 115: 459–464, 1958

Kupfer DJ, Frank E: Relapse in recurrent unipolar depression. Am J Psychiatry 144:86–88, 1987

Leander JD: Fluoxetine, a selective serotonin-uptake inhibitor, enhances the anticonvulsant effects of phenytoin, carbamazepine, and ameltolide (LY201116). Epilepsia 33:573–576, 1992

Liebowitz MR, Quitkin FM, Stewart JW, et al: Antidepressant specificity in atypical depression. Arch Gen Psychiatry 45:129–137, 1988

Lingam VR, Lazarus LW, Groves L, et al: Methylphenidate in treating post-stroke depression. J Clin Psychiatry 49:151–153, 1988

Lydiard RB: Tricyclic-resistant depression: treatment resistance or inadequate treatment? J Clin Psychiatry 46:412–417, 1985

MacKinnon R, Yudofsky SC: Principles of Psychiatric Evaluation. Philadelphia, PA, JB Lippincott, 1991

Marley E, Wozniak KM: Interactions of non-selective monoamine oxidase inhibitor, phenelzine, with inhibitors of 5-hydroxytryptamine, dopamine, or noradrenaline re-uptake inhibitors. J Psychiatr Res 18:191–203, 1984

McGrath PJ, Quitkin FM, Harrison W, et al: Treatment of melancholia with tranylcypromine. Am J Psychiatry 141:288–289, 1984

McGrath PJ, Stewart JW, Harrison WM: Predictive value of symptoms of atypical depression for differential drug treatment outcome. J Clin Psychopharmacol 12:197–202, 1992

Metz A, Shader RI: Adverse interactions encountered when using trazodone to treat insomnia associated with fluoxetine. Int Clin Psychopharmacol 5:191–194, 1990

Mitchell JE, Popkin JE: Antidepressant drug therapy and sexual dysfunction in men: a review. J Clin Psychopharmacol 3:76–79, 1983

Muth EA, Haskins JT, Moyer JA, et al: Antidepressant biochemical profile of the novel bicyclic compound WY-45,030, an ethyl cyclohexanol derivative. Biochem Pharmacol 35:4493–4497, 1986

Neil JF, Licata SM, May SJ, et al: Dietary noncompliance during treatment with tranylcypromine. J Clin Psychiatry 40:33–37, 1979

Nelson JC, Bowers MB: Delusional unipolar depression: description and drug response. Arch Gen Psychiatry 35:1321–1328, 1978

Nelson JC, Mazure CM: Lithium augmentation in psychotic depression refractory to combined drug treatment. Am J Psychiatry 143:363–366, 1986

Nelson JC, Mazure CM, Bowers MB: A preliminary, open study of the combination of fluoxetine and desipramine. Arch Gen Psychiatry 48:303–307, 1991

O'Rourke D, Wurtman JJ, Wurtman RJ, et al: Treatment of seasonal depression with D-fenfluramine. J Clin Psychiatry 50:343–347, 1989

Pande AC, Calarco MM, Grunhaus LJ: Combined MAOI-TCA treatment in refractory depression, in Refractory Depression. Edited by Amsterdam J. New York, Raven, 1991, pp 115–121

Preskorn S: Should bupropion dosage be adjusted based upon therapeutic drug monitoring? Psychopharmacol Bull 27:637–643, 1991

Preskorn SH, Burke M: Somatic therapy for major depressive disorder: selection of an antidepressant. J Clin Psychiatry 53 (No 9, Suppl):5–18, 1992

Preskorn SH, Fast GA: Therapeutic drug monitoring for antidepressants: efficacy, safety, and cost-effectiveness. J Clin Psychiatry 52 (No 6, Suppl):23–33, 1991

Price J, Grunhaus LJ: Treatment of clomipramine-inducedanorgasmia with yohimbine: a case report. J Clin Psychiatry 51:32–33, 1990

Prien RF, Kupfer DJ: Continuation drug therapy for major depression episodes: how long should it be maintained? Am J Psychiatry 143:18–23, 1986

Quitkin F, Rifkin A, Klein DF: Monoamine oxidase inhibitors: a review of antidepressant effectiveness. Arch Gen Psychiatry 35:749–760, 1979

Rabkin JG, Quitkin FM, McGrath P, et al: Adverse reactions to monoamine oxidase inhibitors, Part II: treatment correlates and clinical management. J Clin Psychopharmacol 5:2–9, 1985

Richelson E: Antimuscarinic and other receptor-blocking properties of antidepressants. Mayo Clin Proc 58:40–46, 1983

Roose SP, Glassman AH, Siris SG, et al: Comparison of imipramine- and nortriptyline-induced orthostatic hypotension: a meaningful difference. J Clin Psychopharmacol 1:316–319, 1981

Roose SP, Glassman AH, Walsh BT, et al: Depression, delusions, and suicide. Am J Psychiatry 140:1159–1162, 1983

Roose SP, Glassman AH, Giardina EGV, et al: Tricyclic antidepressants in depressed patients with cardiac conduction disease. Arch Gen Psychiatry 44:273–275, 1987

Roose SP, Dalack GW, Glassman AH, et al: Cardiovascular effects of bupropion in depressed patients with heart disease. Am J Psychiatry 148:512–516, 1991

Satel SL, Nelson JC: Stimulants in the treatment of depression: a critical overview. J Clin Psychiatry 50:241–249, 1989

Schenk CH, Remick RA: Sublingual nifedipine in the treatment of hypertensive crisis associated with monoamine oxidase inhibitors (letter). Ann Emerg Med 18:114–115, 1989

Scher M, Krieger JN, Juergens S: Trazodone and priapism. Am J Psychiatry 140:1362–1363, 1983

Schmauss M, Kapfhammer HP, Meyr P, et al: Combined MAO-inhibitor and tri-(tetra) cyclic antidepressant treatment in therapy resistant depression. Prog Neuropsychopharmacol Biol Psychiatry 12:523–532, 1988

Schweizer E, Weise C, Clary C, et al: Placebo-controlled trial of venlafaxine for the treatment of major depression. J Clin Psychopharmacol 11:233–236, 1991

Seagraves RT: Reversal by bethanecol of imipramine-induced ejaculatory dysfunction (letter). Am J Psychiatry 144:1243–1244, 1987

Seagraves RT: Overview of sexual dysfunction complicating the treatment of depression. J Clin Psychiatry Monogr 10(2):4–10, 1992

Selikoff IJ, Robitzek EH, Ornstein GG: Toxicity of hydrazine derivatives of isonicotinic acid in the chemotherapy of human tuberculosis. Quarterly Bulletin of SeaView Hospital 13(1):17–26, 1952

Sheehan DV, Welch JB, Fishman SM: A case of bupropion-induced seizure. J Nerv Ment Dis 174:496–498, 1986

Silver JM, Yudofsky SC, Kogan M, et al: Elevation of thioridazine plasma levels by propranolol. Am J Psychiatry 143:1290–1292, 1986

Spiker DG, Cofsky Weiss J, Dealy RS, et al: The pharmacologic treatment of delusional depression. Am J Psychiatry 142:430–436, 1985

Spivak B, Ravdan M, Shine M: Postural hypotension with syncope possibly precipitated by trazodone. Am J Psychiatry 144:1512–1513, 1987

Task Force on the Use of Laboratory Tests in Psychiatry: Tricyclic antidepressants—blood level measurements and clinical outcome: an APA Task Force Report. Am J Psychiatry 142:155–162, 1985

Teicher MH, Cohen BM, Baldessarini RJ, et al: Severe daytime somnolence in patients treated with an MAOI. Am J Psychiatry 145:1552–1556, 1988

Teicher MH, Glod C, Cole J: Emergence of intense suicidal preoccupation during fluoxetine treatment. Am J Psychiatry 52:294–299, 1990

Terman M, Terman JS, Quitkin FM, et al: Light therapy for seasonal affective disorder: a review of efficacy. Neuropsychopharmacology 2:1–22, 1989

Thase ME, Kupfer DJ, Frank E, et al: Treatment of imipramine-resistant depressant, II: an open clinical trial of lithium augmentation. J Clin Psychiatry 50:413–417, 1989

Thase ME, Carpenter L, Kupfer DJ, et al: Clinical significance of reversed vegetative subtypes of recurrent major depression. Psychopharmacol Bull 27:17–22, 1991

Thase ME, Frank E, Mallinger AG, et al: Treatment of imipramine-resistant recurrent depression, III: efficacy of monoamine oxidase inhibitors. J Clin Psychiatry 53:5–11, 1992

Tollefson GD: Monoamine oxidase inhibitors: a review. J Clin Psychiatry 44:280–288, 1983

Vaughan DA: interaction of fluoxetine with tricyclic antidepressants (letter). Am J Psychiatry 145:1478, 1988

Vitullo RN, Wharton JM, Allen NB, et al: Trazodone-related exercise-induced nonsustained ventricular tachycardia. Chest 98:247–248, 1990

Ward NG, Davidson RC: Gastric absorption of nifedipine (letter). J Clin Psychiatry 52:188, 1991

Wedin GP, Oderda GM, Klein-Schwartz W, et al: Relative toxicity of cyclic antidepressants. Ann Emerg Med 15:797–804, 1986

Wehr TA, Goodwin FK: Rapid cycling in manic-depressives induced by tricyclic antidepressants. Arch Gen Psychiatry 36:555–559, 1979

Wehr TA, Sack DA, Rosenthal NE, et al: Rapid-cycling affective disorder: contributing factors and treatment responses in 51 patients. Am J Psychiatry 145:179–184, 1988

Weise CC, Stein MK, Pereira-Ogan J, et al: Amitriptyline once daily versus three times daily in depressed outpatients. Arch Gen Psychiatry 37:555–560, 1980

Yager J: Bethanecol chloride can reverse erectile and ejaculatory dysfunction induced by tricyclic antidepressants and mazindol: case report. J Clin Psychiatry 47:210–211, 1986

Yudofsky SC: Electroconvulsive therapy in general hospital psychiatry: a focus of new indications and technologies. Gen Hosp Psychiatry 3:292–296, 1981

Yudofsky SC, Hales RE, Ferguson T: What You Need to Know About Psychiatric Drugs. New York, Grove Weidenfeld, 1991

Zajecka J, Fawcett J, Schaff M, et al: The role of serotonin in sexual dysfunction. J Clin Psychiatry 52:66–68, 1991

Zisook S: A clinical overview of monoamine oxidase inhibitors. Psychosomatics 26:240–246, 1985

Anxiolytics, Sedatives, and Hypnotics

Abernethy DR, Greenblatt DJ, Ochs HR, et al: Benzodiazepine drug-drug interactions commonly occurring in clinical practice. Curr Med Res Opin 8 (suppl 4):80–93, 1984

American Medical Association: Drug Evaluations, 6th Edition. Chicago, IL, American Medical Association, 1986

American Psychiatric Association: Benzodiazepine Dependence, Toxicity, and Abuse: A Task Force Report of the American Psychiatric Association. Washington, DC, American Psychiatric Association, 1990

Angus WR, Romney DM: The effect of diazepam on patients' memory. J Clin Psychopharmacol 4:203–206, 1984

Ansseau M, Doumont A, von Frenckell R, et al: A long-acting benzodiazepine is more effective in divided doses. N Engl J Med 310:526, 1984

Brantigan CO, Brantigan TA, Joseph N: Effect of beta blockade and beta stimulation on stage fright. Am J Med 72:88–94, 1982

Breier A, Charney DS, Heninger GR: Agoraphobia with panic attacks: development, diagnostic stability, and course of illness. Arch Gen Psychiatry 43:1029–1036, 1986

Busto U, Sellers EM, Naranjo CA, et al: Withdrawal reactions after long-term therapeutic use of benzodiazepines. N Engl J Med 315:854–857, 1986

Charney DS, Woods SW: Benzodiazepine treatment of panic disorder: a comparison of alprazolam and lorazepam. J Clin Psychiatry 50:418–423, 1989

Chouinard G, Goodman W, Greist J, et al: Obsessive-compulsive disorder—treatment with sertraline: a multi-center study. Psychopharmacol Bull 26:279–284, 1990

Clomipramine Collaborative Study Group: Clomipramine in the treatment of patients with obsessive-compulsive disorder. Arch Gen Psychiatry 48:730–738, 1991

Cohn J, Wilcox CS: Low-sedation potential of buspirone compared with alprazolam and lorazepam in the treatment of anxious patients: a double-blind study. J Clin Psychiatry 47:409–412, 1986

Cole JO, Orzak MG, Beake B, et al: Assessment of the abuse liability of buspirone in recreational sedative users. J Clin Psychiatry 43:69–74, 1982

Davidson JRT, Ford SM, Smith RD, et al: Long-term treatment of social phobia with clonazepam. J Clin Psychiatry 52 (No 11, Suppl):16–20, 1991

Dixon J, Power SJ, Grundy EM, et al: Sedation for local anaesthesia: comparison of intravenous midazolam and diazepam. Anaesthesia 39:372–378, 1984

Drew PJ, Barnes JN, Evans SJ: The effect of acute beta-adrenoceptor blockade on examination performance. Br J Clin Pharmacol 19:783–786, 1985

Dunner DL, Ishiki D, Avery DH, et al: Effect of alprazolam and diazepam on anxiety and panic attacks in panic disorder: a controlled study. J Clin Psychiatry 47:458–460, 1986

Elie R, Lamontagne Y: Alprazolam and diazepam in the treatment of generalized anxiety. J Clin Psychopharmacol 4:125–129, 1985

Ellinwood EH Jr, Heatherly DG, Nikaido MA, et al: Comparative pharmacokinetics and pharmacodynamics of lorazepam, alprazolam and diazepam. Psychopharmacology (Berl) 86:393–451, 1985

Finkle BS, McCloskey KL, Goodman LS: Diazepam and drug-associated deaths: a survey in the United States and Canada. JAMA 242:429–434, 1979

Flament MF, Rapaport JL, Berg CJ, et al: Clomipramine treatment of childhood obsessive-compulsive disorder: a double-blind controlled study. Arch Gen Psychiatry 42:977–983, 1985

Fyer AJ, Liebowitz JR, Gorman JM, et al: Discontinuation of alprazolam treatment in panic patients. Am J Psychiatry 144:303–308, 1987

Gastfried DR, Rosenbaum JF: Adjunctive buspirone in benzodiazepine treatment of four patients with panic disorder. Am J Psychiatry 146:914–916, 1989

Gelernter CS, Uhde TW, Cimbolic P, et al: Cognitive-behavioral and pharmacologic treatments for social phobia: a preliminary study. Arch Gen Psychiatry 48:938–945, 1991

Goldberg HL, Finnerty RJ: The comparative efficacy of buspirone and diazepam in the treatment of anxiety. Am J Psychiatry 136:1184–1187, 1979

Goodman WK, Price LH, Delgado PL, et al: Specificity of serotonin reuptake inhibitors in the treatment of obsessive-compulsive disorder: comparison of fluvoxamine and desipramine. Arch Gen Psychiatry 47:577–585, 1990

Goodman WK, McDougle CJ, Price LH: Pharmacotherapy of obsessive-compulsive disorder. J Clin Psychiatry 53 (No 4, Suppl):29–37, 1992

Gorman JM, Liebowitz MR, Fyer AJ, et al: Treatment of social phobia with atenolol. J Clin Psychopharmacol 5:298–301, 1985

Greenblatt DJ: Pharmacology of benzodiazepine hypnotics. J Clin Psychiatry 53 (No 6, Suppl):7–13, 1992

Greenblatt DJ, Shader RI: Pharmacokinetics in Clinical Practice. Philadelphia, PA, WB Saunders, 1985

Greenblatt DJ, Allen MD, Noel BJ, et al: Acute overdosage with benzodiazepine derivatives. Clin Pharmacol Ther 21:497–514, 1977a

Greenblatt DJ, Allen MD, Shader RI: Toxicity of high dose flurazepam in the elderly. Clin Pharmacol Ther 21:355–361, 1977b

Greenblatt DJ, Shader RI, Divol M, et al: Adverse reactions to triazolam, flurazepam, and placebo in controlled clinical trials. J Clin Psychiatry 45:192–195, 1984

Herman JB, Rosenbaum JF, Brotman AW: The alprazolam to clonazepam switch for the treatment of panic disorder. J Clin Psychopharmacol 7:175–178, 1987

Hertley LR, Ungapen S, Davie I, et al: The effect of beta-adrenergic blocking drugs on speakers' performance and memory. Br J Psychiatry 142:512–517, 1983

Hewlett WA, Vinogradov S, Agras WS: Clonazepam treatment of obsessions and compulsions. J Clin Psychiatry 51:158–161, 1990

Hoehn-Saric R, McLeod DR, Zimmerli WD: Differential effects of alprazolam and imipramine in generalized anxiety disorder: somatic vs psychic symptoms. J Clin Psychiatry 49:293–301, 1988

Hollander E, DeCaria CM, Schneier FR, et al: Fenfluramine augmentation of serotonin reuptake blockade antiobsessional treatment. J Clin Psychiatry 51:119–123, 1990

Jack ML, Colburn WA, Spirt NM, et al: A pharmacokinetic/pharmacodynamic/receptor binding model to predict the onset and duration of pharmacological activity of the benzodiazepines. Prog Neuropsychopharmacol Biol Psychiatry 7:629–635, 1982

Jenike MA: Approaches to the patient with treatment-refractory obsessive-compulsive disorder. J Clin Psychiatry 51 (No 2, Suppl):15–21, 1990

Jenike MA, Baer L, Summergrad P, et al: Sertraline in obsessive-compulsive disorder: a double-blind comparison with placebo. Am J Psychiatry 147:923–938, 1990

Jenike MA, Baer L, Buttolph L: Buspirone augmentation of fluoxetine in patients with obsessive-compulsive disorder. J Clin Psychopharmacol 12:13–14, 1991

Jonas JM, Coleman BS, Sheridan AQ, et al: Comparative clinical profiles of triazolam versus other short-acting hypnotics. J Clin Psychiatry 53 (No 12, Suppl):19–31, 1992

Kahn RJ, Menair D, Lipman RS, et al: Imipramine and chlordiazepoxide in depressive and anxiety disorders: efficacy in anxious outpatients. Arch Gen Psychiatry 43:79–85, 1986

Klein DF, Fink M: Psychiatric reaction patterns to imipramine. Am J Psychiatry 119:432–438, 1962

Lader M, Olajide D: A comparison of buspirone and placebo in relieving benzodiazepine withdrawal symptoms. J Clin Psychopharmacol 7:11–15, 1987

Liebowitz MR, Gorman JM, Fyer AJ, et al: Social phobia: a review of a neglected anxiety disorder. Arch Gen Psychiatry 42:729–736, 1985

Liebowitz MA, Gorman JM, Fyer AJ, et al: Pharmacotherapy of social phobia: an interim report of a placebo-controlled comparison of phenelzine and atenolol. J Clin Psychiatry 49:252–257, 1988

Liebowitz MR, Hollander E, Schneier F, et al: Fluoxetine treatment of obsessive-compulsive disorder: an open clinical trial. J Clin Psychopharmacol 9:423–427, 1989

Liebowitz MR, Schneier FR, Hollander E: Treatment of social phobia with drugs other than benzodiazepines. J Clin Psychiatry 52 (No 11, Suppl):10–15, 1991

Lucki I: Behavioral studies of serotonin receptor antagonists as antidepressant drugs. J Clin Psychiatry 52 (No 12, Suppl):24–31, 1991

Lucki I, Rickels K, Geller AM: Chronic use of benzodiazepines and psychomotor and cognitive test performance. Psychopharmacology (Berl) 88:426–433, 1986

Mac DS, Kumar R, Goodwin DW: Anterograde amnesia with oral lorazepam. J Clin Psychiatry 46:137–138, 1985

McDougle CJ, Goodman WK, Price LH, et al: Neuroleptic addition in fluvoxamine-refractory obsessive-compulsive disorder. Am J Psychiatry 147:652–654, 1990

Medawarn C, Rassaby E: Triazolam overdose, alcohol, and manslaughter. Lancet 338:1515–1516, 1991

Moskowitz H, Smiley A: Effects of chronically administered buspirone and diazepam on driving-related skills and performance. J Clin Psychiatry 43:45–55, 1982

NIMH [National Institute of Mental Health] Consensus Development Conference: Drugs and insomnia: the use of medication to promote sleep. JAMA 251:2410–2414, 1984

Noyes R Jr, Garvey MJ, Cook BL, et al: Benzodiazepine withdrawal: a review of evidence. J Clin Psychiatry 49:382–389, 1988

Palminteri R, Narbonne G: Safety profile of zolpidem, in Imidazopyridines in Sleep Disorders. Edited by Sauvanet JP, Lange SZ, Morselli PL. New York, Raven, 1988, pp 351–361

Patterson JF: Alprazolam dependency: use of clonazepam for withdrawal. South Med J 81:830–831, 1988

Pigott TA, Pato MT, Bernstein SE, et al: Controlled comparisons of clomipramine and fluoxetine in the treatment of obsessive-compulsive disorders: behavioral and biological results. Arch Gen Psychiatry 47:926–932, 1990

Rakel RE: Long-term buspirone therapy for chronic anxiety: a multicenter international study to determine safety. South Med J 83:194–198, 1990

Regestein QR, Reich P: Agitation observed during treatment with newer hypnotic drugs. J Clin Psychiatry 46:280–283, 1985

Reitan JA, Porter W, Braunstein M: Comparison of psychomotor skills and amnesia after induction of anesthesia with midazolam or thiopental. Anesth Analg 65:933–937, 1986

Rickels K, Case WG, Downing RW, et al: Long-term diazepam therapy and clinical outcome. JAMA 250:767–771, 1983

Rickels K, Schweizer E, Csanelosi I, et al: Long-term treatment of anxiety and risk of withdrawal: prospective comparison of clonazepam and buspirone. Arch Gen Psychiatry 45:444–450, 1988

Rosenberg L, Mitchell AA, Parsells JL, et al: Lack of relation of oral clefts to diazepam use during pregnancy. N Engl J Med 309:1282–1285, 1983

Roth T, Roehrs TA: Issues in the use of benzodiazepine therapy. J Clin Psychiatry 53 (No 6, Suppl):14–18, 1992

Rothschild AJ: Disinhibition, amnestic reactions, and other adverse reactions secondary to triazolam: a review of the literature. J Clin Psychiatry 53 (No 12, Suppl):69–79, 1992

Ruegg EG, Evans DL, Comer WS, et al: Lithium plus fluoxetine treatment of obsessive compulsive disorder, in New Research Program and Abstracts of the 143rd Annual Meeting of the American Psychiatry Association, May 1990; New York, NY, NR92

Salzman C, Shader RI, Greenblatt DJ, et al: Long vs short half-life benzodiazepines in the elderly: kinetics and clinical effects of diazepam and oxazepam. Arch Gen Psychiatry 40:293–297, 1983

Sauvanet JP, Maarek L, Roger M, et al: Open long-term trials with zolpidem in insomnia, in Imidazopyridines in Sleep Disorders. Edited by Sauvanet JP, Lange SZ, Morselli PL. New York, Raven, 1988, pp 339–349

Schneier FR, Liebowitz MR, Davies SO, et al: Fluoxetine in panic disorder. J Clin Psychopharmacol 10:119–121, 1990

Schneier FR, Saoud JB, Campeas RC, et al: Buspirone in social phobia. J Clin Psychopharmacol 13:251–256, 1992

Seidel WF, Cohen SA, Bliwise NG, et al: Buspirone: an anxiolytic without sedative effect. Psychopharmacology (Berl) 87:371–373, 1985

Sellers EM, Schneiderman JF, Romach MK, et al: Comparative drug effects and abuse liability of lorazepam, buspirone, and secobarbital in nondependent subjects. J Clin Psychopharmacol 12:79–85, 1992

Sheehan DV, Ballenger J, Jacobsen G: Treatment of endogenous anxiety with phobic, hysterical, and hypochondriacal symptoms. Arch Gen Psychiatry 39:51–59, 1980

Sheehan DV, Raj AB, Sheehan KH, et al: Is buspirone effective for panic disorder? J Clin Psychopharmacol 10:3–11, 1990

Spier SA, Tesar GE, Rosenbaum JF, et al: Treatment of panic disorder and agoraphobia with clonazepam. J Clin Psychiatry 47:238–242, 1986

Sternbach H: Fluoxetine treatment of social phobia. J Clin Psychopharmacol 10:230–231, 1990

Stroebel CF, Szarek BL, Glueck BC: Use of clomipramine in treatment of obsessive-compulsive symptomatology. J Clin Psychopharmacol 4:98–100, 1984

Tesar GE: High-potency benzodiazepines for short-term management of panic disorder: the U.S. evidence. J Clin Psychiatry 15 (No 5, Suppl):4–10, 1990

Tesar GE, Rosenbaum JF, Pollack MH, et al: Double-blind, placebo-controlled comparison of clonazepam and alprazolam for panic disorder. J Clin Psychiatry 52:69–76, 1991

Tyrer PJ, Lader MH: Response to propranolol and diazepam in somatic anxiety. BMJ 2:14–16, 1984

Tyrer PJ, Owen R, Dawling S: Gradual withdrawal of diazepam after long-term therapy. Lancet 1:1402–1406, 1983

Uhde TW, Tancer ME, Black B, et al: Phenomenology and neurobiology of social phobia: comparison with panic disorder. J Clin Psychiatry 52 (No 11, Suppl):31–40, 1991

Van Ameringen M, Mancini C, Streiner DL: Fluoxetine efficacy in social phobia. J Clin Psychiatry 54:27–32, 1993

Votey SR, Bosse GM, Bayer MJ, et al: Flumazenil: a new benzodiazepine antagonist. Ann Emerg Med 20:181–188, 1991

Walsh JK, Engelhardt CL: Trends in the pharmacologic treatment of insomnia. J Clin Psychiatry 53 (No 12, Suppl):10–17, 1992

Wamsley JK, Hunt MA: Relative affinity of quazepam for type-1 benzodiazepine receptors in brain. J Clin Psychiatry 52 (No 9, Suppl):15–20, 1991

Wheadon DE: Placebo controlled multi-center trial of fluoxetine in OCD. Paper presented at the Fifth World Congress of Biological Psychiatry, Florence, Italy, June 1991

Wysowski DK, Baum C: Outpatient use of prescription sedative-hypnotic drugs in the United States, 1970 through 1989. Arch Intern Med 151:1779–1783, 1991

Yudofsky SC, Silver JM: Beta-blockers in the treatment of performance anxiety. Harvard Mental Health Letter 4(5):8, 1987

Zipursky RB, Baker RW, Zimmer B: Alprazolam withdrawal delirium unresponsive to diazepam: case report. J Clin Psychiatry 46:344–345, 1985

Zitrin CM, Klein DF, Woerner MG, et al: Treatment of phobias: comparison of imipramine and placebo. Arch Gen Psychiatry 40:125–138, 1983

Antimanic Drugs

Akiskal HS, Khani MK, Scott-Strauss A: Cyclothymic temperamental disorders. Psychiatr Clin North Am 2:527–554, 1979

Arana GW, Epstein S, Molloy M, et al: Carbamazepine-induced reduction of plasma alprazolam concentrations: a clinical case report. J Clin Psychiatry 49:448–449, 1988

Baastrup PC, Schou M: Lithium as a prophylactic agent: its effect against recurrent depressions and manic-depressive psychosis. Arch Gen Psychiatry 16:162–172, 1967

Ballenger JC, Post RM: Carbamazepine in manic-depressive illness: a new treatment. Am J Psychiatry 137:782–790, 1980

Battle DC, von Riotte AB, Gaviria M, et al: Amelioration of polyuria by amiloride in patients receiving long-term lithium therapy. N Engl J Med 312:408–414, 1985

Bauer MS, Whybrow PC: Rapid cycling bipolar disorder, II: treatment of refractory cycling with high-dose levothyroxine: a preliminary study. Arch Gen Psychiatry 47:435–440, 1989

Bauer MS, Whybrow PC, Winokur A: Rapid cycling bipolar affective disorder, I: association with grade I hypothyroidism. Arch Gen Psychiatry 47:427–432, 1989

Baxter LR Jr, Liston EH, Schwartz JM, et al: Prolongation of the antidepressant response to partial sleep deprivation by lithium. Psychiatry Res 19:17–23, 1986

Bentsen KD, Gram L, Veje A: Serum thyroid hormones and blood folic acid during monotherapy with carbamazepine or valproate: a controlled study. Acta Neurol Scand 67:235–241, 1983

Bertollini R, Kallen B, Mastroiacovo P, et al: Anticonvulsant drugs in monotherapy: effect on the fetus. Eur J Epidemiol 3:164–171, 1987

Billings PR: Amiloride in the treatment of lithium-induced diabetes insipidus (letter). N Engl J Med 312:1575–1576, 1985

Bone S, Roose SP, Dunner DL, et al: Incidence of side effects in patients on long-term lithium therapy. Am J Psychiatry 137:103–104, 1980

Bowen RC, Grof P, Grof E: Less frequent lithium administration and lower urine volume. Am J Psychiatry 148:189–192, 1991

Brewerton TD: Lithium counteracts carbamazepine-induced leukopenia while increasing its therapeutic effect. Biol Psychiatry 21:677–685, 1986

Brodie MJ, MacPhee GJ: Carbamazepine neurotoxicity precipitated by diltiazem. BMJ 292:1170–1171, 1986

Brotman AW, Fahardi AM, Gelenberg AJ: Verapamil treatment of acute mania. J Clin Psychiatry 47:136–138, 1986

Calabrese JR, Gulledge AD, Hahn K, et al: Autoimmune thyroiditis in manic-depressive patients treated with lithium. Am J Psychiatry 142:1318–1321, 1985

Calabrese JR, Markowitz PJ, Kimmel SE, et al: Spectrum of efficacy of valproate in 78 rapid-cycling bipolar patients. J Clin Psychopharmacol 12:53S–56S, 1992

Camarasa JG: Patch test diagnosis of exfoliative dermatitis due to carbamazepine. Contact Dermatitis 12:49, 1985

Cho JT, Bone S, Dunner DL, et al: The effects of lithium treatment on thyroid function in patients with primary affective disorder. Am J Psychiatry 136:115–116, 1979

Clark JE, Covanis A, Gupta AK, et al: Unwanted effects of sodium valproate in children and adolescents, in The Place of Sodium Valproate in the Treatment of Epilepsy. Edited by Personage MJ, Caldwell ADS. London, Royal Society of Medicine, 1980, pp 223–233

Cohen WJ, Cohen NH: Lithium carbonate, haloperidol and irreversible brain damage. JAMA 230:1283–1287, 1974

Consensus Conference: Electroconvulsant therapy. JAMA 254:2103–2108, 1985

Consensus Development Panel: Mood disorders: pharmacologic prevention of recurrences. Am J Psychiatry 142:469–476, 1985

Cook BL, Smith RE, Perry PJ, et al: Theophylline-lithium interactions. J Clin Psychiatry 46:278–279, 1985

Coopen A, Abou-Saleh MT, Miller P, et al: Lithium continuation therapy following electroconvulsive therapy. Br J Psychiatry 139:284–287, 1981

Coulam CB, Annegers JF: Do anticonvulsants reduce the efficacy of oral contraceptives? Epilepsia 20:519–525, 1979

Cowdry T, Wehr T, Zis A, et al: Thyroid abnormalities associated with rapid-cycling bipolar illness. Arch Gen Psychiatry 40:414–420, 1983

Dean JC, Penry JK: Valproate, in The Medical Treatment of Epilepsy. Edited by Resor SR, Kutt H. New York, Marcel Dekker, 1992, pp 265–278

Deandrea D, Walker N, Mehlmauer M, et al: Dermatologic reactions to lithium: a critical review of the literature. J Clin Psychopharmacol 2:199–204, 1982

Dreifuss FE, Santilli N, Langer DH, et al: Valproic acid hepatic fatalities: a retrospective review. Neurology 37:379–385, 1987

Eichelbaum M, Tomson T, Tybring G, et al: Carbamazepine metabolism in man: induction and pharmacogenetic aspects. Clin Pharmacokinet 10:80–90, 1985

Gelenberg AJ, Wojcik JD, Coggins CH, et al: Renal function monitoring in patients receiving lithium carbonate. J Clin Psychiatry 42:428–431, 1981

Gelenberg AJ, Kane JM, Keller MB, et al: Comparison of standard and low blood levels of lithium for maintenance treatment of bipolar disorder. N Engl J Med 321:1489–1493, 1989

Gerner RH, Stanton A: Algorithm for patient management of acute manic states: lithium, valproate, or carbamazepine? J Clin Psychopharmacol 12 (No 1, Suppl):57S–63S, 1992

Goldfrank LR, Lewin NA, Flomenbaum NE, et al: Antidepressants: tricyclics, tetracyclics, monoamine oxidase inhibitors, and others, in Goldfrank's Toxicologic Emergencies, 3rd Edition. Edited by Goldfrank LR, Flomenbaum ME, Lewis NA, et al. Norwalk, CT, Appleton-Century-Crofts, 1986, pp 351–363

Goldney RD, Spence ND: Safety of the combination of lithium and neuroleptic drugs. Am J Psychiatry 143:882–884, 1986

Gram LM, Bentsen KD: Hepatic toxicity of antiepileptic drugs: a review. Acta Neurol Scand Suppl 97:81–90, 1983

Hart RG, Easton JD: Carbamazepine and hematological monitoring. Ann Neurol 11:309–312, 1982

Hetmar O, Bren C, Clemmesen L, et al: Lithium: long-term effects on the kidney, II: structural changes. J Psychiatr Res 21:279–288, 1987

Hetmar O, Poulsen UJ, Ladefoged J, et al: Lithium: long-term effects on the kidney: a prospective follow-up study ten years after kidney biopsy. Br J Psychiatry 158:53–58, 1991

Hoschl C, Kozeny J: Verapamil in affective disorders: a controlled, double-blind study. Biol Psychiatry 25:128–140, 1989

Hyman NM, Dennis PD, Sinclair KG: Tremor due to sodium valproate. Neurology 29:1172–1180, 1979

Jaeken J, Casaer P, Corbeel L: Valproate, hyperammonaemia and hyperglycinaemia (letter). Lancet 2:260, 1980

Jeavons PM, Clark JE, Harding GFA: Valproate and curly hair. Lancet 1:359, 1977

Joffe RT, Gold PW, Uhde TW, et al: The effects of carbamazepine on the thyrotropin response to thyrotropin releasing hormone. Psychiatry Res 12:161–166, 1984

Jones KL, Lacro RV, Johnson KA, et al: Pattern of malformations in the children of women treated with carbamazepine during pregnancy. N Engl J Med 320:1661–1666, 1989

Julius SC, Brenner RP: Myoclonic seizures with lithium. Biol Psychiatry 22:1184–1190, 1987

Kane JM, Quitkin FM, Rifkin A, et al: Lithium carbonate and imipramine in the prophylaxis of unipolar and bipolar II illness. Arch Gen Psychiatry 39:1065–1069, 1982

Keck PE Jr, McElroy SL, Nemeroff CB: Anticonvulsants in the treatment of bipolar disorder. J Neuropsychiatry Clin Neurosci 4:395–405, 1992

Kemperman CJF, Gerdes JH, DeRooij J, et al: Reversible lithium neurotoxicity at normal serum level may refer to intracranial pathology (letter). J Neurol Neurosurg Psychiatry 52:679–680, 1989

Kramlinger KG, Post RM: Addition of lithium carbonate to carbamazepine: hematological and thyroid effects. Am J Psychiatry 147:615–620, 1990

Labar DR: Antiepileptic drug toxic emergencies, in The Medical Treatment of Epilepsy. Edited by Resor SR, Kutt H. New York, Marcel Dekker, 1992, pp 573–588

Lammer EJ, Sever LE, Oakley GP: Teratogen update: valproic acid. Teratology 35:465–473, 1987

Lassen E, Vestergaard P, Thomsen K: Renal function of patients in long-term treatment with lithium citrate alone or in combination with neuroleptics and antidepressant drugs. Arch Gen Psychiatry 43:481–482, 1986

Leinonen E, Lillsunde P, Laukkanen V, et al: Effects of carbamazepine on serum antidepressant concentrations in psychiatric patients. J Clin Psychopharmacol 11:313–318, 1991

Lewis DA: Unrecognized chronic lithium neurotoxic reactions. JAMA 250:2029–2030, 1983

Lokkegaard H, Andersen NF, Henriksen E: Renal function in 153 manic-depressive patients treated with lithium for more than five years. Acta Psychiatr Scand 71:347–355, 1985

Martin A: Clinical management of lithium-induced polyuria. Hosp Community Psychiatry 44:427–428, 1993

McElroy SL, Keck PE Jr, Pope HG Jr, et al: Valproate in psychiatric disorders: literature review and clinical guidelines. J Clin Psychiatry 50 (No 3, Suppl):23–29, 1989

McElroy SL, Keck PE Jr, Pope HG Jr, et al: Valproate in the treatment of bipolar disorder: literature review and clinical guidelines. J Clin Psychopharmacol 12 (No 1, Suppl):42S–52S, 1992

Mitchell JE, Mackenzie TB: Cardiac effects of lithium therapy in man: a review. J Clin Psychiatry 43:47–51, 1982

Moss GR, James CR: Carbamazepine and lithium synergism in mania. Arch Gen Psychiatry 40:588–589, 1983

Murphy MJ, Lyon IW, Taylor JW, et al: Valproic acid associated with pancreatitis in an adult (letter). Lancet 1:41–42, 1981

Myers DH, Carter RA, Burns BH, et al: A prospective study of the effects of lithium on thyroid function and on the prevalence of antithyroid antibodies. Psychol Med 15:55–61, 1985

Patterson JF: Stevens-Johnson syndrome associated with carbamazepine therapy. J Clin Psychopharmacol 5:185, 1985

Peselow ED, Dunner DL, Fieve RR, et al: Lithium carbonate and weight gain. J Affect Disord 2:303–310, 1980

Placidi GF, Lenzi A, Lazzerini F, et al: The comparative efficacy and safety of carbamazepine versus lithium: a randomized double-blind 3-year trial in 83 patients. J Clin Psychiatry 47:490–494, 1986

Pope HG Jr, McElroy SL, Sathin A, et al: Head injury, bipolar disorder, and response to valproate. Compr Psychiatry 29:34–38, 1988

Pope HG Jr, McElroy SL, Keck PE Jr, et al: Valproate in the treatment of acute mania: a placebo-controlled study. Arch Gen Psychiatry 48:62–68, 1991

Post RM, Uhde TW, Roy-Byrne PP, et al: Antidepressant effects of carbamazepine. Am J Psychiatry 143:29–34, 1986

Post RM, Uhde TW, Roy-Byrne PP, et al: Correlates of antimanic response to carbamazepine. Psychiatry Res 21:71–83, 1987

Ragheb MA, Powell AL: Failure of sulindac to increase serum lithium levels. J Clin Psychiatry 47:33–34, 1986

Ramsey TA, Cox M: Lithium and the kidney: a review. Am J Psychiatry 139:443–449, 1982

Rosa FW: Spina bifida in infants of women treated with carbamazepine during pregnancy. N Engl J Med 324:674–677, 1991

Schou M: Lithium prophylaxis: myths and realities. Am J Psychiatry 146:573–576, 1989

Schatzberg AF, Cole JO: Manual of Clinical Psychopharmacology, 2nd Edition. Washington, DC, American Psychiatric Press, 1991

Shukla S, Cook BL, Miller MG: Lithium-carbamazepine versus lithium-neuroleptic prophylaxis in bipolar illness. J Affect Disord 9:219–222, 1985

Small JG: Anticonvulsants in affective disorders. Psychopharmacol Bull 26:25–36, 1990

Small JG, Small IF, Milstein V, et al: Manic symptoms: an indication for bilateral ECT. Biol Psychiatry 20:125–134, 1985

Takezaki H, Hanaoka M: The use of carbamazepine (Tegretol) in the control of manic-depressive psychosis and other manic-depressive states. J Clin Psychiatry 13:173–183, 1971

Vendsborg PB, Bech P, Rafaelson OJ: Lithium treatment and weight gain. Acta Psychiatr Scand 53:139–147, 1976

Vestergaard P, Amdisen A, Schou M: Clinically significant side effects of lithium treatment. Acta Psychiatr Scand 62:193–200, 1980

Waller DG: Thyroid function and urine-concentrating ability during lithium treatment. J Psychiatr Res 19:569–571, 1985

Warnock JK, Knesevich J: Adverse cutaneous reactions to antidepressants. Am J Psychiatry 145:425–430, 1988

Wehr TA, Sack DA, Rosenthal NE, et al: Rapid cycling affective disorder: contributing factors and treatment responses in 51 patients. Am J Psychiatry 145:179–184, 1988

Yassa R: Hair loss during lithium therapy (letter). Am J Psychiatry 143:943, 1986

Yassa R, Saunders A, Nastase C, et al: Lithium-induced thyroid disorders: a prevalence study. J Clin Psychiatry 48:14–16, 1988

Zubenko GS, Cohen BM, Lipinski JF: Comparison of metoprolol and propranolol in the treatment of lithium tremor. Psychiatry Res 11:163–164, 1984

Antiaggressive Drugs

Angus WR, Romney DM: The effect of diazepam on patients' memory. J Clin Psychopharmacol 4:203–206, 1984

Berridge MJ, Downes CP, Hanley MR: Neural and developmental actions of lithium: a unifying hypothesis. Cell 59:411–419, 1989

Bick PA, Hannah AL: Intramuscular lorazepam to restrain violent patients. Lancet 1:206, 1986

Coccaro EF, Astill JL, Herbert JL, et al: Fluoxetine treatment of impulsive aggression in DSM-III-R personality disorder patients. J Clin Psychopharmacol 10:373–375, 1990

Craft M, Ismail IA, Krishnamurti D, et al: Lithium in the treatment of aggression in mentally handicapped patients: a double-blind trial. Br J Psychiatry 150:685–689, 1987

Dietch JT, Jennings RK: Aggressive dyscontrol in patients treated with benzodiazepines. J Clin Psychiatry 49:184–189, 1988

Fava M, Rosenbaum JF, Pava JA, et al: Anger attacks in unipolar depression, Part 1: clinical correlates and response to fluoxetine treatment. Am J Psychiatry 150:1158–1163, 1993

Feeney DM, Gonzalez A, Lewin A: Amphetamine, haloperidol, and experience interact to affect rate of recovery after motor cortex injury. Science 217:855–857, 1982

Freinhar JP, Alvarez WA: Clonazepam treatment of organic brain syndromes in three elderly patients. J Clin Psychiatry 47:525–526, 1986

Gleason RP, Schneider LS: Carbamazepine treatment of agitation in Alzheimer's outpatients refractory to neuroleptics. J Clin Psychiatry 51:115–118, 1990

Greendyke RM, Berkner JP, Webster JC, et al: Treatment of behavioral problems with pindolol. Psychosomatics 30:161–165, 1989

Haas JF, Cope N: Neuropharmacologic management of behavior sequelae in head injury: a case report. Arch Phys Med Rehabil 66:472–474, 1985

Herrera JN, Sramek JJ, Costa JF, et al: High potency neuroleptics and violence in schizophrenics. J Nerv Ment Dis 176:558–561, 1988

Keats MM, Mukherjee S: Antiaggressive effect of adjunctive clonazepam in schizophrenia associated with seizure disorder. J Clin Psychiatry 49:117–118, 1988

King BH: Fluoxetine reduced self-injurious behavior in an adolescent with mental retardation. Journal of Child and Adolescent Psychopharmacology 1:321–329, 1991

Luchins DJ: Carbamazepine for the violent psychiatric patient. Lancet 2:755, 1983

Luchins DJ, Dojka D: Lithium and propranolol in aggression and self-injurious behavior in the mentally retarded. Psychopharmacol Bull 25:372–375, 1989

Mattes JA: Carbamazepine vs propranolol for rage outbursts. Psychopharmacol Bull 24:179–182, 1988

Mattes JA: Valproic acid for nonaffective aggression in the mentally retarded. J Nerv Ment Dis 180:601–602, 1992

Moskowitz AS, Altshuler L: Increased sensitivity to lithium-induced neurotoxicity after stroke: a case report. J Clin Psychopharmacol 11:272–273, 1991

Mysiw WJ, Jackson RD, Corrigan JD: Amitriptyline for post-traumatic agitation. Am J Phys Med Rehabil 67:29–33, 1988

Pinner E, Rich CL: Effects of trazodone on aggressive behavior in seven patients with organic mental disorders. Am J Psychiatry 145:1295–1296, 1988

Ratey JJ, Sovner R, Mikkelsen E, et al: Buspirone therapy for maladaptive behavior and anxiety in developmentally disabled persons. J Clin Psychiatry 50:382–384, 1989

Ratey JJ, Leveroni CL, Miller AC, et al: Low-dose buspirone to treat agitation and maladaptive behavior in brain-injured patients: two case reports. J Clin Psychopharmacol 12:362–364, 1992a

Ratey JJ, Sorgi P, O'Driscoll GA, et al: Nadolol to treat aggression and psychiatric symptomatology in chronic psychiatric inpatients: a double-blind, placebo-controlled study. J Clin Psychiatry 53:41–46, 1992b

Ratey JJ, Levoroni C, Kilmer D, et al: The effects of clozapine on severely aggressive psychiatric inpatients in a state hospital. J Clin Psychiatry 54:219–223, 1993

Schiffer RB, Herndon RM, Rudick RA: Treatment of pathologic laughing and weeping with amitriptyline. N Engl J Med 312:1480–1482, 1985

Seliger GM, Hornstein A, Flax J, et al: Fluoxetine improves emotional incontinence. Brain Inj 6:267–270, 1992

Sheard MH, Marini JL, Bridges C, et al: The effects of lithium in impulsive aggressive behavior in man. Am J Psychiatry 133:1409–1413, 1976

Silver JM, Yudofsky SC: The Overt Aggression Scale: overview and clinical guidelines. J Neuropsychiatry Clin Neurosci 3:S22–S29, 1991

Silver JM, Yudofsky SC: Aggressive disorders, in Neuropsychiatry of Traumatic Brain Injury. Edited by Silver JM, Yudofsky SC, Hales RE. Washington, DC, American Psychiatric Press, 1994

Silver JM, Yudofsky SC, Kogan M, et al: Elevation of thioridazine plasma levels by propranolol. Am J Psychiatry 143:1290–1292, 1986

Sorbin P, Schneider L, McDermott H: Fluoxetine in the treatment of agitated dementia. Am J Psychiatry 146:1636, 1989

Tiller JWG, Dakis JA, Shaw JM: Short-term buspirone treatment in disinhibition with dementia. Lancet 2:510, 1988

Vetro A, Szentistvanyi L, Pallag M, et al: Therapeutic experience with lithium in childhood aggressivity. Pharmacopsychiatry 14:121–127, 1985

Williams KH, Goldstein G: Cognitive and affective responses to lithium in patients with organic brain syndrome. Am J Psychiatry 136:800–803, 1979

Yatham LN, McHale PA: Carbamazepine in the treatment of aggression: a case report and a review of the literature. Acta Psychiatr Scand 78:188–190, 1988

Yudofsky SC: β-Blockers and depression: the clinicians's dilemma. JAMA 267:1826–1827, 1992

Yudofsky SC, Silver JM, Schneider SE: Pharmacologic treatment of aggression. Psychiatric Annals 17:397–407, 1987

Yudofsky SC, Silver JM, Hales RE: Pharmacologic management of aggression in the elderly. J Clin Psychiatry 51 (No 10, Suppl):22-28, 1990

Electroconvulsive Therapy

Abrams R: Electroconvulsive Therapy, 2nd Edition. New York, Oxford University Press, 1992

American Psychiatric Association: (Task Force Report 14). Washington, DC, American Psychiatric Association, 1978

American Psychiatric Association: The Practice of Electroconvulsive Therapy: Recommendations for Treatment, Training, and Privileging. A Task Force Report of the American Psychiatric Association. Washington, DC, American Psychiatric Association, 1990

Asnis GM, Fink M, Saferstein S: ECT in metropolitan New York hospitals: a survey of practice, 1975–76. Am J Psychiatry 135:479–482, 1978

Avery D, Winokur G: Mortality in depressed patients treated with ECT and antidepressants. Arch Gen Psychiatry 33:1029–1037, 1976

Coppen A, Abou-Saleb MT, Miller P, et al: Lithium continuation therapy following electroconvulsive therapy. Br J Psychiatry 139:284–287, 1981

Dec GW, Stern TA, Welsch C: The effects of electroconvulsive therapy on serial electrocardiograms and serum cardiac enzyme values: a prospective study of depressed hospitalized inpatients. JAMA 253:2525–2529, 1985

Fink M: Efficacy and safety of induced seizures (ECT) in man. Compr Psychiatry 19:1–18, 1978

Glassman AH, Roose SP: Delusional depression: a distinct clinical entity. Arch Gen Psychiatry 38:424–427, 1981

Gomez J: Subjective side effects of ECT. Br J Psychiatry 127:609–611, 1975

Janicak PG, Davis JM, Gibbons RD, et al: Efficacy of ECT: a meta-analysis. Am J Psychiatry 132:297–302, 1985

Malitz S, Sackheim HA: Preface. Ann N Y Acad Sci, Vol 462, 1986

Maltbie AA, Wingfield MS, Volow MR, et al: Electroconvulsive therapy in the presence of brain tumor: case reports and an evaluation of risk. J Nerv Ment Dis 168:400–405, 1980

Sackheim HA, Prudic J, Devanand DP, et al: The impact of medication resistance and continuation pharmacotherapy on relapse following response to electroconvulsive therapy in major depression. J Clin Psychopharmacol 10:96–104, 1990

Sackheim HA, Devanand DP, Prudic J: Stimulus intensity, seizure threshold, and seizure duration: impact on the efficacy and safety of electroconvulsive therapy. Psychiatr Clin North Am 14:803–843, 1991

Sackheim HA, Prudic J, Devanand DP, et al: Effects of stimulus intensity and electrode placement on the efficacy and cognitive effects of electroconvulsive therapy. N Engl J Med 328:839–846, 1993

Salzman C: The use of ECT in the treatment of schizophrenia. Am J Psychiatry 137:1031–1041, 1980

Silver JM, Yudofsky SC, Hurowitz GI: Psychopharmacology and electroconvulsive therapy, in The American Psychiatric Press Textbook of Psychiatry, 2nd Edition. Edited by Hales RE, Yudofsky SC, Talbott JA. Washington, DC, American Psychiatric Press, 1994, pp 897–1007

Squire LR, Slater PC: Electroconvulsive therapy and complaints of memory dysfunction: a prospective three-year follow-up study. Br J Psychiatry 142:1–8, 1983

Squire LR, Slater PC, Chance PM: Retrograde amnesia: temporal gradient in very long-term memory following electroconvulsive therapy. Science 187:77–79, 1975

Weiner RD: The psychiatric use of electrically induced seizures. Am J Psychiatry 136:1507–1516, 1979

Wells DG, Bjorkstein AR: Monoamine oxidase inhibitors revisited. Can J Anaesth 36:64–74, 1989

Yudofsky SC: ECT in general hospital psychiatry: focus on new indications and technologies. Gen Hosp Psychiatry 3:292–296, 1981

Yudofsky SC, Hales RE, Ferguson T: What You Need to Know About Psychiatric Drugs. New York, Grove Weidenfeld, 1991

CHAPTER 28

Brief Dynamic
Individual Psychotherapy

Hanna Levenson, Ph.D.
Stephen F. Butler, Ph.D.

It has now been established in a number of studies with a variety of patients—across a range of settings with diverse agenda—that regardless of the type of outpatient treatment patients receive, the great majority are seen only for 6 to 12 sessions (Phillips 1987; Reder and Tyson 1980). In fact, it has been estimated that 50% of all outpatients drop out of treatment before the eighth session (Phillips 1987). These findings hold even when the treatments are specifically psychodynamic in nature. *Whether planned or not, therefore, most mental health professionals are conducting treatments that are short-term.* However, these treatments seem to be more brief by "default" rather than by "design" (Budman and Gurman 1988). Certainly there should be more to conducting brief dynamic psychotherapy than noting that half of your patients "prematurely" terminate.

■ HISTORICAL PERSPECTIVE

From a historical and conceptual viewpoint, short-term dynamic psychotherapies may be conveniently grouped into "generations" (Crits-Christoph et al. 1991).

☐ The First Generation: Freud and Psychoanalysis

Several of Freud's early treatments were short-term therapies. In 1908 Freud cured Gustav Mahler, the composer, of impotency problems in one single 4-hour session. Even training analyses were conducted in less than 1 year. As psychoanalytic theory became more complex and elaborate, and the goals of analysis became more ambitious, the length of treatments increased.

In 1925, Sandor Ferenczi and Otto Rank advocated time limits, a focus for the treatment, and a frequently active stance for the therapist. Even by today's standards, these authors' contributions to brief dynamic psychotherapy remain innovative and central to modern dynamic approaches. Ferenczi and Rank wished to increase the therapist's activity to counter the patient's passivity. Rank introduced two precursors of modern brief psychotherapy: the issue of separation activated by setting a time limit in advance (Rank's concept of the *birth trauma*), and assessment of the patient's motivation to change (Rank's concept of the *will*). Alexander and French (1946) questioned the presumed relationship between therapeutic outcome and the length of therapy. They advocated therapist flexibility and adjustment of the length and frequency of sessions.

☐ Second Generation: Short-Term Dynamic Psychotherapies

In this phase, from 1960 to 1980, brief dynamic therapy began to emerge as a legitimate therapeutic method. Malan held that "far reaching changes could be brought about in relatively severe and chronic illnesses by a technique of active interpretation containing all the essential elements of full scale analysis" (Malan 1976, p. 20). Malan concentrated on identification of a focal problem—a "nuclear" or childhood conflict that is manifested in some form in the current presentingproblem. He emphasized making interpretations linking recurrent, maladaptive patterns apparent in the therapist-patient relationship (i.e., transference) with patterns evidenced in present and past relationships (i.e., triangle of insight). Mann is credited with deriving a generic theoretical orientation that focuses on the difficulties in dealing with separation and loss (Mann 1973). His *time-limited treatment* (TLT) consists of 12 sessions. It is asserted that the fixed duration forces the patient to face unconscious issues related to the passage of time.

Sifneos developed techniques and a rationale for his *short-term anxiety provoking psychotherapy* (STAPP; Sifneos 1987). He contributed greater specificity to selection and exclusion criteria, focus of inquiry, and anxiety-provoking intervention techniques. His work focuses on the efficacy of brief dynamic therapy with relatively high-functioning patients experiencing conflicts associated with oedipal issues. No number of sessions is agreed upon at the outset, but a length between 6 and 20 sessions is determined as the therapy proceeds.

Davanloo (1978) developed his *intensive short-term dynamic psychotherapy* (ISTDP) approach. ISTDP was designed to break through the patient's defensive barrier using confrontive techniques similar to those of Sifneos. Vagueness, tentativeness, detachment, evasiveness, diversionary tactics, intellectualization, rationalization, rumination, projection, introjection, and weepiness are dramatically pointed out to patients in order to intensify feelings and crystallize the patients' resistance.

☐ Third Generation: Research-Based Interpersonal Therapies

The third generation of brief therapies has done much to provide empirical support for the efficacy of brief dynamic therapy, as well as to elucidate its active therapeutic ingredients. In addition to an empirical emphasis, these therapies herald a move away from *intra*psychic models of theory and practice to more *inter*personal ones. Representatives of this wave are *time-limited dynamic psychotherapy* (TLDP) (Strupp and Binder 1984), *supportive-expressive psychotherapy,* (Luborsky et al. 1988), and *control mastery theory* (Weiss et al. 1986).

The major objective of TLDP is to examine recurrent, maladaptive themes from the patient's range of object relations that are activated in relation to the therapist. Consistent focus is directed to the patient's manner of construing and relating to the therapist both as a significant person in the present and as the personification of past relationships. The patient-therapist relationship is conceived of as a dyadic system in which the behavior of both participants is continually scrutinized and modified. In the tradition of Alexander and French, the goal of TLDP is to provide the patient with a new (i.e., healthier) experience of himself or herself and the other person (i.e., corrective emotional experience). The duration of treatment is approximately 25 sessions and is established very early in treatment.

☐ Fourth Generation: Managed Health Care

The fourth wave, which coexists with the second and third generations of brief dynamic psychotherapies, reflects the powerful major economic and market demands that are affecting the provision of mental health care. Numerous writers have discussed the current state of crisis in the health care industry, the urgent need for cost containment, and the impact and implications of this situation on mental health care providers (Austad et al. 1988).

The current emphasis on brief formats to meet the expectations for service delivery has led researchers and practitioners to address issues such as the ongoing need for more research and training in brief therapy, the necessity of clinicians to rethink their role in the health care field, and the need for mental health care providers to become more flexible in their treatment approaches. Increasing emphasis has been placed on the idea that the psychotherapist should function similarly to the old-fashioned family doctor, who provides "brief, intermittent therapy through the life cycle," treating not only the problems of the individual client but, when indicated, those of other family members as well (Cummings 1987, p. 357).

■ QUALITIES THAT DEFINE BRIEF DYNAMIC PSYCHOTHERAPY

The qualities of brief dynamic psychotherapy can, in general, be organized into two main categories: those qualities pertaining to the *brief features* per se and those germane to the *psychodynamic aspects* (Table 28–1).

☐ Limited Therapeutic Focus

A major concept distinguishing the brief dynamic psychotherapy approaches from long-term psychotherapy or psychoanalysis is the idea of a limited focus of treatment. Brief therapists need a central theme, topic, or problem to serve as a guide to stay on target—a necessity when time is of the essence. Brief therapists cannot pay attention to all clinical data; even fascinating material must sometimes be ignored. Practitioners working with short-term models must learn to use *selective attention* and *benign neglect*, or run the risk of being overwhelmed by the patient's rich intrapsychic and interpersonal life.

Table 28–1.　Qualities that define brief psychodynamic psychotherapy

Brief qualities	Termination
Limited focus (and limited goals)	Optimism
Limited time	Contract
Selection criteria	
Therapist activity	**Psychodynamic qualities**
Therapeutic alliance	Analytic concepts
Rapid assessment/ prompt intervention	Analytic techniques

Note.　Qualities based on frequency mentioned in the literature.

A convergence of findings appears to support the efficacy of establishing a focus and maintaining that focus throughout the treatment. However, rigid efforts to stick to a focus and discourage deviations are likely to damage the therapeutic alliance and result in poor outcome. Paying attention to material directly related to the focus does not mean coercing patients or ignoring what is important to them. Some general guidelines for developing a psychodynamic focus are given in Table 28–2. These guidelines underscore the importance of sensitive and simultaneous attention to patterns of past and present functioning.

The aim of brief dynamic psychotherapy is not "cure" once and for all. Rather the therapy should provide an opportunity to foster some changes in behavior and thinking, permitting more adaptive coping and a better sense of one's self. Brief dynamic therapy is seen as an opportunity to begin a process of change that continues long after the therapy is over.

☐ Time Limits and Time Management

Naturally, time is the critical variable that defines an approach as "short-term," "brief," or "time-limited." Although most clinicians set 25 sessions as the upper limit of brief therapy, the range may be as few as one or as many as 40. Time, like focus, can be conceptualized in a variety of ways. Usually the *limiting* or *rationing* of time is used conceptually to accelerate the therapeutic work, either by raising the patient's awareness of the existential issues of finite time and mortality or by encouraging therapist activity and adherence to a focus.

Although it is most customary for psychodynamically oriented short-term therapists to use the traditional weekly 50-minute "hour," many are experimenting with the frequency of sessions (e.g., frequent initial sessions with more interspersed later sessions), the duration of each therapy session (e.g., the 20-minute "hour"), and even the number

---

Table 28–2.   General principles for developing a psychodynamic focus

1. Gather historical material and other data, but let the patient tell his or her own story.
2. Study the patient's characteristic defensive pattern.
3. Be sensitive to how present patterns have roots in the past.
4. Watch for transference patterns; deal with negative transference reactions rapidly and supportively.
5. Examine possible countertransference feelings and behavior for clues as to repetitive dysfunctional patterns.
6. Constantly look for resistances that threaten to block progress.

Source.   Adapted from Wolberg 1980.

of consecutive brief therapies (e.g., intermittent brief therapy throughout the life cycle). The setting of time limits accomplishes three clinical consequences. First, it emphasizes individuation-separation issues, which commonly underlie presenting problems. Second, it acknowledges the autonomy of the patient. Third, it encourages the patient's independence and self-confidence.

It is important to recall that the brief dynamic psychotherapies have been developed for and researched with highly selected, and usually highly functioning, patients (see subsection on patient selection below). It may be dangerous to make the assumption that brief (especially very brief) courses of treatment can be readily extended to severely disturbed patients with chaotic life-styles. The amount of therapy that is appropriate for the treatment of severe conditions remains an important empirical question.

Variable time limits are used by some therapeutic models that propose altering the time allotted based on various factors such as therapist experience or type and severity of presenting complaint. Recently, however, brief therapists are moving away from conceptualizing therapy just in terms of a specific amount of time, and are instead addressing ways to make every session count regardless of length of treatment. These models are categorized as *time attentive.* Examples of this approach include Binder et al.'s (1987) idea of the therapist's *time-limited attitude* (regardless of the actual length of therapy) and Budman and Gurman's (1988) notion of brief therapy as a "state of mind of the therapist and of the patient" (p. 10).

☐ Selection Criteria

The topic of selection critieria is a controversial subject in the brief dynamic psychotherapy field. Early in the history of psychoanalysis, as psychoanalytic treatments became progressively longer, Freud put forth the possibility that treatment might be shortened with healthier patients. Largely based on this comment, rigorous patient selection to identify the healthiest patients became an early and integral part of virtually all brief dynamic psychotherapies. The problem then arose as to how to determine which patients were the "healthiest" and which ones would respond well to a brief course of treatment. Those credited with bringing brief dynamic psychotherapy into the modern therapeutic arena specify fairly stringent suitability characteristics:

1. Appropriate ego strength
2. Ability to rapidly become involved in and contribute to treatment
3. Adequate motivation
4. A history of meaningful relationships

5. Adequate intelligence or psychological sophistication
6. A relatively circumscribed problem or symptom presentation (as opposed to wide-ranging difficulties in many aspects of the patient's life)

In addition, these authors specify relatively consistent exclusion criteria, such as psychosis, major affective disorders (especially bipolar disorder), drug use, suicidal tendencies (and other acting out) or impulsive tendencies, organic disorders, and some personality disorders (borderline personality disorder, especially in those patients with histories of acting out, and schizoid personality disorder, when interpersonal unresponsiveness on the part of the patient is noted). The inclusion and exclusion criteria for the major short-term dynamic approaches are given in Table 28–3. How do these selection criteria hold up? Research on patient characteristics (e.g., ego functioning, quality of object relations) and on performance criteria (e.g., patient's response to trial interpretation) reveals only modest correlations with outcome (Binder et al. 1987).

Clinically, such selection criteria can only be used to make very qualified predictions of how an individual patient will respond to therapy. As clinicians, we must recognize that patients are not mere passive vessels whom we diagnose and about whom we offer prognoses. Rather, they are responsive to our predictions and may respond to a judgment that they are "too sick" for brief therapy or "not sick enough" for long-term therapy in ways that confound our elegant notions of how psychotherapy is supposed to work. Our position on the use of selection criteria is that, given the present state of knowledge, virtually any psychotherapy with virtually any patient can benefit from a "time-limited attitude" on the part of the therapist. This involves the promotion of a consistent, active engagement of both patient and therapist in the therapeutic relationship. Impediments on the part of the patient to becoming so engaged become an important issue to be addressed in the therapy.

☐ Therapist Activity

Most of those who have written on the qualities that define brief, dynamic psychotherapy have emphasized the need for increased amounts of therapist activity over the essentially passive stance often characterized by psychoanalysts. However, *activity* is only necessary to the extent that one needs to maintain the *focus* and make progress within a certain amount of *time.* Thus, activity is integrally related to the aforementioned aspects of focus and time. It is only through the interventions of the therapist that the focus can be achieved within a specified period.

Many clinicians, when learning brief therapy techniques, become confused that therapist activity means confrontation, advice giving, or

Table 28-3. Criteria for patient selection for brief dynamic psychotherapy

Theorist	Criteria inclusion	Exclusion
Malan Short-term anxiety-provoking psychotherapy	Capacity to form good relationships Good response to trial interpretations	Addictions, serious suicide attempts, ECT Severe major depression, acting out
Sifneos Short-term anxiety-provoking psychotherapy	Intelligence, psychological mindedness History of meaningful relationships Motivation for change beyond symptom relief Appropriate affect during interview One major and specific complaint	Psychosis, major affective syndrome, addiction Suicidal tendencies and acting out Severe personality disorder
Mann Time-limited psychotherapy	Good ego strength, capacity for rapid affective connection Definable focus Mild neurosis and personality disorders	Psychosis, schizoid, and severe obsessional personality disorders Severe psychosomatic disorders
Davanloo Intensive short-term dynamic psychotherapy	Wide range Pass trial therapy	Psychosis, severe major depression, brain damage, suicidal tendencies and acting out, addictions "Decompensation" during or following trial therapy
Luborsky and Mark Supportive-expressive psychotherapy	Coherent, identifiable interpersonal theme Distinction between self and others Capacity for human relationships Ability to form collaborative relationship with therapist	
Strupp and Binder Time-limited dynamic psychotherapy		Psychotics, borderline personality disorder, suicidal acting out, antisocial personality without depression

Horowitz Treatment for stress response syndrome	One or few recent traumatic events	Lack of capacity to be collaborative Unwillingness to enhance strength (e.g, addiction) Value conflict with therapist Normative life crisis Inability to keep acting-out behavior under control Active psychosis, brain damage
Sampson and Weiss **Mt. Zion Group** Plan formulation method	History of positive interpersonal relationships	Psychosis Organic brain syndrome Mental deficiency Serious substance abuse Suicide potential

Source.   Adapted from Barber and Crits-Christoph 1991, pp. 328–330.

directive support. What it more appropriately entails is an awareness of the goals of the work and a plan of how to get there while being sensitive to the patient's presentation and the context of the clinical material. Therapist activity should aid the patient in increasing focally relevant thoughts and behaviors.

☐ Modifications of Psychoanalytic Concepts and Techniques

Brief psychodynamic therapists adhere to many of the psychoanalytically inspired concepts familiar to the various "schools" of psychotherapy such as Freudian, ego analytic, object relations, interpersonal, and self psychology. Specifically, brief dynamic therapeutic work relies on major psychoanalytic and psychodynamic concepts such as the importance of childhood experiences and developmental history, unconscious determinants of behavior, the role of conflicts, the transference relationship between therapist and patient, the patient's resistance to the therapeutic work, and repetitive behavior. Many brief therapists, however, do not feel obliged to adopt elaborate metapsychological models that incorporate highly inferential constructs. Instead, they prefer to stick close to the observable data. Such an inclination may stem from the need to do pragmatic clinical work and from the interest many brief theorists have in conducting research, for which variables must be precisely defined.

Similarly, the techniques used in brief, dynamic psychotherapy have been inspired by those used in psychoanalysis and long-term dynamic therapy. Some classical techniques have been modified to be more compatible with a limited focus and limited time (Crits-Christoph and Barber 1991). Perhaps the most notable of these modifications is that of the *early transference interpretation*. Flegenheimer (1982) sees early interpretation of transference as preventing the occurrence of a transference neurosis: "The early interpretation of transference manifestations brings these phenomena under the scrutiny of the observing portion of the patient's ego, putting the patient on guard, so to speak, against the dangers of dependency and regression which lie ahead" (p. 9). Still others see value in demonstrating to the patient his or her characteristic style of relating.

Another major modification of psychoanalytic technique involves the gathering of psychosocial and historical information. Clearly, in a brief therapy, the amount of time devoted to obtaining background material must be curtailed. Many brief therapists employ the concept of a "focused history," in which the patient begins to tell his or her own story and the therapist asks clarifying questions designed to fill out information relevant to a particular theme that is emerging in the therapy.

With regard to acquiring information, many brief dynamic therapists put less emphasis on knowing factual genetic material. They are more likely to base their focus and interventions on a "here and now" assessment of patients. How are the patients presenting themselves? Why now? What is the nature of the interaction between patient and therapist? What seem to be the characteristic defenses used? What is the therapist's own countertransference?

■ FACTORS RELATED TO THE PRACTICE OF BRIEF DYNAMIC PSYCHOTHERAPY

Levenson et al. (1992) randomly surveyed 1,500 licensed psychologists. With a return rate of 58%, the investigators found over 80% of the therapists to be engaged in some type of brief therapy (i.e., *designed* to be limited in duration and/or focus). As expected, cognitive-behavior therapists did the most brief therapy hours per week, and psychodynamic therapists the least. However, because the psychodynamic therapists constituted 40% of the entire sample, they were responsible for conducting over one-fifth (22%) of all the brief therapy hours done in those two states. Similarly, Kamin (1992) found that 41% of sampled therapists made explicit to 60% of their clients the planned, limited duration of the therapy. Clearly, if these surveys are representative, a great deal of planned brief therapy is being conducted today.

☐ Managed Care, Consumerism, and the Present Zeitgeist

Managed care takes various forms, such as health maintenance organizations (HMOs), preferred provider organizations (PPOs), independent practice associations (IPAs), employee assistance programs (EAPs), and utilization review. Such systems have been established for the ostensible purpose of controlling costs while promoting efficient and effective (but usually limited-access) treatments.

It is no accident that much of the interest in brief approaches has occurred at a time when short-term interventions are being mandated by organizations needing to accommodate consumer needs within fiscal constraints. Austad and Berman (1991) discussed what they call "HMO psychotherapy . . . in which the parameters of treatment have been modified both consciously and unconsciously, to be compatible with the philosophy, theory, and economic and pragmatic conditions of a managed care system" (p. 8). A "good HMO therapist" has been described as someone who has "sound *psychodynamic* training, interest and experience in working in a high-pressure medical setting, interest in a group practice, and commitment to problem-oriented short-term psychotherapy" (Budman et al. 1979, p. 392 [emphasis added]).

Haas and Cummings (1991), focusing on the clinical, ethical, and practical issues in working for managed mental health plans, suggested that "therapists who are not comfortable with a more active, directive role" as well as those who are not competent in using brief therapy should not work for managed mental health care programs (pp. 49–50).

The push for briefer treatments, however, is not solely based on economic considerations. Professionals in the mental health system are concerned about providing more rapid relief of suffering and making services available to more people. Those persons seeking help are demanding the most for their time and money in an age of consumer awareness. Potential patients (more likely called "clients" or "consumers") are questioning therapists ("providers") regarding what results can be expected in what amount of time. A therapist is encouraged to give a client "clear information about the benefits to which he or she is entitled and clear information about the limits of treatment as the clinician envisions them" (Haas and Cummings 1991, p. 50).

☐ Training

From the growing mass of clinical and empirical work, it can be stated emphatically that brief dynamic psychotherapy is not simply a shorter version of long-term therapy. The research literature is clear that brief therapy is a different treatment modality requiring specialized training in its own theories and techniques.

In 1978, the American Association of Directors of Residency Training conducted a survey of psychiatric residency programs and found that 88% of them offered a training experience in brief therapy and 78% required it (Clarkin et al. 1980). Almost two-thirds of the training directors thought their current emphasis on brief psychotherapy would continue, with the remaining 36% expecting growth in brief therapy training. One of the most frequently taught models was focal dynamic psychotherapy (58%), which training directors thought they taught best. Clarkin et al. reasoned that this was because focal dynamic psychotherapy "has the best established theory, widest literature, and most definite technical guidelines" (p. 979).

Despite its importance, training in brief therapy is far less researched and understood than brief therapy techniques and outcome. In one of the few studies to document the extent and type of training in brief dynamic psychotherapy, Levenson et al. (1992) found that of those clinicians who regularly offered brief therapy, over one-third reported having little or no training in it. This is a very distressing statistic, particularly because it is now widely accepted that brief therapy is not "dehydrated" long-term therapy (Cummings 1986) or "just less of the same" (Peake et al. 1988), but requires specialized training in its own methodology. However, the survey data also revealed that professionals with extensive training were doing considerably more brief therapy (16 hours per week) compared with those who received no training (10 hours per week). Also, there was a significant positive relationship between the amount of training and the attitudes about and skill in conducting brief therapy. In the Levenson et al. survey, the most common type of brief therapy training experiences for practicing professionals was reading, followed by workshops and supervision. Supervision was considered by respondents to be the most useful experience.

The parallel processes of supervision and treatment have been observed for years. Frances and Clarkin (1981) noted that the brief therapy "treatment context requires a relatively high level of therapist activity and planning, the setting of clear and limited goals, the focus on a single problem or dynamic conflict, and a quick attachment to and then separation from the therapist. These same conditions are characteristic of the work of brief therapy supervision" (p. 244).

Burlingame et al. (1989) randomly exposed trainee and senior staff of a counseling center to one of three training conditions: no training, self-instructional training, and intensive training (i.e., 10 hours of didactic information, demonstration, role-playing, and discussion). All therapists then conducted an eight-session time-limited therapy. While the more experienced therapists had superior outcomes in general, there were indications that greater amounts of training for *both* the inexperienced and experienced therapists led to greater patient improvements. In other words, even experienced therapists gained significantly from the brief therapy training program.

Training manuals have been one approach to provide more specific descriptions of treatment techniques. One of the best known "manualized" psychodynamic/interpersonal therapies is TLDP (Strupp and Binder 1984). A 5-year study examined the effect of manualized training in TLDP and found that the training program was successful in changing therapists' interventions congruent with the manual (Henry et al. 1993). In addition to manuals, training in brief psychotherapy has emphasized the use of clinical material obtained directly from therapy sessions, including live supervision and use of audio- and videotaping. Students have found watching videotaped sessions of their teachers treating patients invaluable. Supervisors have found few negative effects from such procedures, but have encountered resistance from therapists in training who either consciously or unconsciously fear exposing their work to such close scrutiny. Sifneos (1987) called videotape technology the "microscope" of psychiatry, which underscores both its usefulness and its feared inhibiting effect.

Budman and Armstrong (1992) discussed the lack of training in brief therapy even in such settings as PPOs, HMOs, and EAPs, which have promoted themselves as providing efficient and effective psychotherapeutic services. These authors noted that supervisors and teachers of psychotherapy rarely use adult education principles, which hold that adults 1) have a wealth of previous experience to use when confronted with problems, 2) are autonomous learners who decide what, why, and whether to learn, and 3) want to use their new learning pragmatically and immediately. Budman has trainees apply the skills they are learning in brief psychotherapy in videotaped practice sessions with actors trained to play the roles of patients.

☐ Experience

Experience appears to be another factor that greatly influences the practice of brief dynamic psychotherapy. But how it exerts such influence is somewhat of a paradox. It is widely accepted that brief therapy is a very demanding endeavor—one best suited to be learned after one has already become facile with the basics. Paradoxically, while knowledge and skills learned over the years in doing long-term therapy seem to be a prerequisite for learning brief therapy, one may need to set aside many of the assumptions of long-term therapy in order to make full use of brief therapy techniques and rationale.

The issue of when to train in brief dynamic psychotherapy remains somewhat controversial. However, it seems that the enthusiasm and positive expectation of the neophyte learner may be as valuable as the knowledge and skill of the seasoned clinician. Winokur and Dasberg (1983) found that experienced therapists may suffer from a sense of loss of competence as they experiment with shorter-term treatments. These authors suggested allowing seasoned therapists time to work through negative attitudes they might have toward briefer methods.

Regardless of when brief therapy skills are learned, experience in brief therapy seems to be reliably related to greater skill and confidence in brief therapy techniques. Ursano and Dressler (1977) found that clinicians who were more experienced in brief therapy tended to refer patients to brief therapy more frequently than those who were less familiar. Also, those clinicians who had more brief experience rated themselves as more skilled. Similarly, Levenson et al. (1992) found that the best predictor of self-assessed skill in all types of brief therapy was experience doing brief therapy. For those therapists who were conducting brief therapy but who had little experience in that modality, formal training and amount of brief therapy they were presently conducting were the most potent predictors of skill. For more experienced brief therapists, attitude toward brief therapy played a greater role in predicting skill. Levenson et al. concluded that novice therapists would do well to continue to increase their experience while receiving more training; experienced clinicians, however, might require training that focuses on values and attitudes as well as techniques. Experience alone does not appear to be a sufficient teacher.

☐ Resistances, Attitudes, Expectations

Despite advances in the theory and technique of brief dynamic psychotherapy, as well as a number of research studies demonstrating its overall effectiveness, many therapists are still reluctant to learn these methods as part of their clinical practice. Important variables in understanding this reluctance are therapists' values and assumptions regarding the nature and practice of brief psychotherapy.

Budman and Gurman (1983) proposed that the value systems of the long-term therapist are different from those of the short-term therapist. These authors identified eight dominant values pertaining to the ideal manner in which long-term therapy is practiced, and contrasted these with the corresponding ideal values pertinent to the practice of short-term therapy. For example, Budman and Gurman postulated that one of the ideal value differences between long-term and short-term therapists involves the idea of "cure." Whereas the long-term therapist seeks a change in basic character or "therapeutic perfectionism," the short-term therapist does not believe in the notion of "cure" and prefers pragmatism, parsimony, and the least radical intervention.

Bolter et al. (1990) sought to assess empirically whether, indeed, there were such value differences between short-term and long-term practicing therapists. Two hundred twenty-two psychologists were sent a questionnaire to measure relevant values and preferred therapeutic approaches (short vs. long term). The study provided partial support for Budman and Gurman's proposal: in two of the eight areas long-term and short-term therapists' responses differed significantly. Short-term therapists believed more strongly that psychological change could occur outside of therapy and that setting time limits would intensify the therapeutic work. Furthermore, results indicated that clinicians with a psychodynamic orientation, in contrast to those having a cognitive-behaviorial orientation, were more likely to believe that therapy was necessary for change, that the focus of therapy should be on pathology, that therapy should be open-ended, and that ambitious goals were desirable. Thus, while the findings from Bolter et al.'s study suggest that a short-term orientation is related to therapeutic values, it is important to note that the theoretical orientation of the therapist also plays a significant role in determining values.

The majority of the literature addressing therapists' reluctance to use brief therapy focuses on psychoanalytic or psychodynamic therapists. Bolter (1987) found that 91% of the psychodynamic therapists who responded to an attitude questionnaire indicated that they favored long-term approaches. Speed (1992) similarly found that 87% of those therapists most comfortable with very long-term therapy were psychodynamic in orientation. In a recent random survey of therapists conducting brief psychotherapy (Levenson et al. 1992), psychodynamic brief therapists reported that they had less skill, experience, and training in, and less of a positive attitude concerning the effectiveness of, brief therapy than did their cognitive-behavior therapy colleagues.

Hoyt (1985) proposed that dynamically trained therapists have resistances toward short-term psychotherapy. In trying to answer the question as to why many therapists are not learning and applying short-term dynamic methods as a treatment of choice, Hoyt rejected the idea that it is due chiefly to lack of awareness regarding recent clinical and research developments. Hoyt organized these resistances into six broad categories, as shown in Table 28–4.

Negative attitudes toward briefer modes of intervention could adversely affect therapists' willingness and ability to use brief therapy methods effectively. Flegenheimer (1982) warned that problems could arise during a brief psychotherapy if the therapist's values are "inconsistent with the optimism and confidence that the brief therapist must have in the method and which must be brought to the treatment situation" (p. 13).

Levenson and Bolter (1988) examined the values and attitudes of psychiatry residents and psychology interns before and after a 6-month seminar/supervision in brief dynamic psychotherapy. Findings revealed that after training, trainees were more willing to consider brief therapy for more than minor disorders, more positive about achieving significant insight, more expectant that the benefits would be long-lasting, and less likely to think that an extended "working through" was necessary. Also,

---

Table 28–4. Sources of resistance against short-term dynamic psychotherapy

1. The belief that "more is better" (e.g., treatment must take a long time to be effective)
2. Myth of the "pure gold" of analysis
3. Confusion of patient's interests (in the most efficient, effective help) with the therapist's interests (in uncovering all aspects of the patient's personality)
4. Demanding hard work (to be active and intensely alert)
5. Economic and other pressures (desire to hold onto that which is profitable and dependable)
6. Countertransference and related therapist reactions to termination

---

Source. Adapted from Hoyt 1985.

they were more willing to be active, more likely to see that a time limit was helpful, and more prepared to believe that patients would change significantly after the therapy was over. Levenson and Bolter concluded that attending to philosophical and theoretical differences that determine values and attitudes associated with short-term versus long-term therapy may be a necessary component for the success of any teaching or training program in brief psychotherapy.

■ CLINICALLY RELEVANT RESEARCH ON BRIEF DYNAMIC PSYCHOTHERAPY

☐ The Therapeutic Alliance

The term *therapeutic alliance* typically refers to "the emotional bond and reciprocal involvement that develops between patient and therapist during the course of therapy" (Koss and Shiang 1993). The significance of at least an adequate alliance between patient and therapist extends to long-term therapy, but may be particularly important in brief therapy in which time constraints may preclude extended efforts to correct alliance problems.

Correlational investigations have consistently found the state of the alliance to be a predictor of therapeutic success. Indeed, some studies suggest that the quality of the alliance tends to be established (as good or poor) early in therapy (Strupp and Hadley 1979). Luborsky et al. (1985) reported the existence of a "helping alliance" to far outweigh the contribution of other factors, such as theoretical approach or use of techniques. Indeed, many brief dynamic therapies list the patient's ability to form a collaborative stance with the therapist as a selection criterion (Table 28-3). Such findings raise the question of what happens in cases of poor alliance.

Consistent with the general trend of findings, Marziali et al. (1981) found that patients rated as making a strong positive contribution to the alliance had good outcomes. However, in cases of poor outcome, patients with a "negative disposition to the treatment situation that persisted across the hours of the brief psychotherapy . . . [were] relatively intransigent to the therapist's efforts to shore up the alliance" (Marziali et al. 1981, p. 363). Henry et al. (1986) found that patient communications defined as hostile, withdrawn, or otherwise provocative tended to be met with complementary responses by the therapist. In other words, patient negativity tended to be met with subtly negative responses from the therapist, yielding a negative interaction sequence almost always associated with poor outcome. Rather than concluding that the therapist is helpless in the face of patient negativity or hostility, some authors have proposed the possibility of training therapists to rapidly detect and address such alliance problems (Butler and Strupp 1986; Levenson 1995).

☐ Long-Term Versus Short-Term Therapy

Howard et al. (1986) plotted improvement rates for a large number of studies as a function of time and concluded that 50% of patients show significant improvement by the 8th session and 75% by the 26th session. These figures are consistent with the 10- to 25-session limit of many brief dynamic therapies. Moreover, it should be noted that these 50% and 75% effectiveness marks were derived almost exclusively from studies of long-term or open-ended therapies, rather than of ones that were specifically intended to be brief or time-limited.

When evaluating such findings, one must consider the inherent limitations of research with long-term psychotherapies. For pragmatic reasons, research on long-term therapies usually involves observations of therapies in naturalistic studies, resulting in a loss of the experimental control that is possible in studies of shorter duration. Because more severely disturbed patients often end up in longer-term or more intensive treatment, naturalistic studies may be biased and random assignment to long- or short-term treatment can be hard to implement. Furthermore, it is widely recognized by long-term therapists that symptoms tend to diminish fairly quickly in the treatment process, yet substantive changes in the patient's personality, thought to underlie symptom formation, may take longer. Thus, patients continuing in longer-term therapy are presumably working on issues not directly reflected in the symptom checklists typically used in outcome studies. Any differential effects of long-term treatment may not be detected by standard measures. Although the current literature suggests that brief psychotherapy compares well with long-term therapy, many questions are left unanswered. It is likely premature to conclude that long-term treatment does not add substantially to therapeutic gains. It will be up to researchers in the future to clearly document the benefits of both short-term and longer-term treatments and to specify conditions for maximizing the effectiveness of treatments regardless of treatment length.

Much remains to be learned about who is an "appropriate" brief therapy patient. Attempts to use patient characteristics and performance criteria have not been as helpful as once hoped. We, therefore, take the position that, given the present state of knowledge, virtually any psychotherapy with virtually any patient can benefit from a "time-limited attitude" on the part of the therapist.

One of the most disturbing trends we see is that with the economically based, increased demand for briefer treatments, therapists are being mandated to do shorter-term inventions without adequate training. The future dynamic brief therapist is going to have to be more broadly trained in order to be able to use appropriately and flexibly a variety of intervention techniques and to work collaboratively with other health care providers. What we envision is an emphasis on a psychodynamic understanding of the patient to provide a guide for these appropriate interventions. As stated by Gabbard (1990, p. 4), "Dynamic psychiatry simply provides a coherent conceptual framework within which all treatments are prescribed. Regardless of whether the treatment is dynamic psychotherapy or pharmacotherapy, it is *dynamically informed.*" If brief dynamic therapists of the future emphasize the psychodynamic understanding of patients and their situations, they will have a basis for using any one of a number of specialized techniques, such as cognitive restructuring, hypnosis, psychopharmacology, or more traditionally recognizable psychodynamic interventions. As part of this approach, we predict there will be a liberating movement away from more elaborate metapsychological models, and an increased focus on clinical phenomena and descriptive formulations to guide effective and efficient treatment (Levenson and Hales 1993).

■ REFERENCES

Alexander F, French T: Psychoanalytic Therapy: Principles and Applications. New York, Ronald Press, 1946

Austad CS, Berman WH: Managed health care and the evolution of psychotherapy, in Psychotherapy in Managed Health Care: The Optimal Use of Time and Resources. Edited by Austad CS, Berman WH. Washington, DC, American Psychological Association, 1991, pp 3–18

Austad CS, DeStefano L, Kisch J: The health maintenance organization, II: implications for psychotherapy. Psychotherapy: Theory, Research and Practice 25:449–454, 1988

Barber JP, Crits-Christoph P: Comparison of the brief dynamic therapies, in Handbook of Short-Term Dynamic Psychotherapy. Edited by Crits-Christoph P, Barber JP. New York, Basic Books, 1991, pp 323–356

Binder JL, Henry WP, Strupp HH: An appraisal of selection criteria for dynamic psychotherapies and implications for setting time limits. Psychiatry 50:154–166, 1987

Bolter K: Differences in therapy-related values and attitudes between short-term and long-term therapists. Unpublished doctoral dissertation, California School of Professional Psychology, Berkeley, CA, 1987

Bolter K, Levenson H, Alvarez W: Differences in values between short-term and long-term therapists. Professional Psychology: Research and Practice 21:285–290, 1990

Budman SH, Armstrong E: Training for managed care settings: how to make it happen. Psychotherapy: Theory, Research and Practice 29:416–421, 1992

Budman SH, Gurman AS: The practice of brief therapy. Professional Psychology: Research and Practice 14:277–289, 1983

Budman SH, Gurman AS: Theory and Practice of Brief Psychotherapy. New York, Guilford, 1988

Budman SH, Feldman J, Bennett MJ: Adult mental health services in a health maintenance organization. Am J Psychiatry 136:392–395, 1979

Burlingame GM, Fuhriman A, Paul S, et al: Implementing a time-limited therapy program: differential effects of training and experience. Psychotherapy: Theory, Research and Practice 26:303–312, 1989

Butler SF, Strupp HH: "Specific" and "nonspecific" factors in psychotherapy: a problematic paradigm for psychotherapy research. Psychotherapy: Theory, Research and Practice 23:30–40, 1986

Clarkin JF, Frances A, Taintor Z, et al: Training in brief therapy: a survey of psychiatric residency programs. Am J Psychother 137:978–979, 1980

Crits-Christoph P, Barber JP: Handbook of Short-Term Dynamic Psychotherapy. New York, Basic Books, 1991

Crits-Christoph P, Barber JP, Kurcias JS: Introduction and historical background, in Handbook of Short-Term Dynamic Psychotherapy. Edited by Crits-Christoph P, Barber JP. New York, Basic Books, 1991, pp 1–12

Cummings NA: The dismantling of our health system: strategies for the survival of psychological practice. Am Psychol 41:426–431, 1986

Cummings NA: The future of psychotherapy: one psychologist's perspective. Am J Psychother 41:349–360, 1987

Davanloo H (ed): Basic Principles and Techniques in Short-Term Dynamic Psychotherapy. New York, Spectrum, 1978

Ferenczi S, Rank O: The Development of Psychoanalysis. New York, Nervous and Mental Disease Publication Company, 1925

Flegenheimer WV: Techniques of Brief Psychotherapy. New York, Jason Aronson, 1982

Frances A, Clarkin J: Parallel techniques in supervision and treatment. Psychiatr Q 53:242–248, 1981

Gabbard GO: Psychodynamic Psychiatry in Clinical Practice. Washington, DC, American Psychiatric Press, 1990

Haas LS, Cummings NA: Managed outpatient mental health plans: clinical, ethical, and practical guidelines for participation. Professional Psychology: Research and Practice 22:45–51, 1991

Henry WP, Schacht TE, Strupp HH: Structural analysis of social behavior: application to a study of interpersonal process in differential therapeutic outcome. J Consult Clin Psychol 54:27–31, 1986

Henry WP, Strupp HH, Butler SF, et al: Effects of training in time-limited dynamic psychotherapy: changes in therapist behavior. J Consult Clin Psychol 61:434–440, 1993

Howard KI, Kopta SM, Krause MS, et al: The dose-effect relationship in psychotherapy. Am Psychol 41:159–164, 1986

Hoyt MF: Therapist resistances to short-term dynamic psychotherapy. J Am Acad Psychoanal 13:93–112, 1985

Kamin DJ: Characteristics of brief psychotherapists: a survey of attitudes, training, and effectiveness. Unpublished doctoral dissertation, Ohio University, Athens, OH, 1992

Koss MP, Shiang J: Research on brief psychotherapy, in Handbook of Psychotherapy and Behavior Change, 4th Edition. Edited by Bergin AE, Garfield SL. New York, Wiley, 1993, pp 664–700

Levenson H: Time-Limited Dynamic Psychotherapy: A Guide to Clinical Practice. New York, Basic Books, 1995

Levenson H, Bolter K: Short-term psychotherapy values and attitudes: changes with training. Paper presented at the American Psychological Association Convention, Atlanta, GA, August 1988

Levenson H, Hales RE: Brief psychodynamically informed therapy for medically ill patients, in Medical-Psychiatric Practice, Vol 2. Edited by Stoudemire A, Fogel BS. Washington, DC, American Psychiatric Press, 1993, pp 3–37

Levenson H, Speed J, Budman S: Therapists' training and skill in brief therapy: a survey. Paper presented at the annual meeting of the Society for Psychotherapy Research, Berkeley, CA, June 1992

Luborsky L, McLellan AT, Woody GE, et al: Therapist success and its determinants. Arch Gen Psychiatry 42:602–611, 1985

Luborsky L, Crits-Christoph P, Mintz J, et al: Who Will Benefit from Psychotherapy? Predictive Psychotherapy Outcomes. New York, Basic Books, 1988

Malan DH: The Frontier of Brief Psychotherapy. New York, Plenum, 1976

Mann J: Time-Limited Psychotherapy. Cambridge, MA, Harvard University Press, 1973

Marziali E, Marmar C, Krupnick J: Therapeutic alliance scales: development and relationship to psychotherapy outcome. Am J Psychiatry 138:361–364, 1981

Peake TH, Bordin CM, Archer RP: Brief Psychotherapies: Changing Frames of Mind. Beverly Hills, CA, Sage, 1988

Phillips LE: The ubiquitous decay curve: delivery similarities in psychotherapy, medicine and addiction. Professional Psychology: Research and Practice 18:650–652, 1987

Reder P, Tyson RL: Patient dropout from individual psychotherapy: a review and discussion. Bull Menninger Clin 44:229–252, 1980

Sifneos PE: Short-Term Dynamic Psychotherapy: Evaluation and Technique, 2nd Edition. New York, Plenum, 1987

Speed JL: Therapists' practice, training, and skill in brief therapy: a survey of California and Massachusetts psychologists. Unpublished doctoral dissertation, Wright Institute Graduate School of Psychology, Berkeley, CA, 1992

Strupp HH, Binder JL: Psychotherapy in a New Key: A Guide to Time-Limited Dynamic Psychotherapy. New York, Basic Books, 1984

Strupp HH, Hadley SW: Specific vs nonspecific factors in psychotherapy: a controlled study of outcome. Arch Gen Psychiatry 36:1125–1136, 1979

Ursano RJ, Dressler DM: Brief versus long-term psychotherapy: clinician attitudes and organizational design. Compr Psychiatry 18:55–60, 1977

Weiss J, Sampson H, Mount Zion Psychotherapy Research Group: The Psychoanalytic Process: Theory, Clinical Observations, and Empirical Research. New York, Guilford, 1986

Winokur M, Dasberg H: Teaching and learning short-term dynamic psychotherapy: techniques and resistances. Bull Menninger Clin 47:36–52, 1983

Wolberg LR: Handbook of Short-Term Psychotherapy. New York, Thieme-Stratton, 1980

Psychoanalysis, Psychoanalytic Psychotherapy, and Supportive Psychotherapy

Robert J. Ursano, M.D.
Edward K. Silberman, M.D.

Frequently, psychopathology limits our ability to see options and exercise choices, leading to feelings, thoughts, fantasies, and actions that may be painful, restricted, and repetitive. Psychotherapy addresses these learned forms of behavior that affect health and performance. Originally called the "talking cure," psychotherapy is the generic term for a large number of treatment techniques that are directed toward changing behavior through verbal interchange. Psychotherapy provides understanding, support, new experiences, and new knowledge that can 1) result in learning, 2) increase the range of behaviors available to the patient, 3) relieve symptoms, and 4) alter maladaptive and unhealthy patterns of behavior. In the process of this reorganization, both perception and behavior change.

The target organ of psychotherapy is the brain. Feelings, thoughts, fantasies, and actions are brain functions. If behavior is to change, at some basic level brain function and activity must alter (Kandell 1989). If neuron A used to fire to neuron B, it must now stimulate neuron C. Just as past life experience affects the development and maturation of the brain, and therefore brain activity, so too does present life experience, including the experience of psychotherapy. Our social connectedness, a major focus of psychotherapeutic work, also mediates both morbidity and mortality (House et al. 1988) and serves to regulate bodily function (Hofer 1984). How the "outside" (i.e., life experience) changes what is inside (i.e., our biology) is fundamental to understanding brain function and to the effectiveness of all psychotherapies. Our understanding of these processes, the science of behavior change, is only now emerging (Ursano and Fullerton 1991).

Psychotherapy was defined by Sullivan (1954) as primarily a verbal interchange between two individuals in which one of these individuals is designated an expert and the other a help-seeker. These two persons work together to identify the patient's characteristic problems in living, with the hope of achieving behavioral change. What is dealt with in treatment is what the patient is able to bring into focus, what the patient can tolerate talking about, and what he or she can tolerate the therapist talking about (Coleman 1968).

All medical treatments, including psychotherapy, show the effects of nonspecific curative factors in their outcomes. These nonspecific curative factors, also called "placebo effects," include the presence of a confiding relationship; abreaction (i.e., the expression of intense feelings); the provision of new information; and the provision of a rationale or meaning (i.e., diagnosis) that organizes seemingly unrelated symptoms and events, and maximizes the patient's probability of success experiences (Frank 1971). In addition to these nonspecific factors, most medical treatments also have specific curative factors. Similarly, the psychotherapies identify specific technical interventions and procedures directed toward behavioral change.

The effectiveness of psychotherapy is not argued as it had been in the past (Shapiro and Shapiro 1982). Smith et al. (1980) showed an effect size of psychotherapy of 0.68, a level equivalent to that of several clinical trials that were stopped early because it would have been unethical to withhold such a clearly effective treatment from patients. Recently, Crits-Christoph (1992) demonstrated equivalent effect sizes in a review of well-designed studies of brief psychodynamic psychotherapy. However, the question of which psychotherapy for which patient and by which therapist is still unclear (Parloff 1982).

The cost-effectiveness of psychotherapeutic treatment also remains hotly debated (Krupnick and Pincus 1992). Individual psychotherapy has been shown to result in fewer days of hospitalization for patients on medical and surgical services of a general hospital. In health clinics or health maintenance organizations, brief psychotherapy decreases the number of visits to primary health care providers, reduces the number of laboratory and X-ray studies, decreases the number of prescriptions given, and, overall, reduces direct health care costs (Longobardi 1981;

Sharfstein et al. 1984). Mumford et al. (1984) found that outpatient psychotherapy resulted in a 33% average reduction in medical care utilization. Furthermore, these reductions occurred predominantly in the more expensive, inpatient medical services.

Although at times we speak of psychotherapy beginning as soon as the physician sees the patient, this hyperbole is used primarily to underscore the importance of interpersonal and transferential elements in the initial meeting with the patient. In fact, it is extremely important to distinguish the diagnostic interviews from the ongoing treatment. During the evaluation phase, the physician must assess the diagnosis and the patient's ego strength and physical health. In addition, the clinician must closely consider the selection criteria and the different treatment options, including "no treatment indicated" (Frances and Clarkin 1981). Through negotiation with the patient, a treatment decision is reached and the psychotherapy begins. Many patients, however, do not make it through the evaluation phase of seeking help. Repeatedly, it has been shown that more than 50% of patients drop out by five sessions. It is inappropriate to consider those who drop out as having been in psychotherapy. Clearly, some of these patients experience benefit during their short contact with mental health professionals (Malan et al. 1975)—some through the nonspecific curative factors of help seeking and others through guidance and crisis intervention. In addition, many may drop out because they did not receive what they were looking for.

The psychoanalytically oriented and supportive psychotherapies remain the most commonly used psychotherapies. Many of the principles of the psychodynamic/psychoanalytic treatments have been incorporated into other treatment modalities and into the clinical assessment process and ward milieu work. Understanding the principles and phenomena observed in psychodynamic treatment, therefore, is often critical to successful performance of other treatments and evaluation techniques (Gabbard 1990). In addition, skill in the briefer forms of psychotherapy is related to skill in the longer-term treatments, although these treatment approaches are not the same.

■ PSYCHOANALYTICALLY ORIENTED PSYCHOTHERAPIES

Primary to the psychodynamic (psychoanalytically oriented) treatments is the importance of the patient feeling engaged and involved in the work. Through the exploration of the patient's conflicts evidenced in symptoms, metaphors, and symbols, both defensive patterns and disturbances in present interpersonal relationships can be identified in the treatment setting as well as in the patient's life. The therapist's ability to hear what the patient has to say and to understand its meaning is central to all psychoanalytically oriented treatments. This facet of treatment demands skill in neutral listening and the ability to identify with the patient's perspective and worldview while not losing one's own. The therapist is always listening for the continuity present, but hidden, between each session (Coleman 1968). The therapist operates on the hypothesis that each session is related to the previous one.

In the initial phase of treatment, the therapeutic alliance is developed (Greenson 1965). The therapeutic alliance is the reality-based relationship between the analyst (or the therapist) and the patient that forms the basis of working together in a cooperative manner. The therapeutic alliance is nurtured through the identification of the patient's initial anxieties about beginning treatment.

Few empirical studies of psychoanalytic treatment have been done (e.g., Kantrowitz et al. 1990; Kernberg et al. 1972; Wallerstein 1992). The brief psychodynamic treatments have a somewhat greater empirical data base (e.g., Crits-Christoph 1992; Horowitz et al. 1986; Luborsky et al. 1988; Strupp 1980). In general, the studies that have been conducted support the efficacy of psychoanalytically oriented treatment approaches.

☐ Psychoanalysis

Psychoanalysis was developed by Sigmund Freud beginning in the late 19th century. Originally, Freud used hypnosis to recover forgotten memories related to traumas of early childhood. Historically, he progressed from hypnosis to the "pressure technique" and finally to the modern approach of using free association. Freud found that it was the subjective experience of events in childhood—that is, the psychic reality of the events—rather than the presence or absence of the actual events, that affected development and conflict formation. This discovery led Freud to identify the role of the unconscious and unremembered experiences of childhood and to develop a mechanism, psychoanalysis, to discover and bring these memories into awareness.

Freud identified dreams, slips of the tongue, and free association as important windows on the influence of childhood and the present conflicts of the patient. From the psychoanalytic view, an understanding of the conflicts experienced in childhood is important to gaining knowledge of and changing one's present behavior (Brenner 1976). The conflicts of childhood are called the "childhood neurosis." Conflicts are patterns of feelings, thoughts, and behavior that were "learned" during childhood. "Neurotic" conflicts result in the patient's feelings of anxiety and depression; somatic symptoms; work, social, or sexual inhibition; and maladaptive interpersonal relations. Typically such conflicts are between libidinal (i.e., sexual/bodily) and aggressive wishes. Libidinal wishes can be thought of as longings for sexual and emotional gratification. Aggressive wishes are destructive desires that either are primary or result from frustration and deprivation. The concept of sexual wishes is quite broad in psychoanalysis and is not limited to only genital feelings; sexual wishes include wishes to be held and touched, to control, to eat, and many others.

The goal of psychoanalysis is the elucidation of the childhood neurosis as it presents in the transference neurosis (Table 29–1). This primary focus is what distinguishes psychoanalysis from psychodynamic psychotherapy. Psychoanalysis focuses on the recovery of childhood experiences as they appear in the relationship with the analyst (Freud 1912/1958). This recreation in the doctor-patient relationship of a conflicted relationship with a childhood figure is the *transference neurosis.* Frequently, the transference is paternal or maternal, but it need not be. Sibling, aunt, uncle, and grandparent transferences are all important parts of psychoanalytic work. The transference neurosis (in contrast to transference phenomena) is the sustained appearance of the transference over time. When the transference neurosis is present, the patient experiences the analyst in the same manner as he or she once did the significant figure from the past. Frequently, this experience is accompanied by other elements of the past being experienced in the patient's life.

Several empirical studies support the importance of addressing the transference for a successful outcome of psychodynamic treatment (Fried et al. 1992; Luborsky and Crits-Christoph 1990; Marziali 1984).

Table 29–1. Psychoanalysis

Goal	Resolution of the childhood neurosis as it presents itself in the transference neurosis
Selection criteria	Experiences conflict that is primarily oedipal
	Experiences conflict as internal
	Is psychologically minded
	Is able to obtain symptom relief through understanding
	Is able to experience and observe strong affects without acting out
	Has supportive relationships available in both the present and the past
Duration	Four to five sessions per week; 3 to 6 years, average duration
Techniques	Free association
	Therapeutic alliance
	Neutrality
	Abstinence
	Defense analysis
	Interpretation of transference

Transference is the result of our tendency to see the past in the present, to exclude new information, and to see what is familiar. This "looking for the familiar" results in our reacting and responding in ways that are characteristic of our relationships with significant figures from our past. The analyst's relative abstinence (i.e., avoiding gratifying wishes) and neutrality (i.e., not encouraging one side or another of the patient's conflict—either the wishes or the defenses and prohibitions) help create a setting in which the transference can emerge and, more important, in which it can be observed and understood by the analyst and the patient. It is the contrast between the patient's experience of the analyst in the transference and his or her experience in the therapeutic alliance that facilitates the recognition that the transference thoughts and feelings are self-generated.

Countertransference comprises the analyst's transference responses to the patient. At times, countertransference is also used to describe the analyst's specific neurotic responses to the patient's transference. However, this is not clearly different from the first, more general, definition (Sandler et al. 1973). Countertransference is also a ubiquitous occurrence and not limited to the psychoanalytic setting. Countertransference is increased by life stress and unresolved conflicts in the analyst. It can appear as either an identification with or a reaction to the patient's conscious and unconscious fantasies, feelings, and behaviors (Racker 1957). Through analysis of his or her own countertransference reactions, the analyst recognizes subtle aspects of the transference relationship and is better able to understand the patient's experience (Searles 1965). Skill in recognizing countertransference and transference is an important part of the psychiatrist's armamentarium in all treatment settings. The design of the psychoanalytic treatment situation fosters the patient's observing capacity so that the transference neurosis can be analyzed (Stone 1961).

Modern psychoanalysis continues to require frequent meetings of the analyst and analysand—usually, four to five times per week. This frequency of sessions is continued, on the average, for 3 to 6 years. This intensity of meetings is necessary for the patient to develop sufficient trust to explore his or her inner fantasy life. In addition, frequent meetings enable the patient to explore fantasies rather than only the reality-based perceptions of life events. Individuals in crisis who are very focused on the real events in their life are not good candidates for psychoanalysis. In general, the psychoanalytic patient is encouraged to use the couch so that the patient's focus on fantasies rather than on reality will be further facilitated. In addition, the analyst usually sits out of view, allowing the patient to better elaborate his or her fantasies about the analyst.

Free association is a major element in the technique of psychoanalysis. Freud described free association through an analogy with a train ride (Freud 1913/1958). He suggested that if the analyst and analysand were riding together on a train and the analyst were blind, the analysand would not forget to describe the beautiful mountains or the ugly coal slags. The patient reports all thoughts that come to mind without censorship and without dismissing them as too trivial. In point of fact, free association is difficult to attain, and much of the work of psychoanalysis is based on identifying those places where free association breaks down (i.e., the occurrence of a defense, clinically experienced by the analyst as resistance).

Early in treatment, the analyst establishes a therapeutic alliance with the patient that allows for a reality-based consideration of the demands of the treatment and for a working collaboration between analyst and analysand toward the patient's understanding himself or herself (Greenson 1965). The analyst focuses on analyzing the defenses the patient uses to minimize conflict and disturbing affects (Freud 1913/1958, 1914/1958). Defenses such as intellectualization, reaction formation, denial, repression, and other neurotic cognitive mechanisms are identified and repeatedly interpreted to the patient. Through the analysis of defense, the working alliance strengthens and the patient's ability to observe internal fantasies increases. In addition, the patient's comfort with talking about his or her feelings with the analyst increases. In this way, the transference grows more available and can be analyzed.

The analysis of the patient's dreams is an important element of psychoanalytic treatment (Freud 1911/1958). Dreams, as well as slips of the tongue and symptoms, express the conflicts of the patient in "metaphor." They are a means for the patient to understand the feelings and thoughts that influence his or her life, that are out of awareness, and that often are derived from childhood experiences, beliefs, and views of the interpersonal world and familial behavior (Weiss and Sampson 1986).

The analyst uses a number of techniques in his or her interventions, including interpretation and clarification (Sandler et al. 1973). Classically, an interpretation is the linking together of the patient's experience of an event in the present with the transference experience of the analyst and the childhood-significant figure. Interpretations are rarely actually given in one sentence in one session. More frequently, interpretations occur over a period of time during which the past, the present, and the transference experiences are linked together.

Medications are infrequently used in psychoanalysis, although some analysts are attempting to use psychoanalysis with medication for affective disorders. Psychoanalysis is actually a highly supportive treatment for the individual who experiences frequent contact, quiet inquiry, and intellectual understanding as a supportive environment (de Jonghe et al. 1992; Wallerstein 1986). The analyst operates under several guiding principles that facilitate the analysis of the transference. These principles include 1) neutrality, by which the analyst favors neither the patient's wishes (i.e., id) nor the condemnations of these wishes (i.e., superego); and 2) abstinence, whereby the analyst does not provide gratification to the patient similar to that of the wished-for object (Freud 1915[1914]/1958). It is helpful in understanding the rule of abstinence to recognize a definition of transference used by Joseph Sandler. Sandler (1973) describes transference as the role pressure placed upon the analyst to conform to the behaviors of the significant individual from the past. Abstinence is the avoidance of becoming this figure *in reality* and gratifying these wishes or beliefs.

Psychoanalysis has been useful in the treatment of obsessional disorders, anxiety disorders, dysthymic disorders, and moderately severe personality disorders. Individuals with substantial preoedipal pathology, usually indicated by chaotic life settings and an inability to establish a supportive dyadic relationship, as is often seen in patients with narcissistic, borderline, schizoid, paranoid, and schizotypal personality disorders, are usually not felt to be candidates for traditional psychoanalysis. In the present, cost-effective climate, psychoanalysis is more frequently recommended after a course of brief psychotherapy has proved to be either ineffective or insufficient.

☐ Psychoanalytic Psychotherapy

Psychoanalytically oriented psychotherapy, also known as *psychoanalytic psychotherapy, psychodynamic psychotherapy,* and *explorative psychotherapy,* is a psychotherapeutic procedure that recognizes the development of transference and resistance in the psychotherapy setting (Bruch 1974). Both long-term and brief psychodynamic psychotherapy are possible. "Brief" and "long-term" describe the duration rather than the technique, focus, or goal of the psychoanalytically oriented psychotherapy (Ursano and Dressler 1977). Brief psychotherapy, in particular, requires the therapist to confront his or her own ambitiousness and perfectionism as well as any exaggerated ideal of personality structure and function.

Psychoanalytic psychotherapy is usually more focused than the extensive reworking of personality undertaken in psychoanalysis (Dewald 1978). In addition, psychoanalytic psychotherapy is oriented somewhat more to the here and now, with less attempt to reconstruct the developmental origins of conflicts. Psychoanalytically oriented psychotherapy may take as its entire goal the analysis of a set of defenses that are interfering with the patient's development. The accomplishment of this task may substantially open up the patient's life and development. Psychoanalytic psychotherapy recognizes and interprets transference when it occurs (Table 29–2). However, the entire treatment is not directed toward the establishment and analysis of the transference in the thorough manner of a psychoanalysis.

Table 29–2.   Psychoanalytic psychotherapy

Goal	Defense and transference analysis with limited reconstruction of the past
Selection criteria	When a narrower focus and less comprehensive outcome is acceptable The same selection criteria as in psychoanalysis are used but can include more seriously disturbed patients who can use understanding to resolve symptoms when supportive elements are available in the treatment.
Duration	One to three sessions per week for 1 to 6 years on average
Techniques	Therapeutic alliance Face to face Free association Defense and transference interpretation More use of clarification, suggestion, and learning through experience than in psychoanalysis Medication

Usually, patients in long-term psychoanalytic psychotherapy are seen one, two, or three times per week; twice per week is desirable in order to allow for sufficient intensity for the transference to unfold and to be interpreted. Patient and therapist meet in face-to-face encounters, with free association encouraged. Psychoanalytic psychotherapy may extend from several months to several years, at times being as long as a psychoanalysis. The length of treatment is determined by the number of focal problem areas undertaken in the treatment. Medications can be used in psychoanalytic psychotherapy and provide another means to titrate the level of regression a patient may experience. The therapist uses interpretations and clarifications as in psychoanalysis. In addition, however, the therapist may use other interpretative techniques such as suggestion, manipulation, and confrontation (Bibring 1954). Manipulation in this context refers to learning from experience, such as pointing out that the therapist does not respond in the expected transferential manner. Confrontation is not "fighting" but rather pointing out to the patient when something is being denied or avoided.

Patients with major depression and schizophrenia use psychotherapy to modify illness-onset conditions and facilitate readjustment, recovery, and integration into family and community. In long-term psychoanalytic psychotherapy, the regressive tendencies of such patients can be titrated with greater elements of support, the use of medication as needed, and greater reality feedback through the face-to-face encounter with the therapist. Research has confirmed the importance of interactional variables and support to the outcome in psychotherapy (Luborsky et al. 1988; Strupp and Binder 1984).

The opening phase of psychodynamic psychotherapy is often marked by the activation of the magical expectations of the patient and the belief that past pains will now be resolved. Important aspects of the current problems, the patient's characteristic defense mechanisms and coping styles, and the developmental roots of the central issue become clearer during this phase. In the middle phase of treatment, resistance is likely to appear, as well as the negative transference. The patient experiences the frustration that all of the wished-for changes are not occurring. Defenses are identified and analyzed, and usually the transference is sufficiently evident to be worked with. In the end phase of treatment, termination and the patient's resistances to termination are prominent. Termination is based on having reached a series of life goals that allows the patient to continue on a normal developmental path.

■ INTERPERSONAL PSYCHOTHERAPY

Interpersonal psychotherapy (IPT) is a psychotherapy developed by Klerman et al. (1984). Either brief or longer term, IPT focuses on current interpersonal problems in outpatient nonbipolar, nonpsychotic depressed patients. This psychotherapy has also been used in treating drug abuse. It did not, however, add significantly to outcome when patients were already in a well-run treatment program that included weekly group psychotherapy (Rounsaville et al. 1985). IPT derives from the interpersonal school of psychiatry that originated with Adolf Meyer and Harry Stack Sullivan. The understanding of social supports and of attachment provides further theoretical underpinning for this form of psychotherapy. IPT focuses on reassurance, clarification of feeling states, improvement in interpersonal communication, testing of perception, and interpersonal skills rather than personality reconstruction.

In interpersonal psychotherapy the therapist focuses on the patient's current social functioning (Table 29–3). A complete inventory of current and past significant interpersonal relationships, including the family of origin, friendships, and relations in the community, is a part of the evaluation phase. Patterns of authority, dominance and submission, dependency and autonomy, intimacy, affection, and activities are observed. Cognitions are generally seen as beliefs and attitudes about norms, expectations and roles, and role performance. Defense mechanisms may be recognized, but they are explored in terms of interpersonal relations. Similarly, dreams may be examined as a reflection of current interpersonal problems. The IPT therapist may explore distorted thinking by comparing what the patient says with what he or she does, or by identifying the patient's view of an interpersonal relationship (Klerman et al. 1984).

Table 29–3.   Interpersonal psychotherapy

Goal	Improvement in current interpersonal skills
Selection criteria	Outpatient, nonbipolar, nonpsychotic depression
Duration	Short- and long-term Usually once-weekly meetings
Techniques	Reassurance Clarification of feeling states Improvement of interpersonal communication Testing perceptions Development of interpersonal skills Medication

Interpersonal psychotherapy has been primarily used in the treatment of depressed patients. In the opening phase of IPT, a detailed symptom history is taken, usually using a structured interview. The symptoms are reviewed with the patient, and the patient receives explicit information about the natural course of depression as a clinical condition. A second major task of this phase is the assessment of the patient's interpersonal problem areas. There is an attempt to identify one or more of four problem areas: grief reaction, interpersonal disputes, role transition, and/or interpersonal deficits. Each of these areas is felt to be related to depression.

The middle phase of treatment is directed toward resolving the problem area(s). Clarifying positive and negative feeling states, identifying past models for relationships, and guiding and encouraging the patient in examining and choosing alternative courses of action constitute the basic techniques for handling each problem area.

Clinical trials have demonstrated the advantage of maintenance IPT in enhancing social functioning in recovery from depression and in reducing symptoms and improving functioning during the acute phase of a depressive episode. These effects require 6 to 8 months to become apparent. Depressed patients on combined pharmacotherapy and IPT have the best outcomes (DiMascio et al. 1979; Weissman et al. 1981).

■ SUPPORTIVE PSYCHOTHERAPY

Despite its ubiquitous use by psychiatrists, *supportive psychotherapy* has traditionally been viewed as a residual category to be prescribed for those patients not amenable to other forms of treatment. Its techniques have often been defined negatively, that is, in terms of what to avoid rather than what to do (Wallace 1983; Winston et al. 1986). Supportive psychotherapy can better be defined by its specific goal than by technical procedures. Supportive psychotherapy aims to help the patient maintain or reestablish his or her best possible level of functioning given the limitations of his or her illness, personality, native ability, and life circumstances (Table 29–4). In general, this goal distinguishes supportive psychotherapy from the change-oriented psychotherapies, which aim to reverse primary disease processes and symptoms or restructure personality. However, theorists in self psychology have pointed out that providing a "holding environment," listening empathically, and being a safe and reliable object of identification, which constitute the foundation of supportive therapy, may themselves lead to strengthening of the ego and increased independence of the patient (Ornstein 1986).

☐ Indications

Most often, change or insight-oriented therapy is automatically considered the treatment of first choice, with supportive therapy assigned to those patients who are not considered to be able to change. Some authors, however, have suggested that the two types of treatment should be considered on a more equal basis, because a briefer or less intense treatment may be in many patients' best interest as a treatment of first choice (Pinsker et al. 1991; Rockland 1989b). Such considerations become especially relevant as economic pressures force clinicians to prescribe the most efficient among potentially effective treatments. In common clinical practice, patients at both ends of the health-sickness continuum receive supportive psychotherapy: those who are generally very healthy and

---

Table 29–4.   Supportive psychotherapy

Goal	Support of reality testing
	Provision of ego support
	Maintenance or reestablishment of usual level of functioning
Selection criteria	Very healthy individual faced with overwhelming crises
	Patient with ego deficits
Duration	Days, months, or years—as needed
Techniques	Predictable availability of therapist
	Use of interpretation to strengthen defenses
	Maintenance of reality-based working relationship grounded in support, concern, and problem solving
	Suggestion, reinforcement, advice, reality testing, cognitive restructuring, reassurance, limit setting, and environmental interventions
	Medication
	Psychodynamic life narrative

---

well adapted but who have become impaired in response to stressful life circumstances, and those who have serious illnesses that cannot be cured. The typical candidate for supportive psychotherapy has significant deficits in ego functioning, including the following:

1. Poor reality testing
2. Poor impulse control
3. Poor interpersonal relations
4. Poor balance of affects
5. Lack of ability to sublimate
6. Low capacity for introspection
7. Low verbal ability

A variety of other factors have been proposed as exclusion criteria for insight-oriented psychotherapy and as possible indications for supportive psychotherapy. Motivation has been stressed by many authors as of importance. However, it has yet to be determined whether motivation for symptom change, for behavioral change, for a relationship with the therapist, or for insight (among others) is crucial in assigning patients to explorative/change-oriented (psychodynamic, interpersonal, and cognitive) versus supportive psychotherapy (Bloch 1979). Alexithymic patients are generally referred for supportive rather than insight psychotherapy. Such patients are characterized by an inability to find words to describe their emotions (Sifneos 1975). Patients who are very passive and who lack the conviction that their own efforts are effective may be candidates for supportive rather than insight-oriented psychotherapy (Werman 1981). Patients who derive significant practical benefit from their illness, such as financial or emotional support (i.e., secondary gain), may also be appropriate for supportive psychotherapy rather than an insight-oriented approach (Persson and Alström 1983). Ego strength and the ability to form relationships may be more important than diagnosis in the selection of patients for supportive psychotherapy (Werman 1984). The patient's ability to relate to the therapist and the patient's past history of personal relationships, work and educational performance, and use of leisure time bear importantly on the treatment recommendation.

☐ Techniques

The technique of supportive psychotherapy can be divided into aspects of the therapist-patient relationship and active interventions by the therapist (Pine 1976). The early mother-child relationship has special implications for supportive psychotherapy. The therapist who is predictably available and safe assumes some of the holding functions of the good parent. In such a therapeutic situation, the patient is able to identify with and incorporate the well-functioning aspects of the therapist—such as the capacity for self-observation and the ability to tolerate ambivalence (Pine 1976). The patient's use of the therapeutic relationship to achieve greater autonomy may in some ways parallel the child's growing independence as the child's image of the mothering figure is increasingly internalized (Adler 1982). The use of the mothering figure as a mirror of internal reality or an object of idealization by the child may be necessary to the child's achievement of a cohesive, stable sense of self. Similarly, permitting the patient to see himself or herself "mirrored" in the therapist and part of an idealized parental figure over long periods of time may stabilize new internal structures and behaviors. Such an approach is in contrast to psychoanalytically oriented psychotherapy, in which such attitudes are generally interpreted as a defense.

Patients in supportive psychotherapy frequently develop intensely dependent and ambivalent relationships with the therapist. This relationship often parallels the separation-individuation process of normal child development (Adler 1982). Patients in need of supportive psychotherapy typically fear the destructive power of their rage and envy. They may be helped to modulate their emotional reactions by the reliable presence of the therapist and a therapeutic relationship that remains unchanged in the face of emotional onslaughts.

The therapist uses interpretation to strengthen defenses and fosters the supportive relationship by refraining from interpreting positive transference feelings and waiting until the intensity of feelings has abated before commenting about negative transference feelings (Buckley 1986). Interpretations of the negative transference are limited to those needed to ensure that the treatment is not disrupted. While maintaining a friendly stance toward the patient, the therapist must respect the patient's need to establish a comfortable degree of distance (Robinson and Flaherty 1982). The rapport with the patient, which the supportive psychotherapist tries to establish, differs from the "therapeutic alliance" of insight-oriented therapy. The doctor-patient relationship in supportive psychotherapy does not require the patient to observe and report on his or her own feelings and behavior to the same extent as in the change-oriented, explorative psychotherapies. In addition, the therapist acts more as a guide and a mentor. There is evidence that with more severely ill patients this may take many months, in contrast to work with healthier patients, in which the therapeutic alliance tends to develop early or not at all (Docherty 1989).

The suitability of an interpretation may depend more on the manner in which it is given than on the content (Pine 1986). In supportive psychotherapy, interpretations are phrased to relieve the patient of the pressure to make an immediate response. The patient can be given advance warning that a potentially painful comment is coming. Such techniques are directed toward sufficiently modulating the patient's emotional response so that the interpretation can be tolerated and processed.

The therapist must be available in a way that is regular and predictable. Rather than approaching the patient as a "blank screen," the therapist must actively demonstrate concern, involvement, sympathy, and a supportive attitude. Many of the active interventions of supportive psychotherapy are based on the principle of "substitutive psychotherapy" (Werman 1984): the psychotherapy substitutes for capacities that the patient lacks. This is sometimes stated as the therapist acting as an "auxiliary ego" for the patient. The deficient ego capacities for which substitution is needed may include basic elements of self-perception such as a stable sense of self over time and a clear recognition of boundaries between one's self and others. Techniques that may support the patients' deficient ego functions include suggestion, reinforcement, advice, reality testing, cognitive restructuring, reassurance, clarification, limit setting, environmental interventions, and concurrent use of medication (Rockland 1989b; Werman 1984).

The defenses of denial and avoidance may be handled by encouraging the patient to discuss alternative behaviors, goals, and interpretations of events (Castelnuovo-Tedesco 1986). The therapist tries to reinforce the most adaptive defenses of which the patient is capable while discouraging use of the more primitive defenses. Reassurance has a variety of forms in supportive psychotherapy including supporting an adaptive level of denial, the patient's experience of the therapist's empathic attitude, or the therapist's reality testing of the patient's negatively biased self-evaluations or evaluations of his or her situation (Werman 1984). Reassurance requires a clear understanding of what the patient fears. Overt expressions of interest and concern may be reassuring to a patient who fears rejection, but threatening to one who fears intrusion. In a similar vein, Rockland (1989a, 1989b) stresses the need to tailor interventions to fit the character traits and unconscious transferences of the patient.

Communication of the therapist's knowledge of the patient and his or her circumstances is a "pedagogical" aspect of supportive psychotherapy (Werman 1981). The therapist uses simple, concrete language that has personal meaning to the patient. The therapist may discuss with the highly inhibited patient the advantages of being more assertive or spontaneous, or he or she may point out to the patient with poorly developed social controls the dangers of impulsive behavior. Interpretive comments may be used by the supportive therapist, although the form and content of interpretations usually differ from those in psychoanalytically oriented psychotherapy. Interpretations in supportive psychotherapy are given in a manner consistent with the principle of decreasing (rather than increasing) anxiety and strengthening (rather than loosening) defenses. Thus, they deal with material close to the patient's awareness rather than with unconscious material that might be distressing or frightening, and can often serve to strengthen the defenses of intellectualization and rationalization (Werman 1984).

The "psychodynamic life narrative" can be used as a supportive interpretation (Viederman 1983). The narrative is the formulation of the patient's current difficulties as the inevitable product of previous life experiences. The narrative uses only facts the patient is already aware of and explanations that do not threaten self-esteem. It serves to give the patient a sense of control through understanding, to help him or her accept emotional responses as justifiable and inevitable, and to strengthen the alliance with the therapist, who is seen as giving something valuable. Such a narrative may be contraindicated in patients who can benefit from psychoanalytically oriented psychotherapy, because it will strengthen defensive intellectualization, close off avenues to greater understanding, and possibly stir powerful expectations of gratification from the therapist.

Intellectualized interpretations may be useful in discussing dreams in supportive psychotherapy (Werman 1978). In addition, these interpretations may foster an increased capacity for self-observation (Ermutlu 1977). A technique that has been used for the latter purpose consists of suggesting that pathological behavior is the product of a "sick part" of the patient that is distinct from the patient as a whole. This "induced dichotomy of personality" helps the patient recognize both the pathological behaviors and the better functioning aspects of himself or herself, and fosters his or her identification with more mature, adaptive traits.

The therapist's expression of interest, advice giving, and facilitation of ventilation reinforce desired behaviors. Expressions of interest and solicitude are positively reinforcing. Advice can lead to behavioral change if it is specific and applies to frequently occurring behaviors of the patient. Desired behaviors can be rewarded by the therapist's approval and by social reinforcement. Ventilation of emotions is useful only if the therapist can help the patient safely contain and limit these emotions, thus extinguishing the anxiety response to emotional expression.

Except in the case of brief treatment aimed at supporting the patient through a life crisis or traumatic event, termination in supportive psychotherapy is not a goal in the same sense as it is in change-oriented therapies. In the most usual case, the patient's functional deficits necessitate ongoing, long-term support. In such a case, keeping the patient in treatment might be a more appropriate goal than terminating. A second possibility is that the treatment may gradually evolve to become more change-oriented, including modification of ego structure and improvement in function.

☐ Efficacy

Very little information is available on the effectiveness of supportive psychotherapy. Most data come from studies in which supportive psychotherapy has been used as a control in testing the efficacy of other treatments (Conte and Plutchik 1986). In such studies, the procedures used in supportive psychotherapy tend to be poorly specified, and no attempts are made to correlate individual supportive techniques with outcome. Despite its limitations, the research literature offers some evidence that supportive psychotherapy is an effective treatment. The Menninger Psychotherapy Project assessed long-term explorative and supportive psychotherapy in a group of patients with mixed symptomatic and personality pathology (Wallerstein 1986). A surprising result of the study was that the techniques of supportive therapy produced improvement in functioning and ego strength comparable to that with expressive and insight-oriented techniques. Studies of patients with anxiety disorders have also demonstrated the efficacy of supportive therapy (Klein et al. 1983).

While research on the psychotherapy of schizophrenia has failed to demonstrate the benefit of explorative techniques, the use of supportive techniques appears more promising. May (1968) found that nonchronic schizophrenic inpatients had somewhat better outcomes when treated with supportive psychotherapy and antipsychotic medication than when treated with medication alone. When these approaches were used singly, however, medication was more effective than psychotherapy.

A larger body of research exists indicating that supportive psychotherapy is an effective component of the treatment of patients with a variety of medical illnesses. Forester et al. (1985) assessed the effects of supportive psychotherapy on patients undergoing radiation treatment. The psychotherapy, which consisted of educational clarification of emotional issues and ventilation of feelings, resulted in less emotional distress and fewer complaints of side effects than were evident in the control group, which received no psychotherapy. Mumford et al. (1982) reviewed controlled studies of psychotherapy treatment of patients recovering from myocardial infarction and surgery and found positive effects of the treatment on the experience of pain, cooperation with treatment, incidence of complications, speed of recovery, and number of days in hospital.

■ EDUCATION

The importance of individual psychotherapy to the practicing clinician makes mandatory the inclusion of instruction on psychotherapy in psychiatric residency training. The skills learned in psychotherapy—both the ability to intervene and the ability to recognize transference, counter-transference, and defense—are important in many other treatment modalities. The clinician skilled in recognizing these phenomena is better able to perform a wide array of treatments, including medication management, family therapy, inpatient psychiatric treatment, consultation-liaison, and many others.

Psychiatric residents must develop skills to apply all psychotherapeutic treatment modalities and to understand their indications and contraindications. Psychoanalysis, with its extended intensive training requirements, is essentially a subspecialty area and is now generally pursued postresidency. It offers the opportunity for specific patients to gain broad-based understanding in a generally supportive environment. Supportive psychotherapy, the mainstay of psychiatric treatment, is much more complicated than is often recognized. The understanding of which patient for which treatment at which time is as critical for the prescription of psychotherapy as it is for the prescription of psychopharmacological agents (Frances et al. 1984). With the decrease in the number of psychoanalysts in medical school education, learning the indications for referral for psychoanalysis may be increasingly difficult for future psychiatrists. The brief psychotherapies are best taught in conjunction with the discussion of the principles of long-term psychotherapy, and in the context of learning psychodynamic formulations of pathology and the ways in which defenses, transferences, and countertransferences appear in the psychotherapeutic dyad.

■ REFERENCES

Adler E: Supportive psychotherapy revisited. Hillside J Clin Psychiatry 4:3–13, 1982

Bibring E: Psychoanalysis and the dynamic psychotherapies. J Am Psychoanal Assoc 2:745–770, 1954

Bloch S: Assessment of patients for psychotherapy. Br J Psychiatry 135:193–208, 1979

Brenner C: Psychoanalytic Technique and Psychic Conflict. New York, International Universities Press, 1976

Bruch H: Learning Psychotherapy: Rationale and Ground Rules. Cambridge, MA, Harvard University Press, 1974

Buckley P: [Supportive psychotherapy] A neglected treatment. Psychiatric Annals 16:515–517, 521, 1986

Castelnuovo-Tedesco P: The Twenty-Minute Hour: A Guide to Brief Psychotherapy for the Physician. Washington, DC, American Psychiatric Press, 1986

Coleman JV: Aims and conduct of psychotherapy. Arch Gen Psychiatry 18:1–6, 1968

Conte HR, Plutchik R: Controlled research in supportive psychotherapy. Psychiatric Annals 16:530–533, 1986

Crits-Christoph P: The efficacy of brief dynamic psychotherapy: a meta-analysis. Am J Psychiatry 149:151–158, 1992 de Jonghe F, Rijnierse P, Janssen R: The role of support in psychoanalysis. J Am Psychoanal Assoc 40:475–499, 1992

Dewald P: The process of change in psychoanalytic psychotherapy. Arch Gen Psychiatry 35:535–542, 1978

DiMascio A, Weissman MM, Prusoff BA, et al: Differential symptom reduction by drugs and psychotherapy in acute depression. Arch Gen Psychiatry 36:1450–1456, 1979

Docherty JP: The individual psychotherapies: efficacy, syndrome-based treatments, and the therapeutic alliance, in Outpatient Psychiatry: Diagnosis and Treatment, 2nd Edition. Edited by Lazare A. Baltimore, MD, Williams & Wilkins, 1989, pp 624–644

Ermutlu I: Induced dichotomy of personality as a technique in supportive psychotherapy. Psychiatric Forum 7(1):19–22, 1977

Forester B, Kornfeld DS, Fleiss JL: Psychotherapy during radiotherapy: effects on emotional and physical distress. Am J Psychiatry 142:22–27, 1985

Frances A[J], Clarkin JF: No treatment as the prescription of choice. Arch Gen Psychiatry 38:542–545, 1981

Frances AJ, Clarkin J, Perry S: Differential Therapeutics in Psychiatry: The Art and Science of Treatment Selection. New York, Brunner/Mazel, 1984

Frank JD: Therapeutic factors in psychotherapy. Am J Psychother 25:350–361, 1971

Freud S: The handling of dream-interpretation in psycho-analysis (1911), in The Standard Edition of the Complete Psychological Works of Sigmund Freud, Vol 12. Translated and edited by Strachey J. London, Hogarth Press, 1958, pp 89–96

Freud S: The dynamics of transference (1912), in The Standard Edition of the Complete Psychological Works of Sigmund Freud, Vol 12. Translated and edited by Strachey J. London, Hogarth Press, 1958, pp 97–108

Freud S: On beginning the treatment (further recommendations on the technique of psycho-analysis I) (1913), in The Standard Edition of the Complete Psychological Works of Sigmund Freud, Vol 12. Translated and edited by Strachey J. London, Hogarth Press, 1958, pp 121–144

Freud S: Remembering, repeating and working-through (further recommendations on the technique of psycho-analysis II) (1914), in The Standard Edition of the Complete Psychological Works of Sigmund Freud, Vol 12. Translated and edited by Strachey J. London, Hogarth Press, 1958, pp 145–156

Freud S: Observations on transference-love (further recommendations on the technique of psycho-analysis III) (1915[1914]), in The Standard Edition of the Complete Psychological Works of Sigmund Freud, Vol 12. Translated and edited by Strachey J. London, Hogarth Press, 1958, pp 157–173

Fried D, Crits-Christoph P, Luborsky L: The first empirical demonstration of transference in psychotherapy, J Nerv Ment Dis 180:326–331, 1992

Gabbard GO: Psychodynamic Psychiatry in Clinical Practice. Washington, DC, American Psychiatric Press, 1990

Greenson RR: The working alliance and the transference neurosis. Psychoanal Q 34:155–181, 1965

Hofer MA: Relationships as regulators: a psychobiologic perspective on bereavement. Psychosom Med 46:183–197, 1984

Horowitz MJ, Marmar CR, Weiss DS, et al: Comprehensive analysis of change after brief dynamic psychotherapy. Am J Psychiatry 143:582–589, 1986

House JS, Landis KR, Umberson D: Social relationships and health. Science 241:540–545, 1988

Kandell ER: Genes, nerve cells, and the remembrance of things past. J Neuropsychiatry Clin Neurosci 1:103–125, 1989

Kantrowitz JL, Katz AL, Paolitto F: Followup of psychoanalysis five to ten years after termination, I: stability of change. J Am Psychoanal Assoc 38:471–496, 1990

Kernberg OF, Burstein ED, Coyne L, et al: Psychotherapy and psychoanalysis: final report of the Menninger Foundation's Psychotherapy Research Project. Bull Menninger Clin 36:1–275, 1972

Klein DF, Zitrin CM, Woerner MG, et al: Treatment of phobias, II: behavior therapy and supportive psycotherapy: are there any specific ingredients? Arch Gen Psychiatry 40:139–145, 1983

Klerman GL, Weissman MM, Rounsaville BJ, et al: Interpersonal Psychotherapy of Depression. New York, Basic Books, 1984

Krupnick JL, Pincus HA: The cost-effectiveness of psychotherapy: a plan for research. Am J Psychiatry 149:1295–1305, 1992

Loewald HW: On the therapeutic action of psychoanalysis, in Papers on Psychoanalysis. New Haven, CT, Yale University Press, 1980, pp 221–256

Longobardi PG: The impact of a brief psychological intervention on medical care utilization in an army health care setting. Med Care 19:655–671, 1981

Luborsky L, Crits-Christoph P: Understanding Transference, New York, Basic Books, 1990

Luborsky L, Crits-Christoph P, Mintz J, et al: Who Will Benefit From Psychotherapy. New York, Basic Books, 1988

Malan DH, Heath ES, Bacal HA, et al: Psychodynamic changes in untreated neurotic patients, II: apparently genuine improvements. Arch Gen Psychiatry 32:110–126, 1975

Marziali EA: Prediction of outcome of brief psychotherapy from therapist interpretive interventions. Arch Gen Psychiatry 41:301–304, 1984

May PRA: Treatment of Schizophrenia: A Comparative Study of Five Treatment Methods. New York, Science House, 1968

Mumford E, Schlesinger H, Glass CV: The effects of psychological intervention on recovery from surgery and heart attacks: an analysis of the literature. Am J Public Health 72:141–151, 1982

Mumford E, Schlesinger HJ, Glass GV, et al: A new look at evidence about reduced cost of medical utilization following mental health treatment. Am J Psychiatry 141:1145–1158, 1984

Ornstein A: Supportive psychotherapy: a comtemporary view. Clinical Social Work Journal 14:14–30, 1986

Parloff MB: Psychotherapy research evidence and reimbursement decisions: Bambi meets Godzilla. Am J Psychiatry 139:718–727, 1982

Persson G, Alström JE: A scale for rating suitability for insight-oriented psychotherapy. Acta Psychiatr Scand 68:117–125, 1983

Pine F: On therapeutic change: perspective from a parent-child model. Psychoanalysis and Contemporary Science 5:537–569, 1976

Pine F: [Supportive psychotherapy] A psychoanalytic perspective. Psychiatric Annals 16:526–529, 1986

Pinsker H, Rosenthal R, McCullough L: Dynamic supportive psychotherapy, in Handbook of Short-Term Dynamic Psychotherapy. Edited by Crits-Cristoph P, Barben JP. New York, Basic Books, 1991, pp 220–247

Racker H: Meanings and uses of countertransference. Psychoanal Q 26:303–357, 1957

Robinson MV, Flaherty JA: Self-regulation of distance in supportive psychotherapy. Clinical Social Work Journal 10:209–217, 1982

Rockland LH: Psychoanalytically oriented supportive therapy: literature review and techniques. J Am Acad Psychoanal 17:451–462. 1989a

Rockland LH: Supportive Therapy: A Psychodynamic Approach. New York, Basic Books, 1989b

Rounsaville BJ, Gawin F, Kleber H: Interpersonal psychotherapy adapted for ambulatory cocaine abusers. Am J Drug Alcohol Abuse 11:171–191, 1985

Sandler J, Dare C, Holder A: The Patient and the Analyst: The Basis of the Psychoanalytic Process. New York, International Universities Press, 1973

Searles HF: Collected Papers on Schizophrenia and Related Subjects. New York, International Universities Press, 1965

Shapiro DA, Shapiro D: Meta-analysis of comparative therapy outcome studies: a replication and refinement. Psychol Bull 92:581–604, 1982

Sharfstein SS, Muszynski S, Myers E: Health Insurance and Psychiatric Care: Update and Appraisal. Washington, DC, American Psychiatric Press, 1984

Sifneos PE: Problems of psychotherapy of patients with alexithymic characteristics and physical disease. Psychother Psychosom 26:65–70, 1975

Smith ML, Glass GV, Miller TI: The Benefits of Psychotherapy. Baltimore, MD, Johns Hopkins University Press, 1980

Stone L: The Psychoanalytic Situation: An Examination of Its Development and Essential Nature. New York, International Universities Press, 1961

Strupp HH: Success and failure in time-limited psychotherapy: with special reference to the performance of a lay counselor. Arch Gen Psychiatry 37:831–841, 1980

Strupp HH, Binder J: Psychotherapy in a New Key: Time-Limited Dynamic Psychotherapy. New York, Basic Books, 1984

Sullivan HS: The Psychiatric Interview. Edited by Perry HS, Gawel ML. New York, WW Norton, 1954

Ursano RJ, Dressler DM: Brief versus long-term psychotherapy: clinician attitudes and organizational design. Compr Psychiatry 18:55–60, 1977

Ursano RJ, Fullerton CS: Psychotherapy: medical intervention and the concept of normality, in The Diversity of Normal Behavior: Further Contributions to Normatology. Edited by Offer D, Sabshin M. New York, Basic Books, 1991, pp 39–59

Viederman M: The psychodynamic life narrative: a psychotherapeutic intervention useful in crisis situations. Psychiatry 46:236–246, 1983

Wallace ER: Dynamic Psychiatry in Theory and Practice. Philadelphia, PA, Lea & Febiger, 1983

Wallerstein RS: Forty-Two Lives in Treatment: A Study of Psychoanalysis and Psychotherapy. New York, Guilford, 1986

Wallerstein RS: Followup in psychoanalysis: what happens to treatment gains. J Am Psychoanal Assoc 40:665–690, 1992

Weiss J, Sampson H: The Psychoanalytic Process: Theory, Clinical Observation and Empirical Research. New York, Guilford, 1986

Weissman MM, Klerman GL, Prusoff BA, et al: Depressed outpatients: results one year after treatment with drugs and/or interpersonal psychotherapy. Arch Gen Psychiatry 38:51–55, 1981

Werman DS: The use of dreams in psychotherapy: practical guidelines. Canadian Psychiatric Association Journal 23:153–158, 1978

Werman DS: Technical aspects of supportive psychotherapy. Psychiatr J Univ Ottawa 6:153–160, 1981

Werman DS: The Practice of Supportive Psychotherapy. New York, Brunner/Mazel, 1984

Winston A, Pinsker H, McCullough L: A review of supportive psychotherapy. Hosp Community Psychiatry 37:1105–1114, 1986

Behavior Therapy

W. Stewart Agras, M.D.
Robert I. Berkowitz, M.D.

Behavior therapy has developed as a scientific approach to human behavior change. Among the basic principles underlying the conceptual basis for behavior therapy are the following:

1. Both normal and abnormal behaviors are assumed to be learned and maintained in the same way; thus, procedures that alter normal behaviors will also be useful in altering deviant behaviors. An example of this is positive reinforcement, which affects a wide range of behaviors across a variety of different species and which has proven useful in modifying many problem behaviors.
2. The social environment plays a key role in the development and maintenance of both normal and abnormal behaviors. A consequence of this view is that the patient's environment may need to be altered to maintain newly acquired behaviors and prevent relapse.
3. The major focus of treatment is on the behavior problem itself, and, thus, specification of both the behaviors to be changed and the circumstances presently maintaining those behaviors is an important facet of assessment and treatment. Behaviors requiring treatment will usually be broken up into discrete components, each of which will be treated using individually tailored procedures depending on the behavior and its antecedents and consequences.

4. Behavior therapy is based on a scientific approach to treatment. Treatment procedures must be well specified so that they can be replicated by others; this process of specification involves the development of detailed treatment manuals. Treatment procedures must be evaluated in controlled experiments and the active components of treatment separated from the inactive components by additive clinical experimental designs.

Behavior therapy has changed over the years. In the early days, because it arose in sharp contrast to psychoanalytic theory and practice, there was a distinct tendency for antagonism to arise between the two fields. Yet the contrasting theories—one accentuating environmental effects, the other focusing upon hypothetical internal constructs—gave rise to vigorous and stimulating debate, which in turn shaped the way in which behavior therapy evolved. As the body of research findings developed, behavior therapy became an autonomous field—another, yet distinctive, school of psychotherapy.

More recently, *social-cognitive learning theory* (Bandura 1986) has become the most widely accepted theoretical underpinning for behavior therapy. This theory incorporates elements of both Pavlovian and Skinnerian theories, but goes beyond these in postulating an interaction between environment, behavior, and cognitive processes. Not only does the environment affect the person, but the person can alter his or her personal environment, thus affecting future behavior. Reinforcement is not viewed as the automatic effect of reward, but rather as a source of information about the potential effects of future behavior. Similarly, classical conditioning is no longer viewed as an automatic result of the occurrence of two stimuli occurring closely in time. Recent experimental work has demonstrated that prior experience and recognition of the relatedness of events are often crucial to this type of learning. Therefore, cognitive processes are recognized as important modulators of behavior. Among these processes are expectations, including *outcome expectancies,* defined as the degree of certainty an individual has that a particular behavior will result in a particular outcome, and *efficacy expectancies,* the degree of confidence that individuals have in their ability to carry out a particular behavioral sequence.

It should be recognized that behavior therapy is not a monolithic procedure; rather, it involves the application of a variety of well-specified therapeutic procedures that have been packaged to treat or prevent a variety of disorders. In addition to the developments in theory and practice, behavior therapy has reached into new areas of endeavor. These include the development of behavioral pediatrics and behavioral medicine, which have in turn taken behavior therapy into preventive medicine.

■ THERAPEUTIC PROCEDURES

Systematic desensitization, a procedure introduced by Wolpe (1958), is most used in the treatment of phobias. Following a thorough exploration of the patient's phobia, a hierarchy of feared situations along one dimension is created. The patient is then taught deep-muscle relaxation, and once this has been completed, he or she visualizes the first item in the hierarchy for 20 to 30 seconds, signaling if any anxiety has been aroused. When the visualization of the first scene has produced no anxiety on two repetitions, the therapist moves on to the next item in the hierarchy.

☐ Exposure Therapy (Programmed Practice)

Exposure therapy, sometimes known as programmed practice, is one of the most investigated and frequently used therapies in the treatment of phobias, including agoraphobia. The simplest variant of exposure therapy is known as *exposure instructions.* The therapist helps the patient construct the first few steps in a hierarchy of the feared situation. For example, for the agoraphobic patient who is housebound this involves walking a few yards from the front door, walking half a block, then a block, etc. Using the hierarchy, a course is laid out along which the patient is instructed to walk alone. The instructions are to walk as far as possible until mild anxiety is evident. At least one session, lasting approximately 30 minutes, should be held each day. The patient repeats each walk until the anxiety has dissipated, and then begins to walk further. A diary is kept for each trial. At the next session the diary is reviewed, progress is attended to and praised, and any stumbling blocks are discussed and a solution for them found.

Therapist-assisted exposure consists of the therapist accompanying the patient to the feared situation and providing direct coaching on facing it. In such cases the therapist may challenge the patient to experience maximal anxiety levels. In addition, the therapist may explore the thoughts of the patient during the exposure experience so that distorted cognitions can be directly challenged. *Group exposure therapy* combines individualized exposure instructions and practice with group education concerning the phobia (usually panic disorder with agoraphobia), and with a discussion of the participants' experiences during exposure to the feared situation(s). *Flooding* is a form of exposure therapy in which patients are exposed to the maximal phobic situation and kept in that situation until their fear dissipates. Because this form of treatment, although quicker than graduated exposure, may be associated with much discomfort, it is rarely used today.

☐ Cognitive Therapy

The importance of distorted cognitions has been particularly recognized in the treatment of the anxiety disorders, depression, and the eating disorders. The typical approach to cognitive therapy involves a thorough exploration of the thoughts and feelings preceding, accompanying, and following a particular behavior (e.g., binge eating or purging). For patients who have difficulty recalling such thoughts, self-monitoring is often useful. Once the cognitions have been clearly identified, the reality of such thoughts is considered in detail. When the unrealistic nature of the thoughts is recognized by the patient, such thinking can be challenged in vivo by the patient, or behavioral experiments designed to further test the reality of such thinking can be devised. Cognitive procedures are usually combined with behavior change procedures and that many behavior therapies are now referred to as "cognitive-behavioral" therapies.

☐ Reinforcement

Reinforcement consists of making an event contingent upon the performance of a behavior that one wishes to change. *Positive reinforcement* is said to occur when the contingent application of the event strengthens the behavior. Positive reinforcers are usually viewed as pleasant (e.g., food, attention, praise, and money). Although positive reinforcement forms an aspect of all therapeutic encounters, it is most used to strengthen prosocial behaviors in children with conduct disorder or in schizophrenia. *Negative reinforcement* refers to a process by which a particular behavior removes the reinforcing event, thus strengthening the behavior. The events used in a negative reinforcement paradigm are usually regarded as unpleasant. For example, in the treatment of anorexia nervosa the often-used threat of tube-feeding serves as a negative reinforcer, because the patient can avoid the negative occurrence (i.e., the tube-feeding) by eating and gaining weight.

☐ Extinction

Removal of positive reinforcement weakens behavior and may lead to its total disappearance. This procedure is known as *extinction.* From a clinical viewpoint, extinction can only be used in environments such as an inpatient unit or a classroom in which reinforcement can be controlled, although relatives of patients can be taught to use extinction in the home. It should be noted that the withdrawal of positive reinforcement may lead to an *extinction burst,* in which the unwanted behavior briefly increases in frequency or strength. If the procedure is being applied by relatives in the home setting, it is important to warn them that an increase in the problem behavior may occur at first so that they do not abandon the attempt to control the behavior through extinction.

☐ Punishment

The punishment paradigm consists in applying an aversive stimulus contingent on the unwanted behavior, with the aim of rapidly bringing the behavior under control. Punishment is used infrequently in behavior therapy and only in situations where the behavior in question threatens physical harm and where more benign procedures, such as positive reinforcement or extinction, have failed.

☐ Biofeedback

The principal aim of biofeedback procedures is to magnify a response that is not accessible to a patient and to provide feedback regarding changes in that response over time. For example, small muscle contractions are not usually discriminable by patients. By such responses being amplified through the use of electronic monitoring and displaying a signal, either visually or in the form of a continuous tone, that is proportional to the muscle contraction being measured, the patient is informed about the degree of contraction and can potentially learn to either increase or decrease the contractions depending on the aim of therapy. Biofeedback has many potential applications—for example, in fecal incontinence through training of the anal sphincter, in hypertension by displaying blood pressure and allowing patients to discover methods to control their pressure, and in Raynaud's disease by enhancing temperature control. Through the use of small, portable biofeedback units, patients can practice in their own homes, thus transferring learning from the office to the patients' own environment.

☐ Relaxation Training

Relaxation training is a relatively simple therapeutic technique that is useful in a variety of conditions and that often forms a part of a behavior therapy treatment package. Patients are first presented with a rationale. For example, muscles may tense up as a result of anxiety and may lead to pain (e.g., in the case of tension headache). By learning to relax muscles such pain can be lessened. Patients are then seated comfortably in a chair and are taught to tense and then relax each muscle group systematically. After several treatment sessions with intervening home practice, patients are taught rapid relaxation techniques. In these procedures patients are taught to intermittently scan their bodies for tense muscles and to bring on the relaxation response rapidly using the word "relax," which they have previously paired with a deeply relaxed state. This procedure can then be used during the course of their everyday lives.

☐ Modeling

Modeling refers to a procedure in which a desired behavior is performed by a therapist with the aim of having a patient copy the performance. Modeling has been used in treating children's phobias by encouraging the children to expose themselves to the feared situation; in social skills training in disorders such as schizophrenia; in marital counseling; and in training in better parenting skills.

☐ Social Skills Training

Social skills training is used in the rehabilitation of schizophrenic patients; in the treatment of social phobia, particularly when combined with avoidant personality disorder; and in the treatment of any patient in whom a particular social skills deficit is apparent. The first step is to analyze the social skills deficit in concrete behavioral terms—for example, avoiding eye contact, a slumped body posture that is not conducive to interpersonal communication, or speaking too softly. More appropriate behavior is then gradually developed using modeling and social reinforcement, together with opportunities for the patient to practice the new behaviors.

■ ANXIETY DISORDERS

☐ Panic Disorder With or Without Agoraphobia

Agoraphobia (and the simple phobias) have been a central focus of behavior therapy since Wolpe's (1958) description of systematic desensitization first appeared. Wolpe formulated the hypothesis that if a response inhibiting anxiety occurs in an anxiety-provoking situation, then the anxiety response will be weakened—an example of the principle of *reciprocal inhibition*. In animal experiments, Wolpe used food to inhibit fear while the animal was exposed to gradually intensifying fear-arousing situations. In humans, relaxation was used to inhibit anxiety; thus, in the clinical application of systematic desensitization, deep muscle relaxation was paired with the imagination of feared scenes presented in a graded hierarchy, beginning with those that provoke the least fear and gradually progressing to more fear-arousing scenes.

Findings from analog research challenged the theory on which systematic desensitization was based. Therapeutic instructions were found to be an essential component of desensitization, and removal of such instructions from the therapeutic package weakened the efficacy of treatment. More surprising was the finding that pairing relaxation with feared scenes was not essential for successful outcome, nor was a gradual approach to the feared situation in imagination critical, thus challenging the central notion of reciprocal inhibition. Ultimately, exposure to the feared situation itself was found to be the critical ingredient for successful treatment.

Many controlled clinical trials have demonstrated the effectiveness of graded exposure therapy in the treatment of agoraphobia (Taylor and Arnow 1988). Long-term studies have shown that improvement is maintained for periods of up to 7 years. Overall, exposure therapy is associated with dropout rates of approximately 10%, and over 80% of patients demonstrate marked improvement. However, it appears that exposure therapy is less effective in reducing panic attacks than in reducing or eliminating phobic behavior.

Several studies suggest that the catastrophic interpretation of panic symptoms rather than the frequency of panic attacks is the critical element associated with the severity of agoraphobia. It is hypothesized that persons susceptible to catastrophic cognitions misinterpret either mild symptoms of anxiety or other body changes in a catastrophic manner, leading to spiraling anxiety that culminates in a panic attack. It follows that therapy aimed at correcting such misinterpretations should lead to a reduction in panic. Such therapy consists, first, in identifying the type of cognitions experienced by the patient and, then, having patients expose themselves to situations in which the catastrophic cognitions occur, essentially demonstrating to themselves that the feared consequences do not occur in reality. Controlled studies have demonstrated the effectiveness of this treatment in reducing panic attacks, with reasonable maintenance of effectiveness over time (Craske et al. 1991). Preliminary studies suggest that cognitive-behavior therapy for panic disorder may be as effective as alprazolam in reducing panic (Klosko et al. 1990).

Several controlled studies of the effectiveness of combining medication and exposure therapy in the treatment of agoraphobia with panic have appeared over the past decade. In the majority of these studies, medication was added to exposure treatment, and, therefore, the separate effects of medication and exposure treatment cannot be identified. In general, it appears that the most effective treatment for agoraphobia with panic is a combination of pharmacological treatment and exposure therapy. This conclusion is quite certain for the tricyclic antidepressants, the most studied medications, but few studies are available for the combination of alprazolam and exposure therapy. For agoraphobic patients who have not experienced panic attacks, exposure therapy alone should suffice.

☐ Simple Phobia

Because medication appears to have little place in the treatment of simple phobia, the most used approach to this problem is graded exposure therapy. Most patients with simple phobia respond rapidly to such treatment, and follow-up studies suggest that gains are well maintained.

☐ Social Phobia

Controlled studies suggest that the behavioral treatment of choice for social phobia is a combination of exposure therapy and cognitive restructuring. The principal area of focus for cognitive change is in eliciting the details of the social phobic patient's fears of negative evaluation by others and challenging the reality of these ideas. Exposure therapy is more difficult to arrange than in simple phobia or agoraphobia because social situations are less controllable by the patient than other phobic situations and may become more intense than expected. Careful planning of exposure situations, ensuring a sufficient number of opportunities for exposure and providing support for failure experiences when the social situation is more intense than was planned, is an important aspect of the treatment of social phobia.

☐ Obsessive-Compulsive Disorder

There have been remarkable advances in the treatment of obsessive-compulsive disorder with behavior therapy, although the results of treatment of this difficult disorder are not completely satisfactory. Deriving from basic work concerning the relationship between anxiety and avoidance behaviors such as compulsions, *response prevention* of compulsive rituals has become one of the cornerstones of behavior therapy in obsessive-compulsive disorder (Steketee et al. 1982). The thesis is that the compulsive behavior does not allow for reality testing of the fear.

The main therapeutic procedure is to prevent the patient from engaging in compulsive acts such as hand washing following exposure to "contaminating" situations. This may be accomplished by means of a gradual approach on an outpatient basis in which the patient, perhaps aided by a relative, abstains from engaging in compulsive behavior after exposure to the feared situation. On an inpatient basis, a more intensive approach can be taken—for example, preventing the patient from engaging in hand washing for a period of several days while providing a supportive relationship.

Although response prevention results in marked diminution in compulsive behavior, it does not usually eliminate the dread of contamination. On the other hand, controlled studies have demonstrated that exposure to contaminating situations results in marked diminution in contamination fears but relatively little change in rituals (Steketee et al. 1982). A review of the literature suggests that medication and behavior therapy are about equally effective, and initial controlled studies suggest that the combination of the two therapies may be the most effective way to treat OCD. Baxter et al. (1992) found similar changes in the brains of patients with obsessive-compulsive disorder treated with either fluoxetine or behavior therapy on positron emission tomography (PET) scan posttreatment. Both groups demonstrated decreases in glucose metabolic rate in the head of the right caudate nucleus, which suggests that both therapies produce similar biological changes and share some common mechanism of action.

■ MOOD DISORDERS

The effectiveness of a cognitive-behavioral approach to the treatment of unipolar nonpsychotic depression has been studied extensively in controlled clinical trials. Among the therapeutic procedures used are 1) problem solving combined with the teaching of coping skills to enhance the reinforcement deficit, and 2) an examination of self-defeating cognitions, teaching the patient to recognize such thoughts, challenge them, and substitute more adaptive thinking. Because antidepressant therapy can be viewed as the standard treatment for major depression, research has been aimed at clarifying the relative effectiveness of pharmacological and cognitive-behavior therapies. Elkin et al. (1989) compared cognitive-behavior therapy, interpersonal therapy, and antidepressant medication in a multicenter trial. The results suggested that all three therapies were effective, but that medication was more effective in severe cases of depression. Other studies have found that for patients who respond to therapy, those receiving cognitive-behavior therapy in combination with a tricyclic antidepressant show less tendency to relapse than those receiving antidepressants alone (Simons et al. 1986).

■ DISORDERS OF EATING

☐ Anorexia Nervosa

It is widely agreed that weight restoration in the severely emaciated patient is the first objective of treatment, which should then be followed by

an attempt to deal with whatever problems appear to have precipitated
and are maintaining the eating disorder. Single-case controlled research,
a useful approach when dealing with a relatively rare disorder, has revealed three procedures that promote increased caloric intake: reinforcement of weight gain in small increments, feedback of information
regarding progress (usually accomplished by daily weight and caloric
consumption feedback), and the serving of large meals even though the
patient will at first leave most of the food untouched. These procedures
are used in the context of a carefully negotiated therapeutic contract and
a well-designed ward milieu. Such programs lead to steady weight gain.
Studies suggest that behavior therapy is more efficient than other treatment approaches, resulting in shorter hospital stays for equal amounts of
weight gain.

☐ Bulimia Nervosa

The work of Fairburn (1981), who first described a cognitive-behavioral
treatment for bulimia, has led to the appearance of a relatively large
number of controlled trials in the last decade. It is generally agreed that
the social pressure for women to maintain a thin body shape has increased during the past 15 years. This pressure leads a subgroup of
young women to markedly restrict their caloric intake and to form rigid
food rules, leading to an increased probability of binge eating and eventually, because of threatened weight increase, to purging. It is also probable that the most susceptible young women are those who markedly
restrict their food intake despite being genetically programmed for a
fuller figure.

Cognitive-behavior therapy is aimed at overcoming the dietary restriction and distorted thinking patterns that are believed to maintain
bulimia nervosa. The basic components of such treatment include self-
disclosure to significant others, thus increasing social control over the secretive bulimic behaviors; gradual reintroduction of the consumption of
three adequate meals each day; slow introduction of "feared" binge
foods to the diet; challenge of distorted cognitions regarding food intake;
and a relapse prevention program (Fairburn 1981). Controlled studies
have demonstrated that cognitive-behavior therapy was more effective
in reducing binge eating and purging than were a waiting-list control
condition, psychoeducational treatment, nondirective psychotherapy
combined with self-monitoring of eating behavior, stress management,
and, in some studies, behavior therapy. Overall, some 60% of bulimic patients recover with the use of cognitive-behavior therapy, and some 70%
to 80% maintain their gains over a 1-year follow-up period.

Studies have shown that cognitive-behavior therapy is superior to antidepressant medication in reducing binge eating and purging, and that

the combined treatment is no more effective than cognitive-behavior therapy alone. It appears, however, that the combined treatment more effectively reduces depression and emotionally induced eating; also, there is tentative evidence that, as in depression, the combined treatment leads to better maintenance of improvement (Agras et al. 1992; Mitchell et al. 1990).

☐ Binge-Eating Disorder

The research in bulimia nervosa has resulted in the rediscovery of a subset of the obese who binge-eat but do not purge. The proportion of the overweight who binge-eat increases with increasing levels of adiposity, from 10% in mildly obese persons to over 40% in severely obese persons. Moreover, it appears that these individuals are less successful in their weight loss attempts than are their non–binge-eating counterparts. The similarity of this syndrome to bulimia nervosa suggests that treatments that are effective in bulimia nervosa should be effective in binge-eating disorder.

■ PSYCHOTIC DISORDERS

The behavioral approach to the treatment of psychotic disorders may be viewed as being adjunctive to pharmacological treatment, and directed toward amelioration of specific problem behaviors or, more broadly, toward the social rehabilitation of the disturbed individual. These aims are accomplished with methods deriving from operant conditioning. Thus, precise definition of the problem behavior, combined with the use of reinforcement in various forms, is the core of the approach to patients with either disturbed behavior that does not improve with the use of medication, or limitations in social and vocational skills secondary to the psychotic process.

Social skills training, delivered within complex and sophisticated rehabilitation programs and based on a detailed analysis of each patient's interpersonal deficits, is the most frequently used approach to the schizophrenic patient. Among the skills taught are maintaining eye contact, reacting more quickly to interpersonal communication, varying voice intonation, and reinforcing prosocial responses from others. Techniques such as modeling prosocial behaviors are often used. In addition, the patient and family members may be taught more effective conflict resolution through the use of role playing, video feedback, and practice. A number of controlled studies have demonstrated that clinically meaningful changes in behavior occur as a result of social skills training, with improvements of up to 70% in social functioning and a shortened hospital stay.

In recognition of the fact that environmental stress is a factor affecting the outcome of treatment with schizophrenic patients, the effectiveness of a behavioral family-based treatment has been studied intensively (Falloon et al. 1985). The main focus of such treatment has been problem solving at the family level. When families are unable to successfully use the problem-solving approach, training in communication skills is added to the program. Specific behavior problems impeding the process of therapy are dealt with using appropriate behavior-change techniques. Compared with individual case management, those patients receiving behavioral family therapy showed a 10-fold decrease in the number of days spent in hospital or jail during follow-up. In addition, the number of days spent in residential facilities decreased 30-fold.

■ BEHAVIORAL MEDICINE

Behavior therapy has been usefully applied to a number of medical disorders, including cardiovascular disease risk factors such as essential hypertension, hypercholesterolemia, and overweight; headache; sleep disturbance; gastrointestinal problems; and asthma. In addition, therapeutic procedures have been developed for problems common to many medical disorders such as compliance with medication taking and the response to stress.

One commonly used therapeutic approach to such problems is relaxation training focusing on muscle relaxation and the control of disturbing cognitions. Various procedures appear to have equal benefit, including deep muscle relaxation, different forms of meditation, hypnotically induced relaxation, and biofeedback training. However, at the clinical level, different individuals may respond better to any one of these procedures. Another commonly used procedure is behavior therapy for weight loss. In addition to obesity itself, weight loss is beneficial in a number of medical conditions, including essential hypertension, hypercholesterolemia, cardiovascular disease, Type-II diabetes, sleep apnea, and arthritis.

☐ Obesity

Behavioral treatment for mild to moderate obesity contains the following elements: 1) self-monitoring, 2) reinforcement of an increase in activity levels, 3) slowing of the eating rate, 4) narrowing of the stimuli associated with eating, 5) adherence to a low-fat, high-fiber heart-healthy diet; and 6) the use of reinforcement and self-reinforcement to attain short-term goals. This treatment package has been shown to be more effective than more traditional dietary approaches to weight control, psychotherapy, and even pharmacological treatment in a large number of controlled studies. The degree of weight loss achieved by the average patient is modest, usually averaging about 0.5 kg per week of treatment. Treatment programs of 16 weeks' duration result in a mean weight reduction of 8 to 10 kg.

Maintenance of weight loss appears to depend on the continued practice of behaviors learned during treatment. The most crucial of these are adherence to a healthy diet and eating style, and continued exercise. Patients who continue to practice these behaviors have been shown to maintain or even increase their initial weight losses up to 5 years after treatment. Behavior therapy has also been used to enhance the maintenance of weight loss with a very-low-calorie diet, a treatment regimen used in moderately to severely obese patients. Clinical studies suggest that mean weight losses of 20 kg or more might be expected with this combination of treatments, with marked improvement in cardiovascular risk factors, including blood pressure, serum cholesterol levels, and even sleep apnea.

Several studies involving the combination of appetite-suppressant drugs, such as fenfluramine hydrochloride, and behavior therapy have been reported in recent years. The most impressive of these found an advantage at the end of treatment in terms of weight loss for the groups receiving fenfluramine with or without behavior therapy (Craighead et al. 1981). However, at 1-year follow-up, this result was reversed, with those receiving medication regaining more weight than those receiving behavior therapy. A more recent long-term study of the combination of behavior therapy and two appetite suppressants demonstrated excellent short-term results, as well as reasonable maintenance over nearly 4 years, for patients who continued to take the medication regularly (Weintraub 1992). Additionally, the newer serotonin reuptake inhibitors are associated with at least short-term, and perhaps long-term, weight loss.

☐ Essential Hypertension

Numerous controlled studies have demonstrated that hypertensive patients receiving relaxation training show a greater degree of blood pressure lowering than do patients receiving no treatment, placebo control, or psychotherapy. This finding suggests a specific effect of relaxation training, an effect that is additive to the effects of antihypertensive medication. Studies with 24-hour blood pressure monitoring have shown that the blood pressure lowering induced by relaxation training persists around the clock. Follow-up studies have shown reasonable maintenance of the treatment effects, in one study up to 4 years after treatment (Patel et al. 1981). Other studies have demonstrated that blood pressure lowering induced by relaxation training is accompanied by a decrease in the prescribed amount of antihypertensive medication. The relaxation effect appears to be mediated by decreased sympathetic nervous system arousal. Thus, studies in hypertensive patients have shown that plasma levels of renin, aldosterone, and norepinephrine are reduced significantly more in those patients receiving relaxation training than in untrained individuals.

Overall, however, the results of relaxation training in the treatment of essential hypertension have been somewhat disappointing. Blood pressure lowering varies considerably among individuals, suggesting that relaxation training may be most useful in a subset of hypertensive patients. Unfortunately, it has not been possible to characterize the nature of the subset of individuals who are likely to respond to such therapy. For the overweight hypertensive patient, the use of a behavioral weight control program should also be considered. Controlled studies suggest that modest weight losses lead to blood pressure lowering at all levels of hypertension, and that such losses may be useful in preventing further elevations of blood pressure in the borderline hypertensive patient. The blood pressure lowering due to weight loss does not appear to be a result of the effects of salt restriction that often accompany dietary programs. Moreover, in the borderline hypertensive patient, weight loss is superior to salt restriction in lowering blood pressure (Hypertension Prevention Collaborative Research Group 1992).

☐ Headache

The research literature on the treatment of both tension and migraine headaches suggests that relaxation and biofeedback procedures are equally effective; thus, the preferred treatment, because it is simpler to apply, should be relaxation training. Both relaxation training and biofeedback are more effective in reducing the number and intensity of tension or migraine headaches than either no treatment or various types of placebo control groups (Blanchard 1992).

☐ Primary Insomnia

Two behavior therapy approaches to sleep disturbance, both of which shorten sleep onset time as measured by self-report and polysomnography, have been shown to be effective in controlled studies. The first of these treatments, relaxation training, is based on the rationale that anxiety and other distractions preventing sleep onset can be controlled with such training. The second treatment, stimulus control, is based on the theory that sleep onset should be signaled by a narrow range of stimuli—that is, being in bed in a dark room and feeling drowsy—and that for many patients with sleep onset disturbance the connection between these stimuli and sleep has broken down. Thus, stimulus control treatment consists of removing distractions from the bedroom, such as books, television, and radio. In addition, if patients do not fall asleep within 10 minutes, they are instructed to get up and not to go back to bed until they are drowsy. It has been shown that this treatment is more effective than relaxation training (Lacks et al. 1983).

☐ Stress Management

Relaxation training is useful in ameliorating many symptoms of stress, including anxiety, tension headache, and sleep disturbance. In addition, relaxation training appears to modify the Type A behavior pattern, an independent risk factor for cardiovascular disease. Type A behavior, which may represent a maladaptive response to life stress, consists of aggressive striving, time urgency, irritability, and impatience. A long-term controlled study involving patients who had had myocardial infarction demonstrated that it was possible to modify Type A behavior with an educational treatment regimen based upon relaxation training, and that reduction in this behavior was associated with fewer recurrent myocardial infarctions (Friedman et al. 1984).

■ DISORDERS OF CHILDHOOD

☐ Autism

Although autism is considered organic in its origin, behavioral techniques have been useful in the treatment of the language disturbance, self-injurious and stereotyped behavior, and aggressive behaviors. Lovaas et al. (1979) made an important contribution to our understanding of autism by identifying the perceptual problem of *stimulus overselectivity*. When a variety of stimuli are presented to autistic children, as is the case in almost every social contact, only one portion is attended to, with a lack of response to the complex stimulus and its meaning. Thus, the autistic child's response to situations often appears bizarre. No evidence of sensory deficits is found. When simple cues are presented to autistic children, behavioral responding is more consistent. Using well-defined cues combined with reinforcers—usually immediate and tangible (primary) reinforcers—desired behaviors can be gradually shaped. Behavioral excesses (e.g., tantrums, aggression, self-stimulatory behaviors) may either be punished (using, for example, timeout from reinforcement, in which a child might be put in a room alone for a few minutes contingent upon disruptive behavior) or, if mild, ignored with the aim of weakening them (an example of the removal of reinforcement, i.e., extinction). Therapists and parents can be trained to teach autistic children in this way, and environments can be designed to systematically reinforce desired behaviors.

A controlled study by Campbell et al. (1978) investigated the use of haloperidol or placebo versus contingent or noncontingent reinforcement in a language training program for hospitalized autistic children. Medication reduced stereotypical and withdrawn behavior in older, but not younger, children, while contingency management improved ward behaviors and compliance and imitation in the language training program. The combined haloperidol and contingent reinforcement group showed the best improvement.

☐ Conduct Disorder

Parents often seek help for their children's behavior problems, including aggressiveness, destructiveness, oppositional behavior, temper tantrums, and other negative behaviors (e.g., whining, screaming, threatening, etc.). Numerous studies have described a high rate of what Patterson (1976) described as "coercive interactions" in families of these children. Parents of these children respond with coercive behaviors when attempting to control their children's misbehavior. Patterson described a negative reinforcement model in which the coercive behavior of the parent may be reinforced by the reduction of the aversive behavior of the child. Unfortunately, the parent also models punitive behaviors to the child, who is then trained to behave similarly.

To address such problems, the primary research effort has been in training parents to use social-learning techniques to shape more adaptive and prosocial behaviors in their children. Such programs (Patterson 1976) have taught parents to monitor both prosocial and deviant behaviors, develop positive reinforcement systems (e.g., contingent point systems for obtaining rewards), use extinction (i.e., "ignoring") for minor misbehaviors, and use punishment (e.g., time out) for serious infractions. There are, however, limits to the efficacy of such programs. It has been shown, for example, that marital discord is associated with conduct disorder in children. In such cases improvement is unlikely until the marital discord has been addressed. Other complicating parental factors may include depression, substance abuse, or other psychopathology that require therapeutic attention for the child to improve using behavioral techniques.

Looking beyond the parent-child relationship, one study (Dumas and Wahler 1985) evaluated mother-child dyads participating in a parent-training program for children with conduct disorder. Mothers who had a low level of community contact (i.e., insular mothers) used more aversive control toward their children than did mothers with a higher level of community contact. Children of the insular mothers were more aggressive than those of noninsular mothers in general, and in particular when responding to negative maternal behavior. It is suggested that increasing contacts with friends and social supports in the community may help reduce negative interpersonal interactions.

☐ Attention-Deficit/Hyperactivity Disorder

Behavioral studies using contingent reinforcement of desired behaviors in children with attention-deficit/hyperactivity disorder (ADHD) demonstrate that when teachers differentially attended to and reinforced appropriate classroom behavior, deviant behavior was reduced (Becker et al. 1967). Children who were rewarded for increasing academic work by access to increased free time or to participation in preferred classroom activities made considerable academic gains that were well maintained. Controlled studies have suggested that medication reduces hyperactive behaviors but does little for either the learning deficits or the impulsive and aggressive behaviors associated with ADHD (Gadow 1985). Thus, a combination of behavior therapy and medication is most commonly used in the treatment of this syndrome.

☐ Ruminative Vomiting

Infants with ruminative vomiting regurgitate their food mouthful by mouthful, leading to malnutrition and dehydration, thus posing a threat to life. One approach to treatment is to use the principle of punishment, by making an unpleasant event contingent upon each episode of regurgitation. In one controlled study, a drop of lemon juice on the tongue was used as the unpleasant event. During baseline measurement, before treatment was begun, the infant ruminated between 40% and 70% of the time it was awake (Sajwaj et al. 1974). Once lemon juice was presented contingent upon spitting up food, the rate of ruminative vomiting dropped steadily. Punishment was then briefly removed, and rumination quickly returned to original baseline levels, confirming the effectiveness of lemon juice as a punishing event. Reintroduction of punishment led to disappearance of the behavior and a return to normal weight, with no relapse at 1-year follow-up.

☐ Childhood Depression

The behavioral treatment of childhood depression has been modeled on the demonstratedly successful treatment of adult depression using either social skills training or a more comprehensive cognitive-behavioral treatment package. In one controlled study it was found that some 50% of adolescents no longer met criteria for depression following treatment as compared with little change in the waiting-list control group (Lewinsohn et al. 1990). There was continued improvement over a 2-year follow-up, with less than 10% meeting criteria for depression at 1 year and less than 20% at 2 years, suggesting that while not everyone improves, the effects of treatment are long-lasting.

☐ Behavioral Pediatrics

As in the case of adults, behavioral approaches have been used increasingly in pediatric populations with medical problems. Chronic diseases in childhood often require complex behavior changes for optimal treatment. Such is the case, for example, for the child with insulin-dependent diabetes mellitus who must comply with medications, diet, and exercise. Epstein et al. (1981) developed an educational intervention aimed at increasing knowledge and skills by providing instruction, feedback concerning performance, and reinforcement. The content included insulin dosage, diet, exercise, self-administration of insulin, and the signs and symptoms of hypoglycemia. Parents participated, encouraging child adherence. Significant improvements were made, with negative urine glucose samples changing from 27% to 39% following treatment and increasing to 45% at 2-month follow-up, demonstrating important improvement in diabetic control in these children.

Reinforcement systems have also been used to help children adhere to the demands of hemodialysis (Magrab and Papadopoulou 1977). Children were encouraged to adhere to diet and were rewarded with prizes for improvements in weight and in potassium and blood urea nitrogen levels. Similar reinforcement approaches have been helpful for larger populations, such as for the encouragement of attendance to dental facilities by low-income families (Reiss et al. 1976).

■ REFERENCES

Agras WS, Rossiter EM, Arnow B, et al: Pharmacologic and cognitive-behavioral treatment for bulimia nervosa: a controlled comparison. Am J Psychiatry 149:82–87, 1992

Bandura A: Social Foundations of Thought and Action. Englewood Cliffs, NJ, Prentice-Hall, 1986

Baxter LR Jr, Schwartz JM, Bergman KS, et al: Caudate glucose metabolic rate changes with both drug and behavior therapy for obsessive-compulsive disorder. Arch Gen Psychiatry 49:681–689, 1992

Becker WC, Madsen CH, Arnold CR, et al: The contingent use of teacher attention and praising in reducing classroom behavior problems. Journal of Special Education 1:287–307, 1967

Blanchard EB: Psychological treatment of benign headache disorders. J Consult Clin Psychol 60:537–551, 1992

Campbell M, Anderson LT, Meier M, et al: A comparison of haloperidol and behavior therapy and their interaction in autistic children. Journal of the American Academy of Child Psychiatry 17:640–655, 1978

Craighead LW, Stunkard AJ, O'Brien RM: Behavior therapy and pharmacotherapy for obesity. Arch Gen Psychiatry 38:763–768, 1981

Craske MG, Brown TA, Barlow DH: Behavioral treatment of panic disorder: a two-year follow-up. Behavior Therapy 22:289–304, 1991

Dumas JE, Wahler RG: Indiscriminate mothering as a contextual factor in aggressive-oppositional child behavior: "Damned if you do and damned if you don't." J Abnorm Child Psychol 13:1–17, 1985

Elkin E, Shea MT, Watkins JT, et al. National Institute of Mental Health Treatment of Depression Collaborative Research Program: general effectiveness of treatments. Arch Gen Psychiatry 46:971–982, 1989

Epstein LH, Beck S, Figuera J, et al: The effects of targeting improvements in urine glucose on metabolic control in children with insulin dependent diabetes. J Appl Behav Anal 14:365–376, 1981

Fairburn C[G]: A cognitive behavioural approach to the treatment of bulimia. Psychol Med 11:707–711, 1981

Falloon IRH, Boyd JL, McGill CW, et al: Family management in the prevention of morbidity of schizophrenia: clinical outcome of a two-year longitudinal study. Arch Gen Psychiatry 42:887–896, 1985

Friedman M, Thoresen CE, Gill JJ, et al: Alteration of type A behavior and reduction in cardiac recurrences in postmyocardial infarction patients. Am Heart J 108:237–248, 1984

Gadow KD: Relative efficacy of pharmacological, behavioral, and combination treatments for enhancing academic performance. Clinical Psychology Review 5:513–533, 1985

Hypertension Prevention Collaborative Research Group: the effects of nonpharmacologic interventions on blood pressure of persons with high normal levels: results of the trials of hypertension prevention (Phase I). JAMA 267:1213–1220, 1992

Klosko JS, Barlow DH, Tassinari R, et al: A comparison of alprazolam and behavior therapy in treatment of panic disorder. J Consult Clin Psychol 58:77–84, 1990

Lacks P, Bertelson AD, Gans L, et al: The effectiveness of three behavioral treatments for different degrees of sleep onset insomnia. Behavior Therapy 14:593–605, 1983

Lewinsohn PM, Clarke GN, Hops H, et al: Cognitive-behavioral group treatment of depression in adolescents. Behavior Therapy 21:385–401, 1990

Lovaas OI, Koegel RL, Schreibman L: Stimulus overselectivity in autism: a review of research. Psychol Bull 86:1236–1254, 1979

Magrab PR, Papadopoulou ZL: The effect of a token economy on dietary compliance for children on hemodialysis. J Appl Behav Anal 10:573–578, 1977

Mitchell JE, Pyle RL, Eckert ED, et al: A comparison study of antidepressants and structured intensive group psychotherapy in the treatment of bulimia nervosa. Arch Gen Psychiatry 47:149–157, 1990

Patel C, Marmot MG, Terry DJ: Controlled trial of biofeedback-aided behavioural methods in reducing mild hypertension. BMJ 282:2005–2008, 1981

Patterson GR: The aggressive child: victim and architect of a coercive system, in Behavior Modification and Families. Edited by Mash EJ, Hamerlynck LA, Handy LC. New York, Brunner/Mazel, 1976, pp 93–127

Reiss M, Plotrowski WD, Bailey JS: Behavioral community psychology: encouraging low-income parents to seek dental care for their children. J Appl Behav Anal 9:387–398, 1976

Sajwaj T, Libet J, Agras WS: Lemon juice therapy: the control of life-threatening rumination in a six-month-old infant. J Appl Behav Anal 7:557–563, 1974

Simons AD, Murphy GE, Levine JL, et al: Cognitive therapy and pharmacotherapy for depression: sustained improvement over one year. Arch Gen Psychiatry 43:43–48, 1986

Steketee G, Foa EB, Grayson JB: Recent advances in the behavioral treatment of obsessive-compulsives. Arch Gen Psychiatry 39:1365–1371, 1982

Taylor CB, Arnow B: The Nature and Treatment of Anxiety Disorders. New York, Free Press, 1988

Weintraub M: Long-term weight control: the National Heart, Lung and Blood Institute funded multimodal intervention study. Clin Pharmacol Ther 51:586–594, 1992

Wolpe J: Psychotherapy by Reciprocal Inhibition. Stanford, CA, Stanford University Press, 1958

CHAPTER

31

Cognitive Therapy

Jesse H. Wright, M.D., Ph.D.
Aaron T. Beck, M.D.

Cognitive therapy (CT) is a system of psychotherapy based on theories of pathological information processing in mental disorders. Treatment is directed primarily at modifying distorted or maladaptive cognitions and related behavioral dysfunction. Therapeutic interventions are usually focused and problem-oriented. Although the use of specific techniques is a major feature of this approach, there can be considerable flexibility and creativity in the clinical application of CT.

■ HISTORICAL BACKGROUND

The CT approach to depression was first proposed by Beck in the early 1960s (Beck 1963, 1964). Subsequently, a comprehensive cognitive therapy for depression was articulated, and the treatment model was extended to a variety of other conditions, including anxiety disorders (Beck 1967, 1976; Beck et al. 1979). Therapy interventions were designed to be compatible with the cognitive model of depression and were drawn from several sources including the clinical experiences of Beck and co-workers and the writings of behaviorists and post-Freudian analysts (Beck et al. 1979).

    The phenomenological approach to philosophy significantly influenced the development of cognitive therapy (Beck et al. 1979). Frankl's (1985) logotherapy and Mahoney's (1985) and Guidano and Liotti's (1983) theories on constructivism also played a role in formulating cognitively oriented treatment models. These authors emphasized the importance of cognitive factors in finding meaning in life and in promoting personal growth. The neo-Freudians focused on the importance of perceptions of the self and on the salience of conscious experience (Raimy 1975). Other contributions came from the field of developmental psychology (Bowlby 1985) and from Kelly's (1955) theory of personal constructs.

Cognitive therapy also incorporates theories and treatment methods of behavior therapy. Procedures such as activity scheduling, graded task assignments, exposure, and social skills training play a fundamental role in CT (Beck et al. 1979; Meichenbaum 1977). In addition, Ellis' rational emotive therapy (Ellis 1962, 1973) has helped promulgate CT and related treatments. Investigations in the field of cognitive psychology have solidified the concepts originally proposed by Beck and have led to a refinement of the CT approach (Dobson and Shaw 1986; Hollon and Kendall 1980; Lefebvre 1981).

■ BASIC CONCEPTS

☐ The Cognitive Model

The cognitive model for psychotherapy is grounded on the theory that there are characteristic errors in information processing in depression, anxiety disorders, personality disturbances, and other psychiatric conditions (Beck 1976). Beck (1976) has proposed that there are three major areas of cognitive distortion in depression (the negative cognitive triad of self, world, and future) and that patients with anxiety disorders habitually overestimate the danger or risk in situations. Cognitive distortions such as misperceptions, errors in logic, or misattributions are thought to lead to dysphoric affect and maladaptive behavior. Furthermore, a "vicious cycle" is perpetuated when the behavioral response confirms and amplifies negatively distorted cognitions (Wright 1988).

The CT perspective can be summarized in a working model (Figure 31–1) that expands on the well-known stimulus-response paradigm (Wright 1988). Cognitive mediation is given the central role in this model. However, an interactive relationship between environmental influences, cognition, emotion, and behavior also is recognized. It should be emphasized that this working model does not presume that cognitive pathology is the only cause of specific syndromes or that other factors such as genetic predisposition, biochemical alterations, or interpersonal conflicts are not involved in the etiology of psychiatric illnesses. Instead, the model is used simply as a guide for the actions of the cognitive therapist in clinical practice. It is assumed that most forms of psychopathology have complex etiologies involving cognitive, biological, social, and interpersonal influences, and that there are multiple, potentially useful approaches to treatment (Wright and Thase 1992; Wright et al. 1992b). In addition, it is assumed that cognitive changes are accomplished through biological processes and that psychopharmacological treatments can alter cognitions (Wright and Thase 1992). This position is consistent with outcome research on CT and pharmacotherapy (Blackburn et al. 1981; Imber et al. 1990; Simons et al. 1984) and with other studies that have documented neurobiological changes associated with conditioning in animals or psychotherapy in humans (Baxter et al. 1992; Kandel and Schwartz 1983).

The working model in Figure 31–1 posits a close relationship between cognition and emotion. The general thrust of CT is that emotional responses are largely dependent on cognitive appraisals of the significance of environmental cues. For example, sadness is likely when an event (or memory of an event) is perceived in a negative way, and anger is common when it is judged that there are threats to one's self or loved ones. The cognitive model also incorporates the effects of emotion on cognitive processing. Heightened emotion can stimulate and intensify cognitive distortion (Greenberg and Safran 1984). Therapeutic proce-

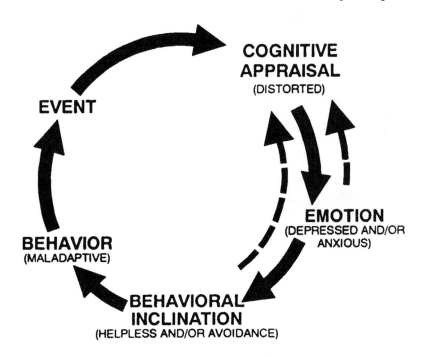

Figure 31–1. A working model for cognitive therapy. Adapted from Wright 1988.

dures in CT involve interventions at all points in the working model diagrammed in Figure 31–1. However, most of the effort is directed at stimulating either cognitive or behavioral change.

☐ Levels of Dysfunctional Cognitions

Beck et al. (1979) have suggested that there are two major levels of dysfunctional information processing: 1) automatic thoughts and 2) basic beliefs incorporated in schemas. *Automatic thoughts* are the cognitions that occur rapidly while a person is in a situation (or is recalling an event). These automatic thoughts usually are not subjected to rational analysis and often are based on erroneous logic. Although the individual may be only subliminally aware of these cognitions, automatic thoughts are accessible through questioning techniques used in CT (Beck et al. 1979; Wright and Beck 1983). The different types of faulty logic in automatic thinking have been termed *cognitive errors* (Beck et al. 1979). Descriptions of typical cognitive errors, such as selective abstraction, arbitrary inference, and absolutistic thinking, are found in Table 31–1.

Schemas are deeper cognitive structures that contain the basic rules for screening, filtering, and coding information from the environment (Beck et al. 1979; Wright and Beck 1983). These organizing constructs are developed through early childhood experiences and subsequent formative influences. Schemas can play a highly adaptive role in allowing rapid assimilation of data and appropriate decision making (Bowlby 1985). However, in psychiatric disorders there are clusters of maladaptive schemas that perpetuate dysphoric mood and ineffective or self-

---

Table 31–1.   Cognitive errors

Selective abstraction (sometimes termed "mental filter"): drawing a conclusion based on only a small portion of the available data.

Arbitrary inference: coming to a conclusion without adequate supporting evidence or despite contradictory evidence.

Absolutistic thinking ("all or none" thinking): categorizing oneself or personal experiences into rigid dichotomies (e.g., all good or all bad, perfect or completely flawed, success or total failure).

Magnification and minimization: over- or undervaluing the significance of a personal attribute, a life event, or a future possibility.

Personalization: linking external occurrences to oneself (e.g., taking blame, assuming responsibility, criticizing oneself) when there is little or no basis for making these associations.

Catastrophic thinking: predicting the worst possible outcome while ignoring more likely eventualities.

Source.   Adapted from Beck et al. 1979; Wright and Beck 1983.

defeating behavior (Beck 1976; Beck et al. 1990). Examples of adaptive and maladaptive schemas are given in Table 31–2.

☐ Cognitive Pathology in Depression and Anxiety Disorders

The role of cognitive functioning in depression and anxiety disorders has been studied extensively. In general, the results of this investigative effort have confirmed Beck's hypotheses (Beck 1963, 1964, 1976; Beck et al. 1979; Wright and Beck 1983; Wright 1988). These findings have played an important role in both confirming and shaping the treatment procedures used in CT. Numerous studies have documented a negative cognitive bias in depression. For example, distorted automatic thoughts and cognitive errors have been found to be much more frequent in depressed persons than in control subjects (Blackburn et al. 1986b; Lefebvre 1981; Watkins and Rush 1983). A selective recall bias also has been described. Depressed individuals are more likely to remember negative than positive self-referent information (Gotlib 1981; Nelson and Craighead 1977; Teasdale and Fogarty 1979).

Substantial evidence has been collected to support the concept of the negative cognitive triad (Haaga et al. 1991; Blackburn et al. 1986b). Also, a large group of investigations has established that one of the elements of the negative cognitive triad, hopelessness, is highly associated with suicide risk (Beck et al. 1975, 1985b; Fawcett et al. 1987; Minkoff et al. 1973).

Table 31–2. Adaptive and maladaptive schemas

Adaptive	Maladaptive
No matter what happens, I can manage somehow.	I must be perfect to be accepted.
If I work at something, I can master it.	If I choose to do something, I must succeed.
I'm a survivor.	I'm a fake.
Others can trust me.	Without a woman, I'm nothing.
I'm lovable.	I'm stupid.
People respect me.	No matter what I do, I won't succeed.
I can figure things out.	Others can't be trusted.
If I prepare in advance, I usually do better.	I never can be comfortable around others.
I like to be challenged.	If I make one mistake, I'll lose everything.
There's not much that can scare me.	The world is too frightening for me.

Beck et al. (1985b) found that hopelessness was the strongest predictor of ultimate suicide in a sample of depressed inpatients followed 10 years after discharge.

Abramson et al. (1978) proposed that attributions to life events are negatively distorted in depression and that misattributions can play a role in the development of this disorder. The relevance of early research on attributions has been questioned, because most investigations were performed with nonclinical experimental subjects (Peterson et al. 1985). Nevertheless, the overall results of research on attributions indicate that clinically depressed individuals are prone to blame themselves for adverse life events, give global meaning to circumscribed occurrences, and believe that negative situations will last indefinitely. In contrast, individuals that do not suffer from depression commonly view noxious events as being due to external forces, as having isolated significance, and as being transient situations (Hammon et al. 1981; Raps et al. 1982; Zimmerman et al. 1986).

Studies of responses to feedback have provided another perspective on dysfunctional information processing. Depressed individuals usually overestimate the amount of negative feedback and underestimate the amount of positive feedback that they receive (DeMonbreun and Craighead 1977; Nelson and Craighead 1977; Wenzlaff and Grozier 1988). Several studies found a "positive self-serving bias" in nondepressed control subjects (Alloy and Ahrens 1987; Gotlib and Olson 1983). The tendency for nondepressed individuals to hear more positive and/or less negative feedback than they actually receive, and to expend extra effort after being told they have not done well, may be an adaptive trait.

Studies of information processing in anxiety disorders have provided additional confirmation for the cognitive model of psychopathology. Anxious patients have been found to have an attentional bias in responding to potentially threatening stimuli (Mathews and MacLeod 1987). Individuals with significant levels of anxiety are more likely than nonanxious persons to have a facilitated intake of information about potential threat; and further, those with anxiety disorders are prone to interpret environmental situations as being unrealistically dangerous or risky (Fitzgerald and Phillips 1991; Mathews and MacLeod 1987). Anxious patients also have been shown to have an enhanced recall for memories associated with threatening situations or past anxiety states (Cloitre and Liebowitz 1991; Ingram and Kendall 1987).

Automatic thoughts associated with themes of danger, threat, uncontrollability, or anticipated incompetence have been observed at much higher rates in patients with elevated levels of anxiety than in those with low anxiety (Ingram and Kendall 1987; Kendall and Hollon 1989). In other studies of cognitive biasing in anxiety disorders, investigators have noted high frequencies of negative self-statements (Glass and Furlong

1990), misinterpretations of bodily stimuli (McNally and Foa 1987), and overestimates of future misfortune (Mizes et al. 1987).

Comparisons of depressed and anxious patients have revealed differences between the two groups and common features of the disorders (Clark DA et al. 1990; Ingram et al. 1987). In depression, cognitions about hopelessness, low self-worth, and failure are more frequent, whereas in anxiety, cognitive themes are usually related to anticipated harm or danger (Clark DA et al. 1990). Although the content of thoughts may be different, depressed and anxious patients both have demoralization, self-absorption, a predominance of automatic information processing, and a reduction in the cognitive capacity needed for problem solving and task performance (Clark DA et al. 1990; Ingram and Kendall 1987; Ingram et al. 1987).

■ THERAPEUTIC PRINCIPLES

Cognitive therapy is usually a short-term treatment, lasting from 10 to 20 sessions. In some instances, very brief treatment courses are utilized for patients with mild or circumscribed problems, or longer series of CT sessions are used for those with chronic or especially severe conditions. After completion of the initial course of treatment, intermittent booster sessions may be useful in some cases, particularly for individuals with a history of recurrent illness.

Although CT is primarily directed at the "here and now," knowledge of the patient's family background, developmental experiences, social network, and medical history helps guide the course of therapy. Collecting a thorough history is an essential component of the early phase of treatment. A problem-oriented approach to treatment is emphasized for several reasons: 1) directing the patient's attention to current problems stimulates the development of action plans that can help reverse hopelessness, avoidance, or other dysfunctional symptoms; 2) data on cognitive responses to recent life events are more readily accessible and verifiable than for events that happened years in the past; and 3) practical work on present problems helps to prevent the development of excessive dependency or regression in the therapeutic relationship.

☐ The Therapeutic Relationship

The therapeutic relationship in CT is characterized by a high degree of collaboration between patient and therapist, and an empirical tone to the work of therapy. The therapist and patient function much like an investigative team. They develop hypotheses about the validity of automatic thoughts and schemas, or alternately about the effectiveness of patterns of behavior. A series of exercises or experiments is then designed to test the validity of the hypotheses and, subsequently, to modify cognitions or behavior. Beck et al. (1979) termed this form of therapeutic relationship *collaborative empiricism*.

The therapist usually is more active in CT than in most other psychotherapies. The degree of therapist activity varies with the stage of treatment and the severity of the illness. Generally, a more directive and structured approach is emphasized early in treatment, when symptoms are severe. As the patient improves and understands more about the methods of CT, the therapist can become somewhat less active. By the end of treatment, the patient should be able to use self-monitoring and self-help techniques with little reinforcement from the therapist.

Collaborative empiricism is fostered throughout the therapy, even when directive work is required. Although the therapist may suggest specific strategies or give homework assignments designed to combat severe depression or anxiety, the patient's input is always solicited and the self-help component of CT is emphasized from the outset of treatment. Also, it is made clear to the patient that CT is not an attempt to convert all negative thoughts to positive ones. In fact, bad things do occur to people, and some individuals have behaviors that are ineffective or self-defeating (Krantz 1985). If cognitive distortions have occurred, then the patient and therapist will work together to develop a more rational perspective. On the other hand, if actual negative experiences or characteristics are identified, they will attempt to find ways to cope or to change.

The development of a collaborative working relationship is dependent on a number of therapist and patient characteristics. The "nonspecific" therapist variables that are important components of all effective psychotherapies (Barrett and Wright 1984; Truax and Mitchell 1971) are equally significant in CT. Professionals who are kind and understanding and can convey appropriate empathy make good cognitive therapists. Other factors of significance are the ability of the therapist to generate trust, to demonstrate a high level of competence, and to exhibit equanimity under pressure (Beck et al. 1979; Thase and Beck 1992; Wright and Davis 1992). Cognitive therapists also must be able to maintain an energetic pace and to sustain their concentration throughout the treatment sessions.

Additional procedures that cognitive therapists use to encourage collaborative empiricism are 1) providing feedback throughout sessions, 2) recognizing and managing transference, and 3) using gentle humor. The therapist gives feedback in order to keep the therapeutic relationship anchored in the "here and now," and to reinforce the working aspect of the therapy process. Comments are made frequently throughout the session to summarize major points, to give direction, and to keep the session on target. Also, questions are asked at several intervals in each session to determine how well the patient has understood a concept or has grasped the essence of a therapeutic intervention. Because CT is highly psychoeducational, the therapist functions to some degree as a teacher. Thus, discreet positive feedback is given to help stimulate and reward the patient's efforts to learn.

A collaborative therapeutic relationship with frequent opportunities for two-way feedback generally discourages the formation of a transference neurosis. Cognitive therapy methodology and the short-term nature of treatment promote pragmatic working relationships as opposed to recapitulations of dysfunctional early relationships. Nevertheless, significant transference reactions can occur. Such reactions are more likely with patients who have personality disorders or other chronic illnesses that require longer-term treatment. When a transference reaction occurs, the cognitive therapist applies CT procedures to understand the phenomenon and to intervene. Typically, automatic thoughts and schemas that pertain to the therapeutic relationship are identified, explored, and modified if possible.

The therapeutic relationship also can be enhanced by using gentle humor during CT sessions. On occasion, the therapist may use hyperbole in a discreet manner to point out an inconsistency or an illogical conclusion. Humor needs to be injected carefully into the therapeutic relationship. Some patients respond quite well to humor; others may be limited in their ability to use this feature of therapy. However, appropriate use of humor can strengthen the therapeutic relationship in CT if patient and therapist are able to laugh *with* each other and to use humor to deflate exaggerated or distorted cognitions.

☐ Structuring Therapy

One of the most important structuring techniques for CT is the use of a *therapy agenda*. At the beginning of each session, the therapist and patient work together to derive a short list of topics, usually consisting of two to four items. Generally, it is advisable to shape an agenda that 1) can be managed within the time frame of an individual session, 2) follows up on material from earlier sessions, 3) allows for a review of any homework from the previous session and provides an opportunity for new homework assignments, and 4) contains specific items that are highly relevant to the patient but are not too global or abstract.

Agenda setting helps to counteract hopelessness and helplessness by reducing seemingly overwhelming problems down into workable segments. The agenda-setting process also encourages patients to take a problem-oriented approach to their difficulties. However, an excessively rigid approach to using a therapy agenda is not advocated. There must be sufficient flexibility to investigate promising new leads or to allow the patient to express significant thoughts or feelings that were unexpected at the beginning of the session.

Feedback procedures described earlier are also used in structuring CT sessions. For example, the therapist may observe that the patient is drifting from the established agenda or is spending time discussing a topic of questionable relevance. In situations such as these, constructive feedback is given to direct the patient back to a more profitable area of inquiry. Commonly used CT techniques add an additional structural element to the therapy. Repeated use of procedures such as thought recording, activity scheduling, and graded task assignments helps to link sessions together, especially if the procedures are introduced in therapy and then assigned as homework.

☐ Psychoeducation

Psychoeducational procedures are a routine component of CT. One of the major goals of the treatment approach is to teach patients a new way of thinking that can be applied in resolving current symptoms and in managing problems that will be encountered in the future. The psychoeducational effort usually begins with the process of socializing the patient to therapy. In the opening phase of treatment, the therapist explains the basic concepts of CT and introduces the patient to the format of CT sessions. Often, reading assignments are given to reinforce learning and to deepen the patient's understanding of CT principles.

The major portion of the psychoeducational work in CT involves brief explanations or illustrations coupled with homework assignments. These activities are woven into treatment sessions in a manner that emphasizes a collaborative, active learning approach. One of the more interesting developments has been to employ computer-based CT in the treatment of depression. Preliminary results suggested that depressed patients show significant improvement after receiving a computerized instructional program on CT (Selmi et al. 1990, 1991). The Selmi et al. program is text-based and requires patients to type responses on a keyboard. A more user-friendly multimedia program with full-screen video has been recently developed by Wright et al. (1995). This form of computer-assisted CT requires no previous experience with computers and thus can be used with a wide variety of patients.

☐ Cognitive Techniques

Identifying Automatic Thoughts

Much of the work of CT is devoted to recognizing and then modifying negatively distorted or illogical automatic thoughts. The most powerful way of introducing the patient to the effects of automatic thoughts is to find an in vivo example of how such thoughts can influence emotional responses. Mood shifts during the therapy session are almost always good places to pause to identify automatic thoughts. The therapist observes that a strong emotion such as sadness, anxiety, or anger has appeared and then asks the patient to describe the thoughts that "went through your head" just prior to the mood shift.

Beck has described emotion as the "royal road to cognition" (Beck 1989). The patient usually is most accessible during periods of affective arousal, and cognitions such as automatic thoughts and schemas generally are more potent when they are associated with strong emotional responses. Hence, the cognitive therapist capitalizes on spontaneously occurring affective states during the interview and also pursues lines of questioning that are likely to produce intense affect.

Socratic questioning (also termed *guided discovery*) is one of the most frequently used procedures in CT. There is no set format or protocol for this technique. Instead, the therapist must rely on his or her experience and ingenuity to formulate questions that will help patients move from having a "closed mind" to a state of inquisitiveness and curiosity. Socratic questioning stimulates recognition of dysfunctional cognitions and development of a sense of dissonance about the validity of strongly held assumptions.

Imagery and *role play* are used as alternate methods of uncovering cognitions when direct questions are unsuccessful in generating suspected automatic thinking (Beck et al. 1979). These techniques also are selected when only a limited amount of automatic thoughts can be brought out through Socratic questioning and the therapist expects that more important automatic thoughts are present. Most patients, particularly in the early phases of therapy, can benefit from "setting the scene" for the use of imagery (Wright 1988). The patient is asked to describe the details of the setting to help bring the scene alive in the patient's mind and facilitate recall of cognitive responses to the situation.

Role play is a related technique for evoking automatic thoughts. When this procedure is used, the therapist first asks a series of questions to try to understand a vignette involving an interpersonal relationship or other social interchange that is likely to stimulate dysfunctional automatic thinking. Then, with the permission of the patient, the therapist briefly steps into the role of the individual in the scene and facilitates the playing out of a typical response set.

Thought recording is one of the most frequently used CT procedures for identifying automatic thoughts. Patients can be asked to log their thoughts in a number of different ways. The simplest method is the two-column technique—a procedure that often is used when the patient is just beginning to learn how to recognize automatic thoughts.

Thought recording is usually explained and illustrated in a therapy session, and then additional exercises are assigned for homework. Depending on the case conceptualization, the therapist may suggest that the patient pay special attention to certain situations or issues. Also, specific assignments may be made to set up an in vivo experience that is likely to generate automatic thoughts.

Modifying Automatic Thoughts

There usually is no sharp division in CT between the phases of eliciting and modifying automatic thoughts. In fact, the processes involved in identifying automatic thoughts often are enough to initiate substantive change. As patients begin to recognize the nature of their dysfunctional thinking, there typically is an increased degree of skepticism regarding the validity of automatic thoughts. Although patients can start to revise their cognitive distortions without specific additional therapeutic interventions, modification of automatic thoughts can be accelerated if the therapist applies Socratic questioning and other basic CT procedures to the change process.

Techniques used for revising automatic thoughts include 1) generating alternatives, 2) examining the evidence, 3) decatastrophizing, 4) using the Daily Record of Dysfunctional Thoughts, and 5) cognitive rehearsal. Socratic questioning is used in all of these procedures.

Examining the evidence is a major component of the collaborative empirical experience in CT. Specific automatic thoughts or clusters of related automatic thoughts are set forth as hypotheses, and the patient and therapist then search for evidence both for and against the hypothesis.

Decatastrophizing involves efforts to reconceptualize feared outcomes in a manner that encourages coping and problem solving. This technique can be effective even if there is a reasonably high likelihood that a negative prediction will actually occur.

The *Daily Record of Dysfunctional Thoughts* (DRDT; Beck et al. 1979) is one of the standard tools used in modification of automatic thoughts. This five-column thought recording device is used to encourage both identification and change of dysfunctional cognitions. Either a stressful event or a memory of event or situation is noted in the first column. Automatic thoughts are recorded in the second column and are rated for degree of belief (i.e., how much the patient believes them to be true at the moment they occur) on a 0-to-100 scale. The third column is used to observe the emotional response to the automatic thoughts. The intensity of emotion is rated on a 1-to-100 scale. The fourth column, rational thoughts, is the most critical part of the DRDT. The patient is asked to stand back from the automatic thoughts, assess their validity, and then write out a more rational or realistic set of cognitions. There are a wide variety of procedures that can be used to facilitate the development of rational thoughts for the DRDT.

Cognitive rehearsal is used to help uncover potential negative automatic thoughts in advance and to coach the patient in ways of developing more adaptive cognitions. First, the patient is asked to use imagery or role play to identify possible distorted cognitions that could occur in a stressful situation. Second, the patient and therapist work together to modify the dysfunctional cognitions. Third, imagery or role play is used again, this time to practice the more adaptive pattern of thinking. Finally, for a homework assignment, the patient is asked to try out the newly acquired cognitive patterns in vivo.

Identifying and Modifying Schemas

The process of identifying and modifying schemas is somewhat more difficult than changing negative automatic thoughts, because these core beliefs are more deeply embedded, may be largely out of the patient's awareness, and usually have been reinforced through years of life experience. However, many of the same techniques described for automatic thoughts are employed successfully in therapeutic work at the schema level (Beck et al. 1979; Thase and Beck 1992; Wright 1988). Procedures such as Socratic questioning, imagery, role play, and thought recording are used to uncover maladaptive schemas.

As the patient gains experience in recognizing automatic thoughts, repetitive patterns begin to emerge that may suggest the presence of underlying schemas. Therapists have several options at this point. A psychoeducational approach can be utilized to explain the concept of schemas (which can be alternately termed "core beliefs" or "basic assumptions") and their linkage to more superficial, automatic thoughts (Dobson and Shaw 1986). Patients may then start to recognize schemas on their own. However, when the patient first starts to learn about basic assumptions, the therapist may need to suggest that certain schemas might be operative and then engage the patient in collaborative exercises that test these hypotheses.

Modification of schemas may require repeated attention, both in and out of therapy sessions. One commonly used procedure is to ask the patient to keep a list in a therapy notebook of all the schemas that have been identified to date. This technique promotes a high level of awareness of schemas and usually encourages the patient to place issues pertaining to schemas on the agenda for therapy. Cognitive therapy interventions that are particularly helpful in modifying schemas include examining the evidence, listing advantages and disadvantages, generating alternatives, and cognitive rehearsal.

☐ Behavioral Procedures

Behavioral interventions are used in CT to 1) change dysfunctional patterns of behavior (e.g., helplessness, isolation, phobic avoidance, inertia, bingeing and purging); 2) reduce troubling symptoms (e.g., tension, somatic and psychic anxiety, intrusive thoughts); and 3) assist in identifying and modifying maladaptive cognitions (Table 31–3).

The Socratic questions used in cognitively oriented procedures have a direct parallel when the emphasis is on behavioral change. The therapist asks a series of questions that help differentiate actual behavioral deficits from negatively distorted accounts of behavior (Wright 1988). Depressed and anxious patients usually overreport their symptomatic distress or the difficulties they have in managing situations. Often, well-framed questions can reveal cognitive distortions and also stimulate change as the patient considers the negative impact of dysfunctional behavior. Two specific behavioral techniques, activity scheduling and graded task assignments, are explained below.

Activity scheduling is a structured method of learning about the patient's behavioral patterns, encouraging self-monitoring, increasing positive mood, and designing strategies for change (Beck et al. 1979; Wright and Beck 1983). A daily or weekly activity log is employed in which the patient is asked to record what he or she does during each hour of the day and then to rate each activity for mastery and pleasure on a 0-to-10 scale. Almost invariably, the patient rates some activities higher than others on mastery and/or pleasure.

Another behavioral procedure, the *graded task assignment,* can be used when the patient is facing a situation that seems excessively difficult or overwhelming. A challenging behavioral goal is broken down into small steps that can be taken one at a time. With depressed individuals, the graded task assignment typically is used as a problem-solving technique. This stepwise approach, coupled with cognitive techniques such as Socratic questioning and thought recording, can reactivate the patient

---

Table 31–3. Behavioral procedures used in cognitive therapy

Questioning to identify behavioral patterns	Response prevention
	Distraction
Activity scheduling with mastery and pleasure recording	Relaxation exercises
	Respiratory control
Self-monitoring	Assertiveness training
Graded task assignments	Modeling
Behavioral rehearsal	Social skills training

---

and focus his or her energy in a productive manner.

Other behavioral techniques used in CT include behavioral rehearsal (a procedure that is usually combined with cognitive rehearsal described earlier), response prevention (a collaborative exercise in which the patient agrees to stop a dysfunctional behavior, such as prolonged crying spells, and to monitor cognitive responses), distraction (alternate activities that can temporarily divert a patient from intrusive thoughts, depressive ruminations, or other dysfunctional cognitions), relaxation exercises and respiratory control, assertiveness training, modeling, and social skills training (Clark DM et al. 1985; Meichenbaum 1977; Thase and Wright 1991; Wright 1988; Wright and Beck 1983).

☐ Selecting Patients for Cognitive Therapy

Cognitive therapy procedures have been described for a broad range of diagnostic categories (Freeman and Dattilio 1992; Freeman et al. 1989; Wright et al. 1992a). Although there are no contraindications to using this treatment approach, CT is usually not attempted with patients who have a substantial degree of organic brain disease (e.g., mental retardation, dementia, or delirium). Cognitive therapy should be considered an adjunctive therapy for disorders such as major depression with psychotic features, bipolar illness, and schizophrenia, for which there is clear evidence for the effectiveness of biological treatments and for which CT has not yet been systematically investigated (Ludgate et al. 1992).

Clinical experience has suggested that patients who are especially suitable for CT are those who are free of severe character pathology (especially borderline or antisocial features), have previously formed strong, trusting relationships with significant others, have a belief in the importance of self-reliance, and have a curious or inquisitive nature (Thase and Beck 1992). Average or above-average intelligence also can be helpful, but CT procedures can be simplified for those patients with subnormal intellectual skills or impaired learning and memory functioning (Casey and Grant 1992; Wright and Salmon 1990).

■ APPLICATIONS OF COGNITIVE THERAPY

Cognitive therapy methods have been outlined for a number of clinical problems, including conditions not covered here, such as eating disorders (Garner 1992), obsessive-compulsive disorder (Emmelkamp and Beens 1991; Salkovskis 1985), alcohol abuse (Barrett and Meyer 1992; Oei et al. 1991), and hypochondriasis (Warwick and Salkovskis 1990). Group CT techniques have been described by Covi and Primakoff (1988). Procedures for marital and family CT have been set forth by Beck (1988) and

Epstein et al. (1988). Specific adaptations of CT for therapeutic work with children and adolescents have been detailed (DiGiuseppe 1989; Schrodt 1993; Wilkes et al. 1994). Also, strategies have been developed for utilizing CT as a comprehensive model for inpatient treatment (Wright et al. 1992a).

☐ Depression

In the opening phase of CT of depression, the cognitive therapist focuses on establishing a collaborative relationship and introduces the patient to the cognitive model. Early in therapy a special effort may be placed on relieving hopelessness because of the close link between this element of the negative cognitive triad and suicide risk. The clinician carefully matches the therapeutic work to the patient's level of cognitive functioning so that learning is encouraged and the patient is not overwhelmed with the material of therapy. Behavioral techniques, such as activity scheduling and graded task assignments, often are a major component of the opening phase of CT for depression (Thase and Wright 1991).

The middle portion of treatment usually is devoted to eliciting and modifying negatively distorted automatic thoughts. Behavioral techniques continue to be used in most cases. By this point in the therapy, patients should understand the cognitive model and be able to employ thought-monitoring techniques to reverse all three elements of the negative cognitive triad.

Work on eliciting and testing automatic thoughts continues during the latter portion of treatment. However, if there have been gains in functioning and the patient has grasped the basic principles of CT, therapy can turn primarily to identifying and altering maladaptive schemas. The concept of schemas usually has been introduced earlier in therapy, but the principal efforts at changing these underlying structures are reserved for the late phase of treatment when the patient is more likely to grasp and retain complex therapeutic initiatives. Before therapy concludes, the therapist helps the patient review what has been learned during the course of treatment and also suggests thinking ahead to possible circumstances that could trigger a return of depression. Problem-solving strategies are developed that can be employed in future stressful situations (Thase 1992).

☐ Anxiety Disorders

Most authors have recommended that a mixture of cognitive and behavioral measures be utilized in patients who suffer from anxiety disorders (Barlow and Cerny 1988; Beck et al. 1985a; Clark DM and Beck 1988). In panic disorder, the emphasis is placed on helping the patient to recognize and change grossly exaggerated estimates of the significance of physiological responses or fears of imminent psychological disaster (Beck et al. 1985a, 1992; Clark DM 1986). The vicious cycle interaction between catastrophic cognitions and physiological arousal can be broken in two complementary ways: 1) by altering the dysfunctional cognitions, and 2) by interrupting the cascading autonomic hyperactivity. Commonly used cognitive interventions include Socratic questioning, imagery, thought recording, generating alternatives, and examining the evidence. Behavioral measures such as relaxation training and respiratory control are used to dampen the physiological arousal associated with panic (Clark DM et al. 1985). Also, when panic attacks are stimulated by specific situations (e.g., driving, public speaking, crowds), graded exposure may be particularly useful in helping patients to both master a feared task and overcome their panic symptoms.

Cognitive therapy of phobic disorders centers on modifying unrealistic estimates of risk or danger in situations and engaging the patient in a series of graded exposure assignments. Generally, cognitive and behavioral procedures are used simultaneously. For example, a graded task assignment for an individual with agoraphobia might include a stepwise increase in experiences in a social setting accompanied by use of the DRDT to record and revise maladaptive automatic thinking. Patients with generalized anxiety disorder usually have diffuse cognitive distortions about many circumstances in their lives (e.g., physical health, finances, loss of control, family issues) coupled with persistent autonomic overarousal (Beck et al. 1985a). The CT approach to generalized anxiety disorder is closely related to methods used for panic disorder and phobias. However, special attention is paid to defining the stimuli that are associated with increased anxiety. Breaking down the generalized state of anxiety into workable segments can help the patient to gain mastery over what initially appears to be an uncontrollable situation.

☐ Personality Disorders

Beck et al. (1990) articulated a CT approach to personality disorders that is based on a cognitive conceptualization of characterological disturbances. These authors suggest that the different personality types have idiosyncratic cognitions in four main areas: basic beliefs, view of self, view of others, and strategies for social interaction.

Several recommendations have been made for modifying CT for treatment of personality disorders (Beck et al. 1990; Linehan 1987). The problem-oriented, structured, and collaborative empirical characteristics of CT are retained in therapeutic work with patients who have personality disturbances, but there is an added emphasis on the therapeutic relationship. In the therapy encounter, persons with characterological disorders often recapitulate the impaired relationships that they have had with significant others in the past.

Treatment of personality disorders with CT may take considerably longer than therapy of more circumscribed problems such as depression or anxiety. Patients with personality disturbances have deeply ingrained schemas that are unlikely to change within the short-term format used for other disorders. When the course of therapy lengthens, there is a greater chance for development of transference and countertransference reactions. In CT, transference is viewed as a manifestation of underlying schemas. Therefore, transferential phenomena are recognized as opportunities for examining and modifying core beliefs.

An individualized case conceptualization is utilized. This formulation includes hypotheses on the role of maladaptive schemas in symptom production. Consideration also is given to the influences of parent-child conflicts, traumatic experiences, and the current social network on cognitive and behavioral pathology. Although an ultimate goal of treatment is to modulate ineffective or maladaptive schemas, initial efforts may be directed at more readily accessible targets such as increasing self-efficacy or decreasing dysphoric mood. Self-monitoring, self-help exercises, and the structuring procedures used in CT may help prevent excessive dependency.

Adherence to treatment recommendations can be a problem in CT for personality disorders. The therapist can use procedures such as Socratic questioning or schema identification to uncover the reasons for noncompliance and help the patient follow through with homework assignments or other therapeutic work. Considerable patience and persistence are required from the therapist as efforts are made to help the patient reverse chronic psychopathology.

☐ Psychosis

Although biological treatments are the accepted form of therapy for psychotic patients, cognitive psychotherapy can help these individuals understand their disorders, adhere to treatment recommendations, and develop more effective psychosocial functioning (Cochran 1986; Eckman et al. 1992; Kingdon and Turkington 1991; Perris 1989). Also, there have been preliminary reports that CT can, in some cases, be used to decrease primary symptoms of schizophrenia (Fowler and Morley 1989; Kingdon and Turkington 1991).

In CT for patients who have psychotic symptoms, the therapist conveys that maladaptive cognitions and reactions to life stress may interact with biological factors in the expression of the illness (Scott et al. 1992). Therefore, attempts to develop more adaptive cognitions or to learn how to cope better with environmental pressures can assist with efforts toward managing the disorder. During the early part of therapy with a psychotic patient, there is a strong emphasis on building a therapeutic alliance (Scott et al. 1992). The rationale for neuroleptic medication is explained, and the therapist tries to stimulate hope by modifying intensely negative cognitions about the illness or its treatment. Usually, attempts to challenge hallucinations or delusions directly are delayed until a solid therapeutic relationship has been established. However, efforts are made to reverse delusional self-destructive cognitions as early as possible in the treatment process.

Reality testing is performed in a gentle, nonconfrontational manner (Kingdon and Turkington 1991). The therapist uses guided discovery as the major intervention, but also may help the patient to record and change disorted automatic thoughts (Scott et al. 1992). Behavioral techniques such as activity scheduling, graded task assignments, and social skills training also are used with psychotic patients. These procedures can be utilized to provide needed structure or to teach adaptive behaviors.

■ EFFECTIVENESS OF COGNITIVE THERAPY

Cognitive therapy for depression has been investigated in many carefully designed outcome trials, and additional studies have tested the effectiveness of CT for other conditions such as anxiety and eating disorders. The most notable area of research has been in comparing CT with pharmacotherapy in the treatment of depression. In a meta-analysis of CT outcome studies, Dobson (1989) concluded that CT was at least as effective as pharmacotherapy for depression and that there was some evidence for superiority of CT when all studies were considered together. However, in a subsequent review, Hollon et al. (1991) argued that some studies have been biased toward either CT or pharmacotherapy, and thus firm conclusions on the relative efficacy of these treatments are still premature. The first major comparison of CT and pharmacotherapy, performed by Rush et al. (1977), found CT to be superior to imipramine in the treatment of depressed outpatients. Two later studies also found CT to be an effective treatment for depression (Blackburn et al. 1981; Teasdale et al. 1984).

Two major investigations attempted to replicate and extend the original study by Rush et al. (1977). Murphy et al. (1984) randomly assigned depressed outpatients to treatment with CT alone, nortriptyline alone, CT plus placebo, or combined CT and nortriptyline. The results of this study indicated that all treatments were effective for short-term symptom reduction. Similar findings were obtained in an outcome trial completed by Hollon et al. (1992).

The National Institute of Mental Health (NIMH) Treatment of Depression Collaborative Research Program (Elkin et al. 1989) also examined the relative efficacy of CT and pharmacotherapy. Additional comparisons were made with interpersonal psychotherapy and with placebo plus clinical management. All four treatments, including placebo plus clinical management, were associated with highly significant improvement in this trial. In the primary statistical analysis, there were no significant differences found between either of the psychotherapies and imipramine (plus clinical management). However, when patients were stratified by level of initial severity, CT was somewhat less effective (in the more severely affected patients) than the other active treatments. This result was unexpected because previous studies of CT failed to find any association between severity of depression (or endogenous subtype) and treatment outcome (Blackburn et al. 1981; Kovacs et al. 1981; Teasdale et al. 1984).

Further evidence for the effectiveness of CT for depression has come in studies of group CT (Covi and Lipman 1987; Free et al. 1991; Zettle and Rains 1989), geriatric depressed patients (Beutler et al. 1987; Riskind et al. 1985; Steuer et al. 1984), and hospitalized depressed patients (Bowers 1990; Miller et al. 1989; Thase et al. 1991).

Several of the investigations reviewed above measured the effects of the short-term therapies 1 and 2 years after treatment was completed. Results of these studies have generally favored CT in preventing relapse. Kovacs et al. (1981) found that patients treated with CT in the Rush et al. (1977) study had a 31% relapse rate at 1 year compared with a 65% relapse rate for those treated with imipramine. An even higher differential relapse rate was described by Blackburn et al. (1986a). A 2-year naturalistic follow-up investigation of patients treated in the Blackburn et al. (1981) study found a substantially lower relapse rate in patients treated with CT alone (23%) or combined therapy (21%) as compared with pharmacotherapy alone (78%). Similar findings were described by Simons et al. (1986), Hollen et al. (1992), and Evans et al. (1992). The only investigation that did not find a superiority for CT in preventing relapse was the NIMH Collaborative Study (Elkin et al. 1989; Shea et al. 1992). However, patients treated with CT were less likely to require treatment in the follow-up period than with any of the other therapies, and relapse rates were lower for CT (36%) than for imipramine plus clinical management (50%) 18 months after the study was completed.

Cognitive therapy also has been found to be an effective therapy for anxiety disorders. Especially strong evidence has been collected to support the usefulness of CT and related therapies in the treatment of panic disorder. Two major forms of therapy have been developed: *panic control treatment* (PCT), a combination of relaxation training, cognitive restructuring, and exposure (Barlow and Cerny 1988); and *focused cognitive ther-*

apy, a more cognitively oriented treatment that utilizes exposure but places less emphasis on behavioral interventions than does PCT (Beck et al. 1985a).

Barlow et al. (1989) reported that 87% of patients who completed a course of PCT were panic-free after treatment and that PCT was significantly more effective than either relaxation training alone or a waiting-list control condition. In a related investigation that compared PCT and alprazolam for panic disorder, this research group observed that PCT was superior to a waiting-list control or placebo (Klosko et al. 1990).

Focused CT, as described by Beck et al. (1985a), also has fared well in outcome studies. Sokol et al. (1989) reported dramatic reductions in panic frequency (mean of 4.5 panic attacks a week before treatment to 0 attacks per week after treatment) in an uncontrolled study of patients treated at the Center for Cognitive Therapy. Subsequently, Beck et al. (1992) studied panic disorder patients who were randomly assigned to CT or supportive psychotherapy. Results strongly favored CT. After 8 weeks, the number of panic-free patients in the CT group was almost three times that of panic-free patients in the supportive therapy group. An additional study by Clark DM et al. (1994) compared focused CT, relaxation training, imipramine, and a waiting-list control in the treatment of panic disorder. All three active treatments were superior to the control condition, but CT led to greater reductions in anxiety levels, catastrophic cognitions, and frequency of panic attacks.

In a trial of CT for generalized anxiety, Power et al. (1990) randomly assigned patients with generalized anxiety disorder to diazepam, placebo, CT, diazepam plus CT, or placebo plus CT. Individuals treated in any of the three CT conditions were substantially improved by the end of the study. Diazepam alone also showed significant treatment effects as compared with placebo, but these were less marked than those seen with CT. Another study of CT for generalized anxiety indicated that CT was clearly superior to behavior therapy or a waiting-list control (Butler et al. 1991). Two well-executed studies noted that CT is also effective for social phobia (Gelernter et al. 1991; Heimberg et al. 1990). Although behavioral treatments have been shown to reduce compulsive symptoms (Salkovskis and Westbrook 1989), as yet there have been no controlled investigations of a fully developed form of CT for treatment of obsessive-compulsive disorder. In several more recently completed trials, CT significantly reduced the symptoms of bulimia (Agras et al. 1992; Fairburn et al. 1991; Garner 1992; Garner et al. 1993).

A number of studies have examined the utility of CT in behavioral medicine. For example, depressed multiple sclerosis patients treated with CT had significantly improved psychological functioning compared with individuals in a no-treatment control condition (Larcombe and Wilson 1984). Also, cancer patients who received mastectomies experienced reduced psychological distress after a course of cognitively oriented therapy (Tarrier and Maguire 1984). Several groups have reported that CT can be a helpful approach in the management of chronic pain (Phillips 1987; Skinner et al. 1990; Turner and Clancy 1986).

Applications of CT for substance abuse, psychotic disorders, and characterological disturbances have been described in treatment manuals or clinically oriented papers, but as yet have been the subject of limited controlled investigations. Two groups of investigators observed that CT can reduce psychotic symptoms in schizophrenic patients (Fowler and Morley 1989; Kingdon and Turkington 1991), and CT has been shown to improve adherence to lithium carbonate regimens in patients with bipolar disorder (Cochran 1986). In addition, CT has been found to be effective in producing enduring gains in self-management skills of schizophrenic patients (Eckman et al. 1992). These studies suggest that CT has a place in the rehabilitation of patients with psychotic illnesses. Outcome research on CT for personality disorders is the beginning stage of development. However, Linehan (1993) demonstrated that a cognitive-behavioral treatment program can have strong effects in reducing symptoms of borderline personality disorder.

■ REFERENCES

Abramson LY, Seligman MEP, Teasdale JD: Learned helplessness in humans: critique and reformulation. J Abnorm Psychol 87:49–74, 1978

Agras WS, Rossiter EM, Arnow B, et al: Pharmacologic and cognitive-behavioral treatment for bulimia nervosa: a controlled comparison. Am J Psychiatry 149:82–87, 1992

Alloy LB, Ahrens AH: Depression and pessimism for the future: biased use of statistically relevant information in predictions for self versus others. J Pers Soc Psychol 52:366–378, 1987

Barlow DH, Cerny JA: Psychological Treatment of Panic. New York, Guilford, 1988

Barlow DH, Craske MG, Cerny JA, et al: Behavioral treatment of panic disorder. Behavior Therapy 20:261–268, 1989

Barrett CL, Meyer RG: Cognitive therapy with alcoholism, in Cognitive Therapy With Inpatients: Developing a Cognitive Milieu. Edited by Wright JH, Thase ME, Beck AT, et al. New York, Guilford, 1992, pp 315–336

Barrett CL, Wright JH: Therapist variables, in Issues in Psychotherapy Research. Edited by Hersen M, Nichelson L, Bellack AS. New York, Plenum, 1984, pp 361–391

Baxter LR Jr, Schwartz JM, Bergman KS, et al: Caudate glucose metabolic rate changes with both drug and behavior therapy for obsessive-compulsive disorder. Arch Gen Psychiatry 49:681–689, 1992

Beck AT: Thinking and depression, I: idiosyncratic content and cognitive distortions. Arch Gen Psychiatry 9:324–333, 1963

Beck AT: Thinking and depression, II: theory and therapy. Arch Gen Psychiatry 10:561–571, 1964

Beck AT: Depression: Clinical, Experimental, and Theoretical Aspects. New York, Harper & Row, 1967

Beck AT: Cognitive Therapy and the Emotional Disorders. New York, International Universities Press, 1976

Beck AT: Love Is Never Enough: How Couples Can Overcome Misunderstandings, Resolve Conflicts, and Solve Relationship Problems Through Cognitive Therapy. New York, Harper & Row, 1988

Beck AT. Cognitive therapy and research: a 25-year retrospective. Paper presented at the World Congress of Cognitive Therapy. Oxford, UK, June 1989

Beck AT, Kovacs M, Weissman A: Hopelessness and suicidal behavior: an overview. JAMA 234:1146–1149, 1975

Beck AT, Rush AJ, Shaw BF, et al: Cognitive Therapy of Depression. New York, Guilford, 1979

Beck AT, Emery GD, Greenberg RL: Anxiety Disorders and Phobias: A Cognitive Perspective. New York, Basic Books, 1985a

Beck AT, Steer RA, Kovacs M, et al: Hopelessness and eventual suicide: a 10-year prospective study of patients hospitalized with suicidal ideation. Am J Psychiatry 142:559–563, 1985b

Beck AT, Freeman A, et al: Cognitive Therapy of Personality Disorders. New York, Guilford, 1990

Beck AT, Sokol L, Clark DA, et al: A crossover study of focused cognitive therapy for panic disorder. Am J Psychiatry 149:778–783, 1992

Beutler LE, Scogin F, Kirkish P, et al: Group cognitive therapy and alprazolam in the treatment of depression in older adults. J Consult Clin Psychol 55:550–556, 1987

Blackburn IM, Bishop S, Glen AIM, et al: The efficacy of cognitive therapy in depression: a treatment trial using cognitive therapy and pharmacotherapy, each alone and in combination. Br J Psychiatry 139:181–189, 1981

Blackburn IM, Eunson KM, Bishop S: A two-year naturalistic follow-up of depressed patients treated with cognitive therapy, pharmacotherapy, and a combination of both. J Affect Disord 10:67–75, 1986a

Blackburn IM, Jones S, Lewin RJP: Cognitive style in depression. Br J Clin Psychol 25:241–251, 1986b

Bowers WA: Treatment of depressed inpatients: cognitive therapy plus medication, relaxation plus medication, and medication alone. Br J Psychiatry 156:73–78, 1990

Bowlby J: The role of childhood experience in cognitive disturbance, in Cognition and Psychotherapy. Edited by Mahoney MJ, Freeman A. New York, Plenum, 1985, pp 181–200

Butler G, Fennell M, Robson P, et al: Comparison of behavior therapy and cognitive behavior therapy in the treatment of generalized anxiety disorder. J Consult Clin Psychol 59:167–175, 1991

Casey DA, Grant RW: Cognitive therapy with depressed elderly inpatients, in Cognitive Therapy With Inpatients: Developing a Cognitive Milieu. Edited by Wright JH, Thase ME, Beck AT, et al. New York, Guilford, 1992, pp 295–314

Clark DA, Beck AT, Stewart B: Cognitive specificity and positive-negative affectivity: complementary or contradictory views on anxiety and depression? J Abnorm Psychol 99:148–155, 1990

Clark DM: A cognitive approach to panic. Behav Res Ther 24:461–470, 1986

Clark DM, Beck AT: Cognitive approaches, in Handbook of Anxiety Disorders. Edited by Last CG, Hersen M. New York, Pergamon, 1988, pp 362–385

Clark DM, Salkovskis PM, Chalkley AJ: Respiratory control as a treatment for panic attacks. J Behav Ther Exp Psychiatry 16:23–30, 1985

Clark DM, Salkovskis PM, Hackmann A: A comparison of cognitive therapy, applied relaxation and imipramine in the treatment of panic disorder. Br J Psychiatry 164(6):759–769, 1994

Cloitre M, Liebowitz MR: Memory bias in panic disorder: an investigation of the cognitive avoidance hypothesis. Cognitive Therapy and Research 15:371–386, 1991

Cochran SD: Compliance with lithium regimens in the outpatient treatment of bipolar disorder. Journal of Compliance in Health Care 1:151–169, 1986

Covi L, Lipman RS: Cognitive behavioral group psychotherapy combined with imipramine in major depression. Psychopharmacol Bull 23:173–176, 1987

Covi L, Primakoff L: Cognitive group therapy, in American Psychiatric Press Review of Psychiatry, Vol 7. Edited by Frances AJ, Hales RE. Washington, DC, American Psychiatric Press, 1988, pp 608–626

DeMonbreun BG, Craighead WE: Distortion of perception and recall of positive and neutral feedback in depression. Cognitive Therapy and Research 1:311–329, 1977

DiGiuseppe R: Cognitive therapy with children, in Comprehensive Handbook of Cognitive Therapy. Edited by Freeman A, Simon KM, Beutler LE, et al. New York, Plenum, 1989, pp 515–534

Dobson KS: A meta-analysis of the efficacy of cognitive therapy for depression. J Consult Clin Psychol 57:414–419, 1989

Dobson KS, Shaw BF: Cognitive assessment with major depressive disorders. Cognitive Therapy and Research 10:13–29, 1986

Eckman TA, Wirshing WC, Marder SR, et al: Technique for training schizophrenic patients in illness self-management: a controlled trial. Am J Psychiatry 149:1549–1555, 1992

Elkin I, Shea MT, Watkins JT, et al: National Institute of Mental Health Treatment of Depression Collaborative Research Program: general effectiveness of treatments. Arch Gen Psychiatry 46:971–982, 1989

Ellis A: Reason and Emotion in Psychotherapy. New York, Lyle Stuart, 1962

Ellis A: Humanistic Psychotherapy: The Rational-Emotive Approach. Edited by Sagarin E. New York, Julian Press, 1973

Emmelkamp PMG, Beens H: Cognitive therapy with obsessive-compulsive disorder: a comparative evaluation. Behav Res Ther 29:293–300, 1991

Epstein N, Schlesinger SE, Dryden W: Cognitive-Behavioral Therapy With Families. New York, Brunner/Mazel, 1988

Evans MD, Hollon SD, DeRubeis RJ, et al: Differential relapse following cognitive therapy and pharmacotherapy for depression. Arch Gen Psychiatry 49:802–808, 1992

Fairburn CG, Jones R, Peveler RC, et al: Three psychological treatments for bulimia nervosa: a comparative trial. Arch Gen Psychiatry 48:463–469, 1991

Fawcett J, Scheftner W, Clark D, et al: Clinical predictors of suicide in patients with major affective disorders: a controlled prospective study. Am J Psychiatry 144:35–40, 1987

Fitzgerald TE, Phillips W: Attentional bias and agoraphobic avoidance: the role of cognitive style. Journal of Anxiety Disorders 5:333–341, 1991

Fowler D, Morley S: The cognitive-behavioral treatment of hallucinations and delusions: a preliminary study. Behavioural Psychotherapy 17:262–282, 1989

Frankl VE: Logos, paradox, and the search for meaning, in Cognition and Psychotherapy. Edited by Mahoney MJ, Freeman A. New York, Plenum, 1985, pp 3–49

Free ML, Oei TPS, Sanders MR: Treatment outcome of a group cognitive therapy program for depression. Int J Group Psychother 41:533–547, 1991

Freeman A, Dattilio FM: Comprehensive Casebook of Cognitive Therapy. New York, Plenum, 1992

Freeman A, Simon KM, Beutler LE, et al (eds): Comprehensive Handbook of Cognitive Therapy. New York, Plenum, 1989

Garner DM: Psychotherapy for eating disorders. Current Opinion in Psychiatry 5:391–395, 1992

Garner DM, Rockert W, Davis R, et al: Comparison of cognitive-behavioral and supportive-expressive therapy for bulimia nervosa. Am J Psychiatry 150:37–46, 1993

Gelernter CS, Uhde TW, Cimbolic P, et al: Cognitive-behavioral and pharmacological treatments of social phobia: a controlled study. Arch Gen Psychiatry 48:938–945, 1991

Glass CR, Furlong M: Cognitive assessment of social anxiety: affective and behavioral correlates. Cognitive Therapy and Research 14:365–384, 1990

Gotlib IH: Self-reinforcement and recall: differential deficits in depressed and nondepressed psychiatric inpatients. J Abnorm Psychol 90:521–530, 1981

Gotlib IH, Olson JM: Depression, psychopathology, and self-serving attributions. Br J Clin Psychol 22:309–310, 1983

Greenberg LS, Safran JD: Integrating affect and cognition: a perspective on the process of therapeutic change. Cognitive Therapy and Research 8:559–578, 1984

Guidano VF, Liotti G: Cognitive Processes and Emotional Disorders: A Structural Approach to Psychotherapy. New York, Guilford, 1983

Haaga DA, Dyck MJ, Ernst D: Empirical status of cognitive theory of depression. Psychol Bull 110:215–236, 1991

Hammon C, Krantz SE, Cochran SD: Relationships between depression and causal attributions about stressful life events. Cognitive Therapy and Research 5:351–358, 1981

Heimberg RG, Dodge CS, Hope DA, et al: Cognitive behavioral group treatment for social phobia: comparison with a credible placebo control. Cognitive Therapy and Research 14:1–23, 1990

Hollon SD, Kendall PC: Cognitive self-statements in depression: development of an automatic thought questionnaire. Cognitive Therapy and Research 4:383–395, 1980

Hollon SD, Shelton RC, Loosen PT: Cognitive therapy and pharmacotherapy for depression. J Consult Clin Psychol 59:88–99, 1991

Hollon SD, DeRubeis RJ, Evans MD, et al: Cognitive therapy and pharmacotherapy for depression: singly and in combination. Arch Gen Psychiatry 49:774–781, 1992

Imber SD, Pilkonis PA, Sotsky SM, et al: Mode-specific effects among three treatments for depression. J Consult Clin Psychol 58:352–359, 1990

Ingram RE, Kendall PC: The cognitive side of anxiety. Cognitive Therapy and Research 11:523–536, 1987

Ingram RE, Kendall PC, Smith TW, et al: Cognitive specificity in emotional distress. J Pers Soc Psychol 53:734–742, 1987

Kandel ER, Schwartz JH: Molecular biology of learning: modulation of transmitter release. Science 218:433–443, 1983

Kelly G: The Psychology of Personal Constructs. New York, WW Norton, 1955

Kendall PC, Hollon SD: Anxious self-talk: development of the Anxious Self-Statements Questionnaire (ASSQ). Cognitive Therapy and Research 13:81–93, 1989

Kingdon DG, Turkington D: The use of cognitive behavior therapy with a normalizing rationale in schizophrenia: preliminary report. J Nerv Ment Dis 179:207–211, 1991

Klosko JS, Barlow DH, Tassinari R, et al: A comparison of alprazolam and behavior therapy in treatment of panic disorder. J Consult Clin Psychol 58:77–84, 1990

Kovacs M, Rush AJ, Beck AT, et al: Depressed outpatients treated with cognitive therapy or pharmacotherapy: a one-year follow-up. Arch Gen Psychiatry 38:33–39, 1981

Krantz SE: When depressive cognitions reflect negative realities. Cognitive Therapy and Research 9:595–610, 1985

Larcombe NA, Wilson PH: An evaluation of cognitive-behaviour therapy for depression in patients with multiple sclerosis. Br J Psychiatry 145:366–371, 1984

Lefebvre MF: Cognitive distortion and cognitive errors in depressed psychiatric and low back pain patients. J Consult Clin Psychol 49:517–525, 1981

Linehan MM: Dialectical behavior therapy for borderline personality disorder: theory and method. Bull Menninger Clin 51:261–276, 1987

Linehan MM, Heard HL, Armstrong HE: Naturalistic follow-up of a behavioral treatment for chronically parasuicidal borderline patients. Arch Gen Psychiatry 50:971–974, 1993

Ludgate JW, Wright JH, Bowers W, et al: Individual cognitive therapy with inpatients, in Cognitive Therapy With Inpatients: Developing a Cognitive Milieu. Edited by Wright JH, Thase ME, Beck AT, et al. New York, Guilford, 1992, pp 91–120

Mahoney MJ: Psychotherapy and human change processes, in Cognition and Psychotherapy. Edited by Mahoney MJ, Freeman A. New York, Plenum, 1985, pp 3–43

Mathews A, MacLeod C: An information-processing approach to anxiety. Journal of Cognitive Psychotherapy: An International Quarterly 1:105–115, 1987

McNally RJ, Foa EB: Cognition and agoraphobia: bias in the interpretation of threat. Cognitive Therapy and Research 11:567–581, 1987

Meichenbaum DB: Cognitive-Behavior Modification: An Integrative Approach. New York, Plenum, 1977

Miller IW, Norman WH, Keitner GI, et al: Cognitive-behavioral treatment of depressed inpatients. Behavior Therapy 20:25–47, 1989

Minkoff K, Bergman E, Beck AT, et al: Hopelessness, depression, and attempted suicide. Am J Psychiatry 130:455–459, 1973

Mizes JS, Landolf-Fritsche B, Grossman-McKee D: Patterns of distorted cognitions in phobic disorders: an investigation of clinically severe simple phobics, social phobics, and agoraphobics. Cognitive Therapy and Research 11:583–592, 1987

Murphy GE, Simons AD, Wetzel RD, et al: Cognitive therapy and pharmacotherapy, singly and together in the treatment of depression. Arch Gen Psychiatry 41:33–41, 1984

Nelson RE, Craighead WE: Selective recall of positive and negative feedback, self-control behaviors, and depression. J Abnorm Psychol 86:379–388, 1977

Oei TPS, Lim B, Young RM: Cognitive processes and cognitive behavior therapy in the treatment of problem drinking. Journal of Addictive Diseases 10(3):63–80, 1991

Perris C: Cognitive Therapy With Schizophrenic Patients. New York, Guilford, 1989

Peterson C, Villanova P, Raps CS: Depression and attributions: factors responsible for inconsistent results in the published literature. J Abnorm Psychol 94:165–168, 1985

Phillips HC: The effects of behavioral treatment on chronic pain. Behav Res Ther 25:365–377, 1987

Power KG, Simpson RJ, Swanson V, et al: Controlled comparison of pharmacological and psychological treatment of generalized anxiety disorder in primary care. British Journal of General Practice 40:289–294, 1990

Raimy V: Misunderstandings of the Self. San Francisco, CA, Jossey-Bass, 1975

Raps CS, Peterson C, Reinhard KE, et al: Attributional style among depressed patients. J Abnorm Psychol 91:102–108, 1982

Riskind JH, Beck AT, Steer RA: Cognitive-behavioral therapy in geriatric depression: comment on Steuer et al. J Consult Clin Psychol 53:944–945, 1985

Rush AJ, Beck AT, Kovacs M, et al: Comparative efficacy of cognitive therapy and pharmacotherapy in the treatment of depressed outpatients. Cognitive Therapy and Research 1:17–37, 1977

Salkovskis PM: Obsessional-compulsive problems: a cognitive-behavioral analysis. Behav Res Ther 25:571–583, 1985

Salkovskis PM, Westbrook D: Behavior therapy and obsessional ruminations: can failure be turned into success? Behav Res Ther 27:149–160, 1989

Schrodt GR Jr: Adolescent inpatient treatment, in Cognitive Therapy With Inpatients: Developing a Cognitive Milieu. Edited by Wright JH, Thase ME, Beck AT, et al. New York, Guilford, 1993, pp 273–294

Scott J, Byers S, Turkington D: The chronic patient, in Cognitive Therapy With Inpatients: Developing a Cognitive Milieu. Edited by Wright JH, Thase ME, Beck AT, et al. New York, Guilford, 1992, pp 357–390

Selmi PM, Klein MH, Greist JH, et al: Computer-administered cognitive-behavioral therapy for depression. Am J Psychiatry 147:51–56, 1990

Selmi PM, Klein MH, Greist JH, et al: Computer-administered therapy for depression. MD Comput 8:98–102, 1991

Shea MT, Elkin I, Imber SD, et al: Course of depressive symptoms over follow-up: findings from the National Institute of Mental Health Treatment of Depression Collaborative Research Program. Arch Gen Psychiatry 49:782–787, 1992

Simons AD, Garfield SL, Murphy GE: The process of change in cognitive therapy and pharmacotherapy for depression: changes in mood and cognition. Arch Gen Psychiatry 41:45–51, 1984

Simons AD, Murphy GE, Levine JL, et al: Cognitive therapy and pharmacotherapy for depression: sustained improvement over one year. Arch Gen Psychiatry 43:43–48, 1986

Skinner JB, Erskine A, Pearce S, et al: The evaluation of a cognitive-behavioral treatment program in outpatients with chronic pain. J Psychosom Res 34:13–19, 1990

Sokol L, Beck AT, Greenberg RL, et al: Cognitive therapy of panic disorder: a nonpharmacological alternative. J Nerv Ment Dis 177:711–716, 1989

Steuer JL, Mintz J, Hammen CL, et al: Cognitive-behavioral and psychodynamic group psychotherapy in treatment of geriatric depression. J Consult Clin Psychol 52:180–189, 1984

Tarrier N, Maguire P: Treatment of psychological distress following mastectomy: an initial report. Behav Res Ther 22:81–84, 1984

Teasdale JD, Fennell MJV, Hibbert GA, et al: Cognitive therapy for major depressive disorder in primary care. Br J Psychiatry 144:400–406, 1984

Teasdale JD, Fogarty SJ: Differential effects of induced mood on retrieval of pleasant and unpleasant events from episodic memory. J Abnorm Psychol 88:248–257, 1979

Thase ME: Transition and aftercare, in Cognitive Therapy With Inpatients: Developing a Cognitive Milieu. Edited by Wright JH, Thase ME, Beck AT, et al. New York, Guilford, 1992, pp 414–435

Thase ME, Beck AT: An overview of cognitive therapy, in Cognitive Therapy With Inpatients: Developing a Cognitive Milieu. Edited by Wright JH, Thase ME, Beck AT, et al. New York, Guilford, 1992, pp 3–35

Thase ME, Wright JH: Cognitive behavioral therapy with depressed inpatients: an abridged treatment manual. Behavior Therapy 22:579–595, 1991

Thase ME, Bowler K, Harden T: Cognitive behavior therapy of endogenous depression, Part 2: preliminary findings in 16 unmedicated patients. Behavior Therapy 22:469–477, 1991

Truax CB, Mitchell KM: Research on certain therapist interpersonal skills in relation to process and outcome, in Handbook of Psychotherapy and Behavior Change: An Empirical Analysis. Edited by Bergin AE, Garfield SL. New York, Wiley, 1971, pp 299–344

Turner JA, Clancy S: Strategies for coping with chronic low back pain: relationship to pain and disability. Pain 24:355–364, 1986

Warwick HM, Salkovskis PM: Hypochondriasis. Behav Res Ther 28:105–117, 1990

Watkins JT, Rush AJ: Cognitive response test. Cognitive Therapy and Research 7:425–435, 1983

Wenzlaff RM, Grozier SA: Depression and the magnification of failure. J Abnorm Psychol 97:90–93, 1988

Wilkes TCR, Belsher G, Rush AJ, et al: Cognitive Therapy for Depressed Adolescents. New York, Guilford Press, 1994

Wright JH: Cognitive therapy of depression, in American Psychiatric Press Review of Psychiatry, Vol 7. Edited by Frances AJ, Hales RE. Washington, DC, American Psychiatric Press, 1988, pp 554–570

Wright JH, Beck AT: Cognitive therapy of depression: theory and practice. Hosp Community Psychiatry 34:1119–1127, 1983

Wright JH, Davis MH: Hospital psychiatry in transition, in Cognitive Therapy With Inpatients: Developing a Cognitive Milieu. Edited by Wright JH, Thase ME, Beck AT, et al. New York, Guilford, 1992, pp 193–218

Wright JH, Salmon PG: Learning and memory in depression, in Depression: New Directions in Theory, Research, and Practice. Edited by McCann CD, Endler NS. Toronto, Wall and Thompson, 1990, pp 211–236

Wright JH, Thase ME: Cognitive and biological therapies: a synthesis. Psychiatric Annals 22:451–458, 1992

Wright JH, Thase ME, Beck AT, et al (eds): Cognitive Therapy With Inpatients: Developing a Cognitive Milieu. New York, Guilford, 1992a

Wright JH, Thase ME, Sensky T: Cognitive and biological therapies: a combined approach, in Cognitive Therapy With Inpatients: Developing a Cognitive Milieu. Edited by Wright JH, Thase ME, Beck AT, et al. New York, Guilford, 1992b, pp 193–218

Wright JH, Salmon P, Wright AS, et al: Cognitive therapy: a multimedia learning program. Paper presented at the annual meeting of the American Psychiatric Association, Miami, FL, May 1995

Zettle RD, Rains JC: Group cognitive and contextual therapies in treatment of depression. J Clin Psychol 45:436–445, 1989

Zimmerman M, Coryell W, Corenthal C, et al: Dysfunctional attitudes and attribution style in healthy controls and patients with schizophrenia, psychotic depression, and nonpsychotic depression. J Abnorm Psychol 95:403–405, 1986

CHAPTER 32

Hypnosis

David Spiegel, M.D.

Hypnosis is a natural state of aroused, attentive focal concentration with a relative suspension of peripheral awareness. It involves an intensity of focus that allows the hypnotized person to make maximal use of innate abilities to control perception, memory, and somatic function. Hypnotic capacity represents both a potential vulnerability to certain kinds of psychiatric illness, such as dissociative disorders, and an asset, a facilitator of various psychotherapeutic strategies. Because it is a normal and widely distributed trait, and because entry into hypnotic states occurs spontaneously, hypnotic phenomena occur frequently. Even psychiatrists who make no formal use of hypnosis can enhance their effectiveness by learning to recognize and take advantage of hypnotic mental states.

Alterations in consciousness occur frequently in the course of ordinary life; indeed, such cyclic variation is the norm, not the exception. Sleep is requisite for normal attention, and it may also be that alterations within wakefulness may optimize attentional processes. Certain variations in consciousness may change the relationship between mental and physical states and alter the degree to which concentration is focused. One of these alterations in consciousness is *hypnosis*, a naturally occurring phenomenon in which focal concentration is intensified at the expense of peripheral awareness. Hypnotic experience involves three main factors—*absorption, dissociation,* and *suggestibility.*

Absorption is an immersion in a central experience at the expense of contextual orientation (Tellegen and Atkinson 1974). When one is intensely involved in a central object of consciousness, one tends to ignore perceptions, thoughts, memories, or motor activities at the periphery. Hypnotized individuals are intensely absorbed in their trance experience. In a hypnotic age regression, subjects act as though they were younger, suspending awareness that they really are decades older than the assumed age. The incongruity is available to them, yet they easily ignore it.

This intense absorption means that many routine experiences that would ordinarily be conscious occur out of ordinary conscious awareness. Even rather complex emotional states or sensory experiences may be dissociated. These experiences may range from the simple, such as a feeling that the hand is not as much a part of the body as usual, to the complex. Some involve memory alterations, such as dissociative amnesia for a traumatic event, while others pertain to identity and motor function, as in a fugue episode in which for a period of hours to months an individual functions as though he or she had a different name and residence. Such experiences can be both induced and reversed with the structured use of hypnosis.

Dissociated information is temporarily and reversibly unavailable to consciousness, but may nonetheless influence conscious (or other unconscious) experience. A rape victim may have no conscious memory of the crime, yet become anxious when exposed to stimuli reminiscent of the event. Absorption and dissociation are complementary constructs. Intense focal attention facilitates putting other information outside of conscious awareness.

Suggestibility is enhanced in hypnosis. Because of their intense absorption in the trance experience, hypnotized individuals usually accept instructions relatively uncritically. They are also less prone to distinguish an instruction as coming from another rather than themselves (i.e., hypnotic source amnesia) and so will tend to act on another person's ideas as though they were their own.

■ CLARIFICATION OF MYTHS

There are a variety of common "mythunderstandings" about hypnosis that are addressed in the following clarifications:

1. **Hypnosis is not sleep.** The hypnotized individual is not asleep, but, rather, awake and alert. Like the sleeping person, a hypnotized individual has suspended peripheral awareness but, in contrast to what occurs in sleep, his or her focal attention is intense and carefully controlled.
2. **Hypnotizability is a trait: not everyone is hypnotizable.** Hypnotizability is a capacity that varies considerably from one individual to another. Indeed, hypnotizability is a stable and measurable trait; it is highest in late childhood and declines gradually throughout adult-

hood. About 1 out of 4 adults is not hypnotizable, and 1 out of 10 is highly hypnotizable (Spiegel and Spiegel 1987).

3. **Hypnosis is not something *done to* a subject or patient.** Recognizing this fact is very helpful in demystifying hypnosis and reducing anxiety on the part of both the doctor inducing hypnosis and the patient. A correctly performed hypnotic induction allows the patient and doctor to assess and explore the patient's hypnotic capacity or lack of it. There are no apparent gender differences in hypnotizability (Stern et al. 1979).

4. **Hypnotizability is *not* a susceptibility or a sign of weak-mindedness.** Rather, it is an intact capacity for focused concentration that is often associated with, if anything, the absence of serious psychotic and neurological disorders.

5. **There is nothing intrinsically dangerous about hypnosis.** Hypnosis is a benign procedure, tolerated well by patients. The same cognitive flexibility that allows patients to enter the trance facilitates their exit from it with clear structure and support from the therapist. There are few serious contraindications for the use of hypnosis. An occasional patient is slow in exiting from the hypnotic state. Calm reassurance never fails to complete the termination of the trance procedure. Rarely, a paranoid patient may incorporate the attempted hypnotic induction into a delusional system, although careful explanation of the procedures in advance and the use of a hypnotizability test as an initial encounter tend to minimize the likelihood of this occurring. A suicidally depressed patient may view the use of hypnosis as a last resort and become dangerously disappointed if he or she perceives it as a failure.

6. **There is nothing intrinsically therapeutic about hypnosis.** Many patients find it a relaxing and comfortable state. The use to which the trance state is put, however, is the crucial issue in determining treatment outcome.

■ MEASURING HYPNOTIZABILITY

A clinical assessment of hypnotizability can be a helpful starting point for the use of hypnosis in treatment (Spiegel and Spiegel 1987). This approach combines a hypnotic induction with a procedure that provides the psychiatrist with a deduction of the patient's hypnotic ability. It has several advantages:

1. Hypnotizability testing helps to clarify the hypnotic interaction. It is the therapist's role to assess systematically patients' ability to respond rather than to push them to respond in a certain manner.

2. The use of such a standardized interaction with a large number of patients allows the psychiatrist to make informed inferences about variations in patient response. Patients' relative ability to allow the therapist to restructure their inner experience via hypnosis, or their inability to do so, also provides helpful information about their general interpersonal style.

3. Hypnotizability testing provides data about the patient's ability to respond to a treatment that employs hypnosis. Nonhypnotizable individuals can be offered an alternative approach that is likely to be more efficacious, such as one of the behavioral therapies, biofeedback, or relevant psychoactive medication.

☐ Hypnotizability Scales

Hypnotizability scales have existed since the early part of the century and have been widely used in research—for example, the Stanford Hypnotic Susceptibility Scales, Forms A and B (SHSS:A) and Form C (SHSS:C) (Hilgard 1965; Weitzenhoffer and Hilgard 1962). These scales involve a structured hypnotic induction and an assessment of the subject's response to a variety of instructions, including alterations in control over movement, sensation, temporal orientation, and perception, such as hallucinatory experiences. More recently, hypnotizability scales have been developed for clinical use (Hypnotic Induction Profile [HIP; Spiegel and Spiegel 1987]; Stanford Hypnotic Clinical Scale [SHCS; Hilgard and Hilgard 1975]). These scales are briefer (5 to 10 minutes for the HIP and 20 minutes for the SHCS, compared with 1 hour for the Stanford research scales) and are designed for comfortable use even with patients who have severe psychiatric disturbances.

The HIP calls for rapid induction commencing with upward gaze and lowering of the eyelids, followed by a series of instructions to the subject to elevate the left hand and keep it in the air, even if the examiner pulls the hand down. Subjects are rated on five items assessing cognitive and behavioral aspects of the hypnotic experience: 1) their ability to experience a sense of *dissociation* of the left hand from the body; 2) *movement* of the hand, floating back up in the air after being pulled down, accompanied by 3) a sense of *involuntariness* while elevating the hand; 4) response to the *cut-off signal* ending the hypnotic experience; and 5) a *sensory alteration* in the hand or elsewhere in the body. The entire procedure can be administered and scored in less than 10 minutes. It predicts responsiveness to a variety of treatments and facilitates differential diagnosis (Spiegel and Spiegel 1987; Spiegel et al. 1982, 1988).

☐ Prediction of Treatment Responsiveness

Because hypnotic trance involves an intensification of concentration and an increase in receptiveness, it would make sense that the capacity to experience hypnosis should be correlated with responsiveness to treatment. Indeed, this has been found to be the case in treatment with hypnosis of problems such as pain (Hilgard and Hilgard 1975), smoking cessation (Spiegel and Spiegel 1987; Spiegel et al. 1993), and asthma (Collison 1975). Hypnotizability is also correlated with the increased likelihood of responding even to treatments that do not explicitly employ hypnosis, such as acupuncture (Katz et al. 1974).

■ HYPNOTIZABILITY AND PSYCHIATRIC DISORDERS

One of the most interesting theoretical areas of research in hypnosis is the relationship between hypnotizability and psychopathology (Figure 32–1). There is accumulating evidence that high hypnotizability is associated with some serious psychiatric disorders.

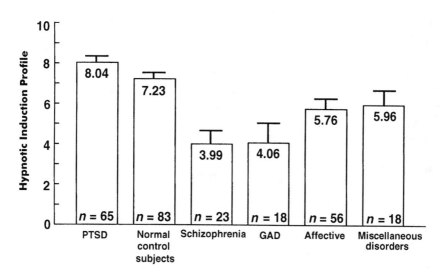

Figure 32–1. Psychopathology and hypnotizability. Hypnotic Induction Profile scores indicate higher than normal responsiveness among patients with posttraumatic stress disorder, but lower responsiveness among other psychiatric patient groups (Spiegel D et al. 1988).

☐ Hypnotizability in Dissociative Identity Disorder

Clinicians have long observed that it is unusual to find a patient with a severe dissociative disorder such as fugue, amnesia, or dissociative identity disorder (i.e., multiple personality disorder) who is not highly hypnotizable (Frischholz 1985). The literature on dissociative identity disorder indicates that most patients with this disorder are highly hypnotizable and report a history of severe physical and sexual abuse in childhood (Braun and Sachs 1985; Kluft 1985). This observation has led to the recognition that the capacity to dissociate—to separate, for example, psychological from physical experience—is mobilized both during and after periods of extreme physical duress such as assault. In some cases, especially of repeated, severe assault in childhood, a temporary dissociation that allows the child to tolerate overwhelming fear and pain becomes an ongoing part of the personality structure.

Hypnosis is useful early in treatment to determine whether patients have a dissociative disorder, and to provide rapid access to these dissociated states. This process can be used to demonstrate for these patients how to control dissociation and to begin a process of communication that in the context of well-structured psychotherapy can eventually lead to a reduction in such spontaneous dissociative symptoms. The capacity for hypnotic dissociation has been found to be relevant to a milder but pronounced cluster of symptoms that has many similarities to the DSM-IV (American Psychiatric Association 1994) Axis II histrionic personality disorder diagnosis. Patients with these symptoms, who are highly hypnotizable, repeatedly establish naive and dependent relationships, often express symptoms in dramatic ways, are sluggish in reorienting to internal rather than external cues, and form intense affiliations with new ideas and persons that tend not to last over time. They require a tightly structured, supportive psychotherapy that recognizes their tendency to unwittingly build relationships in which they are vulnerable to control by others.

☐ Hypnotizability in Schizophrenia and Affective Disorders

Given the complex cognitive tasks involved in tests of hypnotic responsiveness, it makes sense theoretically that patients suffering from delusions, loose associations, and hallucinations might score more poorly on tests of hypnotizability. More than 20 studies have been conducted on the issue, and the findings have generally shown somewhat lower, and the absence of very high, hypnotizability among schizophrenic patients (Lavoie and Sabourin 1980; Pettinati et al. 1990). Schizophrenic patients show a more restricted range of scores, and those who do better on psychological tests such as the Rorschach are more hypnotizable than those who display more thought disorganization.

Studies using the HIP have in particular shown substantially lower hypnotizability scores for schizophrenic individuals compared with normal subjects (Spiegel et al. 1982), while those employing the Stanford scales (SHSS:A and SHSS:C; Weitzenhoffer and Hilgard 1962) have tended to show a restricted range of scores among schizophrenic patients but mean scores that are not significantly lower than those of comparison groups (Lavoie and Sabourin 1980; Pettinati 1982). In addition, patients with major affective disorders have been found to score higher than schizophrenic patients but lower than normal subjects (Spiegel et al. 1982) (Figure 32–1).

These findings on the differential responsiveness for hypnotizability open the possibility that hypnotizability testing can in certain cases be used to clarify differential diagnosis. There is considerable phenomenological overlap among acute psychoses. However, patients with hysterical psychosis and dissociative disorders should be extremely hypnotizable (Steingard and Frankel 1985). On the other hand, patients with chronic or borderline schizophrenia score at the other end of the hypnotizability spectrum (Spiegel et al. 1982).

■ HYPNOSIS IN TREATMENT

Hypnosis has been shown to be an effective adjunct to the treatment of a variety of symptoms and problems (Table 32–1). Hypnosis has an important place in the treatment of dissociative disorders, for example, in identifying and controlling dissociative fugue, amnesia, and identity disorder, and in treating posttraumatic stress disorder and conversion disorder. Hypnosis also has been widely used in the treatment of anxiety disorders and phobias. A number of studies have demonstrated the efficacy of hypnosis in the treatment of pain. It has been useful in the control of such psychosomatic problems as asthma and psoriasis. It has been extensively used in habit control, especially for smoking, and to a lesser extent for weight control.

Consideration should be given to the use of hypnosis if the patient has the requisite hypnotizability, is cooperative with the procedure, and has a problem for which hypnosis has been shown to be of adjunctive use. The first criterion can be met by a brief but frank discussion with the patient about the nature of hypnosis, with clarification of the fact that in hypnosis the doctor does not control the patient but rather explores the patient's capacity to focus and intensify concentration. The therapist should be no more interested in using hypnosis than the patient is, and the extremely rare problems arising from the use of hypnosis can generally be avoided if the procedure is never forced upon an unwilling or ambivalent patient.

Table 32–1.   Uses of hypnosis in psychiatric disorders

Psychiatric disorder	Hypnotic technique(s)	Goals
Bulimia nervosa	Restructuring relationship to body and eating	To control spontaneous dissociative aspects of impulsive behavior.
Conversion disorder	Hypnotizability testing, symptom enhancement, symptom alteration	To help make differential diagnosis and to identify, control, and reduce symptoms.
Dissociative disorder	Hypnotizability testing, symptom elicitation, regression, restructuring	To clarify diagnosis, enhance symptom control, facilitate access to dissociative states, and facilitate working through.
Phobic and anxiety disorders	Dissociate psychological from somatic distress, screen technique, desensitization	To reduce somatic amplification of anxiety, restructure anxiety-inducing stimuli, and separate stimuli from conditioned response.
PTSD	Regression, abreaction, restructuring	To enhance control over access to traumatic memories, reduce spontaneous "flashbacks," and facilitate working through.
Schizophrenia	Hypnotizability testing	To help make differential diagnosis.

☐ Dissociative Disorders

Hypnosis can be a helpful tool in the psychotherapy of dissociative disorders. Patients with these disorders experience their fugue states, dissociated identities, and conversion symptoms as occurring suddenly and beyond their control. The formal use of hypnosis can serve therapeutic as well as diagnostic purposes. The controlled access to the hypnotic state often spontaneously triggers the dissociative symptom (e.g., hysterical pseudoseizures). If not, it is possible to induce the symptom, for example, using age regression and by having the patient reexperience the last time the dissociative symptom was present. In this structured manner the patient can be taught to practice bringing on the symptom and thereby learn to control it.

☐ Posttraumatic Stress Disorder

The use of hypnosis in the psychotherapy of trauma was initially thought to be limited to abreaction, based on Freud's cathartic method. The idea was that some intense affect associated with the traumatic event needed to be released, and that simply repeating the event with its associated emotion in the trance state would suffice to resolve the symptoms. However, it became clear to Freud that conscious, cognitive work must be done on the material for it to be successfully worked through (Freud 1914/1958). For therapy to be effective, the patient must reexperience the traumatic events with an enhanced sense of control over the memories of the experience. This may take the form of a symbolic restructuring of the traumatic experiences in hypnosis (Spiegel and Spiegel 1987), with the use of a grief work model (Spiegel 1981). Hypnosis can be used to provide controlled access to the dissociated or repressed memories of the traumatic experience and then to help patients restructure their memories of the events.

Because there is growing evidence that many people enter a dissociated state during physical trauma (Cardeña and Spiegel 1993), it makes sense that enabling them to enter a structured dissociative state in therapy would facilitate their access to memories of the traumatic experience, memories that must be worked through in order to resolve the posttraumatic symptomatology. Hypnosis can be helpful in allowing the victim to review aspects of the trauma in a controlled manner. In a trance, patients can be quickly taught how to produce a state of physical relaxation despite whatever psychological stress they experience. They can then find a condensation image that symbolizes some aspect of the trauma. It is often helpful to have them do this on an imaginary screen giving them some sense of distance from the event. It is also useful to divide the screen in half, having the patient picture on one side some aspect of the event (e.g., a rape victim's image of the assailant), and on the other side of the screen, something he or she did to protect himself or herself. They can then be taught to practice a self-hypnosis exercise in which they work through traumatic memories while enhancing their sense of control over the process (Spiegel 1981). The principles of this kind of psychotherapy can be summarized with the following eight "C"'s:

1. **Confrontation.** It is important to confront the traumatic events directly rather than attribute the symptoms to some long-standing personality problem.
2. **Confession.** It is often necessary to allow such patients to confess deeds or emotions that are embarrassing to them and at times repugnant to the therapist.
3. **Consolation.** The intensity of these experiences requires an actively

consoling approach from the therapist, lest he or she be perceived as being judgmental or as collaborating in the pain inflicted on the patient.

4. **Condensation.** Finding an image that condenses a crucial aspect of the traumatic experience can make the overwhelming aspects of the trauma more manageable by giving them concrete, symbolic form. This can facilitate restructuring of the experience by joining previously disparate images and allows patients to attenuate their pain.

5. **Consciousness.** Previously dissociated traumatic memories are made conscious in a gradual manner that does not overwhelm the patient.

6. **Concentration.** Use of the intense concentration characteristic of the hypnotic state can reinforce the boundaries of the traumatic experience and the painful affect associated with it. The inference is then made that when the hypnotic state is ended, attention can be shifted away from the traumatic experience.

7. **Control.** Because the most painful aspect of severe trauma is the sense of helplessness and loss of control, it is important that the therapeutic intervention enhance the patient's sense of control over the memories. Allow patients to terminate the working through when they feel they have had enough, feel they can remember as much from the hypnosis as they wish, and feel in charge of their self-hypnosis experience.

8. **Congruence.** The goal is to help patients integrate dissociated or repressed traumatic material into conscious awareness in such a way that they can tolerate experiencing the memories as part of themselves.

■ FORENSIC USES

A major application of hypnosis in the legal setting has been for the purpose of refreshing recollection of witnesses and victims of crimes. There have been some positive results with this technique, for example, the case involving the driver of a hijacked school bus in Chowchilla, California (*People v. Schoenfeld* 1980). Under hypnosis, and not previously, the driver was able to recall the numbers and letters in the license plate on the car that overtook the bus. This led to the arrest and conviction of the kidnappers.

Nonetheless, there has been serious criticism of the use of hypnosis with witnesses and victims. Two charges are leveled at the technique. One is "confabulation"—that a hypnotized witness will make up material and become someone who believes his or her misstatement out of a desire to please the hypnotist or simply as a result of being in the nonrational hypnotic state itself. The other is "concreting"—that having gone through the process of hypnosis, even if new information is not made up, the subject will emerge with an enhanced conviction that his or her memories are correct and that the subject will therefore be more convincing to a jury than he or she should be (Diamond 1980).

From a practical point of view, it is wise to caution attorneys and witnesses that the use of hypnosis might open the possibility of challenge to witnesses' credibility or even to their admissibility as a witness. Taking note of this problem, the California Legislature (1985) passed a law holding that witnesses would be allowed to testify after hypnotic interrogation if certain guidelines were followed. These guidelines include the use of an independent expert psychiatrist or psychologist as a hypnosis consultant, careful documentation of the witness's memory prior to hypnosis, and electronic recording of all interaction preceding, during, and after hypnosis sessions. It is clear that hypnosis is no truth serum and that the courts must weigh the effects of any hypnotic ceremony on a witness. At the same time, hypnosis may in certain cases help a traumatized and amnesic witness to recall details not made available through conventional interrogation methods.

■ BRIEF TREATMENT: SYMPTOM RESTRUCTURING WITH HYPNOSIS

Hypnosis has been used as an adjunctive tool in the treatment of a variety of common psychiatric and medical problems, including habit disorders, anxiety and phobic states, psychosomatic problems, and pain. Because the hypnotic state involves an enhanced and altered state of concentration with an ability to produce changes in perception and certain body functions, it makes sense that it would be an effective tool in managing these psychosomatic problems. A variety of techniques have been employed in symptom-oriented treatment using hypnosis. One is the so-called ego-strengthening approach, in which hypnosis is used to provide positive reinforcement for behavior change (Crasilneck and Hall 1985). Erickson (1967) sought to employ a "therapeutic bind," mobilizing the patient's resistance to treatment by intensifying, or "prescribing," symptoms. The patient would then construe eliminating the symptom as a victory over the therapist. This approach, while not necessary among patients who are well motivated and who have resolved their ambivalence about symptom reduction, has the virtue of demonstrating to patients their ability to modulate symptoms, bypassing defensiveness by worsening rather than lessening them (Erickson 1967).

More recent approaches to the use of hypnosis have emphasized the educational aspects of the experience. In particular, it is most efficient to structure the intervention as a lesson in self-hypnosis that the patient can learn to employ in the service of symptom reduction. Also, it is useful to teach patients a cognitive strategy that alters their perspective on the problem, reinforced by the self-hypnosis. One such approach is called "restructuring" (Spiegel and Spiegel 1987). The principle of restructuring in hypnosis is to use the intense concentration characteristic of the trance state to help patients develop a strategy for change that amounts to an affirmation experience rather than a struggle, focusing on what they are for rather than what they are against.

This kind of restructuring strategy can be applied to other problems as well, such as mild to moderate overeating, and to the treatment of pain. In the latter case patients are taught to transform the pain signal by making the affected body area colder or warmer, or numb, or to focus on a sensation in some other part of their body. The management of anxiety or panic attacks is taught not by an instruction to "relax" or to not be anxious, but rather by teaching patients to affiliate with a physical metaphor that connotes relaxation, such as floating in water. In this way, patients can overcome urges or symptoms not by struggling against them but rather by subsuming them under a commitment to a new way of relating to the body, or through a hypnotically developed capacity to transform sensation (Spiegel and Spiegel 1987).

■ HABIT CONTROL

□ Smoking Cessation

Hypnosis has been employed as an adjunctive tool with a variety of habit control strategies, primarily for smoking cessation. It has been used to 1) provide a kind of substitute physical relaxation for the momentary respite that accompanies inhaling a cigarette, 2) enhance self-observation and self-monitoring, 3) provide positive reinforcement for behavior change, 4) diminish the positive reinforcement provided by smoking itself, and 5) facilitate cognitive restructuring of the smoking habit. Hypnosis has been employed in group and individual settings. Recent emphasis has been on teaching patients self-hypnosis rather than having multiple sessions with a therapist.

One cognitive restructuring model involves emphasizing that smoking is destructive specifically to the patient's body and thereby limits what the patient can do with his or her life. The focus in hypnosis is then placed on protecting the patient's body from poison in the same way that the patient would protect an infant or a pet from ingesting noxious food. This approach enables the patient to balance the urge to smoke against the urge to protect his or her body from damage.

Factors that account for the utility of hypnosis as an adjunct to smoking cessation treatment include 1) enhanced responsiveness to suggestion (Spiegel and Spiegel 1987); 2) alteration of unconscious motivation to smoke (Rabkin et al. 1984); 3) immediate symptom relief (Orne 1977); 4) nonspecific ceremonial, expectational, and placebo factors (Orne 1977); 5) enhanced ability to focus attention on the treatment strategy (Frischholz and Spiegel 1986); and 6) facilitation of ongoing self-administration via self-hypnosis (Spiegel and Spiegel 1987).

The generally accepted criterion for evaluating treatment interventions for smoking is complete abstinence at 6 months rather than reduction in smoking. Results of various trials of hypnosis in treatment indicate quit rates ranging from 13% to 64% with individual interventions and a follow-up time of at least 6 months (Schwartz 1987). The single-session approach is widely used and produces outcomes of 20% to 35% long-term complete abstinence (Frank et al. 1986). Abstinence rates as high as 40% at 6 months have been reported (Williams and Hall 1988). These abstinence rates are superior to the rates of unassisted quitting (Gritz and Bloom 1987). In addition, hypnotizability has been shown to predict better outcome (Spiegel et al. 1993). Thus, while in general there is no evidence that treatments employing hypnosis are more effective than other interventions for smoking, they may well be more efficient in that they enable patients to employ self-hypnosis to reinforce a cognitive restructuring strategy while at the same time providing an episode of physical relaxation.

☐ Weight Control

Hypnosis has been employed as an adjunct to a comprehensive dietary and exercise control program for weight reduction and management. The same restructuring principles discussed above can be applied to overeating: experiencing an excess of food as damaging to the body, and learning to eat with respect for one's body. This again involves focusing on what the patient is *for*—rather than being against food. Indeed, an important component of such an approach can be to teach the patient to use self-hypnosis training to control the urge to overeat by preparing a list of foods that constitute eating with respect and then comparing an urge with the list. If the desired food is on the list, the patient is encouraged to eat it like a gourmet, focusing intently on all aspects of the eating experience. If the food is not on the list, rather than fight the urge, the patient is encouraged to use self-hypnosis to compare it with his or her overall commitment to treat the body with respect and therefore to eat with respect. Patients can therefore deal with the desire to eat not as an occasion to feel deprivation, but rather as one in which they are enhancing their mastery of the urge to eat by focusing on protecting their body. In addition, hypnosis can be used to help patients provide positive self-reinforcement for compliance with a revised eating regimen (Crasilneck and Hall 1985).

Although long-term outcome studies are lacking, clinical experience suggests that persons within 20% of their ideal body weight may obtain some benefit from such restructuring techniques with self-hypnosis in addition to careful attention to diet and exercise. Hypnotizability has been shown to be correlated with weight reduction in some studies (Anderson 1985).

☐ Anxiety Disorders and Phobias

The Epidemiologic Catchment Area study sponsored by the National Institute of Mental Health (NIMH) has demonstrated that anxiety disorders are among the most widely prevalent psychiatric disturbances, affecting as much as 15% of the population (Myers et al. 1984). Anxiety is a state of psychosomatic discomfort experienced by patients largely in physical terms, with elevations in heart rate, gastrointestinal and thoracic discomfort, diaphoresis, and motor restlessness. Hypnosis may be especially helpful as an adjunctive tool for treating these anxiety states because of the ability of the hypnotized person to control somatic response.

There are a variety of treatment strategies employing hypnosis that have in common a restructuring of cognition by combining imagery with physical relaxation. Anxious patients are instructed to maintain such a physical sense of floating relaxation while picturing feared situations on an imaginary screen in the trance state. This approach clearly has elements in common with systematic desensitization (Marks et al. 1968), the difference being that in the former the induction of physical relaxation coupled to a noxious stimulus can be included very quickly without the development and working through of a hierarchy.

The hypnotic session may be used initially to demonstrate to patients that they have a greater degree of control over somatic responsiveness than they had imagined. It may also be useful to teach these patients to picture on the screen a place that they find intrinsically relaxing so that they can use their memory of, for example, a mountain lake or the beach as a means of providing a respite from anxious preoccupation. They may use the same trance state as a means of facing their concerns, placing an image of an upcoming performance, for example, on one side of the screen, while on the other side testing out various strategies for mastering the situation. The pleasant image may be especially useful for medical patients having to undergo procedures. Both in preparation and while in the clinic or hospital they can enter a state of self-hypnosis and imagine being somewhere they enjoy, thereby dissociating their psychological experience from the physical aspects of the procedure.

Special phobias call for variation in cognitive strategy. Individuals with acrophobia can be taught in the trance state to view gravity not as something likely to pull them off a cliff or building but rather something that roots them to the ground. Agoraphobic patients may find it useful to imagine a plastic bubble surrounding them that they can take with them, even when they leave their protective environment. Thus, whatever sense of safety they feel at home can sometimes be carried with them. Patients with animal phobias can be taught to feel more in control of a situation with an animal by first learning to control their own somatic response to it. Cognitively, they can concentrate on the difference between dangerous and tame animals (Spiegel and Spiegel 1988). Other approaches using hypnosis have included instructing patients in a trance to imagine that they are literally somewhere else, away from the fearful stimulus (Erickson 1967), or that their capacity to master the situation and their response to it will improve (Crasilneck and Hall 1985).

■ TREATMENT OUTCOME STUDIES

Outcome studies have generally shown hypnosis to be efficacious and hypnotizability to be predictive of treatment response. A 7-year follow-up of 178 patients treated with a single session of self-hypnosis for flying phobia indicated that 52% were either improved or cured. Hypnotizability predicted responsiveness (Spiegel et al. 1981b). Few well-controlled studies have compared hypnosis as an adjunct with other techniques. Those studies conducted among patient populations tend to show an advantage for hypnosis, especially when patients request it (Glick 1970; Lazarus 1973). Studies among student volunteers who are symptomatic tend to show no clear advantage for hypnosis versus desensitization, while those studies in which stress is induced in normal volunteers show some advantage for relaxation training over hypnosis (Marks et al. 1968). In general, outcome studies show some overlap between behavioral techniques and hypnosis in both structure and outcome. Both approaches involve the use of imagery and restructuring of cognition about the feared stimulus coupled with a means of producing physical relaxation. Hypnosis can be most effective when it is used to enhance patients' sense of mastery and control over psychological experience as well as their somatic response to such experience.

☐ Insomnia

The use of hypnosis to treat insomnia overlaps considerably with the treatment of anxiety disorders. Because hypnosis is not sleep but a form of concentration, it might seem paradoxical to use hypnosis to help people fall asleep. However, it can be helpful for inducing a state of physical relaxation that is at least compatible with sleep, diminishing the sympathetic arousal usually associated with anxious preoccupation. Thus, patients can be instructed to go into a state of self-hypnosis and induce a sense of floating relaxation physically; then, if preoccupied with arousing or uncomfortable thoughts, they can project these thoughts onto an imaginary screen in the trance state. Patients are instructed to become a "traffic director" for their own thoughts, dealing with them on the screen, thereby dissociating them from the evoked physical response (Spiegel and Spiegel 1987). Such approaches can be helpful in conjunction with standard sleep laboratory approaches, which include keeping the bedroom as a place where work and other anxiety-arousing activities do not occur, and avoiding constantly looking at the clock when awakened. It is also important to distinguish routine insomnia due to situational reactions and anxiety from the more severe early morning awakening associated with depression, or from the repeated arousals from sleep that are associated with sleep apnea syndrome.

☐ Psychosomatic Disorders

Because highly hypnotizable individuals show an unusual capacity for psychological control over somatic function, it makes sense that hypnotic phenomena may be involved both in the etiology of some psychosomatic symptoms and in their control (Spiegel 1994). For example, Andreychuk and Skriver (1975) found that hypnotizability not only was a predictor of treatment response for migraine headaches, but also was a correlate of pretreatment symptom severity. That is, more highly hypnotizable individuals complained of more severe migraine symptoms prior to treatment, but responded better to intervention. Highly hypnotizable individuals have been shown to have the capacity to control peripheral skin temperature and blood flow (Grabowska 1971) and to be able to suppress cortical evoked response to a perceptual stimulus while hallucinating an obstruction to that stimulus (Spiegel et al. 1989). It makes sense that certain classical conversion disorders such as hysterical paralysis may well represent dissociative phenomena, because profound alterations in sensation and experience of control over motor function are standard hypnotic phenomena (Spiegel 1994).

In general, hypnosis is useful in two senses, one diagnostic, the other therapeutic. Patients who are highly hypnotizable are more likely to have conversion symptoms, such as hysterical pseudoseizures, than those who are not, especially if hypnotic induction tends to bring on the symptom, worsen, or ameliorate it. Even among highly hypnotizable patients it is rare for a conversion symptom to simply disappear, and, indeed, pushing patients to relinquish it too quickly may humiliate them, since it conveys the message that the problem was "all in their head."

Hypnosis can be quite appropriately used as part of a rehabilitation strategy, particularly insofar as it can help patients master the reactive anxiety that is associated with real physical dysfunction as well as conversion symptoms. A patient can be taught to use a state of self-hypnosis to develop the sense of floating relaxation while picturing bothersome problems on an imaginary screen. The patient can then work on, for example, improving function in a dysfunctional hand by developing tremors that gradually build up strength and circulation. One patient with persistent contractures of the entire hand secondary to a compound fracture of the index finger had been treated with a variety of techniques for 3 years with no improvement. He then used this kind of self-hypnosis exercise to focus on rehabilitation rather than seek further information about causation. At the end of another year of daily exercise, he regained full function of the hand and returned to work (Spiegel and Chase 1980).

Hypnosis has been quite effective in helping asthmatic patients. They can learn to use it as a first resort rather than medication when they begin to feel an attack coming on, thereby interrupting the vicious cycle of anxiety and bronchoconstriction. It is often helpful to have asthmatic patients enter a state of self-hypnosis and imagine that they are somewhere where they naturally breathe easily, for example, inhaling cool mountain or ocean air (Spiegel and Spiegel 1987). Hypnotizability is correlated with treatment response (Collison 1975). Similarly, warts have been treated with hypnosis, and one carefully controlled study demonstrated that simple hypnotic instructions to the effect that the warts would tingle and disappear resulted in a rate of improvement that was significantly better than the spontaneous rate of remission of warts (Surman et al. 1973). Thus, hypnosis can be quite helpful in controlling the psychosomatic interaction that can lead to either deterioration or improvement of somatically related symptoms.

☐ Gastrointestinal System

Relaxation instructions have been helpful for some patients with stress-related bowel disease, such as ulcerative colitis and regional enteritis. Patients have found it helpful to imagine in trance something soothing in their gut, which gives them a sense of control over a symptom that renders them feeling especially helpless, thereby diminishing the cycle of reactive anxiety. A well-conducted randomized trial (Whorwell et al. 1987) showed that 15 patients with irritable bowel syndrome who were treated with hypnosis reported significant improvement in pain, abdominal distension, and diarrhea, as well as emotional well-being, compared with a control group of 15 patients. An 18-month follow-up of 15 of these patients showed continued remission, and the authors reported similar improvement in 35 additional patients. Zeltzer et al. (1984) reported significant reduction in chemotherapy-induced nausea and vomiting among 19 patients who had been taught hypnosis.

Klein and Spiegel (1989) observed significant hypnotic control of gastric acid secretion among 28 highly hypnotizable subjects. When these patients were hypnotized and instructed to eat an imaginary meal, basal acid output rose 89%. In another trial designed to test reduction in acid output, subjects were instructed to use hypnosis to experience deep relaxation. There was a significant 39% drop in basal acid output. In a third trial, subjects were given an injection of pentagastrin, which stimulates maximal parietal cell output. There was still a significant 11% reduction in pentagastrin-stimulated peak acid output during hypnosis. This study further emphasizes the fact that high hypnotizability is a two-edged sword, in that it may increase or decrease a given physiological parameter, depending on the mental content during the hypnotic state. That these observations may have clinical relevance is illustrated by a controlled trial of hypnosis in relapse prevention of duodenal ulcers (Colgan et al. 1988). Thirty patients with rapidly relapsing ulcer disease were randomly assigned after ranitidine to hypnosis or no treatment. All of the control subjects but only 53% of the hypnosis patients relapsed.

☐ Pain Syndromes

Pain is the ultimate psychosomatic phenomenon, always representing both tissue injury and the psychological reaction to such injury. Hypnosis facilitates alteration of the subjective experience of pain (Brose and Spiegel 1992). The techniques most often employed involve physical relaxation coupled with imagery that provides a substitute focus of attention for the painful sensation (Table 32–2). Patients can be taught to develop a comfortable, floating sensation, and highly hypnotizable individuals may simply imagine a shot of novocaine in the affected area, producing a sense of tingling numbness. Some patients prefer to move the pain to another part of their body, or to develop a sensation of floating above their own body, creating distance between themselves and the painful sensation. More moderately hypnotizable patients often prefer to focus on a change in temperature, either warmth or coolness, imagining that they are floating in a warm bath or a mountain stream or immersing a painful hand in a bucket of ice chips. That temperature metaphors are unusually effective may be related to the fact that pain and temperature fibers run together in the lateral spinothalamic tract, separate from other sensory fibers. Less hypnotizable patients may benefit from distraction techniques in which they concentrate hard on sensations in other parts of their body.

Regardless of the metaphor selected, certain general principles can be employed with all uses of hypnosis for pain control. The first principle

Table 32–2. Principles of hypnotic analgesia

1. Induce physical relaxation through a metaphor such as "floating."
2. Alter perception of the pain by:
   Inducing dissociation from current sensory experience
   Altering perception through a sense of warmth, coolness, tingling, or numbness
   Focusing attention on sensation in a nonpainful part of the body
3. Transform the pain.
4. Provide positive reinforcement for symptom improvement.
5. Use a rehabilitation model for treatment.
6. Reduce secondary gain for symptom maintenance.
7. Treat amplifying comorbid conditions:
   Anxiety related to disease progression
   Depression

is to teach patients to "filter the hurt out of the pain." They learn to transform the pain experience by acknowledging that even though it may exist, there is a distinction between the signal itself and the discomfort the signal causes. The hypnotic metaphor helps them transform the signal into one that is less uncomfortable. The second principle is to expand the perceptual options available to patients by having them change from an experience in which either the pain is there or it is not, to one in which they see a third option, which is that the pain is there but transformed by the presence of such competing sensations as tingling, numbness, warmth, coolness, etc. The third principle is to teach patients not to fight the pain. Fighting pain only enhances the pain by focusing attention on it, by enhancing related anxiety and depression, and by increasing physical tension that can literally put traction on painful parts of the body and increase the pain signals generated peripherally.

Hypnotic analgesia seems to work via two mechanisms: *physical relaxation* and *attention control*. Patients in pain tend to splint the painful area instinctively, and yet this enhanced muscle tension around a painful area often increases pain. Most patients find that they can enhance their physical repose by focusing on a variety of images that connote physical relaxation such as a sense of floating. Second, and probably more important, since hypnosis involves an intensification and narrowing of the focus of attention, it allows individuals to place pain at the periphery of their awareness by replacing the pain with some competing metaphor or sensation at the center of their attention. Thus, by focusing on a memory of dental anesthesia and spreading that numbness to the affected area, making the area warmer or cooler, substituting a sense of tingling or lightness, or focusing on sensation in some nonpainful part of the body, hypnotized individuals can diminish the amount of attention they pay to painful stimuli.

That this hypnotic analgesia is not merely social compliance but involves neurophysiological changes in information processing is suggested by the cortical event-related potential studies reviewed earlier. In these studies highly hypnotizable individuals could diminish the P100 and P300 components of their event-related response to a somatosensory stimulus by focusing on a hallucinated image that would block their perception of the stimulus (Spiegel et al. 1989; Figure 32–2). This cortical attention deployment mechanism is at the moment the most plausible explanation, although a number of studies have tested the idea that endogenous opiates are involved in hypnotic analgesia. With one partial exception (Frid and Singer 1979), studies with both volunteers (Goldstein and Hilgard 1975) and patients in chronic pain (Spiegel and Albert 1983)

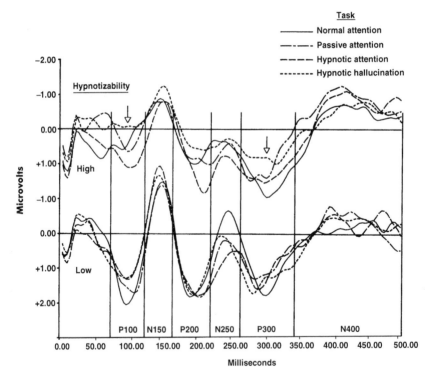

Figure 32–2. Somatosensory event-related potentials among 10 highly hypnotizable and 10 low hypnotizable individuals. Hypnotic obstructive hallucination results in reduction of P100 and P300 amplitude, whereas hypnotic attention is associated with an increase in P100 amplitude.

have shown that hypnotic analgesia is not blocked and reversed by a substantial dose of naloxone given in double-blind, crossover fashion.

Whatever the mechanism, hypnotic analgesia is efficacious. Recent systematic studies have demonstrated that hypnosis is superior to an attentional control condition for analgesia among children undergoing painful procedures (Zeltzer and LeBaron 1982). Furthermore, in a randomized prospective study, a combination of hypnosis and group psychotherapy was shown to result in a 50% reduction in pain among metastatic breast cancer patients (Spiegel and Bloom 1983), and there was a corresponding reduction in mood disturbance (Spiegel et al. 1981a). Hypnotic analgesia has also been shown to be more potent than either placebo analgesia (McGlashan et al. 1969) or acupuncture analgesia (Knox and Shum 1977), although there is a correlation between hypnotizability and responsiveness to acupuncture (Katz et al. 1974). Thus, hypnotic mechanisms of pain control may be mobilized by other treatment techniques, but the explicit use of hypnosis with hypnotizable patients has proved to be a more powerful means of controlling pain.

In a review of studies, Hilgard and Hilgard (1975) estimated a .5 correlation between hypnotizability and treatment responsiveness for pain control. The ability of hypnotizable individuals to focus their attention and alter their response to perception while at the same time producing a physical state of relaxation gives them an unusual way to restructure their experience of pain and thereby develop a sense of mastery over it. Because the pain experience is both psychological and physical, this technique mobilizes and focuses cognitive experience while producing a sense of physical relaxation. It can be especially helpful in giving patients a sense of mastery.

■ REFERENCES

American Psychiatric Association: Diagnostic and Statistical Manual of Mental Disorders, 4th Edition. Washington, DC, American Psychiatric Association, 1994

Anderson MS: Hypnotizability as a factor in the treatment of obesity. Int J Clin Exp Hypn 33:150–159, 1985

Andreychuk T, Skriver C: Hypnosis and biofeedback in the treatment of migraine headache. Int J Clin Exp Hypn 23:172–183, 1975

Braun BG, Sachs RG: The development of multiple personality disorder: predisposing, precipitating, and perpetuating factors, in Childhood Antecedents of Multiple Personality. Edited by Kluft RP. Washington, DC, American Psychiatric Press, 1985, pp 37–64

Brose WG, Spiegel D: Neuropsychiatric aspects of pain management, in American Psychiatric Press Textbook of Neuropsychiatry, 2nd Edition. Edited by Yudofsky SC, Hales RE. Washington, DC, American Psychiatric Press, 1992, pp 245–275

California Legislature: AB 2669 Chapter 7, Hypnosis of Witnesses, added to Chapter 7, Division 6, of the Evidence Code, Enacted January 1, 1985

Cardeña E, Spiegel D: Dissociative reactions to the San Francisco Bay Area earthquake of 1989. Am J Psychiatry 150:474–478, 1993

Colgan SM, Faragher EB, Whorwell PJ: Controlled trial of hypnotherapy in relapse prevention of duodenal ulceration. Lancet 1:1299–1300, 1988

Collison DR: Which asthmatic patients should be treated by hypnotherapy? Med J Aust 1:776–781, 1975

Crasilneck HD, Hall JA: Clinical Hypnosis: Principles and Applications, 2nd Edition. New York, Grune & Stratton, 1985

Diamond BL: Inherent problems in the use of pretrial hypnosis on a prospective witness. California Law Review 68:313–349, 1980

Erickson MH: Advanced Techniques of Hypnosis and Therapy: Selected Papers of Milton H Erickson, M.D. Edited by Haley J. New York, Grune & Stratton, 1967

Frank RG, Umlauf RL, Wonderlich SA, et al: Hypnosis and behavioral treatment in a worksite smoking cessation program. Addict Behav 11:59–62, 1986

Freud S: Remembering, repeating, and working-through (further recommendations on the technique of psycho-analysis II) (1914), in the Standard Edition of the Complete Psychological Works of Sigmund Freud, Vol 12. Translated and edited by Strachey J. London, Hogarth Press, 1958, pp 145–156

Frid M, Singer G: Hypnotic analgesia in conditions of stress is partially reversed by naloxone. Psychopharmacology (Berlin) 61:211–125, 1979

Frischholz EJ: The relationship among dissociation, hypnosis, and child abuse in the development of multiple personality disorder, in Childhood Antecedents of Multiple Personality Disorder. Edited by Kluft RP. Washington, DC, American Psychiatric Press, 1985, pp 99–126

Frischholz EJ, Spiegel D: Adjunctive uses of hypnosis in the treatment of smoking. Psychiatric Annals 16:87–90, 1986

Glick BS: Conditioning therapy with phobic patients: success and failure. Am J Psychother 24:92–101, 1970

Goldstein E, Hilgard E: Failure of opiate antagonist naloxone to modify hypnotic analgesia. Proc Natl Acad Sci U S A 71:1041–1043, 1975

Grabowska MJ. The effect of hypnosis and hypnotic suggestions on the blood flow in the extremities. Kardiol Pol 10:1044–1051, 1971

Gritz E, Bloom J: Psychosocial sequelae of cancer in long-term survivors and their families. Paper presented at the Western Regional Conference of the American Cancer Society, Los Angeles, CA, January 1987

Hilgard ER: Hypnotic Susceptibility. New York, Harcourt, Brace & World, 1965

Hilgard ER, Hilgard JR: Hypnosis in the Relief of Pain. Los Altos, CA, William Kaufmann, 1975

Katz RL, Kao CY, Spiegel H, et al: Pain, acupuncture, and hypnosis. Adv Neurol 4:819–825, 1974

Klein KB, Spiegel D: Modulation of gastric acid secretion by hypnosis. Gastroenterology 96:1383–1387, 1989

Kluft RP. Childhood multiple personality disorder: predictors, clinical findings, and treatment results, in Childhood Antecedents of Multiple Personality Disorder. Edited by Kluft RP. Washington, DC, American Psychiatric Press, 1985, pp 167–196

Knox VJ, Shum K: Reduction of cold-pressor pain with acupuncture analgesia in high- and low-hypnotic subjects. J Abnorm Psychol 86:639–643, 1977

Lavoie G, Sabourin M: Hypnosis and schizophrenia: a review of experimental and clinical studies, in Handbook of Hypnosis and Psychosomatic Medicine. Edited by Burrows GD, Dennerstein L. Amsterdam, Elsevier/North-Holland Biomedical Press, 1980, pp 377–420

Lazarus AA: "Hypnosis" as a facilitator in behavior therapy. Int J Clin Exp Hypn 21:25–31, 1973

Marks IM, Gelder MG, Edwards G: Hypnosis and desensitization for phobias: a controlled prospective trial. Br J Psychiatry 114:1263–1274, 1968

McGlashan TH, Evans FJ, Orne MT: The nature of hypnotic analgesia and the placebo response to experimental pain. Psychosom Med 31:227–246, 1969

Myers JK, Weissman MM, Tischler GL, et al. Six-month prevalence of psychiatric disorders in three communities: 1980 to 1982. Arch Gen Psychiatry 41:959–967, 1984

Orne MT: Hypnosis in the treatment of smoking, in Proceedings of the 3rd World Conference on Smoking and Health, Vol 2 (DHEW NIH 77-1413). Washington, DC, Department of Health, Education and Welfare, 1977, pp 489–507

People v Schoenfeld, 168 Cal Rptr 762, 111 CA3d 671 (1980)

Pettinati HM: Measuring hypnotizability in psychotic patients. Int J Clin Exp Hypn 30:404–416, 1982

Pettinati HM, Kogan LG, Evans FJ, et al: Hypnotizability of psychiatric inpatients according to two different scales. Am J Psychiatry 147:69–75, 1990

Rabkin SW, Boyko E, Shane F, et al: A randomized trial comparing smoking cessation programs utilizing behaviour modification, health education or hypnosis. Addict Behav 9:157–173, 1984

Schwartz JL: Smoking cessation methods: United States and Canada, 1978–85 (USPHS NIH 87-2940). Division of Cancer Prevention and Control, National Cancer Institute, 1987

Spiegel D: Vietnam grief work using hypnosis. Am J Clin Hypn 24:33–40, 1981

Spiegel D: Physiological correlates of hypnosis and dissociation, in Dissociation: Culture, Mind, and Body. Edited by Spiegel D. Washington, DC, American Psychiatric Press, 1994

Spiegel D, Albert L: Naloxone fails to reverse hypnotic alleviation of chronic pain. Psychopharmacology (Berlin) 81:140–143, 1983

Spiegel D, Bloom JR: Group therapy and hypnosis reduce metastatic breast carcinoma pain. Psychosom Med 45:333–339, 1983

Spiegel D, Chase RA: The treatment of contractures of the hand using self-hypnosis. J Hand Surg [Am] 5:428–432, 1980

Spiegel D, Spiegel H: Assessment and treatment using hypnosis, in Handbook of Anxiety Disorders. Edited by Last CG, Hersen M. New York, Pergamon, 1988, pp 401–412

Spiegel D, Bloom JR, Yalom I[D]: Group support for patients with metastatic cancer: a randomized prospective outcome study. Arch Gen Psychiatry 38:527–533, 1981a

Spiegel D, Frischholz EJ, Maruffi B, et al: Hypnotic responsivity and the treatment of flying phobia. Am J Clin Hypn 23:239–247, 1981b

Spiegel D, Detrick D, Frischholz E[J]: Hypnotizability and psychopathology. Am J Psychiatry 139:431–437, 1982

Spiegel D, Hunt T, Dondershine HE: Dissociation and hypnotizability in posttraumatic stress disorder. Am J Psychiatry 145:301–305, 1988

Spiegel D, Bierre P, Rootenberg J: Hypnotic alteration of somatosensory perception. Am J Psychiatry 146:749–754, 1989

Spiegel D, Frischholz EJ, Fleiss JL, et al: Predictors of smoking abstinence following a single-session restructuring intervention with self-hypnosis. Am J Psychiatry 150:1090–1097, 1993

Spiegel H, Spiegel D: Trance and Treatment: Clinical Uses of Hypnosis. Washington, DC, American Psychiatric Press, 1987 [Reprint of Trance and Treatment: Clinical Uses of Hypnosis. New York, Basic Books, 1978]

Steingard S, Frankel FH: Dissociation and psychotic symptoms. Am J Psychiatry 142:953–955, 1985

Stern DL, Spiegel H, Nee JCM: The Hypnotic Induction Profile: normative observations, reliability, and validity. Am J Clin Hypn 21:109–132, 1979

Surman OS, Gottlieb SK, Hackett TP, et al: Hypnosis in the treatment of warts. Arch Gen Psychiatry 28:439–441, 1973

Tellegen A, Atkinson G: Openness to absorbing and self-altering experiences ("absorption"), a trait related to hypnotic susceptibility. J Abnorm Psychol 83:268–277, 1974

Weitzenhoffer AM, Hilgard ER: Stanford Hypnotic Susceptibility Scale, Form C. Palo Alto, CA, Consulting Psychologists Press, 1962

Whorwell PJ, Prior A, Colgan SM: Hypnotherapy in severe irritable bowel syndrome: further experience. Gut 28:423–425, 1987

Williams JM, Hall DW: Use of single session hypnosis for smoking cessation. Addict Behav 13:205–208, 1988

Zeltzer L, LeBaron S: Hypnosis and nonhypnotic techniques for reduction of pain and anxiety during painful procedures in children and adolescents with cancer. J Pediatr 101:1032–1035, 1982

Zeltzer L, LeBaron S, Zeltzer PM: The effectiveness of behavioral intervention for reduction of nausea and vomiting in children and adolescents receiving chemotherapy. J Clin Oncol 2:683–690, 1984

CHAPTER 33

Group Therapy

Sophia Vinogradov, M.D.
Irvin D. Yalom, M.D.

Interpersonal relationships are of crucial importance to human psychological development. It is thus self-evident that a group of people can serve as an immensely specific therapeutic tool. In such a group setting, patients are uniquely provided with a varied array of interpersonal relationships that, with proper guidance, will permit them to identify, explore, and alter maladaptive interpersonal behavior. Because it can provide such a powerful therapeutic experience, the group setting is being used more and more not only by mental health professionals but by laypersons.

A number of specialized groups have been developed to function in a supportive and occasionally highly therapeutic mode in nonpsychiatric medical settings as well. The groundbreaking work of Spiegel et al. (1989) demonstrated a twofold increase in survival rate for patients with metastatic breast carcinoma who participated in a long-term psychodynamically oriented support group. Fawzy et al. (1990) found an improvement both in use of coping strategies and in immune function in patients with malignant melanoma who participated in a short-term group intervention.

■ CLINICAL RELEVANCE OF GROUP THERAPY

□ Efficacy

Multiple outcome studies of varying sophistication and methodological design have been performed since the early 1960s. Investigators over the years have concluded that group treatment is as effective as individual therapy in treating psychological disorders (Shapiro DA and Shapiro D 1982; Smith et al. 1980). More recently, 32 studies that directly contrasted individual and group treatments were analyzed (Toseland and Siporin 1986; Tillitski 1990); in 24 of the studies, no significant differences were found between the two modalities. In the remaining 8 studies, group therapy was found to be more effective than individual therapy.

☐ Numbers of Group Therapy Patients

Enormous numbers of psychiatric patients receive their sole or primary treatment in groups. At least one-half of all psychiatric hospitals and one-quarter of all correctional institutions, not to mention the vast majority of community mental health centers, use group treatments (Shapiro JL 1978). Many health maintenance organizations make substantial use of group therapy as well (Cheifetz and Salloway 1984). Altogether, this represents a potential patient population in the hundreds of thousands.

☐ Nonpsychiatric Groups

New orders of magnitude occur when we consider the staggering number of "nonpsychiatric" clients who receive treatment in specialized therapy groups or in one of the vast number of self-help groups. For example, the use of groups for patients with particular medical conditions—such as cancer support groups, post–myocardial infarction groups, and diabetes education groups—is burgeoning in the health care setting (Stern 1993). In 1983, perhaps 12 to 14 million individuals attended some form of self-help group (Lieberman 1986).

■ COST-EFFECTIVENESS AND EFFICIENCY

In an analysis of nine studies comparing the differential efficiency of individual and group therapy, Toseland and Siporin (1986) concluded that group treatment is more consistently efficient and/or cost-effective. In a future in which cost-containment and third-party payers loom large, these practical considerations of expediency and cost and staff efficiency take on considerable weight. In fact, more than one prescient group therapist has suggested that clinicians may need to justify individual therapy and defend their decision not to use the more cost-effective group therapy (Dies 1986). We wish to point out, however, that although group therapy is more cost-efficient, its advantages transcend simple economic considerations: it is a form of treatment that makes use of unique therapeutic properties not shared by other psychotherapies.

■ SCOPE OF GROUP THERAPY PRACTICE

Therapy groups can be categorized using four interrelated characteristics (Table 33–1): the setting of the group, its duration, its goals, and its techniques.

☐ Setting

A natural line of cleavage among types of groups is their clinical setting. A particularly clear distinction can be made between psychiatric inpatient and outpatient groups. Inpatient groups on a psychiatric ward tend to meet daily, are usually composed of individuals with acute psychiatric problems, and are often mandatory; turnover is great, with membership fluctuating widely because of the short duration of hospitalization. Psychiatric outpatient groups, in contrast, meet once weekly, consist of individuals who show more similar and more stable levels of functioning, and are voluntary in nature; membership tends to be more stable.

Group therapy is also practiced in a myriad of other clinical settings, extending from the daily small groups held in a psychiatric day hospital, to weekly probation groups, to staff retreats or support groups. Specialized groups for medical syndromes, such as diabetes education groups or lupus support groups, are often held in a hospital or clinic setting, whereas other types of specialized groups (e.g., rape crisis groups, Vietnam veterans' groups) may be associated with a center that offers counseling services (e.g., rape trauma center, veterans' outreach center).

☐ Duration

A second consideration for any therapy group is its duration. Most inpatient groups are an indelible part of the treatment program and are thus indefinitely self-sustaining; the ward census may change, different kinds of patients may or may not be hospitalized, but the group is held every day. Outpatient groups have more latitude in their duration. They can exist for one session only, or they can be open-ended and long-term in nature, periodically renewing their membership over the years. A sizable number of groups in the outpatient setting, however, choose a time-limited format, especially if they are focusing on a specific problem.

☐ Goals

A third parameter that can be used to characterize the different kinds of group therapy pertains to the goals of the group, which may be conceptualized as existing along a spectrum. At one end of this spectrum are the ambitious goals of long-term interactional groups: symptom relief and

Table 33–1.   The scope of current group therapy practice

Type of group	Life of group	Attendance	Average patient stay	Goals	Major therapeutic factors/techniques	Membership criteria
Prototypic interactionally oriented groups	Indefinite; as permitted by professional schedule of group leaders	Voluntary but regular attendance essential	1 to 2 years	Character change; symptom relief	Interpersonal learning; corrective recapitulation of primary family group	Higher-functioning patients; interpersonal pathology; desire to change, able to tolerate interpersonal focus; able to attend all sessions
Acute inpatient groups	Indefinite; usually integral part of ward program	Generally mandatory during hospitalization; will show higher turnover	1–2 days to several weeks, depending on length of hospitalization	Restoration of function	Instillation of hope; socialization techniques; altruism; existential factors	Patients may be placed in different groups by level of functioning; membership will fluctuate widely
Follow-up or aftercare groups; discharge planning groups; day hospital groups; probation groups	Indefinite; usually associated with a specific program	Often mandatory	Usually fixed number of sessions	Deinstitutionalization	Instillation of hope; imparting of information; imitative behavior; socializing techniques	Patients require follow-up or aftercare; able to tolerate group setting and attend required sessions
Medication or clinic groups	Indefinite; usually part of clinic program	Voluntary; often occurring on a drop-in basis	Indefinite; depends on patient's enrollment in clinic	Support; education; maintenance of functions	Imparting of information; socializing techniques	Patients on long-term psychiatric medication; able to tolerate group setting

Behaviorally oriented groups (e.g., eating disorders group)	Time-limited, often 6 to 12 sessions; some groups are ongoing	Voluntary but regular attendance generally a prerequisite for group participation	Life of group	Discrete behavior change	Techniques of behavior modification; universality; imitative behavior	Patients with specific behavioral problem; desire to change
Specialized groups for medical disorders (e.g., diabetes, heart disease)	Time-limited, often 6 to 12 sessions; some groups are ongoing	Voluntary; often drop-in basis	Life of group or fixed number of sessions	Education; support; socialization	Universality; cohesiveness; imparting of information; imitative behavior; altruism; existential factors	Patients with specific medical problems; desire for further education, support
Specialized groups for life events: bereavement groups, divorce groups	Tend to be time-limited, 8 to 12 sessions	Voluntary; often flexible	Life of group	Support; catharsis; socialization	Cohesiveness; altruism; existential factors	Patients or clients who have undergone life event; desire for group experience
Specialized support groups: Vietnam veterans' outreach groups, rape crisis groups, student center drop-in groups, professional support groups, professional retreats	Indefinite; ongoing for professional retreats, which usually last 1 to 3 days	Usually drop-in basis; for staff support groups, especially during retreats, all members of staff should attend	Variable	Support; catharsis	Cohesiveness; altruism; occasional interpersonal learning	Patients or clients who belong to specialized situation; desire for support

character change. At the other end, there is the more limited but crucial goal of restoration of function: the deinstitutionalizing role of acute inpatient therapy groups. Between these two extremes lie the goals of the large majority of therapy groups. For some, such as medication clinic groups or inpatient and outpatient groups for chronically mentally ill persons, the most important goal will be maintenance of appropriate psychosocial functioning. Numerous others, including social skills training groups and specialized and self-help groups, attempt to provide education, socialization, and support. Many symptom-oriented short-term groups that are behaviorally focused have the goal of discrete behavior change.

☐ Theoretical Orientation and Techniques

A fourth aspect of any therapy group is its theoretical orientation and the techniques employed by the therapist. This aspect is closely entwined with the goals of the group. An eating disorders group with the goal of discrete behavior change, for example, may have a cognitive-behavioral orientation and may focus on identifying cognitive distortions and triggers to behavioral responses. A wide range of theories and techniques inform the current practice of group therapy (Alonso and Swiller 1993).

☐ Membership Criteria

As can be seen from Table 33–1, the specific membership criteria for a given therapy group can vary widely from one type of group to another and are intimately linked to the goals of the group. Whatever the specific nature of the group, a member must be able to perform the group task as the group works toward its goals. A member must therefore have problem areas that are compatible with the goals of the group and some motivation to change. Exclusion criteria for a potential member include any factors that may interfere with the group task, such as marked incompatibility with group norms or with one or more group members, inability to tolerate the group setting, or a tendency to assume a deviant role in the group. These general criteria are outlined in Table 33–2.

■ THERAPEUTIC FACTORS IN GROUP THERAPY

☐ Identifying the Therapeutic Factors in Group Therapy

Researchers have identified a number of mechanisms of change in group therapy, that is, the curative or therapeutic factors. Yalom (1970) derived an atheoretical, 11-factor inventory of the therapeutic mechanisms operating in group therapy: 1) instillation of hope, 2) universality, 3) impart-

Table 33–2. General membership criteria for group therapy

Inclusion criteria	Exclusion criteria
Ability to perform the group task	Marked incompatibility with group norms for acceptable behavior
Problem areas compatible with goals of group	Inability to tolerate group setting
Motivation to change	Severe incompatibility with one or more of the other members
	Tendency to assume deviant role

ing of information, 4) altruism, 5) development of socializing techniques, 6) imitative behavior, 7) catharsis, 8) corrective recapitulation of primary family group, 9) existential factors, 10) group cohesiveness, and 11) interpersonal learning. Yalom suggests that these primary factors, derived from extensive clinical and research evidence, serve as provisional guidelines for determining how group therapy helps patients to change.

Instillation of Hope

In therapy groups of every ilk, there will be patients who have improved as well as members who are at a low ebb; patients will often remark at the end of therapy how important it was for them to have observed the improvement of others and thus to hope for their own improvement. Many of the self-help groups that have emerged in the past decade also place a heavy emphasis on the instillation of hope. Groups aimed at substance abuse often use the testimonials of ex-alcoholic or recovered addicted persons to inspire hope in new members.

Universality

Many patients go through life with a sense of isolation. In a therapy group, especially in its early stages, the disconfirmation of a patient's sense of uniqueness comes as a powerful sense of relief. Some specialized groups, in fact, are focused on helping individuals for whom secrecy has been an especially important and isolating part of life. As a rule, patients experience a great sense of relief as they discover that they are not alone, that some of their problems are "universal," and that other group members share the same dilemmas.

Imparting of Information

The imparting of information occurs in a group whenever a therapist gives didactic instruction to patients about mental functioning or whenever advice or direct guidance about life problems is offered either by the leader or by other group members. Many self-help groups emphasize *didactic instruction.* Experts are often invited to address the group, and members are strongly encouraged to exchange information among one another. Most, if not all, specialized groups led by professionals rely heavily on this procedure as well; groups aimed at patients with a specific disorder or facing a specific life crisis build in a teaching component and offer explicit instruction about the nature of the patient's illness or life situation.

Unlike explicit didactic instruction from the therapist, *direct advice* from other members occurs without exception in every kind of therapy group. In dynamic interactional therapy groups, it is invariably part of the early life of the group but is generally of limited value to members. Later, when the group has moved beyond an initial "problem-solving" stage and has begun to engage in true interactional work, the reappearance of advice seeking or advice giving around a given issue is an important clue to resistance in the group. In contrast, noninteractionally focused groups often make explicit and effective use of direct suggestions and guidance.

Altruism

In a therapy group, patients become enormously helpful to one another: they share similar problems and offer one another support, reassurance, suggestions, and insight. To the patient starting therapy who is demoralized and who feels that he or she has nothing of value to offer anyone, the experience of being helpful to other members of the group can be surprisingly rewarding. Not only does the altruistic act boost self-esteem, it also distracts patients who spend much of their psychic energy immersed in morbid self-absorption. The therapy group fosters the act of being helpful to others and counters overly solipsistic preoccupation.

Development of Socializing Techniques

Social learning—the development of basic social skills—is a therapeutic factor that operates in all therapy groups, although the nature of the skills taught and the explicitness of the process vary greatly according to the type of group therapy. Role playing is often employed. In groups that are interactionally oriented, patients often learn about maladaptive social behavior from the open feedback they offer one another.

Imitative Behavior

The importance of imitative behavior as a therapeutic factor in groups is difficult to gauge, but there is some evidence from social psychological research that therapists may underestimate its importance. In group therapy we often observe patients who benefit by observing the therapy of another patient with a similar problem constellation, a phenomenon of "vicarious learning."

Catharsis

Catharsis, or the ventilation of emotions, is a complex therapeutic factor that is linked to other processes in the group, particularly universality and cohesiveness. The sheer act of ventilation, by itself, although often accompanied by a sense of emotional arousal and relief, rarely promotes lasting change for a patient. It is the affective sharing of one's inner world, and then the acceptance by others, that is of paramount importance. To be able to express strong emotions and yet still be accepted by others brings into question one's belief that one is basically repugnant, unacceptable, or unlovable. Therapy is both an emotional and a corrective experience; in order for change to take place, a patient must experience something strongly in the group setting and then understand the implications of that emotional experience.

Corrective Recapitulation of the Primary Family Group

Patients often enter group therapy with a history of unsatisfactory experiences in their first and most important group experience, the primary family. Because group therapy offers such a vast array of recapitulative possibilities, patients may begin to interact with leaders or other members as they once interacted with parents and siblings (Baker and Baker 1993). What is of capital importance in interactional group therapy is not only that early familial conflicts are reenacted but that they are understood and corrected. The leader must constantly explore and challenge fixed roles in the group and must constantly encourage members to test new behaviors. By exploring and altering ingrained patterns of behavior with leaders and other group members, the patient is liberated from the yoke of unfinished business from the past.

Existential Factors

An existential approach to the understanding of patients' concerns posits that the human being's paramount struggle is with the givens of our existence: death, isolation, freedom, and meaninglessness (Yalom 1980). In certain kinds of therapy groups, particularly those centered around patients with cancer or chronic and life-threatening medical illnesses, or in bereavement groups, members will often begin to confront some of these "existential" issues. They may find that the ultimate responsibility for the conduct of their lives is their own. They will often learn that, although one can be close to others, there is nonetheless a basic aloneness to existence that cannot be avoided. As they accept some of these issues, many patients who are confronting death learn to face their limitations and their mortality with greater candor and courage. In group therapy, the sound and trusting relationship among members has an intrinsic value as it provides presence and a "being with" in the face of these harsh existential realities (Benioff and Vinogradov 1993).

Group Cohesiveness

Group cohesiveness is one of the more complex and absolutely integral features of a successful therapy group (Dies 1993). Cohesiveness in a group context refers to the affinity that members have for their group and for the other members. The members of a cohesive group are accepting of one another, supportive, and inclined to form meaningful relationships in the group; they are ready to perform the group task. As such, cohesiveness can be conceptualized as a necessary precondition for change rather than a true mechanism of change. And yet, many psychiatric patients have had an impoverished history of "belonging"; never before have they been a valuable, integral, participating member of any kind of group, and the successful negotiation of a group therapy experience may in itself be curative. For these patients, group cohesiveness appears to be a true therapeutic factor. Furthermore, the social behavior required for members to be esteemed by a cohesive group tends also to be adaptive for the individual in his or her social life outside of the group.

Patients are, under cohesive conditions, more inclined to express and explore themselves, to become aware of and integrate hitherto unacceptable aspects of themselves, and to relate more deeply to others. Cohesiveness in a group thus favors self-disclosure, risk taking, and the constructive expression of confrontation and conflict—all phenomena that facilitate successful therapy. Highly cohesive groups are stable groups with better attendance, more active patient commitment and participation, and less membership turnover than groups that have not "cohered." Some groups, such as those specializing in a particular problem or disorder, will by their very nature develop a great deal of cohesiveness. In other kinds of groups, especially those in which membership changes frequently, the leader may need to actively facilitate the development of this important therapeutic factor.

Interpersonal Learning

Surprisingly, this potent mechanism for change in group therapy—interpersonal learning—is often overlooked, misapplied, or misunderstood by leaders, perhaps because the encouragement of interpersonal exploration requires considerable therapist skill and experience. We will examine three underlying concepts: the interpersonal frame of reference, the group as a social microcosm, and learning from behavioral patterns in the social microcosm.

The interpersonal frame of reference. Psychotherapists who utilize an interpersonal frame of reference concentrate on the interpersonal pathology that underlies or arises from a particular symptom complex. The therapist translates symptoms into interpersonal language. For example, the psychotherapist rarely addresses "depression" per se. The typical symptom cluster of dysphoric mood and neurovegetative signs does not in and of itself offer a handhold to begin the process of psychotherapeutic change. Instead, the clinician forms a relationship with the person who is depressed and ascertains the underlying interpersonal problems that arise from the depression and that most certainly also exacerbate it (problems such as dependency, obsequiousness, inability to express rage, hypersensitivity to rejection, and the like). Once these maladaptive interpersonal themes have been identified, the therapist and the patient can undertake the work of understanding and altering them.

The group as a social microcosm. Sooner or later, given enough time and freedom, each person in the group will begin to interact with other group members in the same way that he or she interacts with persons outside of the group. The group becomes a laboratory experiment in which interpersonal strengths and weaknesses unfold "in miniature." Slowly but predictably, each individual's interpersonal pathology comes to be displayed in the group. Arrogance, impatience, narcissism, grandiosity, sexualization—all such traits eventually surface. There is hardly any need for members to describe their past or to report present difficulties with relationships in their outside life. Group behavior provides far more accurate and immediate data. Members act out their interpersonal problems before the eyes of everyone in the group, and a freely interacting group will, in time, develop into a social microcosm of each of the members of that group.

Learning from behavioral patterns in the social microcosm. These preceding concepts interrelate in the process of group therapy to provide the therapist with an extremely powerful tool for change: interpersonal learning. Interpersonal learning is the cardinal mechanism for change in unstructured, longer-term, high-functioning interaction groups; in these settings the elements of interpersonal learning are typically ranked by members as being the most helpful aspect of the group therapy experience (Freedman and Hurley 1980; Yalom 1985). In this process, psycho-pathology emerges from and is embodied in distorted interpersonal interactions, in which the group becomes a social microcosm as each member displays his or her interpersonal pathology, and in which feedback allows members to identify and to change their interpersonal behavior. This process is described below (Yalom 1985, 1986).

1. *Displaying interpersonal pathology*: Members display their characteristic interpersonally distorted behavior.
2. *Providing feedback and self-observation*: Members share observations of each other and discover some of their own blind spots.
3. *Sharing reactions*: Members point out each others' blind spots and point out how each member's behavior makes them feel.
4. *Examining results of sharing reactions:* Each member begins to have a more objective picture of his or her own behavior and of the impact it has on others.
5. *Understanding one's opinion of oneself*: Each member becomes aware of how one's own behavior influences the opinions of others and, hence, one's opinions of oneself.
6. *Developing a sense of responsibility*: As a result of understanding how one's behavior influences one's sense of self-worth, one becomes more fully aware of responsibility for one's interpersonal life.
7. *Realizing one's power to effect change*: With the acceptance of responsibility for life's interpersonal dilemmas, each member begins to realize that one can change what one has created.
8. *Potentiating change through high affect*: The more emotionally laden the events of this sequence, the greater is the potential for change.

☐ Forces That Modify the Therapeutic Factors in Group Therapy

Group therapy is a forum for change whose form, content, and process vary considerably both across groups and within the same group at any given time. In other words, different types of groups will make use of different clusters of therapeutic factors (Table 33–1), and, furthermore, as a group evolves, different sets of factors come into play (Dies 1993). Three modifying forces can influence the therapeutic mechanisms at work in any given group: the type of group, the stage of therapy, and individual differences among patients.

Type of Group

Research on long-term interactional outpatient group therapy indicates that group members consistently select a constellation of three factors—

interpersonal learning, catharsis, and self-understanding—as those elements of group therapy most helpful to them (Yalom 1985). Inpatients tend to identify other mechanisms: the instillation of hope and the existential factor of assumption of responsibility (Leszcz et al. 1985). Groups that are centered around self-help concepts rely on the mechanisms of universality, guidance, altruism, and cohesiveness (Lieberman and Borman 1979).

Stage of Therapy

In its early stages, an outpatient group is most concerned with establishing boundaries and maintaining membership, and factors such as instillation of hope, guidance, and universality loom most important. Other factors, such as altruism and group cohesiveness, will operate throughout the duration of therapy, but their nature changes with the stage of the group. In the case of altruism, for example, early in the group, patients will offer suggestions to each other, ask appropriate questions, and show concern and attention. Later, they will be able to express a deeper caring and "being with" each other or a true sharing of emotion.

Initially, the condition of group cohesiveness operates by means of group support and acceptance, whereas later in the life of the group it facilitates self-disclosure. Ultimately, group cohesiveness makes it possible for members to explore issues of confrontation and conflict, issues so essential to interpersonal learning. The longer patients participate in a group, the more they value the therapeutic factors of cohesiveness, self-understanding, and interpersonal interaction (Butler and Fuhriman 1983).

Differences Among Patients

Higher-functioning patients tend to value interpersonal learning more than do lower-functioning patients in the same group. In one study of inpatient groups, both types of patients chose awareness of responsibility and catharsis as helpful elements of group therapy; however, the lower-functioning patients also valued the instillation of hope, and higher-functioning patients selected universality, vicarious learning, and interpersonal learning as additional useful experiences (Leszcz et al. 1985). Many different mechanisms of change are available, but each individual patient will make the most use out of those particular factors that are most suited to his or her needs and problems. Some patients need to develop very basic social skills through the development of socializing techniques, whereas others benefit from the identification and exploration of much subtler interpersonal issues.

■ THE THERAPIST'S BASIC TASKS IN GROUP THERAPY

Long before the first meeting, the leader will have been hard at work, for the group therapist's initial task is to create a physical entity where none existed. The leader assembles a group and offers the professional help that is the initial raison d'être for the group. The leader selects the members and sets the time, place, and tone for the meetings. In sum, the therapist has the basic tasks of establishing and maintaining the group and of resolving the problems typically encountered in the group setting.

☐ Establishing a Therapy Group

Setting and Size

Before the first group meeting even takes place, the therapist has made certain decisions about its circumstances. The most pragmatic of these involves choosing an appropriate meeting place. A setting that provides privacy and freedom from distraction is essential, of course, but a group meeting room should also be consistently available and of adequate size, and have comfortable seating. The optimal size of a group is a function of its therapeutic goals. Organizations that operate with group settings of up to 80 members rely heavily on inspiration, guidance, and suppression to change members' behavior. But leaders working in a large therapeutic community might wish to make use of a different set of factors, such as group pressure and interdependence to foster reality testing or to instill a sense of individual responsibility to the social community. In this setting, groups of 15 or so members may be more appropriate.

The ideal size for a prototypic interactional group is 7 or 8 members, and certainly no more than 10. Too few members will not provide the necessary critical mass of interpersonal interactions. There will not be enough opportunities for broad consensual validation of different viewpoints, and patients will tend to interact one at a time with the therapist rather than with one another. Anyone who has ever tried to conduct a group with only two or three patients knows the frustration of this enterprise. In a group with more than 10 members, there may be ample fruitful interaction, but some members will be left out. There will simply be insufficient time to examine and understand all of the interactions.

When working with inpatients or when leading specialized outpatient groups, the therapist's focus may not be as explicitly interpersonally oriented as in the prototypic interaction group, but the therapist will still want to aim for an "alive" and engaging group, one that encourages active participation by as many members as possible. In our clinical experience, the optimal group size that allows members to share experiences with one another ranges from a minimum of 4 or 5 to a maximum of 12; groups of 6 to 8 seem to offer the greatest opportunity for verbal exchange among all patients.

Time Constraints

Clinical consensus agrees that the optimal duration for a session in ongoing group therapy is between 60 and 120 minutes (Yalom 1985). Usually 20 to 30 minutes are required for the group to warm up, and at least 60 minutes are needed to work through the major themes of the session. Groups that meet frequently, such as daily inpatient groups, or groups that consist of lower-functioning patients who can only tolerate limited social stimuli, do well with briefer sessions. Groups that meet less often or that are centered on higher-functioning interactional work require at least 90 minutes per session in order to be fruitful.

The frequency of meetings can vary from once a day—typically in the inpatient setting—to the once-a-month medication clinic support group. A once-weekly schedule is most common in outpatient group work and seems well-suited to supportive or specialized groups. Long-term interactional groups also tend to meet once per week, although clinical experience suggests that twice-weekly sessions, when feasible, increase the intensity and productivity of this kind of group.

The Use of Open Versus Closed Groups

The decision to run an open or a closed group is related to the goals of the group and its identified lifespan. A closed group meets for a predetermined number of sessions, begins with a fixed number of members, and, as of the first session, closes its doors and accepts no new members. In such time-limited groups, each session may follow a predetermined protocol. External time constraints can also influence the format of a group. In contrast, open groups either are more flexible about size or may maintain a consistent size by replacing members as they leave the group. Open groups usually have a broader set of therapeutic goals and generally meet indefinitely; although members come and go, the group has a life of its own.

The Use of a Co-Therapist

Co-therapists complement and support each other. A male-female co-therapist team has unique advantages. Many patients can benefit from observing a male and a female therapist working together with mutual respect and without the derogation, exploitation, or sexualizing that the patients too often take for granted in male-female relationships. Moreover, the group is provided with a wider array of transferential possibilities, for patients will differ in their reactions to each of the co-therapists and to the co-therapists' relationship.

In addition to clarifying transference distortions of each other's presentation in the group, co-therapists can support each other in maintaining objectivity in the face of massive group pressure. It is usually the co-therapist who can best help members channel and express their anger in an appropriate manner and who can then lead members to examine the source and the meaning of that anger.

There is some question whether co-therapists should openly reveal their differences of opinion during the group session. Two factors to consider are the level of functioning of the group and the maturity of the group. Patients who are lower functioning and who are more fragile or unstable overall should generally not be exposed to conflict between the co-therapists, no matter how gently it is expressed. Likewise, co-therapist disagreement is not helpful early in the work with even higher-functioning patients, for a beginning group usually is not stable or cohesive enough to tolerate divisiveness in leadership. Later in such a group, however, the therapists' honesty about disagreement can contribute substantially to the potency and honesty of the group. Members observe the leaders they respect disagreeing openly and resolving their differences with honesty and tact. Members also experience the therapists not as infallible authority figures but as humans with imperfections, and they thus learn to differentiate others according to individual attributes rather than stereotyped roles.

Splitting is a phenomenon that often occurs in groups led by co-therapists, and some patients are very perceptive about tensions in the co-therapists' relationship. Occasionally the entire group can become split into two factions, with each co-therapist having a "team" of patients aligned with him or her; this may occur because the patients feel they have a special relationship with one or the other of the therapists or because they feel that one of the therapists is more intelligent, more senior, more attractive, or has a similar ethnic background. Splitting should always be noted and openly interpreted in the group.

☐ Creating a Therapy Group

Formulating Goals

As a first step to creating a therapy group, the therapist must carefully examine all of the clinical facts of life that will bear upon the group. The *intrinsic* factors (e.g., mandatory attendance for patients on legal probation, duration of treatment in a ward group of hospitalized patients with cancer) are built into the clinical situation and cannot be changed; the group leader must adapt to them. The *extrinsic* factors are those that have become tradition or "policy" in a given setting. Extrinsic factors are arbitrary and within the power of the therapist to change.

Once a clear view of the clinical facts of life has been established, the leader's second step is to construct a reasonable set of clinical goals for the group. This is the most important step in creating a therapy group, for the selection of inappropriate or vaguely defined goals is sure to result in failure. The goals of a long-term outpatient group are ambitious: to offer symptomatic relief and also to change character structure. An attempt to apply these same goals to an aftercare group of chronic schizophrenic patients would result in therapeutic nihilism. Goals must be shaped that are appropriate to the clinical situation and achievable in the available time frame. In time-limited, specialized groups, the goals must be focused, achievable, and tailored to the capacity and potential of the group members.

Selecting Patients and Composing a Therapy Group

Once the therapist has a clear idea of the goals of the group—in other words, a clear idea of the group task—he or she must select members who can achieve these goals and perform the group task. The leader's expertise in the selection and preparation of members will greatly affect the group's fate. The therapist must create a group that coheres, and, because nothing threatens a group's cohesiveness more than the presence of a grossly deviant member, the selection of members must be guided by the notion of group integrity and the avoidance of deviancy.

The single most important criterion for member selection, no matter what the group, is ability to perform the group task. The study of group failures reveals that deviancy (i.e., an inability or refusal to engage in the group task) is negatively related to outcome. An individual who considers himself or herself (or is considered by other members) as "out of the group" or as a deviant or mascot has little likelihood of profiting from the group and a fair chance of negative outcome (Lieberman et al. 1973). Selection for group therapy is therefore, in practice, conducted by the process of deselection. Group therapists exclude certain patients from consideration (most often because the therapist predicts the patient will assume a deviant role or because the patient lacks motivation for change) and accept remaining patients.

Above all, the therapist must be concerned about the group's *integrity*. Members must be selected who are committed to the task of therapy and to regular attendance in the group. Perhaps the key concept is group cohesiveness. An effective rule of thumb for longer-term outpatient groups is "homogeneity in ego strength, heterogeneity in problem areas" (Whitaker and Lieberman 1964). In other words, patients profit from a heterodoxy of personality styles, ages, problem areas, but the group co-heres best if all members possess the ego strength necessary to partici-pate equally in the group task.

The situation is different in specialized or symptom-oriented groups; in these cases, members will always share at least one major problem area, but they may be quite heterogeneous in terms of ego strength. Whenever possible, the therapist tries to aim for similar levels of motiva-tion and psychological mindedness in the composition of the group. It impedes the work of a fast-paced, highly motivated group to have one or two members who are fragile, brittle, or work-avoidant. Likewise, a stolid group of more concrete chronically ill psychiatric patients can be-come destabilized if pushed too hard too fast by a confrontative, agi-tated, or manic individual (Kahn 1984; Kanas 1986).

Often the therapist has minimal influence over group membership. At the very least, he or she must exercise the group therapist's preroga-tive and exclude those patients who are markedly incompatible with the prevailing group norms for acceptable behavior. Patients who cannot tol-erate the stress of a group setting, such as the extremely paranoid indi-vidual, and patients who are absolutely incompatible with at least one other member, also should not be included in the group. One reason that it is so difficult to compose an ideal group is because it is extremely diffi-cult to predict subsequent group behavior from information available in the screening procedure. A very important source of information is the candidate's previous experience in groups. Another important source is the screening procedure itself. In the one or two intake interviews, the therapist should focus on the candidate's interpersonal functioning: past, present, and in the interview itself. The therapist must assess the individual's ability to tolerate interpersonal interactions and to reflect on them.

Preparing Patients for Group Therapy

Preparation of the patient for group therapy is another one of the thera-pist's essential tasks. A great deal of research evidence has demonstrated that pregroup preparation decreases the number of dropouts, increases cohesiveness, and accelerates the work of therapy (Piper and Perrault 1989; Yalom 1985). In some settings, such as an inpatient ward or a medi-cation clinic group, this preparation will of necessity be minimal and will consist mainly of orienting the patient to the time, location, composition, procedure, and goals of the group. But even this brief preparation helps to orient patients to the group experience and provides guidelines about how to benefit from the group.

For most outpatient groups, preparation is best accomplished during one or two individual sessions with each patient prior to beginning the group. After deciding during an intake interview that the patient is a suitable candidate for group therapy, the therapist may then proceed to prepare the patient for the group. Providing clarity is the cardinal aim of the pregroup preparatory procedure. The therapist provides patients with a cognitive structure that enables them to participate more effectively in the group from the start.

Many patients hold misconceptions about group therapy's worth and efficacy; they feel that it is cheaper or diluted therapy and therefore not as worthwhile as individual therapy. These negative expectations must be addressed openly and corrected in order to engage the patient fully in treatment. Other patients express concerns about procedure and process: the size of the group, the type of members, the amount of negative confrontation, confidentiality. One of the most pervasive fears is the anticipation of having to reveal oneself and confess shameful transgressions to an audience of hostile strangers.

A cognitive approach to group therapy preparation has several goals:

- To provide a rational explanation to the patient about the group therapy process
- To describe what types of behavior are expected of patients in the group
- To establish a contract about attendance
- To raise expectations about the effects of the group
- To predict some of the problems, discouragement, and frustration that may be encountered in early meetings

☐ Constructing and Maintaining Therapeutic Environment

Building the Culture of the Group

Once the group is a physical reality and the first meeting is under way, the leader must establish behavioral norms that will guide the interactions of the newly formed group. Ideally, *all* of the members in the group will provide support, a sense of universality, and interpersonal feedback. In group therapy it is the leader's task to create a group culture maximally conducive to effective group interaction and to the development of the various therapeutic factors.

Norms constructed early in the group have considerable perseverance and are shaped both by the expectations of the members as they start the group and by the behavior of the therapist during the early sessions. The therapist influences this process of norm setting in two different ways. First, the leader, in the role of technical expert, can *explicitly* shape the group norms. During early preparation of patients for group therapy, for example, patients can be given explicit instructions about the rules for appropriate behavior in the group, such as sharing concerns about body image in an eating disorders group. Once a group gets under way, the leader may reward desirable behavior through social reinforcement. If a usually shy member begins to participate, or if members start to offer one another spontaneous and honest feedback, this new behavior may be shaped and rewarded verbally or nonverbally through changes in the therapist's body language, eye contact, and facial expression.

The second way the therapist shapes therapeutic norms in the group is through model setting. In an acute inpatient therapy group, for example, leaders offer a model of nonjudgmental acceptance and appreciation of members' strengths as well as problem areas, helping to shape a group that is health oriented. In a social skills training group for schizophrenic patients, the leader might choose to model simple, direct, socially rewarding conversation. No matter what the level and functioning of the group, the effective leader sets a model of interpersonal honesty and spontaneity for his or her group members. But the therapist's honesty always transpires against a background of responsibility; nothing takes precedence over the goal of being helpful to the patient.

There are several very basic therapeutic group norms that should be encouraged in any group setting, regardless of its orientation. The first of these is the norm of the *self-monitoring group,* in which the group itself learns to assume responsibility for its own functioning. This can be accomplished by keeping in mind that, initially, only the leader knows when a group has been productive. The therapist must start to share this knowledge with the patients at the very inception of a group and slowly educate them to recognize a good session. The evaluative function can then be shifted to the patients.

General procedural norms must always be actively shaped by the leader. Ideally, the most therapeutic procedural format of a group is one that is unstructured, unrehearsed, and freely flowing. The therapist must intervene actively to preclude the development of a nontherapeutic procedure, for example, a "taking turns" format in which members figuratively line up to discuss specific problems or life crises one after another by rote. In such an instance, the therapist might interrupt and ask how the practice got started or what effect it has on the group. The leader could also indicate that the group has many other procedural options from which to choose.

When *members consider the group important,* group therapy becomes more effective, and the leader who reinforces this norm increases the therapeutic potency of his or her group. Likewise, the therapist augments the power of the group by increasing *the continuity between meetings.* As the group "time-binder," it is the therapist's task to call attention to behavioral patterns developing over several meetings. Finally, a group functions best when it sees its *members as agents of help and support*; a truly therapeutic culture implies that members will learn the most and receive the most help from one another.

Identifying and Resolving Common Problems in Group Therapy

Membership problems.   The early developmental sequence and potency of a therapy group are strongly affected by *membership problems.* Turnover in membership, tardiness, and absence are facts of life in all groups, yet these events will threaten a group's stability and integrity. Tardiness and irregular attendance must be discouraged in all group settings and should be regarded in the same way in which one regards these phenomena in individual therapy.

In the normal course of a long-term outpatient therapy group, leaders should keep in mind that 10% to 35% of the members will drop out in the first 12 to 20 meetings (Yalom 1985). In an open group it is the therapist's task to replace dropouts by adding new members. Dropouts are threatening to the group's stability for two reasons: they impede the development of cohesiveness, and they implicitly (and sometimes explicitly) devalue the group. Dropouts are also threatening to the leader, especially to the neophyte, and the therapist may unwittingly adopt a seductive posture in an effort to keep a patient in the group. The dropout rate can be reduced through vigorous pretherapy selection and preparation (Connelly et al. 1986). If the general problems and frustrations that can arise early in a group are predicted to new members ahead of time, there is less likelihood that dropping out will occur.

Subgrouping.   A second problem commonly encountered in group therapy is *subgrouping*—the splitting off of smaller units. A subgroup usually arises from the belief of two or more members that they can derive more gratification from a relationship with each other than from one with the entire group. Extragroup socializing, which often occurs in outpatient groups (and almost invariably in inpatient groups), is often the first stage of subgrouping. A clique of three or four members will begin to have telephone conversations, to have coffee or dinner, and to share separate observations and interactions with one another. Occasionally, two members will become sexually involved. A subgroup may also coalesce completely within the confines of the group therapy room, as members who perceive themselves to be similar form coalitions based on age, similar values, comparable education, and the like. Remaining group members, excluded from the clique, generally do not possess effective social skills and do not usually coalesce into a second subgroup. This phenomenon of "ingroup" versus "outgroup" can often be strikingly observed in inpatient settings.

It is not subgrouping or extragroup socializing that is crippling to a group per se; rather it is the conspiracy of silence around it that becomes dangerous. The primary task in the group is to examine in depth the interpersonal relationships among all of the members, but extragroup socializing inhibits this examination. Important material—the relationship between members who are interacting outside of the group, feelings of exclusion in patients who are not part of this interaction—remains covert, and the task of the group is sabotaged. Patients who violate group norms through the pursuit of subgrouping or through secret extragroup liaisons are opting for immediate need gratification rather than for involvement in interpersonal learning and change. Subgrouping or extragroup behavior that is not examined in the group session becomes a potent form of resistance.

Conflict.   *Conflict,* a third common problem, is inevitable in the course of a group's development. The task of the therapist is to identify conflict as it arises and to harness it in the service of the group task. Conflict resolution is well-nigh impossible in the presence of off-target or oblique hostility, and, once again, it is the therapist's task to identify and render overt that which has been covert.

One important principle is to find the right level for the group at hand. Too much conflict is threatening and counterproductive for just about any group of individuals, but too little conflict leaves the group stagnant, excessively cautious, and superficial. Here, a judicious amount of confrontation, anger, and conflict resolution can provide an affectively charged learning experience for the group members. Group cohesiveness is the prime prerequisite for the successful management of conflict. Members must have developed a feeling of mutual respect and trust and must value the group sufficiently to be able to tolerate confrontative or uncomfortable interactions. The leader will need to emphasize that open communication must be maintained if the group is to survive; all parties must continue to deal directly with one another, no matter how angry they become.

Not all groups tolerate the same level of conflict. The open, conflictual confrontation that may transpire between two members of a long-term outpatient group would be devastating in a group for schizophrenic patients (Kanas 1986). Gentle, cautious disagreement would be appropriate in a time-limited group for patients with panic disorder, whereas it would be seen as an avoidance of the real issues in the long-term outpatient group. Therapists should remember that conflict can get out of hand, no matter what the group setting. Leaders will often have to intervene vigorously to keep conflict within constructive bounds. Most often, this will include helping patients to express anger more directly and more fairly, and ensuring that everyone "gets a turn" at responding to the anger. As with any affectively charged experience in the group, the therapist will need to encourage active feedback and consensual validation from all of the group members and, more than ever, will need to help patients process the meaning of that experience within the context of the group.

■ TECHNIQUES OF THE GROUP THERAPIST

Although individual and group therapists often use similar psychotherapeutic techniques, a number of interventions are unique to group therapy. These interventions include working in the here and now, using therapist transparency, and employing various procedural aids that can enhance the group work.

☐ Working in the Here and Now

Even in the absence of direct leadership, an environment can develop in which nearly all of the therapeutic factors, from universality to altruism, will operate. There is one important exception, however, and that is the factor of interpersonal learning. Interpersonal learning in group therapy requires the presence of a leader, one who is well versed in the specific therapeutic techniques of working in the "here and now." The principles of working in the here and now and the use of interpersonal learning are of most consequence in prototypic interactional groups, but these fundamental concepts can be modified to suit the needs of other kinds of groups and form an essential part of any group therapist's armamentarium (Dies 1993; Rothke 1986).

Goals

The primary goal of the long-term outpatient therapy group, and, to a lesser extent, of many other kinds of groups, is to help each individual understand as much as possible about his or her interactions with the other members of the group, therapists included. To accomplish this, members must learn to focus on the immediate interpersonal transactions occurring in the group. For the therapist, this means that the most fundamental principle of technique is to focus on the present, on what transpires in the therapy room in the here and now of the group interaction. By directly focusing on the here and now, the leader solicits and engages the active participation of all the members and maximizes the power and efficiency of the group. In other words, the therapy group focus is most powerful if it is basically ahistoric—that is, if it deemphasizes the historical past and even the current outside life of the individual members in favor of the here-and-now events in the group. Deemphasis does not imply that history is unimportant, only that groups work most efficiently on the interactions occurring in the immediate present.

A group experience must, if it is to be therapeutically effective, contain both an affective and a cognitive component. That is, the group members must be involved with one another in an affective matrix: they must interact freely, they must reveal a great deal of themselves, and they must experience and express important emotions. But they must also step outside of that experience and examine, understand, and integrate the meaning of the emotional experience they have just undergone (Yalom and Vinogradov 1993). Thus, a here-and-now focus consists of a rotating sequence of affect evocation followed by affect examination.

Techniques

These two stages of the here-and-now focus—affect evocation followed by affect examination—are different in character and demand two very distinct sets of techniques. For the first stage, the stage of emotional experience, the therapist needs a set of techniques that will plunge the group into the immediate interpersonal interactions. For the second stage, clarification and understanding of the emotional experience, the therapist needs a set of techniques that will help the group transcend itself to examine and interpret its own experience. Let us consider each of these stages in turn.

Plunging the group into the here and now.   The starting place for shaping a group focused in the here and now is in the pregroup preparation. By using straightforward instruction, the leader can offer the patient a rationale of the here-and-now approach through a brief, simplified discussion of the interpersonal approach to therapy. Patients benefit from an explicit description of how various kinds of psychological problems arise from patients' relationships with others and how group therapy is an ideal setting to take a close look at interpersonal relationships. Without this preparation, patients may be confused by the here-and-now focus of the group.

After laying these foundations for the here-and-now focus in the initial pregroup preparation, the leader continues to reinforce this focus throughout therapy. Experienced group therapists think "here and now" at all times and consider themselves as shepherds keeping the group at work grazing on current interactions. All strays into the past, into outside life, or into intellectualization must be headed off or gently herded back into the present. Whenever the group engages in some "there-and-then" discussion, the group leader must think, "How can I bring this back into the here and now?"

Group therapists must be active and continue diligently from session to session to bring the group discussion into the here and now. They must shift the content of the material from outside the group to inside the group, from abstract reflections on problems to specific revelations, from generic statements to personal disclosure. When a patient states that he or she is embarrassed to talk about certain things in the group, the therapist might ask what the patient anticipates happening if he or she were to take the risk and talk about something "embarrassing." Once the group member reveals his or her guesses about others' reactions, the door is open to good interactional work. Other group members can confirm or, as is more often the case, disconfirm those guesses.

Individuals do not engage naturally and easily in the here and now. The experience is new and frightening, especially for the many patients who have not previously had close and honest relationships or who have spent their lives keeping certain thoughts and feelings—anger, pain, intimacy—covert. The therapist must offer much support, reinforcement, and explicit training. A first step is to help patients understand that the here-and-now focus is not synonymous with confrontation and conflict. In fact, many patients have problems not with anger or rage but with closeness and the honest and nondemanding or nonmanipulative expression of positive sentiments. Accordingly, it is important early in the group to encourage the expression of positive feelings as well as critical ones (Yalom and Vinogradov 1993).

Understanding the here and now.   The second stage of the here-and-now focus requires an entirely different set of functions and techniques from the therapist. If the first stage demands "activation" and plunging the group into the present affective experience, the second stage demands reflection, explanation, and interpretation. Often this latter phase of the group work is referred to as "group process." If several individuals engage in a discussion, the content of their discussion consists of the actual words spoken and the substantive issues addressed. The process refers to how this content was expressed and what it reveals about the nature of the relationship of the individuals holding the discussion.

The group therapist must always attend to the process of the communication in the group—that is, he or she must listen to the group discussion with an ear that is examining how the words exchanged shed light on the relationships among the participants. A process-oriented therapist is concerned about "horizontal disclosure" (i.e., disclosure about the disclosure) and, accordingly, will attend to the relational aspects of the disclosure (Vinogradov and Yalom 1989). The recognition of process is part of the art of psychotherapy and often requires a long apprenticeship. To understand process, one needs to continually register all the available data. Who chooses which seats? Who is always late? At whom do members look when talking with each other? Who meets with whom at the end of the group? How does the group change when a particular member is absent? Some of the most valuable data are the therapist's own reactions. Feelings of impatience, frustration, or boredom in a group session represent valuable information and should be put to use. Likewise, when the leader feels engaged or excited by the group interactions, this is often the sign of a potent, hard-working meeting.

☐ Use of Transference and Therapist Transparency

Transference

Group members regard group therapists in an unrealistic light for many reasons. True transference or displacement of affect from some prior object, such as an early parental figure, is one source. Conflicted attitudes toward authority as represented by the leader are another. And still another source is the patient's tendency to imbue therapists with superhuman features so as to use them as a shield against existential anxiety. One final, and realistic, source of strong feelings lies in the members' explicit or intuitive appreciation of the great power that group therapists wield. The therapists' consistent presence and impartiality are essential for group survival and stability. Group therapists cannot be exposed; they can add new members, expel old members, and mobilize enormous group pressure around any issue they wish.

Group therapists have a variety of tasks: they must make good use of any irrational attitudes toward them without at the same time neglecting a leader's many other functions in the group. To work effectively with transference in the therapy group, leaders must help patients recognize, understand, and change their distorted attitudinal sets. Two major approaches or techniques facilitate transference resolution in the therapy group. The first of these involves consensual validation by other group members of the patient's distorted views. The second makes use of increased therapist transparency. In consensual validation, a group leader encourages a patient to validate his or her impressions against those of other members. If many or all of the group members concur in the patient's view of and feelings toward the leader, it can be concluded either that the patient's reaction to the therapist stems from global group forces related to the leader's role, or that the reaction is not an unrealistic one at all and the patient is perceiving the leader quite accurately. If, on the other hand, one member alone of all the group possesses a particular view of the therapist, then this member may be helped to examine the possibility that he or she sees the group leader, and perhaps other persons too, through an internal distorting prism.

Therapist Transparency

Group therapists can also allow a patient to confirm or disconfirm irrational impressions by gradually revealing more of themselves, reacting to the patient as a real person in the here and now. Leaders can thus respond to their patients authentically, share their feelings in a judicious and responsible manner, and acknowledge or refute motives and feelings attributed to them. In this approach, they look at their own blind spots and demonstrate respect for the feedback members offer them. In the face of mounting reality-based data the members have about the therapist, it becomes increasingly difficult for members to maintain their fictitious beliefs about the group leader (Vinogradov and Yalom 1990).

Although therapist self-disclosure generally facilitates the group interaction, it is important to keep in mind that the group therapist's primary raison d'être is not to be fully self-disclosing. Furthermore, leader self-revelation must be guided by the different needs of each group member. Not all patients need the same thing, either from the therapist or from the group. Some patients need to relax controls and to learn how to express their emotions in an honest and responsible manner, whether they be emotions of anger, love, tenderness, envy, or the like. Other patients need quite the opposite: to gain impulse control and to accept limits to the expression of their emotions; their life-styles may already be characterized by labile and immediately acted-upon affect. Even the transparent and authentically self-disclosing therapist must provide some cognitive structuring. Only in this manner can patients learn to generalize their experiences to outside life.

☐ Procedural Aids

A group leader's therapeutic armamentarium can be expanded through the use of procedural aids—specialized techniques that are not essential but may facilitate the course of therapy. Three such approaches are written summaries, videotaping, and structured exercises.

Written Summaries

The course of most outpatient therapy groups, especially the interactionally oriented group, is facilitated by the use of written summaries (Yalom 1985; Yalom et al. 1975). The most useful procedure is for the group leader to dictate a candid, concise description of the group session after each meeting and to have a transcription (of approximately two to three single-spaced pages) sent out to the group members the following day. These summaries provide an extra "contact" with the group's here-and-now interactions during the week between meetings. Patients have been unanimous in their positive evaluation of this technique. Most await the arrival of the weekly summary in the mail with anticipation; they read and consider it seriously. Many members reread the summaries several times, and almost all file them for future review. The patients' therapeutic perspectives and commitment are deepened, and the patient-therapist relationship is strengthened. No serious transference complications, breaks in confidentiality, or other adverse consequences have been noted to occur by practitioners of this method.

The summary serves several functions. It provides an understanding of the here-and-now events of the session and facilitates the integration of powerful affective experiences. It labels good or resistive sessions, notes and rewards patient gains in the group, and predicts undesirable developments in the group, thus minimizing their impact. It increases group cohesiveness by emphasizing similarities among members, by underscoring the expressing of caring or other positive emotions, and by providing continuity from one meeting to another. The summary is also an ideal forum for interpretations, either for repetition of interpretations made during the session or for new interpretations that have occurred to the therapist after the meeting. Finally, the summary provides hope to the patients by helping them realize that the group is an orderly process and that the therapist(s) has some coherent sense of the group's long-term development.

Videotaping

Some therapists make the videotape recording a central feature of therapy; they may arrange for immediate playback of certain segments during a meeting or set up regularly scheduled playback sessions. Other therapists find the technique of value but prefer to use it as a teaching device or occasionally as an auxiliary aid in the therapeutic process.

Videotape provides feedback that is not mediated through a second person. Often a patient's cherished self-image is radically challenged by a videotape playback. It is not unusual for a patient suddenly to recall and to accept previous feedback he or she has gotten from other members. With dramatic impact, the patient realizes that the group has been honest and, if anything, overprotective in previous confrontations. Often profound realizations occur: for the first time, patients observe their full behavior and its impact on others with their own eyes. Many initial playback reactions are concerned with physical attractiveness and mannerisms, whereas in subsequent playback sessions patients begin to make more careful note of their interactions with others, their withdrawal or timidity, and their self-preoccupation or aloofness, or hostility.

Structured Exercises

The term *structured exercises* refers to the many group activities in which members follow some specific set of orders, generally prescribed by the leader. These kinds of exercises play a more important role in brief, specialized therapy groups than in the long-term general outpatient group (Yalom 1985; Yalom et al. 1975). The precise rationale of the procedures varies, but, in general, structured exercises are meant to be accelerating devices. Some structured exercises (warm-up procedures) bypass the hesitant, uneasy first steps of the group; others speed up interaction by assigning individuals interactional tasks that circumvent cautious, ritualized social behavior; still others speed up individual work by helping members "get in touch with" suppressed emotions, with unknown or hidden parts of themselves, and with their physical body.

A structured exercise may require only a few minutes, or it may consume an entire meeting. Though the exercise may be predominantly verbal or nonverbal in nature, there is always a verbal component in that it generates data that subsequently can be discussed by the group. The exercise can involve the entire group as a whole or it can involve one member vis-à-vis the group.

☐ Modification of Basic Techniques for Specialized Clinical Setting: Acute Inpatient Therapy Group

The therapist faced with the task of organizing a therapy group in a specialized clinical situation must learn to modify fundamental group principles and techniques. We suggest these three basic steps:

1. *Assessment of the clinical setting*: Determine the immutable clinical restraints surrounding the group.
2. *Formulation of goals*: Develop goals that are appropriate and achievable within the existing clinical restraints.
3. *Modification of traditional technique*: Retain the basic principles of group therapy but alter techniques to adapt them to the clinical setting and to achieve the specified goals.

We shall illustrate these steps by discussing a highly specialized group setting: the acute inpatient therapy group.

Assessment of the Clinical Setting

The clinical setting facing the inpatient therapist appears highly inhospitable to the practice of traditional group therapy. Intrinsic limitations over which the therapist has no control include the rapid turnover of patients (patients will often be present for only a single group meeting) and the severity and heterogeneity of psychopathology among hospitalized patients. Extrinsic constraints that affect the formation of an inpatient group are represented by such matters as ward policy, staffing, and administrative support (or lack thereof) for group therapy. The therapist must carefully delineate both the intrinsic and extrinsic limitations of the clinical setting and then take steps to change those extrinsic factors that might hinder the group.

Formulation of Goals

Given the clinical facts of life or constraints of the inpatient setting, the therapist must proceed to formulate appropriate goals for an inpatient therapy group. Six achievable goals for the inpatient setting have been highlighted (Yalom 1983):

1. To engage patients in the therapeutic process
2. To teach patients that talking helps
3. To spot problems
4. To decrease patients' sense of isolation
5. To allow patients to be helpful to others
6. To alleviate hospital-related anxiety

Modification of Basic Techniques

Once appropriate goals have been established, therapists must modify their standard group therapy techniques in order to lead effective groups on the acute psychiatric inpatient ward. Four essential modifications that we will discuss are 1) the adoption of an altered time frame, 2) the use of direct support, 3) emphasis on the here and now, and 4) the provision of structure.

Altered time frame.   The first and most fundamental modification the inpatient group leader makes is to adopt a radically shortened time frame. The therapist in an acute inpatient group must consider the life of the group to be only a single session and must strive to offer something useful for as many patients as possible during that session.

Direct support.   Inpatient group therapists must also learn to offer support quickly and directly. The most direct manner is simply to acknowledge openly each patient's efforts, intentions, strengths, positive contributions, and risks. The supportive therapist also makes it a point to help patients—especially objectionable or irritating patients—obtain support from the group. Another approach is to focus on making the group safe. Whereas some conflict and tension are necessary to the therapeutic work in a long-term outpatient group, inpatients are much too vulnerable to tolerate the additional anxiety of group conflict. The group therapist must anticipate and avoid confrontation and conflict whenever possible.

When the therapist leads a group of severely regressed patients, he or she must provide even more support and in an even more direct fashion. The patients' behavior must be examined and then reframed in some positive way. The therapist can, for example, support the mute patient for staying the whole session, compliment the patient who leaves early for even having stayed 20 minutes, or support inactive patients for having paid attention throughout the meeting.

Emphasis on the here and now.   These foregoing considerations of therapist efficiency, activity, and support in the inpatient setting do not make the here-and-now focus any less important than in outpatient therapy. Such a focus helps inpatients learn many important interpersonal skills: to communicate more clearly, to get closer to others, to express positive feelings, to become aware of personal mannerisms that push people away, to listen, to offer support, to reveal oneself, and to form friendships.

Provision of structure.   Finally, work with the acute inpatient group requires structure, and just as there is no place in acute inpatient group work for the inactive therapist, there is also no place for the nondirective therapist. Group leaders provide structure for the inpatient group in several ways: by instructing and orienting patients as to the nature and purpose of the meeting, by establishing very clear spatial and temporal boundaries for the group, and by using a lucid and confident personal style that reassures confused or anxious patients and contributes to a sense of structure. One of the most potent ways of providing structure is to build into each session a consistent, explicit sequence. Although different group sessions will have different sequences depending on the composition and task of the group, the following are natural lines of division:

1. *The first few minutes*: The therapist provides explicit structure for the group. If there are new members, this is the time to orient them to therapy.
2. *Definition of the task*: The therapist determines the most profitable direction for the group to take in a particular session.

3. *Accomplishing the task*: The therapist helps the group to address the broad issues raised at the start of the session and, in the process, attempts to have as many patients participate as possible.
4. *The final few minutes*: The leader indicates that the work phase is over and the remaining time is devoted to review and analysis of the meeting. This is the summing-up period and the "self-reflective" loop of the here-and-now process, in which the therapist attempts to clarify the group interaction that occurred in the session.

■ REFERENCES

Alonso A, Swiller HI: Introduction: the case for group therapy, in Group Therapy in Clinical Practice. Edited by Alonso A, Swiller HI. Washington, DC, American Psychiatric Press, 1993, pp xxi–xxv

Baker MN, Baker HS: Self psychological contributions to the theory and practice of group psychotherapy, in Group Therapy in Clinical Practice. Edited by Alonso A, Swiller HI. Washington, DC, American Psychiatric Press, 1993, pp 49–68

Benioff L, Vinogradov S: Group psychotherapy with cancer patients and the terminally ill, in Comprehensive Textbook of Group Psychotherapy, 3rd Edition. Edited by Kaplan HI, Sadock BJ. Baltimore, Williams & Wilkins, 1993, pp 477–489

Butler T, Fuhriman A: Curative factors in group therapy: a review of the recent literature. Small Group Behavior 14:131–142, 1983

Cheifetz DI, Salloway JC: Patterns of mental health services provided by HMOs. Am Psychol 39:495–502, 1984

Connelly JL, Piper WE, De Carufel FL, et al: Premature termination in group psychotherapy: pretherapy and early therapy predictors. Int J Group Psychother 36:145–152, 1986

Dies RR: Practical, theoretical, and empirical foundations for group psychotherapy, in Psychiatry Update: American Psychiatric Association Annual Review, Vol 5. Edited by Frances AJ, Hales RE. Washington, DC, American Psychiatric Press, 1986, pp 659–667

Dies RR: Research on group psychotherapy: overview and clinical applications, in Group Therapy in Clinical Practice. Edited by Alonso A, Swiller HI. Washington, DC, American Psychiatric Press, 1993, pp 473–518

Fawzy FI, Cousins NI, Fawzy NW, et al: A structured psychiatric intervention for cancer patients, I: changes over time in methods of coping and affective disturbance. Arch Gen Psychiatry 47:720–725, 1990

Freedman S, Hurley J: Perceptions of helpfulness and behavior in groups. Group 4:51–58, 1980

Kahn EM: Group treatment interventions for schizophrenics. Int J Group Psychother 34:149–153, 1984

Kanas N: Group therapy with schizophrenics: a review of controlled studies. Int J Group Psychother 36:339–351, 1986

Leszcz M, Yalom ID, Norden M: The value of inpatient group psychotherapy: patients' perceptions. Int J Group Psychother 35:411–433, 1985

Lieberman M[A]: Self-help groups and psychiatry, in Psychiatry Update: American Psychiatric Association Annual Review, Vol 5. Edited by Frances AJ, Hales RE. Washington, DC, American Psychiatric Press, 1986, pp 744–760

Lieberman MA, Borman L: Self-Help Groups for Coping With Crisis. San Francisco, CA, Jossey-Bass, 1979

Lieberman MA, Yalom ID, Miles MB: Encounter Groups: First Facts. New York, Basic Books, 1973

Piper WE, Perrault EL: Pretherapy preparation for group members. Int J Group Psychother 39:17–34, 1989

Rothke S: The role of interpersonal feedback in group psychotherapy. Int J Group Psychother 36:225–240, 1986

Shapiro DA, Shapiro D: Meta-analysis of comparative therapy outcome studies: a replication and refinement. Psychol Bull 92:581–604, 1982

Shapiro JL: Methods of Group Psychotherapy and Encounter. Itasca, IL, Peacock, 1978

Smith ML, Glass GV, Miller TI: The Benefits of Psychotherapy. Baltimore, MD, Johns Hopkins University Press, 1980

Spiegel D, Bloom JR, Kraemer HL, et al: Effect of psychosocial treatment on survival of patients with metastatic breast cancer. Lancet 2:888–891, 1989

Stern MJ: Group therapy with medically ill patients, in Group Therapy in Clinical Practice. Edited by Alonso A, Swiller HI. Washington, DC, American Psychiatric Press, 1993, pp 185–199

Tillitski CJ: A meta-analysis of estimated effect sizes for group versus individual versus control treatments. Int J Group Psychother 40:215–224, 1990

Toseland RW, Siporin M: When to recommend group treatment: a review of the clinical and the research literature. Int J Group Psychother 36:171–201, 1986

Vinogradov S, Yalom ID: Concise Guide to Group Psychotherapy. Washington, DC, American Psychiatric Press, 1989

Vinogradov S, Yalom ID: Self-disclosure in group psychotherapy, in Self-Disclosure in the Therapeutic Relationship. Edited by Stricker G, Fisher N. New York, Plenum, 1990, pp 191–203

Whitaker DS, Lieberman MAL: Psychotherapy Through the Group Process. New York, Atherton Press, 1964

Yalom ID: The Theory and Practice of Group Psychotherapy. New York, Basic Books, 1970

Yalom ID: Existential Psychotherapy. New York, Basic Books, 1980

Yalom ID: Inpatient Group Psychotherapy. New York, Basic Books, 1983

Yalom ID: The Theory and Practice of Group Psychotherapy, 3rd Edition. New York, Basic Books, 1985

Yalom ID: Interpersonal learning, in Psychiatry Update: American Psychiatric Association Annual Review, Vol 5. Edited by Frances AJ, Hales RE. Washington, DC, American Psychiatric Press, 1986, pp 699–713

Yalom V, Vinogradov S: Interpersonal group psychotherapy, in Comprehensive Textbook of Group Psychotherapy, 3rd Edition. Edited by Kaplan HI, Sadock BJ. Baltimore, Williams & Wilkins, 1993, pp 185–195

Yalom I[D], Brown S, Bloch S: The written summary as a group psychotherapy technique. Arch Gen Psychiatry 32:605–613, 1975

CHAPTER

34

Family Therapy:
Systems Approaches to
Assessment and Treatment

John S. Rolland, M.D.
Froma Walsh, Ph.D.

Family systems theory and family therapy have emerged as major approaches to understanding individual and family problems and the treatment of psychopathology. This approach is not simply another therapeutic method. Rather, it is a conceptual orientation to human problems and processes of change attending to the family context of individual functioning. What distinguishes the family systems orientation is its view of the family as a social system, with assessment and treatment of problems of an individual member in the context of the family as an interactive unit. Also, this approach recognizes the importance of the larger systems context, and especially cultural and socioeconomic factors. From this perspective, individual psychopathology and health cannot be adequately understood apart from their psychosocial context.

■ FAMILY SYSTEMS ORIENTATION

The practice of family therapy is grounded in a set of basic assumptions about the interplay of individual and family processes. The assessment and treatment of psychopathology, or dysfunction, are guided by principles of family systems theory. Family therapy is not simply a therapeutic modality in which all members are treated conjointly. Therapeutic interventions are aimed at modifying dysfunctional family patterns in which symptomatic behavior is embedded. Therapy may focus on a couple relationship, or involve individual sessions with the patient or other family members, combined with direct work with the whole family or part of a system, for instance, parents, siblings, and key extended family members.

Family systems theorists conceptualize the family as an open system that functions in relation to its broader sociocultural context and evolves over the life cycle. The family is composed of subsystems (e.g., adult couple, parental, sibling), and the family interacts with other systems, such as those involving work, health, and education, beyond its own borders. The family operates according to certain rules and principles that apply to all systems (Bertalanffy 1969).

Foremost, family systems theory emphasizes **interaction** and **context.** The concept of interaction encompasses not just the interaction among family members but also that between the family and other systems. Psychiatric problems, events, and processes are evaluated in the context within which they occur rather than in isolation from their environment. From a biopsychosocial perspective, interaction means the interplay between the multiple influences of biological, psychological, and social factors (Engel 1980). Also, transactions occur in relation to time, specifically, how multigenerational and life-cycle influences affect current context and functioning. Family systems approaches take into account multiple system levels, but these approaches choose the level of family as the interactive focal point for assessment purposes—a kind of clearinghouse for this multiplicity of interactive forces. A systems-oriented assessment may lead to a variety of interventions, one of which is family therapy.

Personality development is heavily influenced by social context, especially the interactions within a family system. Family or relationship *processes* are emphasized as much as the *content* of a problem. The interactional patterns that surround, ameliorate, or exacerbate a psychiatric condition are as clinically significant as the description of a disorder. The psychosocial unit becomes the individual in social context. Interventions with the system are seen as a powerful vehicle to bring about individual change. In essence, function and dysfunction, or normality versus pathology, are defined relative to the **fit** between the individual/family and their context and the psychosocial demands of the situation. Most families have strengths and vulnerabilities, in the context of which dysfunction can emerge in stressful situations or stages of family or individual development. Symptoms of family dysfunction may be generated by an overload of external stressors, such as job loss and economic strain; by a crisis, such as traumatic loss; or by the strain of coping with a family member's chronic disorder. *We must be cautious not to equate family distress with family pathology.*

In family systems theory, individuals are interrelated so that change in any one member affects other individuals and the group as a whole, and this, in turn, affects the first individual in a circular chain of influence. Every action in this sequence is also a reaction so that **causality** is seen as circular rather than linear. It is critical to understand the recursive patterns of interaction between symptoms and other parts of the family system that maintain, exacerbate, or improve the problem. This circular tracking process is one of the key elements of a systems-oriented assessment, providing the clinician with a more complete picture of the biological and interactive influences surrounding a symptom or central problem. Skilled therapeutic planning involves choices as to where in a circular sequence an intervention will facilitate changing a repetitive pattern and promote resolution of the central problem. It should be noted that although circular process can reinforce problems, not all participants have equal influence over others.

From a systems perspective, the family as a whole is greater than the sum of its parts; in other words, it cannot be described simply by summing up characteristics of individual members or even of various dyads. According to this basic principle of **nonsummativity**, it is necessary to attend to the *gestalt*—the family as a functional unit, its organization, and interaction patterns that involve the interlocking of behavior among members.

By the term *equifinality,* Watzlawick et al. (1967) refer to the error, or genetic fallacy, in confusing origin with significance in determining outcome. Rather, the same origin may lead to different outcomes and the same outcome may result from different origins. The impact of initial conditions or events (e.g., of early childhood) may be outweighed by the mediating influence of the family organization—its ongoing interactional patterns and responses to events. Thus, one family may be disabled by a particular crisis, whereas another family rallies in response to the same crisis.

Researchers have found no one-to-one correlation between an individual's presenting problem or psychiatric diagnosis and a single pattern of family dysfunction (Grigg and Friesen 1989; Walsh and Anderson 1988). Thus, it would be erroneous to type a family by the diagnosis of a dysfunctional member. Psychiatric problems may be primarily biologically based, as in schizophrenia, or may largely result from social or economic pressures. Therefore, the interaction of influences involving the identified patient, the family, and larger social systems must be carefully assessed in any psychiatric problem.

■ COMPONENTS OF FAMILY FUNCTIONING

☐ Family Organizational Patterns

Drawing from advances in research on normal family processes, we can identify key components of family functioning in the domains of organizational patterns, communication and problem solving, life-cycle development, and belief systems (Walsh and McGoldrick 1991). The functioning of any family must be considered in terms of how effectively it organizes its structure and available resources to master life challenges through the life cycle. At the outset, the *family constellation* needs to be determined. This includes all members of the current household, the extended family system (including noncustodial parents after separation/divorce), and key individuals who function as family insiders (e.g., close friends, professional caregivers).

Family adaptability is one of the chief requisites for well-functioning family systems (Olson 1988). *Stability* (i.e., homeostasis) and *flexibility* (i.e., morphogenesis) are counterbalancing needs in families. The ability of a family to adapt to changing circumstances or life-cycle developmental tasks is balanced by a family's need for enduring values, traditions, and predictable, consistent rules for behavior. Family adaptability or flexibility can vary on a continuum from the dysfunctional extremes of very rigid to chaotic (Olson 1988).

Homeostatic mechanisms are the means by which norms are delimited and enforced to maintain a steady, stable state in the ongoing interactional system. All family members contribute to the homeostatic balance, as in forming or shifting an alliance or rescuing a family member in distress, and through silence or distance. Crisis events, such as significant losses and changing circumstances in relation to the social world, stress the family and require major adaptational shifts of family rules so as to ensure the continuity of family life. A disabled husband may have to flexibly alter traditional gender-based rules to allow himself to assume the role of homemaker while his wife takes a job outside the home.

Cohesion is the other central dimension of family organization. Families must balance needs for closeness and connectedness with a respect for separateness and individual differences. This balance varies with different cultural norms and shifts as families move through the life cycle. For instance, in families with small children, there is relatively greater need for high cohesion. With children entering adolescence, family organization typically shifts to lower cohesion with more emphasis on differentiation and autonomy of adolescent members.

Boundaries, the rules determining who does what, where, and when, are crucial structural requisites. Although family organizational styles vary with cultural norms, dysfunctional families tend to be characterized by extremes of enmeshment or disengagement. An *enmeshed* pattern limits or sacrifices individual differences to maintain a sense of unity. Members are expected to think and feel alike: differences, privacy, and separation are regarded as threats to the survival of the family (Bowen 1978). Typically, identity formation is blocked, there is little sense of self, or a distorted, rigid role assumption is made based on parental needs and projections. A *disengaged* pattern of too low cohesion reinforces individual differences, separateness, and distance at the expense of family relatedness, at the extreme fragmenting the family unit and isolating individual members.

Interpersonal boundaries define and separate individual members and promote their differentiation and autonomous functioning. **Generational boundaries**, the rules differentiating parent and child roles and rights and obligations, maintain hierarchical organization in families. They are established by the parental/marital subsystem, and, in turn, they reinforce the essential leadership of the parental unit as well as the exclusivity of the marital relationship. **Family-community boundaries** are also important; well-functioning families are characterized by a clear sense of the family unit, with permeable boundaries connecting the family with the community. Social networks are important for support and connectedness to the community. In a closed, enmeshed system, family isolation contributes to dysfunction and interferes with peer socialization and emancipation of offspring.

The concept of the **triangle** and the dysfunctional process of **triangulation** are central to the clinical application of systems theory (Bowen 1978; Satir 1983). This term refers to the tendency of two-person systems, especially in marital relationships, to draw in a third person, when tension develops between the two. Three types of triangles most typically occur. In one arrangement, a couple (persons A and B) may avoid or drop their conflict to rally together in a united front of mutual concern about an oppositional child (C), who may be scapegoated in the process. In a second kind of triangle, one member of the dyad (A) may form a coalition with C against or to the exclusion of the other member of the dyad (B). Dysfunctional triangles are formed by the breaching of generational boundaries in a covert parent-child coalition against the other parent, or grandparent-child coalition against a single parent. In a third arrangement, the triangulated member, C, may assume the role of go-between for A and B (e.g., the parents), thereby balancing loyalties and regulating tension and intimacy. In each case, all three members of the triangle are active participants and each benefits in the reduction of family or couple tension. The more dysfunctional a family is, the more rigid these patterns are and the more likely it is that there are multiple interlocking triangles throughout the extended family system.

☐ Communication Processes

Bateson (Ruesch and Bateson 1951) noted that every communication has two functions: 1) a "content" (i.e., report) aspect conveying factual information, opinions, or feelings, and 2) a "relationship" (i.e., command) aspect that defines the nature of the relationship. The statement "Eat your vegetables" conveys an order with expectation of compliance and implies a hierarchical differentiation of status or authority in the relationship, as between parent and child. In an ongoing relationship, communication cannot regularly be left unclear or unresolved without pathological consequences or possibly dissolution.

Family rules organize interaction and function to maintain a stable system by prescribing and limiting members' behaviors. Relationship rules, both explicit and implicit, provide a set of expectations about roles, actions, and consequences that guide family life. A family tends to interact in repetitive sequences so that a relatively small set of patterned and predictable rules govern a family. Relationship rules serve as norms within a family—as baselines or settings on which family behavior is measured and around which it varies to a greater or lesser degree.

Problem solving refers to the family's ability to resolve the normative and nonnormative problems that confront them and to maintain effective family functioning. Well-functioning families are characterized not by the absence of problems but by their joint problem-solving ability. Families can falter at various steps in the problem-solving process. Epstein et al. (1978) identify seven sequential steps in the process:

- Identifying the problem
- Communicating with appropriate people about it
- Developing a set of possible solutions
- Deciding on one alternative
- Carrying such an alternative out
- Monitoring to ensure it is carried out
- Evaluating the effectiveness of the problem-solving process

In a family evaluation, clinicians assess family members' ability to communicate about both pragmatic (i.e., instrumental) and emotional issues (Epstein et al. 1978). Specific patterns to note include toxic or sensitive subjects in which communication falters (e.g., traumatic loss), gender constraints (e.g., males are often good at instrumental tasks but constricted at emotional expression), and specific relationships in which communication is broad and intimate and other relationships in which it is blocked (e.g., anger expressed but not love). Observation of joint problem-solving processes and inquiry about how crucial decisions are arrived at provide important information about shared power and communication processes.

☐ Multigenerational Patterns and the Family Cycle

A family life-cycle perspective views the family as a multigenerational system moving forward over time (Carter and McGoldrick 1989). The individual, family, and culture need to be thought of as systems that co-evolve over time. Each can be represented schematically along two time dimensions, one of which is *historical/intergenerational* (i.e., the vertical axis) and one of which is *developmental and unfolding into the future* (i.e., the horizontal axis). Tracking significant multigenerational family events and patterns guides the formulation of treatment objectives and intervention strategies. It is very useful to note the linkages between the timing of psychiatric symptoms and both past and current critical events that have disrupted or threaten the family (Walsh 1983).

A *genogram* (McGoldrick and Gerson 1985) and family time line are useful to schematize system patterns and focal points for intervention. At the family level, the vertical axis includes the family history—the patterns of relation and functioning that are transmitted down the generations. The horizontal axis describes the stresses impinging on a family as it copes with the transitions posed by individual and family development. These include both the predictable, normative developmental stresses and the unpredictable circumstances that may disrupt the life cycle.

Relationships among family members evolve through stages as the family unit and each member move through the life cycle. Boundaries shift, psychological distance among members changes, and roles are redefined. In the most useful clinical model, that by Carter and McGoldrick (1989), six stages are delineated by key nodal events related to the changes in family structure and relationships. Each stage has key developmental tasks and transitions and corresponding second-order changes in family status that are required to proceed developmentally. Frequently family symptoms and dysfunction coincide with transitions from one stage to another. Although all normative change is to some degree inherently stressful, when the current individual, family, or cultural stressors intersect vulnerable multigenerational themes or issues, there is a tremendous increase in strain on the family system. Many families function well until they reach a critical point in the life cycle at which complications arose a generation earlier.

☐ Family Belief Systems

The responses of families to stressors or psychiatric conditions are strongly influenced by a family's belief system and the meanings attached to the situation, with both immediate and long-term ramifications. Reiss (1981) has described the *family paradigm* as an enduring structure of shared beliefs, convictions, and assumptions about the social world that are shaped by pivotal family experiences and that, in turn, influence basic problem-solving styles and meanings attached to future life challenges. These beliefs contribute to the family's perception of events, the meanings ascribed, and the expectations about their likely consequences.

A family's beliefs about their competence to face and master life challenges are particularly important. In this regard, a family's belief system about what is normal is significant. Family beliefs that define normative as "problem free" or view their own family as deficient in relation to the "ideal family" are shame-inducing and interfere with coping and adaptation (Walsh 1993). Family belief systems are derived from a number of sources. Critical family stories become encoded into family scripts that provide a blueprint and guidelines for behavior when a family is facing a dilemma or crisis. Family rituals convey the family beliefs and provide stabilization and continuity over time; they also can facilitate transformation of beliefs. Family therapists often use rituals as a form of therapeutic intervention to facilitate change or healing (Imber-Black et al. 1988).

Culture, ethnicity, and religion are other basic contributors to family belief systems (McGoldrick et al. 1982). Clinicians should routinely inquire about family beliefs in these areas. This is particularly relevant when the family is a blend of two or more cultural or religious backgrounds, or if the family and clinician hold different cultural values.

■ MAJOR APPROACHES TO FAMILY THERAPY

A number of approaches to family therapy have been developed that can be usefully categorized as *problem-solving approaches*, which are brief, focused, pragmatic interventions; and *intergenerational approaches*, which are more exploratory and growth oriented. Problem-solving approaches include structural, strategic-systemic, behavioral, and psychoeducational models. Intergenerational approaches include psychodynamic, Bowen, and experiential approaches (Table 34–1).

□ Problem-Solving Approaches

Structural Model

Structural family therapy, developed by Minuchin (1974) and his colleagues, emphasizes the importance of family organization for the functioning of the family unit and the well-being of its members. The model focuses on the patterning of transactions in which symptoms are embedded. Problems are viewed as an indication of imbalance in the family's organization, particularly a malfunctioning hierarchical arrangement with unclear parent and child subsystem boundaries. Most commonly, symptoms are a sign of a maladaptive reaction to changing environmental or developmental requirements, such as an inappropriate accommodation to a life-cycle transition. Child-focused problems are seen as symptoms of system problems and are thought to detour conflict between parents or, particularly in single-parent families, between parent and grandparent.

Structural family therapy is action oriented, based on the conviction that change in behavior occurs independently of insight on the part of members. The therapeutic approach centers on strengthening the structural foundation for family functioning: in particular, a generationally appropriate hierarchy, with parents maintaining a strong leadership unit, and with clear boundaries that are neither too diffuse (as in enmeshment) nor too rigid (as in disengagement). The aim of therapy is the repair or modification of dysfunctional organizational patterns so that the family can better perform basic functional tasks and cope with life stresses. It is expected that presenting problems, which are symptoms of family distress, will be resolved as this reorganization is accomplished. Structural family therapy is short term and involves three processes: joining with the family, enactment of the problem situation, and restructuring of the family unit to more effectively handle problems. Particular attention is directed to strengthening the parental subsystem and reinforcing appropriate generational boundaries.

Strategic/Systemic Approaches

In the early development of family therapy, among the most innovative and influential approaches were the strategic and systemic models of the Mental Research Institute in Palo Alto, California, and the problem-solving approach of Haley and Madanes (Haley 1976; Madanes 1981; Selvini-Palazzoli et al. 1978). More recently, solution-focused and constructionist/narrative approaches have been advanced. These systems-oriented problem-solving approaches all focus on the immediate social situation of the identified patient. Assuming that all problems have multiple origins, a presenting problem is viewed as both a symptom and a response to current dysfunction in family interaction. Importance is placed on understanding how a family has attempted to resolve its problems, because a misguided attempted solution may exacerbate the problem or itself become a serious problem. Strategic therapists contend that most families do what they do because they believe it is the right or best way to approach a problem or because it is the only tack they know to take. The therapeutic task is to interrupt ways of handling the problem that do not work—that is, patterns that are dysfunctional. It requires learning the language and conceptualization of each family in order to see the problem through its members' eyes, taking into account their values and ex-

Table 34-1. Major approaches to family therapy

Model of family therapy	View of symptoms or pathology	Goals of therapy	Process of change: strategies and techniques
Problem-solving approaches			
Structural			
Minuchin Philadelphia Child Guidance Center	Symptoms result from current family structural imbalance: a. Malfunctioning hierarchical arrangement and boundaries b. Maladaptive reaction to changing requirements (developmental, environmental)	Reorganize family structure: a. Shift members' relative positions b. Create clear, flexible sub-systems and boundaries c. Promote more adaptive coping	1. Therapist uses power and action to shift interaction patterns a. Joining family b. Enactment of problem c. Map structure, plan stages of restructuring d. Task assignments and paradoxical intervention
Strategic/systemic			
Palo Alto group Haley and Madanes Milan approach Ackerman team Solution focused Narrative	Multiple origins of problems; symptoms maintained by family's unsuccessful problem-solving attempts	Solve presenting problem; set specific behaviorally defined objectives	1. Pragmatic, focused, action oriented: a. Clear plan to change symptom-maintaining sequence to new outcome b. Substitute new behavior patterns to interrupt feedback cycles c. Relabeling, reframing techniques d. Use of consultant-observers 2.
Behavioral			
Patterson Alexander Jacobson Margolin	Maladaptive, symptomatic behavior reinforced by family attention and reward	Concrete, observable behavioral goals, social reinforcement (acknowl-edgment, approval) of adaptive behavior	1. Therapist as social reinforcer, model, educator 2. Change contingencies of reinforcement; interpersonal consequences of behavior 3. Guide family to reward desired behavior 4. Teach negotiation and problem-solving skills

Psychoeducational Anderson Goldstein Falloon	a. Biologically based disorders; stress/diathesis b. Normative and nonnormative adaptational challenges (e.g., remarriage, chronic illness)	a. Family management of chronic illness; stress and stigma reduction b. Reduction of stress c. Mastery of family adaptational changes	(a) and (b): 1. Information 2. Management guidelines/adaptational tasks 3. Social support 4. Respectful collaboration

Intergenerational/growth-oriented approaches

Psychodynamic Ackerman Boszormenyi-Nagy Framo Paul Stierlin	Symptoms due to shared family projection process stemming from unresolved past conflicts or losses in family of origin	1. Resolution of family-of-origin conflict and losses 2. ↓ Family projection processes 3. Relationship reconstruction and reunion 4. Individual and family growth	1. Insight oriented, linking past and present dynamics 2. Assist in resolution of conflicts, losses 3. Facilitate healthier modes of relating

Bowen approach
Bowen
Georgetown Group
Carter
McGoldrick
	Functioning impaired by relationships with family of origin:
	a. Poor differentiation
	b. Anxiety (reactivity)
	c. Triangulation
	d. Cutoffs
		1. Differentiation
		2. ↑Cognitive functioning
		3. ↓Emotional reactivity
		4. Modification of relationships in family system:
		  a. Detriangulation
		  b. Repair cutoffs
			1. Coach individual action outside sessions:
			  a. Survey multigenerational field (use of genogram)
			  b. Plan focused interventions to change self directly with family
			2. Therapist takes cognitive stance, minimizing transference reaction

Experiential
Satir
Whitaker
	Symptoms are nonverbal messages in reaction to current communication dysfunction in system	1. Direct, clear communication
		2. Individual and family growth
			Change here-and-now interaction in conjoint session:
			1. Share feelings about relationships:
			  a. Self-disclosure
			  b. Direct communication
			  c. Experiential techniques: sculpture
			2. Uses therapist's experience with family to model, catalyze process

pectations that determine their approach to handling the problem and their inability to change.

The responsibility of the therapist is limited to initiating change that will get a family "unstuck" from unworkable interactional patterns that maintain symptoms. The goal of therapy is limited to solving the particular problem that is presented. The symptom is regarded as a communicative act that is part of a repetitious sequence of behaviors among family members, serving a function in the interactional network. Therapy focuses on problem resolution by altering the feedback loop that maintains the symptomatic behavior. The therapist's task is to formulate the problem in solvable, behavioral terms and to design an intervention plan to change the dysfunctional family pattern. Techniques of relabeling, reframing, directives, and indirect interventions are employed to this end.

Relabeling and reframing refer to the strategic redefinition of a problem or a situation so as to cast it in a new light. Such redefinition can be particularly useful in shifting a family's rigid view or stereotypical response, in altering an unproductive blaming or scapegoating process, or in overcoming resistance to change. In the reformulation of a problem or set, new solutions can become apparent (Watzlawick et al. 1974).

Directives are carefully designed behavioral tasks assigned to families to be carried out either in a session or between sessions. Directives have several purposes. They are used to gather direct information about the ways family members interact and how they will respond to—and resist—change. Directives are also useful in intensifying the therapist's relationship and influence with the family by involvement in action outside of sessions. Well-formulated and well-timed directives are considered a highly effective way of bringing about a structural modification as well as a behavioral change.

More recent developments of solution-focused (de Shazer 1988; O'Hanlon and Weiner-Davis 1989) and narrative approaches (Anderson and Goolishian 1988; White and Epston 1990) are based in constructivist and social constructionist views of reality (Hoffman 1990). These approaches shift therapeutic attention from problems and the patterns that maintain them to solutions that might work. Proponents of these approaches believe that people are constrained by their narrow, pessimistic views of problems, which limits the range of alternatives for resolution. However, they oppose the earlier view that problems serve ulterior functions for the family and assume that clients really do want to change. The therapeutic relationship is more collaborative, based on trust and respect of clients and oriented toward recognizing and amplifying the positive strengths and resources that clients bring. The uses of narrative and the "restorying" and externalizing of problems serve as means through language to reframe problem situations toward more enabling and empowering constructions that lead to problem resolution.

Behavioral Approaches

Behavioral approaches to family therapy, developed chiefly from behavior modification and social learning traditions, emphasize the importance of family rules and communication processes. They focus on the interactional behaviors and conditions under which social behavior is learned, influenced, and changed. These approaches have been used most successfully with marital conflict (Jacobson 1981) and with families of behaviorally disordered children and adolescents (Barton and Alexander 1981).

Families are viewed as critical learning contexts that are simultaneously created and responded to by members. According to social exchange principles, in well-functioning families the exchange of benefits outweighs costs. Because family relationships involve behavioral exchange over a wide range of possibilities, there are many opportunities for rewarding exchanges that are likely to maintain the relationship. The importance of positive reward for desired behavior is stressed. In well-functioning families, not only is maladaptive behavior not reinforced, but also adaptive behavior is rewarded through attention, acknowledgment, and approval.

Relationship failure is explained by deficient reward exchanges, as in coercive control (Patterson et al. 1975). Symptoms or maladaptive behavior, regardless of origin, are seen as reinforced or rewarded by the family. Treatment problems and goals are specified in concrete and observable behavioral terms. The therapist teaches the couple or family more effective and benign ways of influencing behavior by reinforcing it in a positive manner (Holtzworth-Monroe and Jacobson 1986). Family members learn to give each other approval and acknowledgment for desired behavior instead of rewarding and reinforcing maladaptive behavior with attention and concern.

The therapist analyzes communication processes, including both the informational content and the relational components (i.e., relationship rules implicit in how messages are conveyed). Building skills in negotiation and problem-solving processes are a central focus of interventions. Reciprocity and equitability are especially encouraged in the marital relationship. Adaptability, the capability of using diverse behaviors in different situations, is also an aim of therapy (Weiss 1978).

Psychoeducational Approaches

The development of the psychoeducational model has been the most promising advance in family intervention with schizophrenia and other serious and chronic mental illnesses. Also, this model has been increasingly utilized with a range of chronic physical disorders and stressful life-cycle challenges. These approaches, drawing on elements of behavioral and structural family models, provide family education and offer concrete guidelines and support for crisis management, problem solving, and stress reduction. In contrast to more traditional treatment approaches that have presumed families to be pathogenic influences, the psychoeducational approach engages the family as a valued and essential collaborator in the treatment process.

Goldstein et al. (1978) demonstrated the combined effectiveness of family therapy and drug maintenance to be more effective than either intervention alone in helping schizophrenic patients maintain functioning in the community in the high-risk months following hospitalization. The family therapy model was brief, problem focused, and concrete. The aims of the program were to identify specific stressful events of current concern to the patient and family and then to help them develop coping strategies to prevent the recurrence, and mitigate the destructive impact, of such events. Interactional conflicts and stresses viewed as potential precipitants of a psychotic episode were emphasized. The psychoeducational model developed by Anderson et al. (1986) has been demonstrated to be effective in the treatment of chronic schizophrenia and reduction of family distress. In a carefully controlled study, family intervention combined with drug maintenance and patient social skills training produced the best results with chronic patients, dramatically reducing relapse rates.

The intervention model is based on the assumption that the patient has a core biological deficit and that environmental sources of stress interact negatively with that vulnerability to produce disturbed cognitions and behaviors. Families are viewed as a resource for the long-term management of schizophrenia when given concrete support and information to assist them. A highly structured family-oriented program was designed to avoid treatment dropout, to decrease relapse rates, to return the patient to effective functioning in the community, and to decrease family stress. The basic program goals are twofold: 1) decreasing patient vulnerability to environmental stimulation through maintenance chemotherapy, and 2) increasing stability and predictability of the family environment by decreasing family anxiety about the patient, increasing knowledge about the schizophrenic illness, and increasing confidence about their ability to manage it. As these aims are achieved, pressures between the patient and family are reduced.

The psychoeducational model developed by Falloon et al. (1984) is a cost-effective home-based family intervention approach emphasizing behavioral problem-solving techniques. As in the other psychoeducational approaches, there is an emphasis on lowering expectations to the level of solving daily problems one at a time, measuring success in small increments, and maintaining the morale of the treatment team, the most important members of which are the family (Beels 1988).

☐ Growth-Oriented Intergenerational Approaches

Psychodynamically Oriented Approaches

Psychodynamically oriented approaches conceptualize family interaction in terms of object relations, related internalizations, and introjection and projection processes. The parents are regarded as crucial determinants of healthy or pathological family functioning and of the processes of separation and individuation necessary for the healthy development of offspring. The capacity to function as a spouse and as a parent is largely influenced by each individual's family-of-origin experiences. The relative success or failure in accomplishing developmental tasks is thought to be determined largely by residues of internalized objects and the organization of introjects contributing to identity integration. Spouses are successful in forming a productive shared marital experience to the extent that their relationship is organized in terms of a successfully differentiated and individuated sense of self and not contaminated by pathogenic introjects (Scharff and Scharff 1986).

The interlocking of projection and introjection processes forms a shared projection process based on complementarity of needs (Boszormenyi-Nagy and Spark 1973). Reciprocal relationship bargains involve implicit agreements among family members to relate on the basis of unfulfilled needs. Dysfunctional families are blocked by a greater degree of unconscious, unresolved conflict or loss that interferes with realistic appraisal of and response to other family members. Accordingly, Framo (1970) has viewed symptoms as resulting primarily from unconscious attempts by spouses/parents to reenact, externalize, or master through current relationships the intrapsychic conflicts originating in the family of origin. Current life situations are interpreted in light of the parents' inner object world and role models.

The symptomatic member may serve as a scapegoat for unresolved family conflicts (Ackerman 1958). In some cases, the loss of a significant relationship in the family of origin may disrupt the entire family system, with emotional upheaval and unresolved grief expressed in symptoms by a family member (Paul and Grosser 1991). In other cases, symptoms may express an irrational role assignment, or projective transference distortion, that is reinforced by family myths and ritualized into the family's structural pattern.

Assessment and treatment involve exploration of the complex multigenerational family patterns over time and their connection to resulting disturbances in current functioning and relationships. Extended family members may be included in family sessions, or individual members may be encouraged to work on changing relationships with the family of origin outside of sessions (Framo 1980). Either way, the aim of therapy is for family members to confront and deal with each other directly in order to work through unresolved conflicts. The therapist actively encourages the family's awareness of intense conflictual emotions, interpreting their sources and consequences, as well as identifying shared defense mechanisms. In direct confrontation, the therapist makes covert family processes overt and accessible to resolution through insight and action for emotional working through.

The contextual approach of Boszormenyi-Nagy (1987) emphasizes the importance of covert but powerful family-of-origin loyalty patterns. The therapeutic aim is toward the reconstruction and reunion of relationships in the resolution of grievances. Therapy focuses on the ethical dimension of family relationships, examining the multigenerational legacies of parental accountability and filial loyalty that guide members over the course of the life cycle. Families are thought to be strengthened by moves toward trustworthiness, based on consideration of members' welfare interests for survival, growth, and relatedness.

Bowen Model

Bowen (1978) developed a theory of the family emotional system and a method of therapy. In this model, functioning is thought to be impaired by poorly differentiated relationship patterns characterized by high anxiety and emotional reactivity. This anxiety commonly results in triangulation or cutoffs of highly charged relationships. Stresses on the family system, especially by death, can decrease differentiation and heighten reactivity. Underfunctioning, or symptoms, may be linked with and reinforced by overfunctioning in other parts of the system in a compensatory cycle. Improved functioning is believed to result when emotional reactivity no longer blocks intellectual processes.

The goal of therapy is for individuals to modify their relationships with their families of origin, achieving a higher level of differentiation and reduced anxiety in direct contact. A patient may be seen individually and coached to change himself or herself in relation to other family members in contacts between sessions. When spouses meet together, the focus is on coaching each individual to work separately on his or her own extended family relationships. The therapist serves as consultant or coach, guiding each individual through carefully planned stages of intervention.

The process of change may require a commitment to long-term work in stages (Carter and Orfanidis 1976). First, in engagement, the patient is helped to gain perspective of self-with-others and not set out to change others. The genogram is used to plan steps of intervention. Next, in the reentry phase, the patient begins the process of differentiation by redeveloping personal relationships with key family members, repairing cutoffs, detriangulating from conflicts, and changing the part played in emotionally charged vicious cycles. Techniques of detriangulating and reversals expressing the unacknowledged other side of an issue are two of many means employed to break up rigid communication patterns and to open up a closed system.

Experiential Approaches

Experiential approaches to family therapy were developed by two leading pioneers in the field, Satir (1983), who blended a communication approach with a humanistic frame of reference, and Whitaker (Napier and Whitaker 1978). Their experiential approaches are highly intuitive and relatively nontheoretical forms of therapy. Current behavior and feelings are seen as the natural consequence of one's life experience. Regardless of awareness or intent, old pains are propagated and made stronger by current interaction around them. To explain and change behavior, several important aspects of family process and their mutual influence are taken into account: individual self-worth, communication, system operations, and interactional rules.

The goal of these growth-oriented approaches is a fuller awareness and appreciation of oneself in relation to others through providing an intense, affective experience in the open communication of feelings and differences. Focused on the immediate experience, important information is elicited in current behavior with others, emphasizing the wholistic nature of human interaction in relational systems. The therapist takes a phenomenological approach, characterized by exploration, experimentation, and encouragement of spontaneity of members' responses to each other. Experiential exercises, such as family sculpting and role play, are used to facilitate this process.

■ USE OF SYSTEMS APPROACHES IN PSYCHIATRY

Most clinicians with a family systems orientation combine or integrate elements from the various approaches described above. Regardless of differences in particular techniques, all approaches focus on direct assessment and change of the relationships between individuals. All forms of psychiatric intervention are enriched by a systems lens. In systemic intervention models, the therapeutic transference plays a diminished role, because the therapist can observe patterns and promote change directly among key family members. Transference reactions do occur in family therapy but are redirected for expression and change back into the natural relationship network. Also, systemic models have redefined transference from dyadic to triangular or whole-systems terms and have examined how these relationship patterns are replicated in current systems in the patient's life. Countertransference issues are stimulated as well in family therapy. In fact, the emotional power of a family and the likelihood that some member or relationship in the family may feel too close to "home" for a therapist require that clinicians be aware of the interface issues between their own family experiences and those of the patients/families they are treating.

☐ Assessment

The often-asked question "When is family or couples therapy indicated?" requires reframing from a systems perspective. When problems are conceptualized at the relationship level, an individual's problems cannot be understood or changed apart from the context in which they occur. The question of "indications" becomes a question of what is the symptom-maintaining context of a specific problem in a particular family or couple and how can it most effectively be altered.

The assessment of most problems should therefore include a careful evaluation of the family or couple system, preferably in most cases by convening the family or couple for a conjoint session. It is important to consider all key relationships in the evaluation in order to determine treatment objectives and to decide who to include in subsequent sessions. Accurate history taking is enhanced when other family members are present, especially in terms of the intensity of symptoms, clinical course, or the revealing of behaviors that may be denied by the patient. An initial family or couples assessment can lay the groundwork for timely conjoint sessions even if the therapy remains primarily individual.

At times, some therapists may be reluctant to convene a large family or include small children for fear of being overwhelmed, or because of concern about the impact on a child or vulnerable member. Paradoxically, seeing all members conjointly can be easier, facilitating joint problem solving, and attending to relationship patterns connecting members. For child- and adolescent-focused problems, an initial family assessment places the identified patient's behavior in context. This is particularly true for a variety of conduct, eating, and anxiety-separation disorders (Walsh and Scheinkman 1993). Frequently, the patient is triangulated into a problematic parental relationship. A family assessment can serve several functions. First, family treatment often is the treatment of choice. Second, placing a child or adolescent in individual treatment carries the label of patienthood, which is stigmatizing. Third, a therapist can communicate, "I am a better parent and can do what you couldn't," leaving parents with a profound sense of defeat and shame. Family treatment can avert these toxic side effects by leaving the parents in charge and avoiding singling out a child as an identified patient.

Including a family assessment as part of a standard inpatient intake process serves a number of functions. First, it helps to identify and reduce family resistance. Second, it facilitates mutual familiarization about structure and functioning between the family and a treatment unit. Third, it alerts the treatment team to dysfunctional family patterns that may be replicated within the treatment system. Most important, assessment of the family as a support system is critical for discharge planning.

☐ Therapy

Therapy that focuses on the family system has certain advantages. Therapists can anticipate reactions to change and have more power to alter symptom-maintaining patterns. Since intrapsychic issues are also interpersonal, the systems therapist works under the assumption that change in the system is easier to bring about in behavioral terms and will result in intrapsychic change, regardless of the origin or chronicity of the problem. In addition, direct intervention with significant family members has potential therapeutic benefit for all members, not only the current symptom bearer.

For many problems, an nonsystemic individual treatment may achieve certain individual goals of growth but at the cost of a marriage or family unit. Often individuals presenting relationship difficulties or problems with intimacy are in a troubled relationship at the time of treatment. The decision to work individually without assessment of the couple can leave the therapist with a one-sided view of the problem, a skewed basis for therapy. Often, in these situations, the process of individual therapy becomes increasingly out of touch with a vulnerable real-life relationship. An additional risk is posed by a narrow focus on the individual without remaining attuned to the system: research suggests that individual therapy in distressed marriages skews the couple toward divorce (Gurman et al. 1986). At the same time, research supports the premise that relationship difficulties are well addressed in couples or family treatment (Gurman et al. 1986).

Frequently, couples therapy is followed by individual treatment. Not only can couples therapy preserve and improve a troubled relationship, but the process of such therapy typically leaves each partner with a clearer sense of his or her own issues brought to the relationship, those of the partner, and those that were mutually constructed or due to external factors. Typically, the pace of individual treatment is faster, and relational issues that were initially fused with personal ones have been ferreted out.

The indications for *brief family treatment* need to be distinguished from more open-ended, exploratory ones. Brief treatment is particularly useful when the chief complaint is a focal problem, such as a particular behavior, situation, or normative life-cycle transition. A preventive early-intervention approach with a family can avert a major crisis. Frequently, with focal problems, the therapist and family contract for a certain number of sessions, in which the goals are clearly delineated and progress can be objectively monitored. Depending on the kind of problem, structural, systemic/strategic, behavioral, and intergenerational approaches are all well suited to brief focal treatment. At completion, the therapist and family can renegotiate a new brief contract or shift to a more open-ended exploration.

☐ Systemic Modalities

Family Therapy

A family presenting with a child- or adolescent-focused problem is generally treated conjointly, including parents, siblings, and any other significant members of the household or extended family. In these situations, any marital problems identified during the assessment are best approached by strengthening the coparental alliance around solution of the presenting problem in the child's or adolescent's behavior or functioning. After the presenting child-focused issues improve, the couple will have established a working therapeutic alliance with the clinician and there is a greater likelihood that they will be willing to face their marital difficulties. With child- or adolescent-focused issues, it is often preferable to have a single therapist meet individually with the identified patient and conjointly with the family.

Couples Therapy

When individuals present with problems of intimacy and they are currently in a primary relationship with a partner or spouse, a couples evaluation and treatment are generally indicated. Couples therapy is the treatment of choice for serious relationship conflict and communication problems. Destructive interaction patterns that can escalate into violence or lead to relationship dissolution can be averted by early intervention (Gottman 1992). Couples therapy is also useful when one partner presents with depression, anxiety, or other emotional problems (Rolland 1994).

Individual Systemic Therapy

A particular version of individual systemic therapy, termed *family coaching,* has grown in use and is an outgrowth of Bowen's multigenerational model (Carter and Orfanidis 1976). In this approach, the therapeutic goal is to change relationships with members of one's family of origin. As part of the therapeutic contract, the therapist both connects current problems with unresolved relationship issues and works with the patient toward resolving those relationship issues through planned meetings with key family members, either in or between sessions.

Multifamily Group Therapy

Multifamily group therapy was first developed as an adjunctive treatment for young adults hospitalized with psychotic disorders (Laqueur 1980). Multifamily group interventions have been expanded to address a wider range of psychiatric populations, particularly for the treatment of depression (Anderson et al. 1986) and as an adjunct to or replacement for psychiatric day treatment for patients recovering from psychotic episodes. They have been regularly incorporated into milieu models of inpatient treatment. Groups are typically composed of four or more patients with their families, including parents, siblings, spouses, and sometimes close friends. Objectives include the improvement of communication and structural patterns to reduce interactional stress and to facilitate maximal functioning and problem solving.

The group context provides opportunities for families to learn from other families and support to try out new adaptive patterns of relating. Family members can relate to the experience of their counterparts in other families, gain a cognitive frame for perspective on their own crisis situation, reduce guilt and blame, and feel less stigma and isolation with their problems. Multifamily interventions vary from a single day-long workshop (Falloon et al. 1984) to a specified number of meetings, such as six to eight. Anderson et al. (1986) developed a multiple-family intervention to teach families about schizophrenia as a chronic illness, what to expect, and how to alter the family environment accordingly. This modular, time-limited format is particularly useful for a wide range of chronic psychiatric and physical disorders (Gonzalez et al. 1989) and life-cycle challenges, such as single parenthood.

Combined Modalities

With the expanding range of therapeutic approaches in psychiatry and simultaneous multiple professional system involvement, multiple therapists and modalities are increasingly being combined. For chronic disorders such as schizophrenia or serious physical conditions, at any one time a patient may be involved in individual, group, family, and multifamily group treatments. Treatment models for substance, physical, or sexual abuse also typically use a multimodal approach.

The question is not generally whether these modalities are compatible, but how to make the treatment system work effectively. Two or more therapists need to think systemically about these configurations. An individual therapist may need to incorporate into the therapeutic relationship new information that will change a heretofore skewed presentation of reality. When one partner is already in individual treatment, a couples therapist may find it appropriate for the other partner to begin individual treatment. Many family therapists include individual sessions in their therapeutic approach. Likewise, systems-oriented therapists may include conjoint sessions in the course of an individual therapy.

■ SPECIAL CLINICAL SITUATIONS

□ Serious Mental Disorders

Despite increased awareness of the complicated, mutual influences between biological and social factors in schizophrenia and other major mental disorders, this biopsychosocial perspective has not been well integrated into the treatment of patients and their families. A polarization has persisted between divergent positions—one emphasizing individual biological or dynamic variables and one focusing on family variables—impeding the development of a truly systemic approach that would provide more effective interventions. In recent years, family studies, assuming the mutual, ongoing influence of biological and environmental factors, have emphasized attempts to understand ongoing transactional processes that can influence future course and outcome. The most promising line of inquiry has examined contributions of family attitudes and communication processes. Brown et al. (1972) and Vaughn and Leff (1976) found empirical evidence linking the course of the schizophrenic disorder with certain attitudes expressed by family members, presumably reflecting ongoing family transactions. These authors' concept of "expressed emotion" refers to critical comments and emotional overinvolvement identified as being highly predictive of later symptomatic relapse by the patient.

Whereas psychiatric research to date has concentrated on dysfunctional processes and their reduction, it is important to identify family strengths, resources, and successful coping strategies that can be promoted in family interventions (Walsh 1993). In designing clinical treatment for patients and families, family intervention priorities should include the following:

1. Reduction of the stressful impact of the chronic disorder on the family

2. Provision of information about the illness, the need for psychophar-macological interventions, patient abilities and limitations, and prog-nosis
3. Concrete guidelines for stress reduction and problem solving through different phases of the illness
4. Linkage to supplementary services to support the efforts of families to maintain the patient in the community

The psychoeducational approaches have best demonstrated their ef-ficacy with schizophrenia (Anderson et al. 1986; Falloon et al. 1984). These interventions have been found to delay relapse, reduce family stress, and improve functioning for schizophrenic patients and their families, and to show promise in the treatment of severe affective disor-ders. A number of outcome studies have shown that behavioral treat-ments of affective disorders, phobias, and other anxiety states in which the spouses are included as collaborators in the therapy are superior to individual or group treatments (Coyne 1986; Gurman et al. 1986). It is important to recognize the need for combined intervention strategies in the treatment of serious and chronic disorders. Long-term drug mainte-nance may be necessary to control the severity of symptoms and to pre-vent lengthy and repeated hospitalizations.

Many of the principles of the psychoeducational models have been adapted to fit varied treatment settings and practice with a range of seri-ous and chronic disorders (Bernheim and Lehman 1985). McFarlane (1983) has developed a decision tree to assist clinicians in the determina-tion and sequencing of approaches and priorities in different case situ-ations. Family consultation, an approach advanced by Wynne et al. (1986), shares with psychoeducational approaches a responsiveness to the family's stress as caregivers, and the setting of concrete, realistic ob-jectives in active collaboration with the family.

Brief problem-solving family therapy may be of use to many families with a range of serious disorders, providing structured and focused in-terventions. Improved functioning and reduced stress and relational conflict can be achieved through pragmatic focus on clear, concrete, real-istic objectives that can be met by weekly sessions over several months. Gains can be sustained and setbacks averted in monthly or periodic maintenance sessions or in multiple family therapy groups (McFarlane 1983), or through self-help organizations. Crisis intervention should be available to families in times of acute distress, because most chronic, se-vere disorders involve periodic exacerbation of symptoms. Therapists must be active and provide enough structure to help temporarily disor-ganized and overwhelmed families gain perspective and control of threatening situations. Because patients with serious disorders, espe-cially schizophrenia, may lack motivation for treatment or fail to comply with medication, family collaboration is crucial to keep patients involved in treatment and to help family members cope with acute episodes in ways that will reduce stress to manageable proportions. Stein and Test (1985) documented the importance of continuity of care and community-based management over the long-term course of serious mental illnesses.

☐ Chronic Physical, Psychosomatic, and Organic Brain Disorders

A growing body of research data suggests a strong relationship between family dynamics and the clinical course and exacerbations of conditions such as cancer, diabetes, heart disease, pain syndromes, and end-stage renal disease (Campbell 1986). In the past decade, a multidisciplinary group of health and mental health disciplines have developed a family systems approach to health problems and health care contexts (Griffith and Griffith 1994; Ramsey 1989; Rolland 1994). This preventive approach advocates that near the time of diagnosis a routine family consultation should occur to assess the strengths and vulnerabilities of a family in relation to the practical and emotional demands of a disorder over time.

For clinicians to think in a systemic fashion about the interface of any chronic disorder and the family, the disorder itself needs to be cast in systems terms according to its pattern of psychosocial demands over time. And, to place the unfolding of a chronic disorder into a developmental context, it is crucial to understand the intertwining of three evolutionary threads: the illness, individual, and family life cycles.

The *family systems–illness model* (Rolland 1994) provides a useful framework for evaluation, formulation, and intervention with families who are dealing with chronic illness and disability. The model distinguishes three separate dimensions: 1) "psychosocial types" of illnesses; 2) major developmental phases in their natural history; and 3) key family system variables. On the first dimension, illnesses can be grouped according to key biological similarities and differences that pose distinct psychosocial demands for the patient and his or her family. Illness patterning can vary in terms of *onset* (acute or gradual), *course* (progressive, constant, or relapsing), *outcome* (fatal, shortened life span or possible sudden death, or no effect on longevity), *incapacitation* (none, mild, moderate, or severe), and the *level of uncertainty* about its trajectory. Each type of condition suggests a particular pattern of practical and emotional demands that can be thought about in relation to the practical and affective style, strengths, and vulnerabilities of a family facing a chronic disorder.

On a second dimension, the prime developmental *time phases* in the natural evolution of chronic disorders can be identified. The concept of time phases provides a way for clinicians to think longitudinally and to reach a fuller understanding of chronic illness as an ongoing process with landmarks, transitions, and changing demands. Each phase has its own unique psychosocial developmental tasks that require significantly different strengths, attitudes, or changes from a family. To capture the core psychosocial themes in the natural history of chronic disorders, three major phases can be described: crisis, chronic, and terminal.

The *crisis phase* comprises the initial period of socialization to chronic illness. Developmental tasks include the following:

- Creating a meaning for the disorder that preserves a sense of mastery
- Grieving the loss of the pre-illness family identity
- Accepting, when necessary, the permanency of the condition
- Undergoing short-term crisis reorganization while developing family flexibility in the face of uncertainty and possible threatened loss
- Learning to live with illness-related symptoms and treatments
- Forging a working relationship with professionals and institutional settings

In the *chronic phase,* issues include the following:

- Pacing and avoiding burnout
- Negotiating relationship skews between the patient and other family members
- Sustaining autonomy and preserving developmental goals of the family and of each member within the constraints dictated by the illness
- Sustaining intimacy in the face of threatened loss

By combining the dimensions of psychosocial illness types with the time phase of a disorder, the psychosocial demands of any condition can be thought about in relation to each phase of the disorder. From this vantage point, the significance of different components of family functioning (e.g., communication, problem solving, role flexibility) can be thought about more coherently in relation to specific disorders. This provides a framework for psychiatric consultations and periodic family "psychosocial checkups" over time. At a larger systems level, it provides a lens for a psychiatric consultant to analyze shifts in the relationships between health care institutions, professionals, the patient, and family members.

☐ Substance Abuse

For many years, substance abuse treatment programs, particularly those designed for alcoholism, have included a family component. However, many of these programs have historically treated the family separate from the addicted member. Twelve-step self-help programs (e.g., Alcoholics Anonymous, Al-Anon) and many drug treatment therapeutic communities maintain such philosophies. Innovative models based on family systems concepts are being increasingly utilized to treat alcoholism and drug abuse (Stanton and Todd 1982).

Central to these models is an awareness that chronic substance abuse becomes a central organizing principle in these families' lives, so any long-term solution necessitates family collaboration and involvement in treatment. Family involvement in the development of a comprehensive treatment plan has been successful in reducing the high rate of treatment failure due to dropout of detoxification and early recidivism. A family assessment can help identify substance abuse in other family members and codependent behaviors that undercut successful treatment. A systemic model allows a flexible use of both conjoint family meetings and individual or group interventions for different family members. The current trend in substance abuse treatment focuses less on residential rehabilitation and more on outpatient interventions such as partial hospitalization or evening programs. Because these programs keep the patient at home, family-based treatment will become even more important.

☐ Family Adaptational Challenges: Divorce and Remarriage

With the dramatic changes in family structure over the past three decades, clinical views of the "normal family" have lagged behind emerging realities. The 1950s model of the intact nuclear family, headed by a breadwinning father and supported by a mother who devoted herself to housework, child care, and elder care, now accounts for less than 8% of all households (Walsh 1993). Currently, nearly 70% of mothers of school-age children are in the workplace, either in two-earner families or heading single-parent households, most out of economic necessity. Clinicians need to be alert to the strain and overload that may precipitate symptoms such as child behavior or school problems, parental depression, marital conflict, and divorce.

Single-parent households and stepfamilies are increasingly common, with 50% of marriages currently ending in divorce. By the end of this decade, remarriage families will be the most prevalent family form. Yet stresses inherent in early remarriage contribute to a divorce rate of nearly 60%. These adaptational challenges have important implications for clinical practice, as parents and their children struggle with multiple stressors and attempt to move on with their lives (Hetherington et al. 1993; Walsh 1991).

Clinical intervention and divorce mediation both are highly recommended to help parents work through losses, buffer the stresses and dislocation, plan workable financial and custody arrangements, reorganize to manage the demands of heading a single-parent household, and forge a collaborative coparental arrangement. Therapeutic efforts are usefully directed toward helping families accomplish these adaptational tasks, providing normative information, and helping to establish a viable and flexible postdivorce structure that can be altered over time with changing developmental needs and circumstances. With a parent's further transition to remarriage, clinicians can be helpful in sorting out the complex network of relationships, solidifying the new family unit, and encouraging flexible boundaries to allow children to maintain their relationships with both biological parents and extended families as they develop new step-relations (Carter and McGoldrick 1989; Visher and Visher 1993).

■ REFERENCES

Ackerman NW: The Psychodynamics of Family Life. New York, Basic Books, 1958

Anderson CM: Depression and families, in Chronic Disorders and the Family. Edited by Walsh F, Anderson CM. New York, Haworth, 1988, pp 33–47

Anderson CM, Reiss D, Hogarty G: Schizophrenia and the Family. New York, Guilford, 1986

Anderson H, Goolishian HA: Human systems as linguistic systems: preliminary and evolving ideas about the implications for clinical theory. Fam Process 27:371–393, 1988

Barton C, Alexander JF: Functional family therapy, in Handbook of Family Therapy. Edited by Gurman AS, Kniskern DP. New York, Brunner/Mazel, 1981, pp 403–443

Beels CC: Family therapy, in American Psychiatric Press Textbook of Psychiatry. Edited by Talbott JA, Hales RE, Yudofsky SC. Washington, DC, American Psychiatric Press, 1988, pp 929–949

Bernheim KF, Lehman AF: Working With Families of the Mentally Ill. New York, WW Norton, 1985

Bertalanffy L von: General System Theory: Essays on Its Foundation and Development, Revised Edition. New York, Braziller, 1969

Boszormenyi-Nagy I: Foundations of Contextual Family Therapy. New York, Brunner/Mazel, 1987

Boszormenyi-Nagy I, Spark GM: Invisible Loyalties: Reciprocity in Intergenerational Family Therapy. New York, Harper & Row, 1973

Bowen M: Family Therapy in Clinical Practice. New York, Jason Aronson, 1978

Brown GW, Birley JLT, Wing JK: Influence of family life on the course of schizophrenic disorders: a replication. Br J Psychiatry 121:241–258, 1972

Campbell T: Family's Impact on Health: A Critical Review and Annotated Bibliography (DHHS Publ No [ADM]-86-1461). National Institute of Mental Health Series DN No 6. Washington, DC, U.S. Government Printing Office, 1986

Carter B, McGoldrick M: The Changing Family Life Cycle: Framework for Family Therapy, 2nd Edition. Boston, MA, Allyn & Bacon, 1989

Carter E, Orfanidis M: Family therapy with one person and the family therapist's own family, in Family Therapy: Theory and Practice. Edited by Guerin P. New York, Gardner Press, 1976, pp 193–219

Coyne J: Strategic marital therapy for depression, in Clinical Handbook of Marital Therapy, Vol 2. Edited by Jacobson N, Gurman A. New York, Brunner/Mazel, 1986

de Shazer S: Clues: Investigating Solutions in Brief Therapy. New York, WW Norton, 1988

Engel GL: The clinical application of the biopsychosocial model. Am J Psychiatry 137:535–544, 1980

Epstein NB, Bishop DS, Levin S: The McMaster Model of Family Functioning. Journal of Marriage and Family Counseling 4:19–31, 1978

Falloon IRH, Boyd JL, McGill CW: Family Care of Schizophrenia: A Problem-Solving Approach to the Treatment of Mental Illness. New York, Guilford, 1984

Framo J: Symptoms from a family transactional viewpoint, in Family Therapy in Transition. Edited by Ackerman N. Boston, MA, Little, Brown, 1970

Framo J: Family of origin as a therapeutic resource for adults in marital and family therapy: you can and should go home again. Fam Process 15:193–210, 1980

Goldstein MJ, Rodnick EH, Evans JR, et al: Drug and family therapy in the aftercare treatment of acute schizophrenics. Arch Gen Psychiatry 35:1169–1177, 1978

Gonzalez S, Steinglass P, Reiss D: Putting the illness in its place: discussion groups for families with chronic medical illnesses. Fam Process 28:69–87, 1989

Gottman J: Marital processes predictive of later dissolution: behavior, physiology, and health. J Pers Soc Psychol 63:221–233, 1992

Griffith J, Griffith M: The Body Speaks: Therapeutic Dialogues for Mind-Body Problems. New York, Basic Books, 1994

Grigg DN, Friesen JD: Family patterns associated with anorexia nervosa. Journal of Marital and Family Therapy 15:29–42, 1989

Gurman AS, Kniskern DP, Pinsof W: Research on marital and family therapy, in Handbook of Psychotherapy and Behavior Change, 3rd Edition. Edited by Garfield SL, Bergin AE. New York, Wiley, 1986, pp 565–624

Haley J: Problem-Solving Therapy: New Strategies for Effective Family Therapy. San Francisco, CA, Jossey-Bass, 1976

Hetherington M, Law T, O'Connor T: Divorce: challenges, changes, and new chances, in Normal Family Processes, 2nd Edition. Edited by Walsh F. New York, Guilford, 1993, pp 208–234

Hoffman L: Constructing realities: an art of lenses. Fam Process 29:1–12, 1990

Holtzworth-Monroe A, Jacobson N: Behavioral marital therapy, in Clinical Handbook of Marital Therapy, Vol 2. Edited by Jacobson N, Gurman A. New York, Brunner/Mazel, 1986

Imber-Black E, Roberts J, Whiting R (eds): Rituals in Families and Family Therapy. New York, WW Norton, 1988

Jacobson NS: Behavioral marital therapy, in Handbook of Family Therapy. Edited by Gurman AS, Kniskern DP. New York, Brunner/Mazel, 1981, pp 556–591

Laqueur HP: The theory and practice of multiple family therapy, in Group and Family Therapy. Edited by Wolberg L, Aronson M. New York, Brunner/Mazel, 1980

Madanes C: Strategic Family Therapy. San Francisco, CA, Jossey-Bass, 1981

McFarlane WR (ed): Family Therapy in Schizophrenia. New York, Guilford, 1983

McGoldrick M, Gerson R: Genograms in Family Assessment. New York, WW Norton, 1985

McGoldrick M, Pearce JK, Giordano J (eds): Ethnicity and Family Therapy. New York, Guilford, 1982

Minuchin S: Families and Family Therapy. Cambridge, MA, Harvard University Press, 1974

Napier AY, Whitaker CA: The Family Crucible. New York, Harper & Row, 1978

O'Hanlon WH, Weiner-Davis M: In Search of Solutions in Brief Therapy. New York, WW Norton, 1989

Olson DH: The Circumplex Model. New York, Haworth Press, 1988

Patterson GR, Reid JB, Jones RR, et al: A Social Learning Approach to Family Intervention. Eugene, OR, Castalia, 1975

Paul N, Grosser G: Operational mourning and its role in conjoint family therapy, in Living Beyond Loss: Death in the Family. Edited by Walsh F, McGoldrick M. New York, WW Norton, 1991, pp 93–103

Ramsey RN Jr (ed): Family Systems in Medicine. New York, Guilford, 1989

Reiss D: The Family's Construction of Reality. Cambridge, MA, Harvard University Press, 1981

Rolland JS: Families, Illness and Disability: An Integrative Treatment Model. New York, Basic Books, 1994

Ruesch J, Bateson G: Communication: The Social Matrix of Psychiatry. New York, WW Norton, 1951

Satir V: Conjoint Family Therapy, 3rd Edition. Palo Alto, CA, Science and Behavior Books, 1983

Scharff D, Scharff JS: Object Relations Family Therapy. New York, Jason Aronson, 1986

Selvini-Palazzoli M, Boscolo L, Cecchin G, et al: Paradox and Counterparadox. New York, Jason Aronson, 1978

Stanton MD, Todd T: The Family Therapy of Drug Abuse and Addiction. New York, Guilford, 1982

Stein LI, Test MA: The Training in Community Living Model: A Decade of Experience (New Dir Ment Health Serv No 26). San Francisco, CA, Jossey-Bass, 1985

Vaughn C, Leff J: The measurement of expressed emotion in the families of psychiatric patients. Br J Soc Clin Psychol 15:157–165, 1976

Visher E, Visher J: Remarriage families and stepparenting, in Normal Family Processes, 2nd Edition. Edited by Walsh F. New York, Guilford, 1993, pp 235–253

Walsh F: The timing of symptoms and critical events in the family life cycle, in The Family Life Cycle: Implications for Clinical Practice. Edited by Liddle H. Rockville, MD, Aspen, 1983, pp 120–133

Walsh F: Promoting healthy functioning in divorced and remarried families, in Handbook of Family Therapy, 2nd Edition. Edited by Gurman AS, Kniskern DP. New York, Brunner/Mazel, 1991, pp 525–545

Walsh F: Conceptualization of normal family processes, in Normal Family Processes, 2nd Edition. Edited by Walsh F. New York, Guilford, 1993, pp 3–69

Walsh F, Anderson CM: Chronic disorders and families: an overview, in Chronic Disorders and the Family. Edited by Walsh F, Anderson CM. New York, Haworth, 1988, pp 3–18

Walsh F, McGoldrick M: Loss and the family: a systemic perspective, in Living Beyond Loss: A Framework for Family Therapy. Edited by Walsh F, McGoldrick M. New York, WW Norton, 1991, pp 1–29

Walsh F, Scheinkman M: The family context of adolescence, in Handbook of Clinical Research and Practice With Adolescents. Edited by Tolan P, Cohler J. New York, Wiley, 1993, pp 149–171

Watzlawick P, Beavin J, Jackson D: Pragmatics of Human Communication. New York, WW Norton, 1967

Watzlawick P, Weakland JH, Fisch R: Change: Principles of Problem Formation and Problem Resolution. New York, WW Norton, 1974

Weiss RL: The conceptualization of marriage from a behavioral perspective, in Marriage and Marital Therapy. Edited by Paolino T, McCrady. New York, Brunner/Mazel, 1978

White M, Epston D: Narrative Means to Therapeutic Ends. New York, WW Norton, 1990

Wynne LC, McDaniel S, Weber T: Systems Consultation: A New Perspective for Family Therapy. New York, Guilford, 1986

CHAPTER 35

Treatment of Children and Adolescents

Mina K. Dulcan, M.D.

Until recently, the psychiatric treatment of children and adolescents has been almost exclusively an art, rather than a science. With more rigorous evaluation, development of diagnostic criteria with a stronger empirical base, and greater attention to therapeutic specificity, progress in matching treatments to patients is slow but steady. In contrast to the treatment of adults, a child or adolescent is usually brought by someone else, and in each case there are at least two clients: the parent and the child, whose needs and desires may conflict. In comparison with adults, children are more dependent on others for meeting their basic needs, they have fewer choices of residence or activities, and they are required to attend school.

■ EVALUATION

The components of the evaluation of a child or adolescent are presented in Table 35–1. The child or adolescent patient is interviewed in order to gather data from the clinician's observations and from direct inquiry. Children and adolescents can and should be questioned regarding their lives and their symptoms, although the interview must be adapted for developmental status. In some domains, such as anxiety and depression, or covert conduct problems, children and adolescents are often more accurate reporters than their parents.

    A physical examination within the past 6 months is required, or more recently if the problems are of acute onset, to search for medical causes

Table 35–1. Outline of psychiatric assessment of children and adolescents

Chief complaint and reasons for referral	Academic performance
History of present illness	Peer relations
Development of the symptoms	Relationships with family members
Child's and parents' attitudes	and other significant adults
toward the symptoms	Sexual behavior
Effects on the child and family	**Past history**
Stressors	Medical
Prior psychiatric evaluations and	Psychiatric
treatment and effects	**Developmental history**
Psychotherapy	**Medical review of systems**
Medication	**Family**
Environmental changes	Current family circumstances, con-
Review of behavioral and psycho-	cerns, liabilities, and resources
logical symptoms	Medical history
Current developmental status	Psychiatric history
Motor abilities	**Mental status examination**
Speech and language	

Source. Adapted from Dulcan and Popper 1991.

and to discover and treat any unrelated but coexisting medical disorders. The decision to conduct additional medical evaluations, such as a neurological examination or laboratory tests, is made based on the findings of the medical history and physical exam. Anticipated pharmacological treatment may suggest additional tests to detect possible contraindications and to determine baseline values.

Information from the school is always useful and is essential when there is concern about learning or behavior in school, or peer functioning. With parental consent, the clinician talks with the teacher; obtains records of testing, grades, and attendance; and requests completion of a standardized checklist, such as the Teacher Report Form of the Child Behavior Checklist (Achenbach 1991). Psychological evaluation, including an intelligence test and achievement tests, should be obtained when there is any question about learning or IQ, with additional testing as indicated. Projective tests should not be used diagnostically or in making treatment decisions (Klein 1986).

■ TREATMENT PLANNING

The planning of a treatment regimen takes into consideration psychiatric diagnosis, target emotional and behavioral symptoms, and the strengths and weaknesses of the patient and family. Resources and risks in the school, neighborhood, and social support network, and any religious group affiliation, also influence the selection of treatment strategies.

The clinician must decide which treatment is likely to be the most efficient or have the highest benefit/risk ratio and whether treatments should be administered simultaneously or in sequence. Parents are best included in the choice of treatment strategies, with the strength of the clinician's recommendation depending on the clarity of the indications. The skilled clinician presents the probable course of the disorder if untreated, as well as the best estimate of benefits and risks for a particular child of all available treatments. The child or adolescent patient is included in decision making as appropriate. The motivation and ability of the responsible adults to carry out the treatment should be considered, because the best treatment has little chance of success without the cooperation of the family.

■ CONFIDENTIALITY

It is essential that the guidelines for confidentiality and for sharing information between parent and child be clear. Adolescents are usually more sensitive to this issue than are children. In general, either party should be told when information from one party's session will be relayed to the other. In some situations parents and children may participate in the decision. When children or adolescents are engaged in potentially dangerous activities or have serious thoughts of harming themselves or others, parents must be informed. Carefully planned family sessions in which the therapist coaches and supports parent or child in sharing information may be more useful than secondhand reports.

■ PSYCHOPHARMACOLOGY

Important general principles in the drug treatment of children and adolescents include minimizing polypharmacy and virtually never using medication as the only treatment. Most disorders that require medication are either chronic (e.g., autistic disorder) or likely to have recurrent episodes (e.g., mood disorder), and a long-term relationship with the physician is crucial. It is important to educate the family regarding the disorder, its treatment, and the different needs at each developmental stage.

☐ **Special Issues for Children and Adolescents**

Developmental Toxicology

The term *developmental toxicology* refers to unique or especially severe side effects caused by interaction between a drug and the processes of growth and development. Children and adolescents are growing and developing not only physically but also cognitively and emotionally. It is important that medications not interfere with learning in school or with the development of social relationships within the family or with peers. Behavioral toxicity, the worsening of preexisting behaviors or affective states or the provoking of new ones that are undesirable, often develops before physical side effects are observed, especially in young children.

Metabolism and Kinetics

Dosage may be determined empirically, or by weight or surface area. Ideally, drug doses in children should be derived from studies of children, rather than adults, but this is often not possible. Protocols using normal children are not permitted, and few dosage studies have been done in symptomatic children.

Measurement of Outcome

Both positive therapeutic outcome and side effects are important. The risk/benefit ratio is especially crucial when initiating a possibly long-term treatment for a developing child. These considerations are more difficult in children and adolescents for a variety of reasons: placebo effects (both positive and negative) are substantial, immaturity of cognition and language makes it more difficult for children to report physical or emotional states, and youngsters vary more from day to day and in different situations than adults do. The physician must specify target symptoms and obtain affective, behavioral, and physical baseline and posttreatment data. Therapeutic effects and side effects can be assessed by interviews and rating scales, direct observation, physical examination, and, when appropriate, laboratory tests, or specific tests evaluating attention or learning (Conners 1985). It is important to ask and look actively for side effects, because many young patients will not report them spontaneously and parents may not notice.

Developmentally Disabled Patients

Medication effects are even more difficult to assess in children and adolescents with mental retardation or pervasive developmental disorders. Their impaired ability to verbalize symptoms is relevant to diagnosis, measurement of efficacy, and detection of side effects. These individuals are prone to physical side effects and at risk for idiosyncratic behavioral effects or simply less prominent therapeutic effects. Autistic youngsters often react differently to specific drugs than do children with other psychiatric disorders, even when the target symptoms seem similar.

Compliance

Taking medication as directed is particularly problematic for children and adolescents, because the cooperation of two people, parent and child, and often school personnel as well, is required. Pediatric medications may be incorrectly used because of parental factors such as lack of perceived need for drug, carelessness, lack of money, misunderstanding of instructions, and complex schedules of administration, as well as child refusal (Briant 1978). Administration of psychotropic medications is even more complex, given the emotional, behavioral, and family dynamic issues involved. Educational efforts and improved communication with the parent can improve compliance.

Ethical Issues

The risks of medication must be balanced with the risks of the untreated disorder and with what is known about the relative efficacy of medication and other treatments. In most cases, clinical experience with a drug in adults should be substantial before it is used to treat children and adolescents. Drug companies often do not go to the expense and trouble of testing drugs in children and adolescents. This may result in overly conservative doses and "unapproved" indications.

The interaction between pharmacotherapy and the environment is an important issue for children and adolescents, because their immature developmental status places them in the care of adults, whether parents or teachers, or staff in an inpatient unit or residential treatment setting. There is a danger of misinterpreting the youngster's response to the family, school, or institutional milieu as an exacerbation requiring medication or as improvement due to a medication. Many adults seek to use drugs to control or eliminate troublesome behavior, rather than instituting more time-consuming and difficult therapeutic or behavioral management strategies. The physician must therefore evaluate and monitor the environment as well as the patient.

☐ Stimulants

This category of drugs includes methylphenidate, dextroamphetamine, and magnesium pemoline. Contrary to prevailing mythology, hyperactive boys, normal boys, and normal adults have similar cognitive and behavioral responses to comparable doses of stimulants, except that children report feeling "funny," while adults report euphoria (Donnelly and Rapoport 1985).

Indications and Efficacy

The most established indication is in the treatment of attention-deficit/hyperactivity disorder (ADHD). In preschool-age children, stimulant efficacy is more variable, and the rate of side effects, especially sadness, irritability, clinginess, insomnia, and anorexia, is higher (Campbell 1985). Stimulants remain effective in adolescents with symptoms of ADHD, although response rate is lower than for children (Klorman et al. 1990; Pelham et al. 1991). Some children with attention-deficit disorder (ADD) without hyperactivity may have a positive response to stimulants (Famularo and Fenton 1987).

Stimulants reduce target symptoms of inattention, impulsivity, and overactivity in some children and adolescents with mental retardation (Handen et al. 1992) or autistic disorder (Strayhorn et al. 1988). Stimulants are effective for symptoms of oppositional defiant disorder and conduct disorder, in the presence of ADHD. The use of stimulants in patients with tics or Tourette's disorder is highly controversial.

Global judgments by parents, teachers, and clinicians rate 75% of hyperactive children improved on stimulants, compared with 40% on placebo. The other 25% are rated either unchanged or worse (Barkley 1981). One study using a wide range of doses of methylphenidate and dextroamphetamine found that 96% of the sample improved behaviorally in response to one or both drugs, although some children did not continue on medication because of adverse effects (Elia et al. 1991). Stimulant effects on various domains (cognitive, behavioral, social) are highly variable within and between individuals. A dose that produces improvement in one area may have no effect, or may even lead to worsening, in another. Even more puzzling, the response may differ between measures (e.g., math and reading), even in the same domain.

Initiation and Maintenance

The decision to medicate a child or adolescent with a stimulant is based on the presence of persistent target symptoms that are sufficiently severe to cause functional impairment at school and usually also at home and with peers. Parents must be willing to monitor medication and to attend appointments. Neither neurological soft signs nor electroencephalographic data predict stimulant responsivity (Halperin et al. 1986). Comorbid anxiety disorder may suggest lesser likelihood of improvement, whereas children with more severe inattention may have a greater positive response.

Methylphenidate is the most commonly used and best studied stimulant; dextroamphetamine is less expensive but is not included in many third-party formularies. Disadvantages of dextroamphetamine include negative attitudes of pharmacists, including some who are unwilling to stock it; greater risk of growth retardation; and higher potential for abuse (Table 35–2). Longer-acting preparations of methylphenidate (Ritalin Sustained Release [Ritalin-SR]) and dextroamphetamine (Dexedrine Spansule) are available. For some children, Ritalin-SR is less reliable and less effective than two doses of the standard preparation. Onset of action may be delayed up to 2 hours and may be more variable from day to day (Pelham et al. 1987). On the other hand, Dexedrine Spansule appears to have more consistent results than standard methylphenidate and to be more effective for some children (Pelham et al. 1990). Excessively high doses may result if a child chews an SR tablet or spansule instead of swallowing it. An innovative strategy for difficult-to-manage cases is the combination of short-acting and longer-acting medication forms (Fitzpatrick et al. 1992).

Magnesium pemoline is a longer-acting mild central nervous system (CNS) stimulant that is structurally dissimilar to methylphenidate and

Table 35–2. Clinical use of stimulant medications

	Methylphenidate (Ritalin)	Dextroamphetamine (Dexedrine)	Pemoline (Cylert)
How supplied (mg)	5, 10, 20 Sustained release 20	5, 10 Elixir (5 mg/5 ml) Spansule 5, 10, 15	18.75, 37.5, 75
Single dose range (mg/kg/dose)	0.3–0.7	0.15–0.5	0.5–2.5
Daily dose range (mg/day)	10–60	5–40	37.5–112.5
Usual starting dose (mg)	5–10 daily or bid	2.5 or 5 daily or bid	18.75 or 37.5 daily
Maintenance number of doses per day	2–4	2–4	1–2
Monitor	Pulse Blood pressure Weight Height Dysphoria Tics	Pulse Blood pressure Weight Height Dysphoria Tics	Pulse Blood pressure Weight Height Dysphoria Tics Liver functions

Source. Adapted from Dulcan and Popper 1991.

dextroamphetamine. Pemoline may be able to be given once a day and has the least abuse potential, although absorption and metabolism vary widely, and some children need twice-daily doses. Pemoline, like the other stimulants, has immediate action (Pelham et al. 1990). The possibility of pemoline-induced chemical hepatitis (Nehra et al. 1990), although rare, requires monitoring of liver enzymes and, along with the higher incidence of involuntary movements, limits the usefulness of pemoline.

Stimulant medication should be initiated with a low dose and titrated every week or two according to response and side effects within the recommended range, using body weight as a rough guide (Table 35–2). By 3 years of age, children's absorption, distribution, protein binding, and metabolism of stimulants are similar to those of an adult (Coffey et al. 1983), although adults have more side effects than do children at the same mg/kg dose. Giving medication after meals minimizes anorexia. Preschool-age children or patients with ADHD inattentive type, mental retardation, or pervasive developmental disorders may benefit from and tolerate lower doses than those patients with ADHD. Starting with only a morning dose may be useful in assessing drug effect, by comparing morning and afternoon school performance.

Tolerance is reported anecdotally, but compliance is often irregular, and this should be the first possibility considered when medication appears ineffective. The child should not be responsible for his or her own medication, because these youngsters are impulsive and forgetful at best, and most dislike the idea of taking medication, even when they can verbalize its positive effects and cannot identify any side effects. They will often avoid, "forget," or outrightly refuse medication. Decreased drug effect may also be due to an increase in the patient's weight or a reaction to a change at home or school. Lower efficacy of a generic preparation is another possibility. True tolerance may be more likely with the long-acting formulations (Birmaher et al. 1989); if it occurs, another of the stimulants may be substituted.

Risks and Side Effects

Most side effects are similar for all stimulants (Table 35–3). Insomnia may be due to drug effect, to rebound, or to a preexisting sleep problem. Stimulants may worsen or improve irritable mood (Gadow 1992). Black male adolescents may be at higher risk for elevated blood pressure on stimulants (Brown and Sexson 1989).

Rebound effects, consisting of increased excitability, activity, talkativeness, irritability, and insomnia, beginning 4 to 15 hours after a dose, may be seen as the last dose of the day wears off, or for up to several days after sudden withdrawal of high daily doses of stimulants. This effect may resemble a worsening of the original symptoms.

Table 35–3.   Side effects of stimulant medications

Common initial side effects (try dose reduction)	**Withdrawal effects**
Anorexia	Insomnia
Weight loss	Rebound ADHD symptoms
Irritability	Depression (rare)
Abdominal pain	**Rare but potentially serious side effects**
Headaches	
Emotional oversensitivity, easy crying	Motor or vocal tics
Less common side effects	Tourette's syndrome
Insomnia	Depression
Dysphoria (especially at higher doses)	Growth retardation
Decreased social interest	Tachycardia
Impaired cognitive test performance (especially at very high doses)	Hypertension
	Psychosis with hallucinations
Less than expected weight gain	Stereotyped activities or compulsions
Rebound overactivity and irritability (as dose wears off)	**Side effects reported with pemoline only**
Anxiety	Choreiform movements
Nervous habits (e.g., picking at skin, pulling hair)	Dyskinesias
	Night terrors
Hypersensitivity rash, conjunctivitis, or hives	Lip licking or biting
	Chemical hepatitis–elevated SGOT and SGPT, jaundice, epigastric pain (very rare)[a]

Note.   ADHD = attention-deficit/hyperactivity disorder; SGOT = serum glutamic-oxaloacetic transaminase; SGPT = serum glutamic-pyruvic transaminase.
[a]Patterson 1984.
Source.   Adapted from Dulcan and Popper 1991.

☐ Clonidine

Clonidine is an alpha-noradrenergic agonist approved for the treatment of hypertension.

Indications and Efficacy

Clonidine modestly decreases complex motor and vocal tics (Leckman et al. 1991). Although the effect is less powerful than that of neuroleptics, the side-effect profile is far more benign. Clonidine is most useful in reducing subjective distress and the behavioral symptoms of hyperactivity and impulsivity that often accompany Tourette's disorder. Clonidine may be combined with small doses of haloperidol or pimozide for patients who cannot be satisfactorily treated by either medication alone.

Clonidine is also useful in modulating mood and activity level and improving cooperation and frustration tolerance in children with ADHD, especially those who are very highly aroused, hyperactive, impulsive, defiant, and labile (Hunt et al. 1990). Although not effective in treating inattention per se, clonidine may be used alone in children with tics or in those who are nonresponders or negative responders to stimulants. It may be most useful in combination with a stimulant when stimulant response is only partial or when stimulant dose is limited by side effects; the combination may allow a lower dose of stimulant medication (Hunt et al. 1991). Clonidine often improves the child's ability to fall asleep, whether insomnia is due to ADHD overarousal, oppositional refusal to go to bed, or stimulant effect or rebound.

Initiation and Maintenance

Blood pressure and pulse should be measured and an electrocardiogram (ECG) and baseline laboratory blood studies (especially fasting glucose) should be obtained before starting clonidine. Clonidine is initiated at a low dose of 0.05 mg at bedtime. This converts the side effect of initial sedation into a benefit. Very young children may require lower initial and maintenance doses. The transdermal form (skin patch) may be useful to improve compliance and reduce variability in blood levels (Hunt et al. 1990).

Clonidine has a slow onset of therapeutic action, in part because of the gradual dose increase needed to minimize side effects, and perhaps due to the time required for receptor downregulation (Hunt et al. 1991). Significant clinical response is not seen for as long as a month, and maximal effect may be delayed for another several months. When clonidine is discontinued, it should be tapered rather than stopped suddenly, to avoid a withdrawal syndrome consisting of increased motor restlessness, headache, agitation, elevated blood pressure and pulse rate, and (in patients with Tourette's disorder) exacerbation of tics (Leckman et al. 1986).

Risks and Side Effects

The most troublesome side effect is sedation, although it tends to decrease after several weeks. Dry mouth, nausea, and photophobia have been reported, with hypotension and dizziness possible at high doses. The skin patch often causes local pruritic dermatitis. Depression may occur, most often in patients with a history of depressive symptoms in themselves or their families (Hunt et al. 1991). Glucose tolerance may decrease, especially in those patients at risk for diabetes.

☐ Tricyclic Antidepressants

Indications and Efficacy

Tricyclic antidepressants (TCAs) are indicated for those ADHD patients who do not respond to stimulants or who develop significant depression on stimulants, or for the treatment of ADHD symptoms in patients with tics or Tourette's disorder. Patients with ADHD and comorbid anxiety disorder may respond better to a TCA than to a stimulant (Kutcher et al. 1992). The longer duration of action of TCAs avoids a dose having to be taken at school, and rebound is not a problem. Efficacy in improving cognitive symptoms does not appear to be as great as for stimulants. Drawbacks include possible difficulty maintaining the effect over time; serious potential cardiac side effects, especially in prepubertal children; and the danger of accidental or intentional overdose. Although initial studies used imipramine, desipramine has less anticholinergic effect and well-documented sustained efficacy (Biederman et al. 1989). Nortriptyline produced improved attitude followed by an increase in attention span and a decrease in impulsivity (Saul 1985).

Only one study has documented superiority of a TCA over placebo in treating depression in children. The strongest evidence of efficacy is in hospitalized prepubertal children with major depression who are dexamethasone nonsuppressors (Hughes et al. 1988). Preliminary data suggest that clomipramine is effective in reducing obsessive-compulsive symptoms, and perhaps other symptoms as well, in autistic children and adolescents (Gordon et al. 1992).

Clomipramine, but not other TCAs, is useful in the treatment of obsessive-compulsive disorder (OCD) in children, independent of antidepressant activity (DeVeaugh-Geiss et al. 1992). Symptoms are rarely eliminated entirely, but when the medication is effective, the force of obsessions and compulsions is reduced sufficiently to improve quality of life. Supplemental behavior modification and/or psychotherapy are often necessary.

All of the TCAs have been found to be equally effective in the treatment of nocturnal enuresis. In 80% of patients, within the first week TCAs reduce the frequency of bed wetting.

Initiation and Maintenance

The pharmacokinetics for TCAs are different in children than in adolescents or adults. The smaller fat-to-muscle ratio in children leads to a decreased volume of distribution, and children are not protected from excessive dosage by a large volume of fat in which the drug can be stored. Children have larger livers relative to body size, leading to faster metabolism (Sallee et al. 1986), more rapid absorption, and lower protein binding than in adults (Winsberg et al. 1974). As a result, children are likely to need a higher weight-corrected dose of imipramine than adults. Prepubertal children are prone to rapid dramatic swings in blood levels from toxic to ineffective, and should have divided doses to produce more stable levels (Ryan 1992).

The usefulness of plasma levels is limited by the relative rarity of laboratories able to perform them satisfactorily. Medication cannot be safely titrated by plasma level, as there is no known level below which toxicity can be ensured not to occur. Plasma levels (drawn 9 to 11 hours after the last dose) can identify rapid and slow metabolizers. Determination of levels is recommended for patients who fail to respond to usual doses (possibly low levels) or those who have severe side effects at usual doses (possibly very high levels). Chlorpromazine, even in low doses, increases plasma levels of nortriptyline (Geller et al. 1985).

To treat depression, imipramine is given at a starting dose of 1.5 mg/kg/day, which may be increased to a maximum dose of 5 mg/kg/day (Ryan 1990). Nortriptyline may have fewer side effects and, since it has a longer half-life than imipramine, may be given twice a day in children. Variability in metabolism is greater for nortriptyline than for imipramine (Geller et al. 1986).

To treat ADHD, imipramine therapy is begun with 10 or 25 mg per day, and increased weekly. The maximum dose is 5 mg/kg/day (divided tid in children). Nortriptyline is given at 25 to 75 mg per day in two divided doses (Saul 1985).

For enuresis, daily charting of wet and dry nights is used prior to starting medication to obtain a baseline and subsequently to monitor progress. Much lower doses are needed than for the treatment of depression. Imipramine is started at 10 to 25 mg at bedtime and increased weekly to 50 mg, with a maximum dose of 2.5 mg/kg/day (Ryan 1990). Tolerance may develop, requiring a dose increase. For some children, TCAs lose their effect entirely. If medication is used chronically, the child or adolescent should have a drug-free trial at least every 6 months, because enuresis has a high spontaneous remission rate.

Doses of clomipramine used to treat OCD are generally lower than TCA doses used for depression. Response is delayed for 10 to 14 days, as in the treatment of depression, and unlike the immediate response seen in the treatment of ADHD or enuresis (Rapoport 1986). Clomipramine is started at 25 mg daily (or every other day) and gradually increased over 2 weeks to a maximum of 100 mg/day or 3 mg/kg/day, whichever is less (Green 1991).

Risks and Side Effects

The quinidine-like effect of TCAs slows cardiac conduction time and repolarization. At doses of more than 3 mg/kg/day of imipramine or desipramine, children and adolescents may develop an increased pulse and small but statistically significant ECG changes (Bartels et al. 1991). Prolongation of the QTc interval may be a sensitive indicator of cardiac effect (Wiles et al. 1991). The tendency of prepubertal children to have wider swings in blood levels may place them at higher risk for serious cardiac conduction changes. A minority of the population has a genetic defect in TCA metabolism, increasing risk for toxicity. TCAs should be used only for clear indications and with careful monitoring of therapeutic efficacy and of vital signs and ECG.

Anticholinergic side effects may occur, although less commonly than in adults. Most of these side effects are transient and/or respond to a decrease in dose. Of particular importance for children are dry mouth (which may lead to an increase in dental caries in long-term use [Herskowitz 1987]), drying of bronchial secretions, sedation, anorexia, constipation, nausea, tachycardia, palpitations, and increased diastolic blood pressure. Other reported side effects include abdominal pain, chest pain, headache, syncope, mild tremors of hands and fingers, weight loss, and tics. The seizure threshold may be lowered, with worsening of preexisting EEG abnormalities, and rarely a seizure. Seizures appear to be more common with clomipramine. Side effects with a probable allergic mechanism include rash and worsening of eczema (Campbell et al. 1985).

Behavioral toxicity may be manifested by irritability, worsening of psychosis, mania, agitation, anger, aggression, forgetfulness, or confusion. CNS toxicity may be mistaken for exacerbation of the primary condition. A drug blood level is often required to differentiate the two. As depressed children, especially those who are anergic and withdrawn, improve with TCA treatment, crying and verbalizations of sadness and anger may transiently increase.

Sudden cessation of moderate or higher doses results in a flu-like anticholinergic withdrawal syndrome with nausea, cramps, vomiting, headaches, and muscle pains. Other manifestations may include social withdrawal, hyperactivity, depression, agitation, and insomnia (Ryan 1990). TCAs should therefore be tapered over a 2- to 3-week period. The short half-life of TCAs in prepubertal children produces daily withdrawal symptoms if medication is given only once a day. These symptoms may also indicate that poor compliance is resulting in missed doses. Because of the predictability of TCA-induced electrocardiographic changes, a rhythm strip is useful in monitoring compliance.

☐ Other Antidepressants

Anecdotal reports suggest that fluoxetine may be useful in the treatment of adolescent depression (Boulos et al. 1992), ADHD (Barrickman et al. 1991; Gammon et al. 1991), obsessions and compulsions in OCD or Tourette's disorder (Riddle et al. 1990), and perseverative behaviors in autistic disorder or mental retardation (Cook et al. 1992). Fluoxetine has also been used in combination with low doses of clomipramine in the treatment of OCD that is resistant to either drug alone (Simeon et al. 1990). Although fluoxetine has relatively few somatic side effects (anorexia, weight loss, headaches, nausea, vomiting, tremor), behavioral toxicity is common.

Clinical experience suggests that phenelzine and tranylcypromine may be useful in the treatment of depressed adolescents who do not respond to tricyclics (Ryan et al. 1988b). When using monoamine oxidase inhibitors (MAOIs), suicidal and impulsive outpatients should be excluded because of the risk of severe reactions with dietary indiscretions or drug interaction.

Bupropion is structurally unrelated to other antidepressants. Small open and controlled trials have suggested efficacy of this medication in ADHD and conduct disorder, alone and in combination (Casat et al. 1989).

☐ Lithium Carbonate

Indications and Efficacy

Lithium may be considered in the treatment of children and adolescents with bipolar affective disorder, mixed or manic (Strober et al. 1990; Varanka et al. 1988). Lithium augmentation has been effective in some open trials of adolescents with tricyclic-refractory depression (Ryan et al. 1988a; Strober et al. 1992). In children with severe impulsive aggression, especially when it is accompanied by explosive affect, lithium is equal or superior to haloperidol in reducing aggression, hostility, and tantrums, with fewer side effects (Campbell et al. 1985). Lithium may also be useful in mentally retarded or autistic youths with severe aggression directed toward themselves or others or with symptoms suggestive of bipolar disorder.

Initiation and Maintenance

Lithium should not be prescribed unless the family complies with regular multiple daily doses and with lithium levels. In addition to the usual detailed medical history and physical examination, complete blood count with differential, liver function tests, electrolytes, serum thyroxine and thyroid-stimulating hormone (TSH), BUN, creatinine, and ECG should be determined prior to starting lithium. Some clinicians recommend determination of renal concentrating ability (C. Popper, personal communication, 1992). A patient with a history suggesting increased risk of seizures warrants an EEG. Height, weight, TSH, creatinine, and morning urine specific gravity (or osmolality) should be obtained every 3 to 6 months.

Lithium levels should be obtained twice weekly during initial dose adjustment, and monthly thereafter. Three to four days are required to reach steady-state levels after a dose change. Therapeutic levels are the same as for adults (Campbell et al. 1985). The starting dose is 150 to 300 mg/day, gradually titrated upward in divided doses according to serum levels and clinical effects. Because most children have more efficient renal function than adults, they may require higher doses for body weight (Weller et al. 1986).

Risks and Side Effects

The younger the child, the more likely the occurrence of side effects (Campbell et al. 1991). Autistic children have more frequent and severe side effects than those children with conduct disorder, even at lower doses (Campbell et al. 1991). Children may experience side effects at serum levels that are lower than those in adults: most commonly, weight gain, vomiting, headache, nausea, tremor, enuresis, stomachache, weight loss, sedation, and anorexia (Campbell et al. 1991). Common, early-onset side effects, which seem to be related to rapid increase in serum level, include nausea, diarrhea, muscle weakness, thirst, urinary frequency, a dazed feeling, and hand tremor. Polydipsia and polyuria secondary to vasopressin-resistant diabetes insipidus may result in enuresis, especially in institutionalized retarded patients (Campbell et al. 1985). Electrocardiographic changes, leukocytosis with lymphocytopenia, EEG worsening, and hypothyroidism have also been reported (Campbell et al. 1985). Because of its teratogenic potential, lithium is relatively contraindicated in sexually active girls. Lithium's tendency to aggravate acne may be especially significant for adolescents. Toxicity is closely related to serum levels, and the therapeutic margin is narrow. Symptoms of lithium toxicity include vomiting, drowsiness, hyperreflexia, sluggishness, slurred speech, ataxia, anorexia, convulsions, stupor, coma, and death. Lithium levels may be increased to toxic levels by nonsteroidal anti-inflammatory agents (Fetner and Geller 1992).

☐ Neuroleptic Drugs

Indications and Efficacy

The limited number of existing studies demonstrate modest efficacy of a variety of neuroleptics in schizophrenia (Whitaker and Rao 1992).

Younger schizophrenic patients are less responsive to pharmacotherapy than are adults, and continue to have substantial impairment, even if the more florid symptoms, such as hallucinations, anxiety, and agitation, abate with neuroleptics (Campbell et al. 1985; Realmuto et al. 1984). Children appear to be even less likely than adolescents or adults to respond positively, and they are more likely to have troublesome sedation, especially from low-potency neuroleptics (Campbell et al. 1985). Concerns regarding the development of tardive dyskinesia in long-term use and the prominence of negative symptoms in young schizophrenic patients suggest that clozapine may prove to be useful (Birmaher et al. 1992).

In some hyper- or normoactive autistic children, haloperidol has been found to decrease behavioral target symptoms such as hyperactivity, aggressiveness, temper tantrums, withdrawal, and stereotypies (Anderson et al. 1989). The majority of hypoactive autistic children do not respond well to haloperidol (Campbell et al. 1985), but may do better with pimozide (Ernst et al. 1992).

Efficacy is difficult to evaluate in Tourette's disorder because of the natural waxing and waning of symptoms. Haloperidol in low doses is initially effective for up to 70% of patients (Cohen et al. 1992). Unfortunately, side effects often limit haloperidol's usefulness, and withdrawal of the drug may lead to severe exacerbation of symptoms for up to several months. Pimozide may be useful for patients who do not respond well to either haloperidol or clonidine.

Studies of hospitalized severely aggressive children ages 6 to 12 have demonstrated short-term efficacy of haloperidol and molindone in reducing, although not eliminating, aggression, hostility, negativism, and explosiveness. Chlorpromazine leads to unacceptable sedation at relatively low doses (Campbell et al. 1985).

Initiation and Maintenance

Medication should not be used as the sole treatment in these complex disorders. Prior to initiating medication, a complete physical examination and baseline laboratory workup including complete blood count, differential, liver profile, and urinalysis should be done. Doses must be titrated individually, with careful attention to positive and negative effects. Initial dose should be very low, with gradual increments. In most cases once a therapeutic dosage has been reached, a single daily dose can be used. Children metabolize these drugs more rapidly than do adults, but also require lower plasma levels for efficacy (Teicher and Glod 1990).

Older adolescents with schizophrenia may require doses of neuroleptics in the adult range; for young adolescents doses must be empirically determined. To avoid sedation or cognitive blunting that interferes with learning, one of the higher-potency drugs, such as haloperidol, may be best. It may require several weeks for full efficacy to be achieved.

For Tourette's disorder, careful monitoring for several months prior to starting medication permits the clinician to establish a baseline of symptoms and to assess the need for psychological and educational interventions. An initial dose of haloperidol at 0.5 mg/day may be slowly increased up to 1 to 3 mg per day, divided in twice-daily doses (Cohen et al. 1992). Pimozide, which may be given in a single daily dose, is started at 1 mg per day and may be gradually increased to a maximum of 6 to 10 mg per day (Cohen et al. 1992).

Risks and Side Effects

Acute extrapyramidal side effects, including dystonic reactions, parkinsonian tremor, rigidity and drooling, and akathisia, occur as in adults. Adolescent boys seem to be more vulnerable to acute dystonic reactions than are adult patients, so the physician may be more inclined to use prophylactic antiparkinsonian medication. In children, however, reduction of neuroleptic dose is preferable to the use of antiparkinsonian agents (Campbell et al. 1985). Tardive or withdrawal dyskinesias, some transient but others irreversible, seen in 8% to 51% of neuroleptic-treated children and adolescents (Campbell et al. 1985), mandate caution regarding casual use of these drugs. Tardive dyskinesia has been documented in children and adolescents after as brief a period of treatment as 5 months (Herskowitz 1987), and may appear even during periods of constant medication dose. In children with autism or Tourette's disorder, it may be especially difficult to distinguish medication-induced movements from those characteristic of the disorder. Potentially fatal neuroleptic malignant syndrome has been reported in children and adolescents (Latz and McCracken 1992), with a presentation similar to that seen in adults.

Weight gain may be problematic in the long-term use of the low-potency neuroleptics. Abnormal laboratory findings seem to be reported less often in children than in adults, but the clinician should be alert to the possibility, especially of agranulocytosis or hepatic dysfunction. If an acute febrile illness or easy bruising occurs, medication should be withheld and complete blood count with differential and liver enzymes should be determined (Campbell et al. 1985).

Of particular concern is behavioral toxicity, manifested as worsening of preexisting symptoms or development of new symptoms such as hyperactivity or hypoactivity, irritability, apathy, withdrawal, stereotypies, tics, or hallucinations (Campbell et al. 1985). Low-potency antipsychotic drugs such as chlorpromazine and thioridazine can produce cognitive dulling and sedation that interfere with the patient's ability to benefit from school (Campbell et al. 1985) and are probably best avoided. Children and adolescents are more sensitive than adults to this sedation

(Realmuto et al. 1984). Children may be at greater risk of neuroleptic-induced seizures than adults (Teicher and Glod 1990). Miscellaneous side effects include abdominal pain, enuresis (Realmuto et al. 1984), photosensitivity, and various neuroendocrine effects that may be especially distressing to adolescents.

Side effects are a significant problem in the long-term use of haloperidol for Tourette's disorder. Frequent complaints include lethargy, feeling like a "zombie," dysphoria, personality changes, weight gain, parkinsonian symptoms, akathisia, and intellectual dulling (Cohen et al. 1992). Dysphoria and school avoidance have also been reported (Mikkelsen et al. 1981). Pimozide appears to have a similar but less severe side-effect profile.

☐ Anxiolytics, Sedatives, and Hypnotics

There are very few data on the safety and efficacy of anxiolytics and sedative-hypnotics in children and adolescents. In most cases, psychosocial interventions should precede and accompany pharmacotherapy.

Benzodiazepines. Benzodiazepines may be used in the short-term treatment of children with severe anticipatory anxiety. Preliminary evidence suggests that clonazepam may be useful in the treatment of panic disorder and neuroleptic-induced akathisia in adolescents (Biederman 1987; Kutcher et al. 1992).

Diazepam may be used for severe night terrors, persistent true insomnia, and somnambulism. Infants and children absorb diazepam faster and metabolize it more quickly than do adults (Simeon and Ferguson 1985). When the medication is being discontinued, the dose needs to be tapered gradually to avoid withdrawal seizures or rebound anxiety.

In addition to the risks of substance abuse and physical or psychological dependence, side effects include sedation, cognitive dulling, ataxia, confusion, emotional lability, and worsening of psychosis. Paradoxical or disinhibition reactions may occur, manifested by acute excitation, irritability, increased anxiety, hallucinations, increased aggression and hostility, rage reactions, insomnia, euphoria, and/or incoordination (Reiter and Kutcher 1991).

Antihistamines. Diphenhydramine or hydroxyzine may be used for severe difficulty falling asleep that has not responded to psychological interventions. Medication should be used only for a short time, to break the cycle and to give parents a rest and energy to pursue other solutions. Diphenhydramine is used in the treatment of acute dystonic reactions. The most common side effects of antihistamines are dizziness and oversedation. Some children become paradoxically agitated. Occasionally incoordination, blurred vision, dry mouth, nausea, abdominal pain, or agitation is seen. At high doses the seizure threshold is lowered. Antihistamines have been reported to cause acute dystonic reactions, tics, and possibly tardive dyskinesia. They should not be used for asthmatic patients because of drying of mucous membranes, or in the presence of glaucoma or bladder neck obstruction.

Buspirone.   Buspirone is reported to be less sedating and have less risk of abuse or dependence than do the benzodiazepines. It also has been reported to possibly have weak antidepressant efficacy. Suggested uses are for overanxious disorder, as a supplementary drug in the treatment of OCD, and for the reduction of aggression and anxiety in patients with mental retardation (Ratey et al. 1991), autistic disorder (Realmuto et al. 1989), or conduct disorder. The therapeutic effects may be delayed for 1 to 2 weeks after reaching the proper dose, with maximal effects not seen for an additional 2 weeks. Reported adverse effects in adults include insomnia, dizziness, anxiety, nausea, headache, restlessness, agitation, depression, and confusion (Coffey 1990).

☐ Anticonvulsants

The antiepileptic drugs carbamazepine, valproic acid, and clonazepam are used for a variety of (FDA-nonapproved) psychiatric indications. Efficacy may be unrelated to anticonvulsant effect. Wide variations in bioavailability and rate of absorption of generic products have led to recommendations that the brand name (or at least a single generic) product be prescribed. Data on children and adolescents are generally far more limited than those from studies of adults, but side-effect patterns appear to be similar.

Carbamazepine.   Patients with severe impulsive aggression with emotional lability and irritability who have an abnormal EEG or a strong clinical suggestion of episodic phenomena may deserve a trial of carbamazepine (Evans et al. 1987). Preliminary data suggest this drug's efficacy in children with severe explosive aggression, even in the absence of neurological findings (Kafantaris et al. 1992). Carbamazepine may also be useful in the treatment of psychiatric symptoms associated with temporal lobe epilepsy (Trimble 1990).

Hemoglobin, hematocrit, WBC, platelets, liver function tests, BUN, and creatinine should be measured before starting the patient on carbamazepine. A conservative recommendation for laboratory monitoring includes CBC and liver function studies weekly for the first 4 weeks, monthly for 4 months, and every 3 months thereafter (Silverstein et al.

1983). The initial dose of carbamazepine is 100 mg daily. Children eliminate carbamazepine more rapidly than do adults (Jatlow 1987), and
plasma levels are crucial. Autoinduction of hepatic enzymes may lead to
declining plasma concentration, especially in the first 6 weeks, requiring
an increase in dose.

The most common adverse effects of carbamazepine are drowsiness,
nausea, rash, diplopia, nystagmus, and reversible dose-related leukopenia. Other side effects include vomiting, vertigo, ataxia, tics, muscle
cramps, exacerbation of seizures, rare blood dyscrasias, hepatotoxicity,
severe skin reactions, and inappropriate secretion of antidiuretic hormone
(Trimble 1990). Teratogenic effects have been demonstrated. Adverse
behavioral reactions, such as extreme irritability, agitation, insomnia, obsessive thinking, hallucinations, delirium, psychosis, paranoia, hyperactivity, aggression, and mania, may be seen during the first 1 to 4 weeks of
treatment (Evans et al. 1987).

Valproic acid.   Valproic acid is sometimes used in the treatment of
adolescent mania, when other options have failed. Case reports suggest
the use of valproate for mentally retarded children and adolescents with
mood-related behavioral symptoms that are resistant to lithium and/or
carbamazepine (Kastner et al. 1990). The initial laboratory workup is the
same as for carbamazepine. For children less than 10 years of age,
monthly liver function tests are advisable (Trimble 1990). The most frequent adverse effects are nausea, vomiting, gastrointestinal distress, sedation, weight gain, and tremor (Trimble 1990).

☐ Beta-Blocking Agents

Beta-adrenergic blockers may be useful in patients with otherwise uncontrollable rage reactions and impulsive aggression or self-injurious behavior, especially those with evidence of organicity.

Propranolol was found to be effective in daily doses from 50 to 960
mg (Williams et al. 1982). Propranolol may be effective in the treatment
of agitated, hyperaroused children and adolescents with posttraumatic
stress disorder (PTSD) (Famularo et al. 1988). In an open trial, a single
dose of 40 mg of propranolol appeared to be helpful in reducing test
anxiety and improving performance in a sample of high school students
(Faigel 1991). Pindolol and nadolol, which have fewer side effects and
longer half-lives, have been suggested as alternatives.

Initial workup should include a recent history and physical examination, with particular attention to medical contraindications: asthma, dia-

betes, bradycardia, heart block, cardiac failure, or hypothyroidism. In children and adolescents, the initial dose of propranolol is 10 mg tid, increasing by 10 to 20 mg every 3 to 4 days, monitoring pulse and blood pressure. The short elimination half-life in children may necessitate four doses daily. Maximum improvement at a given dose may not be seen for up to 8 weeks. If a beta-blocker is to be discontinued, it should be tapered gradually to avoid rebound hypertension and tachycardia. Side effects of beta-blockers are generally the same as in adults. Tiredness, mild hypotension, and bradycardia are the most common.

☐ Desmopressin

Desmopressin (DDAVP) is an analog of antidiuretic hormone administered as a nasal spray to treat nocturnal enuresis. Onset of action is rapid (several days) and side effects are negligible (rare nasal mucosal dryness or irritation, and headache) in patients with normal electrolyte regulation. As with the tricyclic antidepressants, few patients become completely dry, and relapse occurs when medication is stopped (Klauber 1989).

■ CATEGORIES OF PSYCHOTHERAPY

☐ Individual Psychotherapy

In the treatment of children and adolescents it is essential to consider the patient's environment and family dynamics. In most cases, work with parents, school, and often pediatrician, welfare agency, courts, or recreation leader must accompany individual therapy. The cooperation of parents, and often teachers, is required to maintain the child or adolescent in treatment and to remove any secondary gain resulting from the symptoms. The therapist must be aware of the patient's level of physical, cognitive, and emotional development in order to understand the symptoms, set appropriate goals, and tailor effective interventions. Behavior modification, cognitive-behavior therapy, and even indirect family therapy can be conducted in individual sessions.

Children use play to express feelings, to narrate past events, to work through trauma, and to regress. It is less threatening and anxiety provoking if the therapist uses the metaphor of the play and bases questions and comments on characters in the play, rather than on the child. Effective communications are tailored to the child's stage of language, cognitive, and affective development. The therapist must be aware that the vocabulary of some bright and precocious children exceeds their emotional understanding of events and concepts. Dramatic play with dolls or puppets, drawing, painting, or modeling with clay, as well as questions about dreams, wishes, or favorite stories or television shows, can provide access to children's fantasies, emotions, and concerns. Adolescents may prefer creative writing or more complex expressive art techniques.

Many children or adolescents do not cooperate in therapy. These young patients have been brought to treatment by adults, often do not wish to change themselves or their behavior, and view their parents' and teachers' complaints as unreasonable or unfair. When a child or adolescent does not talk, whether from anxiety or opposition, the therapist often addresses this reluctance, either directly or through play. Long silences are not generally helpful and tend to increase anxiety or battles for control. Attractive play materials help to make the therapy situation less threatening and to encourage participation while the therapist builds an alliance. One must guard, however, against the danger of the sessions becoming mere play or recreation instead of therapy. Gardner (1979) developed a variety of techniques that incorporate therapeutic activities with story telling, drama, and game boards. Use of behavioral contingencies in the therapy situation may also improve motivation, especially for materially deprived children. A child who is anxious or having difficulty separating from a parent may be helped by initially permitting the parent to remain in the therapy room.

Individual psychotherapy may be useful as a part of a comprehensive treatment plan for children who are schizophrenic or very fragile (Cantor and Kestenbaum 1986). The therapist must be prepared to provide structure, to limit regression and fantasy, and to focus on reality testing and development of stronger defense mechanisms and healthier coping skills. The relationship with the therapist may be especially crucial for these youngsters.

Psychoanalysis

In this relatively infrequently used modality for children and adolescents, neurotic symptoms are viewed as arising from internalized intrapsychic conflict, nonorganic developmental arrest, or regression. The family must be able to sustain a process that is expensive, lasts for years, and requires sessions four to five times a week. The patient must have sufficient intelligence, capacity for verbalization and insight, and frustration tolerance. Psychoanalysis is contraindicated for psychotic youth or those with serious cognitive or ego deficiencies.

Psychodynamically Oriented Therapy

This treatment is grounded in psychoanalytic theory but is more flexible and emphasizes the real relationship with the therapist and the provision of a corrective emotional experience as well as the transference. Frequency is typically once or twice a week, most commonly over a period of 1 to 2 years. Interaction between the parents and the therapist is more active. Goals of therapy include symptom resolution, change in behavior, and return to normal developmental process. Dynamically oriented individual therapy alone is much more likely to be effective for children and adolescents who are in emotional distress or who are struggling to deal with a stressor than for those children with behavior problems. Children and adolescents with attention-deficit, oppositional, or conduct disorders rarely acknowledge their problem behavior and are usually better treated in family or group therapy, by parent training in behavior management, or in a structured milieu. Youngsters with ADHD have little insight into their behavior and its effect on others, and may be genuinely unable to report some of their problems or to reflect on them. Insight-oriented therapy may be useful for some of these youngsters, however, to address comorbid anxiety or depression, or symptoms resulting from psychological trauma.

Supportive Therapy

This type of therapy has less ambitious goals and may be especially useful for children and adolescents who do not have satisfying relationships with adults because parents are unavailable, or unsuitable, or the youngster's symptoms make it difficult to establish a positive relationship. For the patient in crisis, the therapist provides support until a stressor resolves, a developmental crisis has passed, or the patient or environment change sufficiently so that other adults can take on the supportive role. There is a real relationship with the therapist, who facilitates catharsis and provides understanding and judicious advice.

Time-Limited Therapy

All of the various models of time-limited therapy have in common a planned, relatively brief duration; a predominant focus on the present; a high degree of structure and attention to specific, limited goals; and active roles for both therapist and patient. Length of treatment varies among models from several sessions to 6 months. Theoretical foundations include psychodynamic, crisis, family systems, cognitive, behavioral or social learning and guidance, or educational theories (Dulcan and Piercy 1985). A model of interpersonal psychotherapy (IPT) for depressed adolescents has been developed (Moreau et al. 1991). These methods have been recommended for both multiproblem, crisis-oriented families who are unlikely to persist in longer-term treatment, and well-functioning children and families with circumscribed problems of relatively recent onset. Brief treatment is relatively contraindicated for long-standing severe pathology and for children and adolescents who have suffered serious losses and/or deprivation.

Cognitive Therapy

The cognitive therapy techniques developed for the treatment of depression in adults have been adapted for adolescents (Wilkes and Rush 1988). Caution is needed to ensure that the homework assignments that are an integral part of this therapy are not perceived as aversive when added to the homework assigned in school. Children's more concrete cognitive processes make this rather intellectual model impractical, although creative adaptations and the incorporation of behavioral techniques can render this approach accessible (Emery et al. 1983). Cognitive self-control training may be effective in reducing aggressive behavior in adolescents, although compliance with self-monitoring procedures is often poor (Dangel et al. 1989).

☐ Parent Counseling

Parent counseling or guidance is primarily an educational intervention, conducted in a mental health setting. Parents learn about normal child and adolescent development. Efforts are made to help parents understand their child and his or her problems, and to modify practices that seem to be contributing to the current difficulties. The therapist's understanding of the parents' point of view and of the hardships of living with a disturbed child or adolescent is crucial. For some parents who have serious difficulties of their own, parent counseling may merge into or pave the way for individual treatment of the adult or couple.

☐ Behavior Therapy

Behavior therapy is by far the most thoroughly evaluated psychiatric treatment for children. Maximally effective programs require home and school cooperation, focus on specific target behaviors, and ensure that contingencies follow behavior quickly and consistently. Behavior therapy is the most effective treatment for simple phobias, for enuresis and encopresis, and for the noncompliant behaviors seen in oppositional defiant disorder and conduct disorder. For youngsters with ADHD, behavior modification can improve both academic achievement and behavior, if specifically targeted. Both punishment and reward components are required. Behavior modification is more effective than medication in improving peer interactions, but skills may need to be taught first. Many youngsters require programs that are consistent, intensive, and prolonged. A wide variety of other childhood problems, such as motor and vocal tics, trichotillomania, and sleep problems, are treated by behavior modification, either alone or in combination with pharmacotherapy.

The greatest weaknesses of behavior therapy are lack of maintenance of improvement over time and failure of changes to generalize to situations other than the ones in which training occurred. Generalization and maintenance can be maximized by conducting training in the settings in which behavior change is desired, at multiple times and places, facilitating transfer to naturally occurring reinforcers and gradually fading reinforcement on an intermittent schedule.

Parent Management Training

Effective training packages, based on social learning theory, have been developed for parents of noncompliant, oppositional, and aggressive children (Forehand and McMahon 1981) and delinquent adolescents (Patterson and Forgatch 1987). Parents are taught to give clear instructions, to positively reinforce good behavior, and to use punishment effectively. The most powerful parent training programs use a combination of written materials and verbal instruction in social learning principles and contingency management, modeling by the therapist, and behavioral rehearsal of skills to be used. Families with low socioeconomic status, parental psychopathology (such as depression), marital conflict, and lack of a social support network require maximally potent interventions, with attention to parental problems as necessary. Other families may be able to succeed with written materials only, or manuals supplemented by group lectures.

Behavioral intervention can be done in the context of family therapy in which the family learn how to negotiate and to solve problems together. A key technique is parent-child contingency contracting, which entails a written social contract between parent and child to change behaviors in both parties, with specified contingencies (Blechman 1981).

Classroom Behavior Modification

Techniques for behavior modification in schools include token economies, class rules, and attention to positive behavior, as well as response cost programs, in which reinforcers are withdrawn in response to undesirable behavior. One effective program for children with attention and conduct problems required only that the teacher observe every 30 minutes whether the child was on-task and provide verbal feedback (Pelham and Murphy 1986). Reinforcers such as positive recognition or stars on a chart may be dispensed by the teacher, or more tangible rewards or privileges by parents through the use of daily report cards.

Behavioral Treatment of Specific Symptoms

Enuresis and encopresis.   Following an evaluation for psychiatric disorders or sexual abuse and a complete medical history, physical examination, and any necessary laboratory tests to rule out a medical disorder, the treatment of choice for enuresis or encopresis is behavioral. While waiting for the child to outgrow enuresis, the most useful strategy is to minimize secondary symptoms by discouraging the parents from punishing or ridiculing the child. Children can be taught to change their own beds, thus reducing expectable negative reactions from parents. Young children who have never been successfully toilet trained often respond to an intensive behavioral program (see Azrin and Foxx 1974). A simple monitoring and reward procedure using a chart with stars to be exchanged for rewards may be effective for some children who are motivated to stop wetting the bed. If this is not effective, a program using a urine alarm device (Schmitt 1982) results in complete dryness in two-thirds of patients.

The treatment of encopresis is somewhat more complex because encopresis frequently results from chronic constipation and stool withholding, which requires medical treatment. Education of both parents and child in bowel function is essential. Encopresis not associated with constipation may be treated with a behavioral program that rewards first sitting on the toilet and then moving the bowels appropriately. The program may or may not include a negative consequence for soiling. For children with severe stool retention and resulting impaction and loss of bowel tone, an additional program is required, consisting of initial bowel cleanout, followed by a bowel "retraining" program, using oral mineral oil, a high roughage diet, ample fluid intake, development of a regular toileting routine, and a mild suppository if necessary (Levine 1982).

Anxiety disorders.   Desensitization, in vivo or in fantasy, is the treatment of choice for simple phobias, often supplemented by modeling. The techniques are essentially the same as those used with adults, with modification for developmental level. In vivo desensitization, often combined with contingency management and parent guidance, may be effective in the treatment of school avoidance resulting from separation anxiety disorder.

Behavioral Techniques for the Pediatric Setting

A variety of behavioral techniques have been used, in much the same way as in adults, but with adaptations for the child or adolescent's level of cognitive or emotional development. Especially important is an understanding of any misconceptions the youngster may have about the disease state and its treatment. These notions vary according to the patient's stage of cognitive development and his or her unique experience.

Hypnosis. Children are more hypnotizable than adults (Williams 1979). Although hypnosis is occasionally used to remove a behavioral symptom or habit, for children and adolescents the most common uses of hypnosis are in the treatment of physical symptoms with a psychological component or to help a child manage pain or nausea associated with a physical disorder or its treatment. Successful use of hypnosis to reduce pain and anxiety has not been reported in children under the age of 6 (Varni et al. 1986).

Relaxation training. Four types of relaxation procedures are applicable to children and adolescents: progressive muscle relaxation, meditative breathing, autogenics (i.e., silently repeating commands or statements), and imagery-based techniques (Masek et al. 1984). The choice is determined by the characteristics of the child or adolescent and of the disorder being treated. Relaxation training has been used in the treatment of pediatric migraine, juvenile rheumatoid arthritis, and hemophilia. These techniques, also called cognitive-behavioral self-regulation of pain perception, can result not only in decreased subjective experience of pain and reduced need for analgesics, but also in improved mood, self-esteem, and physical and social functioning (Varni et al. 1986). Similar techniques have also been used in the treatment of children and adolescents with asthma or cystic fibrosis.

Pain behavior management. This strategy uses operant techniques in the treatment of chronic pain. For example, the antecedents and consequences of headaches are determined, by observation and by keeping a pain diary (if the child is old enough), and then attempts are made to modify those situations and events that seem to precipitate or positively reinforce pain, working with the patient, parents, teachers, pediatrician, and significant others. Emphasis is placed on functioning normally in spite of pain and on stress management techniques (Masek et al. 1984). These techniques have been adapted to the treatment of respiratory symptoms in children and adolescents with asthma or cystic fibrosis.

Stress inoculation. This multicomponent cognitive-behavioral approach combines education, modeling procedures, systematic desensitization, hypnosis, contingency management, and training and practice in coping skills such as imagery and breathing exercises. It is useful in the prevention of stress and anxiety in children before medical and dental procedures and in chronically ill children for reduction of anxiety, pain, or other discomfort connected to repeated procedures such as spinal taps, bone marrow aspirations, and chemotherapy injections.

☐ Family Treatment

Attempts to treat children and adolescents without considering the persons with whom they live and the patients' relationships with other significant persons are doomed to failure. Any change in one family member, whether resulting from a psychiatric disorder, psychiatric treatment, a normal developmental process, or an outside event, is likely to produce change in other family members and in their relationships.

Evaluation of Families

Data should be gathered on each person living with the patient, as well as others who may be important, or have been so in the past. For families with young children, techniques such as the use of family drawings or puppet play or the assignment of family tasks to be carried out in the session are often useful. A variety of schemas exist by which to assess a family's structure and dynamic functioning. The McMaster Model focuses on the family's current functioning in regard to problem solving, communication, suitability of family roles, ability of family members to respond appropriately to emotional stimuli, extent to which family members are involved in and value each other's interests and activities, and style and success of controlling behavior of family members. Tasks of the initial session of a family assessment include establishing an alliance with family members; gathering data by direct questions, by observing, and by assessing the impact of trial interventions; and proposing a provisional plan for treatment.

Family Therapy

Family therapy is psychological treatment conducted with an identified patient and at least one biological or functional family member. Family therapy addresses primarily the interaction *between* family members, rather than the processes *within* an individual. Although some advocate family therapy as the best treatment for all disorders, most clinicians would agree that there are some situations in which family therapy is preferred over other treatments, others in which it should be combined with other treatments, and still others in which it is not possible or relatively contraindicated.

Family therapy may be particularly useful when there are dysfunctional interactions or impaired communication within the family, especially when these appear to be related to the presenting problem. It may also be useful when symptoms seem to have been precipitated by difficulty with a developmental stage for an individual or the family or by a change in the family such as divorce or remarriage. If more than one family member is symptomatic, family therapy may be both more efficient and more effective than multiple individual treatments. Family therapy should be considered when one family member improves with treatment but another, not in treatment, worsens. When the identified patient is relatively unmotivated to participate or to change, family therapy is likely to be more effective than individual therapy. Attention to family systems issues may also be useful when progress is blocked in individual therapy or in behavior therapy.

Family therapy is contraindicated as a sole treatment method in cases of clearly organic physical or mental illness, or if the family equilibrium is precarious and one or more family members are at serious risk of decompensation. In these situations family therapy may be useful in combination with other treatments, such as medication or hospitalization. It is counterproductive to include in family therapy sessions a patient who is acutely psychotic, violent, or delusional regarding the family. Family sessions may not be helpful when a parent has severe, intractable, or minimally relevant psychopathology, or when the child or adolescent strongly prefers individual treatment. Children and adolescents should not be included in sessions in which parents persist in criticizing the children or in sharing inappropriate information, when the most critical need is for marital therapy, or when parents primarily need specific, concrete help with practical affairs.

Structural family therapy.   This approach to family therapy has been the model most used and studied when a child or adolescent is the identified patient. It has been used extensively with families of children and adolescents with eating disorders and psychophysiological disorders such as asthma. Focus is on the present, in which the identified patient's symptoms serve a function for the family. The process of assessment includes mapping patterns of communication and the structure of the family, including the location and permeability of boundaries between family members and around the family and its subsystems. Other important variables are the character and flexibility of alignments of family members, including alliances and coalitions. Data are gathered on the distribution of power within the family and on the family's sources of stress and support in the environment. The therapist uses assigned tasks and his or her interactions with family members to provoke change in the family structure and thereby its functioning. Relabeling (i.e., redefining a behavior or symptom to have a different, less negative meaning) opens alternative pathways for family interactions.

Multigenerational family therapy.   Multigenerational family therapy emphasizes how current patterns in families are repetitions of the past. Change results from insights gained in the exploration of parents' families of origin and the relationships over several generations of the nuclear family to the extended family. Grandparents are often involved indirectly, or even included in sessions.

Strategic family therapy.   This approach produces change through a complex and indirect plan of action, that is not fully shared with the family. Apparently paradoxical instructions are devised to upset the family equilibrium and permit change, especially in families resistant to more straightforward techniques.

Behavioral family therapy.   Models of behavioral family therapy include Patterson's (1975), based on social learning theory, and Alexander's functional family therapy, both of which are used in the treatment of children and adolescents with conduct disorders. Henggeler and Borduin (1990) extended this model to a multisystemic approach that uses energetic outreach into the home, neighborhood, and school, and adds peer group and school-based interventions to family treatment of adolescent delinquents.

Psychoeducational family therapy.   A psychoeducational approach to family therapy has been most extensively developed in the treatment of families of adult schizophrenic patients (Anderson et al. 1980), but has been extended to a number of childhood disorders, such as eating disorders, ADHD, and depression. Detailed didactic presentations about the disorder, in the setting of a multiple family group, are designed to improve the family's coping skills through increased understanding of the illness and its treatment, to teach home behavior-management techniques, and to enhance family support networks. Ongoing treatment of individual families uses family systems interventions when educational and behavioral techniques are blocked by dysfunctional family structures or processes.

Multiple family therapy.   This multifamily approach combines features of group and family therapy. Sessions include three to five families with similar problems who may be isolated from other supports and who can benefit from the interaction with other families.

☐ Group Therapy

Group therapy is particularly appropriate for children and adolescents, who are often more willing to reveal their thoughts and feelings to peers than to adults. Establishing rewarding social relationships, a crucial developmental task for children and adolescents, is especially difficult for those youths with a psychiatric disorder. Group therapy offers unparalleled opportunities for the clinician to evaluate the youth's behavior with peers, to model and facilitate practice of important skills, and to provide youngsters with companionship and mutual support. Interventions by peers may be far more acute and powerful in their effect than those by an adult therapist. Target symptoms include absent or conflictual peer relationships, aggression, withdrawal, timidity, and deficient social interactive or problem-solving skills. These problems are often not apparent or accessible to intervention in individual therapy sessions. Group therapy can be a powerful modality in the treatment of adolescents with eating disorders or substance abuse.

Group psychotherapy is contraindicated for extremely fragile youngsters and for those who are acutely psychotic or paranoid. Adolescents with sociopathic traits or behaviors should not be included in groups with teenagers who might be victimized or intimidated. Severely aggressive or hyperactive children should probably not be included in outpatient groups because of the difficulty in controlling their behavior, the contagion of problem behaviors, and the intimidation of less assertive children. Groups should *not* be used as a repository for unmotivated, nonverbal, difficult patients. Although group therapy may be used as the sole treatment modality, it is often used in combination with another intervention.

Technical Issues

All of the theoretical models utilized in individual therapy may be used with groups. Therapy may be exclusively verbal, or it may include expressive arts techniques, psychodrama, arts and crafts, and sports activities; behavioral techniques such as modeling or overt practice; or cognitive-behavioral strategies for depression (Lewinsohn et al. 1990). Of all modalities of therapy, the need for co-therapists is most clear in group treatment. In groups of younger children, an extra pair of hands is needed. Co-leaders who differ in age, sex, race, and ethnicity expand the opportunities for different types of patient-therapist relationships.

Groups range from 4 to 10 patients, with the number varying according to the number of leaders, the age and type of pathology of the group members, and the number of suitable candidates available. Patients in support groups are chosen because they share a single stressor—for example, sexual abuse, parental divorce, or the same chronic physical illness. Other groups are specifically targeted to a single disorder. Groups that focus on social skills work best with a mixture of patients. Group members should be in the same or adjacent developmental stage. Children and adolescents change so dramatically as they develop that an age span broader than 2 to 3 years is unlikely to result in a therapeutic group process. In forming groups for pre- and early adolescents, developmental stage is often more important than chronological age, because girls are approximately 2 years ahead of boys in physical and social development. Although some issues are easier to handle in single-sex groups, children and adolescents need to learn to get along with the opposite sex, so mixing boys and girls may be more productive.

The nature of the group and the patients determine the optimal degree of structure. A psychodynamically oriented group composed of depressed or anxious adolescents will need far fewer rules than a group whose goal is to teach social skills to school-age boys with conduct problems. The leaders are responsible for maintaining control of behavior within the group. The leaders must make explicit the rules of confidentiality for the group, as the group setting expands the risk of breach of confidentiality to include the patient's peers.

Involving parents is especially important for preschool- and school-age children, to discover important events in the child's life and to assess progress. Adolescents are more willing and able to report and are also more sensitive to confidentiality issues. All parents should be kept apprised of the goals of the group, both in general and specifically for their child. Parent education in development and behavior management can be efficiently provided by grouping parents together.

Developmental Issues

Young children are less able to verbalize and thus require more structure and planned activities. A group can provide a powerful context for the teaching of social skills and language, especially for children who are autistic or severely delayed.

Because school-age children have great difficulty bringing in outside material for discussion or engaging in introspection, verbal portions of the group are best focused on events that occur in the group itself. Games and craft activities can provide a useful framework, but the leaders must ensure that recreation does not become the only function of the group. Behavior modification and cognitive problem-solving techniques are especially useful for children this age.

Many child patients will not spontaneously attempt to relate to other children. Others have been rejected or scapegoated by peers. If the group is successful, the children will use the skills they have learned to form relationships with peers at school and in their neighborhoods. Children with ADHD are often referred to group therapy because of their difficulty with peer relations and their lack of insight into their difficulties.

Scheidlinger (1985) identified four major categories of group work with adolescents:

1. *Group psychotherapy:* treatment of a balanced selection of patients, using the group as the primary modality, with goals of relief of

psychological distress, modification of pathological modes of functioning, and amelioration of personality dysfunction.

2. *Therapeutic groups for clients in mental health, medical, or residential settings:* used as ancillary treatment or as an aid in rehabilitation.
3. *Human development and training groups:* offered to youths who are not psychiatric patients and focusing on prevention and enrichment.
4. *Self-help and mutual help groups:* these may or may not have professional leaders, and consist of peers working together to satisfy a shared need or overcome a common handicap. This model has been extensively used in the treatment of substance abuse.

Although activities may be useful, many adolescent groups can be conducted in an exclusively verbal format. If both boys and girls are included in the same group, the leaders must be alert to sexual undercurrents and acting out, while facilitating the discussion of sexual concerns and practicing of heterosexual social skills (Scheidlinger 1985).

☐ Hospital and Residential Treatment

Because children and adolescents should be treated in the setting that is least restrictive and disruptive to their lives, hospital or residential treatment is indicated only in emergencies or for youngsters who have not responded to efforts at outpatient treatment, because of severity of disorder, lack of motivation, resistance, or disorganization of patient and/or family. Placement in a residential treatment center may be indicated for children and adolescents with chronic behavior problems such as aggression, running away, truancy, substance abuse, school phobia, or self-destructive acts that the family, foster home, and/or community cannot manage or tolerate. Children and adolescents for whom it is not advisable to return home may be referred to a residential treatment center following a hospital stay.

Short-term hospitalization (7 to 30 days) is more often an acute event, stemming from immediate physical danger to self or others, acute psychosis, a crisis in the environment that reduces the ability of the caregiving adults to cope with the child or adolescent, or the need for more intensive, systematic, and detailed evaluation and observation of the patient and family than is possible on an outpatient basis or in a day program.

Ideally, hospitalization forms part of a comprehensive continuum of care for children and adolescents. With ever-shorter lengths of stay, rapid and efficient planning and execution of evaluation and treatment strategies are essential. The goal is not to eliminate all psychopathology, but to address the "focal problem" that precipitated hospitalization, and then to discharge the patient to home, residential treatment, or foster placement, where he or she can receive outpatient or day treatment (Harper 1989).

The relative emphasis placed on each treatment modality differs according to the philosophy of treatment, the nature of the patient population, the usual length of stay, and the availability of highly specialized staff. All of the following should be present in some form.

Pharmacotherapy

Hospitalization offers an ideal opportunity for systematic trials of medication in children or adolescents who have not responded to conventional treatment, who are diagnostically puzzling, who have medical problems complicating pharmacotherapy, or whose parents are noncompliant, disorganized, or unreliable reporters of efficacy or side effects.

Individual Psychotherapy

As newer treatment methods evolve and hospital stays become ever shorter, individual psychotherapy is less often the primary treatment modality than in the past. Regularly scheduled individual sessions with a therapist with whom the child or adolescent can develop a special relationship continue to be essential, however, in developing a more complete understanding of the patient's intrapsychic, familial, and social dynamics, and to assist him or her in developing more adaptive methods of coping with strong emotions.

Milieu Therapy

This component includes the total environment of a structured schedule for meals, sleep, and so forth, and a program of activities. The patient can be observed over an extended period of time in school, free play with peers, meals, sleep, and self-care. Goals of the milieu include promotion of a feeling of security, by clarity of rules and regularity of schedule, and increased self-esteem and competence through learning of skills.

Group Therapy

In addition to general or special topic groups (e.g., 12-step models, survivors of abuse), many settings include community meetings in which privileges and rules are decided, social skills are practiced, and patients learn to observe their own and others' behavior, and to recognize the impact of their behavior on others.

Education

Virtually all children and adolescents who require psychiatric hospital-ization have had problems in school. The small classes and highly trained teachers of a hospital unit can provide a detailed evaluation of a youngster's academic strengths and weaknesses, incorporating data from intelligence and achievement tests, and special tests for learning disabilities, into direct observation of classroom behavior and learning. Many residential treatment centers have their own schools on the grounds of the program. As youngsters improve, they are gradually inte-grated into special education or mainstream programs in local public or private schools.

Family Treatment

Work with families is an essential part of hospital treatment, which in-cludes intensive evaluation of family functioning and deciding on where the child or adolescent should reside. Interventions may include family therapy, parent counseling in behavior management, and education in the nature of their child's disorder.

Additional Services

Medical evaluation and treatment must be provided. The following, more specialized resources should be available as necessary on a consul-tation basis: neurological evaluation and treatment, speech and language assessment and therapy, physical therapy, and occupational therapy.

Disposition Planning and Follow-Up Care

Disposition planning and follow-up may be the most important part of the treatment, if gains made are to be maintained and continued. A com-plete disposition plan includes consideration of where the child or ado-lescent should live, school placement, and continuation of individual therapy, family therapy, and/or pharmacotherapy.

☐ Day Treatment

A day program may be best for the child or adolescent who requires more intensive intervention than can be provided in outpatient visits, but is able to live at home. Day treatment is less disruptive to patient and family than hospitalization or residential placement, and can offer an op-portunity for more intensive work with parents, who may even attend the program on a regular basis. A day program may be used as a transition for a child or adolescent who has been hospitalized, or to avert a hospitalization. It may be implemented in combination with placement in a foster or group home.

Some programs involve a full day, 5 days a week, and include a school or therapeutic nursery school program. There are decided advantages in being able to integrate the treatment plan and therapeutic focus into the entire day. Other programs may meet in the late afternoon and evening hours, after patients attend community schools. It is desirable to offer all of the treatment modalities that are available on an inpatient unit.

■ REFERENCES

Achenbach TM: Manual for the Teacher's Report Form and 1991 Profile. Burlington, VT, University of Vermont, Department of Psychiatry, 1991

Anderson CM, Hogarty GE, Reiss DJ: Family treatment of adult schizophrenic patients: a psycho-educational approach. Schizophr Bull 6:490–505, 1980

Anderson LT, Campbell M, Adams P, et al: The effects of haloperidol on discrimination learning and behavioral symptoms in autistic children. J Autism Dev Disord 19:227–239, 1989

Azrin N, Foxx R: Toilet Training in Less Than a Day. New York, Simon & Schuster, 1974

Barkley RA: Hyperactive Children: A Handbook for Diagnosis and Treatment. New York, Guilford Press, 1981

Barrickman L, Noyes R, Kuperman S, et al: Treatment of ADHD with fluoxetine: a preliminary trial. J Am Acad Child Adolesc Psychiatry 30:762–767, 1991

Bartels MG, Varley CK, Mitchell J, et al: Pediatric cardiovascular effects of imipramine and desipramine. J Am Acad Child Adolesc Psychiatry 30:100–103, 1991

Biederman J: Clonazepam in the treatment of prepubertal children with panic-like symptoms. J Clin Psychiatry 48 (No 10, Suppl):38–41, 1987

Biederman J, Baldessarini RJ, Wright V, et al: A double-blind placebo controlled study of desipramine in the treatment of ADD, I: efficacy. J Am Acad Child Adolesc Psychiatry 28:777–784, 1989

Birmaher B, Greenhill LL, Cooper TB, et al: Sustained release methylphenidate: pharmacokinetic studies in ADDH males. J Am Acad Child Adolesc Psychiatry 28:768–772, 1989

Birmaher B, Baker R, Kapur S, et al: Clozapine for the treatment of adolescents with schizophrenia. J Am Acad Child Adolesc Psychiatry 31:160–164, 1992

Blechman EA: Toward comprehensive behavioral family intervention: an algorithm for matching families and interventions. Behav Modif 5:221–236, 1981

Boulos C, Kutcher S, Gardner D, et al: An open naturalistic trial of fluoxetine in adolescents and young adults with treatment-resistant major depression. Journal of Child and Adolescent Psychopharmacology 2:103–111, 1992

Briant RH: An introduction to clinical pharmacology, in Pediatric Psychopharmacology: The Use of Behavior-Modifying Drugs in Children. Edited by Werry JS. New York, Brunner/Mazel, 1978, pp 3–29

Brown RT, Sexson SB: Effects of methylphenidate on cardiovascular responses in attention deficit hyperactivity disordered adolescents. J Adolesc Health Care 10:179–183, 1989

Campbell M, Green WH, Deutsch SI: Child and Adolescent Psychopharmacology. Beverly Hills, CA, Sage, 1985

Campbell M, Silva RR, Kafantaris V, et al: Predictors of side effects associated with lithium administration in children. Psychopharmacol Bull 27:373–380, 1991

Campbell SB: Hyperactivity in preschoolers: correlates and prognostic implications. Clinical Psychology Review 5:405–428, 1985

Cantor S, Kestenbaum C: Psychotherapy with schizophrenic children. Journal of the American Academy of Child Psychiatry 25:623–630, 1986

Casat CD, Pleasants DZ, Schroeder DH, et al: Bupropion in children with attention deficit disorder. Psychopharmacol Bull 25:198–201, 1989

Coffey BJ: Anxiolytics for children and adolescents: traditional and new drugs. Journal of Child and Adolescent Psychopharmacology 1:57–83, 1990

Coffey BJ, Shader RI, Greenblatt DJ: Pharmacokinetics of benzodiazepines and psychostimulants in children. J Clin Psychopharmacol 3:217–225, 1983

Cohen DJ, Riddle MA, Leckman JF: Pharmacotherapy of Tourette's syndrome and associated disorders. Psychiatr Clin North Am 15:109–129, 1992

Conners CK: Methodological and assessment issues in pediatric psychopharmacology, in Diagnosis and Psychopharmacology of Childhood and Adolescent Disorders. Edited by Wiener JM. New York, Wiley, 1985, pp 69–110

Cook EH Jr, Rowlett R, Jaselskis C, et al: Fluoxetine treatment of children and adults with autistic disorder and mental retardation. J Am Acad Child Adolesc Psychiatry 31:739–745, 1992

Dangel RF, Deschner JP, Rasp RR: Anger control training for adolescents in residential treatment. Behav Modif 13:447–458, 1989

DeVeaugh-Geiss J, Moroz G, Biederman J, et al: Clomipramine hydrochloride in childhood and adolescent obsessive-compulsive disorder—a multicenter trial. J Am Acad Child Adolesc Psychiatry 31:45–49, 1992

Donnelly M, Rapoport JL: Attention deficit disorders, in Diagnosis and Psychopharmacology of Childhood and Adolescent Disorders. Edited by Weiner JM. New York, Wiley, 1985, pp 179–197

Dulcan MK, Piercy PA: A model for teaching and evaluating brief psychotherapy with children and their families. Professional Psychology: Research and Practice 16:689–700, 1985

Dulcan MK, Popper CW: Concise Guide to Child and Adolescent Psychiatry. Washington, DC, American Psychiatric Press, 1991

Elia J, Borcherding BG, Rapoport JL, et al: Methylphenidate and dextroamphetamine treatments of hyperactivity: are there true nonresponders? Psychiatry Res 36:141–155, 1991

Emery G, Bedrosian R, Garber J: Cognitive therapy with depressed children and adolescents, in Affective Disorders in Childhood and Adolescence: An Update. Edited by Cantwell DP, Carlson GA. New York, Spectrum, 1983, pp 445–471

Ernst M, Magee HJ, Gonzalez NM, et al: Pimozide in autistic children. Psychopharmacol Bull 28:187–191, 1992

Evans RW, Clay TH, Gualtieri CT: Carbamazepine in pediatric psychiatry. Journal of American Academy of Child Psychiatry 26:2–8, 1987

Faigel HC: The effect of beta blockade on stress-induced cognitive dysfunction in adolescents. Clin Pediatr (Phila) 30:441–445, 1991

Famularo R, Fenton T: The effect of methylphenidate on school grades in children with attention deficit disorder without hyperactivity: a preliminary report. J Clin Psychiatry 48:112–114, 1987

Famularo R, Kinscherff R, Fenton T: Propranolol treatment for childhood posttraumatic stress disorder, acute type. Am J Dis Child 142:1244–1247, 1988

Fetner HH, Geller B: Lithium and tricyclic antidepressants. Psychiatr Clin North Am 15:223–241, 1992

Fitzpatrick PA, Klorman F, Brumaghim JT, et al: Effects of sustained-release and standard preparations of methylphenidate on attention deficit disorder. J Am Acad Child Adolesc Psychiatry 31:226–234, 1992

Forehand RL, McMahon RJ: Helping the Noncompliant Child: A Clinician's Guide to Parent Training. New York, Guilford, 1981

Gadow KD: Pediatric psychopharmacology: a review of recent research. J Child Psychol Psychiatry 33:153–195, 1992

Gammon GD, Brown TE, Barua G: Fluoxetine augmentation of methylphenidate for attention deficit and comorbid disorders. Paper presented at the annual meeting of the American Academy of Child and Adolescent Psychiatry, San Francisco, CA, October 1991

Gardner RA: Helping children cooperate in therapy, in Basic Handbook of Child Psychiatry, Vol 3: Therapeutic Interventions. Edited by Harrison SI (Noshpitz JD, Editor-in-Chief). New York, Basic Books, 1979, pp 414–433

Geller B, Cooper TB, Chestnut EC, et al: Preliminary data on the relationship between nortriptyline plasma level and response in depressed children. Am J Psychiatry 143:1283–1286, 1986

Geller B, Cooper TB, Farooki ZQ, et al: Dose and plasma levels of nortriptyline and chlorpromazine in delusionally depressed adolescents and of nortriptyline in nondelusionally depressed adolescents. Am J Psychiatry 142:336–338, 1985

Gordon CT, Rapoport JL, Hamburger SD, et al: Differential response of seven subjects with autistic disorder to clomipramine and desipramine. Am J Psychiatry 149:363–366, 1992

Green WH: Child and Adolescent Clinical Psychopharmacology. Baltimore, MD, Williams & Wilkins, 1991

Halperin JM, Gittelman R, Katz S, et al: Relationship between stimulant effect, electroencephalogram, and clinical neurological findings in hyperactive children. J Am Acad Child Psychiatry 25:820–825, 1986

Handen BL, Breaux AM, Janosky J, et al: Effects and noneffects of methylphenidate in children with mental retardation and ADHD. J Am Acad Child Adolesc Psychiatry 31:455–461, 1992

Harper G: Focal inpatient treatment planning. J Am Acad Child Adolesc Psychiatry 28:31–37, 1989

Henggeler SW, Borduin CM: Family Therapy and Beyond: A Multisystemic Approach to Treating the Behavior Problems of Children and Adolescents. Belmont, CA, Brooks/Cole Publishing Company, 1990

Herskowitz J: Developmental neurotoxicology, in Psychiatric Pharmacosciences of Children and Adolescents. Edited by Popper C. Washington, DC, American Psychiatric Press, 1987, pp 81–123

Hughes CW, Preskorn SH, Weller E, et al: Imipramine vs placebo studies of childhood depression: baseline predictors of response to treatment and factor analysis of presenting symptoms. Psychopharmacol Bull 24:275–279, 1988

Hunt RD, Capper S, O'Connell P: Clonidine in child and adolescent psychiatry. Journal of Child and Adolescent Psychopharmacology 1:87–102, 1990

Hunt RD, Lau S, Ryu J: Alternative therapies for ADHD, in Ritalin: Theory and Patient Management. Edited by Greenhill LL, Osman BB. New York, Mary Ann Liebert, 1991, pp 75–95

Jatlow PI: Psychotropic drug disposition during development, in Psychiatric Pharmacosciences of Children and Adolescents. Edited by Popper C. Washington, DC, American Psychiatric Press, 1987, pp 27–44

Kafantaris V, Campbell M, Padron-Gayol MV, et al: Carbamazepine in hospitalized aggressive conduct disorder children: an open pilot study. Psychopharmacol Bull 28:193–199, 1992

Kastner T, Friedman DL, Plummer AT, et al: Valproic acid for the treatment of children with mental retardation and mood symptomatology. Pediatrics 86:467–472, 1990

Klauber GT: Clinical efficacy and safety of desmopressin in the treatment of nocturnal enuresis. J Pediatr 114:719–722, 1989

Klein RG: Questioning the clinical usefulness of projective psychological tests for children. J Dev Behav Pediatr 7:378–382, 1986

Klorman R, Brumaghim JT, Fitzpatrick PA, et al: Clinical effects of a controlled trial of methylphenidate on adolescents with attention deficit disorder. J Am Acad Child Adolesc Psychiatry 29:702–709, 1990

Kutcher SP, Reiter S, Gardner DM, et al: The pharmacotherapy of anxiety disorders in children and adolescents. Psychiatr Clin North Am 15:41–67, 1992

Latz SR, McCracken JT: Neuroleptic malignant syndrome in children and adolescents: two case reports and a warning. Journal of Child and Adolescent Psychopharmacology 2:123–129, 1992

Leckman JF, Ort S, Caruso KA, et al: Rebound phenomena in Tourette's syndrome after abrupt withdrawal of clonidine: behavioral, cardiovascular, and neurochemical effects. Arch Gen Psychiatry 43:1168–1176, 1986

Leckman JF, Hardin MT, Riddle MA, et al: Clonidine treatment of Gilles de la Tourette's syndrome. Arch Gen Psychiatry 48:324–328, 1991

Levine MD: Encopresis: its potentiation, evaluation, and alleviation. Pediatr Clin North Am 29:315–330, 1982

Lewinsohn PM, Clarke GN, Hops H, et al: Cognitive-behavioral treatment for depressed adolescents. Behavior Therapy 21:385–401, 1990

Masek BJ, Spirito A, Fentress DW: Behavioral treatment of symptoms of childhood illness. Clinical Psychology Review 4:561–570, 1984

Mikkelsen EJ, Detlor J, Cohen DJ: School avoidance and social phobia triggered by haloperidol in patients with Tourette's disorder. Am J Psychiatry 138:1572–1576, 1981

Moreau D, Mufson L, Weissman MM, et al: Interpersonal psychotherapy for adolescent depression: description of modification and preliminary application. J Am Acad Child Adolesc Psychiatry 30:642–651, 1991

Nehra A, Mullick F, Ishak KG, et al: Pemoline-associated hepatic injury. Gastroenterology 99:1517–1519, 1990

Patterson GR: Families: Applications of Social Learning to Family Life. Champaign, IL, Research Press, 1975

Patterson GR, Forgatch M: Parents and Adolescents Living Together. Eugene, OR, Castalia, 1987

Patterson JF: Hepatitis associated with pemoline. South Med J 77:938, 1984

Pelham WE Jr, Murphy HA: Attention deficit and conduct disorders, in Pharmacological and Behavioral Treatment: An Integrative Approach. Edited by Hersen M. New York, Wiley, 1986, pp 108–148

Pelham WE Jr, Sturges J, Hoza J, et al: The effects of sustained release 20 and 10 mg Ritalin bid on cognitive and social behavior in children with attention deficit disorder. Pediatrics 40:491–501, 1987

Pelham WE Jr, Greenslade KE, Vodde-Hamilton M, et al: Relative efficacy of long-acting stimulants on children with attention deficit-hyperactivity disorder: a comparison of standard methylphenidate, sustained-release methylphenidate, sustained-release dextroamphetamine, and pemoline. Pediatrics 86:226–237, 1990

Pelham WE Jr, Vodde-Hamilton M, Murphy DA, et al: The effects of methylphenidate on ADHD adolescents in recreational, peer group, and classroom settings. Journal of Clinical Child Psychology 20:293–300, 1991

Rapoport JL: Antidepressants in childhood attention deficit disorder and obsessive-compulsive disorder. Psychosomatics 27 (No 11, Suppl):30–36, 1986

Ratey J, Sovner R, Parks A, et al: Buspirone treatment of aggression and anxiety in mentally retarded patients: a multiple-baseline, placebo lead-in study. J Clin Psychiatry 52:159–162, 1991

Realmuto GM, Erickson WD, Yellin AM, et al: Clinical comparison of thiothixene and thioridazine in schizophrenic adolescents. Am J Psychiatry 141:440–442, 1984

Realmuto GM, August GJ, Garfinkel BD: Clinical effect of buspirone in autistic children. J Clin Psychopharmacol 9:122–125, 1989

Reiter S, Kutcher SP: Disinhibition and anger outbursts in adolescents treated with clonazepam. J Clin Psychopharmacol 11:268, 1991

Riddle MA, Hardin MT, King R, et al: Fluoxetine treatment of children and adolescents with Tourette's and obsessive-compulsive disorders: preliminary clinical experience. J Am Acad Child Adolesc Psychiatry 29:45–48, 1990

Ryan ND: Heterocyclic antidepressants in children and adolescents. Journal of Child and Adolescent Psychopharmacology 1:21–31, 1990

Ryan ND: The pharmacologic treatment of child and adolescent depression. Psychiatr Clin North Am 15:29–40, 1992

Ryan ND, Meyer V, Dachille S, et al: Lithium antidepressant augmentation in TCA-refractory depression in adolescents. J Am Acad Child Adolesc Psychiatry 27:371–376, 1988a

Ryan ND, Puig-Antich J, Rabinovich H, et al: MAOIs in adolescent major depression unresponsive to tricyclic antidepressants. J Am Acad Child Adolesc Psychiatry 27:755–758, 1988b

Sallee F, Stiller R, Perel J, et al: Targeting imipramine dose in children with depression. Clin Pharmacol Ther 40:8–13, 1986

Saul RC: Nortriptyline in attention deficit disorder. Clin Neuropharmacol 8:382–384, 1985

Scheidlinger S: Group treatment of adolescents: an overview. Am J Orthopsychiatry 55:102–111, 1985

Schmitt BD: Nocturnal enuresis: an update on treatment. Pediatr Clin North Am 29:21–36, 1982

Silverstein FS, Boxer L, Johnson MV: Hematological monitoring during therapy with carbamazepine in children. Ann Neurol 13:685–686, 1983

Simeon JG, Ferguson HB: Recent developments in the use of antidepressant and anxiolytic medications. Psychiatr Clin North Am 8:893–907, 1985

Simeon JG, Thatte S, Wiggins D: Treatment of adolescent obsessive-compulsive disorder with a clomipramine-fluoxetine combination. Psychopharmacol Bull 26:285–290, 1990

Strayhorn JM Jr, Rapp N, Donina W, et al: Randomized trial of methylphenidate for an autistic child. J Am Acad Child Adolesc Psychiatry 27:244–247, 1988

Strober M, Morrell W, Lampert C, et al: Relapse following discontinuation of lithium maintenance therapy in adolescents with bipolar I illness: a naturalistic study. Am J Psychiatry 147:457–461, 1990

Strober M, Freeman R, Rigali J, et al: The pharmacotherapy of depressive illness in adolescence, II: effects of lithium augmentation in nonresponders to imipramine. J Am Acad Child Adolesc Psychiatry 31:16–20, 1992

Teicher MH, Glod CA: Neuroleptic drugs: indications and guidelines for their rational use in children and adolescents. Journal of Child and Adolescent Psychopharmacology 1:33–56, 1990

Trimble MR: Anticonvulsants in children and adolescents. Journal of Child and Adolescent Psychopharmacology 1:107–124, 1990

Varanka TM, Weller RA, Weller EB, et al: Lithium treatment of manic episodes with psychotic features in prepubertal children. Am J Psychiatry 145:1557–1559, 1988

Varni JW, Jay SM, Masek BJ, et al: Cognitive-behavioral assessment and management of pediatric pain, in Handbook of Psychological Treatment Approaches. Edited by Holvman AD, Turk ED. New York, Pergamon, 1986, pp 168–192

Weller EB, Weller RA, Fristad MA: Lithium dosage guide for prepubertal children: a preliminary report. Journal of the American Academy of Child Psychiatry 25:92–95, 1986

Whitaker A, Rao U: Neuroleptics in pediatric psychiatry. Psychiatr Clin North Am 15:243–276, 1992

Wiles CP, Hardin MT, King RA, et al: Antidepressant-induced prolongation of QTc interval on EKG in two children, in Abstracts of the annual meeting of the American Academy of Child and Adolescent Psychiatry, 1991, p 70

Wilkes TCR, Rush AJ: Adaptations of cognitive therapy for depressed adolescents. J Am Acad Child Adolesc Psychiatry 27:381–386, 1988

Williams DT: Hypnosis as a psychotherapeutic adjunct, in Basic Handbook of Child Psychiatry, Vol 3. Edited by Harrison SI (Noshpitz JD, Editor-in-Chief). New York, Basic Books, 1979, pp 108–116

Williams DT, Mehl R, Yudofsky S, et al: The effect of propranolol on uncontrolled rage outbursts in children and adolescents with organic brain dysfunction. Journal of the American Academy of Child Psychiatry 21:129–135, 1982

Winsberg BG, Perel JM, Hurwic MJ, et al: Imipramine protein binding and pharmacokinetics in children, in The Phenothiazines and Structurally Related Drugs. Edited by Forrest IS, Carr CJ, Usdin E. New York, Raven, 1974, pp 425–431

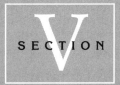

SECTION V

Special Topics

CHAPTER 36

Suicide

T. B. Ghosh, M.D.
Bruce S. Victor, M.D.

The critical issue facing the psychiatric clinician is that of suicide as a "rational" act: can it be a rational act in someone who is suffering from psychiatric illness? The overwhelming majority of suicides, over 90%, are in individuals who are psychiatrically ill at the time of suicide (Black and Winokur 1990).

■ EPIDEMIOLOGY

A knowledge of the demographics and epidemiology of suicide is essential to the clinician for assessing the suicidal patient. Suicide is the ninth leading cause of death in the United States, resulting in 30,000 deaths annually. The rate is almost 11.6 per 100,000 people. Despite suicide prevention programs, more recognition of depression, hospitalization, and advances in biological treatments for depression, the *overall* rate of suicide has not changed over the last several decades: it has remained in the range of 11 to 12 per 100,000 (Sainsbury 1986b; Stevenson 1988). One of the few identified factors that correlate with the *overall* rate of suicide is the availability of the means to suicide.

Although the overall rate of suicide has remained constant over the last several decades, rates among different subgroups of age, sex, and race have changed. The highly publicized increase in adolescent and youth suicide appears to have been offset by a declining rate of suicide among older adults (Robins and Kulbok 1988. The rates for both white and black females are relatively constant and low compared with that for males. The rate for black males peaks between ages 20 and 40, declines, and then increases again after age 75. Finally, and most strikingly, the high rate of completed suicides in white males, initially peaking between ages 20 and 40, levels off between ages 40 and 65 and then rapidly increases after age 65. The suicide rate is extraordinary for white males at ages 85 and over (i.e., 50 suicides per 100,000). The general demographics for persons at low or high risk for completed suicide are presented in Table 36–1.

☐ Parasuicide

Self-destructive behavior and nonfatal suicide attempts, although difficult to categorize, have been conceptualized as *parasuicide*. The distinction between parasuicide and complete suicide is important: parasuicidal patients usually recognize that the means are nonlethal, and these patients have different characteristics than patients who display lethal suicidal behavior. It is estimated that about 23 persons attempt suicide for every 1 who completes it. Suicide attempts are more likely in females, whereas completions are more likely in males. Suicide attempters are more likely to be young (under age 35), whereas completers are more likely to be older (over age 60). The attempter's methods tend to be of low lethality. The patient who makes the suicide attempt in the context of being at home or where he or she can be discovered is in contrast to the patient who chooses an isolated setting where there is a very low chance for rescue. Finally, certain psychiatric diagnoses in suicidal patients have been found to be associated with either suicide attempt or suicide completion. Suicidal patients with adjustment disorders and personality disorders (especially Cluster B personality disorders) are more likely to make nonlethal suicide attempts, whereas suicidal patients with mood disorders, psychoses, and substance abuse problems tend to go on to be completers.

☐ Suicide and Psychiatric Illness

Epidemiological surveys have demonstrated that the vast majority of completed suicides are in patients with diagnosable psychiatric conditions.

Table 36–1. Suicide risk: general demographics

Low risk	High risk
Under age 45	Over age 45
Female	Male
Nonwhite	White
Lives with others	Lives alone
Good health	Poor health

Suicide and Mood Disorders

Mood disorder is the diagnostic category most often represented among persons who suicide. It has been estimated that about 15% of patients with mood disorders will go on to commit suicide (Sainsbury 1986a). Patients with delusional depressive features are at five times greater risk for suicide than patients with other mood disorders (Roose et al. 1983). The rate of suicide completion associated with untreated bipolar disorder has been noted to be as high as 20% (Goodwin and Jamison 1990). Most authors agree that the predisposing factor is not the manic state itself but rather the presence of depression that accompanies a mixed bipolar state. Clinical experience suggests that the mixed bipolar state is associated with a particularly high risk of suicide because of the dangerous combination of highly dysphoric mood and a high level of energy and perturbation. Also, the bipolar II patient group is frequently associated with suicide (Goldring and Fieve 1984). In the absence of frank mania, the bipolar II patient's condition may be underdiagnosed, and the patient may inadvertently be denied a trial of mood stabilizers; consequently, persistent cycling and affective lability may predispose to suicide.

Although sparse data are available on the rate of suicide in a treated population, clinical experience suggests that it is significantly less than 15%. For example, in the National Institute of Mental Health Collaborative Program on the Psychobiology of Depression (Fawcett et al. 1990), the rate of completed suicide was only 3% over 10 years.

Suicide and Anxiety

One of the most important findings of recent years is that anxiety, particularly panic attacks, is a major short-term risk factor in suicide. Fawcett et al. (1990) reported results of a 10-year follow-up of 954 patients with major affective disorders. The authors outlined nine factors that were correlated with suicide. Six of the factors were correlated with suicide within the first year of the follow-up: panic attacks, severe psychic anxiety, diminished concentration, global insomnia, alcohol abuse, and anhedonia. These factors, including the possibility of alcohol as a self-medication for anxiety, demonstrated the importance of anxiety symptoms as markers of short-term suicide risk. The three factors that were found to correlate with suicide *after* the first year, in the subsequent 9 years of the study, were the risk factors that had been identified in prior studies: history of previous suicide attempts, suicidal ideation, and hopelessness. These findings have a major importance clinically because they are factors that can be modified, which highlights the importance of aggressively treating anxiety, panic, and insomnia in patients with mood disorders.

Suicide and Chemical Dependence

Chemical dependence, on either alcohol or drugs, increases the suicide risk in a patient fivefold. It is important to note in this diagnostic group that although alcohol is the single most prevalent substance, the majority of suicides occur in those persons with multiple substance abuse. After mood disorders, chemical dependence represents the most frequently encountered diagnosis among victims of suicide (Marzuk and Mann 1988). There are some general characteristics of chemically dependent persons who complete suicide. These persons tend to be young males who use alcohol and other drugs *concurrently*, who have a history of overdoses, and who have comorbid psychiatric disorders, especially depressive disorders. Although suicide in persons who abuse substances occurs after many years into the illness, it tends to occur abruptly, often within 6 weeks of interpersonal loss.

Depressive disorder and substance abuse constitute a particularly lethal combination (Jaffe and Ciraulo 1986), one that highlights the importance of recognition of depression in the alcoholic patient. These depressive symptoms can be the result of underlying affective illness, but can also result from the direct toxic effects of alcohol, impaired hepatic function, and poor nutrition, as well as organic brain syndromes from head trauma. Another problem is that patients with comorbid psychiatric and substance use disorders exhibit poor compliance with their medication regimen (Drake et al. 1989). Moreover, comorbid psychiatric conditions, especially affective illness, are often undertreated, consequently increasing the likelihood of suicidal behavior.

Acute intoxication also increases suicide risk. Alcohol and drugs may produce disinhibition and remove the remaining constraints to suicide in a given chemically dependent individual, and thus serve as an acute precipitant to suicide. Furthermore, the disinhibition and poor judgment associated with the intoxicated state can result in high-risk behaviors such as auto accidents and drug overdoses. Such events are sometimes considered "accidental" suicidal behavior in this fatalistic population.

Suicide and Schizophrenia

Approximately 10% of patients with schizophrenia complete suicide (Miles 1977). The majority of the suicides in schizophrenic patients are in young males: in a review of studies from the 1980s, 73% of victims were male and the mean age at death was 33 (Weiden and Roy 1992). Also of interest is that in schizophrenia suicide risk is *not* greatest during the active hallucinatory phase; schizophrenic patients are more likely to complete suicide when the psychosis is under control and they are in a depressive recovery phase of the illness. (In this regard, schizophrenia can be contrasted to depression, in which suicide risk is increased during the psychotic delusional phase.) Schizophrenic patients at greatest risk are young men, usually in the first few years of the illness, who are in remission and nonpsychotic, but who remain depressed

A meta-analysis of studies (Breier and Astrachan 1984; Drake et al. 1984; Roy 1982) revealed that of 65 completed suicides among schizophrenic patients, only 2 could be attributed to command hallucinations; however, Weiden and Roy (1992) suggest that these meta-analyses may be biased by secondary treatment effects. These authors note that clinicians are more likely to hospitalize schizophrenic persons for psychotic symptoms than for depressive symptoms. Thus, the schizophrenic person who is actively experiencing command hallucinations gets hospitalized and the suicide is prevented; in contrast, the demoralized psychologically distressed patient tends to not be hospitalized and may not be protected from suicidal behavior.

Suicide risk in schizophrenia, as with other disorders, appears to be greatest during the post–inpatient hospitalization period. This finding is consistent with the observation that the greatest risk occurs not during the psychotic period but more after the psychosis has resolved. At that time patients actually have more insight into their condition and may more clearly recognize the reality of their situation. Later, in their outpatient course, patients may have developed better coping strategies and adapted to their new life circumstance.

Suicide and Borderline Personality Disorder

The incidence of completed suicide in borderline patients ranges from 3% to 8% (McGlashan and Heinssen 1988; Stone et al. 1987). Thus, the overall rate of completed suicide in this group is less than that in patients with primary affective disorders, substance abuse, or schizophrenia.

Jacobs (1992) has proposed a model of assessment of suicide in the borderline patient that focuses on three areas:

1. The specific dynamics of the borderline individual that would place the person at higher risk.
2. The coexistence of other psychiatric disorders that would place the individual at high risk.
3. The suicide perspective, which includes identification of psychological commonalities of suicide and objectification of suicidal intent and behavior.

With regard to specific borderline psychopathology, Kernberg (1984) outlines particular characteristics that are associated with high risk for suicide: impulsivity, hopelessness, despair, antisocial features, and interpersonal aloofness. He also describes characteristics of patients for whom chronic self-mutilation and suicide attempts are a "way of life" and that thus may predispose more to parasuicide than to completed suicide. "Infantile masochistic" patients use suicidal behavior to maintain connection. These behaviors tend to arise at times of intense rage attacks or rage mixed with temporary depressive flare-ups. The behaviors are designed to establish control over the environment by evoking guilt feelings in others, for example, after the breakup of an interpersonal relationship.

The second component of the model is the evaluation of coexisting psychiatric disorders. Although it is unclear whether comorbid disorders, in fact, increase the suicide risk, it is clinically important to recognize and vigorously treat these conditions in borderline patients. Particular attention should be paid to comorbid affective illness, substance abuse, eating disorders, and posttraumatic stress disorder.

The third component of the tripartite assessment model, the suicide perspective, consists of objectification of suicidal intent and the identification of specific psychological commonalities and psychodynamic formulations. After identifying suicidal ideation, it is important to measure actual suicide intent. The clinician needs to determine the patient's ability to control suicidal thoughts, distinguish between active suicidal thoughts and passive suicidal thoughts, determine the patient's reasons for living and dying, determine the degree to which a suicidal plan has been developed, and evaluate the deterrence to carrying out such a plan (e.g., the impact on the family, loved ones).

■ PSYCHOLOGICAL FACTORS IN SUICIDAL BEHAVIOR

There is a high association with hopelessness in long-term suicide risk. Not specific to depression, hopelessness can accompany demoralization with a number of other syndromes: schizophrenia, anxiety disorders, and chronic conditions, including medical conditions. This factor can be measured with the Beck Hopelessness Scale, which assesses the degree to which a person holds negative expectations about the future (Beck and Steer 1988). Hendin (1991) identified desperation as another important factor in suicide. Desperation implies not only a sense of hopelessness about change but a sense that life is impossible without such change. Guilt was also found to be an affective component of desperation.

Classical psychoanalytic theory postulated the importance of aggression toward the self in suicidal behavior. Freud (1917[1915]/1957) described suicide as a murderous attack on an internalized object that had become a source of ambivalence. Thus, from a psychological sense, the introjected love object is the focus of the attack. More recent studies, however, demonstrate that aggression toward others often goes hand in hand with suicidal behavior. Suicide was usually associated with conscious rage in the violent individuals studied, and rage should therefore be viewed as an important psychological factor underlying suicidal behavior (Hendin 1991). Shame and humiliation are two other factors that sometimes underlie suicide. Psychiatrically ill patients may feel shame related to suicidal ideation and may be reluctant to seek treatment or rely on support systems.

■ SUICIDE IN SPECIAL POPULATIONS

□ Suicide and the Elderly

The suicide rate doubles to quadruples in patients over age 65, especially in white males. Factors predisposing to this are social isolation, loss of spouse, anxiety due to financial instability, and, finally, undertreated mood disorders. The prevalence of mood disorders is probably not higher in this age group, but the disorders probably are underrecognized and undertreated. Depression may go underrecognized in elderly persons because of the atypical features in this population, including masked depression and pseudodementia (i.e., the artificially reduced cognitive capacities resulting from a primary depressive condition). Finally, indirect self-destructive behavior is often seen in institutional settings for the elderly, when individuals refuse to accept medications or medical care, refuse to take part in activities, and get into control struggles with caregivers (Morgan 1989).

□ Suicide and Youth

The rate of adolescent suicide has increased dramatically since 1960. The rate of suicide in adolescent males (white and nonwhite) from 1960 to 1980 almost tripled. Adolescent female suicides have increased two- to threefold. Factors that may have contributed to this increase are the rise in depressive disorders among youths, the rise in the divorce rate, the dissolution of the nuclear family, and the availability of firearms (Pfeffer 1988). Males are at greater risk than females, and whites are at greater risk than nonwhites, for *completed* suicide. Exposure to suicide is also an important factor: for certain individuals, experiencing suicide in a family member or friend appears to make suicide more "permissible." This phenomenon may be at play in the "cluster" suicides observed in youth. A suicide in school or one that receives media attention tends to be imitated.

Although there are environmental and sociocultural factors, the importance of psychopathology in youth suicide cannot be overestimated.

In the adolescent the main diagnoses are depression and conduct disorder, especially with antisocial behaviors. Hostility, aggression, and assaultiveness are also correlated with suicide. Suicide in youth, as in other populations, often goes hand in hand with hostility, not only toward the self but toward others.

☐ Suicide in Patients With HIV/AIDS

There is a high prevalence of suicidal ideation among patients afflicted with HIV. Oftentimes suicidal ideation comes in the form of a need to maintain control, especially in a syndrome such as AIDS in which a patient can rapidly develop encephalopathy and dementia. These patients have often seen others in their peer group become, over a short period of time, demented and unable to care for themselves. Patients may develop a view of suicide as a legitimate way out before the demise into debilitation or dementia.

The risk of suicide in persons with AIDS is greater than that in the general population (Zeck et al. 1988). In an epidemiological study of New York City residents, the suicide rate for men with AIDS was 680 per 100,000 persons per year, whereas for a comparison group of men ages 20 to 59 without a diagnosis of AIDS the suicide rate was 18 per 100,000 persons per year. The suicide rate in the AIDS patients was 36 times that in age-matched men without AIDS (Marzuk et al. 1988).

■ BIOLOGICAL ASPECTS OF SUICIDAL BEHAVIOR

The possible importance of biological factors in suicidal behavior was suggested by studies of completed suicide demonstrating a much higher concordance rate for monozygotic twins than dizygotic twins. Later studies examining biological relatives of adoptees who committed suicide found a significantly higher incidence of suicide than in the biological relatives of control subjects (Schulsinger et al. 1979). These results argue for the possible existence of a genetic predisposition toward suicidal behavior.

In the last decade there has been a proliferation of studies detailing more direct examination of the neurochemical functioning of suicidal patients that further distinguishes them from nonsuicidal patients. Although several neurochemical factors have been implicated, the main focus has been on alterations in serotonergic transmission in the central nervous system (CNS).

☐ Postmortem Studies of Suicide Victims

The initial postmortem studies of brains of suicide victims began as a quest to determine underlying biochemical derangements in depressed patients because, at that time, it was assumed that all suicide victims were depressed. Stemming from research involving platelets, it was found that imipramine binding might serve as a measure of presynaptic serotonergic functioning. Four of five studies demonstrated decreased imipramine binding not only in the cortex but also in the hypothalamus (Table 36–2), suggesting decreased presynergetic serotonergic transmission in persons who suicide. Several studies have noted an increase in serotonin$_2$ (5-HT$_2$) receptor binding in the frontal and prefrontal cortex of suicide victims. These findings suggest that there is a postsynaptic compensation for the overall decrease in serotonergic transmission in suicidal patients.

Recent postmortem studies of suicide victims have focused on other neurotransmitter systems. Studies of suicide victims found increases in beta-adrenergic receptor binding not only in the prefrontal cortex but also in the temporal cortex (Mann et al. 1986). One study found that binding sites for corticotropin-releasing factor (CRF) were reduced in the frontal cortex of persons who committed suicide (Nemeroff et al. 1988). This finding is consistent with previous research which found that patients with clinically significant depression have increased CRF in the CSF, suggesting that the reduction of CRF binding sites in the postmortem study represents a downregulation in response to the increase in

Table 36–2.   Postmortem receptor studies of completed suicides: serotonergic receptor findings

Study	Findings
Imipramine binding	
Stanley et al. 1982	⇓ [^{3}H]imipramine binding in cortex
Paul et al. 1984	⇓ [^{3}H]imipramine binding in hypothalamus
Perry et al. 1983[a]	⇓ [^{3}H]imipramine binding in cortex
Crow et al. 1984	⇓ [^{3}H]imipramine binding in cortex
Myerson et al. 1982	⇑ [^{3}H]imipramine binding in cortex
5-HT$_2$ binding	
Stanley and Mann 1983	⇑ 5-HT binding in cortex
Mann et al. 1986	⇑ 5-HT binding in cortex
Meltzer et al. 1987	⇑ 5-HT binding in cortex
Owen et al. 1983	[Nonsignificant increase in 5-HT binding in cortex]
Cheetam et al. 1987	⇓ 5-HT binding in cortex

Note.   5-HT = 5-hydroxytryptamine (serotonin).
[a]Depressed patients dying of natural causes.

CRF (Nemeroff et al. 1984). This finding also dovetails with some studies that suggest an increased capacity for the dysregulation of the hypothalamic-pituitary-adrenal axis as measured by the dexamethasone suppression test (Targum et al. 1983).

☐ Cerebrospinal Fluid Studies of Suicide Attempters

Although the study of biogenic amines and their breakdown products in the CSF reflects a somewhat derivative measure of actual neuronal transmission, a very high positive correlation between 5-HIAA found in the brain at autopsy and in the CSF has been demonstrated. Therefore, the studies of CSF 5-HIAA can be considered reflective of CNS functioning, further corroborating the postmortem literature cited above regarding underlying neurobiological dysfunction in suicidal patients.

The initial studies of CSF in depressed patients also attempted to distinguish between biochemically distinct forms of depression. That patients who had made suicide attempts had low levels of 5-HIAA was significant not only from the standpoint of biochemically distinguishing those patients who had attempted suicide, but also from the perspective of predicting future suicidal behavior. One of the initial studies demonstrated that 21% of patients who had been hospitalized after a suicide attempt and had been found to have low levels of CSF 5-HIAA actually committed suicide within 1 year after the original evaluation (Åsberg et al. 1976). Other studies corroborated the initial finding that depressed patients whose CSF levels of 5-HIAA were subnormal were more likely to have attempted suicide (Banki 1981; Träskman et al. 1981). Interestingly, however, suicidal and nonsuicidal patients with *bipolar* disorder could not be distinguished on the basis of their CSF 5-HIAA (Berrettini et al. 1986).

Decreases in CSF 5-HIAA have also been shown to distinguish between schizophrenic patients who had attempted suicide and those who had not (Roy et al. 1985). This measure also distinguished suicidal patients with personality disorders as well as alcoholic patients with a history of suicide attempts (Brown et al. 1979). These findings further support not only the idea that suicidal behavior is not merely an end result of clinical depression, but also that serotonergic dysfunction may well underlie suicidal behavior in patients across diagnoses. That low levels of 5-HIAA may actually represent a trait disorder is further suggested by the lack of a temporal relationship between the suicide attempt and the CSF 5-HIAA level.

Most recently, a study of violent suicide attempters demonstrated not only lower levels of CSF 5-HIAA but also significantly increased CSF levels of MHPG (3-methoxy-4-hydroxyphenylglycol), the chief metabolic breakdown product of norepinephrine (Träskman-Bendz et al. 1992).

This finding appears to corroborate previous research which suggested that serotonin is an inhibitory neurotransmitter of the noradrenergic system and that heightened noradrenergic turnover in the face of diminished serotonergic input may well represent a significant part of the biochemical underpinnings of violent suicide.

☐ Platelet Studies and Pharmacological Challenge Tests

Because lumbar puncture is generally not performed in the office, investigators have recently searched for alternative methods of assessing the neurochemical functioning. One method of testing the integrity of the serotonergic system is to measure prolactin or cortisol release in response to pharmacological agents such as fenfluramine. Studies have demonstrated that prolactin response to fenfluramine is blunted in patients who have attempted suicide (Coccaro et al. 1989; De Meo et al. 1988).

Other studies have demonstrated that the number of platelet 5-HT$_2$ receptors is increased in suicidal patients (Pandey et al. 1990). This finding is interesting not only because of its consistency with similar changes in the CNS, but also because the relative ease of a venipuncture may provide a more accessible avenue for assessment of serotonergic functioning. However, a recent study (Mann et al. 1992) demonstrated that there was no actual correlation between CSF 5-HIAA and platelet 5-HT$_2$ receptor binding.

Measuring urine metabolites of neurochemicals might provide another peripheral measure of underlying biological differences between suicidal and nonsuicidal patients. Studies have demonstrated increased urinary cortisol, particularly among patients who attempted suicide by violent means. One group found that patients with depression who attempted suicide had significantly lowered levels of dopamine, homovanillic acid (HVA), and DOPAC (dihydrophenylacetic acid) compared with nonsuicidal depressed patients (Roy et al. 1992).

■ ASSESSMENT OF THE SUICIDAL PATIENT

The evaluation of suicidal ideation or behavior is done in a manner similar to the investigation of any symptom cluster that might have adverse medical consequences. First, the clinician maintains an index of suspicion stemming from the demographic characteristics of suicide. Then, the clinician must individualize the assessment to the patient—specifically by considering personal and family history, assessing current medical and psychiatric status, determining psychosocial assets and liabilities, and taking into consideration prior response to treatment.

In taking a personal history of suicidal ideation, it is quintessential to evaluate the patient's level of intention of acting upon such ideation. Furthermore, one must always inquire as to the presence of a plan of suicide action, paying particular attention to the steps already taken to implement such a plan as well as assessing its potential lethality. The availability of means must be assessed, ranging from stockpile medications to firearms. One should also inquire as to whether the patient has taken any specific actions in preparation for death such as purchasing a gun, writing a will, or giving away prized objects. It is also important to inquire about the presence of other symptoms that have been associated with a higher suicide risk: these include delusional symptoms (particular command hallucinations), anhedonia, hopelessness, and severe anxiety.

It is essential to obtain a history of prior suicide attempts as well as a history of violence and impulsivity. In addition, the presence of substance abuse should be assessed, because, as noted earlier in this chapter, it also has been associated with an increased risk of suicide. Patients with a family history of suicide as well as of violence might also alert the clinician to the presence of a liability to more dangerous suicidal behavior. The clinician must also inquire about the circumstances of previous violence as well as whether the patient thinks this behavior is abnormal or unusual. The clinician should also attempt to determine whether the violence is tied to a specific mood state.

A complete evaluation for suicide potential also includes the assessment of an individual's strengths. Despite the presence of suicidal behavior, it may well be that an individual has a proven ability not only to control his or her behavior but also to bring familial or financial resources to bear upon his or her situation. A *motivation to seek help in general,* and meaningful psychiatric treatment in particular, should be determined. As part of this assessment, the clinician should become familiar with the patient's prior responses to treatment, including responses to pharmacotherapeutic intervention as well as psychotherapy and psychosocial support.

Several more formal methods of suicide risk assessment have been used in research settings with varying degrees of success. One of the best developed scales is the Risk Estimator Scale for Suicide (Motto et al. 1985). This scale was the result of a 2-year prospective study of 2,753 patients with depression or suicidality in which completed suicides were noted. Fifteen variables were incorporated into a scale that gives an estimated risk of suicide in 2 years (Table 36–3).

■ TREATMENT OF THE SUICIDAL PATIENT

Suicidal behavior is a syndrome that cuts across rigid diagnostic lines. As such, it is important that this behavior be addressed apart from, and in

Table 36–3. Final set of variables from Risk Estimator Scale for Suicide (Motto et al. 1985)

Variable	High-risk category	Coefficient (weight)	Standard error	P
1. Age	Risk increases with age	0.273[a]	.092	.001
2. Occupation	Executive, administrator, owner of business, professional, semi-skilled worker	0.515	.206	.013
3. Financial resources	Risk increases with resources	0.373	.120	.002
4. Emotional disorder in family	Depression, alcoholism	0.486	.195	.013
5. Sexual orientation	Bisexual, active; homosexual, inactive	0.692	.252	.006
6. Previous psychiatric hospital admissions	Risk increases with number of admissions	0.228	.079	.004
7. Result of previous efforts to obtain help	Negative or variable	0.593	.199	.003
8. Threatened financial loss	Yes	0.674	.271	.013
9. Special stress	Severe	0.676	.191	.000
10. Sleep (hours per night)	Risk increases with number of hours per night	0.395	.161	.014
11. Weight change, present episode	Gain or 1%–9% loss	0.646	.241	.013
12. Ideas of persecution or reference	Yes	0.636	.198	.014
13. Suicidal impulses	Yes	1.071	.227	.000
14. Seriousness of present suicide attempt—intent	Unambivalent or ambivalent but weighted toward suicide	0.943	.201	.000
15. Interviewer's reaction to subject	Risk increases with negativity of reaction	0.454	.163	.006

[a]Applied to square root of age.

addition to, the ostensible underlying psychiatric condition. The clinician must first confront his or her own feelings, however unpleasant or embarrassing, regarding the patient. Initially, it may well seem to the patient that his or her alliance with the clinician is his or her only tie to life.

Ultimately, the patient and clinician must arrive at a mutually agreeable contract regarding further courses of action to be taken based on their alliance.

Principles of acute intervention, as delineated by Blumenthal (1990), begin with adequate supervision of the suicidal patient. If this cannot be sufficiently accomplished in an outpatient setting, hospitalization, whether on a voluntary or involuntary basis, should be considered. It is also necessary to limit the patient's access to potentially self-destructive methods, principal among which is antidepressant medication. It is a poignant irony that medicinal compounds specifically designed to combat conditions leading to suicide are extremely lethal when taken in overdosage. The clinician should be keenly aware of lethal indexes of medications and prescribe only small amounts at a time. Although the clinician cannot eliminate all other potential means to suicide, he or she must make an effort to reduce the risk. This may involve, for example, contracting with the patient for him or her to give up access to firearms that may be in his or her possession, and, at times, even convincing the patient to agree to have knives and other sharp instruments under another person's lock and key.

□ Somatic Treatment

In general, the aim of biological therapy in the treatment of suicidal patients has been to treat the diagnosed psychiatric condition. As a result, there have been few studies describing the response of suicidal behavior, per se, to specific pharmacotherapeutic interventions. With the advent of medications that selectively affect the serotonergic system, one might expect these medications to be associated with more significant amelioration of suicidal behavior than either tricyclic antidepressants or antidepressants that promote noradrenergic transmission.

Teicher et al. (1990) reported six cases of the emergence of severe suicidal preoccupation in patients undergoing treatment with fluoxetine, a selective serotonin reuptake inhibitor (SSRI). Another study noted the emergence of self-destructive behavior in six children and adolescents receiving fluoxetine (King et al. 1991). The dramatic impact of these studies was to draw attention to the possibility of "paradoxical reactions" of antidepressants: the agents appeared to produce or intensify the symptoms that they were ostensibly introduced to treat. Although the above studies seemed to popularize the notion of such paradoxical reactions, the emergency of new-onset suicidality, intensification of previously existing suicidality, and increased assaultiveness had already been reported with tricyclic antidepressants.

Appearance or worsening of suicidal behavior exists with a wide variety of antidepressants, although this phenomenon probably affects fewer than 6% of the patients treated (Mann and Kapur 1991). What mechanisms might explain the production of this paradoxical effect? One explanation is that this phenomenon occurs as a result of drug-induced akathisia. In fact, neuroleptic-induced akathisia, which is initially indistinguishable from that induced by some antidepressants, has been associated with increased acting-out behaviors as well as increased suicide attempts.

Interestingly, other studies suggest that serotonergic agents may selectively decrease suicidality and impulsiveness not only in patients with major depressive disorder but also in patients with borderline personality disorder (Cornelius et al. 1991). A recent study compared the relative effectiveness of serotonergic antidepressants with that of noradrenergic antidepressants in the treatment of patients with major depressive disorders who had already made suicide attempts; the serotonergic antidepressants were found to be significantly more effective in the treatment of these patients (Sacchetti et al. 1991). This is an intriguing finding in light of the posited serotonergic hypofunction in suicidal patients. However, literature to date is too preliminary to support the hypothesis that SSRIs are the antidepressants of choice in the suicidal patient because of their neurotransmitter action. Rather, SSRIs and other new-generation antidepressants may be viewed as more prudent choices over tricyclic antidepressants because of their low lethality index.

Finally, the role of ECT cannot be overemphasized as a safe and relatively rapid somatic treatment for the acutely suicidal depressed patient.

☐ Psychotherapy With the Suicidal Patient

The risk of suicide seems to correlate inversely with the maintenance of ongoing personal and professional relationships. Thus, one of the daunting tasks in the psychotherapy of the suicidal patient is the realization that the psychotherapist may be perceived as the last ballast of hope that human connectedness may be yet something worth striving for. The establishment of the therapeutic alliance, then, is the singularly most important task in the treatment of the suicidal patient.

The establishment of the therapeutic alliance is common to all of the psychotherapeutic traditions. There is no "suicide-specific" psychotherapy, and clinicians are increasingly aware of the value of integrating principles from psychodynamic and cognitive-behavior therapy. An important contribution of cognitive psychology has been the identification of hopelessness as the psychological factor most consistent with suicidal intent—even more so than the subjective experience of depression (Weisman et al. 1979). The emphasis in cognitive therapy of suicidal behavior is the correction of cognitive distortions that may have resulted in the perception of hopelessness, and the therapist strives to instill hope in this process. Also, to the degree that depression or hopelessness has led to deterioration of problem-solving abilities, therapy is geared to the enhancement of those skills, including increasing the patient's capacity to view options and alternatives to suicide.

Psychodynamic psychotherapies have stemmed from an understanding of the dynamics of the individual's suicidal motivation, as well as of the act itself (Dulit and Michels 1992). In addition, the psychodynamic literature offers very useful insights regarding countertransference pitfalls in the treatment of suicidal patients. It is necessary for therapists to address countertransferential feelings in themselves. This is necessary less to expunge oneself of "incorrect" feelings than to realize how one's refusal to acknowledge them might lead to the subversion of the therapeutic alliance (Maltsberger and Buie 1974).

■ REFERENCES

Åsberg M, Thorèn P, Träskman L, et al: Serotonin depression: a biochemical subgroup within affective disorders? Science 191:478–480, 1976

Banki CM: Factors influencing monoamine metabolites and tryptophan in patients with alcohol dependence. J Neural Transm 50:89–101, 1981

Beck AT, Steer RA: Manual for the Beck Hopelessness Scale. San Antonio, TX, Psychological Corporation, 1988

Berrettini WH, Nurnberger JI Jr, Narrow W, et al: Cerebrospinal fluid studies of bipolar patients with and without a history of suicide attempts. Ann N Y Acad Sci 487:197–201, 1986

Black DW, Winokur G: Suicide and psychiatric diagnosis, in Suicide Over the Life Cycle: Risk Factors, Assessment, and Treatment of Suicidal Patients. Edited by Blumenthal SJ, Kupfer DJ. Washington, DC, American Psychiatric Press, 1990, pp 135–153

Blumenthal SJ: An overview and synopsis of risk factors, assessment, and treatment of suicidal patients over the life cycle, in Suicide Over the Life Cycle: Risk Factors, Assessment, and Treatment of Suicidal Patients. Edited by Blumenthal SJ, Kupfer DJ. Washington, DC, American Psychiatric Press, 1990, pp 685–733

Breier A, Astrachan BM: Characterization of schizophrenic patients who commit suicide. Am J Psychiatry 141:206–209, 1984

Brown GL, Goodwin FK, Ballenger JC, et al: Aggression in humans correlates with cerebrospinal fluid amine metabolites. Psychiatry Res 1:131–139, 1979

Cheetam SC, Cross AJ, Crompton MR, et al: Serotonin and GABA function in depressed suicide victims. Abstract of presentation at the International Conference on New Directions in Affective Disorders, Jerusalem, 1987

Coccaro EF, Siever LJ, Klar HM, et al: Serotonergic studies in patients with affective and personality disorders: correlates with suicidal and impulsive aggressive behavior. Arch Gen Psychiatry 46:587–599, 1989

Cornelius JR, Soloff PH, Perel JM, et al: A preliminary trial of fluoxetine in refractory borderline patients. J Clin Psychopharmacol 11:116–120, 1991

Crow TJ, Cross A, Cooper SJ, et al: Neurotransmitter receptors and monoamine metabolites in the brains of patients with Alzheimer-type dementia and depression, and suicides. Neuropharmacology 23:1561–1569, 1984

De Meo MD, McBride PA, Mann JJ, et al: Fenfluramine challenge in major depression, in New Research and Abstracts, 141st annual meeting of the American Psychiatric Association, Montreal, Quebec, May 1988, NR169, p 91

Drake RE, Gates C, Cotton PG, et al: Suicide among schizophrenics: who is at risk? J Nerv Ment Dis 172:613–617, 1984

Drake RE, Osher FC, Wallach MA: Alcohol use and abuse in schizophrenia: a prospective community study. J Nerv Ment Dis 177:408–414, 1989

Dulit RA, Michels R: Psychodynamics and suicide, in Suicide and Clinical Practice. Edited by Jacobs D. Washington, DC, American Psychiatric Press, 1992, pp 43–53

Fawcett J, Scheftner WA, Fogg L, et al: Time-related predictors of suicide in major affective disorder. Am J Psychiatry 147:1189–1194, 1990

Freud S: Mourning and melancholia (1917[1915]), in Standard Edition of the Complete Psychological Works of Sigmund Freud, Vol 14. Translated and edited by Strachey J. London, Hogarth, 1957, pp 237–260

Goldring N, Fieve RR: Attempted suicide in manic-depressive disorder. Am J Psychother 38:373–383, 1984

Goodwin FK, Jamison KR: Manic-Depressive Illness. New York, Oxford University Press, 1990

Hendin H: Psychodynamics of suicide, with particular reference to the young. Am J Psychiatry 148:1150–1158, 1991

Jacobs D: Evaluating and treating suicidal behavior in the borderline patient, in Suicide and Clinical Practice. Edited by Jacobs D. Washington, DC, American Psychiatric Press, 1992, pp 115–130

Jaffe JH, Ciraulo DA: Alcoholism and depression, in Psychopathology and Addictive Disorders. Edited by Meyer RE. New York, Guilford, 1986, pp 293–320

Kernberg OF: Severe Personality Disorders: Psychotherapeutic Strategies. New Haven, CT, Yale University Press, 1984

King RA, Riddle MA, Chappell PB, et al: Emergence of self-destructive phenomena in children and adolescents during fluoxetine treatment. J Am Acad Child Adolesc Psychiatry 30:179–186, 1991

Maltsberger JT, Buie DH: Countertransference hate in the treatment of suicidal patients. Arch Gen Psychiatry 30:625–633, 1974

Mann JJ, Kapur S: The emergence of suicidal ideation and behavior during antidepressant pharmacotherapy. Arch Gen Psychiatry 48:1027–1033, 1991

Mann JJ, Stanley M, McBride PA, et al: Increased serotonin$_2$ and β-adrenergic receptor binding in the frontal cortices of suicide victims. Arch Gen Psychiatry 43:954–959, 1986

Mann JJ, McBride PA, Brown RP, et al: Relationship between central and peripheral serotonin indexes in depressed and suicidal psychiatric inpatients. Arch Gen Psychiatry 49:442–446, 1992

Marzuk PM, Mann JJ: Suicide and substance abuse. Psychiatric Annals 18:639–645, 1988

Marzuk PM, Tierney H, Tardiff K, et al: Increased risk of suicide in persons with AIDS. JAMA 259:1333–1337, 1988

McGlashan TH, Heinssen RK: Hospital discharge status and long-term outcome for patients with schizophrenia, schizoaffective disorders, borderline personality disorder, and unipolar affective disorder. Arch Gen Psychiatry 45:363–368, 1988

Meltzer HY, Nash JF, Ohmori T, et al: Neuroendocrine and biochemical studies in serotonin and dopamine in depression and suicide. Abstract of presentation at the International Conference on New Directions in Affective Disorders, Jerusalem, 1987

Miles CP: Conditions predisposing to suicide: a review. J Nerv Ment Dis 164:231–246, 1977

Morgan AC: Special issues of assessment and treatment of suicide risk in the elderly, in Suicide: Understanding and Response. Edited by Jacobs D, Brown HN. Madison, CT, International Universities Press, 1989, pp 239–256

Motto JA, Heilbron DC, Juster RP: Development of a clinical instrument to estimate suicide risk. Am J Psychiatry 142:680–686, 1985

Myerson LR, Wennogle LP, Abel MS, et al: Human brain receptor alterations in suicide victims. Pharmacol Biochem Behav 17:159–163, 1982

Nemeroff CB, Widerlov E, Bissette G, et al: Elevated concentrations of CSF corticotropin releasing factor–like immunoreactivity in depressed patients. Science 226:1342–1344, 1984

Nemeroff CB, Owens MJ, Bissette G, et al: Reduced corticotropin releasing factor binding sites in the frontal cortex of suicide victims. Arch Gen Psychiatry 45:577–579, 1988

Owen F, Cross A, Crow TJ, et al: Brain 5-HT$_2$ receptors and suicide. Lancet 2:1256, 1983

Pandey GN, Pandey SC, Janicak PG, et al: Platelet serotonin-2 receptor binding sites in depression and suicide. Biol Psychiatry 28:215–222, 1990

Paul SM, Rehavi M, Skolnick P, et al: High affinity binding of antidepressants to a biogenic amine transport site in human brain and platelet: studies in depression, in Neurobiology of Mood Disorders. Edited by Post RM, Ballenger JC. Baltimore, MD, Williams & Wilkins, 1984, pp 845–853

Perry EK, Marshall EF, Blessed G, et al: Decreased imipramine binding in the brains of patients with depressive illness. Br J Psychiatry 142:188–192, 1983

Pfeffer CR: Risk factors associated with youth suicide: a clinical perspective. Psychiatric Annals 18:652–656, 1988

Robins LN, Kulbok PA: Epidemiological studies in suicide. Psychiatric Annals 18:619, 623–627, 1988

Roose SP, Glassman AH, Walsh BT, et al: Depression, delusions, and suicide. Am J Psychiatry 140:1159–1162, 1983

Roy A: Suicide in chronic schizophrenia. Br J Psychiatry 141:171–177, 1982

Roy A, Ninan P, Mazonson A, et al: CSF monoamine metabolites in chronic schizophrenic patients who attempt suicide. Psychol Med 15:335–340, 1985

Roy A, Karoum F, Pollack S: Marked reduction in indexes of dopamine metabolism among patients with depression who attempt suicide. Arch Gen Psychiatry 49:447–450, 1992

Sacchetti E, Vita A, Guarneri L, et al: The effectiveness of fluoxetine, chlomipramine, nortriptyline, and desipramine in major depressives with suicidal behavior: preliminary findings, in Serotonin Related Psychiatric Syndromes. Edited by Cassano GB, Akiskal HS. London, Royal Society of Medicine Services, 1991, pp 47–53

Sainsbury P: Depression, suicide, and suicide prevention, in Suicide. Edited by Roy A. Baltimore, MD, Williams & Wilkins, 1986a, pp 73–88

Sainsbury P: The epidemiology of suicide, in Suicide. Edited by Roy A. Baltimore, MD, Williams & Wilkins, 1986b, pp 17–40

Schulsinger F, Kety SS, Rosenthal D, et al: A family study of suicide, in Origin Prevention and Treatment of Affective Disorders. Edited by Schon M, Stromgren E. New York, Academic Press, 1979, pp 277–287

Stanley M, Mann JJ: Increased serotonin-2 binding sites in frontal cortex of suicide victims. Lancet 1:214–216, 1983

Stanley M, Virgilio JJ, Gerson S: Tritiated imipramine binding sites are decreased in the frontal cortex of suicides. Science 216:1337–1339, 1982

Stevenson JM: Suicide, in The American Psychiatric Press Textbook of Psychiatry. Edited by Talbot JA, Hales RE, Yudofsky SC. Washington, DC, American Psychiatric Press, 1988, pp 1021–1035

Stone MH, Stone DK, Hurt SW: Natural history of borderline patients treated by intensive hospitalization. Psychiatr Clin North Am 10:185–206, 1987

Targum SD, Rosen L, Capodanno AE: The dexamethasone suppression test in suicidal patients with unipolar depression. Am J Psychiatry 140:877–879, 1983

Teicher MH, Glod C, Cole JO: Emergence of intense suicidal preoccupation during fluoxetine treatment. Am J Psychiatry 147:207–210, 1990

Träskman L, Åsberg M, Bertilsson L, et al: Monoamine metabolites in CSF and suicidal behavior. Arch Gen Psychiatry 38:631–636, 1981

Träskman-Bendz L, Alling C, Oreland L, et al: Prediction of suicidal behavior from prologic tests. J Clin Psychopharmacol 12(No 2, Suppl):21S–26S, 1992

Weiden P, Roy A: General versus specific risk factors for suicide in schizophrenia, in Suicide and Clinical Practice. Edited by Jacobs D. Washington, DC, American Psychiatric Press, 1992, pp 75–100

Weisman A, Beck AT, Kovacs M: Drug abuse, hopelessness and suicidal behavior. Int J Addict 14:451–464, 1979

Zeck PM, Tierney H, Tardiff K, et al: Increased risk of suicide in persons with AIDS. JAMA 259:1333–1337, 1988

CHAPTER 37

Violence

Kenneth Tardiff, M.D., M.P.H.

Psychiatrists should be able to evaluate and treat violent patients. A number of studies indicate that approximately 10% of the patients presenting to psychiatric hospitals have manifested violent behavior toward others just prior to being admitted to these hospitals (Davis 1991; Tardiff 1983), a finding that is true for private as well as public hospitals. Learning how to evaluate and manage violent patients is important not only for the safety of society and of patients in treatment settings, but also for the safety of mental health professionals who themselves are at high risk of being assaulted (American Psychiatric Association 1993).

■ CAUSES OF VIOLENCE

The role of the temporal lobe and of epilepsy in violence has been controversial. Delgado-Escueta (1981) conducted a large international collaborative study and found that violence was rare among epileptic patients. Hermann and Whitman (1984) have reviewed the literature and found no overall difference in levels of violence between persons with or without epilepsy. Despite this, some investigators (Monroe 1985; Weiger and Bear 1988) continue to emphasize the importance of epilepsy and limbic ictus in episodic dyscontrol and violence by maintaining that the surface electroencephalogram is a crude and ineffective measurement of subcortical activity and that patients with episodic dyscontrol often respond to anticonvulsant medication. With advances in imaging using magnetic resonance, there is evidence that subtle damage to the amygdaloid nucleus is associated with violence (Tonkonogy 1991).

☐ Genetic Determinants

Schiavi et al. (1984) conducted a double-blind controlled study and found no association between XYY or XXY chromosome abnormalities and violence. The role of these chromosomal abnormalities is doubtful, and any association with arrest for crimes is probably linked to other factors such as low intelligence. Twin studies showing increased criminal behavior in monozygotic twins were subject to a number of methodological problems, and a study by Bohman et al. (1982) of adopted men in Sweden failed to show that the violent crimes committed by these men were related to violence in their biological or adoptive parents. Other studies of twins reared apart have found that inheritance is an important factor in the expression of aggression (Tellegen et al. 1988).

☐ Hormones

Violence may be associated with gross endocrine disease such as Cushing's disease or hyperthyroidism, but the role of androgens, hypoglycemia, and premenstrual syndrome is more controversial. Studies have not found a relationship between androgens and violent behavior (Rada et al. 1983). This leaves us with the probable conclusion that increased rates of violence by men in society are accounted for by other factors such as role expectations in society. Studies of hypoglycemic patients as well as habitually violent defenders have indicated that hypoglycemia may play a role in extreme cases of violence (Virkkunen 1982). Perhaps in some individuals with certain personality and environmental precipitants, the hypoglycemic state may tip the balance toward aggressive behavior. Premenstrual syndrome has been used as a defense in crimes of manslaughter, arson, and assault in Europe (Dalton 1980). Reid and Yen (1981) found little or no research evidence that premenstrual syndrome is a direct contributing factor to criminal activity.

☐ Neurotransmitters

Brown et al. (1982) found that a history of aggressive behavior and a history of suicidal behavior were both related to decreased cerebrospinal fluid (CSF) 5-hydroxyindoleacetic acid (5-HIAA) levels. Lidberg et al. (1985) found that men who were convicted of criminal homicide and a group of men who committed suicide both had lower levels of 5-HIAA in their spinal fluid than did male control subjects. Linnoila et al. (1983) found that among offenders who killed with unusual cruelty, those who were impulsive had significantly lower CSF 5-HIAA concentrations than did nonimpulsive offenders, the latter group defined as those who premeditated their crimes. This finding is in agreement with other studies of suicide and serotonin metabolism (Belfrage et al. 1992). Thus, low CSF 5-HIAA may be a marker of impulsivity rather than of a specific type of violence.

☐ Psychiatric Disorders

Psychiatric patients should not be regarded as a homogeneous group. Diagnosis per se should not be used as an indicator of potential for violence. However, certain categories are overrepresented among groups of patients who are violent. Paranoid schizophrenia is one of these diagnostic categories (Lindqvist and Allebeck 1990; Tardiff 1983). The fact that patients with psychotic disorders pose a higher risk of violent behavior has been confirmed by a number of other studies (Krakowski et al. 1986). In the outpatient setting, nonpsychotic disorders are often associated with violent behavior (Binder and McNeil 1990). Personality disorders, particularly the borderline and antisocial types, are associated with increased rates of violence (Bland and Orn 1986; Hare and McPherson 1984). A number of cognitive impairment disorders with delirium, dementia, or other pathology can be associated with violent behavior (Deutsch et al. 1991).

☐ Alcohol and Drugs

Alcohol is well known for its association with violence through its ability to lessen inhibition against antisocial and violent behavior and to decrease perceptual and cognitive alertness, with resulting impairment of judgment. A number of epidemiological studies have found a strong link between alcohol use and certain types of homicide involving disputes (Goodman et al. 1986; Tardiff et al. 1994). Many street drugs of abuse have been found to be associated with violent behavior, including amphetamines, cocaine, hallucinogens, and minor tranquilizer-sedatives (Swanson et al. 1990). Crack cocaine has become a very important factor, especially in urban settings, in increased rates of homicides. A large proportion of this violence is related to the business of buying and selling cocaine (Goldstein et al. 1989).

☐ Developmental Factors

A prospective cohort study found that being abused and neglected as a child increased one's risk for adult violence (Widom 1989). Furthermore, there are indications that violence need not take place in the home to influence the child and adolescent; for example, television violence could be related to later aggressive behavior (National Institute of Mental Health 1982). In light of the high rate of child abuse, intrafamily violence, and violence depicted in the mass media, there should be great concern that we are raising the next generation of violent adults. Monitoring and regulation of violence in the media are essential to prevent this (Centerwall 1992).

☐ Socioeconomic Factors

The nonwhite population in the United States has high rates of violence as perpetrators as well as victims. This has been explained in terms of the necessity to fight rather than being able to achieve through verbal or economic means, given the widespread poverty in black ghettos. Added to this is the breakup of families, alienation, discrimination, and frustration. Some researchers have courted the hypothesis that blacks and Hispanics live in a violent subculture (Wolfgang 1981). Others have found that in violence there is no difference between blacks and whites when socioeconomic status is taken into consideration (Centerwall 1984). There have been ongoing debates and conflicting findings as to whether economic inequality as opposed to absolute poverty is responsible for high rates of homicide and other crimes among blacks (Williams 1984). Using neighborhoods—rather than metropolitan areas, as in some studies—as units of analysis, Messner and Tardiff (1986) found that economic inequality and race were not related to homicide, but rather the prime determinants were absolute poverty and marital disruption. There appears to be a cycle of poverty, deprivation, disruption of families, unemployment, and further difficulty maintaining personal ties, family structures, and social control.

☐ Firearms

The number of homicides associated with firearms has increased significantly since 1960. It is difficult to determine whether this is due to increased availability of firearms, because the import and export of firearms are not accurately measured. There is evidence, however, that gun control legislation is effective in decreasing the rate of homicides involving firearms (Cook 1982). Knowing whether there is a gun in the home is important in the evaluation of violence potential because it increases the probability of serious violence and death (Saltzman et al. 1992).

☐ Physical Environment

Physical crowding may be related to violence through increased contact and decreased defensible space, while an increased number of persons without crowding may result in increased social control and decrease of violence (Sampson 1983). These principles in society are similar to what is found on psychiatric inpatient units, namely, that increased numbers of patients are associated with increased violence (Palmstierna et al. 1991). The number of bystanders available for surveillance and intervention may prevent the commission of crimes, including homicide (Messner and Tardiff 1985).

Bell and Baron (1981) concluded that there is a curvilinear relationship between heat and aggression: moderately uncomfortable ambient temperatures produce an increase in aggression, whereas extremely hot temperatures decrease aggression. Thus, with overcrowding, inadequate numbers of staff, heat, and disruptive rather than supportive patients, one would anticipate that violence would increase on inpatient units.

■ ACUTE MANAGEMENT

☐ Safety

At one time or another all of us are faced with the situation, whether in the emergency room, the inpatient unit, or even the outpatient clinic, in which we are summoned to deal with a patient who has just struck someone, threw something, or is threatening violence. Often, a group of people—either staff, police, patients, or other observers—have gathered around the patient. The psychiatrist or other professional presiding in that setting is expected to take charge. In defusing the situation and evaluating future potential for violence, the ideal situation is that of being alone with the patient in a closed room. Obviously this may not always be advisable, for safety reasons. The psychiatrist must feel safe with the patient or else this insecurity will interfere with the evaluation and may result in physical injury or death. In talking to the patient, a wide range of options should be considered, from being alone with the patient with the door closed, to being alone with the door open, to being alone with aides outside of the room, to being alone with aides inside of the room, to interviewing the patient while the patient is in physical restraints. In addition to relying on one's feelings concerning safety, one should take into consideration the possibility of countertransference reactions or other inappropriate reactions such as denial that will interfere with the effective management of a particular patient.

☐ Instant Differential Diagnosis

In deciding how to proceed in terms of talking to the patient or using physical means of control, the clinician should make an instant differential diagnosis and categorize the patient's condition into one of three groups:

1. *Organic mental disorders:* For patients with cognitive impairment disorders and substance-related disorders in the middle of a violent episode, it is frequently impossible to intervene effectively through verbal means. One should treat the underlying medical or other physical disorder rather than rely on neuroleptics. If the etiology is unknown, the patient probably should be restrained as the evaluation proceeds.

2. *Psychotic disorders:* Violent patients in this group are usually schizophrenic or manic and are difficult to influence through verbal means. Neuroleptic medication rapidly administered is usually the treatment of choice for these patients, although they may have to be restrained until it takes effect.

3. *Nonpsychotic, nonorganic disorders:* This group primarily includes patients with personality disorders or intermittent explosive disorder who are often amenable to verbal intervention. One may want to offer medication to the patient, thus giving him or her a sense of control in the situation. In deciding to use physical means of control, the psychiatrist can assess the patient's degree of impulse control by the patient's compliance with routine procedures.

☐ Verbal Intervention

Verbal means of intervention and even prevention should receive serious consideration. In terms of prevention, it is essential that an inpatient unit have well-trained staff to ensure implementation of ongoing treatment programs and also for the prevention of violence. In the emergency situation, the staff should be adequate in number and trained to implement seclusion and restraint techniques. Most important, the staff should be caring and nonauthoritarian, yet at the same time act as part of the ward milieu, demonstrating social norms and limits. The staff should talk to patients in a calm, nonprovocative manner and also listen to patients. As tension increases before violence occurs, even the most psychotic schizophrenic patient may respond to nonprovocative interpersonal contact and expression of concern and caring. It is important that the staff recognize for a particular patient the warning signs of violence that have preceded violent acts in the past.

☐ Seclusion and Restraint

Guidelines approved by the American Psychiatric Association (APA) have set reasonable, minimal clinical standards for management of violence using seclusion and restraint in the context of verbal intervention, involuntary medication, and other factors in the treatment environment

(Tardiff 1984). Indications for emergency use of seclusion and restraint are as follows:

1. To prevent imminent harm to others—namely, staff and other patients—if other means are not effective and appropriate
2. To prevent imminent harm to the patient if other means of control are not effective or appropriate
3. To prevent serious disruption of the treatment program or significant damage to the environment
4. As part of an ongoing behavior treatment program
5. To decrease the amount of stimulation that the patient receives (for seclusion)
6. At the patient's request (for seclusion)

These indications for the emergency use of seclusion and restraint state that violence need not actually occur but that these measures may be used for imminent violence if, for example, a patient's past pattern of escalation to violence is known or if it is apparent that a patient is on the verge of exploding. The decision as to whether seclusion, restraint, or involuntary medication is used is a clinical one and should be based on the individual needs of the patient. For example, restraint probably would be preferable if the patient is delirious and the etiology of the delirium is unknown. In this case, one would prefer to keep the patient free of drugs, certainly neuroleptics, until the underlying etiology is determined; seclusion would not be appropriate because sensory deprivation might worsen the patient's delirium. Restraint may also be preferred if close medical monitoring is necessary, as for patients with heart disease, overdoses, or other medical problems. On the other hand, seclusion may be preferred for a manic person who needs decreased stimulation. Involuntary medication may be the choice of control, perhaps with seclusion or restraint, for the paranoid schizophrenic patient who has stopped taking medications and has become violent or is imminently so. A combination of the control measures may be used, for example, for the violent manic patient with a history of epilepsy who may be secluded and given lower doses of involuntary medication (e.g., haloperidol) than are usually prescribed because of the decreased seizure threshold resulting from neuroleptic medication.

As with any medical procedure, there are contraindications as well as indications. Seclusion and restraint should never be used to punish a patient as retribution for a particular act. Seclusion and restraint should never be used solely for the convenience of the staff or of other patients on the inpatient unit, or solely for the sake of the treatment programs on the ward.

☐ Staff Feelings About Violence

The staff should know their own feelings about violence in general and about specific violent patients based on countertransference reactions or other emotional reactions to patients (Lion and Pasternak 1973). In addition, the staff should be constantly monitoring the ward dynamics, particularly in terms of staff conflict that may translate into inappropriate patient care in the management of violence. The staff know their own past experiences with violence and how this may affect their treatment of patients. Anger toward a patient for a particular act may be justified, or it may be the result of countertransference in which the patient resembles an abusive parent or spouse.

A number of defense mechanisms may interfere with the treatment of violent patients and, in fact, may pose a danger to the therapist and others. Denial of a patient's dangerousness may occur because of the therapist's past experiences with violence or because the patient is particularly attractive or interesting. To the contrary, a patient may be viewed as more dangerous than he or she actually is because of staff anxiety projected onto the patient. Displacement can occur from one patient who is really dangerous to another who is not dangerous but who serves as an acceptable scapegoat for a staff member.

Negative emotional reactions about patients may exist on the basis of bias or prejudice. In addition, ward dynamics may result in the inappropriate treatment of violent patients. For example, nursing staff feeling abandoned by the administration or the medical staff may inappropriately seclude or restrain a particular patient so as to activate procedures in which the psychiatrist is required to be on the ward and examine the patient.

☐ Medication in Emergencies

The most common types of medication used are the neuroleptics (Brizer 1988). These are most often used for patients with schizophrenia or mania, but they may be used, with some reservations, for patients with cognitive impairment, organic mental disorders, personality disorders, and mental retardation on an emergency basis. The following concerns should be borne in mind. In terms of cognitive impairment disorders, the sedative or anticholinergic effects of neuroleptics may aggravate delirious or toxic metabolic confusional states. Intoxication with alcohol or sedative drugs is a relative contraindication to the use of neuroleptics, particularly rapid tranquilization, until one can make certain that the patient's level of consciousness is worsening. Overdose with anticholinergic drugs can produce delirium that would be increased by neuroleptics. In such situations and if the etiology of the cognitive impairment disorder is unknown, one should consider using physical restraint until, in the latter case, one can determine the etiology of the disorder. If the patient is restrained one can draw blood for a toxic screen for alcohol and other drugs.

For the schizophrenic or manic patient who is out of control and violent, rapid tranquilization has been found to be safe and effective, in spite of its possible side effects, which include sedation, orthostatic hypotension, anticholinergic effects, seizures, and severe extrapyramidal symptoms. Decrease of violent behavior occurs usually within 20 minutes, and improvement of psychotic symptomatology occurs within 6 hours.

Benzodiazepines are the treatment of choice in withdrawal from alcohol, even with associated psychotic psychopathology, because the use of neuroleptic medications in such patients would decrease seizure threshold and increase the risk of seizures. Restraint or closely monitored seclusion probably would be indicated also in the management of such patients. For the emergency use of benzodiazepines, lorazepam is useful because it produces sedation for a longer period of time than diazepam (the former remaining in the circulation rather than being absorbed into tissues). On the other hand, the half-life of lorazepam is 12 hours, much shorter than that of diazepam, so that accumulation is not as problematic as it is with diazepam. Lorazepam given by intramuscular injection rapidly begins to enter the circulation and produces sedation within an hour. The oral administration of lorazepam produces more gradual effects, with sedation occurring usually longer than 1 hour and less than 4 hours after administration. The dose is 2 to 4 mg by mouth or intramuscularly. A subsequent 2- to 4-mg dose can be repeated if there is continued agitation and aggression, with the timing dependent on the route of administration.

■ POTENTIAL FOR VIOLENCE IN THE NEAR FUTURE

In making a decision about violence potential, one should interview the patient as well as family members, police, and other persons with information about the patient, because patients may minimize threats or violent acts that have preceded the interview. The evaluation of violence potential is analogous to that of suicide potential. If the patient does not express thoughts of violence, one should begin the evaluation by asking a subtle question such as "Have you ever lost your temper?" If the answer is yes, then the evaluation should proceed in terms of how, when, and so on.

Along the same lines as the evaluation of suicide potential, evaluation of violence potential includes an assessment of how well planned the threat is (Tardiff 1989). Vague threats of killing someone are not as serious as saying "I'm going to kill my boss because he doesn't appreciate my work and plans to fire me." As with suicide, the availability of a means of inflicting injury is important. A past history of violence or other impulsive behavior is often predictive of future violence. One should ask about injuries to other persons, destruction of property, reckless driving, reckless spending, sexual acting out, and other impulsive behaviors. One should assess the degree of past injuries, as well as toward whom the violence had been directed and under what circumstances. Often there is a pattern of past violent behavior in specific circumstances—for example, escalation of a dispute between a husband and wife about issues of money, esteem, or sexuality. On an inpatient unit, if a patient has been violent, staff should look for characteristic patterns of behavior before violent episodes or specific situations that have triggered violence. As with suicide, the presence of alcohol or drug abuse should alert the evaluator to an increased risk of violent behavior.

Alcohol, sedatives, and minor tranquilizers decrease inhibition and make it more probable that someone will act on his or her thoughts rather than control his or her behavior. The importance of immediately getting blood and urine samples for assay as soon as possible in the emergency situation, or unannounced in the more prolonged evaluation of the patient, is stressed. As with suicide, the presence of psychosis, in this case usually with paranoid delusional thinking or more disorganized psychosis, should warn the evaluator that threats of violence must be taken very seriously and handled accordingly.

■ MORE EXTENDED EVALUATION OF THE VIOLENT PATIENT

Once the acute violent episode has been managed and the patient is safely in the hospital, one may collect more data in terms of the history, physical examination, laboratory tests, and psychological testing.

☐ Organic Mental Disorders

A number of organic disorders are associated with violent behavior, including substance abuse, central nervous system (CNS) disorders, systemic disorders, and seizure disorders (Eichelman 1992; Elliot 1992). In addition to the usual sensorium disturbances, one should look for dysarthria, nystagmus, unsteady gait, dilated pupils, tachycardia, and tremors, all of which may indicate that a substance use disorder is present. Substances that can produce violent behavior as a result of the intoxicated state as well as during withdrawal include alcohol, barbiturates, other sedatives, and anxiolytics. Other substances that can produce violent behavior when the patient is intoxicated include amphetamines and other sympathomimetics, cocaine, phencyclidine (PCP) and other hallucinogens, anticholinergics, glue (sniffing), and other drugs such as steroids.

☐ Psychotic Disorders

The paranoid schizophrenic patient poses a number of problems. First, paranoid delusions may be very subtle, and the patient may attempt to hide these. Therefore, the evaluator must listen for subtle clues and follow-up regarding the assessment of violence toward others. Other patients with schizophrenia have more disorganized symptomatology, and violence may be the result of that or delusional or hallucinatory symptoms, particularly command hallucinations. It is important to realize that schizophrenic patients can be violent for reasons that have nothing to do with schizophrenia. Manic patients are also disorganized and less intentional in terms of their violent behavior. Depressed patients are rarely violent; when they are, however, it is usually the case of patients who have psychotic depressions and who murder their spouse and/or children and then commit suicide.

☐ Nonorganic, Nonpsychotic Disorders

Among the nonorganic, nonpsychotic patients, a number with personality disorders are associated with violence, and psychodynamic considerations are important. These patients tend to act rather than talk about conflicts. Patients with the best prognosis are those with the diagnosis of intermittent explosive disorder. These patients should be distinguished from persons with other types of personality disorders associated with violent behavior. Intermittent explosive disorder consists of several discrete episodes of loss of control involving violence toward others or destruction of property. The violence may occur for a few minutes or an hour and is often associated with alcohol use. It is followed by remorse and feelings of guilt concerning the beating of a spouse, child, or other family member.

In distinction to intermittent explosive disorder is antisocial personality disorder, in which there are intermittent episodes of violent behavior. Between these violent outbursts there is pervasive antisocial behavior and violence on an ongoing basis. The borderline personality manifests, in addition to episodic violence, a broad instability of interpersonal relationships as well as profound mood and identity problems.

■ LONG-TERM TREATMENT

As with many problems in psychiatry, treatment of violent patients must adhere to the biopsychosocial model. Not all violent patients need medication, but it should be considered in the formulation of the treatment plan. Psychological intervention may be in the form of behavior therapy or psychotherapy. The impact of the patient's violence on various levels of the social order, from the family to society, must be addressed in treatment, as should the role of social factors in causation of the patient's violence.

☐ Medication

There is no medication specific to the treatment of violence. Rather, medication is used to treat the underlying process. The neuroleptics are used for schizophrenia and mania. Fluphenazine and haloperidol have been popular for long-term treatment because they can be given in the depot form if there are problems with compliance, as there usually are with schizophrenic patients. Daily neuroleptic medication should not be given for violent mentally retarded patients in the absence of a clear-cut indication (namely, psychosis), not only because of side effects such as tardive dyskinesia but also because neuroleptic medications decrease learning.

Lithium carbonate is used for aggression and hypersexuality in mania and for the prophylaxis of bipolar disorder. It has been recommended for the management of violent behavior in mentally retarded patients along with haloperidol, for violence by patients with personality and conduct disorders, and even for patients with premenstrual syndrome who are violent. These are case reports, and there have been no convincing controlled studies of the effectiveness of lithium in disorders other than bipolar disorder. Craft et al. (1987) conducted a controlled study of the use of lithium and found that it reduced aggression in mentally handicapped adult patients. Lithium was also found to be effective in decreasing agitation in schizophrenic patients and other psychotic patients in an uncontrolled study (Lee et al. 1992).

Among anticonvulsants, carbamazepine is frequently used in the treatment of violence associated with complex partial seizures and for some aggression in psychiatric patients without epilepsy (Evans and Gualtieri 1985). Even though carbamazepine is not considered the anticonvulsant of first choice for complex partial seizures, it is used because of fewer side effects, such as sedation, compared with phenytoin and barbiturates. In violent psychiatric patients without epilepsy, most notably those with schizophrenia, studies have shown that some of these patients benefited from carbamazepine at doses of approximately 600 mg a day. Many of these patients, although they did not have epileptic disorders, did have temporal lobe abnormalities on the EEG (Luchins 1984; Neppe 1981). Often there are no difficulties in the concurrent use of neuroleptic medication.

Evidence from some studies suggests that propranolol is effective in the treatment of aggressive patients, although controlled studies on its effectiveness have not been done (Silver and Yudofsky 1985; Whitman et al. 1987). Propranolol has been recommended for aggression in patients with head trauma, seizures, Wilson's disease, mental retardation, minimal brain dysfunction, Korsakoff's psychosis, and other organic mental disorders (Silver and Yudofsky 1985). Ratey and his colleagues (1992) have found that nadolol, a beta-blocker that does not act centrally in the brain, is effective in decreasing aggression in chronic psychiatric patients.

☐ Behavior Therapy

Liberman and Wong (1984) have succinctly described the use of behavioral analysis and therapy in the management of violent behavior. They caution that such a program of treatment should be planned and conducted only by clinicians skilled in behavioral analysis and therapy and that there should be standardized policies and review processes to prevent abuse of patients. Programs of behavioral management of violent behavior should definitely not be ad hoc attempts on inadequately staffed and trained general inpatient units.

The target behaviors of the behavioral treatment program must be clearly specified. General terms such as assault or violence are not sufficient; instead, such behaviors as pushing, shoving, hitting, pulling hair, and so forth must be clearly defined. Consequences of such behavior must also be clearly specified. The consequences include a broad spectrum of procedures ranging from a token economy and other means of positive reinforcement and social training skills, to more restrictive procedures such as social extinction, sensory extinction, contingent observation, required relaxation, seclusionary time-out, and contingent restraint. Usually one begins with a positive reinforcement and, later, turns to more restrictive procedures, such as time-out and restraint. However, severe violent behavioral problems usually necessitate use of the more restrictive procedures earlier in the treatment plan.

☐ Long-Term Outpatient Psychotherapy

The frequency of violence among patients in outpatient treatment settings is less than that for patients admitted to inpatient units (Tardiff and Koenigsberg 1985). Although psychotherapy of the violent patient may be on an individual basis, often therapists involve the spouse or family in treatment. This is advisable because of the role of the family in the dynamics of violence. In addition, it is important to get information from persons other than the patient to make certain that problems with violence are not minimized by the patient. Some therapists prefer group therapy for violent patients because it is less threatening to the patient than a one-to-one relationship and allows the patient to appreciate that other people have problems with violence. The group is often supportive, yet, at the same time, the group can confront a patient rather than have the therapist do so. Usually groups are led by two therapists, which makes it less stressful for each leader.

Lion and Tardiff (1987) have reviewed the principles of using psychotherapy for problems with aggression:

1. The motivation of the patient and the patient's reason for psychotherapy must be evaluated.
2. The patient must develop a sense of self-control of emotions and behavior.
3. Verbal communication should be facilitated.
4. The patient should come to have an appreciation of the consequences of violent behavior.
5. The patient should gain insight about the dynamics of violence and early warning signs.

■ SPECIAL CONCERNS IN THE TREATMENT OF VIOLENT PATIENTS

The first concern is that of danger to the therapist. Any threat, even if made in a joking manner, must be taken seriously and evaluated. The therapist should acknowledge to the patient that these threats are frightening, and together they must identify and address the problem if treatment is to continue. There should be some way for the therapist to communicate that he or she is in trouble inside an office or, conversely, for a receptionist to warn the therapist that there is a potential problem with violence before a patient enters the therapist's office. In addition, in emergency rooms patients should be searched for weapons. Offices should not contain heavy objects such as ashtrays and should contain pillows or a light chair that may be used as shields in case of violence, particularly if the patient has a knife or weapon other than a gun.

Another concern is danger to others and the responsibility of the clinician to protect intended victims of violent patients. Mills et al. (1987) have reviewed court decisions and legislation following the *Tarasoff* decision in California. A central issue is a balance between the confidentiality and privileged information given to the physician and the duty to protect the community. Mills et al. point out that the duty to protect need not involve warning the intended victim or the police but rather change of treatment including civil commitments. Appelbaum (1985) has a model for meeting the requirements imposed by the *Tarasoff* doctrine. He recommends viewing the fulfillment of the duty to protect in three stages. First, there must be an assessment of the potential for harm, in that the therapist must gather data relevant to the evaluation of dangerousness and the determination of this dangerousness must be made on the basis of these data. The second part of Appelbaum's model involves formulation of a course of action to protect the intended victim. This may involve a change or increase of medication, hospitalization of the patient, increased security on the inpatient unit, or, lastly, warning the intended victim or the police. The third part of this model is implementation of the plan to protect the intended victim, which may include warning the intended victim.

Beck (1985) has noted, based on a review of cases, especially those outside of California, that the duty to protect or warn exists only if there is evidence that the patient is a serious threat to do bodily harm to a specific person. If careful assessment that is documented in writing fails to reveal such evidence, there is no liability for the therapist. In fact, even if *Tarasoff*-like laws do not exist, such steps should be done as part of good clinical care.

■ REFERENCES

American Psychiatric Association: Clinician Safety: Report of the American Psychiatric Association Task Force on Clinician Safety. Washington, DC, American Psychiatric Association, 1993

Appelbaum PS: Tarasoff and the clinician: problems in fulfilling the duty to protect. Am J Psychiatry 142:425–429, 1985

Beck JC (ed): The Potentially Violent Patient and the Tarasoff Decision in Psychiatric Practice. Washington, DC, American Psychiatric Press, 1985

Belfrage H, Lidberg L, Oreland L: Platelet monoamine oxidase activity in mentally disordered violent offenders. Acta Psychiatr Scand 85:218–221, 1992

Bell PA, Baron RA: Ambient temperature and human violence, in Multidisciplinary Approaches to Aggression Research. Edited by Brain PF, Benton D. Amsterdam, Elsevier/North Holland Biomedical, 1981, pp 76–88

Binder RL, McNeil DE: The relationship of gender to violent behavior in acutely disturbed psychiatric patients. J Clin Psychiatry 51:110–114, 1990

Bland R, Orn H: Family violence and psychiatry. Can J Psychiatry 31:129–137, 1986

Bohman M, Cloninger CR, Sigvardsson S, et al: Predisposition to petty criminality in Swedish adoptees, I: genetic and environmental heterogeneity. Arch Gen Psychiatry 39:1233–1241, 1982

Brizer DA: Psychopharmacology and the management of violent patients. Psychiatr Clin North Am 11:551–568, 1988

Brown GL, Ebert MH, Goyer PF, et al: Aggression, suicide, and serotonin: relationships to CSF amine metabolites. Am J Psychiatry 139:741–746, 1982

Centerwall BS: Race, socioeconomic status and domestic homicide: Atlanta, 1971–72. Am J Public Health 74:813–815, 1984

Centerwall BS: Television and violence: the scale of the problem and where to go from here. JAMA 267:3059–3063, 1992

Cook PJ: The role of firearms in violent crime: an interpretive review of the literature, in Criminal Violence. Edited by Wolfgang ME, Weiner NA. Beverly Hills, CA, Sage, 1982, pp 236–291

Craft M, Ismail IA, Krishnamurti D, et al: Lithium in the treatment of aggression in mentally handicapped patients: a double-blind trial. Br J Psychiatry 150:685–689, 1987

Dalton K: Cyclical criminal acts in premenstrual syndrome. Lancet 2:1070–1071, 1980

Davis S: Violence by psychiatric inpatients: a review. Hosp Community Psychiatry 42:585–590, 1991

Delgado-Escueta AV, Mattson RH, King L, et al: The nature of aggression during epileptic seizures. N Engl J Med 305:711–716, 1981

Deutsch LH, Bylsma FW, Rovner BW, et al: Psychosis and physical aggression in probable Alzheimer's disease. Am J Psychiatry 148:1159–1163, 1991

Eichelman B: Aggressive behavior: from laboratory to clinic. Quo vadit? Arch Gen Psychiatry 49:488–492, 1992

Elliot FA: Violence: the neurologic contribution. Arch Neurol 49:595–603, 1992

Evans RW, Gualtieri CT: Carbamazepine: a neuropsychological and psychiatric profile. Clin Neuropharmacol 8:221–241, 1985

Goldstein PJ, Brounstein HH, Ryan PJ, et al: Crack and homicide in New York City, 1988: a conceptually based event analysis. Contemporary Drug Problems 5:651–687, 1989

Goodman RA, Mercy JA, Loya F, et al: Alcohol use and interpersonal violence: alcohol detected in homicide victims. Am J Public Health 76:144–149, 1986

Hare RD, McPherson LM: Violent and aggressive behavior by criminal psychopaths. Int J Law Psychiatry 7:35–50, 1984

Hermann BP, Whitman S: Behavioral and personality correlates of epilepsy: a review, methodological critique and conceptual model. Psychol Bull 95:451–497, 1984

Krakowski M, Volavka J, Brizer D: Psychopathology and violence: a review of literature. Compr Psychiatry 27:131–148, 1986

Lee HK, Reddy TB, Travin S, et al: A trial of lithium citrate for the management of acute agitation of psychiatric inpatients: a pilot study (letter). J Clin Psychopharmacol 12:361–362, 1992

Liberman RP, Wong SE: Behavior analysis and therapy procedures related to seclusion and restraint, in The Psychiatric Uses of Seclusion and Restraint. Edited by Tardiff K. Washington, DC, American Psychiatric Press, 1984, pp 35–67

Lidberg L, Tuck JR, Åsberg M, et al: Homicide, suicide and CSF 5-HIAA. Acta Psychiatr Scand 71:230–236, 1985

Lindqvist P, Allebeck P: Schizophrenia and crime: a longitudinal follow-up of 644 schizophrenics in Stockholm. Br J Psychiatry 157:345–350, 1990

Linnoila M, Virkkunen M, Scheinin M, et al: Low cerebrospinal fluid 5-hydroxyindoleacetic acid concentration differentiates impulsive from nonimpulsive violent behavior. Life Sci 33:2609–2614, 1983

Lion JR, Pasternak SA: Countertransference reactions to violent patients. Am J Psychiatry 130:207–210, 1973

Lion JR, Tardiff K: The long-term treatment of the violent patient, in Psychiatry Update: Annual Review of the American Psychiatric Association, Vol 6. Edited by Hales RE, Frances AJ. Washington, DC, American Psychiatric Press, 1987, pp 537–548

Luchins DI: Carbamazepine in violent nonepileptic schizophrenics. Psychopharmacol Bull 20:569–571, 1984

Messner S, Tardiff K: The social ecology of urban homicide: an application of the routine activities approach. Criminology 23:241–267, 1985

Messner S, Tardiff K: Economic inequality and levels of homicide: an analysis of urban neighborhoods. Criminology 24:297–317, 1986

Mills MJ, Sullivan G, Eth S: Protecting third parties: a decade after Tarasoff. Am J Psychiatry 144:68–74, 1987

Monroe RR: Episodic behavioral disorders and limbic ictus. Compr Psychiatry 26:466–479, 1985

National Institute of Mental Health: Television and Behavior: Ten Years of Scientific Progress and Implications for the Eighties, Vol 1: Summary Report (DHHS Publ No [ADM] 82-1195). Rockville, MD, National Institute of Mental Health, 1982

Neppe VM: Carbamazepine as adjunctive treatment in nonepileptic chronic inpatients with EEG temporal lobe abnormalities. J Clin Psychiatry 44:326–331, 1981

Palmstierna T, Huitfeldt B, Wistedt B: The relationship of crowding and aggressive behavior on a psychiatric intensive care unit. Hosp Community Psychiatry 42:1237–1240, 1991

Rada RT, Kellner R, Stivastava C, et al: Plasma androgens in violent and nonviolent sex offenders. Journal of the American Academy of Psychiatry and Law 11:149–158, 1983

Ratey JJ, Sorgi P, O'Driscoll GA, et al: Nadolol to treat aggression and psychiatric symptomatology in chronic psychiatric inpatients: a double-blind, placebo-controlled study. J Clin Psychiatry 53:41–46, 1992

Reid RL, Yen SC: Premenstrual syndrome. Am J Obstet Gynecol 139:85–104, 1981

Saltzman LE, Mercy JA, O'Carroll PW, et al: Weapon involvement and injury outcomes in family and intimates assaults. JAMA 267:3043–3047, 1992

Sampson RJ: Structural density and criminal victimization. Criminology 21:276–293, 1983

Schiavi RC, Theilgaard A, Owen DR, et al: Sex chromosome anomalies, hormones, and aggressivity. Arch Gen Psychiatry 41:93–99, 1984

Silver JM, Yudofsky S: Propranolol for aggression: literature review and clinical guidelines. International Drug Therapy Newsletter 20:9–12, 1985

Swanson JW, Holzer CE, Ganju VK, et al: Violence and psychiatric disorder in the community: evidence from the Epidemiologic Catchment Area surveys. Hosp Community Psychiatry 41:761–770, 1990

Tardiff K: A survey of assault by chronic patients in a state hospital system, in Assaults Within Psychiatric Facilities. Edited by Lion JR, Reid WH. New York, Grune & Stratton, 1983, pp 3–19

Tardiff K (ed): The Psychiatric Uses of Seclusion and Restraint. Washington, DC, American Psychiatric Press, 1984

Tardiff K: Concise Guide to Assessment and Management of Violent Patients. Washington, DC, American Psychiatric Press, 1989

Tardiff K, Koenigsberg HW: Assaultive behavior among psychiatric outpatients. Am J Psychiatry 142:960–963, 1985

Tardiff K, Marzuk P, Leon A, et al: Homicide in New York City. JAMA 272:43–46, 1994

Tellegen A, Lykken DT, Bouchard TJ, et al: Personality similarity in twins reared apart and together. J Pers Soc Psychol 54:1031–1039, 1988

Tonkonogy JM: Violence and temporal lobe lesion: head CT and MRI data. Journal of Neuropsychiatry and Clinical Neurosciences 3:189–196, 1991

Virkkunen M: Reactive hypoglycemia tendency among habitually violent offenders: a further study by means of the glucose tolerance test. Neuropsychobiology 8:35–40, 1982

Weiger B, Bear D: An approach to the neurology of aggression. J Psychiatr Res 22:85–89, 1988

Whitman JR, Maier GJ, Eichelman B. β-adrenergic blockers for aggressive behavior in schizophrenia (letter). Am J Psychiatry 144:538–542, 1987

Widom CS: The cycle of violence. Science 244:160–171, 1989

Williams K: Economic sources of homicide: reestimating the effects of poverty and inequality. American Sociological Review 49:283–289, 1984

Wolfgang ME: Sociocultural overview of criminal violence, in Violence and the Violent Individual. Edited by Hoys JR, Robert TK, Solway KS. New York, SP Medical & Scientific Books, 1981, pp 153–170

CHAPTER 38

The Law and Psychiatry

Robert I. Simon, M.D.

■ PSYCHIATRIC MALPRACTICE

Psychiatric malpractice is medical malpractice. *Malpractice* is the provision of substandard professional care that causes a compensable injury to a person with whom a professional relationship existed. Medical malpractice is a tort or civil wrong—that is, a noncriminal or non–contract-related wrong—committed as a result of negligence by a psychiatrist that causes injury to a patient in the psychiatrist's care. *Negligence,* the fundamental concept underlying a malpractice lawsuit, is simply described as doing something that a physician with a duty of care (to the patient) should not have done or failing to do something that a physician with a duty of care should have done. The fact that a psychiatrist commits an act of negligence does not automatically make him or her liable to the patient bringing the lawsuit.

For a psychiatrist to be found *liable* to a patient for malpractice, four fundamental elements must be established by a preponderance of the evidence: 1) that there was a duty of care owed by the defendant, 2) that the duty of care was breached, 3) that the plaintiff (i.e., patient) suffered actual damages, and 4) that the deviation was the direct cause of the damages. Each of these four elements must be met or there can be no finding of liability, regardless of any finding of negligence. Critical to the establishment of a claim of professional negligence is the requirement that the defendant's conduct was substandard or was a deviation in the standard of care owed to the plaintiff. Except in the case of "specialists," the law presumes and holds all physicians to a standard of *ordinary care,* which is measured by its *reasonableness* according to the clinical circumstances in which it is provided.

☐ Somatic Therapies

The use of a somatic therapy, including electroconvulsive therapy (ECT), is evaluated no differently from any other medical treatment or procedure with respect to potential liability. The same general standard of *ordinary* and *reasonable care* will govern the assessment of whether a psychiatrist's use of or failure to use a somatic intervention is legally actionable (Annotation 1979; Annotation 1985).

It is generally acknowledged within the psychiatric profession that there is no *absolute standard* protocol for the administration of psychotropic medication or ECT. Nevertheless, the existence of professional treatment guidelines and procedures that are generally accepted or used by a significant percentage of psychiatrists should alert clinicians to consider such guidelines as practice reference sources. For example, the American Psychiatric Association (APA) has published comprehensive findings and guidelines in the form of task force reports concerning ECT (American Psychiatric Association 1990) and tardive dyskinesia (American Psychiatric Association 1992). Nevertheless, official guidelines must not preempt sound professional judgment in attending to the clinical needs of individual patients.

Official guidelines and procedures publications do not, per se, establish the standard of care by which a court might evaluate a psychiatrist's treatment. They do represent, however, a credible source of information with which a reasonable psychiatrist should at least be familiar and have considered (*Stone v. Proctor* 1963). In addition to expert testimony, courts generally consider official guidelines and the professional literature that establish contemporary psychiatric practices in determining the standard of care.

The "standard" for judging the use of medication is consistent with the general "reasonable care" requirement. The reference source that bears highlighting is the use of the *Physicians' Desk Reference* (PDR) to establish or dispute a psychiatrist's pharmacotherapy procedures. In order to keep abreast of current medication information, psychiatrists should consult publications like the PDR as needed. Although numerous courts have cited the PDR as a credible source of medication-related information in the medical profession, the PDR does not by itself establish *the* standard of care (*Gowan v. United States* 1985). Instead, it may be used as one piece of evidence in order to establish the standard of care in a particular situation (*Doerr v. Hurley Medical Center* 1984). The PDR or any other reference, however, cannot serve as a substitute for the psychiatrist's sound clinical judgment.

The standard of care associated with the use of a somatic therapy to treat a psychiatric patient, *at a minimum*, should include some variation of the following pretreatment considerations and measures:

- Complete clinical history (e.g., medical, psychiatric) (Taylor et al. 1987)
- Complete physical examination, as clinically indicated
- Administration of necessary laboratory tests and review of past test results (Daniel et al. 1992)
- Disclosure of sufficient information to obtain informed consent, including information regarding the risks and benefits both for receiving treatment and for *not* receiving treatment
- Thorough documentation of all decisions, informed consent information, patient responses, and any other relevant treatment data

The following should be considered posttreatment:

- Careful monitoring of the patient's response to treatment, including adequate follow-up evaluations and appropriate laboratory testing (Daniel et al. 1992)
- Prompt adjustments in treatment, as clinically indicated
- Obtainment of additional informed consent when appreciably altering treatment or initiating new treatment

☐ Theories of Liability

A review of the relevant case law indicates that a variety of mistakes, omissions, and poor medication treatment practices commonly result in malpractice actions brought against a psychiatrist.

Failure to Properly Evaluate

Sound clinical practice requires that before any form of somatic treatment is initiated, the patient should be properly examined. The nature and extent of an examination are largely dictated by the type of treatment being contemplated and the medical condition of the patient. A physical examination should be conducted or obtained if clinically indicated. A recently performed physical examination may suffice, or the patient may be referred by a psychiatrist who does not perform physical examinations. Moreover, the duty to ensure that proper informed consent is obtained can also be fulfilled at this time.

Failure to Monitor

Probably the most common act of negligence associated with pharmacotherapy is the failure to monitor the patient's progress on medication, including carefully following the patient for adverse side effects. Once psychotropic medication has been prescribed, it is the psychiatrist's duty to monitor the patient. Consultation or referral may be necessary according to the clinical needs of the patient. A failure to properly supervise patients on psychotropic medication can unnecessarily subject them to harmful side effects and can delay a change to more effective treatment.

Negligent Prescription Practices

In administering psychotropic medication, psychiatrists need only conform their procedures and decision making to those that are *ordinarily* practiced by other psychiatrists under similar circumstances. A review of cases involving allegations of negligent prescription procedures reveals several common practices representing possible deviations from generally accepted treatment practice:

- Exceeding recommended dosages without clinical indications
- Negligently prescribing multiple drugs
- Negligently prescribing medication for unapproved uses
- Negligently prescribing "unapproved" medications
- Negligently failing to disclose medication risks

Any physician who prescribes medication has a duty to first obtain the informed consent of the patient (Table 38–1). Obtaining competent informed consent may be complicated by the fact that a significant number of psychiatric patients have compromised mental capacity for health care decisions due to mental illness. Patients lacking such decision-making capacity require consent for treatment by substitute decision-makers (Table 38–2).

Other areas of negligence involving medication that have resulted in legal action include 1) failure to treat side effects once they have been recognized or should have been recognized, 2) failure to monitor a patient's compliance with prescription limits, 3) failure to prescribe medica-

---

Table 38–1.   Informed consent: reasonable information to be disclosed

Although there exists no consistently accepted set of information to be disclosed for any given medical or psychiatric situation, as a rule of thumb, five areas of information are generally provided:

1. Diagnosis—description of the condition or problem
2. Treatment—nature and purpose of proposed treatment
3. Consequences—risks and benefits of the proposed treatment
4. Alternatives—viable alternatives to the proposed treatment including risks and benefits
5. Prognosis—projected outcome with and without treatment

Source.   Reprinted from Simon 1992a.

Table 38–2. Common consent options for patients lacking the mental
             capacity for health care decisions

Proxy consent of next of kin	Substituted consent of the court
Adjudication of incompetence, appointment of a guardian	Advance directives (living will, durable power of attorney, health care proxy)
Institutional administrators or committees	
Treatment review panels	Statutory surrogates (spouse or court-appointed guardian)[a]

[a]Medical statutory surrogate laws (when treatment wishes of patient are unstated).
Source. Reprinted from Simon 1992a.

tion or appropriate levels of medication according to the treatment needs
of the patient, 4) failure to refer a patient for consultation or treatment by
a specialist, and 5) negligent withdrawal from medication.

☐ Tardive Dyskinesia

Cases involving allegations of negligence after a patient develops tardive
dyskinesia (TD) are based on the same legal elements as any other malpractice action. Moreover, the bases for negligence mirror those that
have been previously identified with general medication cases. These
areas include, but are not limited to, the following:

- Failure to properly evaluate and monitor a patient
- Failure to obtain informed consent
- Negligent diagnosis of a patient's condition
- Wrongful prescription of neuroleptic medication
- Failure to monitor medication side effects

The defenses and preventive measures applicable to TD-related malpractice claims are consistent with those used in any case alleging negligent drug treatment. Generally speaking, the application of sound
clinical practice that is appropriately communicated to the patient and
documented in the medical chart will serve as an effective foil to any allegations of negligence should TD develop.

■ CONFIDENTIALITY AND TESTIMONIAL PRIVILEGE

Confidentiality refers to the right of a patient to have communications
spoken or written in confidence not to be disclosed to outside parties
without implied or expressed authorization. *Privilege,* or more accurately

testimonial privilege, can be viewed as a derivation of the right of confidentiality. Testimonial privilege is a statutorily created rule of evidence that permits the holder of the privilege (e.g., the patient) to exercise the right to prevent the person to whom confidential information was given (e.g., the psychiatrist) from disclosing it in a judicial proceeding.

☐ Confidentiality

Clinical-Legal Foundation

The basis for recognizing and safeguarding patient confidences is derived from four general sources. First, states have acknowledged this right of protection by including confidentiality provisions in either professional licensure laws or confidentiality and privilege statutes. The second source, and probably the most traditional, comprises the ethical codes of the various mental health professions. Third, the common law recognizes an attorney-client privilege, but developing case law also has carved out this source of protection for physicians and psychotherapists. Fourth, the right of confidentiality may be subsumed under the constitutional right of privacy.

Breaching Confidentiality

Regardless of the basis of the right of confidentiality, once the doctor-patient relationship has been created, the professional assumes an automatic duty to safeguard a patient's disclosures. This duty is not absolute, and there are circumstances in which breaching confidentiality is both ethical and legal.

Patients also waive confidentiality in a variety of situations. Medical records are regularly sent to potential employers or to insurance companies for benefits. A limited waiver of confidentiality ordinarily exists when a patient participates in group therapy. Legally, whether one group member can be compelled in court to disclose information shared by another group member during group therapy is still unsettled. Many state confidentiality statutes provide statutory exceptions to confidentiality between the psychiatrist and the patient in one or more situations (Brakel et al. 1985) (Table 38–3).

Patients' access to their own records is normally controlled by statutes. These statutory provisions are found under the heading of "medical records" or the much broader term "privilege."

☐ Testimonial Privilege

The patient—not the psychiatrist—is the holder of the privilege that controls the release of confidential information. Because privilege applies

---

Table 38–3.   Common statutory exceptions to confidentiality between psychiatrist and patient

Child abuse	Intent to commit a crime or harmful act
Competency proceedings	
Court-ordered examination	Civil commitment proceedings
Dangerousness to self or others	Communication with other treatment providers
Patient-litigant exception	

---

only to the judicial setting, it is called *testimonial privilege.* Privilege statutes represent the most common recognition by the state of the importance of protecting information provided by a patient to a psychotherapist. This recognition moves away from the essential purpose of the American system of justice (e.g., "truth finding") by insulating certain information from disclosure in court. This protection is justified on the basis that the special need for privacy in the doctor-patient relationship outweighs the unbridled quest for an accurate outcome in court. Privilege statutes usually are drafted in one of four ways, depending on the type of practitioner:

- Physician-patient (general)
- Psychiatrist-patient
- Psychologist-patient
- Psychotherapist-patient

Cases have been successfully litigated in which the broader physician-patient category has been applied to the psychotherapist when an applicable statute did not exist. Privilege statutes also specify exceptions to testimonial privilege. Although exceptions vary, the most common include the following:

- Child abuse reporting
- Civil commitment proceedings
- Court-ordered evaluations
- Cases in which a patient's mental state is in question as a part of litigation

This last exception, known as the *patient-litigant exception,* commonly occurs in will contests, workers' compensation cases, child custody disputes, personal injury actions, and malpractice actions in which the therapist is sued by the patient.

☐ Liability

An unauthorized or unwarranted breach of confidentiality can cause a patient considerable emotional harm. As a result, a psychiatrist typically can be held liable for such a breach based on at least four theories:

- Malpractice (breach of confidentiality)
- Breach of statutory duty
- Invasion of privacy
- Breach of (implied) contract

■ INFORMED CONSENT AND THE RIGHT TO REFUSE TREATMENT

Informed consent is a legal theory in medical malpractice. It provides a patient with a cause of action for not being adequately informed about the nature and consequences of a particular medical treatment or procedure undertaken. This theory is founded on two distinct legal principles. The first is the right of every patient to determine what will or will not be done to his or her body, often referred to as the *right of self-determination*. The second principle emanates from the fiduciary nature of the doctor-patient relationship. Inherent in a physician's duty of fiduciary care is the responsibility to disclose honestly and in good faith all requisite facts concerning a patient's condition. Included among factors to be disclosed are any treatment risks, alternatives, and consequences. The primary purpose of the doctrine of informed consent is to promote individual autonomy and, secondarily, rational decision making (Appelbaum et al. 1987). There are three essential elements to the doctrine of informed consent:

- Competency
- Information
- Voluntariness

Usually, clinicians provide the first level of screening in identifying patient competency and in deciding whether to accept a patient's treatment decision. The patient or a bona fide representative must be given an adequate description of the treatment. In order to make an informed consent, the patient should be told about the risks, benefits, and prognosis both with and without treatment, as well as alternative treatments and their risks and benefits. In addition, the patient must voluntarily, with a reasonable level of competency, consent or refuse the proposed treatment or procedure.

☐ Competency

It is clinically useful to distinguish the terms *incompetence* and *incapacity*. Incompetence refers to a court adjudication, while incapacity indicates a functional inability as determined by a clinician (Mishkin 1989). Competency is defined as "having sufficient capacity, ability . . . (or) possessing the requisite physical, mental, natural, or legal qualifications" (Black 1990, p. 284). This definition is deliberately vague and ambiguous because the term competency is a broad concept encompassing many different legal issues and contexts. In general, *competency* refers to some *minimal* mental, cognitive, or behavioral ability, trait, or capability required to perform a particular legally recognized act or to assume some legal role.

The legal designation of "incompetent" is applied to an individual who fails one of the mental tests of capacity and is therefore considered *by law* not mentally capable of performing a particular act or assuming a particular role. The adjudication of incompetence by a court is subject or issue specific. In other words, the fact that a psychiatric patient is adjudicated incompetent to execute a will does not automatically render that patient incompetent to do other things, such as consent to treatment, testifying as a witness, marrying, driving, or making a legally binding contract.

The issue of competency, whether in a civil or criminal context, is commonly raised in two situations: when the person is a minor or when he or she is mentally disabled. In many situations, minors are not considered legally competent and therefore require the consent of a parent or designated guardian. However, there are exceptions to this general rule, such as minors who are considered emancipated, or mature, or in some cases of medical need (abortion, mental health counseling). Lack of capacity or competency *cannot* be presumed from either treatment for mental illness or institutionalization of such persons. Mental disability or illness does *not*, in and of itself, render a person incompetent in all areas of functioning. Instead, scrutiny is given to determine whether there are specific functional incapacities that render a person incapable of making a particular kind of decision or performing a particular type of task.

Respect for individual autonomy demands that individuals be allowed to make decisions of which they are capable, even if they are seriously mentally ill, developmentally arrested, or organically impaired. As a rule, a patient with a psychiatric disorder that produces mental incapacity generally must be declared judicially incompetent before that patient's exercise of his or her legal rights can be abridged. The person's current or past history of physical and mental illness is but one factor to be weighed in determining whether a particular test of competency is met.

Legally, only competent persons may give an informed consent. An adult patient will be considered legally competent unless adjudicated incompetent or temporarily incapacitated because of a medical emergency. Incapacity does not prevent treatment; it merely requires the clinician to obtain substitute consent. Legal competence is very narrowly defined in terms of cognitive capacity. This definition derives largely from the laws governing transactions. Important clinical concepts such as affective incompetence are not usually recognized by the law unless cognitive capacity is significantly diminished.

Competency is not a scientifically determinable state and is situation specific. The issue of competency arises in a number of legal contexts. Although there are no hard and fast definitions, legally germane to determining competency is the patient's ability to

- Understand the particular treatment choice being proposed
- Make a treatment choice
- Be able to verbally or nonverbally communicate that choice

The above standard, however, obtains only a simple consent from the patient rather than an informed consent because alternative treatment choices are not provided.

A review of case law and scholarly literature reveals four standards for determining incompetency in decision making (Appelbaum et al. 1987). In order of levels of mental capacity required, these standards include the following:

- Communication of choice
- Understanding of information provided
- Appreciation of options available
- Rational decision making

Psychiatrists generally feel most comfortable with a rational decision-making standard in determining incompetency. Most courts, however, prefer the first two standards. A truly informed consent that considers the patient's autonomy, personal needs, and values occurs when rational decision making is applied by the patient to the risks and benefits of appropriate treatment options provided by the clinician.

A valid consent can be either *express* (oral or in writing) or *implied* from the patient's actions. The competency issue is particularly sensitive when dealing with minors or mentally disabled persons who lack the requisite cognitive capacity for health care decision making. In both cases, it is generally recognized in the law that an authorized representative or guardian may consent for them (Table 38–2).

☐ Information

The standard for exercising a legally sufficient disclosure varies from state to state. Traditionally, the duty to disclose was measured by a professional standard: either what a reasonable physician would disclose under the circumstances or the customary disclosure practices of physicians in a particular community. In the landmark case *Canterbury v. Spence* (1972), a patient-oriented standard was applied. This standard focused on the "material" information that a *reasonable* person in the patient's position would want to know in order to make a reasonably informed decision. An increasing number of courts have applied this standard, and some have expanded "material risks" to include information regarding the consequences of not consenting to the treatment or procedure (*Truman v. Thomas* 1980). Even in patient-oriented jurisdictions, there is no duty to disclose every possible risk. A material risk is defined as one in which a physician knows or should know what would be considered significant by a reasonable person in the patient's position. The issue of how much information a patient has to comprehend for consent to be valid is normally resolved by requiring a doctor to convey all appropriate information in terms that the average patient would understand.

☐ Voluntariness

For a consent to be considered legally voluntary, it must be given freely by the patient and without the presence of any form of coercion, fraud, or duress that impinges upon the patient's decision-making process. In evaluating whether a consent is truly voluntary, the courts will typically examine all of the relevant circumstances, including the psychiatrist's manner, environmental conditions, and the patient's mental state.

☐ Exceptions and Liability

There are four basic exceptions to the requirement of obtaining informed consent. When immediate treatment is necessary to save a life or prevent imminent serious harm, and it is impossible to obtain either the patient's consent or that of someone authorized to provide consent for the patient, the law will typically "presume" that the consent would have been granted. Two distinctions must be understood when applying this exception. First, the emergency must be serious and imminent, and, second, the patient's condition, and not the surrounding circumstances (e.g., adverse environmental conditions), determines the existence of an emergency.

A second exception exists when a patient lacks sufficient mental capacity to give competent consent or is found to be legally incompetent.

Someone who is incompetent is incapable of giving informed consent. Under these circumstances, consent must be obtained from a substitute decision-maker.

The third exception, *therapeutic privilege,* is the most difficult to apply. Informed consent may not be required if a psychiatrist determines that a complete disclosure of possible risks and alternatives might have a deleterious impact on the patient's health and welfare. Jurisdictions vary in their application of this exception. Absent specific case law or statutes outlining the factors relevant to such a decision, a doctor must substantiate a patient's inability to psychologically withstand being informed of the proposed treatment. Some courts have held that therapeutic privilege may be invoked only if informing the patient will worsen his or her condition or so frighten the patient that rational decision making is precluded (*Canterbury v. Spence* 1972). Therapeutic privilege cannot be used as a means of circumventing the legal requirement for obtaining informed consent from the patient before initiating treatment.

Finally, a physician need not disclose risks of treatment when the patient has competently, knowingly, and voluntarily waived his or her right to be informed (e.g., when the patient does not want to be informed of drug risks).

Absent a situation allowing one of the four exceptions, a psychiatrist who physically treats a patient without first obtaining informed consent is subject to legal liability. In some jurisdictions, a lack–of–informed consent action may be defeated if case law or statute provides that a reasonable person under the given circumstances would have consented to treatment. As a rule of thumb, treatment without any consent or against a patient's wishes may constitute a battery (intentional tort), whereas treatment commenced with an inadequate consent will be treated as an act of medical negligence.

☐ Right to Refuse Treatment

The developing concept that an institutionalized mentally disabled person has a right to refuse treatment is probably the most slippery issue in mental health law today. Buttressed by constitutionally derived rights to privacy and freedom from cruel and unusual punishment, the common law tort of battery, and the doctrine of informed consent, mentally disabled persons are increasingly being afforded protections traditionally reserved for the legally competent. This "new freedom" often runs directly counter to the dictates of clinical judgment (i.e., to treat and protect). As a result of this conflict, the courts vary considerably regarding the parameters of this right and the procedures to be followed.

Two landmark cases illustrate this point. In *Rennie v. Klein* (1978), the Third Circuit Court of Appeals recognized a right to refuse treatment in the state of New Jersey. The court, after extended litigation, found that this right could be overridden and antipsychotic drugs administered "whenever, in the exercise of professional judgment, such an action is deemed necessary to prevent the patient from endangering himself or others." In the second case, *Rogers v. Commissioner of Department of Mental Health* (1983), the court decided that in the absence of an emergency, any person who has not been adjudicated incompetent has a right to refuse antipsychotic medication. Incompetent persons have a similar right, but it must be exercised through a "substituted judgment treatment plan" that has been reviewed and approved by the court.

These two decisions are often viewed as legal bookends to the issue of the right to refuse treatment. The cases suggest parameters for other courts attempting to define such a right. The *Rennie* case became the model for subsequent legal decisions that adopted a treatment-driven rationale for the right to refuse treatment. *Rogers* became the basis for rights-driven approaches taken by some courts in litigating the right to refuse treatment.

☐ Right to Die

Legal decisions addressing the issue of a patient's "right to die" fall into one of two categories: those decisions dealing with individuals incompetent at the time that removal of life-support systems is sought (*In re Conroy* 1985; *In re Quinlin* 1976) and those dealing with competent patients.

Incompetent Patients

In what was hoped to be the "final word" on this very difficult and personal question of patient autonomy, the United States Supreme Court ruled, in *Cruzan v. Director, Missouri Department of Health* (1990), that the state of Missouri may refuse to remove a food and water tube surgically implanted in the stomach of Nancy Cruzan without clear and convincing evidence of her wishes. Ms. Cruzan had been in a persistent vegetative state for 7 years. In other words, without clear and convincing evidence of a patient's decision to have life-sustaining measures withheld in a particular circumstance, the state has the right to maintain that individual's life, even to the exclusion of the family's wishes.

The importance of the *Cruzan* decision for physicians treating severely or terminally impaired patients is that they must seek clear and competent instructions regarding foreseeable treatment decisions. For example, psychiatrists treating patients with progressive degenerative diseases should attempt to obtain the patient's wishes regarding the use of life-sustaining measures *while that patient can still competently articulate those wishes.* This information is best provided in the form of a living will or durable power-of-attorney agreement or health care proxy. However, any written document that clearly and convincingly sets forth the patient's wishes would serve the same purpose.

Competent Patients

A small but growing body of cases has emerged involving *competent* patients—usually suffering from excruciating pain and terminal diseases—who seek the termination of further medical treatment. The single most significant influence in the development of this body of law is the doctrine of informed consent. Beginning with the fundamental tenet that "no right is held more sacred . . . than the right of every individual to the possession and control of his own person" (*Schloendorff v. Society of New York Hospital* 1914), courts have fashioned the present-day "informed consent" doctrine and applied it to "right to die" cases.

Notwithstanding these principles, the right to decline life-sustaining medical intervention, even for a competent person, is not absolute. As noted in *In re Conroy* (1985), four countervailing state interests generally exist that may limit the exercise of that right: 1) preservation of life, 2) prevention of suicide, 3) safeguarding the integrity of the medical profession, and 4) the protection of innocent third parties (*In re Conroy* 1985). In each of these situations, and depending on the surrounding circumstances, the trend has been to support a competent patient's right to have artificial life-support systems discontinued (*Bouvia v. Superior Court* 1986; *In re Jobes* 1987; *In re Peter* 1987).

■ THE SUICIDAL PATIENT

The most common legal action involving psychiatric care is the failure to reasonably protect patients from harming themselves. In essence, theories of negligence involving suicide can be grouped into three broad categories: failure to properly diagnose (i.e., assess the potential for suicide); failure to treat (i.e., use reasonable treatment interventions and precautions); and failure to implement (i.e., carry out treatment properly and not negligently). As a general rule, a psychiatrist who exercises reasonable care in compliance with accepted medical practice will not be held liable for any resulting injury. Normally, if a patient's suicide was not reasonably foreseeable, or when the suicide occurred as a result of intervening factors, this rule will apply.

☐ Foreseeable Suicidal Patients

The evaluation of suicide risk is one of the most complex, difficult, and challenging clinical tasks in psychiatry. Suicide is a rare event with low specificity (high false-positive rates). A comprehensive assessment of a patient's suicide risk is critical to a sound clinical management plan. Using reasonable care in assessing suicide risk can preempt the problem of predicting the actual occurrence of suicide, for which professional standards do not yet exist. Standard approaches to the assessments of suicide risk have been proposed (Blumenthal 1990; Simon 1992a). Short-term (24–48 hours) suicide risk assessments are more reliable than long-term assessments.

As an accepted standard of care, an evaluation of suicide risk should be done with all patients, regardless of whether they present with overt suicidal complaints. A review of case law shows that reasonable care requires that a patient who is either suspected of being or confirmed to be suicidal must be the subject of certain affirmative precautions. A failure to either reasonably assess a patient's suicidality or implement an appropriate precautionary plan once the suicide potential becomes foreseeable is likely to render a practitioner liable if the patient is harmed because of a suicide attempt. The law tends to assume that suicide is preventable if it is foreseeable. Foreseeability, however, should not be confused with preventability. In hindsight, many suicides seem preventable that were clearly not foreseeable.

Intervention in an inpatient setting usually requires the following:

- Screening evaluations
- Case review by clinical staff
- Development of an appropriate treatment plan
- Implementation of that plan

Careful documentation of assessments and management interventions with responsive changes to the patient's clinical situation should be considered clinically and legally sufficient psychiatric care. Assessing suicide risk is only half the equation. Documenting the benefits of a psychiatric intervention (e.g., ward change, pass, discharge) against the risk of suicide permits an even-handed approach to the clinical management of the patient. Consideration only of a patient's suicide risk is a manifestation of defensive psychiatry that interferes with good clinical care, possibly further exposing the psychiatrist to a malpractice suit. Psychiatrists are more likely to be sued when a psychiatric inpatient commits suicide. The law presumes that the opportunities to foresee (i.e., anticipate) and control (i.e., treat and manage) suicidal patients are greater in the hospital.

Outpatient therapists face a somewhat different situation. Psychiatrists are expected to assess the severity and imminence of a foreseeably suicidal act. The result of the assessment dictates the nature of the duty-of-care options. Courts have reasoned that when an outpatient commits suicide, the therapist will not necessarily be held to have breached a duty to safeguard the patient from foreseeable self-harm because of the difficulty in controlling the patient (*Speer v. United States* 1981). Instead, the reasonableness of the psychiatrist's efforts will be determinative.

☐ Suicide Prevention Pacts

Suicide prevention "contracts" created between the clinician and the patient attempt to develop an expressed understanding that the patient will call for help rather than act out suicidal thoughts or impulses. These "contracts" have no legal authority. While possibly helpful in solidifying the therapeutic alliance, such "contracts" may falsely reassure the psychiatrist. Suicide prevention agreements between psychiatrists and patients must not be used in place of adequate suicide assessment (Simon 1991b).

☐ Legal Defenses

One legal defense that has created a split in the courts involves the use of the "open door" policy in which patients are allowed freedom of movement for therapeutic purposes. In these cases, the individual facts and reasonableness of the staff's application of the "open door" policy appear to be paramount. Nevertheless, courts have difficulty with abstract treatment notions such as personal growth when faced with a dead patient.

Another defense, the doctrine of sovereign or governmental immunity, may statutorily bar a finding of liability against a state or federal facility. An intervening cause of suicide over which the clinician has no control is another valid legal defense. For example, a court might find that the suicidal act of a borderline patient who experienced a significant rejection between therapy sessions and then impulsively attempted suicide without trying to contact the therapist was caused by the superseding intervening variable of an unforeseen rejection and not by the therapist's negligence. Finally, the best-judgment defense has been used successfully when the patient was properly assessed and treated for suicide risk but he or she committed suicide anyway (Robertson 1991).

■ THE VIOLENT PATIENT

As a general rule, one person has no duty to control the conduct of a second person in order to prevent that person from physically harming a third person (Restatement [Second] of Torts 315(a) [1965]). Applying this rule to psychiatric care, psychiatrists traditionally have had only a limited duty to control hospitalized patients and to exercise due care upon discharge. Within the last two decades, this rule has changed. After *Tarasoff* (*Tarasoff vs. Regents of the University of California* 1976), the therapist's legal duty and potential liability have significantly expanded. In *Tarasoff*, the California Supreme Court first recognized that a duty to protect third parties was imposed only when a special relationship existed between the victim, the individual whose conduct created the danger, and the defendant.

Only a small minority of courts have held that a duty to protect exists for the population at large. Despite the fact that it still is not law in a number of jurisdictions and is subject to different interpretations by individual courts, the duty to protect is, in effect, a national standard of practice. In some jurisdictions, courts have held that the need to safeguard the public well-being overrides all other considerations, including confidentiality. In certain states, a psychotherapist has a duty to act affirmatively to protect an endangered third party from a patient's violent or dangerous acts. Although a few courts have declined to find a *Tarasoff* duty in a specific case, a growing number of courts have recognized some variation of the original *Tarasoff* duty. No court has rejected the duty outright as legally invalid.

A number of states have enacted immunity statutes that protect the therapist from legal liability from a patient's violent acts toward others (Appelbaum et al. 1989). The majority of these statutes define the therapist's duty in terms of warning the endangered third party and/or notifying the authorities. The duty-to-protect language stated in some statutes allows for a greater variety of clinical interventions.

☐ Release of Potentially Violent Patients

Courts closely evaluate decisions made by psychiatrists who treat inpatients that adversely affect the patient or a third party. Liability imposed on psychiatric facilities that had custody of patients who injured others outside the institution following escape or release is clearly distinguishable from the factual situation of *Tarasoff*. Duty-to-warn cases involve patients in outpatient treatment. Liability arises from the inaction of the therapist who fails to take affirmative measures to warn or protect endangered third persons. In negligent-release cases, however, liability may arise from the allegation that the institution's affirmative act in releasing the patient caused injury to the third party. Lawsuits stemming from the release of a foreseeably dangerous patient who subsequently injures or kills himself or someone else are roughly five to six times more common than outpatient duty-to-warn litigation (Simon 1992b).

Psychiatrists must not discharge patients and then forget about them. The patient's willingness to cooperate with the psychiatrist, however, is critical to maintaining follow-up treatment. The psychiatrist's obligation focuses upon structuring the follow-up visits in such a fashion as to encourage compliance. Nevertheless, limitations do exist on the extent of the psychiatrist's ability to ensure follow-up care. These limitations must be acknowledged by both the psychiatric and legal communities (Simon 1992a).

In either the outpatient or inpatient situation, psychiatrists will comply with the responsibility to warn and protect others from potentially violent patients if they reasonably assess a patient's *risk* for violence and act in a clinically appropriate manner based on their findings. Professional standards do exist for the assessment of the risk factors for violence (Simon 1992c). No standard of care exists, however, for the prediction of violent behavior. The clinician should assess the risk of violence frequently, updating the risk assessment at significant clinical junctures (e.g., room and ward changes, passes, discharge). A risk-benefit assessment should be conducted and recorded prior to issuing a pass or discharge.

◼ INVOLUNTARY HOSPITALIZATION

A person may be involuntarily hospitalized only if certain statutorily mandated criteria are met. Three main substantive criteria serve as the foundation for all statutory commitment requirements: that the individual 1) be mentally ill, 2) be dangerous to self or others, and/or 3) be unable to provide for his or her basic needs. Generally, each state spells out which criteria are required and what each means. Terms such as "mentally ill" are often loosely described, thus displacing the responsibility for proper definition onto the clinical judgment of the petitioner.

In addition to individuals with mental illness, certain states have enacted legislation that permits the involuntary hospitalization of three other distinct groups: developmentally disabled (mentally retarded) persons, individuals who are addicted to a substance(s) (alcohol, drugs), and mentally disabled minors. Special commitment provisions may exist governing requirements for the admission and discharge of mentally disabled minors as well as numerous due-process rights afforded these individuals (*Parham v. J.R.* 1979).

Involuntary hospitalization of psychiatric patients usually arises when violent behavior threatens to erupt and when patients become unable to care for themselves. Clinicians must remember that they do not commit patients; this is done solely under the jurisdiction of the court. Commitment statutes do not require involuntary hospitalization but are permissive (Appelbaum et al. 1989). The statutes enable mental health professionals and others to seek involuntary hospitalization for persons who meet certain substantive criteria. On the other hand, the duty to seek involuntary hospitalization is a standard-of-care issue. Patients who are mentally ill and pose an imminent, serious threat to themselves or others may require involuntary hospitalization as a primary psychiatric intervention.

The most common cause of a malpractice action involving involuntary hospitalization occurs when a psychiatrist fails to adhere in good faith to statutory requirements, leading to a wrongful commitment. Often, these lawsuits are brought under the theory of false imprisonment. Other areas of liability that may arise from wrongful commitment include assault and battery, malicious prosecution, abuse of authority, and intentional infliction of emotional distress (Simon 1992a).

■ SEXUAL MISCONDUCT

Therapist-patient sex is usually preceded by progressive boundary violations in treatment (Simon 1989). As a consequence, patients are frequently psychologically damaged by the precursor boundary violations as well as the ultimate sexual misconduct of the therapist (Simon 1991a). An excellent account of the gradual erosion of treatment boundaries leading to near loss of control with a client is given by Rutter (1989).

Awareness of general boundary guidelines for conducting psychiatric treatment and of their transgression may help alert the therapist to progressive boundary violations (Simon 1994). Unfortunately, professional ethics codes are usually silent concerning the boundary violations that often precede therapist sexual misconduct. Sexual misconduct does not occur in isolation but usually involves a variety of negligent acts of omission and commission.

□ Civil Liability

Psychiatrists who sexually exploit their patients are subject to civil and criminal actions as well as ethical and professional licensure revocation proceedings (see Table 38–4). Malpractice constitutes the most common area of liability.

Table 38–4. Legal and ethical consequences of sexual exploitation

Civil lawsuit	Civil action for intentional tort
Negligence	(e.g., battery, fraud)
Loss of consortium	License revocation
Breach-of-contract action	Ethical sanctions
Criminal sanctions (e.g., adultery,	Dismissal from professional
sexual assault, rape)	organizations

Source.   Reprinted from Simon 1992a.

An increasing number of states have statutorily made sexual activity both civilly and criminally actionable. The number of states enacting civil statutes is constantly increasing (Simon 1992a). Moreover, a number of states make therapist sexual misconduct a crime. Some states prosecute sexual exploitation suits using their sexual assault statutes. Legislatures in a number of states have enacted statutes that provide civil or criminal remedies to patients who were sexually abused by their therapists (Appelbaum 1990; Strasburger et al. 1991).

Three basic types of remedies have been codified: reporting, civil liability, and criminal statutes. *Reporting statutes* require the disclosure to state authorities by a therapist who learns of any past or current therapist-patient sex. A few states have *civil statutes* proscribing sexual misconduct. Civil statutes incorporate a standard of care and make malpractice suits easier to pursue. *Criminal sanctions* may be the only remedy for exploitative therapists without malpractice insurance, who are unlicensed, or who do not belong to professional organizations.

☐ Criminal Sanctions

Sexual exploitation of a patient, under certain circumstances, may be considered rape or some analogous sexual offense and may therefore be criminally actionable. Typically, the criminality of the exploitation is determined by one of three factors: the practitioner's means of inducement, the age of the victim, or the availability of a relevant state criminal code.

Sex with a current patient may be criminally actionable under sexual assault statutes if the state can prove beyond a reasonable doubt (i.e., with 90% to 95% certainty) that the patient was coerced into engaging in the sexual act. Typically, this type of evidence is limited to the use of some form of substance (e.g., medication) to either induce compliance or reduce resistance. Anesthesia, electroconvulsive treatment, hypnosis, drugs, force, and threat of harm have been used to coerce patients into sexual submission (Schoener et al. 1989). To date, claims of "psychological coercion" via the manipulation of transference phenomena have not been successful in establishing the coercion necessary for a criminal case. In cases involving a minor patient, the issue of consent or coercion is irrelevant, because minors and incompetent persons (including adult incompetent persons) are considered unable to provide valid consent. Therefore, sex with a child or an incompetent person is automatically considered a criminal act.

☐ Professional Disciplinary Action

For the purposes of adjudicating allegations of professional misconduct, licensing boards are typically granted certain regulatory and disciplinary authority by state statutes. As a result, state licensing organizations, un-like professional associations, may discipline more effectively and puni-tively an offending professional by suspending or revoking his or her license. Patients may bring ethical charges against psychiatrists before the district branches of the American Psychiatric Association. Ethical vio-lators may be reprimanded, suspended, or expelled from the APA. All national organizations of mental health professionals have ethically pro-scribed sexual relations between therapist and patient. Ethical charges can only be filed against members of a professional group.

■ ASSESSMENT OF SEXUAL HARASSMENT

Civil suits alleging sexual harassment are burgeoning. Psychiatrists are being called upon to testify in these cases that present emerging, com-plex psychological and social issues. The statutory basis for sexual harass-ment claims is found in Title VII of the Civil Rights Act of 1964. Section 703(a)(1) of Title VII, 42 U.S.C. § 2000e-2(a), provides:

> It shall be an unlawful employment practice for an employer . . . to fail or refuse to hire or to discharge any individual, or otherwise to discriminate against any individual with respect to his compensation, terms, condi-tions, or privileges of employment, because of such individual's race, color, religion, sex, or national origin.

In 1980, the Equal Employment Opportunity Commission (EEOC) is-sued guidelines that declared sexual harassment to be a violation of Sec-tion 703 of Title VII. The guidelines propounded criteria for determining unwelcome conduct of a sexual nature that constituted sexual harass-ment, defined the circumstances under which an employer may be held liable, and suggested affirmative steps that an employer should take to prevent sexual harassment (Guidelines on Discrimination Because of Sex, 29 C.F.R. § 1604.11).

In defining sexual harassment, Title VII does not proscribe all con-duct of a sexual nature in the workplace. Only unwelcome sexual con-duct that is a term or condition of employment constitutes a violation. The EEOC's guidelines define two kinds of sexual harassment: "quid pro quo" and "hostile environment." Sexual conduct constitutes sexual har-assment when "submission to such conduct is made either explicitly or implicitly a term or condition of an individual's employment" (29 C.F.R. § 1604.11[a][1]). "Quid pro quo" harassment takes place whenever "sub-mission or rejection of such conduct by an individual is used as the basis for employment decisions affecting such individual" (29 C.F.R. § 1604.11[a][2]). The EEOC guidelines also recognize that unwelcome sexual conduct that "unreasonably interfere[es] with an individual's job performance" or creates an "intimidating, hostile, or offensive working environment" can constitute sex discrimination, even if it causes no tangible or economic job consequences (29 C.F.R. § 1604.11[a][3]).

The United States Supreme Court, in *Harris v. Forklift Systems, Inc.* (1993), ruled unanimously that a woman who claims she was sexually harassed on the job need not prove she was psychologically injured to win money damages. The Court defined unlawful harassment as creating a work environment that a reasonable person would find "hostile or abusive." The broadly written ruling will likely make it easier for employees to bring suits for sexual harassment.

Psychiatrists who become involved in sexual harassment litigation usually are asked to determine the veracity of harassment complaints, the psychological consequences of harassment, and the treatment needs and prognosis for women or men who have been sexually harassed.

■ SECLUSION AND RESTRAINT

The psychiatric legal issues surrounding seclusion and restraint are complex. Seclusion and restraint have both indications and contraindications as clinical management modalities (see Tables 38–5 and 38–6). The legal regulation of seclusion and restraint has become increasingly more stringent over the past decade. Legal challenges to the use of restraints and seclusion have been made on behalf of the institutionalized mentally ill and the mentally retarded. Normally, these lawsuits do not stand alone, but are part of a challenge to a wide range of alleged abuses within a hospital.

Generally, courts hold, or consent decrees provide, that restraints and seclusion can be implemented only when a patient presents a risk of harm to self or others and no less restrictive alternative is available. Additional considerations include the following:

1. Restraint and seclusion can only be implemented by a written order from an appropriate medical official.
2. Orders are to be confined to specific, time-limited periods.
3. A patient's condition must be regularly reviewed and documented.
4. Any extension of an original order must be reviewed and reauthorized.

In addition to these guidelines, some courts and state statutes outline certain due-process procedures that must be followed before a restraint or seclusion order can be implemented. Typical due-process considerations include some form of notice, a hearing, and the involvement of an

---

Table 38–5.   Indications for seclusion and restraint

1. Prevent clear, imminent harm to the patient or others.
2. Prevent significant disruption to treatment program or physical surroundings.
3. Assist in treatment as part of ongoing behavior therapy.
4. Decrease sensory overstimulation (seclusion only).
5. Respond to patient's voluntary reasonable request.

Source.   Reprinted from Simon 1992c.

Table 38–6.   Contraindications to seclusion and restraint

1. Extremely unstable medical and psychiatric conditions[a]
2. Delirious or demented patients unable to tolerate decreased stimulation[a]
3. Overtly suicidal patients[a]
4. Patients with severe drug reactions or overdoses or those patients requiring close monitoring of drug dosages[a]
5. For punishment or for convenience of staff

---

[a]Unless close supervision and direct observation are provided.
Source.   Reprinted from Simon 1992c.

---

impartial decision-maker. Notably, patient due-process protections are only required in cases in which restraint and seclusion are used for disciplinary purposes. Absent language to the contrary, these procedures may be eased in cases of emergency.

The acceptability of restraint or seclusion for the purposes of training was recognized in the landmark case *Youngberg v. Romeo* (1982). *Youngberg* involved a challenge to the "treatment" practices at the Pennhurst State School and Hospital in Pennsylvania. The United States Supreme Court held that patients could not be restrained except to ensure their safety or, in certain undefined circumstances, "to provide needed training." While recognizing that the defendant had a liberty interest in safety and freedom from bodily restraint, the Court added that these interests were not absolute and in conflict with the need to provide training. The Court also held that decisions made by appropriate professionals regarding restraining the patient would presumptively be considered correct. *Youngberg* is viewed as the first step in the right direction by advocates for the developmentally disabled. In addition, psychiatrists and other mental health professionals have lauded the decision because the Court recognized that professionals, rather than the courts, are best able to determine the needs of patients, including determining when restraint is appropriate.

Most states have enacted statutes regulating the use of restraints, normally specifying the circumstances in which restraints can be used. Most often, those circumstances occur only when a risk of harm to self or danger to others is imminent. Only about one-half of the states have laws relating to seclusion. National guidelines for the proper use of seclusion and restraints have been established by the American Psychiatric Association Task Force on the Psychiatric Uses of Seclusion and Restraint (1984). The Joint Commission on Accreditation of Healthcare Organizations (JCAHO) has promulgated detailed guidelines for hospitals regarding seclusion and restraint requirements (JCAHO 1990, SC.2.1– SC.2.10, pp. 146–147). Unless precluded by state freedom from restraint and seclusion statutes, a variety of uses for seclusion can be justified on both clinical and legal grounds (Simon 1992a).

■ ADVANCE DIRECTIVES

The use of advance directives such as a living will, health care proxy, or a durable medical power of attorney is recommended in order to avoid ethical and legal complications associated with requests to withhold life-sustaining treatment measures (Simon 1992a; Solnick 1985). The Patient Self-Determination Act, which took effect on December 1, 1991, requires hospitals, nursing homes, hospices, managed care organizations, and home health care agencies to advise patients or family members of their right to accept or refuse medical care and to execute an advance directive (LaPuma et al. 1991). These advance directives provide a method for individuals, while competent, to choose proxy health care decision-makers in the event of future incompetency. A living will can be contained as a subsection of a durable power-of-attorney agreement. In the ordinary power of attorney created for the management of business and financial matters, the power of attorney generally becomes null and void if the person creating it becomes incompetent.

Generally, durable power of attorney has been construed to empower an agent to make health care decisions. Such a document is much broader and flexible than a living will, which covers just the period of a diagnosed terminal illness, specifying only that no "extraordinary treatments" be utilized that would prolong the act of dying (Mishkin 1985). To rectify the sometimes uncertain status of the durable power of attorney as applied to health care decisions, a number of states have passed or are considering passing health care proxy laws. The health care proxy is a legal instrument akin to the durable power of attorney but specifically created for health care decision making.

In a durable power of attorney or health care proxy, general or specific directions are set forth about how future decisions should be made in the event one becomes unable to make these decisions. The determination of a patient's competence, however, is not specified in most durable power-of-attorney and health care proxy statutes. Because this is a medical or psychiatric question, the examination by two physicians to determine the patient's ability to understand the nature and consequences of the proposed treatment or procedure, the ability to make a choice, and the ability to communicate that choice, is usually minimally sufficient.

Because durable-power-of-attorney agreements or health care proxies can be easily revoked, the treating psychiatrist or institution has no choice but to honor the patient's refusal, even if there is reasonable evidence that the patient is incompetent. Legal consultation also should be considered at this point. If the patient is grossly disordered and is an immediate danger to self and others, the physician or hospital is on firmer ground medically and legally to temporarily override the patient's treatment refusal. Otherwise, it is generally better to seek a court order for treatment than risk legal entanglement with the patient by attempting to enforce the original terms of the advance directive. Typically, unless there are compelling medical reasons to do otherwise, courts will generally honor the patient's original treatment directions given while competent.

■ GUARDIANSHIP

Guardianship is a method of substitute decision making for individuals who have been judicially determined to be unable to act for themselves (Brakel et al. 1985). In some states, there are separate provisions for the appointment of a "guardian of one's person" (e.g., health care decision making) and for a "guardian of one's estate" (e.g., authority to make contracts to sell one's property) (Sale et al. 1982). This latter guardian is frequently referred to as a *conservator*. A further distinction, also found in some jurisdictions, is *general (plenary)* and *specific* guardianship (Sale et al. 1982). As the name implies, the specific guardian is restricted to exercising decisions about a particular subject area. General guardians, in contrast, have total control over the disabled individual's person, estate, or both (Sale et al. 1982).

Guardianship arrangements are increasingly utilized with patients suffering from dementia, particularly AIDS-related dementia and Alzheimer's disease (Overman and Stoudemire 1988). Under the Anglo-American system of law, an individual is presumed to be competent unless adjudicated incompetent. Thus, incompetence is a legal determination made by a court of law based on evidence provided by health care providers and others that the individual's functional mental capacity is significantly impaired.

Generally, the appointment of a guardian is limited to situations in which the individual's decision-making capacity is so impaired that he or she is unable to care for personal safety or provide such necessities as food, shelter, clothing, and medical care, likely resulting in physical injury or illness (*In re Boyer* 1981). The standard of proof required for a judicial determination of incompetency is *clear and convincing evidence.* Although the law does not assign percentages to proof, clear and convincing evidence is in the range of 75% certainty (Simon 1992a).

■ SUBSTITUTED JUDGMENT

Psychiatrists often find that the time required to obtain an adjudication of incompetence is unduly burdensome and that the process frequently interferes with the provision of quality treatment. Moreover, families are often reluctant to face the formal court proceedings necessary to declare their family member incompetent, particularly when sensitive family matters are disclosed. A common solution to both of these problems is to seek the legally authorized *proxy consent of a spouse or relative serving as guardian* when the refusing patient is believed to be incompetent. Proxy consent, however, is not available in every state (Simon 1992a).

There are clear advantages associated with having the family serve as decision-makers (Perr 1984). First, use of responsible family members as surrogate decision-makers maintains the integrity of the family unit and relies on the sources that are most likely to know the patient's wishes. Second, it is more efficient and less costly. There are some disadvantages, however. Proxy decision making requires synthesizing the diverse values, beliefs, practices, and prior statements of the patient for a given specific circumstance (Emanuel and Emanuel 1992). Ambivalent feelings, conflicts within the family and with the patient, and conflicting economic interest may make certain family members suspect as guardians (Gutheil and Appelbaum 1980). Also, relatives may not be available or want to get involved.

A number of states permit proxy decision making by statute, mainly through informed-consent statutes (Solnick 1985). Some state statutes specify that another person may authorize consent on behalf of the incompetent patient, while others mention specific relatives. Unless proxy consent by a relative is provided by statute or by case law authority in the state where the psychiatrist practices, it is not recommended that the good-faith consent by next of kin be relied upon in treating a patient believed to be incompetent (Klein et al. 1983). The legally appropriate procedure to follow is to seek judicial recognition of the family member as the substitute decision-maker.

For the patient who continues to lack mental capacity for health care decisions, an increasing number of states provide administrative procedures authorized by statute that permit involuntary treatment of the incompetent and refusing mentally ill patients who do not meet current standards for involuntary civil commitment (Zito et al. 1984). In most jurisdictions, a durable power-of-attorney agreement permits the next of kin to consent through durable power-of-attorney statutes (Solnick 1985).

■ CRIMINAL PROCEEDINGS

Individuals charged with committing crimes frequently display significant psychiatric and neurological impairment. A history of severe head injury may be present. The possibility of a neuropsychiatric disorder must be thoroughly investigated. For example, Lewis et al. (1986) examined 15 death-row inmates who were chosen for examination because of imminent execution rather than evidence of neuropathology. In each case, evidence of severe head injury and neurological impairment was found.

☐ Criminal Intent (*Mens Rea*)

Under the common law, the basic elements of a crime are 1) the mental state or level of intent to commit the act (known as the *mens rea*, or guilty mind), 2) the act itself or conduct associated with committing the crime (known as *actus reus*, or guilty act), and 3) a concurrence in time between the guilty act and the guilty mental state (*Bethea v. United States* 1977). To convict a person of a particular crime, the state must prove beyond a reasonable doubt that the defendant committed the criminal act with the requisite intent. All three elements are necessary in order to satisfy the threshold requirements for the imposition of criminal sanctions.

The question of intent is a particularly vexing problem for the courts. For example, everyone would agree that killing another person is deplorable conduct. But should the accidental death of child in a car accident, the heat-of-passion shooting by a husband of his wife's lover, and the "cold blooded" murder of a bank teller by a robber all be punished the same? The determination of the defendant's intent, or *mens rea*, at the time of the offense is the law's mechanism for deciding criminal culpability and appropriate retribution. For instance, a person who deliberately plans to commit a crime is more culpable than one who accidentally commits one.

There are two classes of intent used to categorize *mens rea*: specific and general. Specific intent refers to the *mens rea* in those crimes in which a *further intention* is present beyond that which is identified with the physical act associated with an offense. For instance, the courts will frequently state that the intent necessary for first-degree murder includes a "specific intent to kill," or a person might commit an assault "with the intent to rape" (Melton et al. 1987). Unlike general criminal intent, specific criminal intent cannot be presumed from the unlawful criminal act but must be proved independently. General criminal intent is more elusive. Such intent may be presumed from commission of the criminal act. It usually is used by the law to explain criminal liability in which a defendant was merely conscious or should have been conscious of one's physical actions at the time of the offense (Melton et al. 1987).

Persons with certain mental handicaps or impairments represent an interesting challenge for prosecutors, defense counsel, and judges in determining what, if any, retribution is justifiable. Mental impairment often raises serious questions about the intent to commit a crime and the appreciation of its consequences. In addition to *mens rea,* a person's mental status can play a deciding role in whether the defendant will be ordered to stand trial to face the criminal charges, be acquitted of the alleged crime, be sent to prison, be hospitalized, or, in some extreme cases, be sentenced to death. Before any defendant can be criminally prosecuted, the court must be satisfied that the accused is competent to stand trial, that is, understands the charges brought against him or her and is capable of rationally assisting counsel with the defense.

☐ Competency to Stand Trial

In every situation in which competency is a question, the law seeks to reiterate a common theme: that only the acts of a rational individual are to be given recognition by society (*Neely v. United States* 1945). Throughout involvement with the trial process, the defendant must have "sufficient present ability to consult with his lawyer with a reasonable degree of rational understanding and whether he has a rational as well as factual understanding of the proceedings against him" (*Dusky v. United States* 1960).

Typically, the impairment that raises the question of the defendant's competence will be associated with a mental disease or defect. However, a person may be held to be incompetent to stand trial even if the defendant does not suffer from a mental disease or defect as defined by the American Psychiatric Association (1994) in DSM-IV. For example, children under a certain age ordinarily are deemed incompetent to stand trial. Although the majority of impairments implicated in competency examinations are functional rather than organic (Reich and Wells 1985), various forms of neuropsychiatric impairments will typically raise questions about a defendant's competency to stand trial. It is the actual *functional* mental capability to meet the minimal standard of trial competency, and not the severity of the deficits, that determine whether an individual is cognitively capable to be tried.

The Competency to Stand Trial Instrument (CSTI) was designed to standardize, objectify, and qualify relevant criteria for the determination of an individual's competency to stand trial. The following are the recommended 13 functions to be assessed (McGarry 1973):

- Ability to appraise the legal defenses available
- Level of unmanageable behavior
- Quality of relating to attorney
- Ability to plan legal strategy
- Ability to appraise the roles of various participants in the courtroom proceedings
- Understanding of court procedure
- Appreciation of the charges
- Appreciation of the range and nature of possible penalties
- Ability to appraise the likely outcome
- Capacity to disclose to attorney available pertinent facts surrounding the offense
- Capacity to challenge prosecution witnesses realistically
- Capacity to testify relevantly
- Capacity to manifest self-serving versus self-defeating motivation

The degree of a defendant's impairment in one particular function, however, does not automatically render the accused incompetent. For example, the fact that the defendant is manifesting certain deficits because of damage to the parietal lobe does not necessarily mean that he or she lacks the requisite cognitive ability to aid in his or her own defense at trial (Tranel 1992). The ultimate determination of incompetency is solely for the court to decide (*United States v. David* 1975). Moreover, the impairment must be considered in the context of the particular case or proceeding. Mental impairment may render an individual incompetent to stand trial in a complicated tax fraud case but not incompetent for a misdemeanor trial.

☐ Insanity Defense

Defendants with functional or organic mental disabilities who are found competent to stand trial may seek acquittal on the basis that they were not criminally responsible for their actions because of insanity at the time the offense was committed. The vast majority of criminals commit crimes for many reasons, but the law presumes that all of them do so rationally and with their own free will. As a result, the law concludes that they are deserving of some form of punishment. Some offenders, however, are so mentally disturbed in their thinking and behavior that they are thought to be incapable of acting rationally. Under these circumstances, civilized societies have deemed it unjust to punish a "crazy" or insane person. While the insanity defense is rarely used, a successful insanity defense is even rarer.

A generally accepted, precise definition of legal insanity does not exist. Over the years, tests of insanity have been subject to much controversy, modification, and refinement (Brakel et al. 1985). The development of the insanity defense standard in the United States has had four basic elements: presence of a mental disorder, presence of a defect of reason, lack of knowledge of the nature or wrongfulness of the act, and an incapacity to refrain from the act (Simon 1994).

The threshold issue in making an insanity determination is not the existence of a mental disease or defect per se, but the lack of substantial mental capacity because of it. Therefore, the lack of capacity due to mental defects other than mental illness may be sufficient. For instance, mental retardation may represent an adequate basis for the insanity defense under certain circumstances.

The impulse disorders—intermittent explosive disorder, kleptomania, pathological gambling, and pyromania—generally have not fared well under an insanity defense. These conditions would not meet the cognitive prong of an insanity defense. Presumably, the volitional prong would be applicable but is usually insufficient by itself. Moreover, courts and juries tend to view criminal acts arising from impulse disorders as impulses not resisted rather than irresistible impulses.

☐ Diminished Capacity

It is possible for a person to have the required *mens rea* and yet still be declared legally insane. For instance, a defendant's actions may be considered so "crazy" as to convince a jury that he or she was criminally insane and therefore not legally responsible. Yet his or her knowledge of the criminal act was relatively intact. From this distinction, the law recognizes that there are "shades" of mental impairment that obviously can affect *mens rea*, but not necessarily to the extent of completely nullifying it. In recognition of this fact, the concept of *diminished capacity* was developed (Melton et al. 1987).

Broadly viewed, diminished capacity permits the accused to introduce medical and psychological evidence that relates directly to the *mens rea* for the crime charged, without having to assert a defense of insanity (Melton et al. 1987). For example, in the crime of assault with the intent to kill, psychiatric testimony would be permitted to address whether the offender acted with the purpose of committing homicide at the time of the assault. When a defendant's *mens rea* for the crime charged is nullified by psychiatric evidence, the defendant is acquitted only of that charge. In the above example, the prosecutor may still try to convict the defendant of another offense requiring a lesser *mens rea*, such as manslaughter (Melton et al. 1987). Patients suffering from psychiatric disorders who commit criminal acts may be eligible for a diminished capacity defense.

☐ Guilty but Mentally Ill

In a number of states, an alternative verdict of *guilty but mentally ill* (GBMI) has been established. Under GBMI statutes, if the defendant pleads not guilty by reason of insanity, this alternative verdict is available to the jury (Slovenko 1982). Under an insanity plea, the verdict may be not guilty, not guilty by reason of insanity, guilty but mentally ill, or guilty. The problem with GBMI is that it is an alternative verdict without a difference from finding the defendant plain guilty.

☐ Exculpatory and Mitigating Disorders

Psychotic disorders of differing etiology form the most common basis for an insanity defense. But in addition to the major psychiatric and organic brain disorders, a number of other conditions may provide a foundation for an insanity or diminished capacity defense.

Automatisms

For conviction of a crime, there must be not only a criminal state of mind (*mens rea*) but also the commission of a prohibited act (*actus reus*). The physical movement necessary to satisfy the *actus reus* requirement must be conscious and volitional. A defense claiming the commission of a crime was an involuntary act usually is referred to as an "automatism defense." A conscious, reflexive action carried out under stressful circumstances may qualify for an automatism defense. For example, a driver who is being attacked in his car by a bee loses control in attempting to swat the insect. The car strikes a pedestrian, who is killed. An automatism defense exists to charges of vehicular homicide.

Intoxication

Ordinarily, intoxication is not a defense to a criminal charge. Because intoxication, unlike mental illness, mental retardation, and most neuropsychiatric conditions, is usually the product of a person's own actions, the law is naturally cautious about viewing it as a complete defense or mitigating factor. Most states view voluntary alcoholism as relevant to the issue of whether the defendant possessed the *mens rea* necessary to commit a specific intent crime or whether there was premeditation in a crime of murder. Generally, however, the mere fact that the defendant was voluntarily intoxicated will not justify a finding of automatism or insanity. A distinct difference does arise when, because of chronic, heavy use of alcohol, the defendant suffers from an alcohol-induced organic mental disorder, such as alcohol hallucinosis, withdrawal delirium, amnestic disorder, or dementia associated with alcoholism. If competent psychiatric evidence is presented that an alcohol-related neuropsychiatric disorder caused significant cognitive or volitional impairment, a defense of insanity or diminished capacity could be upheld.

Temporal Lobe Seizures

Another "mental state" defense occasionally raised by defendants regarding assault-related crimes is that the assaultive behavior was involuntarily precipitated by abnormal electrical patterns in the defendant's brain. This condition is frequently diagnosed as temporal lobe epilepsy (Devinsky and Bear 1984). Episodic dyscontrol syndrome (Elliott 1982) has also been advanced as a neuropsychiatric condition causing involuntary aggression.

Metabolic Disorders

Defenses based on metabolic disorders have also been tried. The so-called Twinkie defense was used as part of a successful diminished capacity defense of Dan White in the murders of San Francisco Mayor George Mosconi and Supervisor Harvey Milk. This defense was based on the theory that the ingestion of large amounts of sugar contributed to a state of temporary insanity (*People v. White* 1981).

■ PERSONAL INJURY LITIGATION

Civil litigation in psychic injury and head trauma cases may require the evaluation and testimony of psychiatrists as well as neurologists, other physicians, psychologists, neuropsychologists, and allied mental health professionals. Psychiatrists can become involved in litigation as witnesses in one of two ways: as treaters or as forensic experts.

Psychiatrists who venture into the legal arena must be aware of the fundamentally different roles that exist between a treating psychiatrist and the forensic psychiatric expert. Treatment and expert roles do not mix. For example, unlike the orthopedist who possesses objective data such as the X ray of a broken limb to demonstrate orthopedic damages in court, the treating psychiatrist must rely heavily on the subjective report-ing of the patient. In the treatment context, psychiatrists are interested primarily in the patient's perception of his or her difficulties, not neces-sarily the objective reality. As a consequence, many treating psychiatrists do not speak to third parties or check pertinent records to gain additional information about a patient or to corroborate the patient's statements. The law, however, *is* interested only in that which can reasonably be established by facts. Uncorroborated, subjective patient data are fre-quently attacked in court as being speculative, self-serving, and unreli-able. The treating psychiatrist usually is not well equipped to counter these charges.

Credibility issues also abound. The treating psychiatrist is, and must be, a total ally of the patient. This bias toward the patient is a proper treatment stance that fosters the therapeutic alliance. In court, opposing counsel will take every opportunity to portray the treating psychiatrist as a subjective mouthpiece for the patient-litigant. Also, court testimony by the treating psychiatrist may compel the disclosure of information that may not be *legally* privileged, but nonetheless is viewed as intimate and confidential by the patient. This disclosure by the previously trusted therapist is bound to cause psychological damage to the therapeutic rela-tionship (Strasburger 1987). In addition, psychiatrists must be careful to inform patients about the consequences of releasing treatment informa-tion, particularly in legal matters.

The American Academy of Psychiatry and the Law (1989), in its eth-ics statement, advises that "a treating psychiatrist should generally avoid agreeing to be an expert witness or to perform an evaluation of his pa-tient for legal purposes because a forensic evaluation usually requires that other people be interviewed and testimony may adversely affect the therapeutic relationship." The treating psychiatrist should attempt to re-main solely in a treatment role. If it becomes necessary to testify on be-half of the patient, the treating psychiatrist should testify only as a fact witness rather than as an expert witness. As a fact witness, the psychia-trist will be asked to describe the number and length of visits, diagnosis, and treatment. Generally, no opinion evidence will be requested con-cerning causation of the injury or extent of damages. In some jurisdic-tions, however, the court may convert a fact witness into an expert at the time of the trial. Psychiatrists must remain ever mindful of the many double agent roles that can develop when mixing psychiatry and litiga-tion (Simon 1987, 1992a).

The forensic expert, on the other hand, is usually free from these en-cumbrances. No doctor-patient relationship is created during forensic evaluation, with its treatment biases toward the patient. The expert can review a variety of records and can speak to a number of people who know the litigant. Furthermore, the forensic expert is not as easily distracted from considering exaggeration or malingering because of a clear appreciation of the litigation context and the absence of treatment bias. Finally, the forensic psychiatrist is not placed in a conflict-of-interest position of recommending treatment from which he or she would personally benefit.

■ FORENSIC PSYCHIATRY

Forensic psychiatry is defined as "a subspecialty of psychiatry in which scientific and clinical expertise is applied to legal issues in legal contexts embracing civil, criminal, correctional or legislative matters" (American Academy of Psychiatry and the Law 1989, 1991). The American Board of Forensic Psychiatry has certified a number of psychiatrists in forensic psychiatry since its first examination in 1978. In addition, the American Board of Medical Specialties has recognized forensic psychiatry as a subspecialty of psychiatry.

Just a few of the major areas in which forensic psychiatrists evaluate cases and provide testimony include malpractice litigation, will contests, personal injury litigation, competency determinations (both civil and criminal), criminal responsibility, and presentencing hearings. Many other areas of law and psychiatry also require the professional services of the forensic psychiatrist. In the course of practice, the forensic psychiatrist often sees very unusual, challenging cases that are not ordinarily found in the general outpatient or inpatient practice of psychiatry.

The forensic psychiatric evaluation of the injured *claimant* differs in a number of significant ways from the traditional psychiatric evaluation. In the litigation context, the distinction between the role of treating psychiatrist versus forensic evaluator must be firmly maintained. Problems invariably arise for the clinician when these roles are confused. The psychiatrist who enters the legal arena must understand that equities usually exist on both sides of a legal case, otherwise the case would probably not have been brought to litigation. The fact that opposing experts disagree does not necessarily mean that one side or the other is wrong. The opinions of opposing experts should be carefully considered.

□ Team Approach

The comprehensive forensic psychiatric evaluation requires cooperation with a number of other practitioners and specialists. Usually, the forensic psychiatrist who is evaluating the claimant may require the input of a neurologist, psychologist, neuropsychologist, and an internist or general practitioner. Depending on the complexities of the case, a number of other disciplines may need to be consulted. The forensic evaluator must also consider the findings of other examinations performed at the request of opposing counsel. The burgeoning number of ever-more-complicated brain studies currently available makes consultation with a qualified neurologist virtually a necessity in cases involving claims of brain injury.

☐ Absence of Doctor-Patient Relationship

The psychiatrist should inform the claimant at the time of examination that no doctor-patient relationship will be formed. The psychiatrist should explain that he or she has been retained to perform an independent psychiatric examination. The sole purpose of the examination is to provide information to the party retaining the psychiatrist.

☐ Absence of Confidentiality

The claimant must be informed that, unlike the usual doctor-patient relationship, confidentiality surrounding the forensic evaluation may not exist. Once the retaining attorney decides to disclose the findings of the evaluation in litigation, the information will be available to both sides and will likely become public record.

☐ Standard Diagnostic Schema

The diagnostic evaluation of claimants should be made according to the multiaxial classification system contained in the DSM-IV (American Psychiatric Association 1994). All five axes should be employed. Axis I permits the clinician to consider the major clinical psychiatric syndromes, either single or multiple. It is not unusual for the claimant to have concurrent Axis I diagnoses. Concurrent Axis I disorders may have preexisted or been exacerbated.

Axis II forces the clinician to consider personality disorders that are often overlooked or ignored in the forensic evaluation of a claimant. The occurrence of significant head injuries is high among the violent criminal population among which there is a higher incidence of antisocial personality disorder (Lewis et al. 1986). On Axis III, the relationship of medical disorders and their treatments to the patient's clinical presentation on Axis I must be carefully evaluated. The claimant may have a number of injuries requiring extensive pharmacotherapy that may further complicate the clinical picture. Moreover, a host of medical disorders may present with or have associated symptoms of cerebral dysfunction. Prior head injuries or preexisting CNS disorders must be considered.

Axis IV permits the evaluation of a psychosocial stressor or multiple psychosocial stressors occurring within the year preceding the current evaluation that may have contributed to the development of a new mental disorder, recurrence of a prior mental disorder, or exacerbation of an already existing psychiatric disorder. Posttraumatic stress disorder is the only exception to the 1-year rule. The search for multiple psychosocial stressors must be carefully conducted. Finally, functional impairment should be assessed on Axis V according to the Global Assessment of Functioning Scale in combination with other standard methods of evaluation of psychiatric impairment.

☐ Collateral Sources of Information

In the treatment situation, the psychiatrist relies almost exclusively on the subjective reporting of the patient. The patient, who is suffering from a disorder, is presumed to be candid. No conscious, hidden agendas are usually present. In litigation, however, the claimant must naturally be expected to favor his or her own legal case. The possibility of malingering must always be kept in mind. Malingering is not limited to the fabrication of symptoms; more often it is manifested by the *exaggeration* of symptoms.

The forensic examiner should request that the retaining lawyer provide *all* relevant information. Proceeding to court with incomplete information will likely be exposed by opposing counsel, undercutting the psychiatrist's testimony and damaging the claimant's case irreparably. The forensic psychiatrist should review all data carefully before coming to a conclusion. Collateral sources of information include other physicians and health care providers; hospital, school, police, and military records; family; witnesses; and prior medical and psychiatric records (Simon 1994).

☐ Traumatic Brain Injury

In evaluating the mental status of the traumatic brain injury (TBI) claimant, the psychiatrist must be able to conduct a thorough and reliable mental status examination. Moreover, the mental status assessment is an integral part of the psychiatric examination that cannot be delegated to others. Usually, it is better to conduct the examination in divided sessions over the course of 2 days because of possible fluctuations in the mental status of the TBI claimant. The practice of performing a perfunctory mental status examination or relying solely on the neuropsychological assessment of the neuropsychologist is unwarranted. Neuropsychological assessment can be a valuable adjunct to the neuropsychiatric assessment of the TBI claimant (Becker and Kay 1986). Nevertheless, the psychiatrist will have little basis for critically reviewing the neuropsychological findings unless he or she can perform a competent mental status examination.

The role of neuropsychological testing must be critically evaluated in each case. Neuropsychological tests are not totally objective. The qualifications and experience of the neuropsychologist constitute a critical variable. Thus, the consideration of motivation is critical. Also, low test scores may be caused by factors other than brain damage (e.g., environment, physical health, psychological distress, medications, errors in scoring or interpretation).

A number of psychiatric disorders may mimic traumatic brain injury. Some of the more common traumatic brain injury mimics include conversion, factitious, somatization, and depressive disorders presenting with symptoms of neurological and cerebral dysfunction. Conversion disorder symptoms classically mimic neurological disease. Dissociative symptoms may present with amnesia or atypical memory loss. Depressive pseudodementia is a commonly recognized clinical disorder in elderly patients. Posttraumatic stress disorder manifesting symptoms of difficulty in concentration and psychogenic amnesia may also mimic brain injury.

To complicate matters, litigants may be receiving psychoactive substances. Neuroleptics, antidepressants, lithium, and particularly benzodiazapines can produce side effects that mimic neurological and brain disorders. Psychoactive substances may produce serious memory difficulties, either directly by acting on brain chemistry or indirectly through sedation. Comorbidity and drug effects also must be considered when evaluating the results of neuropsychological test assessments. Questionable results will be obtained in the neuropsychological testing if the impact of concurrent psychiatric disorders and medications on the neuropsychological data is not considered.

☐ Disability Determinations

In addition to the psychiatric diagnosis, an assessment of functional impairment and disability must be made. In litigation, it is the degree of functional impairment, not the psychiatric diagnosis per se, that determines the amount of the monetary damage award. The psychiatrist also must understand the difference between impairment and disability. An impaired individual may not necessarily be disabled. Psychiatric impairment is considered disabling only when a psychiatric disorder limits a person's capacity to meet the demands of living.

Standard impairment assessment methods should be used in combination with the DSM-IV (American Psychiatric Association 1994) Axis V global assessment of functioning. The credible psychiatric assessment of functional impairment will avoid strictly subjective, idiosyncratic, *ex cathedra* pronouncements about the claimant's impairment and the need for future treatment. Instead, whenever possible, the claimant's functional impairment and future treatment needs should be evaluated according to the American Medical Association's *Guide to the Evaluation of Permanent Impairment* (1988). Assessment of permanent impairment should not be made until maximum medical improvement has been achieved.

■ REFERENCES

American Academy of Psychiatry and the Law: Ethical Guidelines for the Practice of Forensic Psychiatry. Adopted May 1987. Revised October 1989, 1991

American Medical Association: Guide to the Evalution of Permanent Impairment, 3rd Edition. Chicago, IL, American Medical Association, 1988

American Psychiatric Association: The Psychiatric Uses of Seclusion and Restraint (APA Task Force Report No 22). Washington, DC, American Psychiatric Association, 1984

American Psychiatric Association: Diagnostic and Statistical Manual of Mental Disorders, 4th Edition. Washington, DC, American Psychiatric Association, 1994

American Psychiatric Association: The Practice of Electroconvulsive Therapy: Recommendations for Treatment, Training, and Privileging: A Task Force Report of the American Psychiatric Association. Washington, DC, American Psychiatric Association, 1990

American Psychiatric Association: Tardive Dyskinesia: A Task Force Report of the American Psychiatric Association. Washington, DC, American Psychiatric Association, 1992

Appelbaum PS: Statutes regulating patient-therapist sex. Hosp Community Psychiatry 41:15–16, 1990

Appelbaum PS, Lidz CW, Meisel A: Informed Consent: Legal Theory and Clinical Practice. New York, Oxford University Press, 1987; see pp 84–87

Appelbaum PS, Zonana H, Bonnie R, et al: Statutory approaches to limiting psychiatrists' liability for their patients' violent acts. Am J Psychiatry 146:821–828, 1989

Becker B, Kay GG: Neuropsychological consultation in psychiatric practice. Psychiatr Clin North Am 9:255–265, 1986

Black HC: Black's Law Dictionary, 6th Edition. St Paul, West Publishing Company, 1990

Blumenthal SJ: An overview and synopsis of risk factors, assessment, and treatment of suicidal patients over the life cycle, in Suicide Over the Life Cycle. Edited by Blumenthal SJ, Kupfer DJ. Washington, DC, American Psychiatric Press, 1990, pp 685–733

Brakel SJ, Parry J, Weiner BA: The Mentally Disabled and the Law, 3rd Edition. Chicago, IL, American Bar Foundation, 1985

Daniel DG, Zigun JR, Weinberger DR: Brain imaging in neuropsychiatry, in The American Psychiatric Press Textbook of Neuropsychiatry, 2nd Edition. Edited by Yudofsky SC, Hales RE. Washington, DC, American Psychiatric Press, 1992, pp 165–186

Devinsky O, Bear D: Varieties of aggressive behavior in temporal lobe epilepsy. Am J Psychiatry 141:651–656, 1984

Elliott FA: Neurological findings in adult minimal brain dysfunction and the dyscontrol syndrome. J Nerv Ment Dis 170:680–687, 1982

Emanuel EJ, Emanuel LL: Proxy decision making for incompetent patients—an ethical and empirical analysis. JAMA 267:2067–2071, 1992

Gutheil TG, Appelbaum PS: Substituted judgement and the physician's ethical dilemma: with special reference to the problem of the psychiatric patient. J Clin Psychiatry 41:303–305, 1980

Joint Commission on Accreditation of Healthcare Organizations: Consolidated Standards Manual, 1991. Chicago, IL, JCAHO, 1990

Klein J, Onek J, Macbeth J: Seminar on Law in the Practice of Psychiatry. Washington, DC, Onek, Klein & Farr, 1983

LaPuma J, Orentlicher D, Moss RJ: Advance directives on admission: clinical implications and analysis of the Patient Self-Determination Act of 1990. JAMA 266:402–405, 1991

Lewis DO, Pincus JH, Feldman M, et al: Psychiatric, neurological, and psychoeducational characteristics of 15 death row inmates in the United States. Am J Psychiatry 143:838–845, 1986

McGarry AL: Competency to stand trial and mental illness [a monograph sponsored by the Center for Studies of Crime and Delinquency, National Institute of Mental Health] (DHEW Publ No HSM 73-910). Washington, DC, U.S. Government Printing Office, 1973, p 73

Melton GB, Petrila J, Poythress NG, et al: Psychological Evaluations for the Courts: A Handbook for Mental Health Professionals and Lawyers. New York, Guilford, 1987; see p 128

Mishkin B: Decisions in Hospice. Arlington, VA, The National Hospice Organization, 1985

Mishkin B: Determining the capacity for making health care decisions, in Issues in Geriatric Psychiatry (Advances in Psychosomatic Medicine Vol 19). Edited by Billig N, Rabins PV. Basel, S Karger, 1989, pp 151–166

Overman W Jr, Stoudemire A: Guidelines for legal and financial counseling of Alzheimer's disease patients and their families. Am J Psychiatry 145:1495–1500, 1988

Perr IN: The clinical considerations of medication refusal. Legal Aspects of Psychiatric Practice 1:5–8, 1984

Reich J, Wells J: Psychiatric diagnosis and competency to stand trial. Compr Psychiatry 26:421–432, 1985

Robertson JD: The trial of a suicide case, in American Psychiatric Press Review of Clinical Psychiatry and the Law, Vol 2. Edited by Simon RI. Washington, DC, American Psychiatric Press, 1991, pp 423–441

Rutter P: Sex in the Forbidden Zone: When Therapists, Doctors, Clergy, Teachers and Other Men in Power Betray Women's Trust. Los Angeles, CA, JP Tarcher, 1989

Sale B, Powell DM, Van Duizend R: Disabled Persons and the Law: State Legislative Issues. 1982; see p 461

Schoener GR, Milgrom JH, Gonsiorek JC, et al: Psychotherapists' Sexual Involvement With Clients. Minneapolis, MN, Walk-In Counseling Center, 1989

Simon RI: The psychiatrist as a fiduciary: avoiding the double agent role. Psychiatric Annals 17:622–626, 1987

Simon RI: Sexual exploitation of patients: how it begins before it happens. Psychiatric Annals 19:104–112, 1989

Simon RI: Psychological injury caused by boundary violation precursors to therapist-patient sex. Psychiatric Annals 21:614–619, 1991a

Simon RI: The suicide prevention pact: clinical and legal considerations, in American Psychiatric Press Review of Clinical Psychiatry and the Law, Vol 2. Edited by Simon RI. Washington, DC, American Psychiatric Press, 1991b, pp 441–451

Simon RI: Clinical Psychiatry and the Law, 2nd Edition. Washington, DC, American Psychiatric Press, 1992a

Simon RI: Clinical risk management of suicidal patients: assessing the unpredictable, in American Psychiatric Press Review of Clinical Psychiatry and the Law, Vol 3. Edited by Simon RI. Washington, DC, American Psychiatric Press, 1992b, pp 3–63

Simon RI: Concise Guide to Clinical Psychiatry and the Law. Washington, DC, American Psychiatric Press, 1992c

Simon RI: Treatment boundaries in psychiatric practice, in Forensic Psychiatry: A Comprehensive Textbook. Edited by Rosner R. New York, Van Nostrand Reinhold, 1994

Slovenko R: Commentaries on psychiatry and law: "guilty but mentally ill." Journal of Psychiatry and Law 10:541–555, 1982

Solnick PB: Proxy consent for incompetent nonterminally ill adult patients. J Leg Med 6:1–49, 1985

Strasburger LH: "Crudely, without any finesse": the defendant hears his psychiatric evaluation. Bull Am Acad Psychiatry Law 15:229–233, 1987

Strasburger LH, Jorgenson L, Randles R: Criminalization of psychotherapist-patient sex. Am J Psychiatry 148:859–863, 1991

Taylor MA, Sierles FS, Abrams R: The neuropsychiatric evaluation, in American Psychiatric Press Textbook of Neuropsychiatry. Edited by Hales RE, Yudofsky SC. Washington DC, American Psychiatric Press, 1987, pp 3–16

Tranel D: Functional neuroanatomy: neuropsychological correlates of cortical and subcortical damage, in The American Psychiatric Press Textbook of Neuropsychiatry, 2nd Edition. Edited by Yudofsky SC, Hales RE. Washington, DC, American Psychiatric Press, 1992, pp 70–75

Zito JM, Lentz SL, Routt WW, et al: The treatment review panel: a solution to treatment refusal? Bull Am Acad Psychiatry Law 12:349–358, 1984

■ LEGAL CITATIONS

Annotation 94 ALR 3rd 317 (1979)

Annotation 42 ALR 4th 586 (1985)

Bethea v United States, 365 A2d 64, (DC 1976), cert denied, 433 US 911 (1977)

Bouvia v Superior Court, 179 Cal App 3d 1127, 225 Cal Rptr 297 (1986)

Canterbury v Spence, 464 F2d 772 (DC Cir), cert denied, Spence v Canterbury, 409 US 1064 (1972)

Cruzan v Director, Missouri Department of Health (110 S Ct 284 1990)

Doerr v Hurley Medical Center, No 82-674-39 NM Mich Aug (1984)

Dusky v United States, 362 U.S. 402 (1960)

Gowan v United States, 601 FSupp 1297 (D Or 1985)

Harris v Forklift Systems, Inc., 62 USLW 4004 (1993)

In re Conroy, 98 NJ 321, 486 A2d 1209, 1222–23 (1985)

In re Boyer, 636 P2d 1085, 1089 (Utah 1981)

In re Jobes, 108 NJ 394 (1987)

In re Peter, 108 NJ 365, 529 A2d 419 (1987)

In re Quinlin, 70 NJ 10, 355 A2d 647, cert denied, 429 US 922 (1976)

Neely v United States, 150 F2d 977 (DC Cir), cert denied, 326 US 768 (1945)

Parham v JR, 442 US 584 (1979)

People v White, 117 Cal App 3d 270, 172 Cal Rptr 612 (1981)

Rennie v Klein, 462 FSupp 1131 (D NJ 1978), remanded, 476 FSupp 1294 (D NJ 1979), affd in part, modified in part and remanded, 653 F2d 836 (3d Cir 1980), vacated and remanded, 458 U.S. 1119 (1982), 720 F2d 266 (3rd Cir 1983)

Rogers v Commissioner of Dept of Mental Health, 390 Mass 489, 458 NE2d 308 (Mass 1983)

Schloendorff v Society of New York Hospital, 211 NY 125, 105 NE 92 (1914), overruled, Bing v Thunig, 2 NY2d 656, 143 NE2d 3, 163 NYS2d 3 (1957)

Speer v United States, 512 FSupp 670 (ND Tex 1981), affd, Speer v United States, 675 F2d 100 (5th Cir 1982)

Stone v Proctor, 259 NC 633, 131 SE2d 297 (1963)

Tarasoff v Regents of the University of California, 17 Cal 3d 425, 551 P2d 334, 131 Cal Rptr 14 (1976)

Truman v Thomas, 27 Cal 3d 285, 611 P2d 902, 165 Cal Rptr 308 (1980)

United States v David, 511 F2d 355 (DC Cir 1975)

Youngberg v Romeo, 457 U.S. 307 (1982), on remand, Romeo v Youngberg, 687 F2d 33 (3rd Cir 1982)

■ CRIMINAL STATUTES

CAL BUS & PRO CODE § 729 (Supp 1989)

COLO REV STAT § 18-3-405.5 (1989)

FLA 1990 SESS LAWS SERV 490.0112 § 1(1) (tentative assignment) (West 1990)

GA CODE ANN § 16-6-5.1 (Michie 1992) (amended)

MAINE REVISED STATUTES, Title 17-A, § 253(2)(I) (Supp 1989)

MICH COMP LAWS ANN §§ 750.520(b) (1) (d) (i); 750.90 (West Supp 1984–85)

MINN STAT ANN § 609.344(g,)(v),(h-j) (West Supp 1985)

MINN STAT ANN § 609.344 (West 1989)

MINN STAT § 609.341 et seq (Supp 1990)

ND CENT CODE § 12.1-20-06.1 (1) (Michie Supp 1989)

NH REV STAT ANN § 632-A:2 Part VIII (Supp 1986)

WIS STAT ANN § 940.22(2) (West 1989)

WYO STAT § 6-2-303 (1988)

■ CIVIL STATUTES

CAL CIV CODE § 43.93(b) (West Supp 1990)

FLA STAT ANN § 458.329, 331 (West Supp 1986)

ILL ANN STAT ch 70, 802 (Smith-Hurd 1989)

MINN STAT ANN § 148 A.02 (West 1989)

WISC STAT § 895.70 (1991)

CHAPTER 39

Ethics and Psychiatry

William L. Webb, Jr., M.D.
Bruce S. Rothschild, M.D.
Lee Monroe, M.S.

Ethical principles are essential to the practice of psychiatry. Every clinical decision has a moral dimension, often requiring the physician to weigh one value against another. Without clear-cut ethical codes and a strong moral philosophy, decisions of this nature are difficult to make and may result in harm to both physician and patient. The process of treatment in psychiatry is arguably more dependent on ethical codes of conduct than in any other branch of medicine.

■ ETHICAL CODES OF CONDUCT IN THE MEDICAL PROFESSION

The modern version of the Hippocratic tradition is *The Principles of Medical Ethics of the American Medical Association* (American Medical Association 1992; Table 39–1). The AMA (1992) defines ethics as "matters involving (1) moral principles or practices; (2) customs and usages of the medical profession; and (3) matters of policy not necessarily involving issues of morality in the practice of medicine." The AMA's code of ethics was adopted in 1847 and received major revisions in 1903, 1912, 1947, 1956, and 1980. In 1973 the American Psychiatric Association (APA) first published *The Principles of Medical Ethics With Annotations Especially Applicable to Psychiatry*. When the AMA's Principles were revised in 1980, the APA incorporated its annotations into the revised Principles and printed

---

Table 39–1.   The Principles of Medical Ethics

PREAMBLE

The medical profession has long subscribed to a body of ethical statements developed primarily for the benefit of the patient. As a member of this profession, a physician must recognize responsibility not only to patients but also to society, to other health professionals, and to self. The following Principles, adopted by the American Medical Association, are not laws but standards of conduct, which define the essentials of honorable behavior for the physician.

SECTION 1

A physician shall be dedicated to providing competent medical service with compassion and respect for human dignity.

SECTION 2

A physician shall deal honestly with patients and colleagues, and strive to expose those physicians deficient in character or competence, or who engage in fraud or deception.

SECTION 3

A physician shall respect the law and also recognize a responsibility to seek changes in those requirements which are contrary to the best interests of the patient.

SECTION 4

A physician shall respect the rights of patients, of colleagues, and of other health professionals, and shall safeguard patient confidences within the constraints of the law.

SECTION 5

A physician shall continue to study, apply, and advance scientific knowledge, make relevant information available to patients, colleagues, and the public, obtain consultation, and use the talents of other health professionals when indicated.

SECTION 6

A physician shall, in the provision of appropriate patient care, except in emergencies, be free to choose whom to serve, with whom to associate, and the environment in which to provide medical services.

SECTION 7

A physician shall recognize a responsibility to participate in activities contributing to an improved community.

---

its version in 1981, with revisions in subsequent printings (American Psychiatric Association 1993).

In the past the Principles have emphasized a primary responsibility to patients. The current preamble calls upon the physician to recognize a responsibility not only to patients but also to society and other professionals. This modern broadening of the physician's perspective immediately raises the prospect of ethical priorities and potential conflicts. The

Principles draw an ideal picture of the modern physician, competent in his or her professional skill, honest in his or her dealings with others, compassionate, law abiding, respectful of the rights of others, oriented to learning, free to choose whom he or she will treat, and mindful of his or her responsibilities to society.

A more pragmatic document, published by the Ethics Committee of the APA, is the *Opinions of the Ethics Committee on The Principles of Medical Ethics With Annotations Especially Applicable to Psychiatry* (American Psychiatric Association 1992a). Each year the committee gets requests from clinicians for opinions on ethical problems that arise in their psychiatric practice. A brief analysis of the kinds of questions asked of the committee provides a reasonably accurate picture of the ethical concerns of practitioners in the field. Issues involving direct patient care are numerous. They include questions about competent psychiatric practice, confidentiality, exploitation of the doctor-patient relationship, "do no harm," honesty, and informed consent. Other major areas of concern include interrelationships among psychiatrists, and those among psychiatrists, institutions, and the law.

■ BENEFICENCE IN THE DOCTOR-PATIENT RELATIONSHIP

In recent years the Hippocratic oath has come under criticism as encouraging a paternalistic attitude in the doctor-patient relationship, ignoring patient rights, and neglecting the doctor's responsibility to society. Pelligrino and Thomasma (1988) suggested shifting the balance toward an egalitarian relationship that emphasizes an appreciation of the doctor's professional integrity and respect for the patient's rights of self-determination. These authors describe a model for the doctor-patient relationship that is based on a concept they term "beneficence," defined as "the principle that prompts physicians to cite their moral commitments and personal support for patients beyond just respecting their [the patients'] rights" (p. 35).

This reconceptualization of the doctor-patient relationship sensitizes the psychiatrist to the inequity in the power structure between patient and psychiatrist. For those patients who are not truly autonomous or capable of responding in a completely rational manner to informed consent, the psychiatrist is under special obligation to engage the patient's emotional as well as intellectual collaboration in a "partnership," as described by Redlich and Mollica (1976).

■ ETHICAL ISSUES IN DAILY PSYCHIATRIC PRACTICE

☐ Competent Psychiatric Care

The first Principle puts a high premium on competence and its annotation specifically recommends that the ethical psychiatrist submit his work for peer review. In the *American Psychiatric Association Ethics Newsletter* (1986), incompetence is defined as being unable to perform professional functions that someone occupying that particular position ought to be able to perform satisfactorily. Incompetence may be the result of a physical, mental, or volitional disability, but more often it is due to lack of training or practicing outside of one's area of expertise. Incompetence resulting from a physical or mental impairment, particularly if the impairment is outside the psychiatrist's awareness, may have the paradoxical effect of producing unethical behavior that is not the physician's intent. This points to the importance of reporting our colleagues who are impaired or incompetent to the impaired physician committee of the local medical society.

☐ Exploitation of the Doctor-Patient Relationship

Trust is the basic therapeutic element in the psychiatric doctor-patient relationship. The psychiatric annotations to the Principles take special note of the vulnerability of the patient and the patient's need to trust the integrity of the psychiatrist not to gratify his or her own needs by exploiting the relationship established with the psychiatrist (American Psychiatric Association 1993). The most sensationalized form of exploitation is undue intimacy or sexual activity between a psychiatrist and his or her patient. A 1986 survey of psychiatrists reported that 6.4% of respondents admitted to having sexual or inappropriately intimate relationships with patients (Gartrell et al. 1986). The overwhelming majority of these relationships occur between male psychiatrists and female patients. Webb (1986) has summarized the destructive nature of sexual exploitation as follows: "Not only does it defy the intent of the therapeutic relationship but it perverts it into a real intrusion into the patient's world of fears, hopes, and guilt" (p. 1149).

Sexual misconduct does not occur only in the context of current or ongoing doctor-patient relationships. On the issue of sexual contact with former patients, until very recently the psychiatric annotations to the Principles read as follows: "Sexual involvement with one's former patients generally exploits emotions deriving from treatment and therefore almost always is unethical" (American Psychiatric Association 1992b, p. 4). The APA has recently been engaged in debate as to whether or not to remove the qualifying phrase "almost always," thus making it clear that this behavior is never ethical; the most recent edition of the annotations states simply and forcefully, "Sexual activity with a current or former patient is unethical" (APA 1993, p. 4).

Although somewhat less spectacular, ethical questions of undue influence in financial matters are numerous and important. On occasion, a very grateful patient will offer some major financial benefit to a therapist. Examples include the patient's offering a relative of the therapist a job, making an outright bequest of money, or offering to include the therapist in his or her will. Not only do these offerings place major obstacles in the therapeutic process, but they also represent an exploitation of the relationship.

☐ Breach of Confidentiality

Appelbaum et al. (1984), in a study of 58 patients, revealed that most had implicit trust that their confidentiality would be protected by their therapist and were quite upset that it might be breached against their will, particularly to courts or family members. Psychiatric practice in the United States offers many opportunities for breach of confidentiality. The first source is the psychiatrist himself or herself, with the breach of confidentiality occurring most often with colleagues and others as a result of carelessness. Many psychiatrists assume multiple roles (e.g., consultant, therapist, forensic evaluation), offering access to private information about patients and families that can easily be shared without consent. Educational activities (e.g., case conferences, videotapes, case reports, and one-way mirrors) may not offer protection of privacy.

Information systems and computerized records may lack appropriate safeguards to protect confidentiality. A serious and insidious infringement on privacy comes from insurance carriers, peer review activities, and case management reviews related to payment for psychiatric services. With permission from the patient in the form of a signed release, a psychiatrist may ethically convey information to third-party payers. This information should be limited to the diagnosis, course, and treatment of the patient's illness, and should avoid unnecessary personal detail.

Special problems arise around the protection of confidentiality after a patient's death. The psychiatrist may be tempted to breach confidentiality in an effort to console a grieving relative, but usually the psychiatrist is not in a position to know how the information might be used or abused. The AMA, in *Current Opinions of the Council on Ethical and Judicial Affairs*, recognizes only one exception to the ban on violating confidentiality after death, and that is in order to prevent others from imminent harm, or under legal compulsion (American Medical Association 1992).

Treating minors also poses special problems in confidentiality. The APA, in its "Guidelines on Confidentiality" (American Psychiatric Asso-

ciation 1987), noted that parents and legal guardians are entitled to information to make informed decisions, but that the therapist has an obligation to protect the confidences of minors, particularly adolescents. In
child custody cases the rule of confidentiality is waived because it is
deemed to be in conflict with the best interest of the child.

Other conflicts arise when a patient voices information in therapy
that is self-destructive or dangerous and destructive to others. Since the
Tarasoff decision in 1976, psychiatrists are under legal constraint to warn
an intended victim of a potentially homicidal patient (Karasu 1991). Privacy is waived when the patient is acutely suicidal or reports child abuse.

☐ Accountability and Informed Consent

Karasu (1991) made the point that there is an increasing expectation that
psychiatrists be accountable. The issue of informed consent is as important in establishing the treatment contract in the clinical setting as it is in
the research setting, where it is mandated by law. The ethicality of the
psychiatrist's actions in many treatment situations depends on whether
or not he or she has discussed the situations with the patient and received the patient's knowing consent as part of the treatment contract.

The psychiatric patient is seldom in a position to be an enlightened
consumer who can really evaluate in a rational manner all aspects of a
treatment contract. This is most apparent in the psychotic patient, whose
illness may severely impair his or her capacity to consent. The issue is
further complicated if the patient's legal status is compromised by being
under commitment, a prisoner, or a minor. Various attempts to resolve
this ethical dilemma have included the use of guardians, advocates, or
the courts. Ultimately the best results are obtained in a negotiated partnership between patient and therapist that maximizes the patient's per-
sonhood and freedom of choice. Usually the refusal of treatment is time
limited, and the patient's cooperation can be obtained. If this cannot be
achieved, a review can be conducted by an outside psychiatrist or an external review board.

☐ Primum Non Nocere

The principle of *primum non nocere* ("first do no harm") is the backbone of
the Hippocratic tradition. Although much of our previous discussion
touches on aspects of potential harm in the doctor-patient relationship,
three kinds of intervention bring it into bold relief: hospitalization
against the patient's will, psychopharmacotherapy, and the use of other
somatic treatments. Any of these interventions may be life-saving. On
the other hand, all may be harmful or have been accused of being harmful. Hospitalization is potentially harmful because it constrains the pa-

tient's fundamental right to freedom and forces him or her into an environment that is seldom pleasant. Medications may produce permanent side effects, habituation, and addiction, or may be employed in a suicide attempt. The somatic therapies, principally electroconvulsive therapy (ECT) and psychosurgery, have been the object of public and legal criticism and constraint.

Therapeutic decisions nearly always involve a balancing of risk and benefit to the patient. The decision to hospitalize a patient who has made a suicide attempt will weigh the lethality of the situation against the negative effects of hospitalization on the patient. Prescribing a phenothiazine to a young psychotic patient is always clouded with the aura of possible tardive dyskinesia over time. Knowledge about the risk-benefit ratio for ECT and psychosurgery is especially important. In the past, both of these therapies were overused without proper safeguards and have received a bad reputation with the public. Yet the current data on ECT document that with the use of modern techniques and safeguards, it is a very safe treatment with practically no mortality and minimum morbidity.

☐ Duty to Not Abandon the Patient

A final important area of accountability is the question of how and when the psychiatrist's therapeutic responsibility for a patient ends. The determination of this is rather straightforward in those circumstances where there is mutual agreement. Therapy is terminated with the explicit understanding that the patient can return if necessary. What about circumstances in which termination is more abrupt? The Principles clearly state that the physician shall be free to choose whom to serve, but that it is unethical to abandon. Patients should be forewarned, either before the consultation begins or well in advance, that the psychiatrist is leaving. Adequate efforts should be made to refer the patient elsewhere.

■ ETHICS AND THE PROFESSIONAL ENVIRONMENT

Psychiatrists are brought into contact with different patient populations (some for therapy, some not), as well as a broad range of institutions and mental health professionals (their relationships with whom are sometimes collaborative, sometimes competitive). Moreover, we are witnessing a revolution in the economics of health delivery. Fanned by rising costs that now total 14% of the gross national product, the corporate sector, government, and third-party payers have launched major new cost-saving initiatives. These relationships raise many ethical issues and a number of ethical conflicts.

☐ Relationship of Psychiatrists to Hospitals

Psychiatric hospitals once again figure prominently in the psychiatrist's professional life. There has been a proliferation of for-profit psychiatric hospitals throughout the country. At the same time there has been increased emphasis on shortened length of hospital stay. The average length of stay in private hospitals is now about 14 days. Although there is no hard evidence of widespread unethical activity accompanying these developments, there are a number of areas of potential ethical conflict. These include excessive ordering of tests, financial reward to the physician by the hospital for admitting patients, and "perks" offered for exclusive admitting agreements. Some of these practices are clearly more unethical than others, but all impact on the free choice of physician and patient that has been a strong ethical tradition of medical practice in the past.

☐ Managed Care

Relationships between psychiatrists and managed care companies skirt ethical issues in a number of areas, including problems of double agentry, informed consent, and confidentiality. The APA's 1992 Opinions of the Ethics Committee, however, identified several additional issues that fall outside these categories. For example, the Opinions define a psychiatrist's participation in managed care systems as ethical if patients or their employers are informed of "a. their other options; b. benefit limits; c. the pre- and current authorization process; d. their right to appeal a utilization decision; e. the limits as to whom they can see without having to make a greater financial investment; and f. the potential invasion of their privacy by the review process" (American Psychiatric Association 1992a, p. 49). It is unethical, however, for reviewers and practitioners to be financially rewarded for denying care. Psychiatrists who function as reviewers or clinicians in managed care networks must avoid setting limits on clinical care in order to further their own financial gain or that of the company.

☐ The Problem of Double Agentry

The proliferation of health maintenance organizations, preferred provider organizations, employee assistance programs, and independent practice organizations suggests that the psychiatrist of the future will, in part, be salaried and that his or her flow of patients will come largely from these affiliations rather than from other private practice professionals. Not only does this structure further constrain the free access of patient and doctor, but it also presents additional ethical dilemmas. Most of these systems operate by sharing the financial risk of health care with the provider. Ultimately, it will be the psychiatrist who will be forced to make very difficult and ethically strenuous decisions about the allocation of treatment resources.

In institutions where psychiatrists are employed full- or part-time for consultation or treatment services, the problem of double agentry is generic. A psychiatrist in student mental health services must make a very clear distinction between those students who are treated and those who are seen for administrative purposes. The first are entitled to full confidentiality; the latter are not and should be so informed. The two should not be mixed.

Psychiatrists working in prisons are called upon both to do therapy and to make parole evaluations. Again, the two functions should be carefully separated. The prisoner who is being evaluated should be aware that the evaluation will be fully accessed by the parole board. Evaluations of any kind, whether for the court or for workmen's compensation, place the psychiatrist in a peculiar adversarial role. We are, by nature and ethic, healers, not adversaries. We compensate for this dilemma by making certain that the evaluated client understands the nature and purpose of the evaluation and that he or she is an agreeing participant.

☐ The Psychiatrist and the Law

Waithe et al. (1982) pointed out that in many instances a psychiatrist who assists the legal system stands in jeopardy of ethical conflicts. The adversarial nature of the legal process creates numerous ethical conflicts between the rights of the individual and the right of the court to know. Appelbaum (1984) suggested that the yardstick of honesty is the best measure for the ethical forensic psychiatrist. The psychiatrist honestly does a careful examination and honestly reports the results, taking care to provide only information relevant to the legal question at hand. The psychiatrist takes pains to inform the examinee that what the examinee says will appear in the report to the court. The psychiatrist remains neutral in the adversarial process and fulfills his or her role as expert witness to his or her best degree. The psychiatrist is honest about what he or she doesn't know. If the psychiatrist is testifying from a medical record or other materials and has not personally examined the defendant, he or she makes this clear to the court.

A psychiatrist's relationship with an institution carries with it an obligation to reconcile his or her professional ethics with the rules and regulations of the institution. Examples of the kinds of questions that emerge around this issue include the following:

- How much influence should a community board of a mental health center exert on treatment policy?

- When moving from a practice in a public clinic to private practice, is it ethical for the psychiatrist to carry patients with him or her?
- What are the ethical conditions for terminating an uncooperative patient from a community mental health center?

☐ Economic Pressures and Relationships With Fellow Professionals

Mental health care will continue to be influenced by new cost-saving initiatives. Competition for patients will increase, and the temptation to develop unethical practice arrangements may also intensify. An example is the payment of one physician to another for the referral of patients. This transaction, called *fee-splitting*, is unethical on the grounds that it violates the requirement to deal honestly with patients and colleagues.

Competition, on the other hand, among practitioners is not only ethical but encouraged. The AMA's Council on Ethical and Judicial Affairs, in its Current Opinions, asserted that "ethical medical practice thrives best under free market conditions when prospective patients have adequate information and opportunity to choose freely between and among competing physicians and alternate systems of medical care"(American Medical Association 1992, p. 31). What the free market does not address is the problem of chronic illness. In a pure market environment, the emphasis is on the less costly forms of illness whose treatment produces the best financial return. The most severe forms of mental illness are chronic, producing a population that is out in the cold in a free market situation. Similarly, a large, disenfranchised American "underclass" has limited access to the medical system, pointing out the maldistribution of care that currently exists in this country. The appropriate advocacy for the underserved chronically mentally ill in America remains an ethical responsibility for psychiatry.

The modern psychiatrist commonly works closely with nonmedical mental health professionals. This may occur in the context of a multidisciplinary team or group practice. Referrals may be made to a nonmedical colleague, or the psychiatrist may function in a supervisory role. The ethical relationship in these associations rests on several principles. Professionals should not practice outside their level of competency. Also, no referral should be made to a nonmedical colleague when there are medical responsibilities involved.

■ ENFORCEMENT OF THE ETHICAL CODE

Ethical misbehavior is generally viewed as being the province of the profession's Ethics Committee. If a psychiatrist is suspected of being impaired, however, the Ethics Committee may take more serious action by referring the case to the state's medical licensing board. Complaints regarding a psychiatrist's ethical behavior may also be brought directly to the state licensing board by a patient, and the board will determine whether or not to investigate further. If the licensing board takes action, including the possibility of license revocation, the psychiatrist or the complainant may appeal to the state superior court through the process of judicial oversight.

Increasingly, various states are enacting legislation designed to enhance the government's role in remedying unethical behavior. Having sex with a patient, for example, can be a misdemeanor or a felony, depending on the jurisdiction (Appelbaum and Jorgenson 1991). Another example of governmental involvement in the enforcement process was the formation of the National Practitioner Data Bank in 1990 (Johnson 1991). This organization plays a centralizing role in the reporting of disciplinary actions by local medical societies, hospital boards, and state medical societies. It is meant to diminish the possibility that clinicians found guilty of unethical or illegal behavior in one state can simply move to another state with impunity.

How successful is the profession in policing itself? Zitrin and Klein (1976) expressed considerable skepticism about the process as it is presently organized. They pointed out that it is entirely a voluntary process, with little staff support, and noted the limitations of the investigatory process. For example, often it is a question of the doctor's word against the patient's complaint. Despite these obvious limitations, Moore (1985) reported that from 1972 to 1983, 382 members were charged, 86 were found unethical, and 27 were expelled, a quantum leap over the previous 20 years when only 82 were charged, 12 found unethical, and 6 expelled.

■ ETHICS AND PSYCHIATRIC RESEARCH

A growing concern about the rights of human research subjects led to the appointment of a National Commission for the Protection of Human Subjects of Biomedical and Behavioral Research. What has evolved is an Institutional Review Board and a set of ethical guidelines in every institution where research is conducted. Deliberations concern such issues as informed consent, risk to the patient, quality of research design, and confidentiality.

Issues of informed consent and confidentiality in research are essentially the same as those encountered in clinical practice. Research, however, bears the additional burden that therapeutic experimentation involves the possibility of harm. This becomes particularly significant when the experiment may be of no direct benefit to the experimental subject. Matters become even more complicated if the subject's mental capacity to consent is impaired because of illness or if his or her civil status is compromised because he or she is a prisoner or is committed to a hospital for mental illness. An additional area of concern occurs when the researcher is also the patient's therapist. The potential then exists for losing sight of the patient's best interests in order to further the goals of the study.

■ REFERENCES

American Medical Association: Current Opinions of the Council on Ethical and Judicial Affairs of the American Medical Association. Chicago, IL, American Medical Association, 1992

American Psychiatric Association: American Psychiatric Association Ethics Newsletter. Washington, DC, American Psychiatric Association, 1986

American Psychiatric Association: Guidelines on confidentiality. Am J Psychiatry 144:1522–1526, 1987

American Psychiatric Association: Opinions of the Ethics Committee on The Principles of Medical Ethics With Annotations Especially Applicable to Psychiatry. Washington, DC, American Psychiatric Association, 1992a

American Psychiatric Association: The Principles of Medical Ethics With Annotations Especially Applicable to Psychiatry. Washington, DC, American Psychiatric Association, 1992b

American Psychiatric Association: The Principles of Medical Ethics With Annotations Especially Applicable to Psychiatry. Washington, DC, American Psychiatric Association, 1993

Appelbaum PS, Jorgenson L: Psychotherapist-patient sexual contact after termination of treatment: an analysis and a proposal. Am J Psychiatry 148:1466–1473, 1991

Appelbaum PS, Kapen G, Walters B, et al: Confidentiality: an empirical test of the utilitarian perspective. Bull Am Acad Psychiatry Law 12:109–116, 1984

Gartrell N, Herman J, Olarte S, et al: Psychiatrist-patient sexual contact: results of a national survey, I: prevalence. Am J Psychiatry 143:1126–1131, 1986

Johnson ID: Reports to the National Practitioner Data Bank. JAMA 265:407, 411, 1991

Karasu T: Ethical aspects of psychotherapy, in Psychiatric Ethics, 2nd Edition. Edited by Bloch S, Chodoff P. New York, Oxford University Press, 1991, pp 135–166

Moore RA: Ethics in the practice of psychiatry: update on the results of enforcement of the code. Am J Psychiatry 142:1043–1046, 1985

Pelligrino ED, Thomasma DC: For the Patient's Good. Oxford, UK, Oxford University Press, 1988

Redlich F, Mollica RF: Overview: ethical issues in contemporary psychiatry. Am J Psychiatry 133:125–136, 1976

Waithe ME, Rappeport JR, Weinstein HC (Chairman), et al: Ethical issues in the practice of forensic psychiatry. Journal of Psychiatry and Law 10:7–43, 1982

Webb WL Jr: The doctor-patient covenant and the threat of exploitation (editorial). Am J Psychiatry 143:1149–1150, 1986

Zitrin A, Klein H: Can psychiatry police itself effectively? The experience of one district branch. Am J Psychiatry 133:653–656, 1976

CHAPTER 40

Women and Psychiatry

Nada L. Stotland, M.D.

■ WOMEN'S DEVELOPMENT AND PSYCHOLOGY IN SOCIAL CONTEXT

□ Historical and Anthropological Perspectives

In no area of scholarship has the nature/nurture controversy been more salient than in the discussion of gender development and psychology. Investigators have attempted to highlight the relevant factors by examining child-rearing and gender-linked behaviors in Western and non-Western societies. LeVine (1991) concluded that "the more we know about human gender roles and differences through cross-cultural and historical research, the less support we can find for unqualified innatism or environmentalism" (p. 4).

The majority of societies are patriarchal, with family lineage and place of residence determined by the father. Women almost everywhere are responsible for the care of very young children, although few cultures center child care so closely in the nuclear family as our own. As children grow, the care and education of boys move toward schools and the male community. The extent to which males and females are separated and expected to manifest differing behaviors varies widely.

In modern Western society, women have occupied a subordinate role in the decisions and formal activities of society, simultaneously perceived as exalted beings to be cherished and protected, and as sources of sexual temptation and pollution. Women's institutionalized roles have been largely limited to household maintenance and reproduction, and their formal identities have derived from their fathers and husbands. Fatherless and unmarried women have occupied a sometimes more independent, but deviant, role. Because recorded history is based almost entirely on formal, nondomestic activities, and women's contributions in other areas tend to be marginalized, there is little record of what women have done.

The tradition of maternal lives devoted to child rearing is a modern one. Historically, most people have had to struggle to attain the basic necessities of life, and relatively few have enjoyed great wealth. The mother in an impoverished family was often forced to seek paid work and, in any event, spent most hours of the day at physically demanding domestic labor. She was repeatedly pregnant and breast-feeding, and at risk of death from complications of pregnancy, abortion, and delivery. As soon as families acquired some affluence, servants were hired to nurse and care for the children. Women's roles have been defined, and their behavior determined, by their wifehood and motherhood. Women are expected to facilitate the fulfillment of others' desires and needs. Although a desire for physical attractiveness may be allowed or expected, educational and professional ambition are not fully compatible with the feminine role. Men are socialized to be aggressive and competitive, women to be compliant and collaborative.

☐ Foundations of Psychodynamic Theory

Sigmund Freud did not claim to be an expert on women's development and psychology, but attempted to extrapolate or reason from his observations about males' developmental stages and dynamics. The perception of the anatomic differences between the sexes occurs during toddlerhood and precipitates differing lines of development for male and female children. According to Freud, boys believe that girls have lost their penises, fear that they will be castrated by their fathers as punishment for their libidinous wishes toward their mothers, and identify with their fathers instead. Girls believe that their mothers have failed to endow them with penises, and live ever after with a sense of deprivation, resentment, and resignation. Women grow into adult roles by substituting a husband for the father, and their husband's child for the penis they lack. Freud believed that because they already see themselves as castrated, girls lack the dynamic motivation to develop strong superegos. At the same time, Freud realized that all human beings have admixtures of "male" and "female" qualities (Freud 1933/1964).

Subsequent generations of psychoanalytic theorists have both elaborated and challenged Freud's original formulations (Okey 1991). Both Karen Horney and Helene Deutsch wrote books devoted to female psychology. Horney disputed Freud's contention that young girls experienced their genitalia only as lacking. Her work with women patients led her to believe that toddler girls are aware of their vaginas, their inner procreative and valuable spaces. It is male children who have the greater challenge; the healthy development of male children requires rebellion against and rejection of the early parental figure (Williams 1983).

Deutsch (1984) posited female masochism—that is, sexual pleasure derived from pain—to account for women's tolerance for defloration, impregnation, pregnancy, childbirth, and breast-feeding. She underscored the centrality of these experiences in women's lives and psychology. She poignantly described the outpouring of love that a mother experiences for her baby when the fear and pain of childbirth end just as she greets the infant for the first time.

☐ Feminist Criticism, Scholarship, and Research

Feminist scholars have mounted substantive arguments against many facets of traditional female psychology. They have related Freud's characterizations of female psychology to the child-rearing styles and gender expectations of the geographic area, historical era, and social stratum in which Freud, his family, and his patients lived. They have attributed "penis envy" to women's feelings about men's dominance over them in society, or dismissed it altogether, affirming women's pleasure in their own anatomy and generative and nurturing abilities. They have criticized the positing of men's interests, skills, styles, and development as normative and superior and women's as deviant or derivative. Gilligan (1982) demonstrated that girls and women were more likely to ground an ethical decision on its implications for others' well-being, whereas men were more likely to base theirs on rigid moral rules. Neither style of behavior is necessarily superior; they are simply different.

☐ Neuropsychology

As increasingly sophisticated studies address the methodological complications, the curves describing male and female cognitive abilities and styles increasingly overlap. At the neural level, nature and nurture are indistinguishable; circulating sex hormones can be construed as either genetic or environmental. In the brains of adults of both sexes, both androgen and estrogen receptors are active, but their effects differ. Therefore, male and female brains may differ in their responses to neurotransmitters and psychoactive medications. This is known to be true of amphetamines, antidepressants, and major tranquillizers (Hamilton 1989). We must be careful not to make unsupported connections between studies of brain function, such as lateralization, and gender differences.

□ Social Influences

There is clear evidence of differences between male and female infants from birth onward. Male and female infants are treated differently. Parents are rougher with male babies, whose motor skills and explorations they differentially encourage. Powerful social expectations make it difficult to determine whether there are biologically derived, genetic differences in cognition between men and women or girls and boys. Girls excel in school during the early primary years and then fall behind boys in some parameters. Female children are reared to be physically, emotionally, and socially pleasing to others. They are at high risk for sexual, physical, and psychological abuse (Hamilton 1989).

In many settings, neither parents, peers, nor teachers encourage or reward girls' school performance, whether in the classroom or on the playing fields, areas that serve as central models for competitive adult work situations. Girls recognize that the qualities they have fostered—closeness, nurturing, cooperation, self-sacrifice—are devalued. Ambition and assertiveness are necessary for women's advancement, but these qualities are experienced by women as not being consonant with their gender. Women tend to attribute their self-made successes to others or to luck. The tendency of boys and girls, men and women, to experience and think in different ways is also, ironically, an obstacle to their intimate, social, and professional communication with each other.

Women are significantly underrepresented at higher levels of management and in the professions, even when corrections are made for year of entry into the system (Nadelson 1989). They earn less for the same work (Calandra 1992). Women's participation in leadership roles has actually declined over the last 10 or 15 years. There is little social support for their dual roles (i.e., workplace and domestic), with the United States notable among Western countries for its lack of day care, parental leave, and financial benefits for parents. Women's outside employment has little impact on the traditional division of domestic responsibilities; women carry out almost all the managerial and operational tasks of running households and caring for children and other dependent relatives (Tesch et al. 1992).

■ PSYCHIATRIC ASPECTS OF FEMALE REPRODUCTIVE FUNCTIONS AND TREATMENTS

Reproductive symptoms, dysfunctions, complications, and interventions form a nidus around which psychological conflicts and pathology crystallize. Sexual issues carry great emotional weight, often associated with taboos and shame. Psychiatrists have powerful feelings about these issues as well. They may project onto the patient their unconscious, unexamined assumptions and affects about sexual and reproductive events. Psychologically important reproductive events are often not inquired after or acknowledged in the diagnostic process. At other times, psychiatric illnesses have been inappropriately attributed to reproductive milestones such as menopause or hysterectomy.

Because of the psychological and sociological significance of reproductively linked events and treatments, and the likelihood of their being omitted by patients and psychiatrists in standard diagnostic procedures, it is important to take a careful, specific sexual and reproductive history with every patient. Take nothing for granted: sexual inactivity in the elderly or unmarried, virginity in the pious, heterosexuality in the married. An understanding of the patient's sexual and contraceptive practices is relevant to her psychology. It is useful to ask, "Tell me about your past and current sexual life—by yourself and with others." It is best to phrase inquiries with the assumption that behaviors and events have occurred; it is easier for a reticent patient to correct that assumption when inaccurate than to volunteer the fact that she has engaged in behavior she considers embarrassing or improper. It is also best not to reveal assumptions about a patient's feelings or reactions to a given event.

The same is true when a patient, either in the course of an ongoing therapeutic relationship or in a specific consultation, seeks help making a decision about a reproductive choice or intervention. It is absolutely essential to facilitate the patient's consideration of her own background, values, religious heritage, beliefs and practices, circumstances, financial and social resources, preferences, and plans for the future, as well as her feelings about the views and responses of her significant others. Psychiatrists must make themselves aware of their own strong feelings about reproductively related choices so as to provide a therapeutic environment in which a woman can make the kind of autonomous, supported decision that is associated with the most favorable psychiatric outcome. A psychiatrist unable to be neutral about an issue is bound by professional ethics to disclose this situation to the patient and offer referral to a more neutral practitioner.

☐ Menstrually Related Symptoms

The menstrual cycle, a perfectly normal female physiological function, has been a focus of taboo and ritual throughout history. Disability was thought to occur mainly during menstrual bleeding, until the late 1930s, when techniques for measuring female hormones were developed. Over the years, attention has shifted to the premenstrual phase. Premenstrual dysphoric disorder was included in DSM-IV (American Psychiatric Association 1994) after heated controversy. Diagnostic legitimacy may facilitate funding for research and treatment, and relieve symptomatic women, but it may also exacerbate the general tendency to associate normal female physiological functions with disability.

☐ Pregnancy and Childbirth

The state of pregnancy demands adjustments in self-image, relationships, priorities, and plans but does not cause significant dysfunction or constitute an illness. Pregnancy and childbirth preparation classes now offered in many settings can reflect and enhance women's knowledge, comfort, and mastery of these experiences but may also occasion anxiety about the "right" approach and the patient's ability to achieve it (Notman 1990). The possibility of pregnancy and the effects of psychotropic medication must be considered in all female patients at all times.

Rates of admission to psychiatric inpatient units decrease during pregnancy and increase during the postpartum period. Psychotic illness is associated with an increased rate of obstetrical complications and poor neonatal outcomes, and successful psychiatric treatment with improved obstetrical status. There is sometimes pressure to commit pregnant women whose behavior, such as substance abuse or noncompliance with obstetrical care, endangers the fetus's well-being. Unless the behavior poses an immediate danger to the woman herself, involuntary institutionalization or interventions are contrary to the canons of medical ethics.

Mild, self-limited "baby blues," starting within a day or two of delivery and lasting a few days, affect up to 50% of new mothers in America. Both hormonal and social factors probably play etiological roles; the incidence of this condition in non-Western cultures is not known. Approximately 10% of women with newly delivered babies suffer a major mood disorder postpartum, with less than 0.2% suffering a psychosis (Apfel and Handel 1993). Symptoms may be depressive, manic, and/or psychotic. Postpartum psychiatric illness may be associated with symptoms related to other reproductive events and tends to recur with subsequent pregnancies. The treatment approach is dictated by the signs, symptoms, and circumstances of the patient. The patient's wish to breast-feed the infant, and the physiological advantages for both mother and infant, must be weighed against the need for psychotropic medications. Mother-infant inpatient units have proved highly successful both in this country and elsewhere (Apfel and Handel 1993). Such units preserve the mother-infant attachment and the patient's confidence in her parental skills while permitting round-the-clock professional observation and enhancement of maternal behaviors.

☐ Infertility and Reproductive Technology

Infertility, which is thought to affect 10% of couples, is a grievous narcissistic injury (Kraft et al. 1980). Psychiatric problems that should be considered include anorexia nervosa and sexually unconsummated relationships. Psychologically, women who have difficulty conceiving tend to feel empty, hollow, worthless, unfeminine, and undesirable. In their search for an explanation, they relive guilt over past sexual behavior and regret over past induced abortions. They may lose interest in sexual activity, or engage in it frantically in an unconscious attempt to act out their worthlessness or deny it. Women who fulfill career plans before attempting conception experience infertility as their first encounter with a challenge that they cannot conquer. Women frequently report that infertility is the most stressful situation they have ever encountered. Men are more reticent about their responses to infertility. Tension often develops between partners when the woman feels the need to share her problem with friends and relatives while the man insists on keeping it secret (Dickstein 1990).

In vitro fertilization, the transfer of gametes and embryos between couples, the induction of fertility in postmenopausal women, and other new interventions have led the public to believe that virtually any woman can conceive and/or bear a child. The new developments that offer hope also complicate the ethical and psychological challenges of infertility. Both care providers and patients must grapple with difficult questions: how to evaluate treatment outcome, who qualifies for treatment, what to do with frozen embryos, how to protect the legal rights of those involved, and when to stop trying to achieve pregnancy. The process postpones acceptance and grieving. Some women who do conceive and deliver suffer a paradoxical depression; the reality of ordinary parenthood is a letdown after years of fantasy and single-minded effort. Support groups have proven extremely helpful to otherwise psychiatrically well infertility patients who simply need to mobilize their own coping skills and share their experiences (Stewart 1992).

☐ Induced Abortion

Induced abortion has been practiced throughout history, evoking profoundly mixed emotions, wrenching social conflict, and political crisis. Reproductive choice is fundamental to women's autonomy. The reality of many women's lives severely restricts their access to contraceptives and contraceptive services, and their ability to articulate and enforce stipulations on sexual relationships. This leaves them vulnerable to pregnancies that may threaten their support of existing children, their educations, their life plans, or their own safety and support. Russo and Zierk

(1992) found that abortion's positive effect on a woman's well-being was related to its role in controlling fertility and the woman's coping resources. Pregnant women may consult psychiatrists when they cannot resolve their ambivalence about the continuation of the pregnancy. The object of therapy under these circumstances is to facilitate the woman's review of her own values, plans, and circumstances, to enable her to make an informed choice.

The decision to have an abortion is a deeply felt and considered one for nearly all women. It is made in the context of the situation that makes the pregnancy untenable, of medical time constraints, and of social ambivalence manifest in geographic, financial, chronological, and other restrictions. Even when abortion is chosen, it represents a loss. After an abortion, some women experience transient feelings of guilt. Most are relieved (Russo and Zierk 1992). The process of making and following through on the decision improves these women's self-esteem and sense of control over their lives. The incidence of severe psychiatric illness after childbirth far exceeds that following induced abortion (Zolese and Blacker 1992). Women who are not permitted to make an autonomous choice, women aborting because of genetic defects diagnosed in the fetus, and women with prior or current psychiatric illness are at greatest risk (Herz 1991).

☐ Menopause

Menopause was viewed in past generations as an (or *the*) etiological factor in midlife psychiatric disorders. It was seen as a developmental crisis during which a woman had to face her loss of youth, fertility, and desirability just as her daughters were enjoying theirs. Research has established the centrality of the psychosocial context in the response to menopause. Within our predominant culture, menopause is significantly problematic only for those who have defined themselves largely through childbearing and child rearing, and who have not moved toward other interests and gratifications as their children grew independent. There is some evidence for an association between the so-called "replacement" hormones and depression (Palinkas and Barrett-Conner 1992).

☐ Breast Pathology

One of every 12 women in the United States will be diagnosed with a malignancy of the breast during her lifetime. Women whose first-degree female relatives have suffered from breast cancer are at a two- to three-fold higher risk (Wyngaarden et al. 1992). Empirical evidence does not support the belief that breast cancer is a psychogenic disease; the treating psychiatrist should be aware of the harmful consequences of the implication that the patient caused her own life-threatening illness (Hiller 1989). Psychiatrists may encounter women whose terror of the disease has become a disabling obsession, but it is far more common for women to deny the danger. Psychotherapy may help the patient to overcome irrational fears.

Some women have felt that the medical profession has not fully appreciated the sense of mutilation they suffered after radical mastectomy. Advances in the treatment of breast cancer often allow the preservation of breast tissue without compromising prognosis. Breast reconstruction, with or without the placement of an artificial implant, is often offered. Patients may need help to decide whether the cosmetic effect warrants the additional risk, pain, and expense. The concerns of some women who claim to have suffered severe medical and psychiatric complications following the implantation of silicone breast inserts have ignited a controversy within the Food and Drug Administration (FDA) and in the media.

☐ Pelvic Pain

Patients with pelvic pain require a thorough gynecological examination and a careful history. Past pelvic infections or surgery may have led to pelvic adhesions. Psychiatric diagnoses may include any of the somatization disorders. Patients with a history of past or current abuse are at greater risk. Surgery can further complicate the symptoms and diagnosis. In addition, minor pathology that is discovered by sophisticated technology may be unrelated to the symptoms, but may precipitate major interventions. Some patients complain of perineal itching, burning, and pain. Diagnosis and treatment are currently controversial. Some gynecologists are convinced that the symptoms are caused by significant pathology that has simply not yet been identified and classified, and report that their patients are cured by vulvectomy.

☐ Hysterectomy and Gynecological Malignancies

In the United States hysterectomies were performed at a rate of 3.9 per 1,000 women in 1989. Linguistic confusion about the procedure is common; the term "hysterectomy" is used to denote removal of the uterus alone, or removal of the uterus, fallopian tubes, and ovaries. The patient herself may not know what organs are to be or have been removed. Some doctors see hysterectomy as a benign intervention; others are extremely reluctant to perform the operation. Therefore, some women who feel debilitated and inconvenienced by dysfunctional bleeding and are desperate to be rid of their uterus are unable to obtain the surgery, whereas others have it urged upon them without any inquiry into its psychological consequences. Studies of psychological and psychiatric outcome have yielded conflicting results; confounding variables include the length of the follow-up period, the preoperative psychological preparation and expectations of the patient, the attitudes of her significant others, and the attitudes and methods of the researchers.

Gynecological malignancies tend to evoke feelings of shame in addition to the fear, anger, and grief precipitated by most malignancies. Attempts to explain their affliction reawaken in women patients conflicts and guilt related to past autoerotic and interpersonal sexual behavior, and concerns about the adequacy of gynecological care they have undergone in the past. Most women are neither knowledgeable about nor comfortable with their reproductive anatomy, which is mostly internal, and do not have regular pelvic examinations and Pap smears. Diagnosis of cervical malignancy is therefore often delayed, resulting in many preventable deaths. Providers of mental health care may contribute significantly to women's health by helping them to become comfortable with gynecological care and by helping gynecologists to provide care that is more sensitive to women's feelings and fears.

■ WOMEN AS PATIENTS

☐ Epidemiology and Diagnosis

Gender roles influence the outward manifestations of psychiatric illness, its visibility, and the reactions of others to the ill person, thereby affecting epidemiological data. Alcoholism is a case in point. Diagnostic criteria derive from male patterns of alcohol abuse and the impact of men's drinking on their social roles, including paid employment, violence, and interactions with the criminal justice system. Clinicians' perception of psychopathology is demonstrably influenced by the concordance or dissonance between a patient's symptoms and social gender role expectations.

☐ Disorders of Childhood and Development

Two factors are significant in gender differences in psychiatric disorders in childhood and development. Girls may acquire verbal skills earlier than do boys. Children must be brought to treatment by adults. Childhood disorders that produce conflict with other people and with institutions, such as attention-deficit hyperactivity disorder (ADHD), conduct disorder, oppositional defiant disorder, encopresis and enuresis, stuttering, and others, are probably diagnosed and treated more often than are disorders such as depression, which may actually make the child less demanding. Boys outnumber girls with respect to the former; girls suffer more depressions (American Association of University Women 1992).

☐ Substance Abuse and Addiction

Women's consumption of alcohol is frowned upon in most societies; this complicates both the diagnosis of individual patients and epidemiology in general (Oppenheimer 1991). In most cultures studied, men outnumber women among alcohol users and abusers. How genetics and culture figure in the etiology of the difference is not definitively known. Women are more sensitive to the effects of alcohol. Although women abuse illicit drugs less frequently than do men, significant numbers of women engage in illicit drug use. In a household survey conducted by the National Institute on Drug Abuse (1991), 53% to 57% of women between the ages of 18 and 34 reported that they had used an illicit drug at least once (Horton 1992).

The media and the medical profession have focused on cocaine-abusing women as vectors of infection and as mothers of affected newborns and neglected children, rather than as suffering individuals, thus alienating potential patients and decreasing compliance with treatment. Substance-abusing women who are pregnant and/or mothers fear that their seeking treatment will result in prosecution and/or the loss of custody (Blume and Russell 1993). Outrage against women for engaging in behavior detrimental to their unborn children resulted in attempts in several states to criminalize crack cocaine use during pregnancy. The American Psychiatric Association adopted a position objecting to this approach and encouraging the development of sorely needed treatment resources instead. Women seeking treatment outnumber the available places by hundreds to one.

The AIDS epidemic has added a deadly dimension to the problems of women who use illicit substances. Addiction to crack cocaine drives many women into prostitution, increasing their risk of infection; other women acquire HIV from husbands or lovers. The rate of HIV infection is going up faster among women and children than among any other group. Preventive strategies have been largely aimed at males (Wiener 1991). The prevention of HIV spread to women requires that they assert themselves to deny sexual intercourse or to demand the use of condoms, both of which are behaviors that run counter to the socialization and circumstances of the women most at risk (Guinan 1992).

☐ Use of Prescription Psychoactive Medication

Women receive two times more prescriptions for psychoactive medications such as sedatives, stimulants, tranquilizers, and analgesics than do men (Ashton 1991). Women may be more likely to use the medications in ways other than those prescribed, and they are more likely to become addicted to them.

☐ Trauma-Related Syndromes

Recent years have seen an explosion in the recognition of interpersonal abuse of girls and women and of its role in the genesis of a number of psychiatric disorders, including personality disorders, multiple personality, somatizing disorders, and posttraumatic stress disorder (Koss 1990). There has been debate over the classification of disorders in which early life and ongoing abuse may play a major role; is it appropriate to apply a descriptive label, or does that stigmatize the sufferer? Reliance on retrospective data can skew studies of incidence in either direction.

It is estimated that 26% of women are raped at least once in their lives (Hamilton 1989). Thirty-eight percent of female children are sexually abused (including exposure). It is estimated that anywhere between 25% and 50% of wives or female domestic partners are physically and/or sexually attacked (Hamilton 1989).

The abuse of girls and women has been hidden within the family, officially or unofficially socially accepted, and poorly investigated, publicized, and prosecuted. Women who claimed they had been raped were, and in many instances still are, subjected to degrading interrogations implying their invitation of or complicity with the act. Society's reaction to rape victims mirrors the victim's response to the trauma with feelings of being dirty, guilty, and/or tainted. Natural reactions to these feelings, such as failure to report the crime, and intense bathing and cleaning, may eradicate forensic evidence, delay investigation, and decrease the victim's credibility. Assault predisposes victims to long-term psychiatric sequelae that are exacerbated by denial, isolation, shame, and secrecy (American Medical Association 1992).

Rape crisis teams and self-help organizations, often including former victims, have fostered educational efforts to increase the sensitivity of law enforcement and health care professionals to the reactions and needs of rape victims and to develop protocols that increase the likelihood of successful prosecution of perpetrators (Koss 1990).

☐ Anxiety Disorders

Anxiety disorders are common in both men and women. Agoraphobia is diagnosed more often in women than in men, which is not the case with panic disorder. It has been hypothesized that this difference is related to gender role and environment, in that women are more likely to be housebound than are men.

☐ Somatizing Disorders

Hysteria, or *conversion disorder*, is the ancient prototype of a disorder directly related to female reproductive organs. The psychological use of bodily experiences and metaphors to express feelings and conflicts is highly culture bound (Dunk 1989). In our society, the female condition itself has been seen as disabling, with complaints and dysfunction related to menstruation, childbearing, and menopause expected and accepted. Women are often seen as complainers, and their symptoms may not be taken as seriously as men's. When women and men complain of the same symptoms, men are more likely to be referred for diagnostic tests (Ayanian and Epstein 1991).

☐ Depression

Both community studies and studies of clinical populations indicate that the prevalence of major depression among women is twice that of men. Major depression is the most common major psychiatric disorder in women; it is estimated that seven million women in the United States currently qualify for the diagnosis. More women than men suffer from other varieties of depression as well. The sex difference prevails across boundaries of race, ethnicity, and socioeconomic status (Horton 1992). Depression is most common in women between the ages of 25 and 44, with some evidence of a shift to younger ages at onset. Women are more likely to attempt suicide, but men account for 8 of every 10 completed suicides. Most suicidologists attribute the difference to men's tendency to use more lethal and immediate methods, whereas women choose methods, such as the ingestion of pills, that allow more time for effective intervention (Shaffer 1988). The underdiagnosis of depression in women is a significant public health problem, and the psychiatric community is making a major effort to bring this problem to the attention of primary care providers, health care policy-makers, and the population at large.

No biological factors explaining women's increased vulnerability to depressive illness have been identified. Although menopause, hysterectomy, and abortion are psychologically meaningful, they are not associated with significant increases in the incidence of depression or psychosis. The only reproductive event reliably linked to psychiatric illness is childbirth. As many as 50% of women who have newly delivered a child experience a mild, self-limited syndrome, "baby blues." The incidence of clinical depression postpartum may be as much as 10%. Many of these women are also depressed during pregnancy, when the hormonal milieu is very different. The demands of infant care in a society that has lost much traditional support and has failed to institute governmental support for parenthood may play a role in the etiology of postpartum psychiatric illness.

☐ Eating Disorders: Anorexia and Bulimia Nervosa

Eating disorders are so much more prevalent in women than in men that clinicians may fail to consider the diagnosis in male patients. Most patients with anorexia nervosa are white, middle-class women in their teens or early adult years. Estimates of incidence are complicated by patients' failure to seek treatment, but may be about 1% (Jones et al. 1980). Gender role factors considered to be significant in the etiology of anorexia include the emphasis on physical appearance and slimness for women in American culture, their tendency to be dissatisfied with their bodies and to diet, and issues of control between the young woman and her family.

Because bulimia nervosa is a condition in which body weight remains within normal limits, its prevalence is even more difficult to ascertain. Reported prevalence ranges from 1% to 18% (Drewnowski et al. 1988). Both anorexia and bulimia have been associated with histories of abuse in childhood. Obesity is also more common in girls and women than in boys and men.

☐ Personality Disorders

The relationship between gender and environmental factors and the diagnosis of personality disorders has sparked major controversies. There is first the question of sexual stereotypes in the formulation and application of diagnoses of character disturbances. Both histrionic and dependent personality disorder as described in DSM-IV can be construed as portraits of traditional forms of feminine behavior. It is extremely difficult to decide when the behaviors reach a pathological degree.

One approach to this problem is to specify that the traits must be disabling. However, this judgment is largely context-dependent as well. If subjective distress is a requisite, the diagnostic category becomes not all individuals who exhibit the described behaviors, but only those who are not pleased with the behaviors. From the perspective of the diagnostician, the application of the diagnosis will be largely dependent on attitudes about gender roles.

☐ Sexual Dysfunction

Clinicians should be alert to the possibility of undisclosed, perhaps repressed, past sexual abuse in the histories of women with functional sexual dysfunction, and in all women patients.

■ THE PSYCHIATRIC TREATMENT OF WOMEN

☐ Psychotherapy

The therapist's gender-related assumptions interact in complex ways with those of the patient. A clash can produce implicit disapproval, narcissistic injury, and therapeutic stalemate. A shared, but unexamined, assumption can deprive the patient of the opportunity to explore a full range of life options. The gender of the therapist raises similar issues. A therapist of dissimilar anatomy, physiology, and gender-related experience must make a special effort to develop therapeutic empathy for a patient. However, this effort may, in fact, contribute to the therapeutic process. The assumption that a therapist of the same sex can and will understand the patient simply on that basis can also lead to therapeutic difficulties. The therapist may ignore differences and/or overidentify with the patient.

☐ Pharmacotherapy

Medications may be metabolized differently in women and men, and, in women, over the menstrual cycle, during pregnancy, and during other cycles in their reproductive life span. Women patients may take for granted oral contraceptive or hormonal "replacement" therapy to the extent that they neglect to mention them when asked about their medications. Oral contraceptives interact with minor tranquilizers, barbiturates, and phenytoin. There is evidence of varying response to antidepressants over the menstrual cycle (Cotton 1990). Side effects of psychoactive agents may include sexual dysfunction. This is true of monoamine oxidase inhibitors and serotonin reuptake inhibitors, which have been associated with anorgasmia (Lesko et al. 1982). Women tend not to be asked about these effects and not to volunteer the information, although the symptoms may affect compliance.

The use of psychotropic medication during pregnancy and breast-feeding deserves special consideration. Although only lithium has been clearly shown to have deleterious effects on the fetus and newborn, there are few data demonstrating the absence or safety of subtle and long-term effects of other agents.

☐ Special Management Issues

The treatment of women patients often necessitates attention to their life circumstances and to both deprivations and resources related to gender. Women are more likely than men to be poor and to lack health insurance. They are more likely to be responsible for the care of children, disabled persons, and elderly individuals, and those groups are likely to suffer from the same deprivations. The need to arrange care for others often hinders women's ability to undergo their own outpatient and inpatient psychiatric care. Women may need empowerment and substantive help to delegate some of those responsibilities so as to take care of themselves. When the dependent is an infant or young child, mother-child inpatient and outpatient units have proven extremely effective in enhancing psychiatric well-being, maternal function, and outcome for both mother and child.

Self-help or professionally led groups focusing on specific or general issues affecting women are also an effective adjunct to psychiatric treatment. The psychiatrist should be familiar with the philosophy and effectiveness of the particular group so as to enhance its effectiveness for the patient and to forestall conflicts. The ethos of some groups fosters the feeling that all of the adverse events and circumstances of a woman's life are attributable to the experience or trait shared by the group.

Past or current abuse by family members, health care providers, and others in positions of power and responsibility is always a possibility. Increased risk during pregnancy is a counterintuitive reality. Care may necessitate interactions with state and federal agencies and the legal/judicial system. Issues that arise include child abuse and child custody, domestic violence, and the reporting of patient abuse by a previous therapist. Laws vary widely across geographic regions; often the district branch and/or state government office of the American Psychiatric Association can supply information.

■ WOMEN AS PSYCHIATRISTS

☐ Women in Psychiatric Training

Psychiatry has traditionally been one of the preferred specialty choices for women medical graduates. As the percentage and absolute numbers of women medical students has risen dramatically over the last 25 years, so have the opportunities for women in specialties previously closed to them, notably the surgical subspecialties. Women medical students receive less financial support from their families than do men, and graduate with major debt loads, which may affect specialty choice (DeAngelis 1991). Many women medical graduates marry and bear children during residency and fellowship training. Of these, approximately 85% marry professionals and 50% marry fellow physicians (Tesch 1992).

Few programs offer part-time residency or child care. Few provide a sufficient array of female role models who can share their experiences of various styles of professional and personal life with younger colleagues. Many prejudices persist—for example, a resident who is a mother may not be considered eligible for research or leadership opportunities. Residents and young psychiatrists who have not married may face fewer conflicts of schedule and commitment, but encounter other problems instead. Women who wish to marry and bear children become concerned about the "biological clock." Women who do not wish to marry, whether they are heterosexual or homosexual, must repeatedly explain themselves. Lesbian residents are subject to prejudice and discrimination.

Recent revelations have highlighted the incidence of sexual harassment of female medical students, residents, and practicing physicians/faculty. The vulnerability of students and residents to exploitation has led the American Medical Association and the American Psychiatric Association to refine their codes of ethics to address the issue of romantic and sexual relationships between teachers and trainees. The responsibility of the teacher or clinical supervisor to evaluate the trainee and to facilitate or impede advancement, and the powerful emotions inherent in the teacher and student roles, prevent the parties from entering into a genuinely mutual, consenting relationship. Should romantic or sexual feelings and behaviors intrude into the educational setting, consultation should immediately be sought and discipline may be indicated. Both trainees and faculty must be informed of these mandates and the reasons for them.

☐ Career Development

Social gender roles have a significant impact on the career planning and development of women psychiatrists. Women tend to be less comfortable than men with ambition and competition. They seldom acquire faculty mentors who encourage them to plan for leadership positions and advise them on how to attain them. Their interest and skills in nurturing, facilitating, and cooperating are often exploited in positions (e.g., advising medical students, working on committees) that they discover only later to be irrelevant or even deleterious to career advancement (Nadelson 1989). If their scholarly and research interests lie in "women's issues," their work tends to be regarded as "unfocused" and "soft" by recruiters and promotions committees.

Participation in professional associations offers women residents and psychiatrists a wider exposure and acquaintanceship. Unfortunately, it is often the very residents who could most use support and advice from regional and national networks of colleagues who feel unable to attend meetings because of their heavy commitments. Because mothers continue to assume most responsibility for the care of children, physicians who are mothers often prioritize flexibility in their hours and location over other aspects of possible positions.

Career development patterns have been predicated on a model demanding intense work and long hours during the very phase of life when most women are bearing and caring for children. Women remain professionally active, on average, longer in life than do men. Rather than scaling down later in life, they are often eager to pursue their careers with renewed vigor after their children are independent. Despite the value of their maturity and life experience, entry into subspecialty training, research fellowships, or organizational positions finds them in a peer group in their 20s and 30s, with entry-level salaries. The entry of women into the higher levels of psychiatric leadership has not kept pace with their increasing representation at lower levels. The percentage of women attaining department chairs, tenured academic positions, and executive positions has stabilized or even dropped over the last 15 years. This phenomenon has become known as the "glass ceiling."

☐ Psychiatric Practice

There has been considerable speculation about the relationship between gender and either psychotherapeutic skill or the suitability of a particular therapist for a particular patient and problem. However, individual traits and talents outweigh gender differences.

Some practice issues are limited to female psychiatrists. A psychiatrist's pregnancy precipitates powerful feelings in herself and in her patients. Patients experience envy of both the pregnant therapist and her unborn child. The pregnancy is visible evidence of the therapist's sexual activity and emotional closeness with a person in her private life. Patients fear abandonment, by virtue of the therapist's decreasing or interrupting of her working schedule before or after delivery, and/or because her emotional energy will be consumed by the mother-child relationship. Should the psychiatrist make few professional concessions to parenthood, patients may be concerned that she is generally uncaring, or that they are receiving attention to which her baby is entitled.

Women psychiatrists may be especially sought after by patients who have been abused in childhood and/or exploited by former therapists, employers, or others in positions of power and responsibility. The subsequent treating psychiatrist faces many issues, including reporting, helping the patient decide whether to bring a lawsuit and/or complaint before a licensing or ethics board, and dealing with the powerful emotions evoked by the patient's ordeal and helplessness. Women physicians, who have coped actively with prejudice and often with harassment in order to function, may have an especially difficult time remaining empathic to a patient who tolerates abuse and who often unconsciously attempts to provoke it in the treatment setting. Should the patient decide to bring charges against a former victimizer, the attorney who defends the victimizer may accuse the subsequent (female) psychiatrist of causing or exacerbating the harm that has befallen the patient.

■ REFERENCES

American Association of University Women: How Schools Shortchange Girls: A Study of Major Findings on Girls and Education. Washington, DC, American Association of University Women Education Foundation and the National Education Association, 1992

American Medical Association, Council on Scientific Affairs: Violence against women: relevance for medical practitioners. JAMA (Council Reports) 267:3184–3189, 1992

American Psychiatric Association: Diagnostic and Statistical Manual of Mental Disorders, 4th Edition. Washington, DC, American Psychiatric Association, 1994

Apfel RJ, Handel MH: Madness and Loss of Motherhood: Sexuality, Reproduction, and Long-Term Mental Illness. Washington, DC, American Psychiatric Press, 1993

Ashton H: Psychotropic-drug prescribing for women. Br J Psychiatry 158 (suppl 10):30–35 1991

Ayanian JZ, Epstein AM: Differences in the use of procedures between women and men hospitalized for coronary heart disease. N Engl J Med 325:221–225, 1991

Blume SB, Russell M: Alcohol and substance abuse in the practice of obstetrics and gynecology, in Psychological Aspects of Women's Health Care: The Interface of Psychiatry and Obstetrics and Gynecology. Edited by Stewart DE, Stotland NL: Washington, DC, American Psychiatric Press, 1993, pp 391–409

Calandra B: Closing the gap. Scott-Levin's Pallas Athena 1(1):27–30, 1992

Cotton P: Examples abound of gaps in medical knowledge because of groups excluded from scientific study. JAMA 263:1051–1055, 1990

DeAngelis C: Women in medicine. Am J Dis Child 145:49–52, 1991

Deutsch H: The menopause. Int J Psychoanal 65:55–62, 1984

Dickstein LJ: Effects of the new reproductive technology on individuals and relationships, in Psychological Aspects of Reproductive Technology. Edited by Stotland NL. Washington, DC, American Psychiatric Press, 1990, pp 123–139

Drewnowski A, Yee DK, Krahn DD: Bulimia in college women: incidence and recovery rates. Am J Psychiatry 145:753–755, 1988

Dunk P: Greek women and broken nerves in Montreal. Med Anthropol 11:29–45, 1989

Freud S: Femininity (1933), in The Standard Edition of the Complete Psychological Works of Sigmund Freud, Vol 22. Translated and edited by Strachey J. London, Hogarth Press, 1964, pp 112–135

Gilligan C: In a Different Voice. Cambridge, MA, Harvard University Press, 1982

Guinan M: HIV, heterosexual transmission, and women. JAMA 268:520–521, 1992

Hamilton JA: Emotional consequences of victimization and discrimination in "special populations" of women. Psychiatr Clin North Am 12:35–51, 1989

Herz EK: Issues in decision making: psychotherapeutic work with women who have problem pregnancies, in Psychiatric Aspects of Abortion. Edited by Stotland NL. Washington, DC, American Psychiatric Press, 1991, pp 108–110

Hiller JE: Breast cancer: a psychogenic disease? Women and Health 15(2):5–18, 1989

Horton JA (ed): The Women's Health Data Book: A Profile of Women's Health in the United States. Washington, DC, Jacobs Institute of Women's Health, 1992

Jones DJ, Fox MM, Babigian HM, et al: Epidemiology of anorexia nervosa in Monroe County, New York: 1960–1976. Psychosom Med 42:551–558, 1980

Koss MP: The women's mental health research agenda: violence against women. Am Psychol 45:374–380, 1990

Kraft AD, Palombo J, Mitchell D, et al: The psychological dimensions of infertility. Am J Orthopsychiatry 50:618–628, 1980

Lesko LM, Stotland NL, Segraves RT: Three cases of female anorgasmia associated with MAOIs. Am J Psychiatry 139:1353–1354, 1982

LeVine RA: Gender differences: interpreting anthropological data, in Women and Men: New Perspectives on Gender Differences. Edited by Notman MT, Nadelson CC. Washington, DC, American Psychiatric Press, 1991, pp 1–8

Nadelson CC: Professional issues for women. Psychiatr Clin North Am 12:25–33, 1989

National Institute on Drug Abuse: National Household Survey on Drug Abuse: Population Estimates, 1991 (DHHS Publ No. [ADM]-92-1887). Washington, DC, Alcohol, Drug Abuse, and Mental Health Administration, 1991

Notman MT: Reproduction and pregnancy: a psychodynamic developmental perspective, in Psychiatric Aspects of Reproductive Technology. Edited by Stotland NL. Washington, DC, American Psychiatric Press, 1990, pp 13–24

Okey JL: Is psychoanalytic theory relevant to the psychology of women? J Am Acad Psychoanal 19:396–402, 1991

Oppenheimer E: Alcohol and drug misuse among women: an overview. Br J Psychiatry 158 (suppl 10):36–44, 1991

Palinkas LS, Barrett-Conner E: Estrogen use and depressive symptoms in postmenopausal women. Obstet Gynecol 80:30–36, 1992

Russo NF, Zierk KL: Abortion, childbearing, and women's well-being. Professional Psychology: Research and Practice 23:269–280, 1992

Shaffer D: The epidemiology of teen suicide: an examination of risk factors. J Clin Psychiatry 49 (No 9, Suppl):36–41, 1988

Stewart D: A prospective study of the effectiveness of brief professionally-led infertility support groups, in Reproductive Life: Advances in Research in Psychosomatic Obstetrics and Gynaecology. Edited by Wijma K, von Schoultz B. NJ, Parthenon Publishing Group, 1992, pp 540–545

Tesch BJ, Osborne J, Simpson DE, et al: Women physicians in dual-physician relationships compared with those in other dual-career relationships. Acad Med 67:542–544, 1992

Wiener LS: Women and human immunodeficiency virus: a historical and personal psychosocial perspective. Social Work 36:375–378, 1991

Williams JH: Psychology of Women: Behavior in a Biosocial Context, 2nd Edition. New York, WW Norton, 1983

Wyngaarden JB, Smith Jr LH, Bennett JC (eds): Cecil Textbook of Medicine. Philadelphia, PA, WB Saunders/Harcourt Brace Jovanovich, 1992

Zolese G, Blacker CVR: The psychological complications of therapeutic abortion. Br J Psychiatry 160:742–749, 1992

CHAPTER 41

Essentials of
Cultural Psychiatry

Ezra E. H. Griffith, M.D.
Carlos A. González, M.D.

■ DEFINITIONS OF CULTURAL PSYCHIATRY

Certain key concepts have been consistently critical to the understanding of cultural psychiatry. First is *society*, which Leighton and Murphy (1965) defined as a group of human beings who live together in a system of social relationships. A second crucial concept is *culture*, considered by Leighton and Murphy (1965) to be an abstract concept that describes a particular society's entire way of living. The notion encompasses shared patterns of belief, feeling, and knowledge that ultimately guide everyone's conduct and definition of reality. Culture refers to a multiplicity of elements that define human life, such as social relationships, religion, technology, and economics. Furthermore, it is an ever-changing concept, one that is learned, taught by one generation to the next, and obviously an integral part of all societies. *Ethnicity* is a somewhat narrower term, in that it encompasses the notion that people identify with each other because of a shared heritage. In a technical sense, distinctions exist between social structure and cultural processes. However, it is often the case in the psychiatric arena that social and cultural components are combined to facilitate conceptualizations.

Another important definition centers on *environment*, which refers to physical circumstances of climate, altitude, natural resources, and the presence or absence of noxious agents. In this context, it is to be understood that, for example, a tropical climate has considerable influence on the games played by adolescents and favors the use of the outdoors. Similarly, a severely cold climate influences the dating practices of young lovers, because activities outdoors would be circumscribed.

These definitions lead to a clearer appreciation of the notion that cultural psychiatry concerns itself with the relationship between psychiatric disorders and the matrix created by the interplay of society, culture, and environment. The more restrictive term *cross-cultural* (or *transcultural*) implies that a psychiatric problem in two different cultures is being compared in some way, or that a psychiatric question in a particular culture is being studied or approached by someone who is from another culture.

Another important consideration in cultural psychiatry is the difference between the *emic* and the *etic* perspective. Simply stated, the term *emic* refers to the conceptually narrow view by people in a given culture of a phenomenon occurring within that culture. The term *etic* refers to a culture-general or universal approach to the viewing of psychiatric problems. Westermeyer (1985) warned against thinking that a diagnosable phenomenon is either emic or etic in nature, but rather states the issue as the extent to which a given diagnostic entity is emic versus the extent to which it is etic. Consequently, observers from culture A may impose their cultural perspectives on their observations about culture B. The result is a "pseudoetic" or "imposed etic" view that may very well include a number of distortions about culture B. Berry (1975) argued that an observer from culture A should temper this imposed etic view with emic considerations acquired through observation of culture B in order to eventually achieve a "derived etic" view of the specific psychiatric issue that is being considered within culture B.

■ SCOPE OF THE DISCIPLINE

Interest in cultural psychiatry has spread around the globe and has led to significant widening of its scope. Broadly speaking, the discipline now includes such themes as the study of people in their natural habitats; the relationship of cultural factors to specific psychiatric disorders; the relationship of psychiatric disorders and processes to human universals such as gender and age; culture and personality development; culture-bound syndromes; comparative studies of diagnostic entities; culture and healing systems; culture and social roles; culture and psychotherapy; and the impact of race and ethnicity on response to psychotropic medications (Draguns 1981; Kiev 1964; Leighton and Murphy 1965).

■ CULTURE AND PERSONALITY

☐ Developmental Issues

The role of culture in the development of long-standing personality traits is paramount. Misunderstandings will occur if cultural factors are not considered in our view of children's development and personality formation. Stoller and Herdt (1982) described at length the socially prescribed way of raising male children by the Sambia, a tribal people of New Guinea who hold in the highest esteem the maleness and warriorhood of their men. The authors outlined the ways in which the Sambia established first a strong and prolonged bond between mother and son, then went through unique and elaborate rituals to break that bond and ultimately develop strong heterosexual males. The clarity of the cultural expectation and reinforcing value of the rituals ensured the social outcome of heterosexual maleness. Other researchers have addressed issues such as the influence of culture on the development of dependency traits among West Indians (Allen 1985) and the culturally determined socialization toward trance and dissociative states among particular groups (Bateson 1975; Koss 1975).

In the inner cities, the cultural milieu often includes poverty, chronic exposure to crime, street and domestic violence, and substance abuse, as well as a predominance of young, undersupported single mothers who are heads of households. The impact of this upbringing cannot be overlooked when viewing a child from these origins. Although it has been stated that traits that are routinely characterized as antisocial may be culturally appropriate and defensive in nature within this culture (Reid 1985), others (Cohen and Brook 1987) found such phenomena as family instability and parental inconsistency to be risk factors for later psychopathology in children, such as immature behavior and conduct disorder, the latter a known precursor to antisocial personality disorder. It is unclear what the long-term effects will be of protracted exposure to the chronic stress of such an environment. The role of the extended family on the development of otherwise disadvantaged youth has been cited as an important compensatory factor whose long-term effect has yet to be ascertained (Wilson 1989).

☐ Effect on Intrapsychic Development

The impact of culture on intrapsychic development has been an important theme, and nowhere has this been more evident than in the work generated about the development of self-concept. As would be expected, this has been of special interest to minority groups in this country. It is an old hypothesis that, for example, American blacks possess significant self-hatred. This negative self-concept has been thought to be reinforced by the white dominant American culture that defines blackness as bad and inferior. Spurlock (1986) reviewed research focused on the development of self-concept in African-American children, pointing out how the early conclusions have been subsequently challenged.

Other equally important issues have been studied in regard to the effect of culture on intrapsychic development. Considerable work has been done on the cultural stimuli in American society that lead women to conceptualize their status as secondary to the male's position (Carmen et al. 1981). The assumption has been that cultural values and stereotypes have been at the core of the notions that women are, for example, unable to be first-rate airplane pilots or surgeons. In general, many researchers have taken the position that restructuring of such distorted values could lead to significant change in the way future generations of women will think about themselves.

☐ Effect on Interpersonal Relationships

It should follow that the work on culture and its effect on developmental and intrapsychic tasks might be extrapolated to conclusions or hypotheses about interpersonal relationships. Consequently, observations that led to assertions about the development of masculinity in particular societies were ultimately used also to clarify theories about homosexual and transsexual behavior. In the Sambia observations, the powerful and intense initiation rituals, coupled with the values and behavioral interventions of the males, led to the exclusion of transsexual behavior in that culture.

Similarly, females in American culture, who have thought of themselves as unable to perform certain jobs that have traditionally been held by males, have then in turn related hesitantly to the males, who have naturally been viewed as having all the power. Delgado et al. (1985) pointed out that in the business world it has long been assumed that females are submissive, dependent, not adventurous, suggestible, noncompetitive, excitable when facing crises, likely to have their feelings hurt, emotional, and conceited about their appearance. The expectation has also been that such traits render a woman unable to make decisions with confidence and dispatch. Alternatively, it has been argued that the female who, in effect, behaves like a man in this type of job would be considered a "castrating woman."

It is in fact fairly easy to demonstrate that society, through its enunciation of values and beliefs, can affect and order the nature of interpersonal relationships. However, it cannot be assumed that one can draw a straight line of linkage from a baby's early experiences with his or her mother, who is the very embodiment of that culture's values, to the specific type of personality that characterizes the adult the baby has become.

Schweder (1979) pointed out that it is indeed difficult to be sure how specific child-rearing practices can lead to adult behavior that is predictable in a multiplicity of contexts. Such caution is a useful reminder that culture, as a single element, should never be taken as the only determinant of thinking or behavior.

■ FREQUENCY OF PSYCHIATRIC DISORDERS

Attempts to establish the frequency of psychiatric disorders across cultures have been fraught with difficulties. In the United States, significant problems have been associated with health care surveys of all the minority populations, specifically those of Native American, Hispanic, African, and Asian heritage. Much has been said about the task of identifying and sampling such groups, the complexity of achieving their cooperation, the tendency among many of the subgroups simply to answer yes to any interviewer's questions, the difficulty in designing valid interview protocols, and the complexity of controlling the bias of interviewers. In addition, there have often been technical difficulties associated with the preparation of interviewers who may not use the language of their respondents. The survey instruments may have been developed and validated using populations other than the minority groups. Even in the U.S., much of the work done has reflected contradictory results, some of which seem related to either the sampling or the methodologies used.

Williams (1986), reviewing the epidemiology of mental illness in African Americans, noted emerging difficulties in the NIMH-sponsored Epidemiologic Catchment Area (ECA) program. For example, the ECA surveys attempted to obtain good samples of African Americans by including inner-city communities. However, Williams suggested this was biased in favor of low-income African-American males. Consequently, he questioned whether middle-class and other African Americans would be surveyed. There were early claims that depression was rare among American blacks (Schwab 1978), and, indeed, conclusions have been drawn from these original data that few African Americans commit suicide (Prudhomme 1938). More recent work consistently contradicted such earlier findings (King 1982) and suggested that those earlier conclusions were a function of the bias of the observers who were conducting such work. Serious consideration of all this cross-cultural scholarship leads inevitably to the conclusion that relatively little is understood about the incidence and prevalence of psychiatric disorders across different nations and cultures.

It is hoped that the efforts to make DSM-IV a more culturally informed work have led to diagnostic categories that will retain more of their meaning in cross-cultural diagnostic endeavors.

■ CULTURE, SYMPTOMS, AND DIAGNOSIS

□ Symptom Expression

The International Pilot Study of Schizophrenia (IPSS) was a transcultural psychiatric investigation of 1,202 patients in nine countries: Colombia, Czechoslovakia, Denmark, India, Nigeria, Taiwan, the Soviet Union, Great Britain, and the United States. Although it was not an epidemiological survey, a major task of the project was to engender methods that might be used in different cultures to evaluate patients (Strauss et al. 1976). Specific interview schedules were used to collect data on patients who had already been admitted to treatment facilities.

Some conclusions from the IPSS merit consideration. Certain symptoms (i.e., phenomena reported by patients, such as hallucinations and delusions) were the object of greatest inter-rater reliability, although the reliability was better for raters from the same center than for raters from different centers. In contrast to this finding, the data showed that the rating of signs gathered by observation rather than by self-report, such as flatness of affect or incongruity of affect, was below acceptable reliability ranges. Historical information, such as that having to do with patients' prior level of functioning, personality traits, work history, and social relationships, showed even more cross-cultural variability. This work suggested that some cross-cultural psychiatric information might be reliable, although it depended on what type of information one was collecting. Symptoms reported by patients would be a more useful reference point for comparison than signs rated by observers, and premorbid history may be misleading when viewed by a clinician from a culture different from the patient's. Consequently, the cross-cultural diagnosis of paranoid schizophrenia (for which there is substantial reliance on symptomatology) might be more reliable than the cross-cultural diagnosis of catatonic schizophrenia (for which the physician relies on observation of signs).

Marsella (1988) elaborated a view of the interplay of biology, psychology, and culture that describes an inverse relationship between the extent that a disorder is biologically based (i.e., internal) and the impact of environmental (external) factors on a disorder's clinical presentation (Table 41–1). Marsella posited that a disorder primarily shaped by biological forces will have less variability between cultures than a disorder whose primary causation is social or environmental. Such a model predicts that the presentation of a cerebrovascular accident, for example, would have much less cross-cultural variability than would a dissociative disorder, the latter having a much larger presumed component from the social and environmental sphere. Psychotic and mood disorders, thought to have a sizable biological determinant but also to be strongly

Table 41–1. Hypothesized impact of internal (biological) and external
(psychosocial) factors on cross-cultural variability of clinical
presentation

Clinical entity	Biological factors	Psychosocial factors	Cross-cultural variability
Cerebrovascular accident	***	*	Low
Psychotic disorders	**	**	Moderate
Dissociative disorders	*	***	High

influenced by the sociocultural milieu, should fall between these two extremes with regard to their degree of cross-cultural variability.

The Epidemiologic Catchment Area (ECA) study, conducted in the
last decade, appeared to confirm that Puerto Ricans reported somatic
symptoms out of proportion to the rest of the population, resulting in a
higher mean number of somatization symptoms detected by the Diagnostic Interview Schedule (Escobar 1987). Guarnaccia et al. (1989b)
subsequently reviewed these data after having created a measure to
quantify the existence of *ataques de nervios,* a culturally accepted syndrome used to express personal distress. Their results implied that the
"excessive" somatic symptoms picked up by the structured interview
were related to the presence of *ataques de nervios* in this population, a syndrome that the interview schedule was not looking for, and consequently did not find. Caution therefore suggests that the use of etic
diagnostic systems that are not tempered by knowledge of indigenous
(i.e., emic) categories may lead to unexplainable or meaningless results.
Not only does culture affect the expression of distress, but it can also act
to hamper one's ability to identify distress in an individual from another
culture.

☐ Culture and Diagnostic Classification

The categorization or definition of normal behavior is, of course, a culture-bound phenomenon. Consequently, someone who suffers from
hysterical drop attacks might be considered in one culture to be an individual who has received a special blessing, rather than someone in need
of medical or psychiatric attention. Another such example has centered
on the phenomenon of homosexuality. Even within the United States,
the question of whether homosexuality is abnormal behavior has been
the topic of significant discussion and disagreement among the lay public. Psychiatrists have not been exempt from this disagreement, eventually changing the "diagnosis" from homosexuality to "ego-dystonic"
homosexuality (American Psychiatric Association 1980, p. 281), until arriv-

ing at the classification of "persistent and marked distress about one's sexual orientation" as a sexual disorder not otherwise specified in DSM-III-R (American Psychiatric Association 1987, p. 296), which did not change in DSM-IV. An important criterion that has been reaffirmed by such changes is that any syndrome must be associated with subjective distress and/or help-seeking behavior in order to be classified as a disorder.

Such differences over the definitions of normal and abnormal are not simply academic and do not relate only to settling what appears at first to be a straightforward disagreement. There are other important implications that flow from the resolution of this basic question. As mentioned above, general health behavior and help-seeking behavior are products of the process that defines normality. Waxler (1974) has reminded us that the views of the society not only influence the diagnosis of the disorder but, in fact, also condition the treatment and even the prognosis of what might be ultimately diagnosed as normal.

There are, of course, limitations to the power of redefining emotions and behavior in the context of the person's culture in order to "depathologize" them. The idea that all pathology stems from cultural incongruities is just as implausible as attributing all psychopathology to biological processes while ignoring social and environmental influences. Several studies (Levy et al. 1979; Neutra et al. 1977) followed the lives of Navajo persons with epilepsy who presented with "hand-trembling," a symptom viewed by the Navajo as a positive sign of power and ability to become a "shaman-like diagnostician" (Neutra et al. 1977, p. 256). These authors discovered no evidence that the culture provided any protection from physical suffering, or that it allowed the sufferer continued privileged status or problem-free function within Navajo society.

Culture has possibly influenced diagnostic practices in ways that still await further clarification. For example, little attention has been given to how sociocultural factors such as poverty might influence the expression of psychiatric disorders. Poverty can produce malnutrition that in turn could potentially influence the expression of psychiatric illness. Poverty can lead to exposure to a multitude of stressors besides that of material need. Inner-city neighborhoods have more than their share of violence, chemical dependence, and crime, all of which can affect an individual's view of life, and all of which need to be taken into consideration by a culturally informed clinician.

☐ Race and Diagnosis

Race differs from culture in that, by definition, it is generally outwardly evident and therefore may be the first thing that a clinician usually knows about a patient (and that a patient knows about a clinician). If these two individuals happen to reside in a setting where the race of one is privileged in comparison with the race of the other, then differences take on further clinical significance.

Adebimpe (1981) described how African-American patients in the United States were overdiagnosed in some categories and underdiagnosed in others. It is an important claim that was suggested earlier by Bell and Mehta (1980) and amplified and reviewed by Jones and Gray (1986). Adebimpe had reviewed several studies and concluded from the data that the apparent misdiagnosis of African Americans in comparison with whites resulted in African Americans being found more often to be schizophrenic and less often to have mood disorders. However, Adebimpe realized that the data did not provide an answer to whether African-American clinicians made the errors less often than white clinicians. There are also obvious implications here that erroneous diagnosing ultimately suggests the execution of inappropriate treatment plans and the communication of negative prognoses to the African-American patients. In addition, the overdiagnosis of schizophrenic disorders in bipolar African-American patients may result in their undue exposure to long-term treatment with antipsychotics, thereby increasing these patients' risk of developing tardive dyskinesia.

Several reasons have been given for these alleged errors in diagnosis (Adebimpe 1981; Jones and Gray 1986), all of which are related to the amount of social and cultural distance between patient and clinician, which in part is dependent on race. These differences are manifested in the areas of vocabulary, styles of interaction, values, and modes of communicating distress. Stereotypes of African-American psychopathology have also been evoked as partially responsible. For example, Jones and Gray (1986) reminded us of the long-held belief that African Americans are always cheerful and that having so little, they are unable to experience object loss. Also, differences in African Americans' expression of depression may lead to missing the diagnosis. It has been suggested that African Americans somatize a great deal more than white patients. Racial differences can also lead to misperceptions of the clinician by the patient. It is not unlikely that a patient from a nondominant race will react to a clinician from the majority race with feelings of suspicion and anger, which in turn may be interpreted by the clinician as paranoia, lability, or avoidance.

Considerable emphasis has been placed on the bias inherent in the instruments that are used to aid clinicians in making diagnostic conclusions. African Americans have been noted to score higher than whites on several scales, including the schizophrenia scale (Gynther 1972). This finding has been used to raise questions about the conclusions clinicians may reach from the use of scales that have not been originally validated on African-American populations (Greene 1987). Dana and Whatley (1991) cited a number of reasons that the Minnesota Multiphasic Personality Inventory has limited utility in interracial diagnosis. These include the lack of social, economic, and political considerations; the intrinsic limitations of comparative norms; the use of stereotypes; and neglect of the impact of the assessor's role on interpretation.

Indeed, there have been extensive arguments on the topic of intelligence testing in the African-American community, and a most incisive summary has been provided by Samuda (1973). Williams (1987) summarized the general issues relating to the psychological testing of minority patients. On the one hand, it has been pointed out that the definition of the intelligence quotient is precise and that there is nothing wrong with the use of intelligence tests, even if the tests do nothing but measure the adaptation of a black individual to a white middle-class view of American life. Others have taken opposing views and emphasized that intelligence testing of blacks should be discontinued because the tests were standardized and normalized on white middle-class individuals. Furthermore, such opponents of the utilization of intelligence testing often have pointed to the fact that the test results are misapplied and that the reference bases for the tests are obscure. Finally, they have frequently underlined the point that the test scores are inappropriately applied to predictions about African Americans that often spell a dim future for this already disadvantaged subgroup of the population.

☐ Culture-Specific Syndromes

Considerable work has been done on the description of syndromes that psychiatrists consider either to be unique to certain cultures or to occur with special frequency among a defined group of people. As would be expected, questions remain as to whether there are special elements in a given culture that favor the development of unique clinical entities. It also remains to be clarified whether the unusual clinical syndromes seen in one culture have corresponding clinical counterparts in other cultures. Furthermore, the comparable clinical states in the two cultures could conceivably take different external clinical forms even though the core biopsychological elements remain the same.

DSM-IV defines a "mental disorder" as a "clinically significant behavioral or psychological syndrome or pattern that . . . is associated with present distress (a painful symptom) or disability (impairment in . . . functioning) or with a significantly increased risk of suffering death, pain, disability, or an important loss of freedom" (American Psychiatric Association 1994). Questions have arisen about why clinically significant and distressing symptom patterns seen as "bound" to non-Western cultures retain the status of syndrome while other symptom patterns, seen as clearly bound to Western culture, are reified as "disorders." With this in mind, it is important to understand that the separate discussion of culture-bound syndromes is arbitrary, because, at the present time, there is no good reason for some of the entities discussed below to be excluded as disorders from the current diagnostic schema used in the United States.

It is also interesting that many of the syndromes classified as "culture-bound" have components of either somatization, dissociation, or both. Of all diagnostic categories in the DSM, those of somatoform and dissociative disorders are the ones that are most likely to be influenced by environmental and social forces. To make the diagnosis of a somatoform disorder, one must first exclude any biological component. History of social or environmental trauma or conflict predisposes an individual to dissociative disorders. It therefore makes sense that phenomena which demonstrate either dissociative or somatoform pathology would show the most cross-cultural variability, as theorized by Marsella (1988) (Table 41–1).

The following are some examples of culture-bound syndromes:

Ataques de nervios.   Described in Puerto Ricans and other Hispanic groups (Guarnaccia et al. 1989a, 1989b), *ataques de nervios* refers to a socially sanctioned display of grief or great conflict characterized by "diffiulty moving limbs, loss of consciousness or mind going blank, memory loss, [and symptoms of hyperventilation in which] . . . the person begins to shout, swear and strike out at others, [then] falls to the ground and either experiences convulsive body movements or lies 'as if dead'" (Guarnaccia et al. 1989b, p. 280). Generally, the episode is self-limited and may last only minutes. At other times, it is severe and extends to a few days, or the victim may suffer frequent attacks with few precipitating stressors, leading to distress and help-seeking behavior. González et al. (1992) advocated the classification of this syndrome under the general category of dissociative disorders, whereas others have focused on the somatic and pseudoepileptiform aspects to favor its being classified as a somatoform disorder. The mere fact that a syndrome exists that straddles these two categories questions the wisdom of making hard distinctions between somatoform and dissociative disorders.

"Falling-out."   Seen among black Americans but also called "blacking out" by Bahamians and *indisposition* by Haitians in Miami (Philippe and Romain 1979), "falling-out" characteristically occurs in response to a high degree of emotional excitement, such as may occur in the setting of a religious ceremony, during an argument, in fear-producing situations, or in "profound sexual conflict" (Weidman 1979, p. 99). Those who manifest this syndrome often simply collapse but without biting the tongue or losing the contents of bowel or bladder. There is an accompanying lack of ability to speak or move, even though the individual hears and understands. Although some have favored the addition of trance and possession trance disorder to the section on dissociative disorders in DSM-IV (González et al. 1992), the present decision to include the syndrome's description under dissociative disorder not otherwise specified is still a substantial improvement in the manual's cross-cultural scope.

Amok.   This phenomenon was traditionally associated with Malaya (Carr 1978), but has been described as occurring also in Africa and more rarely in Papua, New Guinea (Burton-Bradley 1968). Often, there is a prodromal period of brooding after an incident during which the victim (almost always male) has felt slighted or humiliated. What follows is a sudden, uncontrollable rage that leads to the individual's aimlessly running around with a weapon that is ultimately used to kill a number of people or animals. Sometimes the perpetrator then kills himself. Those captured alive have claimed no memory of the killing (Schmidt et al. 1977). While some studies have shown the syndrome to be associated with psychotic disorders (Tan and Carr 1977), this does not appear to be a uniform finding. Although recent studies (Gaw and Bernstein 1992; Spiegel D and Cardeña 1991) favored the inclusion of *amok* as an impulse control disorder, the final outcome of discussions is its mention under dissociative disorder not otherwise specified in DSM-IV; a cardinal feature of the syndrome is a temporary alteration in consciousness.

"Running" syndromes.   Simons (1985) used the term "running taxon" to describe several similar syndromes characterized by prodromal lethargy, depression, or anxiety, followed by a high level of activity, a trancelike state, potentially dangerous behavior in the form of running or fleeing, and ensuing exhaustion, sleep, and amnesia for the episode. Among such syndromes are *pibloktoq* among native peoples of the Arctic (Gussow 1960), *chakore* in the Ngawbere of Panama (Bletzer 1985), *grisi siknis* among the Miskito of Nicaragua (Dennis 1985), and Navajo "frenzy" witchcraft (Neutra et al. 1977). Although present diagnostic schema are only able to place such syndromes in the sphere of dissociative disorder not otherwise classified, it is possible that future versions of the DSM will allow for the diagnosis of psychogenic fugue in some of these cases.

Koro.   Various reports from Asia, including Hong Kong (Yap 1965), Singapore (Ngui 1969), India (Nandi et al. 1983), China (Tseng et al. 1988), and Malaysia (Adityanjee et al. 1991), referred to the syndrome of *koro*, or *suo-yang*. This syndrome occurs either singly or in epidemics and is characterized by acute and prominent panic-like symptoms brought about by the sudden onset of fear that one's genitalia are retracting into the abdomen and that this will result in death. Although similar syndromes have also been described in Western settings, these have always been associated either with major (Axis I) diagnoses such as schizophrenia (Ede 1976; Edwards 1970) or with neurological/organic etiologies such as brain tumor (Lapierre 1972) or toxic states (Dow and Silver 1973). In contrast to this, reports from Asia suggest that *koro* presents as a generally benign, time-limited illness without association to additional psychopathology, and with a good prognosis. Bernstein and Gaw (1990) outlined a classification scheme for *koro* as a "genital retraction disorder" under the section of somatoform disorders. The proposed criteria would exclude organic factors and Axis I disorders other than somatoform disorders, and would ask for the determination of whether the case occurred within or outside of the cultural context.

Anorexia nervosa; bulimia nervosa.   Bulimia nervosa has been argued to be most common among middle-class American white females, although it seems to be appearing also among black females from a similar socioeconomic background. This syndrome is characterized by excessive food intake that is then followed by self-induced vomiting. It is often associated with depression and anorexia. Although classified among the eating disorders by United States psychiatrists, these disorders are thought to represent American culture-bound syndromes, because they exist rarely, if at all, in other parts of the world. British psychiatrists have also been struck by the infrequent appearance of black subjects among their cases of anorexia nervosa or bulimia nervosa (Thomas and Szmukler 1985).

Spirit possession; multiple personality disorder.   Globally, there are a number of syndromes of "spirit possession," or possession trance (Akhtar 1988; Chandrashekar 1989; Kleinman 1980; Stoller 1989; Suryani 1984; Yap 1960). These syndromes, which are characterized by the belief that the victim's body is taken over by a spirit, are manifested by identity confusion, an inability to control one's actions, a temporary change in the personality of the victim, and partial or total amnesia for the episode. In India, this disorder appears to be more prevalent among women (Chandrashekar 1989) and among individuals having experienced chronic or acute interpersonal conflict or a recent loss. It is often reversible, with the longest episodes lasting days to weeks. In many cases, an episode of possession trance makes the person in such a trance more likely to be possessed again in the future.

Hwa-byung.   This syndrome of somatic complaints, ascribed by Korean folklore to excess anger—the word *hwa* means "fire" or "anger," and the word *byung* means illness—is typically characterized by a sensation of an epigastric mass, anorexia, anxiety, dyspnea, and epigastric pain (Lin 1983). It is said to be primarily an illness of women and to be attributed by the affected persons themselves to adverse social circumstances such as "disappointments, sadness, miseries, hostility, grudges, and unfulfilled dreams and expectations" (Pang 1990, p. 496). Partial response of the syndrome to antidepressants has been reported (Lin 1983).

Generalized somatic syndromes. This term *generalized somatic syndromes* is meant to cover several illness behaviors that have in common the symptoms of low energy, poor ability to concentrate, poor sleep, headaches, and vague somatic complaints. The Nigerian syndromes of "brain-fag," described by Prince (1985) in students, and *Ode Ori*, described by Makanjuola (1987) among the Yoruba, qualify as part of this group. Sufferers of *Ode Ori* who were examined with the Present State Examination commonly exhibited depressed mood, "tension pains," complaints of ill health, delayed sleep, anxiety, and low energy.

Another generalized somatic syndrome with a strong component of mood dysregulation is that of "neurasthenia" in China (Kleinman 1982; Lin 1989), also known in Japan by the name of *shinkeisuijaku*, or "ordinary" *shinkeishitsu* (Russell 1989; Suzuki 1989). The term neurasthenia was used in the late 19th century by American physician George M. Beard to describe a syndrome of headaches, insomnia, gastrointestinal symptoms, and vague somatic complaints, which Beard believed derived from an exhaustion of the victim's nervous system.

■ MIGRATION AND PSYCHIATRIC DISORDERS

☐ Effect on Families and Individuals

It is no secret that migration has for many years been regarded as a cause of pathology. The movement of individuals from a cultural context in which they have been surrounded by family, friends, and familiar institutions to a different geographic area that distances these people from their usual support systems has generally been seen as seriously stressful. Such dislocation of human beings from their own cultural groups has frequently been a contributory element to the emergence of psychopathology in the individual who has moved. Clinicians have been so confident of this that they have often recommended that the patient then be sent back to his or her hometown or country, presumably with the idea that reentry into the home context would have a therapeutic effect on the patient. However, Hickling (1991) suggested that this reentry into the home environment may also be stressful and problematic.

The problem of migration is most easily conceptualized in terms of movement of families or individuals from one country to another. But clinicians need to remember that it is also an issue at home in the United States. On several occasions, the lead author has observed clinicians dealing with African-American university students studying in predominantly white universities. The African-American students previously only frequented predominantly African-American institutions. In moving to the white university, they felt dislocated, rootless, and overwhelmed by a sensation of inferiority and of being an outsider. This in turn led to their becoming increasingly suspicious, defensive, and withdrawn. Obviously, their academic performance suffered. Once the therapist understands the role that is being played by cultural dissonance, he or she can then set about structuring ways of facilitating the adjustment of the student to the new culture.

☐ Process of Acculturation

Anthropologists worked in the early years on the concept of *acculturation* as a way of studying how two groups with different cultures come in contact and interact with each other. Often, one of the groups was numerically, politically, and economically stronger than the other. In recent years, it has been noted that groups, families, and individuals participate in this process of adaptation to a different culture.

Berry and Kim (1988) theorized that there is a systematic course to acculturation characterized by contact of the two groups, conflict between them, and adaptation to the interaction. Conflict occurs especially when there is resistance to the process by either of the two groups. Such stress ultimately influences the type of acculturative outcome.

The result of acculturation for the groups and the individuals concerned depends on a number of interacting factors, such as the phase of acculturation, the mode of acculturation, the type of acculturating group, the nature of the dominant cultural group, social and cultural characteristics of the less dominant group, and psychological characteristics of the individuals involved in the process.

Berry and Kim constructed a theoretical model (Table 41–2) that is useful when attempting to understand how the various outcomes of the acculturation process differ in the level of stress that they generate for the individual and the group. These theorists suggested that when a nondominant group comes in contact with a dominant group, members of the nondominant group must respond to two important questions. The first is whether the nondominant individual's cultural identity has such value that it should be retained. The second question is whether positive relations with the majority dominant group ought to be sought. Potentially, the varieties of answers to these two questions would influence the extent of stress present in the acculturative process, both for the individual and for the group.

In the application of this model to acculturation, Berry and Kim carefully asserted that this theoretical framework is still subject to influence

Table 41–2.   Potential outcome of acculturative interaction between
              dominant and nondominant groups

Nondominant individual's cultural identity valuable	Positive relations sought with dominant group	Outcome of acculturation
Yes	Yes	Integration
No	No	Marginality
Yes	No	Resistance
No	Yes	Assimilation

Source. Data adapted from Berry and Kim 1988.

by elements such as the psychology of the individuals, economics, and politics. Thus, for example, the minority group may seek to pursue a strategy of *integration* by answering yes to both questions. In doing this, they may be purposefully looking for a style of acculturative adjustment that has minimal stress. Nevertheless, the majority group may simultaneously be following a political goal of blocking such integration because of a wish to deny the importance of the minority group's identity. In such a case, the integration approach would indeed produce significant stress for the nondominant group.

Another possible adaptive response is *marginality.* In this case, both of the questions would be answered in the negative. Marginality represents a hopeless and negative view of life, and individuals who subscribe to this position are most likely to be functioning on the very periphery of the society. By answering no to both questions, these individuals reject any compromise with the dominant group and also see no value in their individual or group identity. It would seem evident that a consequence of this position would be intense identity conflict and confusion, both personally and politically.

There are two other possibilities of adaptive response to the difficulties of acculturation: *resistance* and *assimilation.* In the context of the theory described above, both of these would be predictive of considerable acculturative stress. In the case of resistance, the individual answers affirmatively to the question of whether his or her nondominant group's identity is of value, and answers in the negative to the question of whether positive relations should be sought with the majority group. In this situation, resistance implies a state of perpetual conflict with the dominant group. Although it is true that resistive acculturation could provide group support and enhancement of self-esteem, opposition to the seeking of positive relations with the dominant group would be expected to take its toll in the political and economic arena. One could argue that the Black Panther party was an example, par excellence, of the resistance pattern.

The posture of assimilation is an adaptive response in which the individual responds in the negative to the question of whether the nondominant group's identity is of value and answers affirmatively to the question of whether positive relations should be sought with the dominant group. While resistive acculturation would seem to lead potentially to caustic and difficult interactions with the dominant group, the assimilation stance still leads to a repudiation of the nondominant group's self-esteem and potentially results in what Bush (1976) considered to be the "depreciated character." Clearly, Bush would argue that any refutation of a nondominant group's sense of self would inevitably lead to a pervasive feeling of hopelessness.

■ ETHNOCULTURE, RACE, GENDER, AND PSYCHIATRIC TREATMENT

☐ Culture and Psychotherapy

All societies have developed ways of confronting physical and psychological suffering. Psychotherapy in its broadest sense should be seen as a curing system for psychological ills. The technical ways in which psychotherapy is applied or practiced obviously vary from one culture to another. However, Frank (1963) postulated that six elements lie at the core of all nonmedical healing and should exist independently of the cultural context in which the healing is practiced: 1) the emotional stirring of the individual, 2) the existence of a healer on whom the individual depends for help and who holds out hope of relief, 3) the arousal of the individual's expectations by the healer's personal attributes, 4) the evocation of hope in the individual, 5) the bolstering of the individual's self-esteem, and 6) the strengthening of the individual's ties with a supportive group.

More recently, Blue and González (1992) commented on the fallacy of seeing psychodynamic psychotherapy as being independent of culture, noting that psychodynamic thinking is rather a culture unto itself, and intimating that even psychodynamic psychotherapy that is intraracial and intraethnic is vulnerable to cross-cultural distortions. Comas-Díaz and Jacobsen (1991) examined the notable impact of ethnic, racial, and cultural differences on the psychotherapeutic relationship, from the view of both transference and countertransference. Possible signs of interethnic transference include overcompliance, denial of ethnocultural differences, and the more understandable feelings of mistrust and hostility in a patient from an oppressed group. Intraethnic transference, in turn, can be characterized by idealization of the therapist, by viewing the therapist as a "traitor" to his or her race or culture, or by fear of merging with the therapist. Countertransferential reactions in an interethnic psychotherapeutic relationship can be characterized by denial of differences, excessive cultural curiosity, and guilt or pity when the patient is from a highly disadvantaged group. Intraethnic relationships are susceptible to countertransference reactions such as overidentification and collusion, as well as anger, especially when work with the patient touches on the therapist's unresolved feelings about oppression and prejudice.

The successful resolution of many of the difficulties resulting from cultural differences requires from therapists openness, flexibility, curiosity, and a willingness to acknowledge and explore the cross-cultural components of transference and countertransference. Not all therapists may be capable of such stances. The traditional stance of having the therapist leave value choices ultimately and completely to the patient may only be theoretically possible in a vacuum. As the therapy unfolds, the therapist may indeed be sneaking into exercising his or her own value representations. Ultimately, the emphasis on individualism and autonomy that is so much a part of American psychotherapy may have to be replaced by what J. P. Spiegel (1976) considered to be horizontal, collaborative decision making.

☐ Race and Psychotherapy

While researchers such as Jones (1982) provided significant research impetus to the area of race and psychotherapy, Bradshaw (1982) emphasized effectively the clinical problems that have emerged as a function of the role that race plays in psychotherapy. He concentrated entirely on the problems of the black-white dichotomy. However, the issues that he outlined are applicable to other potential dichotomies in the patient-therapist context. Certain errors seem specific to the white therapist–black patient dyad. Bradshaw showed how the therapist could be influenced by common myths such as that of the African-American family as a repository of severe pathology, the one-parent family as leading unavoidably to psychopathology, African Americans as having a poor self-image, African Americans as being sexually promiscuous, and African-American patients as unable to be treated by traditional psychotherapy.

The maintenance of such myths seems partly related to the fact that white therapists are frequently ignorant of the reasons that African-American patients present themselves as passive and inarticulate. In addition, the situation can be rendered more complex if the therapist's position is countenanced and reinforced by a white supervisor. Obviously, a white therapist's countertransference can be stimulated by anti-white hostility coming from the patient.

Bradshaw also saw the black therapist–white patient dyad as having the potential for certain difficulty. In this context, both individuals may be unable to deal with the meaning of race in the therapeutic relationship. Blue and González (1992) viewed the stress on African-American therapists as the result, in part, of their sense of distance from both their culture of origin and the dominant culture, as represented by the patient. For the therapist, they advocated careful self-examination and reliance on supervision, with the intent of focusing on racial transference as a way of addressing the patient's conflict, rather than as something to be avoided or ignored.

The black therapist–black patient dyad is not exempt from having specific difficulties. African-American therapists may also accept the myth that African-American patients are "bad" patients. The patient may be seen as having so many social problems that he or she cannot benefit from psychotherapy. African-American therapists who are not of the same social class as the African-American patient may also react negatively to the patient's mannerisms and style that reflect a linkage to the lowest social and educational level. Black therapists and black patients may also establish a quick relationship that can lead to taking certain things for granted. For example, they may collude in attributing all the problems to the white society. Another possibility may be that the black therapist becomes angry at the black patient who expresses negative feelings about black people in general.

The white clinician–black patient dyad has served as a useful model for reflecting on countertransference problems in cross-cultural psychotherapy. Indeed, this dyad has been a framework for others, the most recent of which has been the example of Jewish therapist and Arab patient. Gorkin (1986) outlined how to manage certain types of countertransference that emerge in this unique situation. In particular, he noted how a Jewish therapist might experience guilt and aggression while in the process of treating an Arab patient.

☐ Race, Gender, and Pharmacotherapy

Lin et al. (1991) reviewed the response of Asians to various psychotropics. They mentioned the well-known enzyme polymorphisms of alcohol dehydrogenase and aldehyde dehydrogenase, more prevalent in Asian populations, which are responsible, respectively, for some of the increased sensitivity to alcohol and the flushing response observed in many people of Asian descent or origin. A great majority of Asians are estimated to be "fast acetylators," in comparison with approximately 50% of Caucasians and African Americans. This may have an impact on Asians' metabolism of such drugs as clonazepam, caffeine, and phenelzine. In addition, differences in the activity of catechol-O-methyltransferase have been linked to the higher incidence of dyskinesia in Asian parkinsonian patients treated with L-dopa. Racial differences in metabolism have also been confirmed as being responsible for the increased susceptibility of Asians to antipsychotics, antidepressants, and benzodiazepines.

Mendoza et al. (1991) reviewed studies on psychopharmacological treatment of Hispanic and Native Americans, finding that although some interesting differences have been found in various pathways of drug metabolism (debrisoquine and S-mephenytoin metabolism, acetylation, protein binding), little in the way of clinical correlation has occurred.

Strickland et al. (1991) reviewed psychopharmacological studies in African-American populations and commented on the replicated finding that black Americans develop higher plasma levels and faster clinical responses to tricyclic antidepressants than do white populations. Lithium metabolism appears to be less efficient in black populations, and this may necessitate the use of lower doses in the treatment of bipolar disorder in this group. Studies looking at differences in the metabolism of antipsychotics, however, have been inconclusive, in part because of what seems to be a bias toward blacks being diagnosed as schizophrenic more often than whites.

■ REFERENCES

Adebimpe VR: Overview: white norms and psychiatric diagnosis of black patients. Am J Psychiatry 138:279–285, 1981

Adityanjee [], Zain AM, Subramaniam M: Sporadic koro and marital disharmony. Psychopathology 24:49–52, 1991

Akhtar S: Four culture-bound psychiatric syndromes in India. Int J Soc Psychiatry 34:70–74, 1988

Allen EA: Psychological dependency among students in a "cross-roads" culture. Wis Med J 34:123–127, 1985

American Psychiatric Association: Diagnostic and Statistical Manual of Mental Disorders, 3rd Edition. Washington, DC, American Psychiatric Association, 1980

American Psychiatric Association: Diagnostic and Statistical Manual of Mental Disorders, 3rd Edition, Revised. Washington, DC, American Psychiatric Association, 1987

American Psychiatric Association: Diagnostic and Statistical Manual of Mental Disorders, 4th Edition. Washington, DC, American Psychiatric Association, 1994

Bateson G: Some components of socialization for trance. Ethos 3:143–155, 1975

Bell CC, Mehta H: The misdiagnosis of black patients with manic-depressive illness. J Natl Med Assoc 72:141–145, 1980

Bernstein RL, Gaw AC: Koro: proposed classification for DSM-IV. Am J Psychiatry 147:1670–1674, 1990

Berry JW: Ecology, cultural adaptation and psychological differentiation: traditional patterning and acculturative stress, in Cross-Cultural Perspectives on Learning. Edited by Brislin R, Bochner S, Lonner W. New York, Wiley, 1975, pp 207–231

Berry JW, Kim U: Acculturation and mental health, in Health and Cross-Cultural Psychology: Toward Applications. Edited by Dasen P, Berry JW, Sartorius N. Newbury Park, CA, Sage, 1988, pp 207–236

Bletzer KV: Fleeing hysteria (chakore) among Ngawbere of northwestern Panama: a preliminary analysis and comparison with similar illness phenomena in other settings. Med Anthropol 9:297–318, 1985

Blue HC, González CA: The meaning of ethnocultural difference: its impact on and use in the psychotherapeutic process, in Treating Diverse Disorders With Psychotherapy (New Dir Ment Health Serv No 55). Edited by Greenfeld D. San Francisco, CA, Jossey-Bass, 1992, pp 73–84

Bradshaw WH Jr: Supervision in black and white: race as a factor in supervision, in Applied Supervision in Psychotherapy. Edited by Blumenfeld M. New York, Grune & Stratton, 1982, pp 200–220

Burton-Bradley BG: The amok syndrome in Papua and New Guinea. Med J Aust 1:252–256, 1968

Bush JS: Suicide and blacks: a conceptual framework. Suicide Life Threat Behav 6:216–219, 1976

Carmen E[H], Russo NF, Miller JB: Inequality and women's mental health: an overview. Am J Psychiatry 138:1319–1330, 1981

Carr JE: Ethno-behaviorism and the culture-bound syndromes: the case of amok. Cult Med Psychiatry 2:269–293, 1978

Chandrashekar CR: Possession syndrome in India, in Altered States of Consciousness and Mental Health. Edited by Ward CA. Newbury Park, CA, Sage, 1989, pp 79–95

Cohen P, Brook J: Family factors related to the persistence of psychopathology in childhood and adolescence. Psychiatry 50:332–345, 1987

Comas-Díaz L, Jacobsen FM: Ethnocultural transference and countertransference in the therapeutic dyad. Am J Orthopsychiatry 61:392–402, 1991

Dana RH, Whatley PR: When does a difference make a difference? MMPI scores and African-Americans. J Clin Psychol 47:400–406, 1991

Delgado AK, Griffith EEH, Ruiz P: The black woman mental health executive: problems and perspectives. Administration in Mental Health 12:246–251, 1985

Dennis PA: Grisi Siknis in Miskito culture, in The Culture-Bound Syndromes: Folk Illnesses of Psychiatric and Anthropological Interest. Edited by Simons RC, Hughes CC. Dordrecht, The Netherlands, D Reidel, 1985, pp 289–306

Dow TW, Silver DA: Drug-induced koro syndrome. J Fla Med Assoc 60:32–33, 1973

Draguns JG: Cross-cultural counseling and psychotherapy: history, issues, current status, in Cross-Cultural Counseling and Psychiatry. Edited by Marsella J, Pedersen P. New York, Pergamon, 1981, pp 3–27

Ede A: Koro in an Anglo-Saxon Canadian. Canadian Psychiatric Association Journal 21:389–392, 1976

Edwards JG: The koro pattern of depersonalization in an American schizophrenic patient. Am J Psychiatry 126:1171–1173, 1970

Escobar JI: Cross-cultural aspects of the somatization trait. Hosp Community Psychiatry 38:174–180, 1987

Frank JD: Persuasion and Healing: A Comparative Study of Psychotherapy. Baltimore, MD, Johns Hopkins Press, 1963

Gaw AC, Bernstein RL: Classification of amok in DSM-IV. Hosp Community Psychiatry 43:789–793, 1992

González CA, Lewis-Fernández R, Griffith EEH, et al: The impact of culture on dissociation: suggested modifications to DSM-IV, in Cultural Proposals for DSM-IV. Submitted to the DSM-IV Task Force by the NIMH-sponsored Group on Culture and Diagnosis. Edited by Mezzich JE, Kleinman A, Fabrega H, et al. 1992, pp 144–153

Gorkin M: Countertransference in cross-cultural psychotherapy: the example of Jewish therapist and Arab patient. Psychiatry 49:69–79, 1986

Greene RL: Ethnicity and MMPI performance: a review. J Consult Clin Psychol 55:497–512, 1987

Guarnaccia PJ, de la Cancela V, Carrillo E: The multiple meanings of ataques de nervios in the Latino community. Med Anthropol 11:47–62, 1989a

Guarnaccia PJ, Rubio-Stipec M, Canino G: Ataques de nervios in the Puerto Rican Diagnostic Interview Schedule: the impact of cultural categories on psychiatric epidemiology. Cult Med Psychiatry 13:275–295, 1989b

Gussow Z: Pibloktoq (hysteria) among the polar Eskimo. The Psychoanalytic Study of Society 1:218–236, 1960

Gynther MD: White norms and black MMPIs: a prescription for discrimination? Psychol Bull 78:386–402, 1972

Hickling FW: Double jeopardy: psychopathology of black mentally ill returned migrants to Jamaica. Int J Soc Psychiatry 37:80–89, 1991

Jones BE, Gray BA: Problems in diagnosing schizophrenia and affective disorders among blacks. Hosp Community Psychiatry 37:61–65, 1986

Jones EE: Psychotherapists' impressions of treatment outcome as a function of race. J Clin Psychol 38:722–731, 1982

Kiev A: The study of folk psychiatry, in Magic, Faith and Healing. Edited by Kiev A. London, Free Press of Glencoe, 1964, pp 3–35

King LM: Suicide from a "black reality" perspective, in The Afro-American Family: Assessment, Treatment, and Research Issues. Edited by Bass BA, Wyatt GE, Powell GJ. New York, Grune & Stratton, 1982, pp 221–236

Kleinman A: Patients and Healers in the Context of Culture: An Exploration of the Borderland Between Anthropology, Medicine, and Psychiatry. Berkeley, CA, University of California Press, 1980

Kleinman A: Neurasthenia and depression: a study of somatization and culture in China. Cult Med Psychiatry 6:117–189, 1982

Koss JD: Therapeutic aspects of Puerto Rican cult practices. Psychiatry 38:160–171, 1975

Lapierre YD: Koro in a French Canadian. Canadian Psychiatric Association Journal 17:333–334, 1972

Leighton AH, Murphy JM: Cross-cultural psychiatry, in Approaches to Cross-Cultural Psychiatry. Edited by Murphy JM, Leighton AH. New York, Cornell University Press, 1965, pp 3–20

Levy JE, Neutra R, Parker D: Life careers of Navajo epileptics and convulsive hysterics. Soc Sci Med 13B:53–66, 1979

Lin K-M: Hwa-Byung: a Korean culture-bound syndrome? Am J Psychiatry 140:105–107, 1983

Lin K-M, Poland RE, Smith MW, et al: Pharmacokinetic and other related factors affecting psychotropic responses in Asians. Psychopharmacol Bull 27:427–439, 1991

Lin T: Neurasthenia revisited: its place in modern psychiatry. Cult Med Psychiatry 13:105–129, 1989

Makanjuola ROA: "Ode Ori": a culture-bound disorder with prominent somatic features in Yoruba Nigerian patients. Acta Psychiatr Scand 75:231–236, 1987

Marsella AJ: Cross-cultural research on severe mental disorders: issues and findings. Acta Psychiatr Scand Suppl 78 (No 344):7–22, 1988

Mendoza R, Smith MW, Poland RE, et al: Ethnic psychopharmacology: the Hispanic and Native American perspective. Psychopharmacol Bull 27:449–461, 1991

Nandi DN, Banerjee G, Saha H, et al: Epidemic koro in West Bengal, India. Int J Soc Psychiatry 29:265–268, 1983

Neutra R, Levy JE, Parker D: Cultural expectations versus reality in Navajo seizure patterns and sick roles. Cult Med Psychiatry 1:255–275, 1977

Ngui PW: The koro epidemic in Singapore. Aust N Z J Psychiatry 3:263–266, 1969

Pang KYC: Hwabyung: the construction of a Korean popular illness among Korean elderly immigrant women in the United States. Cult Med Psychiatry 14:495–512, 1990

Philippe J, Romain JB: Indisposition in Haiti. Soc Sci Med 13B:129–133, 1979

Prince R: The concept of culture-bound syndromes: anorexia nervosa and brain-fag. Soc Sci Med 21:197–203, 1985

Prudhomme C: The problem of suicide in the American Negro. Psychoanal Rev 25:372–391, 1938

Reid WH: The antisocial personality: a review. Hosp Community Psychiatry 36:831–837, 1985

Russell JG: Anxiety disorders in Japan: a review of the Japanese literature on Shinkeishitsu and taijinkyofusho. Cult Med Psychiatry 13:391–403, 1989

Samuda RJ: Psychological Testing of American Minorities. New York, Harper & Row, 1973

Schmidt K, Hill L, Guthrie G: Running amok. Int J Soc Psychiatry 23:264–274, 1977

Schwab JJ: Nineteenth-century studies of mental illness in Southern blacks. Interaction 1(4):21–25, 1978

Schweder RA: Rethinking culture and personality theory, Part 1. Ethos 7:255–278, 1979

Simons RC: Sorting the culture-bound syndromes, in The Culture-Bound Syndromes: Folk Illnesses of Psychiatric and Anthropological Interest. Edited by Simons RC, Hughes CC. Dordrecht, The Netherlands, D Reidel, 1985, pp 25–38

Spiegel D, Cardeña E: Cultural diversity of dissociative and somatoform disorders. Paper presented at the NIMH Conference on Culture and Diagnosis, Pittsburgh, PA, April 1991

Spiegel JP: Cultural aspects of transference and countertransference revisited. J Am Acad Psychoanal 4:447–467, 1976

Spurlock J: Development of self-concept in Afro-American children. Hosp Community Psychiatry 37:66–70, 1986

Stoller P: Fusion of the Worlds. Chicago, IL, University of Chicago Press, 1989

Stoller RJ, Herdt GH: The development of masculinity: a cross-cultural contribution. J Am Psychoanal Assoc 30:29–59, 1982

Strauss JS, Carpenter Jr WT, Bartko JJ: A review of some findings from the international pilot study of schizophrenia, in Annual Review of Schizophrenic Syndrome, Vol 4. Edited by Cancro R. New York, Brunner/Mazel, 1976, pp 74–88

Strickland TL, Ranganath V, Lin K-M, et al: Psychopharmacologic considerations in the treatment of black American populations. Psychopharmacol Bull 27:441–448, 1991

Suryani LK: Culture and mental disorder: the case of bebainan in Bali. Cult Med Psychiatry 8:95–113, 1984

Suzuki T: The concept of neurasthenia and its treatment in Japan. Cult Med Psychiatry 13:187–202, 1989

Tan EK, Carr JE: Psychiatric sequelae of amok. Cult Med Psychiatry 1:59–67, 1977

Thomas JP, Szmukler GI: Anorexia nervosa in patients of Afro-Caribbean extraction. Br J Psychiatry 146:653–656, 1985

Tseng W-S, Kan-Ming M, Hsu J, et al: A sociocultural study of koro epidemics in Guangdong, China. Am J Psychiatry 145:1538–1543, 1988

Waxler NE: Culture and mental illness: a social labeling perspective. J Nerv Ment Dis 159:379–395, 1974

Weidman HH: Falling-out: a diagnostic and treatment problem viewed from a transcultural perspective. Soc Sci Med 13B:95–112, 1979

Westermeyer J: Psychiatric diagnosis across cultural boundaries. Am J Psychiatry 142:798–805, 1985

Williams CL: Issues surrounding psychological testing of minority patients. Hosp Community Psychiatry 38:184–189, 1987

Williams DH: The epidemiology of mental illness in Afro-Americans. Hosp Community Psychiatry 37:42–49, 1986

Wilson MN: Child development in the context of the Black extended family. Am Psychol 44:380–385, 1989

Yap PM: The possession syndrome: a comparison of Hong Kong and French findings. Journal of Mental Science 106:114–137, 1960

Yap PM: Koro—a culture-bound depersonalization syndrome. Br J Psychiatry 111:43–50, 1965

CHAPTER

Geriatric Psychiatry

Dan Blazer, M.D., Ph.D.

Psychiatrists who work with older adults encounter diagnostic and therapeutic problems that are more complex than those encountered in young adult and middle-aged patients. Most elderly patients with psychiatric disorders do not fit easily into the diagnostic categories of DSM-IV (American Psychiatric Association 1994), for they experience multiple symptoms that affect both physical and psychiatric functioning.

Multiple system involvement and functional impairment are not unique to geriatric psychiatry. Geriatricians must manage equally complex disease presentations that involve a range of dysfunctions, from the molecular to the psychosocial. Psychiatrists working with older adults can benefit from the syndromal approach to impairment, a paradigm shift developed by geriatricians to structure diagnostic and therapeutic strategies for elderly patients. Geriatricians deemphasize specific "diagnosis" and concentrate instead on "geriatric syndromes," which include incontinence, dizziness, falling, failure to thrive, and constipation. Seven psychiatric syndromes are most prevalent among elderly individuals: acute confusion, memory loss, insomnia, anxiety, suspiciousness, depression, and hypochondriasis.

■ ACUTE CONFUSION

Acute confusion, or delirium, is a transient organic brain syndrome characterized by acute onset and global impairment of cognitive function. Thinking is disorganized and speech becomes rambling. Emotional disturbances accompany acute confusion and include anxiety, fear, irritability, and anger.

Acute confusion in late life is the common outcome of a cascade of biological, cognitive, and environmental contributors. Biological brain function declines with age, although functional capacity varies greatly within age groups. Degenerative changes, such as those characteristic of Alzheimer's disease, render the elderly person more susceptible to physiological changes secondary to aging and disease. Cognitive contributors to delirium include a predisposition to hallucinations and delusions, such as with an aging patient who has a history of schizophrenia. Environmental contributors include unfamiliar surroundings.

General therapy for the confused elder begins with medical support. Vital signs and level of consciousness should be closely monitored. Vasopressor agents may be needed to increase blood pressure, and excessive fever should be treated with ice baths and alcohol sponges. Once the syndrome of acute confusion is recognized and the precipitant of the confusion is established through history, physical examination, and laboratory studies, the clinician can begin therapy. The initial treatment should include the establishment of an adequate airway to ensure that the patient is breathing, and the administration of 100 ml of 50% dextrose plus 100 mg of thiamine intravenously if hypoglycemia and Wernicke's encephalopathy cannot be ruled out.

The clinician must also pay special attention to reducing the demands that excess and conflicting environmental stimuli make on the patient's cerebral function. Order and simplicity in the environment are critical to the management of the confused elderly patient. Physicians, nurses, and other hospital personnel should explain all procedures. Restraints should be kept to a minimum. Behavioral agitation can generally be managed by judicious use of antipsychotic medications, such as haloperidol, in low doses.

■ MEMORY LOSS

Late-life memory loss is usually accompanied by a more or less sustained decline in cognitive function from a previously obtained intellectual level, usually with an insidious onset. Other cognitive capacities that decline with memory include language, spatial or temporal orientation, judgment, and abstract thought. There is usually no alteration of state of consciousness until very late in the memory loss syndrome, which is in contrast with acute confusion.

Disabling memory loss may begin in midlife but is much more frequent in persons over the age of 75 than in persons between the ages of 65 and 74. Prevalence estimates from community samples of memory impairment are generally 5% to 15%, with most investigators estimating memory impairment in at least 5% of elderly persons in the community and in 30% to 50% of institutional residents (Katzman and Jackson 1991). Memory loss is usually progressive. Until age 75, persons experiencing Alzheimer's disease or multi-infarct dementia usually have their life expectancy reduced by about one-half.

Alzheimer's disease is the most common cause of memory loss. More than 50% of persons experiencing chronic memory loss will, at autopsy, exhibit the changes of Alzheimer's disease only. The next most common contributors to the syndrome are the vascular dementias, especially multi-infarct dementia. Multi-infarct dementia is also frequently comorbid with Alzheimer's disease (Tomlinson et al. 1970). Many patients with Parkinson's disease develop brain changes late in the course of their disease similar to those changes found in Alzheimer's disease. Approximately 5% of elderly persons experience memory loss as a result of alcohol amnestic disorder (Lishman 1981).

The primary risk factor for Alzheimer's disease is age; other risk factors include Down's syndrome, a family history of Alzheimer's disease, head trauma, and possibly a lack of education. Male sex, hypertension, and possibly the black race are risk factors for multi-infarct dementia.

The diagnostic workup of the older adult suffering memory loss begins with a history, which should be obtained from both family members and the patient. The nature and degree of the cognitive dysfunction should be assessed by both a thorough mental status examination and objective cognitive testing, using standardized mental status examinations such as the Mini-Mental State Examination (MMSE; Folstein et al. 1975). The in-office or hospital-based initial assessment of memory and cognitive functioning is followed by a more in-depth evaluation of cognition using instruments such as the Reitan Battery, the Trail Making Test, and tests of functions such as delayed recall and spatial ability (Reitan 1955). Laboratory tests to assess memory loss, such as that seen in Alzheimer's disease, are listed in Table 42–1. The purpose of the comprehensive diagnostic workup of the older adult suffering memory loss is to establish the baseline functional impairment as well as to rule out reversible causes of the dementia syndrome.

Though no definitive treatment for cognitive decline in Alzheimer's disease has been discovered, many clinical trials are currently under way to establish the efficacy of agents that might retard the progression of memory problems in older persons. Most of these therapies are based on the cholinergic hypothesis of memory and include the use of cholinergic precursors such as 1) lecithin, dietary supplements rich in choline; and 2) cholinergic agonists such as tetrahydroaminoacridine (THA) and physostigmine. Psychotropic medications are used extensively in patients suffering from memory loss, primarily because of secondary symptoms such as verbal or physical aggression, anxiety, depression, psychoses, and severe agitation or regressive behavior. Other secondary behaviors,

Table 42–1.   Laboratory tests to assess memory loss

Standard diagnostic tests	Elective tests
Complete blood count, electrolyte panel, screening metabolic panel, thyroid function test (T_3, T_4, FTI, thyroid-stimulating hormone)	Magnetic resonance imaging or computed tomography
	Electroencephalogram
Vitamin B_{12} and folate levels	Formal neuropsychological assessment
Tests for syphilis	Cerebral blood flow studies
Urinalysis	Lumbar puncture
Electrocardiogram	Event-related potentials
Chest X ray	

however, such as wandering, inappropriate verbalization, repetitive activities (touching), obstinacy in following suggestions or commands, hoarding materials, stealing, and inappropriate voiding, are not amenable to medication. Therefore the first step for the clinician treating the patient with memory loss is to assess what symptoms might be responsive to a medication.

Agitation and anxiety can be treated with antianxiety agents (such as short-acting benzodiazepines), neuroleptics (generally the high-potency neuroleptics are preferred in low doses), anticonvulsants (such as carbamazepine), beta-blockers, lithium, buspirone, and occasionally low doses of antidepressant agents (such as trazodone) at night. Clonazepam has been reported to be of benefit in agitated patients with multi-infarct dementia; however, the episodic mood swings and acute confusion that often accompany such dementia are not as responsive to medications.

The neuroleptics are the most effective psychotropics for controlling severe agitation, aggressive behavior, and psychoses. Most neuroleptics are effective but produce side effects, and, therefore, the selection of a drug is usually determined by the side-effect profile least adverse for a given patient. The most troublesome side effects that ensue from using neuroleptic agents are postural hypotension (and the risk of falling) and tardive dyskinesia. These side effects may be avoided by using agents such as buspirone and carbamazepine.

Because depression is frequent among patients with chronic memory loss, the use of an antidepressant agent is often indicated. In general, the antidepressant agent will not lead to an improvement in memory. Postural hypotension is a major concern when using the antidepressant medications. Despite theoretical concerns regarding anticholinergic effects, most tricyclic antidepressants with low to moderate anticholinergic effects can be prescribed to demented elderly patients without the risk of increasing their memory dysfunction.

The behavioral management of the patient with memory loss not only is useful to the patient but provides the family with the sense of accomplishment in the presence of an illness that tends to leave the family helpless and bewildered. The family and the physician should develop behaviors that promote both patient and family security. Familiar routines and consistent repetition of instructions usually enhance security. Families must also compensate for the loss of impulse control that accompanies memory loss. One means is distraction; the patient who is about to remove his or her clothes or masturbate in public can be distracted by getting the patient's attention through conversation or asking the patient to walk with a family member.

Management of memory loss must include a review of the patient's environment for problems in safety. Typical safety problems include becoming lost, wandering into busy traffic, erratic or accidental use of medicines, falls, accidents while driving, and leaving things unattended. Home visits by geriatric nurse specialists are most hopeful in reviewing the household for potential problems.

Perhaps the most important long-term component for managing the older adult with memory loss is support of the family. Families are the primary caregivers of elderly persons with memory loss until the memory loss becomes severe enough to lead to institutionalization. Education of the family regarding the expected progression of memory loss and the many behaviors that accompany such loss, but which may not be intuitively recognized as resulting from the illness, is key to family support. Excellent educational materials are available and support groups are located throughout the world to assist the family of the patient with memory loss. Families must be monitored for caregiver stress.

■ INSOMNIA

Insomnia is more frequent in the elderly population than in any other age group. The most common sleep disturbances leading to insomnia in the elderly are

1. Primary insomnia
2. Sleep-disordered breathing
3. Nocturnal myoclonus
4. Sleep-wake schedule disorder

Secondary causes of insomnia are frequent in late life and include anxiety disorders, depressive disorders, dementing disorders, and physical illnesses such as chronic or obstructive pulmonary disease and, most frequently, nocturia.

Sleep changes characteristic in late life include decreased total sleep time, frequent arousals, increased percentages of Stage 1 and Stage 2 sleep, decreased percentages of Stage 3 and Stage 4 sleep, decreased rapid eye movement (REM) latency, decreased absolute amounts of REM sleep, and a tendency to exhibit a redistribution of sleep across the 24-hour day (e.g., napping during the day). Older persons are also more likely to phase-advance in the sleep cycle, with a tendency toward "morningness."

Nearly 35% of older persons report sleep-related problems in community surveys. Even though older persons comprise only 11% of the United States population, they are estimated to take between 25% and 40% of the sedative-hypnotics prescribed (National Institutes of Health Consensus Development 1990). Sleep apnea is more prevalent in elderly men than women, with the apnea index (i.e., the number of apneas per hour of sleep) being 5 or greater in 25% to 35% of elderly persons in the community (Berry and Phillips 1988). The prevalence of myoclonus probably ranges from 25% to 50% among healthy elderly persons in the community (Dickel et al. 1986).

The diagnostic workup of an older person experiencing insomnia begins with a recognition of the severity of the sleep disturbance. Screening questions during the interview should include an assessment of the patient's satisfaction with his or her sleep, daytime napping, fatigue during usual daily activities, and complaint by a bed partner or other observer of unusual behavior during sleep (such as snoring, pauses in breathing, or periodic myoclonic movements).

Medication history is essential in determining the etiology of insomnia. Prescribed medications, especially sedative-hypnotics and anxiolytics, as well as alcohol, have significant effects on sleep and also may impair cardiopulmonary function. Symptoms of the major psychiatric disorders affecting older persons, such as dementia, depression, or severe anxiety, may also lead to insomnia.

Although primary care physicians can usually recognize most sleep disorders and manage them effectively, specialized evaluation of sleep disorders is sometimes required. Referral to a psychiatrist or neurologist with special interest in sleep disorders is indicated. Upon referral, most patients, after a thorough history/physical examination and withdrawal from medication, are evaluated by polysomnography. The clinician must distinguish between the causes of insomnia in the elderly patient, many occurring simultaneously in the same patient. These include

- Normal age-dependent changes in sleep
- Sleep-disordered breathing and nocturnal myoclonus
- Sleep-phase alterations
- Psychiatric disorders such as Alzheimer's disease or major depression

- Medical problems contributing to sleep difficulties such as chronic pain
- Effects of medications such as the prolonged use of a sedative-hypnotic agent
- Poor sleep hygiene such as excessive stimulation prior to bedtime
- Environmental factors that prevent sleep such as excessive heat or noise
- Psychological factors such as loneliness or boredom

The cornerstones of effective treatment of insomnia in late life are the management of the underlying causes of the sleep disturbance and improved sleep hygiene. Both of these conditions are responsive to therapy. Physical problems such as hypothyroidism or arthritis may not be reversed, but the symptoms can be relieved with medications or other therapeutic interventions. Nocturnal myoclonus or restless leg syndrome may respond to medication such as tryptophan or clonazepam. Sleep-apnea syndrome that does not respond to conservative management may require surgery to improve flow in the nasopharyngeal region. Institution of good sleep hygiene is the next step in managing insomnia among elderly patients. Methods of relaxation training can be used successfully in enabling the insomniac elderly patient to initiate sleep.

A number of medications can be used to facilitate sleep in the elderly population, yet these medications should be used with care. The antidepressant agents not only are useful in managing the older adult with insomnia secondary to depression but can be used as sedative agents as well, especially if prescribed in low dose. For example, 25 to 50 mg of trazodone or 25 mg of amitriptyline may be preferable to using a benzodiazepine on a long-term basis if chronic use of a sedative is indicated. In general, the benzodiazepines that are short- to medium-acting are preferred over those that are more extended in length of action.

■ ANXIETY

Anxiety is a frequent symptom among older persons, either secondary to other problems, such as hyperthyroidism, or as the primary symptom of a disorder such as generalized anxiety disorder. Many of the anxiety disorders, however, are relatively less frequent in late life. Although phobia disorders can affect persons at all stages of the life cycle, the more severe phobias, such as agoraphobia and social phobia, begin early in life and are more common in children and young adults than in older persons. Panic disorder is relatively frequent and severe among younger persons but much less so among elderly persons. Obsessive-compulsive traits are common throughout the life cycle, although the severe manifestations of this disorder are less likely to be observed in older persons. Therefore, the management of anxiety symptoms in older persons usually consists of managing the symptoms of generalized anxiety that are the primary problem or comorbid with other disorders.

Community surveys of anxiety symptoms estimate that approximately 5% of older persons have generalized anxiety disorder. Approximately 20% of elderly persons report some cognitive or somatic symptoms of anxiety in community surveys, with somatic symptoms being more prevalent than cognitive symptoms. Simple phobia was found in 10% of persons 65 years of age or older compared with 13% of persons in middle age. Agoraphobia was found in 5% of the 65-or-over age group compared with 7% of the middle-age group (Blazer et al. 1991).

Anxiety results from a number of medical and psychiatric conditions. Hyperthyroidism, with an atypical presentation, may be mistaken for a psychogenic anxiety disorder. Cardiac arrhythmias may produce palpitations and shortness of breath in older persons. Pulmonary emboli, if not severe, may present as shortness of breath and subjective anxiety. Many medications lead to symptoms of anxiety. Caffeine is a frequent cause of anxiety. Over-the-counter sympathomimetic medications may lead to palpitations and subsequent subjective symptoms of anxiety. Anticholinergic agents, when they impair memory, lead to anxiety that is secondary to the memory loss and confusion. Older persons may also experience significant anxiety upon withdrawal from certain medications, especially alcohol and anxiolytic agents.

Many psychiatric disorders are manifested, in part, by symptoms of anxiety. Moderate to severe acute confusion is usually associated with anxiety and agitation. Anxiety is a common accompaniment of major depression, with elderly patients who are experiencing major depression also meeting the criteria for generalized anxiety disorder in over 50% of the cases. Hypochondriasis is associated with anxiety, especially when dependency needs are not met by family and health care professionals. Dementing disorders, especially in the early and middle stages, are associated with anxiety and agitation. Late-life schizophrenia with acute paranoid ideation is usually accompanied by agitation and anxiety. The clinician must not overlook the possibility that the anxiety symptoms may be secondary to appropriate fear. Many elderly persons must expose themselves daily to situations that threaten their security. Elderly persons with memory loss who live alone may fear that they will get lost driving to the doctor's office.

The use of nonpharmacological therapies for the treatment of anxiety in older adults has not been studied extensively. Nevertheless, the danger of medication, coupled with the successful application of cognitive-behavioral therapies to other psychiatric disorders in late life, especially depression, suggests that these therapies may also be applicable to anxiety disorders. Older persons who do not suffer cognitive dysfunction are good candidates for relaxation training and biofeedback. Cognitive restructuring has not been adapted for anxiety in older adults to date.

The cornerstone of pharmacological therapy for the anxiety disorders is the use of benzodiazepines. These drugs have repeatedly been demonstrated to be effective for the control of anxiety. They are generally well tolerated by persons of all ages but present unique problems when prescribed to older persons. For example, the half-life of the benzodiazepines may be increased dramatically in late life. Older persons are also more susceptible to potential side effects of benzodiazepines such as fatigue, drowsiness, and memory impairment. Therefore, the shorter-acting benzodiazepines have been preferred agents in late life. Other agents are generally less effective in controlling late-life anxiety. Buspirone is relatively safe, with few side effects, and does not appear to lead to abuse or dependency. Nevertheless, it takes 3 to 4 weeks for the therapeutic effect to manifest itself, and the drug is generally not as well accepted as being effective for anxiety as the benzodiazepines. Older adults who perceive that they have benefited from benzodiazepines generally do not accept buspirone as an alternative. Beta-blockers may be more effective in controlling agitation and behavioral problems in dementia patients than in controlling generalized anxiety.

■ SUSPICIOUSNESS

A frequent symptom in older adults, especially older adults experiencing cognitive impairment, is suspiciousness, which may range from increased cautiousness and distrust of family and friends to overt paranoid delusions. Of the suspicious or paranoid elderly persons, a unique group has been described: "late-life paraphrenia" is characterized by marked paranoid delusions in older adults who nevertheless maintain function in the community for months. Persons experiencing paraphrenia are predominantly women and often live alone.

The predominant delusions encountered in older persons are persecutory delusions and somatic delusions. Persecutory delusions often revolve around a single theme, such as family and neighbors conspiring against the delusional elderly person. Suspiciousness and paranoid behavior were found in 17% of persons in one community survey (Lowenthal 1964), and a sense of persecution was reported in 4% in another survey (Christenson and Blazer 1984). Among persons in the community, fewer than 1% suffer from schizophrenia or a paranoid disorder.

Many different disorders may lead to suspiciousness, delusions, and agitation. Chronic schizophrenic disorder, which has its onset earlier in life and persists into late life, is perhaps the most easily identified cause of late-life suspiciousness. As schizophrenia tends to be characterized by a decline in social function over the life cycle and a shorter life expectancy, chronic schizophrenia that persists into late life and yet leaves the elderly person relatively free of other symptoms is uncommon. Schizophrenic-like illness may have its first onset in late life. Organic mental disorders and late-onset depression are frequently associated with some psychotic symptoms.

Delusional disorder, with mild to moderate symptomatology, is a more frequent cause of suspiciousness in late life. Delusions, often of being persecuted by family and friends, usually center on a single theme or a connection of themes. These delusions may lead to a withdrawal of affection, financial support, and social contact. Another common cause of suspiciousness in late life is organic delusional syndrome. These delusions, in contrast to delusional disorder, wax and wane through time in severity and in content. Persecutory delusions are most common and often emerge when the elderly person's environment is changed. For some persons experiencing Alzheimer's disease, paranoid thoughts may dominate other symptoms of the dementing illness, especially in the early stages. Perhaps the most common encounter psychiatrists have with suspicious elderly persons is the encounter with the demented patient who has become a management problem because of suspiciousness and agitation.

The key to the diagnostic workup of the suspicious elderly person is the psychiatric evaluation. Delusional thinking and agitation usually render the patient's history inaccurate, and therefore family members should be interviewed to review the patient's behavior, especially any change in behavior. Previous psychotic or delusional episodes should be documented, as well as previous treatment.

The management of suspiciousness and agitation in older adults requires 1) ensuring a safe environment; 2) initiating a therapeutic alliance; 3) considering and, if appropriate, instituting pharmacological therapy; and 4) managing acute behavioral crises. In general, paranoid elderly persons do not adapt well to the hospital. Change from familiar surroundings and interaction with strange persons tend to exacerbate the suspiciousness. Nevertheless, elderly patients often are so disabled that hospitalization is necessary.

Once the elderly patient is hospitalized, the clinician must initiate a therapeutic alliance. With elderly patients, this alliance is best accomplished by taking a medical approach to the patient and expressing concern about all of the patient's physical as well as emotional concerns. Most suspicious elderly patients are quite accepting of medical care and are trusting of physicians. It is rarely necessary for clinicians to confront the patient regarding suspicions or delusional thinking.

The cornerstone of the management of the moderately to severely suspicious elderly patient is the use of medication, especially antipsychotic agents. Medications most frequently used to treat older persons are thioridazine, haloperidol, thiothixene, and loxapine. Dosage of these agents is relatively small initially, and one-half of the dose should be given during the evening. Physicians who prescribe antipsychotic medications for the treatment of suspiciousness in an older adult should carefully monitor the success of these agents. If the drug is deemed not successful—for example, if the target symptoms do not change with the medication—then it should be discontinued, given the significant side effects that may result.

Finally, the physician must be prepared to deal with severe agitation and violent behavior. Medications alone will not control these behaviors. Physicians must work with the nursing staff in order to prevent such behavior in patients at risk while they are in the hospital and to instruct families regarding methods of prevention when these patients are at home. Suggestions for preventing violent behavior are listed in Table 42–2.

■ DEPRESSION

Depression is one of the more frequent and probably the second-most disabling geriatric psychiatry syndrome experienced by older adults. Late-life depression is characterized by symptoms similar to those experienced at earlier stages of the life cycle, with some significant differences. The depressed mood is usually apparent in the older adult but may not be a spontaneous complaint. Older persons are more likely to experience weight loss during a major depressive episode and are less likely to report feelings of worthlessness or guilt. Persistent anhedonia associated with a lack of response to pleasurable stimuli is a common and central symptom of late-life depression. Older persons are also more

Table 42–2. Suggestions for preventing aggressive and violent behavior in the suspicious older adult

Psychologically disarm the elderly patient by assisting him or her to express his or her fears.	Communicate clearly and concisely.
	Communicate expectations.
Distract the attention of the elderly patient.	Avoid arguing and defending.
	Avoid threatening body language.
Provide directions to the elderly patient in simple terms for even the most simple behaviors.	Remain at a safe distance from the agitated elderly patient until help is available.

likely to exhibit psychotic symptoms during a depressive episode than are younger persons.

In community surveys, older adults are less likely to be diagnosed with major depression than are persons in young adulthood or middle age. Standardized interviews reveal 1% to 2% of persons in the community diagnosed as experiencing major depression, while an additional 2% are diagnosed with dysthymia (Blazer et al. 1987). Major depression is much more prevalent among older persons in the hospital and in long-term–care facilities, ranging from 10% to 20% (Koenig et al. 1988).

Late-life depression fits well the biopsychosocial model of psychiatric disorders. Although a hereditary predisposition to depression is less likely among persons in late life experiencing a first onset of depression, a number of biological factors are associated with late-life depression. Poor regulation of the hypothalamic-pituitary-adrenal axis as well as disruption of the sleep cycle and other circadian rhythms is more likely to be present among older persons than among younger persons. Both of these problems have also been associated with major depression. Most older persons are satisfied with their lives and are not psychologically predisposed to depression. Nevertheless, some experience a demoralization and a despair resulting not only from incapacities due to aging but also from a sense of not having fulfilled their life expectations. Older persons must adapt to many adverse life experiences, especially losses of relatives and friends, yet they are often more likely to respond to these losses without difficulty than are persons who are younger.

As with other geriatric psychiatry syndromes, the patient's history and a collateral history from a family member are the keys to making the diagnosis of depression in late life. The history should be complemented by a thorough mental status examination with attention directed to disturbances of motor behavior, perception, presence or absence of hallucinations, disturbances of thinking, and thorough cognitive testing. The laboratory workup of the depressed older adult is presented in Table 42–3.

Major depression is relatively infrequent among older persons yet is the most challenging of the late-life mental disorders to manage. Clinical management involves pharmacotherapy, ECT, psychotherapy, and work with the family. Most geriatric psychiatrists still prefer to begin the older adult with one of the secondary amines, such as nortriptyline or desipramine. Each has relatively low anticholinergic effects and is known to be an effective antidepressant. Postural hypotension is the most troublesome side effect that older adults usually encounter when treated with the tricyclic antidepressants. The selective serotonin uptake inhibitors, such as fluoxetine, sertraline, and paroxetine, can be used at a somewhat lower dose than is prescribed at earlier stages of the life cycle. The most common adverse effects that limit the use of the selective sero-

Table 42–3. Laboratory workup of the depressed older adult

Routine	Elective
Complete blood cell count (CBC)	Dexamethasone suppression test
Urinalysis	Polysomnography
T_3, T_4, FTI, thyroid-stimulating hormone (TSH)	Magnetic resonance imaging (or computed tomography)
VDRL	Cerebrospinal fluid assays
Vitamin B_{12} and folate assays	Thyroid-releasing hormone (TRH) stimulation test
Chemistry screen (Na, Cl, K, BUN, Ca, glucose, creatinine)	
Electrocardiogram	

tonin uptake inhibitors are agitation and persistent weight loss. The older person who does not respond to the antidepressant medications or who experiences significant side effects may be a candidate for ECT therapy. Candidates for ECT should be experiencing a severe depressive episode. They are especially likely to respond to ECT if they are experiencing psychotic symptoms.

A number of studies have demonstrated the effectiveness of cognitive and behavioral therapies for treating older persons with major depression without melancholia as outpatients. Cognitive and behavior therapy is well tolerated by older people because of its limited duration and educational orientation, as well as the active interchange between the therapist and the patient. Any effective therapy for depression with older persons must include work with the family. Families should be informed as to the danger signs, such as potential for suicide, in a severely depressed elderly family member. In addition, the family can provide structure for reengaging a withdrawn and depressed older person into social activities.

■ HYPOCHONDRIASIS

Hypochondriasis among older persons is one of the more common and frustrating of the somatoform disorders encountered by health care professionals. An essential feature of hypochondriasis in older persons is a belief by the elderly person that he or she has one or a number of serious illnesses. The medical workup often will reveal some physical abnormality but does not support a medical diagnosis that can account for the severity and breadth of symptoms experienced.

In community surveys, exaggerated concern about health is found among 10% of older persons (Blazer and Houpt 1979). In contrast, another

10% usually perceive their health as being significantly better than it actually is. The majority of elderly persons assessed their health accurately.

A number of mechanisms may contribute to hypochondriasis in older persons. First, the symptoms may be used to shift anxiety from specific psychological conflicts to more concrete problems with body functioning. An older person may fear the loss of his or her mind, the loss of a spouse, the loss of personal capabilities, or the loss of a social role. Fear of these losses is then replaced by a preoccupation with physical health in hypochondriasis. Social factors are probably the major reason that aging persons are at risk for developing hypochondriasis. Older persons often have difficulty meeting personal and/or social expectations. Failure to meet these expectations, or perhaps anger at the family for insisting that these expectations be met, can lead the elderly person to focus on his or her physical problems to the exclusion of facing the issue directly. Older persons also use hypochondriasis as a means of adapting to the real problem of isolation.

The clinician must be vigilant for the presence of more severe psychopathology. Depression is frequently accompanied by exaggerated physical concerns, regardless of age. Suicide has been demonstrated to be more common in persons exhibiting both depression and exaggerated physical concerns. Hypochondriasis may also mask emerging difficulties with memory.

Hypochondriacal elderly patients are best managed by a primary care physician as opposed to a psychiatrist. Following the initial evaluation, the hypochondriacal elderly patient should be seen for relatively brief but regularly scheduled visits. Medications that can be used for treating the hypochondriacal elderly patient include those with relatively few side effects and those that have been demonstrated to be at least minimally effective for alleviating the symptoms expressed by the patient.

Whatever treatment plan is instituted, it, in fact, is a management plan with the goals of 1) controlling and decreasing the use of health services, 2) decreasing the concern and anxiety expressed by the hypochondriacal older person about the availability and commitment of health care professionals, 3) decreasing strain on the family, 4) increasing the capabilities of the family to provide a supportive environment to the hypochondriacal older person, 5) decreasing conflicts within the family, and 6) decreasing anxiety expressed by the hypochondriacal elderly person. Given these goals, it is essential that the hypochondriacal elderly person be treated within the context of the family when family members are available. As elderly persons resolve conflicts with family, and as they accept their one and only life for what it is, anxiety decreases and appropriate social interactions increase.

■ REFERENCES

American Psychiatric Association: Diagnostic and Statistical Manual of Mental Disorders, 4th Edition. Washington, DC, American Psychiatric Association, 1994

Berry DTR, Phillips BA: Sleep-disordered breathing in the elderly: review and methodological comment. Clinical Psychology Review 8:101–120, 1988

Blazer DG, Houpt JL: Perception of poor health in the healthy older adult. J Am Geriatr Soc 27:330–336, 1979

Blazer D, Hughes DC, George LK: The epidemiology of depression in an elderly community population. Gerontologist 27:281–287, 1987

Blazer DG, George L, Hughes D: The epidemiology of anxiety disorders: an age comparison, in Anxiety Disorders in the Elderly. Edited by Salzman C, Lebowitz B. New York, Springer, 1991, pp 17–30

Christenson R, Blazer D: Epidemiology of persecutory ideation in an elderly population in the community. Am J Psychiatry 141:1088–1091, 1984

Dickel MJ, Sassin J, Mosko S: Sleep disorders in an aged population: preliminary findings of a longitudinal study. Sleep Research 15:116–123, 1986

Folstein MF, Folstein SE, McHugh PR: Mini-Mental State: a practical method for grading the cognitive state of patients for the clinician. J Psychiatr Res 12:189–198, 1975

Katzman R, Jackson JE: Alzheimer's Disease: Basic and Clinical Advances. J Geriatr Psychiatry 39:516–525, 1991

Koenig HG, Meador KG, Cohen HJ, et al: Self-rated depression scales and screening for major depression in the older hospitalized patient with medical illness. J Am Geriatr Soc 36:699–706, 1988

Lishman WA: Cerebral disorder in alcoholism: syndromes of impairment. Brain 104:1–20, 1981

Lowenthal MF: Lives in Distress. New York, Basic Books, 1964

National Institutes of Health Consensus Development: The Treatment of Sleep Disorders in Older Persons. Washington, DC, U.S. Government Printing Office, 1990

Reitan RM: The distribution according to age of a psychologic measure dependent upon organic brain functions. J Gerontol 10:338–340, 1955

Tomlinson E, Blessed G, Roth M: Observations on the brains of demented old people. J Neurol Sci 11:205–242, 1970

CHAPTER

43

Public Psychiatry
and Prevention

H. Richard Lamb, M.D.

Public psychiatry in the 1990s is far different from the much publicized and much criticized community psychiatry of the 1960s. This changing role has given rise to the need for a new term—hence the widespread and increasing use of the term "public psychiatry." Community psychiatry of the 1960s generally neglected the chronically and severely mentally ill and instead focused on less sick patients, primary prevention, and community activism in efforts to change the basic fabric of society. That focus gave rise to criticisms such as that community psychiatry "has branched out well beyond mental illness into problems that it is not especially qualified to handle—community, national, and international affairs; poverty, politics, and criminality" (Kety 1974, p. 962). Moreover, issues such as the homeless mentally ill population have demonstrated the major problems in the way that deinstitutionalization was implemented, problems for which the community psychiatry of past decades has to share the blame.

■ BRIEF HISTORICAL REVIEW

Out of the experience of military psychiatrists in World Wars I and II (Cozza and Hales 1991) came principles that were to have a major impact on public psychiatry for the civilian population. These included a) proximity (i.e., treatment as close as possible to the combat zone); b) immediacy (i.e., early identification and treatment of psychiatric disorder);

c) simplicity (i.e., rest, food, and social support); and d) expectancy (i.e., the expectation of prompt return to duty). It was found that this approach was far more effective than evacuation of all psychiatric casualties to far-away hospitals from which few returned to duty. The principle of treatment close to home became central to public psychiatry, as did the principles of early diagnosis and active treatment to effect prompt remission of acute psychiatric problems and avoid regression. The military experience also demonstrated that selected mental disorders are precipitated by stress and that identifying the precipitating stressors and finding ways of resolving them are very important.

For more than half of the 20th century, the state hospitals fulfilled the function for society of keeping mentally ill persons out of sight and thus out of mind. Moreover, the controls and structure provided by the state hospitals, as well as the granting of almost total asylum, may have been necessary for many of the chronically and severely mentally ill patients before the advent of modern psychoactive medications. Unfortunately, the ways in which state hospitals achieved this structure and asylum led to everyday abuses that left scars on the mental health professions as well as on the patients.

The stage was set for deinstitutionalization by the periodic public outcries about the deplorable conditions that were documented by journalists such as Albert Deutsch (1948). The process of deinstitutionalization was considerably accelerated by two significant federal developments in 1963. First, categorical Aid to the Disabled (ATD) became available to mentally ill persons, making them eligible for the first time for federal financial support in the community. Second, the community mental health centers legislation was passed. The second significant federal development of 1963 was the passage of the Mental Retardation Facilities and Community Mental Health Centers Construction Act, amended in 1965 to provide grants for the initial costs of staffing the newly constructed centers. The centers were defined as requiring five basic services: 1) inpatient treatment, 2) emergency services, 3) partial hospitalization, 4) outpatient services, and 5) consultation-education.

In 1975 Congress passed the Community Mental Health Centers Amendments, which established the principle of continuing federal responsibility for the treatment and prevention of mental disorder, with community mental health as the basic federal activity in this area. This law established the requirement for 12 services instead of the previous 5 services. The added services were 1) services for children, 2) services for the aged, 3) follow-up services for patients who were formerly in institutions, 4) screening before admission to state hospitals, 5) alcoholism services, 6) drug abuse services, and 7) transitional housing. It further required that quality assurance programs and utilization review be built into each center.

In 1977 the President's Commission on Mental Health was formed. Its report, which was completed in 1978, led to the Mental Health Systems Act, which was passed in 1980 but never implemented. The act emphasized coordination of services, patients' rights and advocacy, and a number of grant programs for underserved populations.

■ PUBLIC PSYCHIATRY PRINCIPLES

A number of community (i.e., public) psychiatry "principles" were proposed in the 1960s (Caplan and Caplan 1967). These principles, listed in Table 43–1, have proven to be useful and valid, although only to varying degrees, and have undergone considerable rethinking and change in the succeeding decades.

☐ Responsibility to a Population

The concept of a *catchment area*—that is, a community mental health center taking responsibility for a total population in a geographic area—has great appeal. This approach was adopted by federal legislation and defined as a geographic area that includes 75,000 to 200,000 people. Theoretically, a community mental health center would identify all the mental health needs of its catchment area, formulate a plan to meet these needs, and provide services based not on the staff's preferences with regard to the kind of mental health activity in which it wants to engage, but rather on the actual needs of the population. These needs would be determined by both citizens and staff and would take into account the cultural backgrounds of the population.

The catchment area concept has worked well when the catchment area includes a discrete area, both politically and geographically. There have, however, been many problems when this concept has been used in large metropolitan or sparsely populated rural areas, where a minimum population of 75,000 may result in a catchment area so large geographically that great distances make the rational provision of services unwieldy.

Table 43–1. Community psychiatry "principles" as conceptualized in the 1960s

Responsibility to a total population (catchment areas)	Consumer participation
	Program evaluation and research
Treatment close to the patient's home	Prevention
Comprehensive services	Mental health consultation
Multidisciplinary team approach	Linkages to health and human services
Continuity of care	

☐ Multidisciplinary Team Approach

Each mental health discipline has something unique to add to the treatment of mentally ill patients. In the early days of community mental health, there was much emphasis on role blurring—that is, minimizing the differences between the disciplines and having professionals from the different disciplines tending to fulfill similar roles. This approach caused considerable confusion to both staff and patients, encouraged turf battles, and often resulted in inefficient utilization of skilled staff. Although some role blurring is inevitable in a multidisciplinary team approach, there has in recent years been a greater recognition of the importance of taking full advantage of the unique skills of each discipline.

☐ Consumer Participation

Mental health services can be more effective and relevant to a population when there is input from community members rather than having mental health needs and programs defined only by professionals. This is, however, a much more complex issue than it might appear at first. The involvement of the citizens of a small city or town with their mental health center may indeed be very positive. The mental health staff become known and trusted in the community, the needs of the community are articulated to the professionals, and the services become more relevant. Mental health concepts become better understood and accepted, and citizens may provide important assistance to the center and to its patients.

Consumer participation has not been as successful in many large cities. Citizen advisory boards may seem to be representative of a city or a part of a city in terms of ethnicity, race, geographic area, and a host of other factors. However, these groups may not be as cohesive in the cities as is often assumed, and persons representing them may, in fact, be representing primarily themselves and not their group or the city as a whole. Or the mental health director may "pack" the citizens advisory board with persons known to be sympathetic to his or her policies, and such a group may represent not the community but instead the mental health director.

In recent years an important source of citizen input has been from families of patients with major mental illness (i.e., schizophrenia, schizoaffective disorder, bipolar disorder, and major depression). Families have organized, developed a new self-concept, and effectively devoted themselves to advocacy for the needs and rights of the chronically mentally ill population (Lefley and Johnson 1990). The formation of the National Alliance for the Mentally Ill has caused community treatment centers to give higher priority to chronically and severely mentally ill persons.

☐ Program Evaluation and Research

Program evaluation—the use of scientific techniques to measure the value of an agency's work—is a major concern in public psychiatry. Every program—national, regional, state, or local—needs to be objectively evaluated. Objectivity must be stressed, because without it we become dependent on our subjective impressions and are influenced by our biases. Most health and welfare workers feel that their work is important and has a positive influence on their patients. One of the purposes of scientific research methods is to minimize such subjective bias so that conclusions can be based on hard data.

Evaluative research that has determined the effectiveness with which a program serves its particular patients still has not done enough. Effort must be directed toward objectively examining the overall efficacy of the program. The research must examine not only how well patients are served but also how great a contribution the program makes to solving a particular mental health problem or to meeting a particular need. Ideally, evaluation should be conducted within a controlled research framework. At a minimum, program goals must be explicit and formulated in a manner that permits objective evaluation of the program. We must be prepared to terminate programs that do not produce evidence of their worth.

■ PROBLEMS IN PUBLIC PSYCHIATRY

☐ Chronically and Severely Mentally Ill Patients

Interest in working with persons who are chronically and severely mentally ill has revived in recent years (Talbott 1987). The term *chronically and severely mentally ill* refers to patients with chronic and severe major mental illness—schizophrenia, schizoaffective disorder, bipolar disorder, or major depression—and the resulting functional impairment, social and/ or vocational. Another way to define this population is those persons who, before deinstitutionalization, would have lived out their lives in state hospitals. Psychiatry has had the technology to treat and rehabilitate these patients for some years. Thus, we know about the importance of case management; of supervised housing; of adequate, comprehensive, and accessible psychiatric and rehabilitation services; of having less restrictive laws governing involuntary treatment; of having better coordination of community services; and of providing structured, ongoing 24-hour care for that small proportion of patients in need of it. What has been lacking has been the willingness of both society and the mental health professions to devote the resources necessary to employ this technology.

☐ Needs Formerly Met by State Hospitals

In the midst of very valid concerns about the shortcomings and anti-therapeutic aspects of state hospitals, it was not appreciated that these hospitals fulfilled some essential functions for patients who were chronically and severely mentally ill. The term "asylum" was in many ways an appropriate one, for these imperfect institutions did provide asylum and sanctuary from the pressures of the world with which, in varying degrees, most of these patients were unable to cope (Lamb and Peele 1984). Further, these institutions provided services such as medical care, patient monitoring, respite for the patient's family, and a social network for the patient, as well as food, shelter, and needed support and structure (Wing 1990).

In the state hospitals, the treatment and services that did exist were in one place and under one administration. In the community, the situation is very different. Services and treatment are under various administrative jurisdictions and in various locations. Even mentally healthy individuals have difficulty dealing with a number of bureaucracies, both governmental and private, and getting their needs met. Further, patients can easily get lost in the community as compared with a hospital, where they may have been neglected but at least their whereabouts were known.

☐ Homeless Mentally Ill Persons

Homeless mentally ill persons have become one of the greatest challenges to public mental health, and to society generally. The two American Psychiatric Association (APA) task forces on the homeless mentally ill (Lamb 1984; Lamb et al. 1992) concluded that this problem is the result not of deinstitutionalization per se, but of the way it has been implemented. Homelessness among chronically and severely mentally ill persons is symptomatic of the grave problems facing them generally in this country. Thus, the problem of homelessness will not be resolved until the basic underlying problems of the chronically and severely mentally ill population generally are addressed and a comprehensive and integrated system of care for them is established. The solutions, then, for homelessness among the mentally ill are the same solutions enumerated later in the subsection on community treatment for persons who are chronically and severely mentally ill.

Chronically and severely mentally ill persons are not proficient at coping with the stresses of this world; therefore, they are vulnerable to eviction from their living arrangements, sometimes because of an inability to deal with difficult or even ordinary landlord-tenant situations, and sometimes because of circumstances in which they play a leading role. In the absence of an adequate case management system, these individuals are out on the streets and on their own. Many, especially the young, have a tendency to drift away from their families or from a board-and-care home; they may be trying to escape the pull of dependency and may not be ready to come to terms with living in a sheltered, low-pressure environment. If they still have goals, they may find an inactive life-style extremely depressing. Or they may want more freedom to drink or use street drugs.

Once mentally ill persons are out on their own, they will more than likely stop taking their medications and after a while will lose touch with the Social Security Administration and will no longer be able to receive their SSI checks. The lack of medical care on the streets and the effects of alcohol and other drug abuse are further serious complications. Evidence is beginning to emerge that homeless mentally ill persons have a greater severity of illness than do mentally ill persons in general. At Bellevue Hospital in New York City, approximately 50% of inpatients who were homeless are transferred to state hospitals for long-term care as opposed to 8% of other Bellevue psychiatric inpatients (Marcos et al. 1990).

☐ Criminalization

As a result of deinstitutionalization, there are now large numbers of mentally ill persons in the community. At the same time, there is a limited amount of community psychiatric resources, including hospital beds. Rather than hospitalization and psychiatric treatment, mentally ill persons often are subject to inappropriate arrest and incarceration. Legal restrictions placed on involuntary hospitalization also probably result in a diversion of some patients to the criminal justice system.

Studies of county jail inmates referred for psychiatric evaluation (Lamb and Grant 1982) found that this population was characterized by severe acute and chronic mental illness, and generally functioned at a low level. Homelessness was common; at the time of arrest, 39% had been living on the streets, on the beach, in missions, or in cheap hotels. Almost half of the men and women charged only with misdemeanors had been living on the streets, compared with one-fourth of those charged with felonies.

☐ Problems in Treating Chronically and Severely Mentally Ill Patients

It is essential that mental health professionals have realistic expectations in their clinical work with chronically and severely mentally ill patients. If, instead, professionals proceed as if these patients can function at levels beyond their capabilities, the result will often be exacerbations of psychosis, dysphoria, and perhaps homelessness (Lamb 1986).

Ideology must often give way to pragmatism. For example, although we all want chronically and severely mentally ill patients to experience the self-esteem and gratification from a life of employment, our ideology must not obscure the clinical reality that most such patients cannot handle the stress of competitive employment and that, for the minority who can, entry-level, low-stress jobs most often should be the initial goal. Otherwise the patient is simply given another experience of failure, which further lowers his or her self-esteem. Moreover, the gratification that can be derived from working with chronically and severely mentally ill patients must not be overlooked. Without achieving high levels of functioning for their patients, psychiatrists can help to change chaotic, dysphoric life-styles into lives characterized by greater stability.

☐ Dependency and Asylum

The fact that chronically and severely mentally ill persons have been de-institutionalized does not mean they no longer need social support and protection, and relief, either periodic or continuous, from the pressures of life. In short, they need asylum and sanctuary *in the community* (Lamb and Peele 1984). Unfortunately, because the old state hospitals were called "asylums," the word took on a pejorative connotation. Only in recent years has the word again become one that denotes the function of *providing asylum*, rather than *conceiving of asylum as a place*.

Professionals must realize that whatever degree of rehabilitation is possible for each patient cannot take place unless support and protection are provided. It has been shown that the treatment of chronically and severely mentally ill patients cannot be time limited; if it is not ongoing most patients will regress (Stein and Test 1985). Thus, it is important to guard against termination of treatment of chronically and severely mentally ill patients with the idea that they are cured; their need for a support system has not ended even though they may appear intact.

☐ Families of the Chronically and Severely Mentally Ill

Psychiatrists have learned that chronically and severely mentally ill persons and their families need advice. Many of the patients themselves lack the ability to cope with the routine stressors of life and need tutelage and specific guidance about what to do in many areas of their lives. Managing major mental illness in a relative at home is an immensely difficult task. Families can learn by trial and error over a period of years how to help stabilize their mentally ill relative by encouraging the avoidance of excessive stress, having realistic expectations, setting appropriate limits, understanding the patient's problem in tolerating social stimulation, learning how to react to psychotic symptoms, and encouraging the taking of medications. But families learn this at great emotional cost that could have been avoided had they been assisted by knowledgeable professionals.

Psychiatrists can also utilize families' abilities to play an important role in the treatment process. Psychiatrists have to learn to help families set limits and take charge of their households (Kanter 1985); psychiatrists have to feel comfortable in telling the family that schizophrenia and other major mental illnesses are biological illnesses and that the family has not caused them; psychiatrists have to be unambivalent about the use of psychoactive medications and in advising families to urge their relatives to take them; psychiatrists have to work with the families and the patients to determine what are realistic goals. Psychiatrists need to help relatives understand that social withdrawal may be a necessary defense for patients against too much stress or social stimulation, but that excessive withdrawal may lead to a form of institutionalism in the home.

☐ Model Programs: A Solution?

Much attention has been paid to glamorous, innovative pilot treatment and rehabilitation programs. The publicizing of these demonstration programs has led to one proposed remedy for the problems of the deinstitutionalized chronically and severely mentally ill patient: the mass cloning of these "model programs." However, what works in one community may not work in another. Some programs are well suited to urban areas but not to rural areas, and vice versa; some programs that work well in small- or medium-sized cities are not feasible in inner-city settings. Even beyond this, programs that are highly successful in one community may fail or be rejected in what appears to be an entirely comparable set of circumstances elsewhere. Cultural, political, and socioeconomic factors specific to each community must be taken into account. Furthermore, it is more exciting to develop and run one's own innovative and pioneering program than to replicate someone else's. It is instructive for program planning to look at the eight elementary principles common to successful model programs as conceptualized by Bachrach (1980) (Table 43–2).

☐ Community Treatment for Chronically and Severely Mentally Ill Patients

A comprehensive and integrated system of care for chronically and severely mentally ill patients, with designated responsibility, accountability, and adequate fiscal resources, must be established. Adequate, comprehensive, and accessible psychiatric and rehabilitative services must be available and, when necessary, be provided assertively through

Table 43–2.   Elementary principles common to successful model programs

1. Assigns top priority to the care of the most severely impaired.
2. Provides realistic linkage with other resources in the community.
3. Provides out-of-hospital alternatives for the full range of functions performed in hospital settings.
4. Individually tailors treatment for each patient.
5. Provides cultural relevance and specificity—that is, tailoring programs to conform to the local realities of the community in which they are located.
6. Involves trained staff who are attuned to the unique survival problems of chronic mental patients living in noninstitutional settings.
7. Provides access to a complement of hospital beds, because there are some patients for whom periods of hospital care continue to be a necessity.
8. Incorporates an ongoing internal assessment mechanism that permits continuous self-monitoring.

outreach services. First, there must be an adequate number of direct psychiatric services that provide 1) outreach contact with the mentally ill persons in the community; 2) psychiatric assessment and evaluation; 3) crisis intervention, including hospitalization; 4) individualized treatment plans; 5) psychotropic medication and other somatic therapies; and 6) psychosocial treatment. Second, there must be an adequate number of rehabilitative services that provide socialization experiences, training in the skills of everyday living, and social and vocational rehabilitation. Third, both treatment and rehabilitative services must be provided assertively—for instance, by going out to patients' living settings if they do not or cannot come to a centralized program location.

Crisis services must be available and accessible. An adequate number of professionals and paraprofessionals must be trained for community care of chronically and severely mentally ill persons. An adequate number and ample range of graded, stepwise, supervised community housing settings must be established. Some small proportion of chronically and severely mentally ill persons can graduate to independent living. For the majority, however, mainstream low-cost housing is not appropriate. There must be settings that offer different levels of supervision, both more and less intensive, including quarterway and halfway houses, board-and-care homes, satellite housing, foster or family care, and crisis or temporary hostels.

A system of responsibility for chronically and severely mentally ill persons living in the community must be established, with the goal of ensuring that each patient ultimately has one mental health professional or paraprofessional who is responsible for care. In such a case management system, each patient's case manager would ensure that the appropriate psychiatric and medical assessments are carried out; formulate, together with the patient, an individualized treatment and rehabilitation plan, including the proper pharmacotherapy; monitor the patient; and assist the patient in receiving services.

For the more than 50% of the chronically and severely mentally ill population living at home or for those with positive ongoing relationships with their families, programs and respite care must be provided to enhance the family's ability to provide a support system. When the use of family systems is not feasible, the patient must be linked with a formal community support system.

For outpatients who are so gravely disabled and/or who have such impaired judgment that they cannot care for themselves in the community without legally sanctioned supervision, it must become easier to obtain conservatorship status (Lamb and Weinberger 1992). Involuntary commitment laws must be made more humane to permit prompt return to active inpatient treatment for patients when acute exacerbations of their illnesses make their lives in the community chaotic and unbearable. Involuntary treatment laws should be revised to allow the option of outpatient civil commitment (Miller 1992); in states that already have provisions for such treatment, that mechanism should be more widely used. Finally, advocacy efforts should be focused on making available competent care in the community, rather than simply focusing on "liberty" for patients at any cost.

A system of coordination among funding sources and implementation agencies must be established. Because the problems of chronically and severely mentally ill persons must be addressed by multiple public and private authorities, coordination, which was so lacking in the deinstitutionalization process, must become a primary goal. Territorial and turf issues have often been at the root of this problem, and different agencies serving the same patients have often worked at cross purposes.

General social services must be provided. In addition to the need for specialized social services, such as socialization experiences and training in the skills of everyday living, there is a pressing need for generic social services. Such services include arranging for escort services to accompany the patient to agencies and potential residential placements, helping the patient with applications to entitlement programs, and assisting the patient in mobilizing the resources of his or her family.

Ongoing structured 24-hour care should be available for that small proportion of chronically and severely mentally ill persons who do not respond to current methods of treatment and rehabilitation. Some persons, even with high-quality treatment and rehabilitation efforts, remain dangerous or gravely disabled. For these persons, there is a pressing need for ongoing structured 24-hour care in long-term settings, whether in hospitals or in locked, highly structured community facilities (Lamb 1980).

☐ Underserved Populations: Rural Areas

It is generally held that the risks of psychiatric illness are at least as great in rural places compared with urban settings and that rural individuals tend to be exposed to a variety of stressors that can result in a need for psychiatric care (President's Commission on Mental Health 1978). Physical isolation, low levels of education, inadequate funding, and ignorance of psychiatric problems and of techniques for addressing them further inhibit optimal psychiatric service utilization. Thus, rural populations in the United States are considered to have a substantial need for, but generally poor access to, psychiatric services (Bachrach 1983).

In terms of space, the sheer dimensions of rural service areas can be overwhelming. Most rural mental health catchment areas, for example, exceed 5,000 square miles. The largest mental health catchment area in the United States, located in Arizona, consists of 60,000 square miles. In conjunction with conditions of physical isolation, low population density, a limited tax base, and personnel shortages, space may create major barriers to providing care. Urban residents typically have at least potential access to a multiplicity of private and public psychiatric services, but rural residents may have only one psychiatric facility available within a reasonable distance. Even when such facilities exist in rural areas, the scope of available treatment modalities may be limited by a small staff. Residential facilities for persons discharged from state hospitals may be particularly scarce.

Working in a rural area can present many problems for psychiatrists and other mental health professionals. They may have to provide a variety of services and thus be service generalists. They may be cultural outsiders, and that, together with the fact that they are mental health professionals, may make them suspect in the local community. They may experience professional isolation with the problems of lack of peer support and lack of ability to learn from fellow mental health professionals. Further, rural service agencies tend to be understaffed, and as a result workloads may be excessive.

There are also advantages in rural areas. The rural sense of community may provide a potential source of support for mental health efforts that is rarely found in urban areas. Tolerance of deviance may also be greater. There must, of course, be sensitivity to the local culture, but the rural social organization, when properly utilized, may well be an advantage in the delivery of psychiatric services (Bachrach 1983). There is evidence that rural mental health centers may be most helpful by providing brief therapy for immediate short-term interventions (Mooney and Johnson 1992). This approach also maximizes use of limited staff. Seriously ill psychiatric patients may have high visibility in a rural area, causing these patients to get help sooner. Moreover, rural psychiatrists may learn more about their patients in the normal course of conversation in a rural community.

☐ Governance Problems

There is a tendency today for fewer mental health directors to be psychiatrists, but instead to be psychologists, social workers, and psychiatric nurses. This has come about in part because of the reluctance of psychiatrists to assume purely administrative positions, in part because nonpsychiatrists command a considerably lower salary, and in part because of interdisciplinary rivalries and the active seeking out of administrative positions by nonpsychiatrists. There is also a tendency to appoint to high administrative mental health posts persons who may not be mental health professionals, but who were primarily trained as professional managers. This situation presents problems because persons without training and experience in actually providing treatment cannot begin to appreciate the enormity, variety, and complexity of the task of caring for mentally ill patients.

☐ Unstable Funding

In the process of deinstitutionalization, the numbers of patients in state hospitals have been dramatically reduced, but the funding of the state hospitals has not been transferred to community programs to provide treatment to the hundreds of thousands of patients who now live in the community (Talbott 1985). In many cases, state hospital budgets have not decreased because of the state's attempts to bring the hospitals up to the standards of the Joint Commission on Accreditation of Healthcare Organizations in order to achieve accreditation and because of union pressures to maintain hospital jobs. Another factor is the state's desire to save money. The result is insufficient funds and services to treat chronically and severely mentally ill patients in the community.

☐ Fewer Psychiatrists

The number of psychiatrists working in public psychiatry has decreased both in actual numbers and as a percentage of the total number of public mental health professionals. One factor is the reluctance to offer competitive salaries to psychiatrists. Often there is resentment from other professionals at the high salaries of psychiatrists. Conversely, these salaries cannot compete with the remuneration that psychiatrists receive in areas such as the private sector. Many times community programs believe that they can save money by hiring nonpsychiatrists instead of psychiatrists. This short-sighted approach overlooks what is often a sacrifice in quality of both leadership and clinical work when psychiatrists are not actively recruited and adequately compensated. Another major problem has been a tendency in many community programs to use psychiatrists primarily where they cannot be substituted for, namely, to write prescriptions, instead of utilizing their clinical skills for the full range of treatment and consultation to other staff. Still another problem has been that of role blurring, the notion that all of the mental health professions have similar skills in the evaluation and management of mental disorder.

■ PREVENTION

Mental health practitioners divided preventive activities into primary, secondary, and tertiary forms (Caplan 1964). *Primary prevention* refers to the actual avoidance of the occurrence of cases of mental illness. *Secondary prevention* (i.e., treatment) involves enabling people to regain their normal level of functioning and preventing further development of illness after its occurrence; early diagnosis and treatment is a sine qua non. *Tertiary prevention* (i.e., rehabilitation) involves preventing or reversing the sequelae of illness—in other words, disability.

□ Primary Prevention

Many past and present primary prevention efforts have been attempted through indirect services, as exemplified by consultation to teachers or welfare workers, or to the police who have actual contact with the patient or the potential patient (Talbott 1988), as opposed to direct services, in which the professional works directly with and treats the patient. Although techniques, such as mental health consultation, have proven useful, there is no evidence that the incidence of mental illness has decreased with their use. As a result, there has been a tendency for the goals of primary prevention to become more realistic—that is, preventing exacerbations in persons who have already suffered mental illness rather than preventing the underlying illness itself, and focusing on areas in which primary prevention has been shown to be effective (see subsection below on prevention, proven and probable). In any case, the disillusionment with primary prevention that occurred in the early 1970s has given way to another upsurge of interest (Price et al. 1988).

□ A Field in Disarray

Much of the debate over primary prevention relates to the lack of clarity of the concepts and definitions underlying the issues (Lamb and Zusman 1981). Unless care is taken to distinguish prevention of mental illness from prevention of unhappiness, feelings of distress, or social incompetence, discussants will often be examining several different phenomena while thinking that they are focusing on one. Interest in prevention undoubtedly stems from the expectation of reducing the number of seriously ill and disabled individuals, and not simply from the belief that prevention may lead to a happier life for the average person. It is only on the basis of preventing mental illness and thereby reducing the need for treatment resources that the allocation of a large proportion of limited mental health funds and personnel for "preventive" efforts can be justified.

Those professionals concerned with primary prevention in the mental health field face a complex problem of definition: determining the boundaries of mental health. Public health practitioners almost always use the word *prevention* in regard to illness. Mental health services, on the other hand, usually deal not only with individuals who have a diagnosable illness but also with those who have no recognized psychiatric illness but want help instead with interpersonal problems and concerns of everyday living that cause them distress and unhappiness. Meaningful and reasonable objective exploration of "prevention" and "mental illness" requires that the discussion be confined to diagnosable mental illness, including the neuroses and personality disorders.

Can investigators actually demonstrate that primary prevention is effective? Without knowledge of cause, primary prevention programs can only be shots in the dark. Modern research has increasingly suggested the operation of genetic and biochemical factors in the causation of mental illness. Both adoption studies (Kety 1987) and twin studies (Kendler 1988) have indicated that schizophrenia is, for the most part, genetically determined. The same is true for bipolar disorder and major depression (Tsuang and Faraone 1990). The effect of genetic traits can be reduced, of course, through measures such as genetic counseling, but that is not what most proponents of primary prevention have in mind. It also seems possible that the expression of genetic traits—the actual precipitation of the full-blown illness—may be related to environmental conditions. It is not yet clear that measures to prevent the expression of a genetic trait should be labeled primary prevention and directed at entire populations rather than only toward known mentally ill individuals, who are either overtly ill or in remission.

☐ Crisis Intervention as Prevention

The lack of knowledge about specific causation as well as the mounting genetic evidence for etiology has probably laid the conceptual groundwork for more recent trends in prevention. Some leading proponents of primary prevention have come to believe that a patient's current reality may be a more important determinant of mental disorders than his or her past traumas (Bloom 1981). They question whether there should not be a movement away from consideration of causative and predisposing factors in mental illness toward a focus on precipitating factors—that is, stressful life events thought to be associated with the precipitation of mental illness. Thus crisis intervention has been considered a fertile area for efforts in primary prevention. Although focusing on precipitating stressors might often avert acute exacerbations in persons already known to be mentally ill, it should be recognized that crisis intervention with only this segment of the population is really secondary prevention, the provision of treatment services to persons whose ability to cope with stress is known to be impaired.

☐ Mental Health Promotion

Primary prevention has been subdivided into two categories: activities that promote health generally and thereby increase resistance to disease, and activities that are aimed against the occurrence of specific illnesses. Promotion of general physical health is an easily understood concept; yet in the area of mental health, most, if not all, successful primary preventive activities have been aimed at specific diseases. In contrast to physical health, there is no evidence that "general mental health" can be promoted or strengthened and thus that resistance to mental illness can be increased by preventive activities. Despite massive efforts to combat poverty, to increase social welfare and Social Security benefits, and to change the educational systems and methods of child rearing, there is no indication that the incidence of any of the functional (i.e., nonorganic) mental illnesses has decreased. Nor is there evidence that other countries with stronger social welfare systems and different child-rearing practices have different rates of mental illness. Thus, the major functional mental illnesses (as well as the frequently occurring diagnosable minor illnesses) remain untouched by efforts to strengthen mental health.

☐ Social Problems and Prevention

The relationship between environment and the causation of mental illness has been strongly argued by some researcher-clinicians. For example, there can be no doubt that the prevalence of symptoms associated with mental illness and the rates of admission to state hospitals and of diagnosis of the major mental illnesses are higher among the poor. What remains to be unequivocally demonstrated, however, is that poverty is somehow causative. For instance, persons who are ill or on the verge of illness may gravitate toward poverty-stricken neighborhoods (i.e., downward drift).

☐ Prevention: Proven and Probable

Some primary prevention techniques in psychiatry have been shown to be extremely effective. Psychiatric complications of syphilis and vitamin deficiency are seldom seen today in developed nations. Decreased rates of birth injury and improved prenatal care have lowered the incidence of major psychiatric problems that result from congenital brain damage. Other common neuropsychiatric disorders such as stroke and head injury have been shown to be highly preventable. Elimination of lead from house paint has reduced the number of children suffering from organic brain syndromes, and control of industrial toxins has virtually eliminated "mad hatters" and other such problems.

More recent preventive programs should also reduce the incidence of certain illnesses. For instance, counseling prospective mothers not to delay pregnancy until the later childbearing years is likely to reduce the incidence of mongolism. Other programs show promise but await solid research findings demonstrating their effectiveness. Interventions directed toward abusing parents, such as Parents Anonymous, seem likely to prove effective in breaking the cycle of child abuse, which has been shown to be socially transmitted from generation to generation. Raising infants in impersonal institutions or without a consistent mother figure over a long period of time has been demonstrated to be deleterious. Programs to replace institutions for homeless children with long-term, high-quality foster care or adoption should help to prevent personality disturbance. With the mounting evidence of genetic influence on the occurrence of schizophrenia and manic-depressive psychosis, the appropriate use of birth control and genetic counseling should be effective in preventing the births of individuals who would be at high risk for development of these illnesses.

■ REFERENCES

Bachrach LL: Overview: model programs for chronic mental patients. Am J Psychiatry 137:1023–1031, 1980

Bachrach LL: Psychiatric services in rural areas: a sociological overview. Hosp Community Psychiatry 34:215–226, 1983

Bloom BL: The logic and urgency of primary prevention. Hosp Community Psychiatry 32:839–843, 1981

Caplan G: Principles of Preventive Psychiatry. New York, Basic Books, 1964

Caplan G, Caplan RB: Development of community psychiatry concepts, in Comprehensive Textbook of Psychiatry. Edited by Freedman AM, Kaplan HI. Baltimore, MD, Williams & Wilkins, 1967, pp 1499–1516

Cozza KI, Hales RE: Psychiatry in the Army: a brief historical perspective and current developments. Hosp Community Psychiatry 42:413–418, 1991

Deutsch A: The Shame of the States. New York, Harcourt Brace Jovanovich, 1948

Kanter JS (ed): Clinical Issues in Treating the Chronic Mentally Ill (New Directions for Mental Health Services, No 27). San Francisco, CA, Jossey-Bass, 1985

Kendler KS: The genetics of schizophrenia: an overview, in Handbook of Schizophrenia, Vol 3. Edited by Tsuang MT, Simpson JC. New York, Elsevier, 1988, pp 437–462

Kety SS: From rationalization to reason. Am J Psychiatry 131:957–963, 1974

Kety SS: The significance of genetic factors in the etiology of schizophrenia: results from the National Study of Adoptees in Denmark. Journal of Psychiatric Research 4:423–429, 1987

Lamb HR: Structure: the neglected ingredient of community treatment. Arch Gen Psychiatry 37:1224–1228, 1980

Lamb HR (ed): The Homeless Mentally Ill: A Task Force Report of the American Psychiatric Association. Washington, DC, American Psychiatric Association, 1984

Lamb HR: Some reflections on treating schizophrenics. Arch Gen Psychiatry 43:1007–1011, 1986

Lamb HR, Grant RW: The mentally ill in an urban county jail. Arch Gen Psychiatry 39:17–22, 1982

Lamb HR, Peele R: The need for continuing asylum and sanctuary. Hosp Community Psychiatry 35:798–802, 1984

Lamb HR, Weinberger LE: Conservatorship for gravely disabled psychiatric patients: a four-year follow-up study. Am J Psychiatry 149:909–913, 1992

Lamb HR, Zusman J: A new look at primary prevention. Hosp Community Psychiatry 32:843–848, 1981

Lamb HR, Bachrach LL, Kass FI (eds): Treating the Homeless Mentally Ill: A Report of the Task Force on the Homeless Mentally Ill. Washington, DC, American Psychiatric Association, 1992

Lefley HP, Johnson DL (eds): Families as Allies in Treatment of the Mentally Ill: New Directions for Mental Health Professionals. Washington, DC, American Psychiatric Press, 1990

Marcos LR, Cohen NL, Nardacci D, et al: Psychiatry takes to the streets: the New York City initiative for the homeless mentally ill. Am J Psychiatry 147:1557–1561, 1990

Miller RD: An update on involuntary civil commitment to outpatient treatment. Hosp Community Psychiatry 43:79–81, 1992

Mooney DK, Johnson RD: Rural mental health appointment adherence: implications for therapy. Community Ment Health J 28:135–139, 1992

Price RH, Cowen EL, Lorion RP, et al (eds): 14 Ounces of Prevention: A Casebook for Practitioners. Washington, DC, American Psychological Association, 1988

President's Commission on Mental Health: Report of the Task Panel on Rural Mental Health, Vol 3. Washington, DC, U.S. Government Printing Office, 1978

Stein LI, Test MA (eds): The Training in Community Living Model: A Decade of Experience (New Directions for Mental Health Services, No 26). San Francisco, CA, Jossey-Bass, 1985

Talbott JA: The fate of the public psychiatric system. Hosp Community Psychiatry 36:46–50, 1985

Talbott JA: The chronically mentally ill: what do we now know, and why aren't we implementing what we know? in The Chronic Mental Patient II. Edited by Menninger WW, Hannah GT. Washington, DC, American Psychiatric Press, 1987, pp 1–29

Talbott JA: The Perspective of John Talbott (New Directions for Mental Health Services, No 37). San Francisco, CA, Jossey-Bass, 1988

Tsuang MT, Faraone SV: The Genetics of Mood Disorder. Baltimore, MD, Johns Hopkins University Press, 1990

Wing JK: The functions of asylum. Br J Psychiatry 157:822–827, 1990

Administration in Psychiatry

Stephen Rachlin, M.D.
Stuart L. Keill, M.D.

■ EDUCATION AND TRAINING

Most psychiatric administrators do not obtain formal education leading to a graduate degree in business, public, or hospital administration, although some complete Master of Public Health programs that have significant administrative components. One can enroll in individual courses at a nearby university to learn the basics. For the average level of interest, "minicourses" in administrative psychiatry are given periodically in several geographic locations. Self-study should be viewed not as a substitute but as a supplement.

Organizations concerned with the education and training of clinicians in management are another source of seminars. The American Association of Psychiatric Administrators, which, like the American Psychiatric Association (APA), was an outgrowth of a network of former state hospital directors, has open membership to psychiatrists interested in the field, and several local chapters. That there is a body of knowledge in psychiatric administration is also attested to by various symposia, workshops, papers, and lectures at the two annual meetings sponsored by the APA.

For the past 40 years, the APA has had a structure for credentialing psychiatrists in administration. Under the auspices of the Committee on Administrative Psychiatry, a 2-hour written examination is administered, and, for those who pass, the 4-hour oral examination is conducted immediately prior to the annual meeting in May. Several hundred psychiatrists have achieved certification. Both the written and the oral examinations cover four generic areas. *Administrative theory* details personnel issues, management structures, and the like. *Psychiatric care management* includes such matters as managed care, utilization review, and quality assurance, among others. The third section is *law and ethics*. Finally, *fiscal management* includes but is not limited to such issues as budgeting, sources of revenue, and other related topics.

■ THE ADMINISTRATOR AS LEADER

Barton and Barton (1983) stated that the psychiatrist-administrator should be able to do planning, organizing, staffing, directing, controlling, communicating, innovating, and representing. They went on to characterize the capacity for leadership as including the abilities to decide, prioritize, resolve conflicts, coordinate the work of others, expedite task completion, motivate staff, use power wisely, and delegate authority to others.

Talbott (1987) distinguished the related concepts of management, administration, and leadership. Management is a hands-on process, designed to keep the organization running smoothly. It refers, by and large, to those persons occupying "middle management" positions and concerns itself with procedures. Administration is best conceptualized as a broader function, one of overseeing and taking executive charge. It is concerned with policy and ensuring that tasks of the organization are performed well.

Leadership, in contrast, involves giving direction (as opposed to providing directions), with something of a visionary component. The leadership role includes promoting and protecting the values of the organization and, if it is to survive and grow, involving, inspiring, and nurturing other staff. In an oft-repeated saying, the administrator does things right while the leader does the right things. The effective leader does not get bogged down in all the day-to-day crises, but rather delegates this job to subordinates, whom he or she then helps develop toward additional responsibility.

It is well to remember that while a chairman, chief of service, or department head may well be "the front office" to staff working on the clinical service, that same person is middle management to the chief executive officer, dean, commissioner, or others to whom he or she is accountable. Managing the many exchanges across these boundaries is yet another challenge to those persons in executive positions.

☐ Administrative Styles and Skills

The personality and style of the individual directing an organization will affect its tone and output. Staff will, by and large, adjust to a variety of personal styles and traits, although extremes are likely to create problems. Some common traits, however, characterize effective leaders. As with all positive relationships, the staff and the supervisor's relationship is based on mutual respect and trust. The leader's behaviors consistently convey ethical integrity, a commitment to the goals of the organization and a primary focus on the needs and the rights of patients as well as a valuing of staff performance. Staff members work with more security when they believe in the reliability of the leader and his or her intentions to seek the resources that are needed to carry out the work. Commitments for action must be honored and breaches explained. Excellent performance is valued, poor performance rejected.

Administrators make decisions with a sense of timeliness. Many day-to-day decisions can be made quickly and easily, because occasional errors can be corrected. Major decisions require more data and deliberation, including input from those affected by them. A fine balance needs to be maintained between the need for input and the need for timeliness of decision making. The leader's actions and decisions have credibility when they are rooted in a broad body of knowledge about the clinical aspects of psychiatric treatment, rehabilitative systems, patients' and family needs, gaps in the resources, the community, the strengths and weaknesses of staff members' performance, and the effectiveness of the program.

The successful psychiatric administrator has insight into his or her own behavior and its motivations, dynamics, and impact on others, as in one's clinical utilization of transference-countertransference phenomena. The supervisor also teaches, directs, and provides a role model for the staff. He or she seeks input from the staff about patients' needs and ways to improve services to patients and families. Inculcating the concept of genuine *collaboration* among the staff fosters commitment to a common goal. This differs from *cooperation,* which is a willingness to help each other. Collaboration means sharing a responsible concern for outcome. Departmental structures for ongoing communication about planning, patient care, and other functions should foster the concept of shared ownership of programs and problems.

Optimism is another important quality for a leader. He or she also must maintain positive expectations for change even in the face of setbacks. Staff members need to experience the optimism of their leader. The competent leader has confidence in his or her abilities and is not threatened by, but indeed welcomes, the fact that some of his or her subordinates will be more competent in many activities. The leader cannot be expert in all areas, but learns from and looks to the other experts in his or her program.

■ PLANNING

The accepted starting point in the planning process is the development of a mission statement. Actions by subdivisions must reflect these goals of the parent body. Basic to shaping the organization's future is a *strategic plan*. By definition, this is long-range in nature, often 5 years, and it provides the guideposts that are to be adhered to as overarching principles. Budgets, to be discussed in a succeeding section, should reflect the strategic plan and may be rejected if they do not. Due recognition is, of course, given to the fact that no plan is so static as to be immune from change, as long as direction remains intact.

Change may come from a variety of sources, both internal and external. Examples of the latter are alterations in state mental health laws, modifications in the requirements of accrediting bodies, community demands, and the availability of funding for special projects. Internal stimuli include, among others, the hiring of a new staff member with special interests (or the development of such skills by existing personnel), a crisis on existing units or programs, and the appointment of a new leader. Barriers to effective planning include lack of resources, either in dollars or staff, and also regulatory constraints and unavailability of other supports. The kinds and numbers of staff directly affect the process as well.

A useful way to conceptualize and describe how one goes about planning, especially for the shorter term with which most of us are more familiar and involved, is the acronym DIME. This four-stage cycle refers to **D**esign, **I**nitiation, **M**anagement, and **E**valuation. It can be used for a new program or for modification of one that is ongoing.

The first stage, *design*, includes a study of the mission and a measurement of available resources. Based on an appropriate balance, a draft plan is articulated. The next step is *initiation*, the point at which the actual structure is created. This is a particularly rewarding time, with high levels of staff excitement and enthusiasm. Managers select and train staff. Old procedures are modified and support is developed, in part, by dissemination of information to interested collaborating services. *Management* oversees the program in ongoing operation and determines its success or failure. Many clinical and administrative decisions will need to be made, dealing with foreseen and unforeseen difficulties.

The process of *evaluation*, in reality, needs to be introduced from the very beginning of the management phase. Records are kept and data collected; resources are balanced and reports made. This component is known as program evaluation and represents the measurement of effectiveness and efficiency of the defined program. Through the analysis of this information, judgments can be made in continuing management and in setting a course for the future.

■ ACCOUNTABILITY

All mental health agencies, and, indeed, human services in general, are accountable in a variety of ways to the three branches of government. The legislature enacts laws that govern the operations of hospitals, clinics, and the like, and provide for the licensing of professional staff. The executive component, operating through state and/or local departments of mental health or hygiene, has the authority to issue regulations for many aspects of psychiatric treatment, and these have the force of law. And if we are unfortunate enough to be the subject of a lawsuit, judicial decrees may have a substantial influence on how the job gets done. Even absent this degree of intervention, it is the courts that interpret the foregoing laws and regulations and, in so doing, directly impact on what we do.

☐ To the Government

Depending on the institution's auspices, program directors may be accountable to municipal, state, or federal officials. One or another of these has statutory responsibility for approving and licensing of institutions or components thereof, both initially and throughout their operation. Obtaining such certification from government, to which funding is tightly tied, involves a process of external evaluation of mission, staffing patterns, recruiting techniques, life safety factors, patients' rights, quality assurance, fiscal responsibility, and the all-important documentation of what it is we are doing in the individual clinical record.

Evaluation site visits can be helpful. The identification of service gaps and operating problem areas serves the useful purpose of gaining allies for their correction. Sometimes the visibility of such problem areas to regulatory bodies motivates and mobilizes additional administrative support and resources for their correction.

☐ To the Community

For many years, both providers and consumers have perceived that the major systems for the delivery of health care in this country are *of* the community as well as *in* the community. It is therefore helpful for the program, educational for the staff, and significant for the executive to work with informed and interested consumers and advocates. A comfortable way to begin such dialogue is with sophisticated groups such as the Alliance for the Mentally Ill or local and state mental health associations.

Most large organizations, including hospitals and other health care institutions, are directed by a board of directors, trustees, managers, or governors. Prominent members of the community are appointed or elected to serve. In other than public programs, they may have significant responsibility for raising funds. In government-sponsored facilities, while such boards may exist, the chief executive is additionally accountable to an appointed or elected official. Many board members are able, knowledgeable, and administratively well versed. Mutual respect, plus continuing and open communications, can provide major benefits to patients.

☐ To the Media

Because the press, radio, and television influence the public, and therefore governmental figures, they can have a powerful effect on programs. The populace is interested in coverage of new techniques for dealing with psychiatric and other health care problems. Given the nature of many public psychiatric facilities, there is always a potential for various kinds of scandal. It is essential, therefore, that the psychiatrist-administrator maintain a mutually respectful relationship with key figures in the media.

■ FISCAL PRACTICES

For health care organizations, personnel account for the lion's share of expenditures. The percentage will vary by type of service provider, but can be as much as 80% of annual outlays. Staff salaries, plus the cost of fringe benefits, make up this component. Other costs include rent, utilities, janitorial services, travel, postage, telephone, and so forth. These monies must be monitored, and a budget is the mechanism for doing this, much as it may be in a family.

☐ The Budget

First and foremost, a budget is a financial plan. It flows from, and is consonant with, the overall mission statement and strategic plan. It thus supports the goals and objectives of the organization and recognizes that resources are finite. It is the overall plan that drives the budget, and not the reverse.

Warren (1992) discussed other functions of the budget. It is a policy document, balancing competing priorities and providing a framework for their implementation. Performance can be studied and measured against allocations, and any type of variance noted. This also allows feedback to program directors so that "midstream" corrections may be made.

Various types of operational budgets are in use. Governmental entities commonly operate from a *fixed ceiling, or lump sum, appropriation*. The executive has some flexibility in moving dollars from one purpose to another, as long as he or she does not exceed the preset limit. By contrast, the *line item, or object, budget* provides a specific amount for each particular expenditure, and perhaps also for every staff position in the agency. A *program budget* defines what is to be accomplished, by unit or division. This budget, also known as a PPBS (i.e., planning programming budget system), is a complicated process, producing a matrix-like structure containing objectives allowing for measurable units of performance. A *zero base budget* requires that all expenditures be looked at each year. Finally, the *incremental budget* simply adjusts upward or downward from the prior year, depending on service demand and utilization, cost-of-living allowances, and the like.

All institutions have both *direct* and *indirect costs*. Direct costs are those that arise out of operation of the programs, such as salaries and supplies. On the other hand, indirect costs, housekeeping and utilities being examples, are necessary but not unique to the program.

Once the budget is prepared, it must be submitted for approval to a higher authority, to a board of directors, to a governmental entity, or perhaps to all, depending on the type of facility. The executive, or the financial officer with whom he or she is working, must be careful to avoid the trap of saving money by cutting staff if, in fact, a program generates more in reimbursement than it costs to operate.

☐ Financing of Services

By long tradition, state governments have financed mental health care through wholly owned and operated hospitals and clinics, as well as grants to other agencies to care for psychiatric patients. Although many state systems are presently downsizing, partly in response to deinstitutionalization, they still provide an enormous amount of direct care.

The federal government provides a significant amount of the money used to fund programs for the elderly, the poor, and the disabled populations. Medicare and Medicaid were created by the 1965 amendments to the social security law. Medicare was originally enacted to provide medical care for the elderly. Medicaid is a federally sponsored program in association with the various states. Overall, the federal government pays half the costs, with states (and perhaps localities) picking up the other half, but the exact proportions vary depending on the relative wealth, or lack thereof, of the states. Beneficiaries of public assistance are categorically eligible for Medicaid, as may be others whose income is above that required for welfare payments but insufficient to take care of their medical needs, rendering them "medically indigent." Medicaid also has special exclusions relative to psychiatry. It does not pay for psychiatric hospital treatment of adults under age 65, but general hospitals can be reimbursed for such care. Freestanding psychiatric hospitals, state facilities, and psychiatric skilled nursing homes may receive federally funded Medicaid only for those inpatients under age 21 or older than 65.

Psychiatric facilities have come to rely a great deal on these sources of income, and virtually all health care entities are supported by multiple streams of revenue. Commercial insurers cover many workers and their dependents. Some employers self-insure, a few patients are wealthy enough to do the same, and a huge number of Americans have no insurance whatsoever. Each plan or program of insurance has different benefit levels, creating a bewildering array for any reimbursement manager or program administrator. Further complicating the picture is that payment may be made retrospectively or prospectively. The traditional fee-for-service indemnity insurance pays after the services are rendered, based on a bill submitted. Various prospective plans, however, impose limits, up front, on what will be paid for and at what level. For example, many prepaid health maintenance organizations limit inpatient care to 30 days annually, and outpatient treatment to 20 visits per year.

☐ Cost Control

Society in general, and elected officials in particular, are expressing an ever-increasing amount of concern about the cost of health care and the percentage of the gross national product it is consuming. In response to this perception, the Health Care Financing Administration developed the payment system known as diagnostic related groups (DRGs) for Medicare-funded hospital care. All illnesses are classified into one of several hundred diagnostic categories, and a fixed amount is paid for the hospital treatment of that illness. This scheme proved extremely difficult to implement for psychiatric patients, because diagnosis alone serves to explain only a small amount of the variability in resources consumed or length of stay.

One positive step psychiatric administrators can take is marketing of services. This is of ever-increasing importance. Consumer groups, insurers, and any other payers on the horizon must be made aware of and encouraged in the appropriate use of those services, both general and special, that we provide, in order to maximize our resource utilization and avoid "down time."

■ MANAGED CARE

Cost containment is not only a priority for government-sponsored methods of payment for health care, but almost a national obsession. Private insurers and other payers are equally concerned, as the cost of health insurance continues to rise. Obviously, one of the major reasons for this increase is the availability of expensive technology, but, again, staff are necessary to provide treatment, and their numbers and salaries continue to rise. One common method of cutting insurance costs is by increasing the annual deductible that the individual and family must pay out-of-pocket before the company will reimburse expenses. In addition, and this is all too frequently applied to mental health care, there is the technique of increasing the copayment for which the insured is personally responsible. This is accomplished either by simply raising the percentage of copayment or by lowering the maximum amount that will be reimbursed per treatment visit.

Utilization review has been around, in part as a cost control, for many years. Originally required for Medicare, it is now applied to all payers and patients and is necessary for hospital accreditation. Performance of this function may be prospective (i.e., preadmission certification), concurrent (i.e., while the patient is hospitalized), or retrospective (i.e., after discharge). Utilization review serves to ensure that the treatment is indicated and that the services are provided in an efficient manner.

The use of resources is more tightly overseen by those third-party payers such as insurance companies and now by so-called fourth parties (i.e., utilization management companies under contract to approve, deny, and monitor care rendered to beneficiaries). A system of case-by-case allocation, known as *utilization management*, is created. When utilization management is combined with a select network of providers, institutions and individuals both, we have what is generally called *managed care* (American Psychiatric Association, Committee on Managed Care 1992). The tightest form of control is that of the *health maintenance organization* (HMO): a preset amount is paid to the organization, which is then responsible for all necessary care and treatment.

A second, and rather powerful, trend, which may cost a bit more than the HMO but will likely still be less expensive than traditional fee-for-service indemnity, is what is known as a PPO (i.e., *preferred provider organization*). Subscribers must receive all of their medical services from a defined group of practitioners and must use a participating hospital when inpatient care is necessary. In both types of arrangements, there is usually a primary physician "gatekeeper" who must authorize referrals to specialists and hospitalization.

Preadmission certification under managed care provides an advance evaluation of proposed services in terms of both the site (hospital, office) and the level of intensity. Duration of treatment and the particular modalities to be used must be specified. Even then, the authorization can be for no more than initial procedures for evaluation and creation of a treatment plan. Only those procedures that are consistent with the treatment plan are approved, and finite intervals for additional review are delineated. Greater scrutiny is generally given to more expensive items such as inpatient admission, but ambulatory services are subjected to the procedures as well.

While the patient is receiving care, it is reviewed in a concurrent fashion. On the inpatient side, this could be as frequently as every few days but rarely exceeding a week, while for psychiatric outpatients it might, for example, be every 10 sessions. The provider needs to demonstrate that progress toward treatment goals is being made and that, regardless of modality, the patient is moving in the direction of fulfilling the criteria for discharge readiness. Some review organizations provide "case managers" to assist this process.

In order to ensure the approval of treatment, the provider must demonstrate "medical necessity." This is defined as being that which is adequate and essential for evaluation and/or treatment of disease, reasonably expected to improve the patient's condition or level of functioning, and in keeping with accepted standards of psychiatric practice (American Psychiatric Association, Committee on Managed Care 1992). Implicit in managed care is the possibility of a denial. If the provider fails to follow the plan guidelines or contractual procedures, an administrative denial will result. More usual is the clinical denial, in which the reviewer disagrees with one or another aspect of treatment, likely based on a written protocol. The provider, on appeal, can supply additional documentation, elaborate upon the treatment plan, and further explain the reasons for the chosen interventions. A psychiatrist will most probably be consulted, and only such a peer should be permitted to make an ultimate and final disapproval decision.

Managed care companies save money through their reimbursement procedures. Although there may still be a fee-for-service system, the reimbursed fee almost always is at a discount from that which the provider usually charges. Another payment method, as in the HMO, is *capitation*, in which a pre-agreed-upon amount is paid periodically and in advance, in exchange for which all necessary services will be provided for the specified patient population. Should the managed care organization suffer total financial collapse, the psychiatrist may still be liable to continue the patients' treatment (American Psychiatric Association, Committee on Managed Care 1992).

Insurers will continue to be held to a legal standard of good faith and fair dealing, and they will be required to do their reviews responsibly and in accordance with accepted standards. The professions, however, are held to a higher standard, that of ethics. This makes it the responsibility of the psychiatrist not to abandon his or her patient, but to continue to provide necessary care, at least until another acceptable arrangement can be made, even if no reimbursement whatsoever is forthcoming.

Some states have enacted legislation to control various aspects of managed care. Among the provisions proposed (local law, if any, should be consulted) are publication of protocols, required review by a physician in the same specialty, specified appeal processes, prohibition of payment to the fourth party based on a percentage of the money "saved," and mandatory consultation with the treater before denial of payment.

Hospitals have been forced to expand their departments or divisions of utilization review simply to respond to the demands and inquiries of third and fourth parties. They are not, however, reimbursed for this function. Another problem is the vulnerability of public-sector services to these private-sector cost-containment activities (Rachlin 1992). If, for example, continued hospitalization is indicated by the staff of a private facility but the managed care company disagrees and refuses to pay, the options for the facility are to continue to treat while incurring significant financial loss, or to attempt to arrange a transfer to a government-sponsored hospital. It may safely be presumed that the latter course will be pursued more often than not.

■ QUALITY ASSESSMENT AND IMPROVEMENT

Despite the fiscal constraints just delineated, patients and payers both want to know that the treatment they receive is of high, or at least professionally acceptable, quality. The ethics of medicine require no less of us as psychiatrists. The very finest care possible cannot truly be delivered for pennies, but we owe it to our patients to strike an equitable balance. The process of quality assurance seeks, in part, to approach this goal.

Quality assessment is required not only by third and fourth parties but also by virtually every accrediting or regulatory agency with which we come into contact. It has not been a static entity, having had a series of modifications over the years, which are destined to evolve further. Utilization review was perhaps the first phase of quality management, looking at the necessity for, and efficiency and utilization of, health care resources. Federally mandated peer review organizations came on the scene not only to ensure quality where taxes were funding treatment, but to attempt to contain costs as well.

Understanding quality assurance requires the learning of a new vocabulary. Fauman (1989) and Wilson and Phillips (1992) provided valuable dictionaries and other information on the process. *Quality care* indicates that there is optimal outcome through the use of appropriate and available resources, that the provider meets explicit or implicit standards, and that the type of facility and kinds of services are relevant to the patient's diagnosis and clinical needs. *Standards,* in turn, are established principles that are expected or required and against which measurement may be made. *Norms* are qualitative or quantitative measures of aspects of practice. In turn, standards and norms combine to produce the criteria used to make quality-of-care judgments, because they define the appropriateness of care. These criteria need to be elucidated by professionals, from experience and the literature, and applied by peers once a review is triggered. Criteria can pertain to structure (Does the provider have appropriate resources and mechanisms?), process (How is care actually provided?), or outcome (What are the actual results for the patient?).

A clear trend in quality assurance is occurring away from process toward outcome monitoring—that is, do you actually provide a high level of care? Mirin and Namerow (1991) argued that despite difficulty in design and implementation, outcome study is essential so that we modify our clinical practices in accordance with knowledge of which modalities are essential, which are useful, and which are ineffective. There are many treatment-related variables and a complicated system of mental health delivery.

Risk management is that subdivision of quality improvement concerned with identification, analysis, and actions to deal with potential legal liability, hopefully before suits are filed and in order to prevent them. Kinzie et al. (1992) reviewed deaths, major medical complications, seclusion and restraint, extended length of stay, early readmission, suicide attempts, and violence, and presented the first 100 undesirable outcomes. A fair number of these events were judged at least potentially avoidable; the authors stressed that this is just one component of their overall program.

A related aspect of this work is the development of *clinical practice guidelines.* Also known as *practice parameters,* these guidelines are defined as detailed strategies and pathways for the treatment of disease. Although practice guidelines might well reduce variations in treatment and enhance quality, they may not result in lowered utilization or costs. Such guidelines are under development by the federal government, researchers, and medical specialty societies, including the APA.

On the horizon is movement in the direction of total quality management, or continuous quality improvement. This new element, which is based on industrial quality management techniques first used in postwar Japan, aims to assess the full range of services and processes that affect patient outcome and satisfaction (Taylor 1992). The quality improvement process attempts to take a broad view of the overall system rather than focusing on individual practitioner aberrances. Thus, there is less emphasis on the occasional, unusual event and more of a focus on common problems.

The new monitoring and evaluation processes are overseen by the organization's leaders (as opposed to departments or services), and it is the superordinate body that delineates scope of care, identifies high priorities, and enumerates key functions. Teams of experts, without necessary regard to discipline or department, identify indicators and establish levels for each that will trigger intensive evaluation. The leaders then seek opportunities for improvement, set priorities, assign teams to evaluate patient care, ensure that improvement is sustained over time, and disseminate information as necessary. Continuous quality improvement is a requirement for accreditation by the Joint Commission on Accreditation of Healthcare Organizations (1994).

■ REFERENCES

American Psychiatric Association, Committee on Managed Care: Utilization Management: A Handbook for Psychiatrists. Washington, DC, American Psychiatric Association, 1992

Barton WE, Barton GM: The psychiatrist-administrator, in Psychiatric Administration: A Comprehensive Text for the Clinician-Executive. Edited by Talbott JA, Kaplan SR. New York, Grune & Stratton, 1983, pp 179–185

Fauman MA: Quality assurance monitoring in psychiatry. Am J Psychiatry 146:1121–1130, 1989

Joint Commission on Accreditation of Healthcare Organizations: 1995 Comprehensive Accreditation Manual for Hospitals. Oakbrook Terrace, IL, Joint Commission on Accreditation of Healthcare Organizations, 1994

Kinzie JD, Maricle RA, Bloom JD, et al: Improving quality assurance through psychiatric mortality and morbidity conferences in a university hospital. Hosp Community Psychiatry 43:470–474, 1992

Mirin SM, Namerow MJ: Why study treatment outcome? Hosp Community Psychiatry 42:1007–1013, 1991

Rachlin S: The psychiatrist-administrator in the economic crossfire, in American Psychiatric Press Review of Clinical Psychiatry and the Law, Vol 3. Edited by Simon RI. Washington, DC, American Psychiatric Press, 1992, pp 209–218

Talbott JA: Management, administration, leadership: what's in a name. Psychiatr Q 58:229–242, 1987

Taylor D: The Joint Commission quality assessment and improvement model, in Manual of Psychiatric Quality Assurance: A Report of the American Psychiatric Association Committee on Quality Assurance. Edited by Mattson MR. Washington, DC, American Psychiatric Association, 1992, pp 69–77

Warren SJ: Budget, in Textbook of Administrative Psychiatry. Edited by Talbott JA, Hales RE, Keill SL. Washington, DC, American Psychiatric Press, 1992, pp 287–312

Wilson GF, Phillips KL: Concepts and definitions used in quality assurance and utilization review, in Manual of Psychiatric Quality Assurance: A Report of the American Psychiatric Association Committee on Quality Assurance. Edited by Mattson MR. Washington, DC, American Psychiatric Association, 1992, pp 23–30

CHAPTER

Psychiatric Education

Jonathan F. Borus, M.D.
William H. Sledge, M.D.

Psychiatric education is a broad area involving many different teachers and learners. It utilizes didactic and experiential opportunities to help learners acquire 1) a knowledge base about normal and abnormal human behavior, 2) clinical skills to understand and therapeutically intervene to relieve suffering and restore function, and 3) appropriate attitudes and empathic sensitivity to successfully interact with patients to understand and treat their emotional disorders. Many forces impact psychiatric education, including the academic settings in which much of the education occurs, organizations accrediting individual learners and educational programs, professional and public interest groups concerned about both the education itself and its products, and economic and political influences on the profession that shape its educational possibilities.

■ LEARNING PRINCIPLES IN MEDICAL AND PSYCHIATRIC EDUCATION

As in other areas, education in medicine is the product of an interactive process between teachers and learners based on educational principles. A first principle is that there are many different teaching and learning methods and styles, making the alliance and the congruence between teacher and learner important variables—for example, a teacher who insists on lecturing to a visual learner will not be successful. Too often in psychiatry, as in other medical disciplines, exposure to information is considered sufficient to produce learning. The fact that most curricula only require that learners sit through a course of lectures, attend a defined seminar series, and/or see a specific number of patients to ensure that they, the learners, have been exposed to important knowledge and practice issues betrays a naive conception of how people learn.

Second, learners not only must be exposed to new information but must also incorporate it (a process often aided by multimodal exposure and repetition); integrate the new material with prior ideas and skills; and master the newly integrated learning through utilizing it in their professional and personal activities (Borus 1993).

Third, medical education is also based on the principle of progressively increasing the learner's responsibility as he or she gains knowledge, skills, and experience (Accreditation Council for Graduate Medical Education [ACGME] 1992; Association of American Medical Colleges [AAMC] 1984; Ludmerer 1985). In medical education this progression begins with presentation of basic information to provide a knowledge base for the learner to understand a problem, demonstration of the problem and its treatment by an experienced clinician, work by the learner under direct supervision, individual work by the learner with collateral (indirect) supervision, and, finally, when the learner is sufficiently educated and trained, working alone without ongoing supervision but with life-long, self-initiated, continuing education. A specific problem in this paradigm for psychiatric education is that psychiatrists, unlike other physicians, in order to ensure confidentiality often work in a dyadic relationship without a supervisor directly observing the patient-doctor interaction. Whether in psychotherapy, consultation on a medical ward, or an emergency room setting, there is danger that a neophyte psychiatric learner may be put into a situation in which he or she will be overwhelmed by or toxic to the patient. Psychiatry needs to develop new ways to directly monitor, as well as collaterally supervise, its trainees in order to avoid this pitfall.

In medicine, the terms "education" and "training" are often used interchangeably but actually refer to different kinds of learning that should be distinguished (Eaton 1980). *Education* is the development of the capacity for understanding, analysis, problem solving, and dealing with unique and novel circumstances. It may involve the study of topics and areas that seem to have little direct relevance to particular clinical problems. *Training,* also a type of learning, refers to the capacity to carry out certain behaviors and apply certain skills in a prescribed and standardized manner. Surgeons are trained to make precise incisions and educated about infection, anatomy, and physiological function. Psychiatrists are educated to understand depression and trained to prescribe antidepressants and carry out electroconvulsive therapy (ECT).

A fourth principle of medical education, with special implications for psychiatry, is the professionalization of intimacy (Parsons 1951). Physicians are sanctioned to explore intimate bodily areas and functions; in addition, psychiatrists are expected to share in patients' most intimate thoughts and feelings. Therefore psychiatric educators must help their learners understand the powerful emotional issues in the patient-doctor relationship and how to monitor, control, and utilize them to the advantage of the patient's treatment. The psychiatric professional also has to become more intimately acquainted with himself or herself as an important evaluative and therapeutic "instrument" in order to understand, and intervene in, a patient's disturbed behavior and emotions. Facilitating the concurrent learning by trainees about themselves and their patients is a major task in psychiatric education.

■ REGULATION OF PSYCHIATRIC EDUCATION

Psychiatric education, like all other medical specialties, is embedded in regulatory systems established to create public accountability and maintain professional standards through regular review and certification. In addition to medical licensing, which is administered at the state level, this regulatory thrust is aimed toward individuals through certification by the American Board of Psychiatry and Neurology, Inc. (ABPN), and other psychiatry subspecialty boards, and toward programs through accreditation by the Liaison Committee on Medical Education (LCME) for undergraduate, the Residency Review Committee (RRC) in Psychiatry of the Accreditation Council for Graduate Medical Education (ACGME) for residency, and the Accreditation Council for Continuing Medical Education (ACCME) for continuing education programs.

Certification is the means by which individuals demonstrate that their skills and knowledge meet the standards of competency of the profession. Certification is voluntary, but it is increasingly linked to compensation in institutional settings. The ABPN performs this certification function for the specialty fields of general psychiatry, child and adolescent psychiatry, and neurology, and has begun certifying "added qualifications" in some subspecialty areas such as geriatric psychiatry and addictions psychiatry. The ABPN is an independent board whose members are nominated by its sponsoring organizations, the American Medical Association (AMA), the American Psychiatric Association (APA), the American Neurological Association (ANA), and the American Academy of Neurology (AAN) (American Board of Psychiatry and Neurology 1992). The ABPN is a member of the American Board of Medical Specialties (ABMS), which sets standards and serves as an advocacy organization for all medical specialty boards. The ABPN offers graduates of accredited residency programs in general psychiatry or child and adolescent psychiatry a written test of knowledge and a clinical test of skills, knowledge, and attitudes for those who pass the written test. Effective

October 1, 1994, all ABPN certifications in psychiatry and its subspecialties will be limited and require recertification every 10 years. The ABPN also has provisions for double certification in neurology and psychiatry, and internal medicine and psychiatry, and a "triple board" pilot project whereby highly selected applicants may become eligible for board certification in pediatrics, psychiatry, and child psychiatry with a 5-year training program at one of six approved training centers.

Accreditation is the process whereby programs are reviewed and measured against programmatic standards and requirements set by independent accrediting agencies. The LCME sets standards for accreditation of schools granting medical degrees in the United States and Canada and monitors accredited medical schools with written reviews and site visits every 7 years (Liaison Committee on Medical Education 1991). The ACGME sets general standards for all institutions providing medical specialty training programs and conducts periodic institutional reviews to see that these standards are met. It has specialty-specific RRCs that write and monitor residency program requirements for the appropriate specialty (ACGME 1992). The RRCs set specialty-specific requirements and carry out accreditation reviews of residency training programs; however, the ACGME has the final authority for policy and accreditation actions. The Psychiatry RRC is composed of 10 members: 4 from the ABPN (three directors and ABPN's executive vice president), 3 from the APA, and 3 from the AMA's Council on Medical Education. Finally, the ACCME is the agency that sets policy and reviews programs that are seeking to offer continuing medical education credits.

■ UNDERGRADUATE MEDICAL EDUCATION IN PSYCHIATRY

The psychiatric curriculum in undergraduate education has two basic domains of knowledge to convey to medical students (Lidz and Edelson 1970; Werkman 1966): the teaching of psychopathology and the psychological and social aspects of medicine in general. Psychiatry is unique within the medical school curriculum in being responsible for both *basic science material* (social and behavioral sciences such as psychology, sociology and anthropology, as well as basic biological sciences such as molecular genetics and neurobiology of behavior) and *clinical material* (psychopathology, psychopharmacology, normative response to illness, doctor-patient relationship, etc.). Psychiatry has its own domain of pathological conditions (i.e., severe mental illness) that virtually no other medical discipline shares, as well as a range of conditions that also belong to other areas of medicine (e.g., dementias, normative responses to illness, the nature of the doctor-patient relationship, etc.). Psychiatry is often allied with other departments (e.g., pharmacology, pediatrics, internal medicine, neurology) and functions as an integrative and problem-solving discipline. Most skills, knowledge, and professional attitudes proffered by psychiatry are low in technology and frequently process oriented. Psychiatry's domain represents some of the most cherished ideals of modern medical education, namely, that the student will learn to think for himself or herself and relate helpfully to distressed patients.

The National Board of Medical Examiners (NBME), in its role as developer of the national student evaluation and licensing examinations, exerts substantial informal influence on what is included in the average curriculum (National Board of Medical Examiners 1992). With the emphasis on the need to teach and learn massive quantities of biomedical information, some medical faculties and students are intolerant of the process orientation of modern psychiatry. The 1984 General Professional Education of the Physician (GPEP) Report focused medical educators on the need to reexamine the educational process and stimulate active faculty and student participation in general medical education (Association of American Medical Colleges 1984). Medical schools have begun exploring problem-based small-group teaching that integrates basic science and clinical materials, and psychiatrists have played prominent roles in several of these new ventures (Tiberius 1990; Tosteson 1990). Generally, however, the medical school curriculum is still divided into 1) preclinical material that provides the basic science underpinnings for medical practice, 2) introduction to clinical medicine courses, and 3) clinical rotations that involve both required and elective clerkships.

☐ The Psychiatric Curriculum

In the preclinical curriculum, departments of psychiatry are frequently tasked with providing an introduction to the behavioral sciences. Such courses typically address phenomenology such as anxiety and depression, human development from the perspective of emerging psychological capacities and social roles, and social science material on the impact on behavior of culture, race, family, and social roles. A psychodynamic or psychoanalytic perspective may also be presented. With the growth of biological psychiatry, psychiatry often also collaborates with pharmacology in the presentation of material that addresses the effects of agents on the brain, and with neurology and basic neuroscience faculties in the presentation of information that relates neurobiology to particular affective states and motivated behavior. Changes in general medical education since the GPEP report have also stimulated collaborations between psychiatrists and primary care internists in courses focused on the sick role, the patient-doctor relationship, and psychosocial development throughout the life cycle.

In the introduction to the clinical medicine portion of the medical school curriculum, psychiatrists are responsible for teaching psychopathology, diagnostic skills necessary to recognize mental illness, and knowledge of appropriate treatment approaches. During this segment of the curriculum, psychiatrists are frequently called upon to provide basic instruction in patient interviewing techniques and mental status assessment.

The LCME lists psychiatry as a required clinical clerkship. This experience is usually conceptualized as a means to convey to the future nonpsychiatric medical practitioner knowledge of the manifestations of defined mental illness and its available treatment approaches, as well as the skills to recognize and diagnose mental disorders and refer mentally ill patients for specialty treatment (Reiser et al. 1988). The clerkship also offers opportunities to practice psychiatric interview techniques and initiate brief treatment efforts under close supervision. Students who are considering psychiatry for a career, or who want to learn more psychiatric skills, may take advanced elective clerkships that provide more clinical responsibility, independence, and opportunities to learn about the field.

In general, the process-oriented material of psychiatry fares better in settings where it can be demonstrated, discussed, and applied. A combination of lectures, small discussion groups, seminars, workshops, and supervised clinical experiences can be an effective and well-accepted means of conveying much of the material taught by psychiatry in the undergraduate curriculum.

If a department of psychiatry is fortunate, 5% to 10% of its graduating students will become future psychiatrists. This means that the bulk of undergraduate psychiatric education is oriented toward students who will not become psychiatrists. It is important for the psychiatric educator to deal with this issue by constantly considering the view of psychiatry through the eyes of the primary care practitioner. Psychiatric concepts and terminology should be made accessible and not exotic, overly jargonistic, or pedantic; issues of recognition, diagnosis, and treatment or referral for psychiatric specialist care of primary care patients with mental disorders should be emphasized; and time should be devoted to demonstrating the roles of personality, defenses, and coping styles in patients presenting with medical and surgical illness. Furthermore, the psychiatrist educator should demonstrate the value of psychological knowledge and skills in caring for nonpsychiatric patients.

■ GRADUATE PSYCHIATRIC EDUCATION (RESIDENCY TRAINING)

Residency in general psychiatry is a 4-year program of learning and experiential education and training through supervised clinical practice that begins after graduation from medical school. In its "Special Essentials" for psychiatry training, the RRC provides both broad and specific guidelines for residency program design. A minimum of 4 months of training in a primary medical care specialty and 2 months of training in neurology are required during the 4-year residency, preferentially during the first postgraduate year (PGY I) after medical school. Psychiatry programs alternately may choose to devote the full PGY I to medicine and neurology and begin formal training in psychiatry in PGY II. Also specified by the RRC are minimum FTE requirements of 9 months of inpatient psychiatry, 1 year of outpatient psychiatry, 2 months of child psychiatry, 2 months of consultation psychiatry, and a variety of clinical experiences with different patient populations and settings, the lengths of which are not specified. The latter include experiences in public-community psychiatry; emergency psychiatry; individual, group, couple, and family psychotherapy; psychopharmacology; treatment of substance abuse; psychiatric investigation, and so forth. In many programs the curriculum is structured to provide most of the required clinical experiences in the first 3 years to achieve a broad foundation in psychiatry, while allowing time in PGY IV for the senior resident to selectively focus on particular areas of interest.

☐ Resident Selection in Psychiatry

Residents are selected almost exclusively through the National Residency Matching Plan (NRMP), which runs a computerized match for postgraduate medical training in the United States. Under a single entry agreement implemented in 1988 and monitored by the national Psychiatry Match Review Board, medical students applying for residency positions in psychiatry at either the PGY I level (in 4-year programs) or the PGY II level (after obtaining their own PGY I internship, or after completing another medical specialty training program) do so through the NRMP, which performs a two-stage match for psychiatry in late February and announces the results in mid-March.

☐ Residency Design

The usual configuration of psychiatry residencies includes PGY I with between 4 and 10 months of internal medicine, 2 months of neurology, and any remaining months (if not in medicine) devoted to inpatient psychiatry or other activities at the interface of psychiatry and medicine. PGY II in most programs is an inpatient psychiatry year in which residents, often in more than one setting, learn to undertake a comprehensive evaluation of inpatients, make descriptive and dynamic diagnoses and formulations of patient problems, and design and implement inpatient treatment plans related to follow-up outpatient care. In many programs a small number of outpatients are begun in treatment during PGY II to allow a modest 3-year longitudinal outpatient psychiatry experience. PGY III is often an outpatient year with focus on a variety of long- and short-term individual, group, couple, and family psychotherapies. In PGY III many programs also have major rotations in consultation-liaison and child psychiatry. In the former rotation, residents under supervision provide psychiatric expertise and interventions for medical, surgical, and obstetric/gynecological inpatients. Child psychiatry training is often outpatient based and usually focuses on diagnostic evaluation of children and their families rather than longitudinal treatment.

PGY IV in most programs combines continued longitudinal outpatient clinical experiences with elective or selective opportunities to focus more intensively on a particular area or areas of psychiatry. Many residents also use part of this year to take on senior or chief residency responsibilities that provide experiences in psychiatric clinical administration and teaching. Others undertake research during PGY IV as a transitional step toward becoming psychiatric investigators. With the increasing trend toward subspecialization in psychiatry, PGY IV provides an opportunity to solidify areas of interest as a bridge to a formal subspecialty fellowship after residency. The opportunity for residents to use their final year of residency to select an area of focus from the broad psychiatric foundation gained in the first 3 years of residency is an important developmental step toward choosing a practice area. Transition-to-practice seminars in the PG IV year are valuable opportunities in which residents are encouraged to explore a variety of practice possibilities within themselves and the external world prior to committing to a postresidency position (Borus 1978, 1982; Hales et al. 1982, 1985).

☐ Teaching and Supervision in Residency

The excellent residency will offer a series of core didactic learning experiences to provide the resident with knowledge about modern psychiatry as well as the opportunity to become skilled in applying such knowledge through clinical practice under the close supervision of experienced faculty members. More so than in other fields of medicine, the psychiatry resident himself or herself is a vital interpersonal "instrument" in understanding, diagnosing, and treating the patient, making close supervision of the resident's clinical practice a crucial component of the resident's professional learning and development (Thorbeck 1992). Supervision in psychiatry can be direct or collateral. Opportunities for a supervisor to directly observe the interactions of resident and patient most often occur in inpatient and emergency room settings as well as during consultations on medical and surgical inpatients. In outpatient and intensive inpatient psychotherapeutic clinical experiences, which are usually based on the dyadic relationship between the (resident) therapist and patient, most supervision occurs on a collateral basis. After the clinical encounter, a verbal, audiotaped, and/or videotaped presentation is made to the supervisor who provides feedback, increased understanding, and direction to the resident (Betcher and Zinberg 1988). It is important for residents to receive supervision from faculty with differing orientations and expertise who can help the residents integrate a multiplicity of perspectives and potential interventions into a specific treatment plan for each patient.

☐ Evaluation

Regular evaluation of residents, faculty, and the training program itself is a crucial step in the development of high-quality psychiatric practitioners (Borus and Yager 1986). Evaluation of residents should be both formative and summative. Ongoing informal formative feedback to the resident from his or her clinical unit chiefs and supervisors about strengths and weaknesses should occur throughout the course of a clinical rotation or supervised psychotherapy. Intermittent scheduled summative evaluation should occur through formal supervisory reports, end-of-service unit chief evaluations, and tests of cognitive and clinical skills. The RRC requires annual examinations of cognitive knowledge and an evaluation of clinical skills at least twice during the PG II–IV years (ACGME 1992).

Most programs use the Psychiatry Resident In-Training Examination (PRITE), a national examination of residents' knowledge, to meet the cognitive examination requirement. Sponsored by the American College of Psychiatrists, the PRITE provides residents and their training directors with feedback on each resident's performance in nine content areas as well as a comparison of the resident's performance with others in his or her residency class, the total residency program, and other residents throughout the country who have had similar amounts of training (Smeltzer and Jones 1990). To meet the second requirement, most programs conduct a "Mock Board" clinical examination in which residents are directly observed by faculty examiners evaluating a patient and asked to discuss their evaluation, diagnosis, formulation, and treatment plan for this patient and similar cases. The RRC also requires that a summative yearly evaluative statement of the progress of each resident be discussed directly with the resident and recorded in his or her training file.

In a similar fashion, training programs should require regular resident feedback and evaluation of teachers, supervisors, clinical rotations, and the overall structure and content of the residency program. Such formal evaluations by their students can be used as one criterion of teaching quality by faculty promotions committees (Borus 1993). Residents' feedback about deficiencies in the training program should be viewed by faculty as important information that can improve the program (Sledge 1978).

◼ PSYCHIATRIC EDUCATION OF NONPSYCHIATRIC RESIDENTS

Nonpsychiatric physicians are notoriously poor at recognizing and correctly diagnosing defined mental disorders in their patients (Borus et al. 1988), yet studies have shown that they provide the vast majority of care for patients with mental disorders in this country (Shapiro et al. 1984). Nonpsychiatric physicians need teaching to recognize when their patients have a mental disorder, to correctly diagnose the disorder, and to learn when to treat this disorder within their practice or refer the patient for treatment to a psychiatrist or other mental health specialist. Much of this teaching to primary care residents has been by psychologists who have focused on improving interviewing skills (Burns et al. 1983), while paying inadequate attention to teaching psychiatric diagnosis or psychopharmacological treatment (Borus 1985).

Nonpsychiatric residents should be trained how, within the time limitations of general medical practice, to assess patients for psychiatric disorders and make definitive diagnoses. It is also important in working with nonpsychiatric residents to discuss the presentation of prevalent mental disorder in their patient population, to stress the importance of these disorders to the patient's overall health, and to emphasize that there are successful treatments for many psychiatric disorders, some of which can be provided as part of general medical care. Stemming from the APA's desire to make DSM-IV (American Psychiatric Association 1994) more relevant for primary care physicians, psychiatry has developed an interspecialty collaboration with the major professional organizations of internists, family practitioners, pediatricians, and obstetricians/gynecologists to write a DSM for primary care medical practice (DSM-PC) emphasizing the most prevalent mental disorders that can be incorporated into the residency training and continuing education of nonpsychiatric physicians. This emphasis should raise the priority of primary care physicians' recognition of psychiatric disorders, and DSM-PC should provide a schema for diagnosing such disorders within their practices.

The psychiatric education of the nonpsychiatric resident should also include a basic course in psychopharmacology so that physicians understand the appropriate uses of antidepressant, antianxiety, neuroleptic, and sedative medications. General physicians often overuse antianxiety medications and underutilize and underdose antidepressive and neuro-leptic medications. The vital role of the general physician in longitudi-nally monitoring and treating the physical health problems of patients with mental disorders should be emphasized. In addition, primary care residents should be taught to recognize difficulties in the doctor-patient relationship, specifically the roles played by patients' fear, shame, hu-miliation, demoralization, and character style, as well as the resident's own subjective response to caring for very ill patients (Sledge et al. 1987).

■ FELLOWSHIPS AND SUBSPECIALIZATION

As the knowledge base in psychiatry expands and as reimbursement po-tential is increasingly linked to expertise in ever-narrowing areas, sub-specialization has become a fact of our field. The recent moratorium on the creation of new medical subspecialty boards may slow down the rate of development of subspecialty areas within psychiatry but is unlikely to halt the process. The current subspecialty areas with ABPN certification are child and adolescent psychiatry, geriatric psychiatry, and addictions psychiatry. Administrative psychiatry has an APA-sponsored certifying ex-amination, and forensic psychiatry has a certifying process administered by the American Academy of Psychiatry and the Law. Both consultation-liaison and community psychiatry have a strong cadre of psychiatrists but, to date, lack a formal certifying process.

Subspecialization is linked to the provision of formal fellowship pro-grams leading to eligibility for certification within a particular subspe-cialty area. Child and adolescent psychiatry has the oldest subspecialty training accreditation and certification processes. The 2-year child and adolescent psychiatry training requirements are established by a sub-committee of the Psychiatry RRC. Residents may elect to enter child psychiatry training as early as the PG IV year and, after successfully com-pleting two additional years of child training, are eligible for board certi-fication in child and adolescent psychiatry. Other subspecialty areas developing formal fellowship requirements for eligibility for certification of "added qualifications" include geriatric psychiatry and addictions psy-chiatry. In addition, other less formal fellowship programs offer in-depth postresidency experience within a particular circumscribed area of the field as well as opportunities for research over a 1- or 2-year period. Al-though a PGY IV elective may resemble a PGY V fellowship, the ABPN and the RRC are quite clear that except for child psychiatry, PGY IV sub-specialty experiences will not count toward eligibility for subspecialty certification.

Psychoanalytic training, the oldest formal subspecialty area of psy-chiatry, is carried out as a part-time training activity under the auspices of independent educational institutes. Psychoanalytic training has three components: a formal didactic curriculum addressing the basic theoretical, technical, historical, and clinical aspects of psychoanalysis; close supervision of selected cases; and a personal analysis. Many psychoanalytic institutes also sponsor continuing education activities that address assessment and treatment of patients from a psychoanalytic or psychodynamic perspective for psychiatrists and other mental health professionals who do not pursue full psychoanalytic training.

■ PSYCHIATRIC EDUCATION OF NONPHYSICIAN MENTAL HEALTH PROFESSIONALS

Increasingly the practice of psychiatry has become a multidisciplinary undertaking. With the development of community-based services, the delivery of mental health care is carried out in a wide range of settings in which providers from the disciplines of psychiatry, psychology, social work, and nursing must work together in a harmonious, collaborative manner. Much of this work is carried out in teams in which each discipline fulfills some functions specific to that discipline as well as functions and roles that overlap those of other disciplines. Psychiatrists can be of assistance in educating and training members of these disciplines through either formal or in-service, on-the-job training programs that teach general mental health skills as well as areas of particular psychiatric expertise, such as the use of psychoactive medications, the interface between medical and psychological processes, and some forensic and legal issues.

■ CONTINUING PSYCHIATRIC EDUCATION (CME)

Psychiatric practitioners must stay up to date on meaningful developments in the field to avoid obsolescence. This has become an increasingly important issue as managed care monitors and third-party insurers "change the rules" of psychiatric practice and shift the focus to short-term interventions rarely emphasized in residencies in the past. The rapidly growing neuroscience knowledge base in psychiatry; refinements in traditional psychotherapeutic, psychopharmacological, and psychosocial techniques; and exciting new imaging aids to diagnosis of serious mental disorder all require sophisticated education and, for some, additional training for the clinician to understand and appropriately integrate into his or her clinical repertoire. Many states require CME for licensure renewal. An added impetus to continuing psychiatric education has been the decision by the ABPN to provide only time-limited certifications after 1994; this will require the psychiatrist to demonstrate continuing competence for recertification every 10 years. Finally, the ultimate reason for continuing psychiatric education is the desire of practitioners to continue to learn and develop professionally to maintain an up-to-date understanding of the field and the best possible treatment armamentarium.

With the rapid development of our field, CME limited to didactic information transfer may not be able to provide an adequate educational experience to enable the practicing psychiatrist to avoid clinical obsolescence. One might question whether periodic retraining, with both intensive acquisition of new knowledge and supervised practice of new diagnostic and treatment methods, should be a required part of the continuing education of psychiatrists. Providing such opportunities requires major additional teaching and supervisory efforts by faculty. The faculty costs of such efforts might be offset by the clinical care provided by retraining psychiatrists as they expand their expertise, or might be funded by special institutional initiatives. Although there are many obstacles to such required, periodic (perhaps the equivalent of 6 months every decade) retraining of psychiatrists, it is unclear whether practitioners will be able to provide their patients with the most effective treatment without it.

■ REFERENCES

Accreditation Council for Graduate Medical Education: Directory of Graduate Medical Education Programs 1992–1993. Chicago, IL, American Medical Association, 1992

American Board of Psychiatry and Neurology: Information for Applicants. Deerfield, IL, American Board of Psychiatry and Neurology, 1992

American Psychiatric Association: Diagnostic and Statistical Manual of Mental Disorders, 4th Edition. Washington, DC, American Psychiatric Association, 1994

Association of American Medical Colleges: Physicians for the Twenty-First Century: The GPEP Report: Report of the Panel on the General Professional Education of the Physician and College Preparation for Medicine. Washington, DC, Association of American Medical Colleges, 1984

Betcher RW, Zinberg NE: Supervision and privacy in psychotherapy training. Am J Psychiatry 145:796–803, 1988

Borus JF: The transition to practice seminar. Am J Psychiatry 135:1513–1516, 1978

Borus JF: The transition to practice. J Med Educ 57:593–601, 1982

Borus JF: Psychiatry and the primary care physician, in Comprehensive Textbook of Psychiatry/IV, 4th Edition, Vol 2. Edited by Kaplan HI, Sadock BJ. Baltimore, MD, Williams & Wilkins, 1985, pp 1302–1308

Borus JF: Teaching and learning psychiatry. Academic Psychiatry 17:3–11, 1993

Borus JF, Yager J: Ongoing evaluation in psychiatry: the first step toward quality. Am J Psychiatry 143:1415–1419, 1986

Borus JF, Howes MJ, Devins NP, et al: Primary health care providers' recognition and diagnosis of mental disorders in their patients. Gen Hosp Psychiatry 10:317–321, 1988

Burns BJ, Scott JE, Burke JD, et al: Mental health training of primary care residents: a review of recent literature (1974–1981). Gen Hosp Psychiatry 5:157–169, 1983

Eaton JS Jr: The psychiatrist and psychiatric education, in Comprehensive Textbook of Psychiatry/III, 3rd Edition, Vol 3. Edited by Kaplan HI, Freedman AM, Sadock BJ. Baltimore, MD, Williams & Wilkins, 1980, pp 2926–2946

Hales RE, Baker FW, Borus JF, et al: Preparing Army physicians for practice, I: a survey of hospital commander and physician attitudes. Milit Med 147:554–557, 1982

Hales RE, Baker FW, Borus JF: Preparing Army physicians for practice, II: a transition to practice seminar. Milit Med 150:91–96, 1985

Liaison Committee on Medical Education: Functions and Structure of a Medical School. Chicago, IL, and Washington, DC, American Medical Association/Association of American Medical Colleges, 1991

Lidz T, Edelson M (eds): Training Tomorrow's Psychiatrist: The Crisis in Curriculum. New Haven, CT, Yale University Press, 1970

Ludmerer K: Learning to Heal: The Development of American Medical Education. New York, Basic Books, 1985

National Board of Medical Examiners: Test development committees for USMLE and NBME examinations. The National Board Examiner, Summer, 1992, pp 1–6

Parsons T: Social structure and dynamic process: the case of modern medical practice, in Social System. Edited by Parsons T. New York, Free Press, 1951, pp 428–479

Reiser LW, Sledge WH, Edelson M: Four-year evaluation of a clerkship: 1982–1986. Am J Psychiatry 145:1122–1126, 1988

Shapiro S, Skinner EA, Kessler LG, et al: Utilization of health and mental health services: three Epidemiologic Catchment Area sites. Arch Gen Psychiatry 41:971–978, 1984

Sledge WH: Resource identification: a use of psychiatric residents' evaluation of faculty. J Med Educ 53:149–151, 1978

Sledge WH, Lieberman PB, Reiser L: Teaching about the doctor-patient relationship in the first postgraduate year. J Med Educ 62:187–190, 1987

Smeltzer DJ, Jones BA: Reliability and validity of the Psychiatry Resident In-Training Examination. Academic Psychiatry 14:115–121, 1990

Thorbeck J: The development of the psychodynamic psychotherapist in supervision. Academic Psychiatry 16:72–82, 1992

Tiberius RG: Small Group Teaching. Toronto, Ontario Institute for Studies in Education Press, 1990

Tosteson DC: New pathways in general medical education. N Engl J Med 332:234–238, 1990

Werkman SL: The Role of Psychiatry in Medical Education: An Appraisal and a Forecast. Cambridge, MA, Harvard University Press, 1966

Index

*Page numbers printed in **boldface** type refer to tables or figures.*

Behavior therapy *(continued)*
  for conversion disorder, 563
  for depression, in geriatric patients,
    1319
  for eating disorders, 999–1001
      anorexia nervosa, 999–1000
      binge-eating disorder, 1001
      bulimia nervosa, 1000–1001
  for enuresis, 758
  for gender identity disorders of
    childhood, 611
  for mood disorders, 999, 1319
  for obsessive-compulsive disorder,
    506–507
  for paraphilias, 622
  for pathological gambling, 646
  with pharmacotherapy, for phobic
    disorder, 997–998
  for pica, 749
  for posttraumatic stress disorder, 517
  for psychotic disorders, 1001–1002
  for rumination disorder, 751–752
  for simple phobia, 997–998
  for social phobia, 998
  for stereotypic movement disorder,
    768
  therapeutic procedures in, 993–996.
    See also specific techniques
      biofeedback, 995
      cognitive therapy, 994
      exposure therapy, 993
      extinction, 994–995
      modeling, 996
      punishment, 995
      reinforcement, 994
      relaxation training, 995–996
      social skills training, 996
  for transsexualism, 609–610
  for violent patients, 1203
Belief systems, of families, 1103–1104
Benadryl. *See* Diphenhydramine
Beneficence, 1253
Benton Face Recognition Test, 256
Benton Line Orientation Test, 256
Benton Test of Visual Retention, 255
Benzodiazepines, 881, **882,** 883. *See also
    specific drugs*
  abuse and dependence on, 359–361
      clinical features of, 360–361
      treatment of, 361

  for aggression, acute, 915–916
  for agitation
      acute, 915–916
      in geriatric patients, 1310
  for alcohol withdrawal, 357
  for Alzheimer's disease, 327
  amnesia due to, 337
  with antidepressants, 865–866
  for anxiety disorders, in geriatric
    patients, 1315
  for bipolar disorder, 461
  during breast-feeding, 895–896
  for children and adolescents, 1144
  chronic use of, 780–781
  for delirium, 319
  dependence on, 893
  for dissociative identity disorder,
    599
  drug interactions of, 895
  for generalized anxiety disorder,
    881, **885,** 885–886
  for insomnia, 883
  for intermittent explosive disorder,
    638
  overdose of, 895
  for pain disorders, 831
  for panic disorder, 485, 881, 883,
    887–888
  for parasomnias, 787
  pretreatment evaluation for, 283
  rebound anxiety with, 894
  for schizophrenia, 422
  for sedative-hypnotic abuse and
    dependence, 361
  for separation anxiety disorder, 762
  side effects of, 889, 892, 894
  for violence, in emergencies, 1199
  withdrawal from, 893
Benztropine, for extrapyramidal
    disorders, **847**
Bereavement, uncomplicated, mood
    disorders differentiated from,
    464
Beta-adrenergic blocking drugs
    (beta-blockers), 884
  for aggression, chronic, 919–920,
    920
  for agitation, in geriatric patients,
    1310
  for anxiety disorders, 485–486